Current
Reconstructive
Surgery

Current Reconstructive Surgery

Editors

Joseph M. Serletti, MD, FACS
Henry Royster—William Maul Measey
Professor of Surgery and Chief
Division of Plastic Surgery
Vice Chair (Finance), Department of Surgery
University of Pennsylvania
Philadelphia, Pennsylvania

Peter J. Taub, MD, FACS, FAAP
Professor, Surgery and Pediatrics
Chief, Craniomaxillofacial Surgery
Co-Director, Mount Sinai Cleft and
Craniofacial Center
Division of Plastic and Reconstructive Surgery
Mount Sinai Medical Center and
Kravis Children's Hospital
New York, New York

Liza C. Wu, MD, FACS
Assistant Professor
Director of the Microsurgery Program and
Clinical Research Program
Division of Plastic Surgery
University of Pennsylvania Health Systems
Philadelphia, Pennsylvania

David J. Slutsky, MD
Clinical Assistant Professor
Department of Orthopedics
Chief of Reconstructive Surgery
Harbor-UCLA Medical Center
Los Angeles, California
Private Practice
The Hand and Wrist Institute
Torrance, California

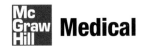

New York   Chicago   San Francisco   Lisbon   London   Madrid   Mexico City
Milan   New Delhi   San Juan   Seoul   Singapore   Sydney   Toronto

Current Reconstructive Surgery

1 2 3 4 5 6 7 8 9 0   CTP/CTP   17 16 15 14 13 12

ISBN 978-0-07-147723-9
MHID 0-07-147723-3

This book was set in Berling by Thomson Digital.
The editors were Brian Belval and Regina Brown.
The production supervisor was Sherri Souffrance.
Project management was provided by Charu Bansal, Thomson Digital.
The interior designer was Mary McKeon; the cover designer was Anthony Landi.
China Translation & Printing, Ltd. was printer and binder.

Library of Congress Cataloging-in-Publication Data

Current reconstructive surgery / editors, Joseph M. Serletti ... [et al.].
  p. ; cm.
 Includes bibliographical references and index.
 ISBN 978-0-07-147723-9 (softcover : alk. paper)
 ISBN 0-07-147723-3 (softcover : alk. paper)
 I. Serletti, Joseph M.
 [DNLM: 1. Reconstructive Surgical Procedures. WO 600]
 617.9'52—dc23
                                                    2011050201

McGraw-Hill books are available at special quantity discounts to use as premiums and sales promotions, or for use in corporate training programs. To contact a representative please e-mail us at bulksales@mcgraw-hill.com.

I dedicate this to my wife Bonnie and my daughters
Lacey and Tate for their immeasurable support.
—Joseph M. Serletti, MD, FACS

To Dylan, Justin, and Joey for their support and understanding
especially when work occasionally takes me away from my family.
—Peter J. Taub, MD, FACS, FAAP

To my best friends Brett and Jesse for all of the joy
and love that you bring to my life.
—David J. Slutsky, MD

To my mentors who have taught me and to my family who
support me in the practice of plastic surgery.
—Liza C. Wu, MD, FACS

Contents

Contributors

Ahmed M. Afifi, MD
Assistant Professor
Division of Plastic Surgery
University of Wisconsin
Madison, Wisconsin
Associate Professor
Department of Plastic Surgery
Cairo University
Cairo, Egypt

Richard L. Agag, MA, MD
Division of Plastic Surgery
University of Pennsylvania School of Medicine
Philadelphia, Pennsylvania

Gretchen Ahrendt, MD, FACS
Associate Professor of Surgery
Division of Surgical Oncology
Co-Director Comprehensive Breast Cancer
  Program of University of Pittsburgh Medical Center
Magee-Womens Hospital of University of Pittsburgh
  Medical Center
Pittsburgh, Pennsylvania

Naveen K. Ahuja, MD
Fellow, Microvascular Reconstructive Surgery
Division of Plastic Surgery
University of Pittsburgh Medical Center
Pittsburgh, Pennsylvania

Robert J. Allen, MD
Clinical Professor
Department of Plastic Surgery
New York University
New York, New York

Stephan Ariyan, MD, MBA
Clinical Professor of Surgery
  (Plastic Surgery, Otolaryngology)
Yale University School of Medicine
New Haven, Connecticut
Associate Chief
Department of Surgery
Yale-New Haven Hospital
New Haven, Connecticut

Christopher E. Attinger, MD
Professor
Department of Plastic Surgery
Georgetown University School of Medicine
Washington, District of Columbia
Chief
Division of Wound Healing
Georgetown University School of Medicine
Washington, District of Columbia

Stephen B. Baker, MD, DDS, FACS
Professor and Program Director
Department of Plastic Surgery
Georgetown University Hospital
Washington, District of Columbia
Co-Director
Craniofacial Anomalies Program
Inova Fairfax Hospital
Falls Church, Virginia

Sameer Bashey, MD
Division of Plastic and Reconstructive Surgery
Mount Sinai School of Medicine
New York, New York

John D. Bauer, MD
Associate Professor
Department of Surgery
University of Texas Medical Branch at Galvetson
Galveston, Texas

Stephen P. Beals, MD, FACS, FAAP
Associate Professor of Plastic Surgery
Mayo Clinic
Medical Director
Barrow Cleft and Craniofacial Center
St. Joseph's Hospital and Medical Center
Phoenix, Arizona

Michael L. Bentz, MD, FACS, FAAP
Professor and Chairman
Division of Plastic Surgery
University of Wisconsin School of Medicine
  and Public Health
Madison, Wisconsin
Vice Chairman for Clinical Affairs
Department of Surgery
University of Wisconsin
Madison, Wisconsin

Christopher J. M. Brooks, MD
Attending Physician
Department of Plastic Surgery
Joe DiMaggio Children's Hospital
Hollywood, Florida
Adjunct Professor
Division of Plastic Surgery
Cleveland Clinic Florida
Weston, Florida

Steven R. Buchman, MD, FACS
M. Haskell Newman Professor in Plastic Surgery
Professor of Neurosurgery
University of Michigan
Medical School
Chief
Pediatric Plastic Surgery
CS Mott Childrens Hospital
Director
Craniofacial Anomalies Program
University of Michigan
Medical Center
Ann Arbor, Michigan

Louis P. Bucky, MD, FACS
Clinical Professor
Plastic and Reconstructive Surgery
The Hospital of the University of Pennsylvania
Philadelphia Pennsylvania
Chief
Plastic and Reconstructive Surgery
Pennsylvania Hospital
Philadelphia, Pennsylvania

Jamal M. Bullocks, MD, FACS
Assistant Professor
Division of Plastic Surgery
Baylor College of Medicine
Houston, Texas

James Chang, MD
Professor and Chief
Division of Plastic Surgery
Stanford University Medical Center
Palo Alto, California

Benjamin Chang, MD, FACS
Associate Professor of Clinical Surgery
Division of Plastic Surgery
University of Pennsylvania School of Medicine
Philadelphia, Pennsylvania
Senior Surgeon
Division of Plastic Surgery
The Children's Hospital of Philadelphia
Philadelphia, Pennsylvania

Mark Warren Clemens, MD
Assistant Professor
Department of Plastic Surgery
MD Anderson Cancer Center
University of Texas
Houston, Texas

Meredith S. Collins, MD
Resident
Division of Plastic Surgery
Mount Sinai School of Medicine
New York, New York

Matthew J. Concannon, MD
Owner
Concannon Plastic Surgery
Columbia, Missouri

Richard W. Dabb, MD
Associate Professor
Department of Surgery
Johns Hopkins University
Baltimore, Maryland
Clinical Professor
Department of Surgery
Milton S. Hershey/Penn State Medical Center
Hershey, Pennsylvania

Lisa R. David, MD, FACS
Professor
Department of Plastic Surgery
Program Director
Department of Plastic Surgery
Wake Forest University
Winston-Salem, North Carolina

Edward H. Davidson, MA (Cantab), MBBS
Resident
Division of Plastic Surgery
University of Pittsburgh Medical Center
Pittsburgh, Pennsylvania

Frederic W.-B. Deleyiannis, MD, MPhil, MPH, FACS
Associate Professor
Chief, Deptartment of Pediatric Plastic Surgery
Director, Cleft Lip and Palate Clinic
Director, Craniofacial Microsurgery and Trauma
Departments of Surgery and Otolaryngology
The Children's Hospital and University of Colorado
    School of Medicine
Aurora, Colorado

Christopher A. Derderian, MD
Assistant Professor
Department Plastic Surgery
UT Southwestern Medical Center
Children's Medical Center
Dallas, Texas

Joseph J. Disa, MD, FACS
Attending Surgeon
Plastic and Reconstructive Surgery
Memorial Hospital for Cancer and Allied Diseases
New York, New York
Professor of Surgery
Weill Medical College of Cornell University
New York, New York

Howard D. Edington, MD, MBA
Associate Professor
Department of Surgery
Associate Professor
Department of Dermatology
University of Pittsburgh School of Medicine
Pittsburgh, Pennsylvania

Jeffrey A. Fearon, MD, FACS, FAAP
Director
The Craniofacial Center
Medical City Dallas
Dallas, Texas

Derek Fletcher, MD
Resident
Plastic Surgery
University of Pittsburgh Medical Center
Pittsburgh, Pennsylvania

Joshua Fosnot, MD
Housestaff
Division of Plastic Surgery
University of Pennsylvania School of Medicine
Philadelphia, Pennsylvania

Allen Gabriel, MD, FACS
Assistant Professor
Plastic Surgery
Loma Linda University Medical Center
Loma Linda, California
Chief of Plastic Surgery
Department of Plastic Surgery
Southwest Washington Medical Center
Vancouver, Washington

Jesse A. Goldstein, MD
Chief Resident
Department of Plastic Surgery
Georgetown University
Washington, District of Columbia

Vijay S. Gorantla, MD, PhD
Associate Professor of Surgery
Administrative Medical Director,
    Reconstructive Transplant Program
Director, Veterans Affairs Pittsburgh
    Hand Transplant Program
Department of Plastic and Reconstructive Surgery
Veterans Affairs Hospital
Pittsburgh, Pennsylvania

Lawrence J. Gottlieb, MD, FACS
Professor of Surgery
Director of Burn and Complex Wound Center
Section of Plastic and Reconstructive Surgery/
    Department of Surgery
University of Chicago
Chicago, Illinois

Alexander J. Gougoutas, MD
Resident
Division of Plastic Surgery
University of Pennsylvania
Philadelphia, Pennsylvania

Mark S. Granick, MD
Professor and Chief of Plastic Surgery
Division of Plastic Surgery
New Jersey Medical School-UMDNJ
Newark, New Jersey

Joseph S. Gruss, MD, FRCS[C]
Professor
Department of Surgery
Marlys C. Larson Endowed Chair and
    Professor in Pediatric Craniofacial Surgery
University of Washington School of Medicine
Seattle, Washington
Attending Surgeon
Division of Plastic and Craniofacial Surgery
Seattle Childrens Hospital and Harborview Medical Center
Seattle, Washington

Laurence M. Hausman, MD
Associate Professor
Department of Anesthesiology
Director
Ambulatory Anesthesiology
Mount Sinai Medical Center
New York, New York

Christoph Heitmann, MD, PhD
Associate Professor
Aesthetic of Plastic Surgery
University of Heidelberg
Heidelberg, Germany

James P. Higgins, MD
Chief
Curtis National Hand Center
MedStar Union Memorial Hospital
Baltimore, Maryland

William Y. Hoffman, MD
Professor and Chief
Division of Plastic and Reconstructive Surgery
Stephen J. Mathes Endowed Chair
Vice Chair, Department of Surgery
University of California
San Francisco, California

Richard A. Hopper, MD, MS
Associate Professor
Department of Surgery
University of Washington
Seattle, Washington
Chief
Surgical Director
Division of Plastic Surgery, Craniofacial Center
Seattle Children's Hospital
Seattle, Washington

Ronald E. Hoxworth, MD
Assistant Professor
Department of Plastic Surgery
University of Texas Southwestern Medical Center
Dallas, Texas
Chief of Plastic Surgery
North Texas VA Medical Center
Dallas, Texas

Bradley A. Hubbard, MD
Resident
Division of Plastic Surgery
University of Missouri, Columbia
Columbia, Missouri

Helen G. Hui-Chou, MD
Resident
Department of Plastic and Reconstructive Surgery
Johns Hopkins University and University
   of Maryland School of Medicine
Baltimore, Maryland

Tara Lynn Huston, MD
Instructor in Surgery
Department of Surgery, Division of Plastic Surgery
New York Presbyterian Hospital—Weill
   Cornell Medical Center
New York, New York

Scott D. Imahara, MD
Plastic and Reconstructive
Hand and Cosmetic Surgery
Palo Alto Medical Foundation—Santa Cruz
Soquel, California

Oksana Jackson, MD
Assistant Professor
Department of Surgery
Perelman School of Medicine at
   the University of Pennsylvania
Philadelphia, Pennsylvania
Attending Physician
Division of Plastic Surgery
Children's Hospital of Philadelphia
Philadelphia, Pennsylvania

Jeffrey M. Jacobson, MD
Resident
Curtis National Hand Center
Union Memorial Hospital
Baltimore, Maryland

Keith Jeffords, MD, DDS
Private Practice
Paramount Plastic Surgery
Smyrna, Georgia

M. Renee Jespersen, MD
Assistant Professor
Department of Plastic Surgery
Children's Hospital of Philadelphia
Philadelphia, Pennsylvania

Suhail Kanchwala, MD
Assistant Professor of Surgery
Division of Plastic and Reconstructive Surgery
Hospital of the University of Pennsylvania
Philadelphia, Pennsylvania

Hahns Y. Kim, MD
Resident
Division of Plastic Surgery
Mayo Clinic
Phoenix, Arizona

Richard E. Kirschner, MD, FACS, FAAP
Chief, Section of Plastic and Reconstructive Surgery
Director, Cleft Lip and Palate Center
Nationwide Children's Hospital
Columbus, Ohio
Professor of Clinical Plastic Surgery and Pediatrics
The Ohio State College of Medicine
Columbus, Ohio

Zinon T. Kokkalis, MD
Senior Fellow
Reconstructive Microsurgery
Department of Surgery, Division of Plastic and
   Reconstructive Surgery
Eastern Virginia Medical School
Norfolk, Virginia

Angela Song Landfair, MD
Division of Plastic Surgery and
   Department of Epidemiology
University of Pittsburgh
Pittsburgh, Pennsylvania

Jeffrey D. Larson, MD
Chief Resident
Division of Plastic Surgery
University of Wisconsin Hospital and Clinics
Madison, Wisconsin

Michele A. Leadbetter, OTL, CHT
Senior Hand Therapist
Hand Therapy Department
Curtis National Hand Center
Baltimore, Maryland

W. P. Andrew Lee, MD
The Milton T. Edgerton, MD
   Professor and Chairman
Department of Plastic and Reconstructive Surgery
Johns Hopkins University School of Medicine
Baltimore, Maryland

Christopher Lentz, MD, FACS, FCCM
Professor of Surgery
University of New Mexico
Albuquerque, New Mexico

Lawrence S. Levin, MD, FACS
Paul B. Magnuson Professor of Orthopaedic Surgery
Chairman, Department of Orthopaedic Surgery
Professor of Surgery (Plastic Surgery)
University of Pennsylvania School of Medicine
Philadelphia, Pennsylvania
Attending Physician
Orthopaedic Surgery
Hospital of the University of Pennsylvania
Philadelphia, Pennsylvania

Joseph E. Losee, MD, FACS, FAAP
Professor of Surgery and Pediatrics
Chief, Division of Pediatric Plastic Surgery
University of Pittsburgh Medical Center
Pittsburgh, Pennsylvania

David W. Low, MD
Professor of Surgery
Division of Plastic Surgery
Perelman School of Medicine at
   the University of Pennsylvania
Philadelphia, Pennsylvania
Attending Surgeon
Division of Plastic Surgery
Children's Hospital of Philadelphia
Philadelphia, Pennsylvania

Daniel Y. Maman, MD, MBA
Private Practice
Millennium Aesthetic Surgery
Division of Plastic and Reconstructive Surgery
Mount Sinai School of Medicine
New York, New York

Ernest K. Manders, MD
Professor of Surgery
Division of Plastic and Reconstructive Surgery
University of Pittsburgh Medical Center
Pittsburgh, Pennsylvania

Alexandre Marchac, MD
Chef de Clinique–Assistant des Hôpitaux de Paris
Department of Plastic Surgery
Hôpital Européen Georges Pompidou, Assistance Publique
   des Hôpitaux de Paris
Paris, France

Paul A. Martineau, MD, FRCSC
Assistant Professor
Head Section of Upper Extremity Surgery
Division of Orthopaedic Surgery
McGill University Health Center
Montreal, Quebec

G. Patrick Maxwell, MD, FACS
Clinical Professor
Department of Plastic Surgery
Loma Linda University
Loma Linda, California
Clinical Assistant Professor
Department of Plastic Surgery
Vanderbilt University
Nashville, Tennessee

Walter B. McClelland, Jr., MD
Fellow–Hand, Microvascular & Upper Extremity Surgery
Curtis National Hand Center
Union Memorial Hospital
Baltimore, Maryland

Michael N. Mirzabeigi, MD
Resident Physician
Division of Plastic Surgery
University of Pennsylvania
Philadelphia, Pennsylvania

Suhail K. Mithani, MD
Chief Resident
Department of Plastic Surgery
Johns Hopkins Medical Institutions
Baltimore, Maryland

Fernando Molina, MD
Professor of Plastic and Reconstructive Surgery
Universidad Nacional Autonoma de Mexico
Mexico City, Mexico
Chief of Plastic and Reconstructive Surgery
Hospital General Dr. Manuel Gea Gonzalez
Mexico City, Mexico

Lisa C. Moody, MD
Resident
Department of Surgery
Division of Plastic Surgery
University of Texas Medical Branch
Galveston, Texas

Robert J. Morin, MD
Craniofacial Fellow
Plastic Surgery
Miami Children's Hospital
Miami, Florida

Thomas A. Mustoe, MD
Lucille and Orion Stuteville Professor of Plastic Surgery
Division of Plastic Surgery
Feinberg School of Medicine
Northwestern University
Chicago, Illinois

Wesley T. Myers, MD
Private Practice
The Woodlands, Texas

Sanjay Naran, MD
Resident
Division of Plastic Surgery
University of Pittsburgh
Pittsburgh, Pennsylvania

Vu T. Nguyen, MD
Assistant Professor
Associate Program Director
Division of Plastic Surgery, Department of Surgery
University of Pittsburgh School of Medicine
Pittsburgh, Pennsylvania

Adam J. Oppenheimer, MD
Resident
Section of Plastic Surgery
University of Michigan
Ann Arbor, Michigan

Kristina D. O'Shaughnessy, MD
Department of Surgery
Division of Plastic Surgery
Feinberg School of Medicine
Northwestern University
Chicago, Illinois

Srdjan A. Ostric, MD
Attending Physician
Department of Plastic Surgery
Resurrection Medical Center
Chicago, Illinois

Brian M. Parrett, MD
Attending Physician
Division of Plastic Surgery and Microsurgery
The Buncke Clinic
San Francisco, California

Aaron T. Pelletier, MD
Zaccone Family Fellow in Reconstructive Microsurgery
Section of Plastic and Reconstructive Surgery
Department of Surgery
University of Chicago Medical Center
Chicago, Illinois

Linda G. Phillips, MD
Professor and Chief
Division of Plastic Surgery
University of Texas Medical Branch at Galveston
Galveston, Texas

Brian A. Pinsky, MD
Associate
Long Island Plastic Surgical Group, P. C.
Garden City, New York

Julian J. Pribaz, MD
Professor
Division of Plastic Surgery
Harvard Medical School
Boston, Massachusetts

Eduardo D. Rodriguez, MD, DDS
Associate Professor and Chief
Plastic, Reconstructive and Maxillofacial Surgery
University of Maryland School of Medicine
R. Adams Cowley Shock Trauma Center
Baltimore, Maryland

Rod J. Rohrich, MD, FACS
Professor and Chairman
Department of Plastic Surgery
Crystal Charity Ball Distinguished Chair in Plastic Surgery
Betty and Warren Woodward Chair in Plastic and
    Reconstructive Surgery
Distinguished Teaching Professor
University of Texas Southwestern Medical Center
Dallas, Texas

S. Alex Rottgers, MD
Integrated Plastic Surgery Resident
Division of Plastic and Reconstructive Surgery
University of Pittsburgh School of Medicine
Pittsburgh, Pennsylvania

J. Peter Rubin, MD
Chief of Plastic and Reconstructive Surgery
Director
Life After Weight Loss Body Contouring Program
University of Pittsburgh
Pittsburgh, Pennsylvania

Roee E. Rubinstein, MD
Hand Surgery Fellow
Department of Orthopedic Surgery
David Geffen UCLA School of Medicine
Los Angeles, California

Rachel A. Ruotolo, MD
Diplomate
American Board of Plastic Surgery
Craniofacial & Pediatric Plastic Surgery
Long Island Plastic Surgical Group, P.C.
Garden City, New York

Claire Sanger, DO
Assistant Professor, Surgery
University of Kentucky
College of Medicine
Lexington, Kentucky

Adam D. Schaffner, MD, FACS
Director
Plastic Surgery Institute of New York
Clinical Assistant Professor,
Weill Cornell Medical College
New York, New York

Mark B. Schoemann, MD
Craniofacial and Pediatric Plastic Surgery Fellow
Children's Healthcare of Atlanta
Atlanta, Georgia

Norman H. Schulman, MD, FACS
Clinical Professor of Surgery
Department of Surgery, Division of Plastic Surgery
Weil-Cornell Medical College
New York, New York
Director of Plastic Surgery
Lenox Hill Hospital
New York, New York

Scott M. Schulze, MD
Hand Surgeon
Attending Physician, Department of Surgery
Beebe Medical Center
Lewes, Delaware

Joseph M. Serletti, MD, FACS
Henry Royster—William Maul Measey
    Professor of Surgery and Chief
Division of Plastic Surgery
Vice Chair (Finance), Department of Surgery
University of Pennsylvania
Philadelphia, Pennsylvania

Mitchel Seruya, MD
Resident Physician
Department of Plastic Surgery
Georgetown University Hospital
Washington, District of Columbia

Kenneth C. Shestak, MD
Professor
Department of Plastic Surgery
University of Pittsburgh School of Medicine
Pittsburgh, Pennsylvania

Jaimie T. Shores, MD
Assistant Professor
Department of Plastic and Reconstructive Surgery
Johns Hopkins University School of Medicine
Baltimore, Maryland

Ronald P. Silverman, MD, FACS
Associate Professor
Department of Surgery
University of Maryland School of Medicine
Baltimore, Maryland

Devinder P. Singh, MD
Assistant Professor
Division of Plastic Surgery
University of Maryland School of Medicine
Baltimore, Maryland
Chief
Section of Plastic Surgery
Veterans Affairs Hospital—Baltimore
Baltimore, Maryland

Wesley N. Sivak, MD, PhD
Resident
Division of Plastic and Reconstructive Surgery
Department of Surgery
University of Pittsburgh School of Medicine
Pittsburgh, Pennsylvania

David J. Slutsky, MD
Clinical Assistant Professor
Department of Orthopedics
Chief of Reconstructive Surgery
Harbor-UCLA Medical Center
Los Angeles, California
Private Practice
The Hand and Wrist Institute
Torrance, California

Mark L. Smith, MD, FACS
Assistant Professor
Department of Surgery
Albert Einstein College of Medicine
Bronx, New York
Director
Plastic and Reconstructive Surgery
Continuum Cancer Centers of New York
Beth Israel Medical Center
New York, New York

Scott L. Spear, MD
Professor and Chairman
Department of Plastic Surgery
Georgetown University Hospital
Washington, District of Columbia

Geoffrey H. Sperber, BDS, MSc, PhD, FICD
Professor Emeritus
School of Dentistry
Faculty of Medicine and Dentistry
University of Alberta
Edmonton, Alberta, Canada

Samuel Stal, MD
Professor and Chief, Plastic Surgery
Baylor College of Medicine
Houston, Texas

Matthew G. Stanwix, MD
Clinical Fellow
Department of Plastic and Reconstructive Surgery
Johns Hopkins University School of Medicine
Baltimore, Maryland
Clinical Fellow
Division of Plastic and Reconstructive Surgery
R. Adams Cowley Shock Trauma Center
University of Maryland School of Medicine
Baltimore, Maryland

Matthew R. Swelstad, MD
Physician
Colorado West Otolaryngologists, P.C.
Grand Junction, Colorado

Amir H. Tahernia, MD
Fellow
Division of Plastic Surgery
Duke University School of Medicine
Durham, North Carolina
Private Practice
Plastic and Reconstructive Surgery
Los Angeles, California

Peter J. Taub, MD, FACS, FAAP
Professor, Surgery and Pediatrics
Chief, Craniomaxillofacial Surgery
Co-Director, Mount Sinai Cleft and Craniofacial Center
Division of Plastic and Reconstructive Surgery
Mount Sinai Medical Center and
Kravis Children's Hospital
New York, New York

Julia K. Terzis, MD, PhD, FACS, FRCS(C)
Clinical Professor
Department of Plastic Surgery
New York University Medical Center
New York, New York
Medical Director
International Institute of Reconstructive Microsurgery
Long Island City, New York

Jonathan W. Toy, MD, FRCS(C)
Attending Physician
Division of Plastic Surgery
University of Alberta
Edmonton, Alberta, Canada

Thomas Trumble, MD
Professor and Chief
Division of Hand and Microvascular Surgery
Department of Orthopaedics & Sports Medicine
University of Washington School of Medicine
Seattle, Washington

Anthony P. Tufaro, DDS, MD, FACS
Associate Professor
Departments of Plastic and
    Reconstructive Surgery and Oncology
Johns Hopkins University
Baltimore, Maryland
Attending Surgeon
Department of Plastic and Reconstructive Surgery
Johns Hopkins Hospital
Baltimore, Maryland

Jon P. Ver Halen, MD
Assistant Professor
Department of Plastic Surgery
University of Tennessee
Memphis, Tennessee

Stephen M. Warren, MD
Associate Professor
Department of Plastic Surgery
New York University Medical Center
New York, New York

Andrew J. Watt, MD
Department of Surgery
Division of Plastic and Reconstructive Surgery
Stanford University Hospital & Clinics
Palo Alto, California

Jeffrey Weinzweig, MD, FACS
Chief of Craniofacial Surgery
Director
Craniofacial Anomalies Program
Division of Plastic Surgery
Advocate Illinois Masonic Medical Center
Chicago, Illinois
Director
The Chicago Center for Plastic & Reconstructive Surgery
Chicago, Illinois

Bradon J. Wilhelmi, MD, FACS
Leonard J. Weiner Professor and Chief
Plastic Surgery Residency Program Director
Plastic Surgery
University of Louisville School of Medicine
Louisville, Kentucky
Attending Physician
Plastic Surgery
University of Louisville Hospital
Jewish Hospital, Norton Hospital,
    Kosair's Children's Hospital
Louisville, Kentucky

Ian F. Wilson, MD, MPH
St. Petersburg, Florida

Liza C. Wu, MD, FACS
Assistant Professor
Director of the Microsurgery Program and Clinical
    Research Program
Division of Plastic Surgery
University of Pennsylvania Health Systems
Philadelphia, Pennsylvania

Michael J. Yaremchuk, MD
Professor
Department of Surgery
Harvard Medical School
Boston, Massachusetts
Chief of Craniofacial Surgery
Department of Surgery, Division of Plastic Surgery
Massachusetts General Hospital
Boston, Massachusetts

Jack C. Yu, DMD, MD, MS Ed, FACS
Milford B. Hatcher Professor and Chief
Section of Plastic Surgery
Medical College of Georgia
Augusta, Georgia

Elvin G. Zook, MD
Professor Emeritus
Division of Plastic Surgery
Southern Illinois University
Springfield, Illinois

Principles of Wound Healing and Fundamentals of Wound Repair

Kristina D. O'Shaughnessy, MD / Thomas A. Mustoe, MD

● INTRODUCTION

Achievement of adequate wound repair, resolution of healing, and prevention of pathologic scarring is dependent not only on a complete understanding of this process but also on an understanding of wound biomechanics. This chapter will first focus on certain features of wound biology and biomechanics where early intervention may prevent healing complications and problem scarring. The fundamentals of wound repair, emphasizing choice of incision, suture, and technique will be explored to further enhance decision making at the time of tissue restoration. In some cases, failure of resolution of the normal proliferative response, which occurs at the resolution phase of normal wound healing, can lead to proliferative scarring; however, prevention steps are possible provided the surgeon is knowledgeable about the pathogenesis of hypertrophic scars. Due to the challenging treatment of hypertrophic scars and keloids, both surgical and nonsurgical treatments will be discussed in addition to prevention strategies.

● PRINCIPLES OF WOUND HEALING

Wound Biomechanics

The plastic surgeon must plan each case relative to the biomechanical properties of skin. The principle constituent of skin is collagen, which is a structural protein organized in sheets with distinct spatial structural components. Elastin fibers are also present in smaller amounts, giving the skin both elasticity and viscoelastic properties. In other words, in response to constant force, the skin will stretch and not fully return to its unstretched state.

Skin Tensions. Placement of skin incisions and resultant scar formation are dependent on both static and dynamic skin tensions. Static tension is the inherent force which stretches the skin over the underlying structures when the body is motionless.[1] The static tension varies enormously within individuals based on anatomic location—for instance, it is quite high over the sternum and minimal in the groin. As a person ages, not only does skin relax and lose elasticity, but the magnitude of tension also changes. As mentioned earlier, the collagen fibers have a spatial orientation, and this organization is reflected in static lines of maximal skin tension called Langer lines. An incision along one of these lines will result in a tension-free closure with minimal static forces pulling against the scar. The outcome is a narrow, fine, camouflaged scar. In contrast, placing an incision against the directional orientation of static skin tension will result in a wider, more visible scar. This is the sequela of continuous high-magnitude forces pulling at the healing wound margins.[2]

There has been an increased understanding at the cellular level of the impact of mechanical forces on signal transduction mediated through fibroblast attachments to the collagen matrix via integrin receptors.[3,4] Fibroblasts respond to tension with cellular proliferation, and collagen synthesis, while fibroblasts relieved of tension undergo programmed cell death (apoptosis).[5] If tension is sustained within a healing wound over several weeks, the excessive fibrosis may lead to pathologic scarring. Dynamic skin tensions are caused by a variety of changing forces such as voluntary muscle activity and movement across joints. These tensions may cause contractures in areas of high skin mobility if incisions are placed perpendicular to Langer lines.[2] The skin in these areas must offer a significant amount of extensibility and, since scars lack elasticity, mobility is restricted.

Tensile Strength. The breaking strength of a wound is a measure of the maximum amount of stress that a wound can withstand without dehiscing. Tensile strength is breaking strength per unit of cross-sectional area. The rate of which a wound gains tensile strength has served as a useful index of wound healing.[6] Tensile strength is dependent on collagen accumulation and its organization. Although collagen accumulation is maximal at 17 to 20 days postwounding, tensile strength is only a fraction of its original value. This can be attributed to lack of cross-linking and organization. Over 6 months, collagen synthesis and breakdown occurs, with a gradual improvement in collagen organization and increase in wound strength. At 2 weeks, wounds have gained less than 10% of their eventual strength, and at 6 weeks, wound strength is still only 30% to 50% of normal. Wounds never completely gain the strength of unwounded skin. In fact, at the end of a year, a wound is only about 80% of its original strength.[7] Most absorbable sutures retain their tensile strength for only 3 weeks, and if the incisions are closed under tension, scar widening will not be prevented. An alternative, more effective strategy is to place permanent sutures which will stay in at least 6 months.

Biology of Wound Healing

Inflammation, epithelization, and contraction are all normal processes essential to the tissue repair process. However, prolonged inflammation and contraction or delayed epithelization can have deleterious effects on wound healing and ultimately scar formation.

Inflammation. Excessive inflammation contributes to scar formation through increased expression of fibrogenic growth factors, most importantly, transforming growth factor beta (TGF-β). Though TGF-β is necessary for the repair process, its sustained presence promotes fibrosis by inducing fibroblast production of collagen and other extracellular matrix (ECM) components, and by inhibiting expression of collagenases, slowing collagen turnover.[8] Any process that delays wound healing will contribute to prolonged inflammation, including reaction to absorbable or retained sutures, wound margin necrosis, wound infection, and imprecise wound coaptation leading to delayed epithelization. Proper wound evaluation, appropriate debridement, meticulous tissue coaptation with gentle handling of tissues, and semiocclusive dressings applied at the time of wound closure are a few simple strategies to avoid a prolonged inflammatory phase.[9]

Epithelization. Epithelization of a wound bed occurs through keratinocyte migration from wound margins and epidermal appendages. The epithelial layer of a healing wound serves a critical barrier function to protect the underlying tissues from bacteria and water loss. When barrier function is restored, experimental evidence and

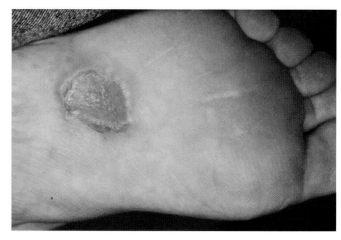

FIGURE 1-1. This patient had skin grafting to repair a defect on the plantar surface of his foot after wide local excision of a lesion. At 20 days, a rim of hypertrophic scar at the periphery of the healing wound signifies delayed epithelization.

clinical observations indicate that inflammation is down-regulated and the underlying granulation tissues undergo apoptosis.[10] The critical role of the epidermis in regulating scar formation has been under appreciated. The faster this protection is initiated, the less chance of pathologic scarring. The amount of time required to re-epithelize a wound is a critical factor in determining risk of scar formation (Figure 1-1). The burn, dermabrasion, and chemical peel literature has shown an absence of scarring with partial thickness wounds that epithelize at less than 2 weeks.[11]

Contraction. Contraction of healing wounds narrows the distance between wound edges and reduces the overall surface area at a rate much faster than the maximal rate for re-epithelization. Much of our knowledge on wound contraction comes from animal studies; however, the proportion of wound closure by contraction varies from species to species.[12] For example, loose skin animals such as rodents and rabbits heal up to 95% by contraction. In contrast, humans can heal by as much as 80% to 90% by contracture where there is a great deal of tissue laxity such as the groin, but only 30% over the tibia. The human has many attachments of the overlying skin to the underlying fascia, and there is limited tissue laxity in most areas of the body. The greater the degree of skin slack, the greater the degree of contraction.

The myofibroblast is the predominant cell responsible for contraction. Myofibroblasts are mesenchymal cells that have characteristics of both the fibroblast and smooth muscle cell, exhibiting bundles of microfilaments which express alpha-smooth muscle actin (α-SMA). The actin filaments interact with ECM components, exerting contractile forces on the granulation tissue. Myofibroblasts also produce ECM components, such as collagen, which stabilizes these forces. After epithelization of the healing wound is complete, myofibroblasts disappear from the granulation tissue through apoptotic cell death. A failure of this process likely contributes to hypertrophic scar formation and debilitating contractures, as persistent myofibroblasts produce excessive ECM components and continue to exert contractile forces on the wound.[13]

On a molecular level, myofibroblast differentiation is largely dependent on TGF-β. TGF-β has also been shown to stimulate fibroblast-populated collagen lattice contraction in vitro, and TGF-β antagonists reduce wound contraction in vivo.[14] Proteases and inhibitors of proteases are active in ECM turnover. Because contracture is dependent on the ECM wound environment, wound contraction is reduced when certain matrix metalloproteinases are inhibited.[15]

● FUNDAMENTALS OF WOUND REPAIR

The ultimate goals of wound repair are to achieve an adequately healed wound which preserves function and results in an aesthetically acceptable scar. To accomplish this goal, the surgeon must conduct a detailed wound evaluation, formulate a repair plan, and appropriately prepare the wound bed. In addition, the choice of both suture material and closure technique is paramount in obtaining a successful result. These choices are dependent on a variety of wound characteristics, including depth, tension, surface, and anatomic location. In formulating a decision tree for wound repair, each step must be thoughtfully executed based on the biomechanics and biologic principles of wound healing as discussed above.

Patient Evaluation and Selection

Plastic surgeons often repair acute wounds secondary to trauma. Most of these wounds will require suturing; however, there are several antecedent factors to consider. First, the surgeon must obtain a thorough history, including associated medical problems, allergies, approximate time of injury, source of trauma, and any history of tetanus immunization. Next, the location and size of the wound are examined, taking into account the length, width, and depth of the lesion. Superficial lacerations may be repaired with simple tape strips, tissue adhesive, or conventional suturing techniques. However, larger, deeper wounds require a much more complex layered closure, especially if they are under tension or if there is fascia or muscle involvement. Evaluate the surrounding tissues for evidence of contamination or local tissue damage, such as edema, erythema, or drainage. Heavily damaged or contaminated tissues will need to be extensively prepped and treated prior to closure. Closely examine the quality of the wound margins and gaping of the defect. If the wound edges are irregular or appear to be under tension, then undermining or rearrangement of the tissue and incision lines may be required to ensure a healthy, well-vascularized, tension-free closure. However, if debridement would result in a substantially more severe defect, it may be prudent to leave marginal tissue in place and accept the need for secondary scar revision or secondary closure. If bleeding seems significant, look for involvement of large blood vessels or other vital structures, such as tendons or nerves, which would take precedence and necessitate additional repair.

Patient Preparation

Wound preparation is the most critical step in the wound repair process. Minimizing bacterial burden positively influences the rate and quality of wound healing. Most traumatic wounds will have some element of contamination; however, this does not necessarily translate into infection. Wound preparation through cleansing, irrigation, and debridement reduces the risk of wound infection, delayed healing and unfavorable scar formation. Cleansing of the wound with normal saline is sufficient. It is important to avoid betadine scrubs, hydrogen peroxide, or alcohol, as these solutions are harmful to tissues. Debris and foreign materials can be loosened and removed from the wound bed by gentle scrubbing or irrigation through an 18-gauge plastic catheter attached to a 10-cc syringe, which gives sufficient pressure to lower bacteria count and effectively reduce contamination in tissue. Alternatively, pulsed lavage may also be used and is quite effective at lowering bacterial load. If wound edges are irregular, ischemic, or necrotic, then debridement will be necessary to achieve clean, well-vascularized margins. Likewise, if debris remains despite scrubbing and irrigation, then debridement will be necessary to avoid unwanted tattooing. Debridement is best accomplished with a sharp scalpel blade or tissue scissors.

Wound healing may be separated into three types: primary, secondary, and tertiary, also referred to as delayed primary. Wound edges that are acutely approximated using sutures, tape, or tissue adhesives heal by primary intention. This type of closure is best suited for wounds that have minimal contamination and tissue loss. Contraindications to primary closure consist of several local and systemic factors. Some local factors include excessive bacterial counts or the presence of infection, which may be seen in puncture wounds, animal bites, or contaminated, aged wounds. The age of the wound in regard to timing of wound repair remains controversial. Instead of memorizing a timeline, it is best to weigh the risk of infection, location of the wound, and vascularity of the tissues. For example, the head and neck have an excellent blood supply and often tolerate higher bacterial loads. On the other hand, if wound edges appear dusky, necrotic, or inflamed, it is best to delay closure. Absolute systemic contraindications to primary closure include persistent fevers or signs of sepsis. Patients with uncontrolled diabetes or diseases requiring high-dose steroids may receive primary closures; however, the surgeon and patient should be aware that risk of infection and wound-healing complications are much more likely to occur. Often, many of the local contraindications can be corrected in a timely manner allowing a delayed primary closure. If a wound is effectively irrigated in the emergency room, delayed closure can occur safely up to 24 hours later.

Secondary closures heal secondarily by granulation and contraction. These wounds are left open because of infection, severe tissue trauma, or excessive tissue loss. Clinically, this type of closure has advantages over primary intention healing when used on certain areas of the face. Contraction occurs in a centripetal fashion, producing circular scars which can be much smaller than primary closure in a linear fashion, resulting in an elongated scar. For example, the defect left by Mohs micrographic surgery in certain concave areas, such as the nasal ala, heals rapidly and with little scar compared with primary closure, which would entail a much longer incision to encompass the defect or require use of a skin graft or flap.

Tertiary closures, also known as delayed primary closures, are reserved for wounds that cannot be closed acutely, usually as a result of extensive trauma or contamination. The wound is initially left open for several days, after which the skin edges are brought together as in a primary closure. Wound closure delay by 4 to 5 days results in faster gains in tensile wound strength due to a shortening of the lag phase of wound healing and increased resistance to infection.[16] This strength is attributed to the existing rate of collagen synthesis at the time of closure. The increased resistance to infection is due to the accelerated phase of wound healing at the time of closure. Interestingly, the scar is often aesthetically comparable to that of a primary closure. However, if delay is extended past a week to 10 days, the result is a progressively wider and more raised scar. Regardless, the result is favorable when compared with an incision left to heal by secondary intention.

Techniques of Wound Closure

A thorough understanding of the properties of anesthetic solutions and injection techniques is required prior to suturing. The choice of anesthetic and technique are individualized for every patient in relationship to the severity of wounds, location of wounds, and allergic reactions. Lidocaine is the most commonly used local anesthetic, usually used with epinephrine, except in vital end organs such as the fingertips. It is usually used at a strength of 0.5% to 1% with 1:100,000 epinephrine not exceeding a dose of 5 mg/kg without epinephrine and 10 mg/kg with epinephrine. The approximate duration of lidocaine action is 70 minutes. Because, epinepherine causes vasoconstriction, it not only decreases bleeding but also prolongs the anesthetic effect of lidocaine. If a long period of anesthesia is required for an extensive repair, then bupivacaine may be used at a strength of 0.25%, not to exceed 3 mg/kg. However, it does have a slow onset of action, approximately 10 to 15 minutes.

The purpose of sutures in wound closure is to effectively splint the wound until it has regained adequate tensile strength. In addition, maintaining wound closure enhances rapid wound healing, minimizing the risk of excessive scar formation. The ideal suture handles well, glides easily through tissues, maintains knot security, causes minimal tissue reactivity, has high resistance to infection, and has enough elasticity to accommodate tissue edema while maintaining adequate strength. Absorption rate of sutures must also be considered when deciding on the appropriate suture material.

Sutures can be divided into several classes: absorbable or nonabsorbable, natural or synthetic, and monofilament or multifilament. They also come in a variety of sizes based on the diameter of the suture, which is vital to proper wound closure, depending on the anatomic area of repair. For wound repair, the reverse cutting needle is usually used due to its sharp cutting edges. This type of needle cuts through tissues smoothly, avoiding tearing and stretching.

Tissue adhesives are a popular alternative to sutures in certain cases of wound closure. Composed of cyanoacrylate, tissue adhesives polymerize upon contact with fluid at opposed wound edges, creating a water-resistant protective layer. Use of a tissue adhesive in acute, superficial, linear, low-tension wounds has similar cosmesis, dehiscence, and wound infection rates when compared with standard suturing techniques.[17] Advantages of tissue adhesives include faster closure times and significantly decreased pain. In addition, they are bacteriostatic and do not require a dressing. Tissue adhesives should not be applied to wounds in areas of high tension or friction to avoid dehiscence. To prevent foreign body reaction, inflammation, and possible wound dehiscence, it is important to avoid inadvertent leakage of tissue adhesive into the wound bed by approximating the wound margins prior to application, which often requires a deeper layer of sutures. A major advantage of tissue adhesives is the lack of need for suture removal, which makes them particularly useful for children and in the emergency room. In areas where wounds are more complex in shape or in extent of injury, tissue adhesives are less useful.

The suturing technique chosen for repair depends largely on wound tension, anatomic location, and depth of the wound. All wound closures should display uniform tensile strength along skin edges that are precisely approximated and maximally everted. Eversion is necessary to counteract the inward rotation imparted on wound edges by contractile forces during the healing process, and also to maximize dermis-to-dermis contact resulting in early gains in tensile strength which minimizes scar spreading. Sutures should be placed to obliterate dead space and maintain wound tensile strength until healing is complete. These splinting sutures should be placed evenly through the dermis, which is the strongest skin layer. Sutures placed across the epidermis should not be so tight that they strangle the tissue, causing ischemia and tissue damage. Furthermore, closure under tension should be avoided whenever possible to prevent wound-healing problems or fibroproliferative scarring. If necessary, sharp undermining of the tissues may be used to relieve tension.

Running continuous sutures are quick but require precision to properly evert and approximate the wound edges. Usually this type of suture technique evenly distributes tension along the closure line, allowing for postrepair

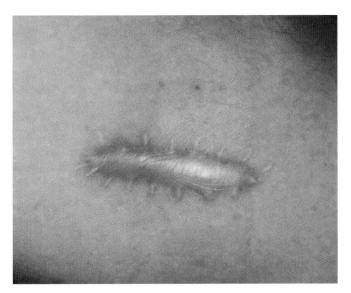

● **FIGURE 1-2.** This patient underwent excision of a chest lesion with primary repair. Tight sutures in areas of tension not only cause localized ischemia, but also leave track marks. A combination of significant tension, ischemia, and subsequent delayed epithelization all led to hypertrophic scar formation in this healing wound.

edema. Simple interrupted sutures take more time, but allow for wound-edge height adjustments, especially after placement of mattress sutures. These types of sutures are also ideal for repairing superficial stellate lacerations. Care must be taken to avoid tying these sutures too tight. Excess tension will cause tissue strangulation and ischemia, also leaving suture marks (Figure 1-2). The vertical mattress technique is a more challenging suture to achieve wound-edge approximation; however, this stitch is excellent at attaining eversion. The horizontal mattress technique can be used to oppose skin of different thickness. Many surgeons do not use this stitch due to risk of skin-edge necrosis. The corner suture, or half-buried horizontal mattress suture, is used on skin flap tips. By placing a suture through the dermis of a skin flap as opposed to the tip, there is less risk of damaging the blood supply. The running intradermal suture, or subcuticular technique, is used for closures where splinting will need to be maintained for a prolonged period of time until adequate wound healing has occurred. Since the entire suture is run within the dermis, risk of suture marks is avoided. Wound eversion is more difficult with the subcuticular stitch, but approximation can be easily attained with precise, evenly placed dermal tissue bites along the length of the incision. The ends may either be knotted or locked to maintain tension. For clean incisions, such as those created surgically, subcuticular closure avoids any risk of suture marks; and, if absorbable sutures are used, they do not need removal. Permanent sutures, such as Prolene, can be left in for months, minimizing scar spreading if there is tension on the suture line. Although a subcuticular closure can be technically more demanding, it has become the most commonly used technique for closure by plastic surgeons.

Timing of suture removal will vary depending on the amount of suture layers, anatomic location, and depth of the wound. If the wound was under any amount of tension, then the splinting sutures will need to remain in place until healing is complete to avoid dehiscence. The health of the patient must also be considered, as certain diseases, such as diabetes or ones that require high-dose steroids, delay wound healing.

Some known causes of fibroproliferative scarring include genetic predisposition, wound tension, excess inflammation, and delayed epithelization, which lead to excess cell proliferation and collagen synthesis. An understanding of each of these principles translates into application of prevention strategies at the time of initial consult or surgical insult. Many of these factors were introduced at the beginning of this chapter and we will now expand on ways to avoid or minimize these variables in order to prevent pathologic scarring.

Avoiding Tension

When an incision is closed in an area of cutaneous laxity within natural skin folds, a fine linear scar is minimally visible. Inevitably, repair of many surgically created wounds will result in a closure under some degree of tension. Likewise, traumatic wounds with even minimal tissue loss can result in a gaping defect that, if closed, primarily would produce tension on the wound margins. Fortunately, several techniques are available to minimize or alleviate tension and thereby circumvent unsightly scarring.

Analyzing the degree of wound-edge retraction in a cutaneous defect prior to restoration aids in planning the repair technique and in choosing materials which will avoid undue closing tension. Simply undermining, while being mindful to preserve vascular integrity, can resolve minor tension but should be minimal in most cases as most of the gain from undermining occurs by releasing a limited area at the skin margins. Aggressive undermining results in more devascularization, bleeding, and raw surfaces, which is usually a poor trade-off for the limited reduction in tension. In more moderate or severe cases, suturing techniques must be utilized to effectively splint the wound until adequate tensile strength is attained; otherwise, the vectors of tension will need to be rearranged through application of flap techniques.

Choice of suture material must be carefully thought out. Buried absorbable sutures not only eliminate dead space but, by bringing together the deep layers, relieve tension on the more superficial areas, allowing good blood flow to the wound margins. Unfortunately, most absorbable sutures lose their tensile strength within 3 weeks, when wound strength is only about 10% of normal skin. The most long-lasting suture, polydioxanone, retains 50% of its tensile strength for 6 weeks, but scar widening can occur for 6 months.[18] Therefore, a nonabsorbable, superficial intradermal suture is necessary to effectively splint the wound until adequate tensile strength is achieved if the wound is under significant tension for an optimal outcome. If sutures are removed too early from wounds under tension, mechanical forces will cause hypertrophic scarring or, worse, dehiscence. This has to be balanced by the potential for suture extrusion and resulting inflammation.

Original width of a scar under tension at 3 weeks will increase fourfold by 6 months. In specific plastic surgery cases, such as abdominoplasty, where tension is concentrated at the incision line, using a polypropylene superficial intradermal suture for up to 6 months in addition to deep dermal polylactate or lactomer absorbable sutures significantly improves scar appearance. Another alternative to polypropylene is clear nylon, interrupted intradermal sutures, which are sometimes used in the face where the dermis is thin. If the sutures are 5-0 or 6-0, then inflammation and late suture extrusion are minimal. Polypropylene continuous sutures can be relatively easily removed at the 6-month time point if they are near the surface. However, in order to prevent slippage through the dermis, the ends must either be knotted, which can cause spitting and inflammation; or they may be locked and brought up through normal skin just past the boundary of the incision.

Tissue rearrangement with transposition flaps, such as z-plasty or w-plasty, can better align scars within relaxed skin tension lines. These techniques break up long, linear incisions which camouflage the scar, improving cosmesis. Function can also be improved due to a decrease in contraction. Tension redistribution is accomplished using adjacent areas of skin laxity and redirecting tension vectors. Disadvantages include possible delayed healing at triangle margins and increased length of incisions. If performing a z-plasty with 60-degree angles on each side, the scar will be lengthened 75%.[19] Many general textbooks on plastic surgery describe excellent, detailed, operative techniques for performing these and other types of transposition flaps.[20]

Reducing Inflammation

Exercising good surgical technique, abstaining from unnecessary retraction on the wound margins, and avoiding excessive handling of skin edges with improper instruments will minimize tissue trauma, and therefore inflammation. Toothed forceps should always be used on the skin when placing sutures, as nontoothed forceps can lead to crush injury and decreased blood flow. Adequate vascular inflow is essential to efficient wound healing. The ischemia produced by prolonged retraction or improper tissue handling is followed by subsequent reperfusion, causing an influx of leukocytes, complement activation, oxidative stress, and microvasculature dysfunction. The resultant tissue damage not only prolongs the inflammatory phase but also lengthens the rate of epithelization.

Rapid Epithelization

A wound should be closed primarily whenever possible to optimize rapid epithelization, rather than prolonging the inflammatory process and allowing granulation tissue to form. The excess collagen matrix produced by granulation tissue is predisposed to fibroproliferative scar formation. Meticulous placement of superficial dermal sutures allows for optimal wound coaptation, which accelerates epithelization. While waiting for wound re-epithelization, healing tissues should be covered with a semi-occlusive dressing which will enhance the wound-healing environment by acting as a water-barrier substitute for the protective stratum corneum of the keratinized epithelial layer. Paper tape, polyurethane film, silicone gel sheeting, or even an occlusive ointment can accomplish this goal. Furthermore, occlusion of healing wounds decreases pain and discomfort.

● COMPLICATIONS

Keloids and Hypertrophic Scarring

Two types of fibroproliferative scarring, hypertrophic scars and keloids scars, are the result of excess collagen deposition above that which normally occurs in an adequate wound-healing environment. Although keloids and hypertrophic scars are both the result of excessive scar formation, they have very distinct clinical and histopathologic findings. Therefore, it is not surprising that they differ in their pathophysiology, which has yet to be fully elucidated. Much of the existing knowledge concerning fibroproliferative scar pathogenesis is based on fibroblast activity and impaired matrix homeostasis during the inflammatory and maturation phases of wound healing. Prolonged inflammation stimulates many cytokines and growth factors, namely TGF-β, which activates collagen and extracellular matrix synthesis and inhibits breakdown of these constituents.[8] Prolonged inflammation can be due to technical reasons, such as reaction to sutures, necrotic skin edges, excess bacteria, poor skin apposition, or ingrown hairs. The inflammatory process is muted with aging, and so hypertrophic scarring and keloids occur predominantly in children and adults younger than 40 years of age. In addition, an exaggerated inflammatory phase can delay epithelization.

Fibroproliferative scars have several similar gross characteristics, such as erythema, rigidity, and a raised appearance. Patients also tend to report similar subjective findings, such as pain, burning, and itching. Increased collagen causes these scars to be raised and rigid, while excessive presence of mast cells which release histamine are thought to be responsible for the pruritis reported by many patients. However, fibroproliferative scars also have a distinct gross appearance, which makes them easily distinguishable from one another. Hypertrophic scars remain within the borders of the original wound, whereas keloid scars extend beyond the boundaries of injury. While histologically both types of scars display increased collagen deposition, increased cellularity, and increased angiogenesis compared with normal scar, the collagen organization is very different. Collagen bundles within hypertrophic scars, although flatter, wavy, and less distinct, are still similar to normal skin dermis in that they run parallel to the epidermis. Keloid collagen fibers, on the other hand, lack any type of discernable orientation relative to the epidermis and bundles are virtually absent.[21]

Both types of scars occur more often in sites of tension like the anterior chest and shoulders. Keloids have a predilection for the upper back, chest, upper arms, and shoulders. However, the most common location for keloids is the earlobe, which is likely the result of prolonged irritation and minor trauma from repeated insertion of earrings and inevitable presence of bacteria along the piercing tract in the setting of a patient who is genetically prone. Trauma in the form of a laceration, vaccination, or tattooing often is the inciting event in many keloid scars, regardless of location. Other inciting events may include surgery, burns, and many types of inflammation, such as insect bites, infections, and acne.

Demographically, fibroproliferative scars lack gender predominance and occur most frequently in patients between 10 and 30 years of age. Keloids are more common in dark-skinned individuals with a reported incidence of up to 16%, but which varies widely in many reports.[22] In our own clinical experience, true keloids in African Americans occur in no more than a very few percent, but are more common in some African populations. Hypertrophic scar incidence is less well documented and in some groups may occur in up to 50% of scars. However, the incidence of hypertrophic scars can be dramatically reduced with attention to scar prevention techniques discussed below. Obtaining a family history of fibroproliferative scarring is a requirement prior to any plastic surgery case, as genetic inheritance among patients with keloids has demonstrated both autosomal dominant and recessive patterns. However, personal history of scars is the most reliable. Because so many women have pierced ears, the presence or absence of ear keloids is a quick and useful history to obtain.

Understanding the known causes of fibroproliferative scarring translates into applying appropriate prevention strategies. Likewise, using the above-stated characteristics to distinguish between keloid and hypertrophic scars is paramount in applying the appropriate treatment regimens. Because the pathophysiology of these types of scars is so complex and not yet fully understood, treatment has had to focus on the few known causes. We will thus discuss several methods, although not one has proven to be superior to the others. Due to the challenging therapeutic dilemma facing plastic surgeons today, the best way to treat fibroproliferative scars is to prevent them.

Treatment of Fibroproliferative Scars

Hypertrophic scars start to appear several weeks after surgery. Fortunately, they tend to partially regress spontaneously or with nonsurgical, local treatment measures. In contrast, keloids scars may not appear until several months or even years after surgery and do not tend to spontaneously regress. The key to treatment is early recognition and prompt intervention.

Nonsurgical Management

Due to a lack of large prospective randomized clinical trials, efficacy of nonsurgical treatments is in large part due to surgeon experience and extensive use. Injection of insoluble steroids and application of silicone gel are the two most widely accepted forms of nonsurgical treatment; however, pulsed dye lasers, cryotherapy, and radiation are other scar therapies that have been used with success.

Intralesional Steroid Injections. Insoluble steroid injections may be used in both prevention and treatment of fibroproliferative scarring. In addition, these injections offer symptomatic relief of pain and pruritis. The 50% to 100% scar response rate of intralesional steroid injections is quite variable, and recurrence rates may approach 50%.[23] Steroids act directly to suppress collagen synthesis and increase collagen breakdown, and indirectly reduce collagen by reducing inflammatory mediators. The most common injectable steroid for scar treatments is triamcinolone acetonide; however, dosage and frequency of administration depend on the surgeon and severity of the lesion. For prevention, steroid may be layered into the wound just prior to closure. Good surgical technique, appropriate suture selection, and prolonged maintenance of wound splinting will protect the wound from the delayed gain of tensile strength secondary to steroid effects. Most adverse events, such as extensive wound-healing delay, depigmentation, atrophy, and telangiectasias, occur with inadvertent injection of the tissues surrounding the scar or use of too high a dose. In the treatment of scars, small amounts should be injected while withdrawing the needle through scar tissue to optimize delivery.

Occlusive Dressings. Occlusive dressings made from silicone are manufactured and packaged in many forms: sheeting, ointment, gel, or spray. There has been ample debate regarding the mechanism of action of silicone occlusion. Through recent studies and research in our laboratory, we believe that silicone occlusion of a wound mimics the stratum corneum, providing a moist environment and hydration of the healing tissue layers, which reduces inflammation and promotes early epithelization. Occlusion further provides symptomatic relief of pain and pruritis and decreases scar elevation. Silicone occlusion may also be used as prevention applied after taping or approximately 2 weeks after surgery; however, it must be used at least 12 hours per day for 2 to 3 months to impart an effect. All fresh surgical wounds should be treated with occlusive dressings, such as Steri-Strips, for approximately 2 weeks. Occlusion provides a moist healing environment which enhances rapid epithelization.

Radiation. Use of radiation remains controversial due to risk of carcinogenesis. However, with improved technology and precision dosimetry, radiation may be delivered directly to the lesion with minimal radiation to surrounding tissue. Radiation restricts the growth of new blood vessels and inhibits proliferation of fibroblasts. When combined with surgery, radiation treatment can have up to a 37% recurrence rate.[24] In our opinion, the use of radiation should be restricted to keloids recalcitrant to other treatments.

Lasers. Carbon dioxide, Nd:YAG, and argon lasers have all been shown to decrease erythema and provide symptomatic relief; however, these modalities have minimal effect on scar reduction with high rates of recurrence.[25] Although anecdotal reports support the efficacy of laser, there is a lack of prospective randomized studies. Scars improve spontaneously over time, so it is difficult to judge how effective lasers are.

Pressure Dressings. Compression of fibroproliferative scars with pressure dressings should begin as soon as epithelization is complete. The exact mechanism of action is unknown; however, histological observations of decreased fibroblast content are attributed to local tissue hypoxia. Clinically, scars partially reduce in size and soften in most patients; however, garments must be worn 18 to 24 hours a day for 6 to 12 months. Further disadvantages include lack of comfort, especially if worn in warm weather or over areas of mobility such as joints. These areas are best treated by other means, as maintenance of sufficient compression necessary for success is not usually achieved. Pressure earring clips for ear keloids can be effective, and pressure garments for burn scars are still widely used; but the duration of treatment, the pressure needed for efficacy and other variables are not known, so treatment protocols are largely empiric.

Cryosurgery. Cryosurgery with substances such as liquid nitrogen induces microvascular damage resulting in ischemia. Three treatments have shown volume reduction greater than 80% in many keloids scars.[26] These treatments may need to be repeated to reduce recurrence risk; and the freezing process causes pain, hypopigmentation, and atrophic depressed scars. Furthermore, this modality is only used in a few centers.

Future Treatments. Novel scar therapies are based on the molecular pathophysiology of fibroproliferative scarring. The two most studied regimens consist of interferons and TGF-β. In culture, interferons reduce fibroblast production of collagen and increase collagenase activity.[27] When injected, scar height may be reduced up to 50%. Furthermore, when injected at the time of keloid excision, it may reduce recurrence rates.[28] TGF-β is a key mediator in the pathogenesis of fibroproliferative scarring. It therefore is not surprising that studies have shown a reduction in hypertrophic scarring with antibodies against TGF-β.[29]

Surgical Management

Surgical excision as a single modality treatment for keloids has a high failure rate, with recurrences reported in up to 90% of cases.[20] Hypertrophic scars can also be very difficult to treat. Therefore, a combination of surgical excision and local scar treatment using nonsurgical techniques is essential in obtaining an aesthetically pleasing result with low risk of recurrence. Keloids pose the most challenging problem and are quite resistant to spontaneous regression. Therefore, adjuvant therapy in addition to combination treatments is often necessary (Figure 1-3A,B) Since these types of scars are usually the result of inflammation, removal of stimulating factors such as foreign bodies and infection are a priority.

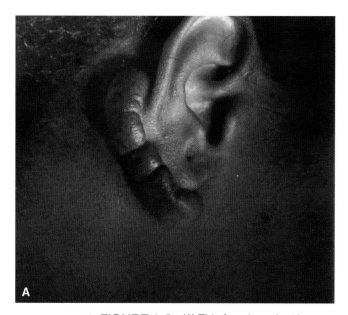
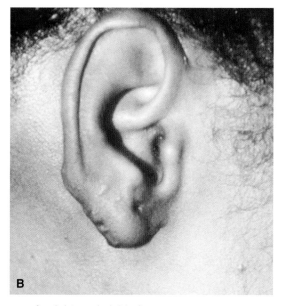

● **FIGURE 1-3.** (A) This female patient has recurrence of a right ear keloid after surgical excision and steroid injections. (B) Several months later, the lesion was again surgically removed with skin grafting to repair the defect. Adjuvant therapy with radiation was begun the day of surgery. Combination therapy is often required to successfully treat earlobe keloids.

When formulating a treatment plan for fibroproliferative scars, causative factors should first be explored. If the fibroproliferative scar was caused by any of the factors discussed above, such as excessive tension with failure to effectively support the wound with appropriate nonabsorbable intradermal sutures for a period up to 6 months, prolonged inflammation, or delayed epithelization, then these variables can be addressed at the time of repair after simple scar excision. Following wound closure, application of early postoperative occlusion and subsequent use of local nonsurgical treatment measures will further decrease the risk of recurrence.

Use of transposition flaps, such as the z-plasty or w-plasty, should be reserved for scar contractures or for scars under excessive tension. The beneficial results from reorientation of tissues will outweigh the increased scar length and potentially negative effects of delayed epithelization at the flap tips.

REFERENCES

1. Thacker JG, Stalnecker MC, Allaire PE, et al. Practical applications of skin biomechanics. *Clin Plast Surg.* 1977;4(2):167.

2. Edlich RF, Becker DG, Long WB, et al. Excisional biopsy of skin tumors. *J Long Term Eff Med Implants.* 2004;14(3):201.

3. Zamir E, Geiger B. Molecular complexity and dynamics of cell-matrix adhesions. *J Cell Sci.* 2001;114:3583.

4. Katsumi A, Orr AW, Tzima E, et al. Integrins in mechanotransduction. *J Biol Chem.* 2004;279(13):12001.

5. Niland S, Cremer A, Fluck J, et al. Contraction-dependent apoptosis of normal dermal fibroblasts. *J Invest Dermatol.* 2001;116(5):686.

6. Van Winkle W Jr. The tensile strength of wounds and factors that influence it. *Surg Gynecol Obstet.* 1969;129(4):819.

7. Levenson SM, Geever EF, Crowley EW, et al. The healing of rat skin wounds. *Ann Surg.* 1965;161:293.

8. Shah M, Foreman DM, Ferguson MW. Neutralisation of TGF-beta 1 and TGF-beta 2 or exogenous addition of TGF-beta 3 to cutaneous rat wounds reduces scarring. *J Cell Sci.* 1995;108:985.

9. Mustoe TA, Cooter RD, Gold MH, et al. International clinical recommendations on scar management. *Plast Reconstr Surg.* 2002;110(2):560.

10. Bartak P. The epidermal permeability barrier and its function in immune reactions. *Cas Lek Cesk.* 2001;140(9):259.

11. Deitch EA, Wheelahan TM, Rose MP, et al. Hypertrophic burn scars: analysis of variables. *J Trauma.* 1983;23(10):895.

12. Hayward PG, Robson MC. Animal models of wound contraction. *Prog Clin Biol Res.* 1991;365:301.

13. Desmouliere A, Chaponnier C, Gabbiani G. Tissue repair, contraction, and the myofibroblast. *Wound Repair Regen.* 2005;13(1):7.

14. Liu XD, Umino T, Ertl R, et al. Persistence of TGF-beta1 induction of increased fibroblast contractility. *In Vitro Cell Dev Biol Anim.* 2001;37(3):193.

15. Mirastschijski U, Haaksma CJ, Tomasek JJ, et al. Matrix metalloproteinase inhibitor GM 6001 attenuates keratinocyte migration, contraction and myofibroblast formation in skin wounds. *Exp Cell Res.* 2004;299(2):465.

16. Fogdestam I. A biomechanical study of healing rat skin incisions after delayed primary closure. *Surg Gynecol Obstet.* 1981;153(2):191.

17. Coulthard P, Worthington H, Esposito M, et al. Tissue adhesives for closure of surgical incisions. *Cochrane Database Syst Rev.* 2004;(2):CD004287.

18. Mustoe TA. Surgery of scars: hypertrophic, keloid and aesthetic sequellae. In: Teot L, ed. *Surgery in Wounds.* Heidelberg, Germany: Springer-Verlag; 2004:504.

19. Hove CR, Williams EF, Rodgers BJ. Z-plasty: a concise review. *Facial Plast Surg.* 2001;17(4):289.

20. Aston S, Beasley R, Thorne C. *Grabb & Smith's Plastic Surgery.* 5th ed. Philadelphia, PA: Lippincott-Raven Publishers; 1997.

21. Ehrlich HP, Desmouliere A, Diegelmann RF, et al. Morphological and immunochemical differences between keloid and hypertrophic scar. *Am J Pathol.* 1994;145(1):105.

22. Rahban SR, Garner WL. Fibroproliferative scars. *Clin Plast Surg.* 2003;30(1):77.

23. Berman B, Flores F. Recurrence rates of excised keloids treated with postoperative triamcinolone acetonide injections or interferon alfa-2b injections. *J Am Acad Dermatol.* 1997;37(5 Pt 1):755.

24. Ogawa R, Mitsuhashi K, Hyakusoku H, et al. Postoperative electron-beam irradiation therapy for keloids and hypertrophic scars: retrospective study of 147 cases followed for more than 18 months. *Plast Reconstr Surg.* 2003;111(2):547.

25. Norris JE. The effect of carbon dioxide laser surgery on the recurrence of keloids. *Plast Reconstr Surg.* 1991;87(1):44.

26. Rusciani L, Paradisi A, Alfano C, et al. Cryotherapy in the treatment of keloids. *J Drugs Dermatol.* 2006;5(7):591.

27. Duncan MR, Berman B. Gamma interferon is the lymphokine and beta interferon the monokine responsible for inhibition of fibroblast collagen production and late but not early fibroblast proliferation. *J Exp Med.* 1985;162(2):516.

28. Larrabee WF, East CA, Jaffe HS, et al. Intralesional interferon gamma treatment for keloids and hypertrophic scars. *Arch Otolaryngol Head Neck Surg.* 1990:116(10):1159.

29. Lu L, Saulis AS, Liu WR, et al. The temporal effects of anti-TGF-beta1, 2, and 3 monoclonal antibody on wound healing and hypertrophic scar formation. *J Am Coll Surg.* 2005;201(3):391.

chapter 2

Perforator Flaps

Christoph Heitmann, MD, PhD / *Robert J. Allen, MD*

● INTRODUCTION

As the twentieth century drew to a close, it seemed as if there was little left in the way of fundamental flap design to be discovered. The reconstructive microsurgeon had numerous musculocutaneous and fasciocutaneous flaps at hand and the operative microscope enabled him/her to use those flaps to reconstruct the most challenging defects. The musculocutaneous free flaps, however, were bulky because of the obligatory muscle and often imposed a greater morbidity on the donor site when compared to their fasciocutaneous counterparts. In 1989, Koshima presented his work with a skin flap based only on a perforating vessel of the deep fascia that emanated from the deep inferior epigastric artery. Koshima became the first surgeon to name a "perforator flap." With this information, it became apparent that vessels previously thought to be too small to sustain a flap by themselves now needed to be reconsidered. Allen also targeted the perforators of the deep inferior epigastric artery. By 1992, Allen showed that it was possible to dissect musculocutaneous perforators and trace them to their underlying source vessel to provide a sleeker flap and at the same time to preserve muscle function. Thus the deep inferior epigastric perforator (DIEP) flap was introduced for autologous breast reconstruction. The success of the DIEP flap stimulated re-examination of other musculocutaneous flaps. The concept of "perforator flaps" evolved and was expanded to include the direct fasciocutaneous vessels. The current information about existing perforator flaps are gathered in one comprehensive work. The book *Perforator Flaps* by Blondeel, Morris, Hallock, and Neligan is unique in its coverage and contains all pioneers who blazed the trails to bring us to this point in the development of the perforator flap technique.[1]

Perforator flaps represent the latest milestone in the evolution of reconstructive flap surgery. They provide the reconstructive microsurgeon with more freedom to select a donor site that most closely matches the recipient site skin color, thickness, texture, and subcutaneous fat quality. More attention can be paid to the aesthetic quality of the reconstruction.

We have progressed from the era of simply closing defects to that of customizing our reconstructions to achieve the best functional and aesthetic result in the reconstructed site as well as the donor site. If one masters the technique for freeing the perforator vessels from surrounding tissues, the only limitations to the development of new perforator flaps will be the individual surgeons' ingenuity, creativity, and surgical skill. We firmly believe that by learning about perforator flaps, one will gain access to a vast array of new reconstructive options that will benefit his or her practice and patients.

However, within the first years of the development of perforator flaps, confusion was already present. Soon it became clear that in a totally new field of flap surgery, many surgeons were taking initiative to develop new flaps. Myriads of so-called "perforator flaps" have been published. Different authors were using different names for the same flap, leading to much confusion. Soon there was a European point of view, a Canadian proposal, and a statement by the Asian microsurgical community on the nomenclature of perforator flaps. Blondeel and colleagues proposed a global standard nomenclature as follows.

Definition of a Perforator Flap

A perforator vessel starts where it branches off its source vessel that has a common anatomic name and ends in the subdermal plexus. Generally, perforators do not have a name. To classify perforator flaps it is necessary to differentiate between three types of perforator vessels. The schematic drawing (Figure 2-1) shows direct perforators, indirect muscle perforators, and indirect septal perforators. Direct perforators perforate only the deep fascia after they branch of

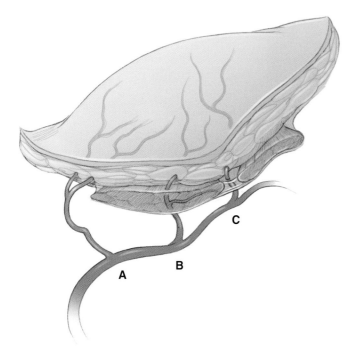

● **FIGURE 2-1.** Schematic drawing of the abdominal wall as a cross-section. (A) Direct perforator. (B) Indirect muscle perforator. (C) Indirect septal perforator.

the source artery, pass through loose fatty tissue, and supply the blood to a distinct area of skin and subcutaneous fat (eg, SIEA [superficial inferior epigastric artery] flap, groin flap). Indirect perforators will run through a specific anatomic structure such as muscle or septum before piercing the deep fascia. Skin flaps vascularized by a muscle perforator are called musculocutaneous perforator flaps, such as DIEP, the superior gluteal artery perforator (S-GAP), and the inferior gluteal artery perforator (I-GAP).

Skin flaps vascularized by septal perforators are called septocutaneous perforator flaps. By these definitions, it is possible to classify most of the perforator flaps used in daily practice as indirect musculocutaneous, indirect septocutaneous, or direct perforator flaps.

To give a perforator flap a name, certain rules should be followed. A perforator flap should be named after the nutrient artery, and not after the underlying muscle. Muscle perforator flaps are named by their nutrient or source vessel. The letters *AP* always follow the abbreviation of the source vessel (for example, S-GAP stands for superior gluteal artery perforator flap). Inclusion of the *A* of artery makes pronunciation and semantics easier in most cases. If the nomenclature is not specific enough, the muscle origin of the perforators is abbreviated and italicized to indicate the anatomic origin of the flap. For example, LCFAP-VL stands for the lateral circumflex femoral artery perforator-vastus lateralis muscle, and LCFAP-TFL stands for the lateral circumflex femoral artery perforator-tensor fascia lata muscle.

The goal of this nomenclature is to end the Babel of language and create a universal scientific language. Another advantage of the nomenclature is that the term "perforator

flap" indicates to the surgeon involved that a specific surgical technique is needed to harvest the flap. The adjuncts of indirect musculocutaneous, indirect septocutaneous, and direct perforator flap clearly describe which surgical technique is needed. Indirect musculocutaneous perforator flaps will have to be raised by opening the deep fascia, splitting the donor muscle, preserving its other vascularization and motor innervation, and eventually, exposing its source artery. In a direct perforator flap, like the groin flap, the perforators do not run through a specific intermuscular septum. A specific septum is not looked for and the microsurgical technique is different from the technique used to harvest a septocutaneous flap.

Perforator flaps have allowed the transfer of the patients' own skin and fat in a reliable manner with minimal donor site morbidity for more than a decade. However, these techniques have brought new difficulties and problems that must be addressed. First and foremost, these techniques require microsurgical expertise.

What is the learning curve for a perforator flap breast reconstruction? Some say perhaps 50 to 100 procedures. Variability of vascular anatomy contributes to the difficulties with the procedures. Judgment as to how many and what size and location of perforators to select affect factors such as length of operation and incidence of fat necrosis. It is amazing how little blood supply is actually necessary to adequately perfuse skin and fat, but how little is enough? It is beyond the scope of this chapter to give an overview of all the existing perforator flaps. The authors will rather present the perforator flaps they are most confident with, such as DIEP, SIEP, S-GAP, I-GAP, LCFAP-VL (former ALT), and TDAP flap.

● DEEP INFERIOR EPIGASTRIC PERFORATOR FLAP

The DIEP flap arose as a refinement of the conventional transverse rectus abdominis myocutaneous (TRAM) flap. The DIEP flap can carry the same tissue as the TRAM flap without the sacrifice of the rectus muscle or fascia, thereby minimizing donor site morbidity including bulge, hernia, weakness and shortening recovery time. The DIEP flap is commonly used for breast restoration to provide a soft, naturally shaped, long-lasting result.[2]

Patient Evaluation and Selection

An excellent source of soft tissue for free flap reconstructions is the lower abdomen in women. Generally speaking, women who would benefit from an abdominoplasty are possible candidates for a DIEP flap and in fact most women who have had or will have mastectomies for breast cancer are candidates for the DIEP flap. In the case of breast reconstruction, we prefer to have the patient complete any radiation therapy and a delay of 6 months prior to the free flap procedure. While the perforator flaps usually tolerate radiation well, a superior long-term result is typically obtained in reconstructions performed after rather than before chest wall radiation. Abdominal scarring is probably the most important risk factor for raising a DIEP flap and can cause major problems during the dissection of perforators and epigastric vessels.

Intramuscular scarring is not always diagnosed on preoperative ultrasound and can spread out further than suspected from the place and length of a previous incision. Smoking is considered a relative contraindication to raising a DIEP flap. Smokers who request elective, delayed reconstructions are required to stop smoking at least 3 months before becoming a candidate for surgery. Absolute contraindications for a DIEP procedure in our practice are history of previous abdominoplasty or abdominal liposuction.

Patient Preparation

The patient is usually seen in the office on the day prior to surgery for preoperative markings and Doppler studies. The patient should assume a standing position and an elliptical skin island is drawn on the abdomen. The borders of a DIEP flap are generally located at the level of the suprapubic crease, the umbilicus, and both ASI spines. A DIEP flap generally measures 12 cm in height and extends 20 to 24 cm from the midline. The tension of the donor site following closure should be estimated, as this ultimately limits the size of the flap that can be harvested. The side of the abdomen contralateral to the side to be reconstructed is preferred, as this provides for easier insetting at the time of surgery. With the patient in supine position, a Doppler probe is used to identify the main perforators of the deep inferior epigastric artery. This road map of the largest perforators helps the surgeon make decisions intraoperatively. The superficial inferior epigastric artery and vein are likewise found with the Doppler and marked. The operation is performed under general anesthesia, with the patient in supine position and the arms positioned beside the trunk. Preoperatively placement of intravenous lines, an indwelling urinary catheter and deep vein thrombosis prophylaxis with low dose heparin and sequential pressure hose.

Technique

A two-team approach is used, with simultaneous raising of the flap and preparation of the recipient vessels. For breast reconstruction, internal mammary artery (IMA) and vein (IMV) are the recipient vessels of choice and are used in more than 90% of our cases. The central positions of IMA and IMV in the chest wall make medial placement of the flap easier on insetting. The vessels are dissected between second and third rib space. A distance of 2 to 3 cm width is enough space to enable anastomosis. If the rib space is less than 3 cm in width, the removal of a portion of the lower rib is performed. The thoracodorsal vessels are used alternatively when the internal mammary vessels prevent proper flap insetting and geometry, such as in cases of partial breast reconstruction. While making the inferior skin incision, care is taken to preserve the superficial epigastric vein. If venous drainage of the flap is insufficient or

thrombosis of the perforator veins occurs after the anastomosis, the superficial epigastric vein can be used as an additional venous conduit. The vein is dissected over a length of 4 to 5 cm and ligated with clips to make them easily retrievable later, if needed. If the inferior epigastric vessels are found to be sufficient in size and quality, they are followed down to their origin from the common femoral artery and an SIEA perforator flap can be performed.

For the DIEP flap, the abdominal incisions are continued down to the fascia. Beveling is avoided unless extra volume is required, as this may later lead to a depressed scar in the abdomen. However, the flap may be beveled laterally to include more fat and reduce residual dog ears. The dissection of the vascular pedicle of a DIEP flap can be divided into three different technical stages: suprafascial, intramuscular, and submuscular. The most demanding stage is the intramuscular dissection of the vascular pedicle.

At first, the abdominal skin island is carefully elevated from lateral to medial until the lateral row of perforators is encountered. If a large perforator is found, the flap may be based on this vessel. Additional perforators in the same row may also be dissected and included with the flap for additional perfusion.

If no large perforator is found, the medial row is approached in a similar fashion. If no dominant single perforator is found, two or even three smaller perforators in the same medial or lateral row may be taken to carry the flap. In cases where more than one large perforator is present, the perforator with a more central location to the proposed flap is used. In our experience, approximately 25% of DIEP flaps are based on one perforator, 50% on two, and 25% on three and more perforators. We prefer a flap to be based on a single large perforator. The abdominal muscles must be relaxed at all times and the perforating vessels kept moist with normal saline. Complete dissection of a perforator helps prevent vessel damage when raising the flap from the contralateral side. In the case of a unilateral DIEP flap reconstruction, if the medial and lateral row perforators on the initially approached side of the abdomen are found to be less than optimal, the perforators on the opposite side of the abdomen are investigated as the contralateral side often yields a perforator of better quality.

Once the appropriate perforators are chosen, the anterior rectus fascia is incised with a pair of microscissors, following the direction of the rectus abdominis muscle fibers at the rim of the tiny gap in the fascia through which the perforating vessel passes. If more than one perforator is dissected, the different gaps can be connected. The division of the fascia is continued superiorly for a distance of 2 to 4 cm, and inferiorly to the lateral border of the rectus abdominis muscle. It is advisable to fully complete the dissection of the DIEP flap on one side before progressing to the other. This precaution provides a lifeboat in the form of a contralateral DIEP flap to be performed if the perforator is inadvertently damaged. As dissection progresses, the DIEP flap should be secured to the abdominal wall or carefully held by an assistant. The rectus abdominis muscle is spread apart in the direction of the fibers and care is taken to identify and preserve any intercostal nerves. Dissection continues through the muscle down to the deep inferior epigastric vessels. By doing so the perforator is liberated from the muscle by blunt dissection, staying close to the vessel at all times, as it remains covered by a thin layer of loose connective tissue.

As a general rule, if resistance to dissection is encountered, a side branch or a nerve is identified. Using bipolar coagulation diathermy and small hemoclips, one continues to ligate all side branches until the inferior epigastric artery is reached on the posterior surface of the rectus abdominis muscle. If two perforators have been selected that run in adjacent perimysial planes, the muscle fibers between the two must be divided.

In submuscular dissection, the lateral border of the rectus abdominis muscle is raised to open the plane posterior to the rectus abdominis muscle. The main pedicle of the deep inferior epigastric vessels is exposed and side branches of the main stem are ligated. The length of the pedicle can be tailored to meet the needs of different recipient sites, or the demands of the shape of the flap. If one is certain that the blood flow through the deep inferior epigastric vessels is sufficient, the remainder of the flap can be raised. The umbilicus is released and the entire skin flap is raised. The artery and the veins of the pedicle are then clipped and the pedicle slid out underneath any crossing intercostal nerves. Sometimes, it is necessary to divide a crossing motor intercostal nerve to release the vascular pedicle. In these cases, the nerve is repaired with two interrupted 8-0 nylon sutures prior to closure of the abdominal fascia. The flap is then weighted and transferred to the recipient site. Great care is taken to lay the donor pedicle to the recipient vessels without any twists or kinks. While the overall incidence of vascular complication is low, experience has shown that many cases of venous compromise can be traced to a twisted pedicle. Temporary stay sutures are placed in the flap with the orientation of the 180 degrees with the umbilicus inferiorly. This allows for the thicker part of the flap to lie medially on the chest wall. The operating microscope is brought into position.

For the venous anastomosis, we use an anastomotic coupling device. The coupling device makes the anastomosis easier and faster, and has the additional benefit of stenting the vein open after the vessels are joined.

The arterial anastomosis is typically performed manually with interrupted sutures. After the anastomosis is complete, the flap is checked for bleeding and capillary refill.

The insetting and closure are performed over a suction drain and great care is used to monitor the integrity of the pedicle during the insetting of the flap at all times. If a contralateral flap is used, the flap is turned between approximately 90 to 120 degrees, such that the medial portion of the abdominal flap becomes the base of the reconstructed breast. Excess skin is de-epithelialized superiorly and inferiorly, and the flap inset with a visible skin paddle is left in place. The external Doppler probe is used to identify the

locations on the flap with good arterial and venous signals, and these locations are marked for postoperative monitoring in the postanesthesia care unit and on the floor with a hand held Doppler. For monitoring, it is also possible to use an implantable Doppler probe. This is especially helpful in cases where a smaller skin paddle is left or no dominant point can be found on the exposed skin portion of an otherwise healthy flap. Also, in nipple sparing mastectomies where no skin island is left, the implantable probe is used. Care must be taken with the placement of these probes. A Doppler sleeve placed too loosely around the vessel may result in loss of signal despite the presence of good blood flow, while a tight sleeve or wire connection may kink or otherwise compromise the vessel's patency.

The abdominal fascia is closed and securely tied with a running size 1-0 absorbable suture. Mesh or other synthetic materials are not used in abdominal wall closures. The edges of the umbilicus are tacked down to the fascia with a 2-0 Vicryl suture. The upper abdominal flap is undermined to the level of the xiphoid and costal margin. The patient is then flexed and the wound closed in layers over two closed suction drains. As in an abdominoplasty, the umbilicus is brought out through the abdominal flap and secured in place (Figure 2-2A,B).

Complications

Complications are infrequent. In the published series by the senior author of over 750 DIEP flap reconstructions, 6% of patients returned to the operating room for flap-related problems. Partial flap loss occurred in 2.5% and total flap loss in less than 1%. Problems with the vein or venous anastomosis were almost four times more likely than problems with the arterial anastomosis. Fat necrosis appeared in 12% of flaps. Seroma formation at the abdominal donor site was approximately 3.5% and abdominal hernia occurred in 0.7% of cases.

● THE SUPERFICIAL INFERIOR EPIGASTRIC ARTERY PERFORATOR FLAP

An SIEA flap could be an ideal flap for breast reconstruction concerning both the donor site morbidity and the quality and volume of the tissue. This technique was first used by us for breast reconstruction in 1989. However, the SIEA flap has never been very popular because of its variable vascular anatomy, often small arterial vessel diameter, and insufficient blood supply for the contralateral abdomen.

Patient Evaluation and Selection

The SIEA flap provides the same abdominal skin and fat for reconstruction as the DIEP flap. Of the two flaps, the SIEA flap causes the least donor site morbidity as no incision must be made in the abdominal fascia and no vessel dissection performed through the rectus abdominis muscle.

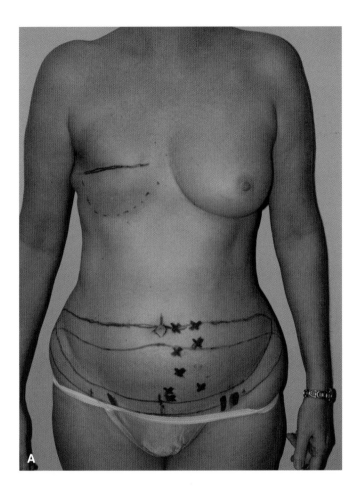

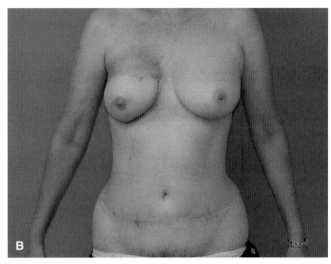

● **FIGURE 2-2.** (A) Preoperative view of a patient marked for DIEP (*upper ellipse*) and SIEA (*lower ellipse*). (B) Results at 1 year after DIEP and nipple-areola reconstruction.

There is minimal to no risk of a new abdominal hernia and even less abdominal pain than with other abdominal flaps. The amount of skin and fat which may be safely carried by an SIEA flap is limited to zones 1 and 2 and any tissue taken more than 1 to 2 cm past the midline will often demarcate and necrose in hours or days after the initial reconstruction. Because the vascular pedicle extends from one side of the flap, insetting at the donor site may be more difficult compared to the DIEP flap. The indications for the SIEA flap are the same as for the DIEP flap.

Patient Preparation

The markings, preoperative preparation and operating room set up are the same for the SIEA flap as with the DIEP flap and therefore the SIEA flap is marked using the standard abdominoplasty pattern.

An advantage is that sometimes the pattern can be shifted lower on the abdomen. According to the skin and volume requirements, the SIEA flap needs to be planned, keeping in mind that only half of the lower abdominal region has adequate blood perfusion unless the artery is located more medial than usual in which case contralateral abdominal tissue can be used.

Rather than taking too much tissue across the midline, a more lateral design is recommended. For identification of the superficial inferior epigastric vessels, the midpoint between the anterior iliac spine and pubic tubercle is marked. Often the superficial inferior epigastric artery pedicle can be found lateral to this point.

Technique

During flap harvest, the superficial inferior epigastric vessels are approached first. If these vessels are found to have sufficient caliber (approx. 1.0–1.5 mm) at the level of the inferior flap incision, they are followed down to their origin from the common femoral artery and saphenous bulb. The origin of the superficial inferior epigastric vessels is found 1 to 3 cm below the inguinal ligament. The pedicle pierces the cribriform fascia one finger width beneath the inguinal ligament and ascends in the subcutaneous tissue to the level of the umbilicus. Only the surgical dissection itself at the level of the inguinal ligament confirms the presence and caliber of the pedicle, although preoperative Doppler can suggest the size. After the skin is incised, the superficial epigastric vein is typically identified under loupe magnification, lying superficially and medially. Next, the dissection is continued more laterally and deeply, but superficial to the Scarpa fascia, to find the superficial inferior epigastric artery pedicle. Two veins are used to drain an unilateral SIEA flap. One is a superficial vein, which is medial and superficial to

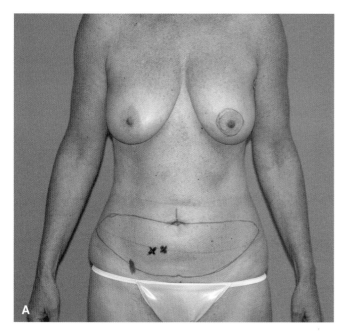
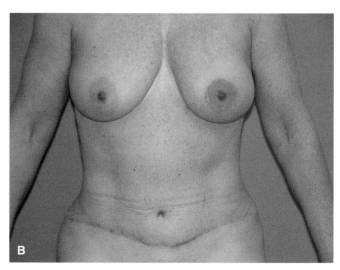

● **FIGURE 2-3.** (A) Preoperative view of a patient marked for SIEA breast reconstruction. (B) Result after immediate breast reconstruction with SIEA flap and secondary nipple-areola reconstruction.

the superficial inferior epigastric artery pedicle and always has a large diameter. The other vein is a comitant vein of the superficial inferior epigastric pedicle. The venae comitantes should have an acceptable diameter for microvascular anastomoses. If it becomes apparent that the superficial inferior epigastric artery on one side of a lower abdominal flap is inappropriate with respect to diameter, the contralateral artery should be explored in the same way.

The vascular anatomy of each side is usually different. After identification of a sufficient pedicle, the incisions of the flap edges are completed to the level of the external oblique fascia, from which the entire flap can be harvested in the plane superficial to the aponeurosis of the abdominal muscles.

When an SIEA is dissected to the common femoral artery, there is usually a common trunk with the superficial circumflex iliac artery. This common trunk matches the IMA best. If neither superficial inferior epigastric artery pedicle is satisfactory, the next flap to consider is the DIEP flap (Figure 2-3A,B).

Complications

Complications for the SIEA flap are similar to those for the DIEP flap. In a review on more than 200 SIEA flap breast reconstructions, rates of return to the operating room and arterial and venous insufficiency are similar to those found with DIEP flap reconstructions. The rate of abdominal seroma formation was slightly higher, approximately 9% vs 3.5% for the DIEP flap, due to the increased dissection around the inguinal lymphatics as required by this procedure. A hernia or bulge is not a possibility for the SIEA flap.

● SUPERIOR GLUTEAL ARTERY PERFORATOR FLAP

The gluteal artery perforator flaps are a good choice for breast reconstruction in women whose abdomen is not a choice. The donor site morbidity is minimal and no sacrifice of muscle is required.[3,4]

Patient Evaluation and Selection

Patients who require large volume tissue transfer may be candidates for GAP flaps. Patients in whom the abdomen cannot be used as a donor site or who have more tissue in the buttocks area than in the abdomen are the best candidates.

Absolute contraindications specific to GAP flap breast reconstruction include history of previous liposuction at the donor site or active smoking. Patients should be informed about possible contour deformities and the future location of a scar at the buttock.

The horizontal, or preferably, the upwardly slanted oblique designs are superior to other designs in the gluteal area in terms of concavity of the donor site and concealing the scar. Closure of the superficial fascial system is also important to avoid contour irregularity.

Patient Preparation

Markings are placed while the patient is placed in lateral position for unilateral reconstruction and prone for bilateral reconstruction. The Doppler probe is used to find perforating vessels from the superior gluteal artery. These are usually found approximately one third of the distance on a line from the posterior superior iliac crest to the greater trochanter.

Additional perforators may be found slightly more lateral from above. The skin paddle is marked in an oblique pattern from inferior medial to superior lateral to include these perforators. Hence, the outline of the flap may be customized to almost any orientation, as long as it contains the perforating vessels. The width of the skin paddle is 8 to 10 cm. The length of the flap is usually 20 to 24 cm.

Patient positioning is very important when using the S-GAP flap. In a lateral decubitus position, a two-team approach is possible. Normally, the arm ipsilateral to the breast being reconstructed is prepared and draped into the field so that it can be maneuvered to provide adequate exposure. The patient is returned to a supine position after harvesting of the flap, closure of the donor site, and before flap anastomosis. When breast reconstruction is being performed, the mastectomy specimen is weighed to gauge the volume needed. The flap dimensions are measured and flap weight (g) is estimated as follows: width (cm) × one half of the length (cm) × height or thickness (cm). For example, an S-GAP flap that is 20 cm long, 10 cm wide, and 4 cm thick would have an appropriate weight of 400 g. These weights and estimates are important to avoid over or under harvest.

Technique

An incision is made and carried down to the fascia of the gluteus maximus muscle. Beveling is used as needed in the superior and inferior direction to harvest enough tissue. The flap is elevated from the muscle in the subfascial plane and the perforators approached beginning from medial to lateral. It is preferred to use a single large perforator, if it is present, but two perforators which lay in the same plane and the direction of the gluteus muscle fibers can be taken together as well. Subfascial elevation is also performed from lateral to medial to ensure that the largest perforator is found before the flap is islanded out. The muscle is then spread in the direction of the muscle fibers, and the perforating vessels are dissected free. The dissection proceeds until both the artery and vein are of sufficient size to be anastomosed. The artery usually is the limiting factor in this dissection. The artery and vein diameter for anastomosis is 2.0 to 2.5 mm and 3.0 to 4.0 mm, respectively. Excellent exposure is required throughout the procedure but becomes critically important when ligating tributaries to the superior gluteal vein. Without adequate exposure, the risk of injury to the gluteal vein is significant. To avoid this damage, we recommend placing the retractor so that it holds the piriformis and gluteus minimus muscle apart. Ligation of the venous tributaries is performed only when the gluteal vein is clearly visualized as it exits the pelvis. The pedicle length is usually 7 to 9 cm. The donor defect should be closed with great care. After undermining the skin flaps, a single suction drain is placed over the muscle. The superficial fascial system is identified and closed with sutures before final skin closure. At the end of the procedure the patient should be placed in a supporting girdle, which we recommend be worn for 2 weeks as well as leaving the drain for 2 weeks (Figure 2-4A–D).

Complications

In a review of 394 GAP flaps done by the senior author for breast reconstruction, the incidence of complications was low. The overall take-back rate was approximately 8% with 6% rate of vascular complication.

The total flap failure rate was approximately 2%. Donor site seroma occurred in 6% of patients and approximately 10% of patients required revision of the donor site.

● INFERIOR GLUTEAL ARTERY PERFORATOR FLAP

The technique of the S-GAP flap was applied to the inferior gluteal vasculature practically at the same time in 1993. However, in the early experiences with the I-Gap flap, surgeons felt the donor sight contour and scar location of the I-GAP flap was inferior to the S-GAP procedure.[3,4] In 2004, we began placing the scar in the lower gluteal crease and harvesting fat from the trochanter area. This preserves the round shape of the upper buttock. Although the sciatic nerve is adjacent to the inferior gluteal vessels, we have had no case of sciatic verve damage in approximately 100 I-GAP procedures.

Patient Evaluation and Selection

As for the S-GAP, the I-GAP flap is the better choice for patients with inadequate tissue in the abdomen. For some patients with excess tissue in the saddle bag area, an I-GAP flap may be chosen over an S-GAP flap to make use of this extra tissue and provide desirable body contouring. Many women with excess buttock tissue will automatically point to the inferior buttock when asked where excess tissue might preferably be removed. The flap is designed as a horizontal ellipse with the axis centered above the gluteal crease. The gluteal crease is marked with the patient in the standing position and forms the inferior aspect of the skin paddle ellipse. Then, with the patient in the lateral decubitus position, a handheld Doppler probe is used to find the strongest perforator vessels to the skin. The superior aspect of the skin island ellipse is then marked to capture these perforators. The direction of the skin paddle usually parallels the inferior gluteal crease. The dimensions of the flap are around 8 × 20 cm, depending on the amount of skin needed and the amount of excess buttock tissue available.

Technique

A two-team approach is used with the patient in the lateral decubitus position and the ipsilateral chest wall and buttock prepped and draped for unilateral breast reconstruction. The ipsilateral arm and leg are prepped into the field as well to facilitate exposure at the surgical sites. For bilateral procedures the flaps are harvested prone. Incisions are made along the previously drawn marks and Bovie electrocautery is used to divide the flap down to the muscle. The fat is beveled superiorly and inferiorly to include the maximum amount of fat and soft tissue in the flap as deemed necessary.

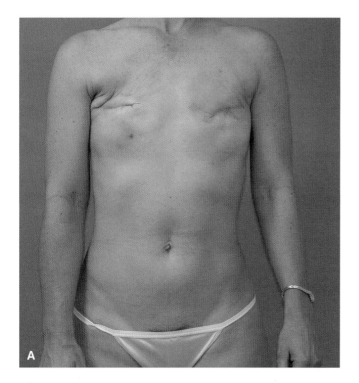
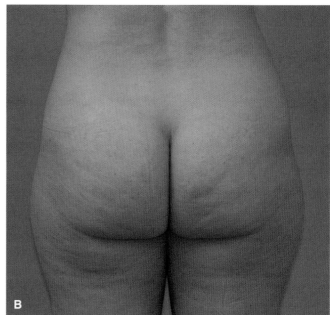
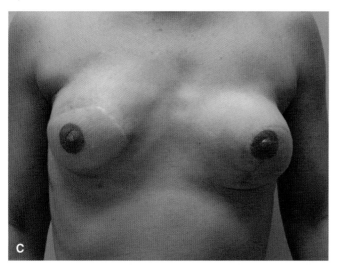
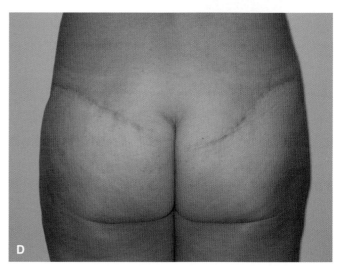

● **FIGURE 2-4.** (A,B) Preoperative view of a patient for secondary double S-GAP reconstruction. (C,D) Result and donor site.

When harvesting the I-GAP flap, care must be taken to preserve the lighter colored medial fat pad that overlies the ischium. Preservation of the fat pad will prevent possible donor site discomfort when sitting. The fascia of the gluteus maximus is incised laterally and the dissection proceeds in the subfascial plane to allow easier visualization of the perforators. The perforator dissection proceeds through the muscle until a pedicle of sufficient length and with sufficient vessel caliber is obtained to allow microsurgical anastomosis. This usually occurs when the perforating vessels join the descending branch of the inferior gluteal artery. The sciatic nerve is usually not visualized. Some small sensory branches of the posterior femoral cutaneous nerve may be divided in pedicle dissection. The typical pedicle length is

8 to 11 cm, the arterial diameter greater than 2 mm and the venous diameter is 3 to 4 mm. The buttock wound is closed in three layers over a suction drain with a resulting scar in and slightly lateral to the buttock crease (Figure 2-5A–E).

Complications

In a series of 70, in-the-crease, I-GAP flap reconstructions, there was one flap loss due to venous thrombosis. Four more patients were returned to the operating room for successful treatment of venous insufficiency. These were both thought to be secondary to twisting or kinking of the flap vein and were probably inset related. Two patients had wound breakdowns at the recipient site.

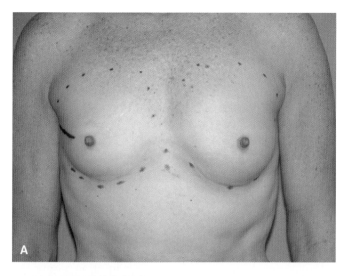

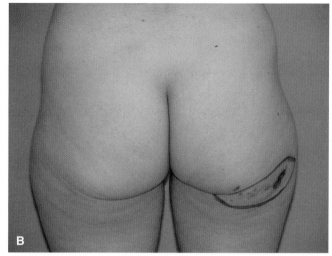

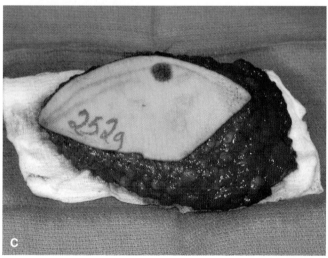

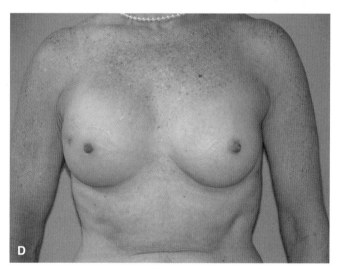

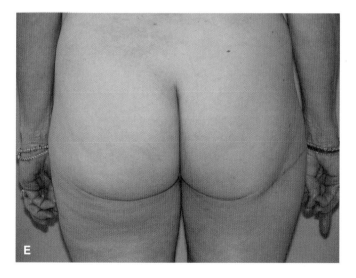

● FIGURE 2-5. (A,B) Preoperative view of a patient with a failed implant reconstruction Baker IV on the right side. (C) I-GAP flap. (D,E) Result after I-GAP breast reconstruction.

Both patients had undergone previous radiation therapy to the chest wall and both eventually healed their wounds. No patients had complains about discomfort on sitting position after 6 weeks.

Our experience with the in-the-crease, I-GAP donor site is that the donor site defect is more aesthetically favorable and less noticeable in the great majority of patients. The aesthetic unit of the buttock is preserved and the scar falls in the inferior gluteal crease. Significant soft tissue depression at the donor site occurs less often and appears less noticeable than with the typical S-GAP donor site. This results both in an improved postoperative appearance and also allows a greater amount of beveling and fat harvest with the flap in thin patients. However, this scar is more exposed with high-cut swimsuits.

The I-GAP flap, as is the S-GAP flap, is a thick flap and is sometimes difficult to inset in the irradiated chest after skin excision. If irradiated skin will be removed, and there will be a large skin requirement, the abdomen may be the better choice for patients who have the tissue available.

Overall, the DIEP, SIEP, S-GAP, and I-GAP flaps allow reliable and aesthetic reconstructions of the breast without the sacrifice of the muscle at the donor site. Patient satisfaction has been very high. With these four perforator flaps, the plastic surgeon should have a treatment plan ready for the vast majority of patients who consult for breast reconstruction.

● THE THORACODORSAL ARTERY PERFORATOR FLAP

The thoracodorsal artery perforator (TDAP) flap is a skin flap from the lateral thoracic region that leaves the muscle compartment of the latissimus dorsi intact. The vascular territory of the TDAP flap essentially lies on top of and anterior to the latissimus dorsi muscle. The extent of the skin flap is limited mainly by the need of primary closure. Skin flaps up to 14 × 25 cm have been used without complications. The skin island can be oriented in different directions, thus the perforator does not need to be centered to reliably perfuse the flap.[5-7]

Patient Evaluation and Selection

As a pedicled flap with a longitudinally oriented skin island, the TDAP flap reaches the upper arm and elbow, neck, shoulder, and upper back area to provide reliable skin coverage. When it is transversely oriented, the skin flap takes advantage of a natural fold in the skin and subcutaneous tissue of the back. The classic latissimus dorsi musculocutaneous flap for breast reconstruction is designed with this orientation. The flap is outlined with its anterior corner just reaching the beginning of the inframammary crease. The main indications for use in breast surgery are either partial breast reconstruction after ablative surgery or autologous augmentation for hypoplasia. We have used the TDAP for total breast reconstruction in two patients. As a free flap, the indication is any defect that requires skin coverage. In this respect, the TDAP flap rivals other flaps such as the scapular, ALT, radial for arm, and lateral arm flap. The greatest advantage of the TDAP flap lies in the versatility of tissue options provided by the thoracodorsal pedicle. A compound flap can be created with a split latissimus dorsi muscle component, a serratus anterior muscle, or the anterior margin of the scapular, or scapular or parascapular skin islands. Through its suprafascial and intramuscular course, the perforator has an independent range of motion of approximately 4 to 6 cm.

Technique

The patient is placed in a lateral decubitus position with the upper arm in 90-degree abduction and 90-degree flexion at the elbow. In this position, the anterior border of the latissimus dorsi muscle is palpated through the skin and marked. The anterior border of the flap should lie in front of the latissimus dorsi border at the level of the hilus, which is about 8 cm below the axillary crease. For a free flap, the TDAP flap is outlined as a vertical ellipse over the latissimus dorsi muscle. Flaps measuring 14 × 25 cm have been raised reliably on a single perforator.

The perforators run posteriorly, on top of the muscle fascia, for a variable distance (2−6 cm) after exiting the muscle over the course of the descending branch of the thoracodorsal artery. The initial incision is made at the anteroinferior border of the flap. This location allows the surgeon to identify the anterior border of the latissimus muscle and eventually reposition this border accordingly. Dissection proceeds upward on top of the fascia in a loose areolar plane between fascia and the overlying fat. When a suitable perforator is identified, it is dissected free from the underlying muscle to the point of its entry into the skin. The perforator can be easily freed from the surrounding muscle fibers because it is enveloped in a fatty layer that allows for its excursion during contraction. To support the flap, the perforator does not need to be centrally located in the flap. The pedicle length of 14 to 18 cm may be obtained. As the dissection proceeds proximally, care should also be taken not to miss a cutaneous branch of the thoracodorsal artery, either as a direct cutaneous branch or as a perforator following the anterior border of the latissimus dorsi muscle.

The motor nerves to the latissimus dorsi muscle run on a deeper plane, making it possible to dissect the pedicle without injuring the nerves. At the end of the procedure, the anterior border of the latissimus dorsi muscle is sutured back into its original position to retain its strength (Figure 2-6A–D).

Complications

When the TDAP flap is oriented longitudinally, a rather unattractive donor scar remains. In women patients, the tension of primary closure can temporarily displace the nipple-areola complex. Nevertheless the donor defect is far less unsightly than the traditionally musculocutaneous latissimus dorsi flap and preserves function of the latissimus muscle.

● LATERAL CIRCUMFLEX FEMORAL ARTERY PERFORATOR-VASTUS LATERALIS FLAP

The LCFAP-VL flap, or the anterolateral thigh flap, as it is most universally known, has gained acceptance as a soft tissue flap since it was introduced by Song in 1984 and became popularised by Fu-Chan Wei. The Taiwan group gained experience with more than 2000 LCFAP-VL perforator flaps and found it to be an "ideal" soft tissue flap for a variety of indications.[8]

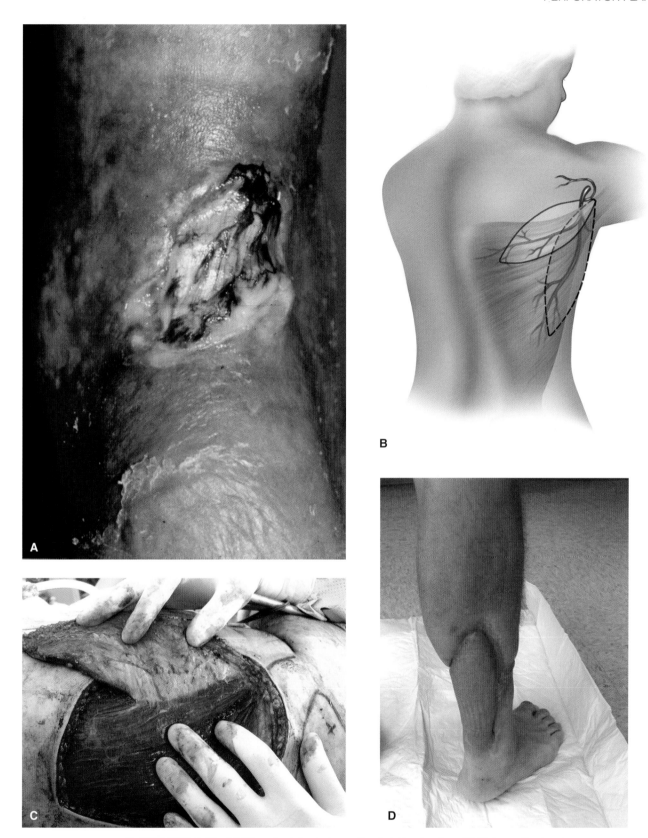

● FIGURE 2-6. (A) Chronic defect above the Achilles tendon. (B) Schematic drawing of the skin island of the TDAP flap. (C) Intraoperative view of the TDAP flap with the main perforator emerging through the latissimus dorsi muscle. (D) Result at 6 months postoperatively.

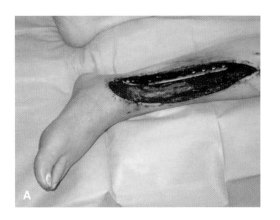

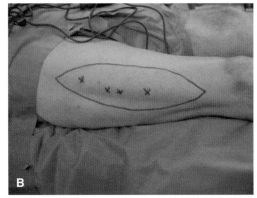

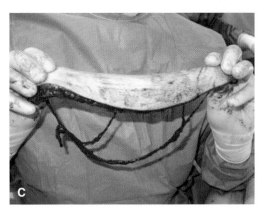

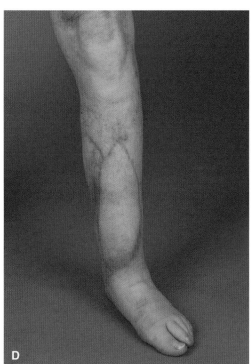

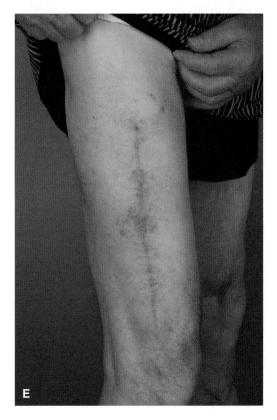

● **FIGURE 2-7.** (A) Classic lower extremity defect after open tibial fracture fixed with a plate. (B,C) Marking of the ALT flap and harvest of the flap. (D,E) Result at 1 year postoperatively.

Patient Evaluation and Selection

In the series of 2000 LCFAP-VL flap procedures, the flap has been used for head and neck including the oral cavity, esophagus, scalp, lip and cheek, upper extremity, hand, abdominal wall, lower extremity, breast, and many other locations throughout the body. Our main indication is lower extremity trauma or exposed hardware at the lower extremity. For this indication, the donor site of the anterior lateral thigh is our primary choice with all the advantages such as two-team approach, pliability of the flap, skin to skin wound closure, long pedicle, and large caliber anastomosis with hardly any donor side morbidity. If several skin vessels are included in the flap, the flap can be split into two skin islands, each separately supplied by one of the identified skin vessels.

For preoperative marking, the patient is placed in the supine position. We use the markings as suggested by Donald Serafin in *Atlas of Microsurgical Composite Tissue Transplantation*.[9] The central axis of the flap is a line drawn from the anterior superior iliac spine to the superolateral border of the patella. At the midpoint of this line, a circle with a 3 cm radius is drawn. A transcutaneous Doppler probe is then used to locate the perforators within the circle, especially in the lower outer quadrant. When the perforators are located, a flap of appropriate size is drawn with its base overlying these perforators. If no vessels are found, localization proceeds in a caudal to cephalic direction along the marked line or slightly posterior to the intermuscular septum.

If the Doppler signal remains weak, attention should be directed toward the anteromedial aspect of the thigh where the cutaneous perforator of the innominate branch of the lateral femoral circumflex artery is sought.

Technique

The leg is circumferentially prepped. A large skin paddle (up to 35 × 25 cm) can be reliably based on one dominant perforator. When such a large skin flap is needed, it is preferable to include more than one perforator. In general, a flap 8 to 9 cm × 22 cm can be harvested with a single skin vessel without problems. The plane of dissection can be either subfascial or suprafascial. The subfascial dissection is thought to be simpler to perform with an easier identification of the skin vessels in a relatively bloodless plane, and a better exposure of the intermuscular septum with the descending branch of the lateral circumflex femoral artery. If, however, a thin flap is required, and sensory innervation to parts of the thigh are to be preserved, a suprafascial dissection is preferred. For these reasons, we mainly end up using the suprafascial dissection to cover lower extremity defects. An incision along the medial border of the designed flap is made through the skin and subcutaneous tissue down to the level of the fascia of the thigh. The dissection continues above the fascia in a lateral direction until the skin vessels previously located by audible Doppler are encountered. When a suitable skin vessel that has pierced the fascia is identified, the lateral border skin incision is made down to the same suprafascial plane as the medial border. At this point, it becomes evident if one traces down a septal or muscle perforator vessel. In case of a septal perforator, the dissection becomes quick and easy. The perforator is followed through the septum until enough pedicle length is encountered. However, it is much more likely to see muscle perforators. In these cases, an incision is made near the skin vessel, and the vessel is traced in a retrograde fashion through the muscle fibers of the vastus lateralis until adequate vessel length and caliber are achieved. Manipulation of the skin vessel should be done gently and only when necessary to avoid spasm. If spasm does occur, it can be relieved with topical application of xylocaine (Figure 2-7A–E).

Complications

If the vessels supplying the skin island of the LCFAP-VL flap appear to be too small for the surgeon to perform the intramuscular dissection comfortably and safely using loupe magnification, a mapping with an audible Doppler of the region medial to the incision should be performed. Usually, there will be an inverse correlation between the number and caliber of vessels in the lateral, anteromedial, and medial thigh region. In most cases of lacking skin vessels in the lateral thigh, good quality anteromedial or medial thigh vessels exist. Therefore, if a promising skin vessel is detected medially, the dissection should proceed medially. If the skin vessel is injured during dissection, it is better not to rely on that perforator and to search for another more suitable perforator. If the donor site cannot be closed primarily, the only alternative in our hands is skin grafting with the result of an unsightly donor area. This should be discussed with the patient beforehand as well as alternatives in flap selection.

REFERENCES

1. Blondeel PN, Morris SF, Hallock GG, Neligan PC. *Perforator Flaps: Anatomy, Technique, & Clinical Application*. St. Louis, MO: Quality Medical Publishing; 2006.
2. Gill P, Hunt J, Guerra A. A 10-year retrospective review of 758 DIEP flaps for breast reconstruction. *Plast Reconstr Surg*. 2004;113:1153.
3. Guerra A, Metzinger S, Bidros R, et al. Breast reconstruction with gluteal artery perforator (GAP) flaps: a critical analysis of 142 cases. *Ann Plast Surg*. 2004;52:118.
4. Babineaux K, Granzow JG, Bardin E, et al. Microvascular breast reconstruction using buttock tissue: the preferred scar location and shape. *Plast Reconstr Surg*. 2005;116:174.
5. Heitmann C, Guerra A, Metzinger SW et al. The thoracodorsal artery perforator flap: anatomical basis and clinical application. *Ann Plast Surg*. 2003;51:23.
6. Kim JT. Latissimus dorsi perforator flap. *Clin Plast Surg*. 2003;30:403.
7. Tsai FC, Yang JY, Mardini S, et al. Free split cutaneous perforator flaps procured using a three dimensional harvest technique for the reconstruction of postburn contracture defects. *Plast Reconstr Surg*. 2004;113:185.
8. Wei FC, Jain V, Celik N, et al. Have we found the ideal soft tissue flap? An experience with 672 anterolateral thigh flaps. *Plast Reconstr Surg*. 2002;109:2219.
9. Serafin D. The anterolateral thigh flap. In: Serafin D, ed. *Atlas of Microsurgical Composite Tissue Transplantation*. Philadelphia, PA: W.B. Saunders; 1996:421.

chapter 3

Alloplastic Craniofacial Implants

Michael J. Yaremchuk, MD

● INTRODUCTION

Alloplastic implants are used as substitutes for autogenous tissues in plastic and reconstructive surgery. This chapter will focus on their use for reconstruction of the craniofacial skeleton. Reconstruction with autogenous bone has the conceptual advantage that it will, in time, become revascularized and incorporated into the skeleton, thereby resisting migration, extrusion, and infection. Revascularization, however, may also predispose the graft to resorb with a concomitant change in volume and shape, thereby making the end result less predictable. The use of synthetic material avoids donor area morbidity and simplifies the procedure in terms of time and complexity. Furthermore, the use of alloplastic implants in facial reconstruction often provides a superior result. With the exception of interposition grafts used to reconstruct segmental load-bearing defects of the maxilla and mandible where only autogenous bone is appropriate for reconstruction, the majority of cranial replacement, internal orbit reconstruction, and, particularly, facial skeleton augmentation, is done with alloplastic implants (Figure 3-1).

● BIOCOMPATIBILITY

The implant materials used are biocompatible. Biocompatibility implies that there is an acceptable reaction between the implant material and the host. In general, the host has little or no enzymatic ability to degrade the implant with the result that the implant tends to maintain its materials properties, volume, and shape. Likewise, the implant has a minimal and predictable effect on the host tissue which surrounds it. This type of relationship is an advantage over the use of autogenous bone or cartilage which, when revascularized, will be remodeled to varying degrees, thereby changing volume and shape.

Surface Characteristics

Current alloplastic implants used for facial reconstruction have not shown to have any toxic effects on the host.[1] The host responds to these materials by forming a fibrous capsule around the implant, which is the body's way of isolating the implant from the host. The most important implant characteristic which determines the nature of the encapsulation is the implant's surface characteristics. Smooth implants result in the formation of smooth-walled capsules. Porous implants allow varying degrees of soft tissue ingrowth, which results in a less dense capsule.

Animal studies have demonstrated that implant pore sizes of larger than 100 µg encourage tissue ingrowth.[2–4] Pore sizes smaller than 100 µg limit tissue ingrowth; whereas materials with large pore sizes (>300 µg) have drawbacks associated with material breakdown.[5,6] It is a clinical observation that porous implants, as a result of fibrous tissue ingrowth, have less tendency to erode underlying bone, to migrate, due to soft tissue mechanical forces, and, perhaps, to be less susceptible to infection when challenged with an inoculum of bacteria.

● MATERIALS

Three basic categories of alloplastic materials are used as implants in facial reconstruction. Polymers and ceramics are used to replace or augment bone. Metals are used as fixation or support devices.

Polymers

Polymers are long molecules composed of repeating subunits. Structure of the subunit, chain length, and crosslinks, all determine physical properties of the material. Eppley[7] has summarized the attributes of these materials.

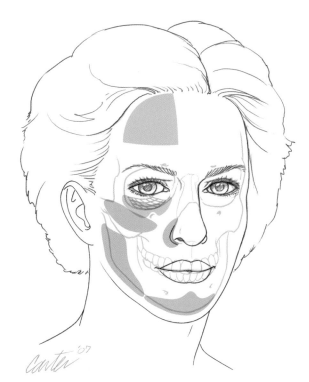

● **FIGURE 3-1.** A diagrammatic survey of the alloplastic implants used for craniofacial skeletal reconstruction and enhancement.

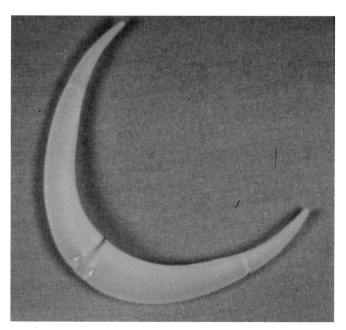

● **FIGURE 3-2.** Examples of silicone chin implants. These implants have a smooth surface and are relatively flexible, depending on the thickness of the implant.

Polysiloxane (Silicone)

Polysiloxane is a polymer created from interlinking silicon and oxygen [SiO(CH$_3$)$_2$] with methyl side groups. Solid silicone or the silicone rubber used for facial implants is a vulcanized form of polysiloxane. Silicone implants are used to augment the contours of the facial skeleton.

Solid silicone has the following advantages: it can be sterilized by steam or irradiation; it can be carved with either a scissors or scalpel; and it can be stabilized with a screw or a suture. Because it is smooth, it can be removed quite easily. Disadvantages include the tendency to cause resorption of underlying bone, particularly when used to augment the chin; the potential to migrate if not fixed; and the potential for its fibrous capsule to be visible when placed under a thin soft tissue cover. Figure 3-2 shows examples of silicone chin implants.

Acrylic

Acrylic biomaterials are made from polymerized esters of either acrylic or methyl acrylic acids (methyl methacrylate). Acrylic implants have smooth surfaces, are strong, and are inflexible. The most commonly used material for skull reconstruction is polymethyl methacrylate (PMMA). PMMA is radiolucent and therefore does not affect postoperative imaging. It is unaffected by temperature and is strong. When used for full-thickness defects, it can fill intracranial dead space—a problem with bone cranioplasty. When used as an onlay, bony overcorrection can compensate for overlying soft tissue deficiencies resulting in a smooth skin surface contour. Because it is encapsulated by the host rather than incorporated by surrounding soft tissues, PMMA is believed by some to be more susceptible to infection and late complications (Figure 3-3).

Porous Polyethylene

Polyethylene is a simple carbon chain of ethylene monomer. The high-density, porous variety, Medpor, is used for facial implants because of its higher tensile strength. Polyethylene has a firm consistency which resists material compression while still permitting some flexibility. It has an intramaterial porosity between 125 and 250 μg,

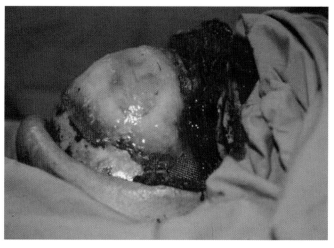

● **FIGURE 3-3.** Example of a PMMA frontal cranioplasty. Intraoperative view shows completed PMMA cranioplasty.

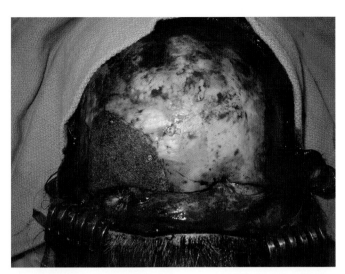

● **FIGURE 3-4.** Example of a porous polyethylene implant used to reconstruct the right frontal area. This implant was fabricated using 3D CT scan data.

which allows fibrous ingrowth. The porosity of Medpor has both advantages and disadvantages. The advantages of porous polyethylene include its tendency to allow extensive soft tissue ingrowth, thereby lessening its tendency to migrate and to erode underlying bone. Its firm consistency allows it to be easily fixed with screws and contoured with a scalpel or power equipment without fragmenting. However, its porosity causes soft tissue to adhere to it, making placement more difficult and requiring a larger pockets to be made than with smoother implants. The soft tissue ingrowth also makes implant removal more difficult than with smooth surface implants. This material is the implant material of choice for this author. A porous polyethylene implant is shown in Figure 3-4.

Polymethyl Methacrylate/ Polyhydroxyethyl Methacrylate

HTR derives its name from the acronym for hard tissue replacement. It is a porous composite of polymethyl methacrylate and polyhydroxyethyl methacrylate, which allows some soft tissue ingrowth. A calcium hydroxide coating imparts a negative surface charge to encourage bony ingrowth and deter adhesion of bacteria to the implant.[8] HTR is not flexible.

Ceramics

Ceramic materials are usually heated to high temperatures (sintered) to fuse their crystal-like components.

Hydroxyapatite

The ceramic material most commonly used in craniofacial surgery is hydroxyapatite. Hydroxyapatite is a calcium phosphate salt found as a major component of bone

matrix. Dense hydroxyapatite can be produced synthetically. Porous hydroxyapatite can be entirely synthetic, or formed by chemically converting the naturally porous calcium carbonate skeleton of marine coral. Unlike the other biomaterials presented in this chapter, which have no osteoactivity, calcium phosphates have the theoretical advantage of being osteoinductive and osteoconductive. Osteoinduction is the ability of the biomaterial to initiate osteogenesis without ingrowth from adjacent bone. Osteoconduction is the ability for the biomaterial to act as a bridge for the ingrowth of bone from an adjacent osseous bed. These attributes have been shown experimentally,[9,10] but have not demonstrated clinical relevance in the craniofacial skeleton.

Porous hydroxyapatite is available as granules for injection and as brittle blocks. Although hydroxyapatite is osteoactive and has the potential to be replaced by bone, this has been an inconsistent clinical finding.

Hydroxyapatite is also available in a cement paste that has been advocated as a material to be used for cranioplasty (Figure 3-5). The cement paste has an advantage over the ceramic form in that it can be shaped during surgery. To date, there is no histologic evidence of significant bone ingrowth or resorption of this material in humans over a follow-up period of up to 3 years.[7] These findings are consistent with animal studies.[11,12]

Metals

The three types of metals currently used as fixation devices are stainless steel, cobalt-chromium alloy (Vitallium), and titanium (either pure Ti or as an alloy with aluminum and vanadium). Titanium has largely replaced the use of the other two metals for craniofacial use because of its high strength and reduced artifact on CT and MR imaging studies.[13–15]

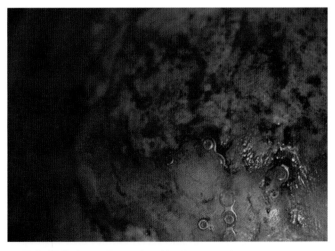

● **FIGURE 3-5.** Example of hydroxyapatite cement cranioplasty performed to augment a traumatically deformed supraorbital rim.

● CLINICAL APPLICATIONS

Alloplastic materials have three main uses in craniofacial reconstruction. These include cranioplasty, internal orbit reconstruction, and onlay augmentation of the facial skeleton.

Cranioplasty

Patient Selection. Acquired cranial bone deformities are usually full-thickness defects of the skull. Cranioplasty is performed not only to normalize appearance, but also, and more importantly, to provide protection for the brain. The most common etiology of full-thickness cranial defects is the infectious loss of a craniotomy graft created by the neurosurgeon to access the brain for neurosurgical treatment. Cranial defects may also result from bone loss after trauma.

Patient Preparation

Computer-aided Design/Computer-aided Manufacturing (CAD/CAM). CT imaging of skull defects provides digitized information that can be transferred to design software. Data describing the contour along the edge of the defect and the surface characteristics of the normal cranium surrounding the defect can be used to design a custom-fit implant. The electronic data describing the newly designed prosthesis are then used by a computer-controlled manufacturing system to create a wax model, which is then cast, or to directly mill raw material into the finished implant.[16,17] An alternative method is for anatomically precise stereolithographic (SL) biomodels (ie, exact physical replicas) of the cranium to be constructed. Subsequently, each SL biomodel is used as a template for the construction of preliminary implant, which is then inspected physically or online by the surgeon who either approves the implant or requests further modifications. If approved, the final implant is then prepared and packaged sterilely (Figure 3-6). Prefabricated implants of various materials, including polymethyl methacrylate–polyhydroxalmethyl methacrylate (HTR),[18] porous polyethylene,[19] and polymethyl methacrylate,[20] are available. The use of custom prefabricated implants can reduce operative time significantly.

Technique. Cranioplasty is performed when acute infection and risk factors for recurrent infection are eliminated. It requires that any potential communications between the sinuses and the planned cranioplasty graft be eliminated. Communications between the sinuses and the anterior cranial fossa, require placement of a vascularized barrier for effective isolation. A galea frontalis flap, if available and adequate, or a free tissue transfer may be required. Finally, the adequacy of the soft tissues to provide secure closure at the time of elective cranioplasty must be assured. This may require a preliminary scalp expansion or flap reconstruction before or at the time of cranioplasty.

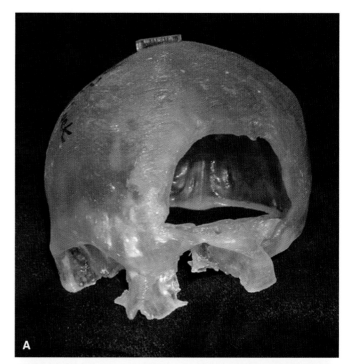

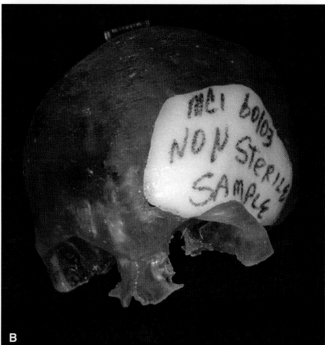

● **FIGURE 3-6.** 3D CT data was used to construct an exact replica of the skull on which a custom implant was fabricated. (A) Skull model shows left frontal defect. (B) Custom implant fabricated from CT scan data.

A significant reduction in incidence of infection has been shown when 1 year is allowed to elapse between the initial injury or infection and the subsequent reconstruction.[21-23] In my experience, a 6-month, infection-free period has been sufficient to assure that infection has been adequately treated.

At surgery, the patient is positioned so that a panoramic view of the skull and, if appropriate, the upper face can be draped into the field. This position allows the surgeon to mimic the contralateral anatomy and to avoid unnatural transitions.

Unless prefabricated implants are used, the exposed bone edge is saucerized by removal of the outer table with rongeurs or a high-speed burr. The resultant inner table ledge provides a ledge for implant placement and stabilization Craniofacial surgeons usually advocate the use of bone for cranioplasty; while the vast majority of neurosurgeons use PMMA. In reviewing their experience of 42 posttraumatic reconstructions of frontal defects in which both bone and acrylic were used, Manson et al.[21] found that the material employed was not as important as the timing of reconstruction and the treatment of sinus disease. In the past, I had used bone when there had been recurrent infection or when overlying soft tissues were compromised (eg, after radiation therapy). Presently, I use alloplastic materials for almost all cranioplasty.

The most commonly used material for skull reconstruction is polymethylmethacrylate. PMMA reconstruction is technically less demanding than reconstruction with autogenous bone and the aesthetic results are far superior. Cranioplasty kits are available that contain a single dose of 30 g of powdered polymer and 17 mL of liquid monomer. The elements are mixed with a spatula in a bowl. The mixing should be conducted under ventilation so that the person mixing is not overcome by fumes.

Two techniques are used to shape the implant. One method places the doughy mixture in a plastic sleeve provided in the cranioplasty kit. The sleeve containing the still pliable implant mixture is placed onto the skull defect and molded by digital compression (Figure 3-7). The other technique for PMMA cranioplasty requires first placing a wire mesh into the skull defect (Figure 3-8). PMMA is then cured directly on the mesh. This technique allows more

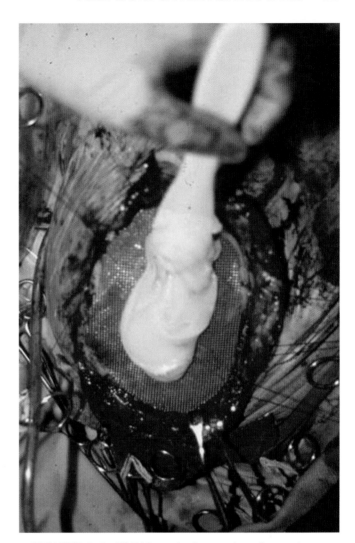
● FIGURE 3-8. PMMA cranioplasty using wire mesh technique.

risk for burn damage to the dura during the exothermic reaction, which, unlike the sleeve technique, takes place in the surgical field. Irrigation of the implant during the exothermic reaction can avoid heat injury to the dura.[21,24]

Complex curvatures, particularly in the supraorbital area, are formed by adding material to an initial construct. Final adjustments can be made with a contouring burr on a high-speed drill. The implants may be fixed with wires or, more simply and rapidly, with microscrews. The screws are used to fix the position of the implant in one of two ways. In both techniques, the implant must overlie intact skull. Screws may be driven through the acrylic and into underlying bone before it is completely hardened. Another technique, particularly useful in augmenting contour depressions, is first to place the screw in the area to be augmented, leaving the head and two or three threads above the bone surface. The acrylic is then poured over the screw so that it is incorporated in the construct.

The implant may be perforated to allow the dura to be tented up to it. This method lessens the potential for

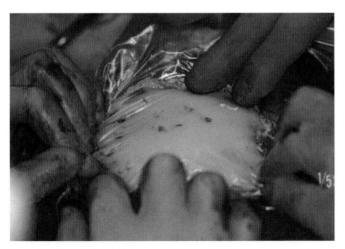
● FIGURE 3-7. PMMA cranioplasty performed using the sleeve molding technique.

epidural collection. Perforations in the implant also allow drainage and soft tissue ingrowth, which also aids in implant fixation.

Complications. Hydroxyapatite cement has been shown to be osteoconductive and therefore became a popular implant material for cranioplasty with the expectation that, in time, the implant would be repopulated with host bone. However, only minimal direct bone or vascular ingrowth occurs because of the implant's extremely small pore size.[25–28] Any bone ingrowth that occurs is a direct turnover of hydroxyapatite to bone at the periphery of the implant. Implant volume is thought to remain stable because the implant remains largely avascular. Because of its low flexural resistance, it is recommended for use as an onlay material to improve contour. It has been used with metallic mesh to reconstruct defects. In this application, Moreira-Gonzalez and Zins reported a major complication rate of 42.8%, with some complications occurring as late as 4 years postoperative. The main problems observed at reoperation were fragmentation of the hydroxyapatite cement, exudation, and severe soft tissue inflammatory reaction (Figure 3-9).[29] Others have cautioned about the use of this material for vault reconstruction.[30]

Internal Orbit Reconstruction

Patient Selection. Disruption of the skeletal architecture of the orbit usually results in globe malposition. Enophthalmos, the inward sinking of the eye, may result from fractures involving only the orbital floor or medial orbital wall. These are termed "pure blowout" fractures. More often, enophthalmos is part of an orbital deformity whereby not only the internal orbit is disrupted, but also the adjacent facial skeleton. The internal orbit disruption is referred to as an "impure blowout" fracture in these situations.

Because posttraumatic enophthalmos is primarily due to alterations in the configuration of the bony internal orbit rather than to changes in the amount or character of its soft tissue contents, the treatment strategy for restoring eye position is the anatomic reconstruction of the internal orbit. This is best accomplished by defining the location and extent of injury preoperatively with CT scans, widely exposing the injured area, retrieving displaced orbital soft tissues, and reconstructing the invariably comminuted fractured skeleton.[31–33]

Technique. I prefer a transconjunctival retroseptal incision, often with a lateral canthotomy extension, to approach the orbital floor and lower medial and lateral walls. Using loupe magnification, the soft tissue contents of the orbit are freed from the injured skeleton by subperiosteal dissection. Ideally, intact bony edges are identified for orientation and to provide stable constructs on which to position grafts or implants. This dissection can be exceedingly difficult in extensive injuries, particularly when surgery has been delayed and prolapsed orbital soft

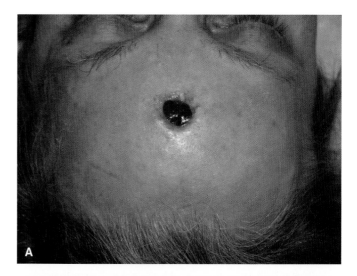

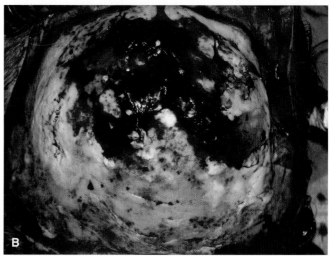

● **FIGURE 3-9.** Example of hydroxyapatite cement onlay cranioplasty complication. (A) Draining sinus. (B) Intraoperative appearance. Note fragmentation of construct.

tissues have healed to damaged mucosa in the maxillary or ethmoid sinuses, or to the temporalis muscle in the temporal fossa. The orbital contents must be separated from these structures and replaced in the orbit. An inferior orbitotomy increases internal orbit access and thereby simplifies soft tissue mobilization.[34] This maneuver is frequently used for secondary or late reconstructions.

The size of the defect and the normal configuration of the injured area will dictate the dimensions, thickness, and number of grafts. For example, a small floor defect is usually reconstructed with a single, thin graft, thereby replicating the relatively flat shape of the orbital floor. A similarly dimensioned inferomedially located defect usually requires a thick graft or stacked grafts to recreate the convex shape of the orbit in this area. Failure to replicate this convexity effectively increases the volume of the orbit from normal and tends toward enophthalmos. Similarly, placement of an overly thick graft to reconstruct the floor would also create an internal orbit shape different from normal. In this case, the abnormal convexity beneath the globe would elevate it resulting in an ocular dystopia.

To avoid changes in graft shape and volume, as well as to avoid the morbidity and operative time associated with autogenous graft harvest, alloplastic implants have long been used for orbital floor reconstruction. These include polytetrafluoroethylene, silicone, dense and porous polyethylene, resorbable materials, metal plates, and polymethyl methacrylate.

Porous polyethylene is the author's preferred nonmetallic orbital implant. In personal experience with more than 200 patients since 1987, there has been no known instance of infection or graft extrusion using this material. Clinical experience suggests that the soft tissue ingrowth into the material limits the tendency for migration seen with smooth surfaced implants. Others have presented anecdotal data, suggesting that this soft tissue ingrowth has the potential to include adjacent ocular motility muscles with the possibility of ocular motility disorder. To avoid this potential problem polyethylene implants are now available with a smooth surface on one side and a porous surface on the other. The smooth surface is intended to face the orbital soft tissue contents and the porous side to face the sinuses. The smooth surface is intended to prevent soft tissue ingrowth and possible motility problems, while the porous side allows soft tissue ingrowth with concomitant immobilization and mucosalization.

For injuries involving only the floor, I routinely use an alloplastic implant. Most often it is a sheet of porous polyethylene or titanium mesh. To assure stability of the construct, I routinely immobilize the implant with a screw. Injuries involving two or more walls of the orbit are problematic. Rigid fixation techniques allow these complex injuries to be subdivided into a series of smaller, more manageable areas for reconstruction. Titanium metal implants are attached to the orbital rim and are used to span large defects.[35-37] The implant alone may be used to restore the internal orbital contour or may serve as a platform on which to place grafts or implants. Laminated implants of titanium metal and polyethylene are available. A titanium mesh infrastructure is sandwiched between a sheet of smooth polyethylene on one side and a sheet of porous polyethylene on the other. The metal facilitates implant conformability and screw fixation. The smooth laminate is intended to interface with the soft tissues contents preventing their prolapse into the metallic mesh. The porous laminate is intended to interface with the mucosal surface. Figure 3-10 shows an example of a patient who underwent secondary reconstruction of posttraumatic orbital deformities with alloplastic implants.

When injuries are devastating and mucosalization of an alloplastic implant is thought unlikely, I prefer to reconstruct the internal orbit with a combination of autogenous bone and metallic mesh.

Complications. High rates of extrusion have been documented for the rigid, smooth-surfaced implants made of silicone (3.1%) and nylon (12%). There are also many reports of late complications, especially with silicone, polytetrafluoroethylene, and nylon plates. These have been noted to occur as late as 21 years after placement, and include infection, extrusion, migration with hematoma formation, and lower eyelid deformity.[1] Clinical experience obtained from treating these complications suggest that these problems are related to capsule formation around smooth surfaced implants with the concomitant tendency toward implant migration.

Facial Skeleton Augmentation

Patient Selection. Alloplastic implants can be used as onlays to restore symmetry during reconstruction of posttraumatic or postablative facial deformities. Most often, facial skeletal augmentation is done electively to improve facial aesthetics. The most commonly used and commercially available materials today for facial skeletal augmentation are solid silicone and porous polyethylene.

Patient Preparation

Anesthesia. Facial skeletal augmentation can be performed under local or general anesthesia. It is routinely done on an outpatient basis. The surgical site is infiltrated with a solution containing Marcaine for postoperative pain control and epinephrine to minimize bleeding.

Incisions. Facial implants are placed through inconspicuous remote incisions borrowed from craniofacial and aesthetic surgery. These include coronal, intraoral, transconjunctival, and submental approaches.

Implant Shape. The external shape of the implant should mimic the shape of the bone it is augmenting. Its posterior surface should mold to the bone to which it is applied. Gaps between the bone and implant result in a relative increase in augmentation and a potential site for seroma and hematoma formation. The implant margins must taper imperceptibly into the bone they are augmenting so that they are neither visible nor palpable.

Positioning. Although some surgeons prefer to place implants in a soft tissue pocket, clinical experience has led me to adopt a policy of strict subperiosteal placement. Placement in a subperiosteal pocket involves a dissection that is safe to peripheral nerves and relatively bloodless. It allows visualization and more precise augmentation of the skeletal contour desired for augmentation. The size of the pockets is determined by the type of implant used and its immobilization. The long-standing teaching when using smooth silicone implants is to make a pocket just large enough to accommodate the implant so as to guarantee its position. Porous implants require a larger pocket because they adhere to the soft tissue during their placement. When using smooth or porous implants, I dissect widely enough to have a perspective of the skeletal anatomy being augmented, which allows more precise and symmetric implant positioning.

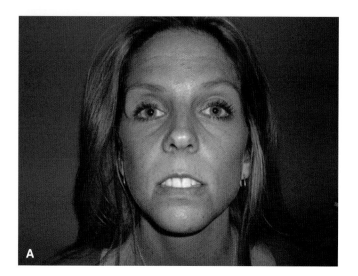

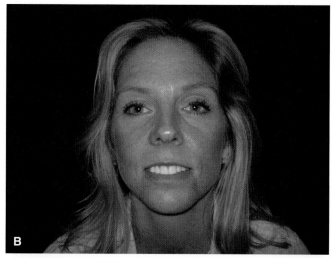

● **FIGURE 3-10.** A 40-year-old woman developed enophthalmos as well as a loss of malar prominence after initial treatment of a right orbital injury. Surgery was performed through a transconjunctival retroseptal with lateral canthotomy and intraoral incisions. The internal orbit was reconstructed with porous polyethylene immobilized with titanium screws. The lateral and inferior orbital rims were augmented with screw immobilized porous polyethylene. (A) Preoperative frontal view. (B) Postoperative frontal view. (C) Preoperative 3D CT showing initial reconstruction. The artist has depicted the placement of screw-fixed porous polyethylene implants used to reconstruct three walls of the internal orbit and the depressed malar area.

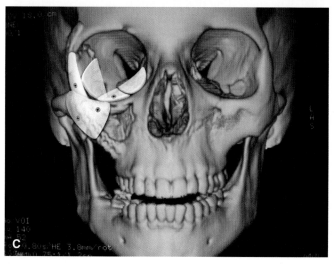

Immobilization. Many surgeons stabilize the position of the implant by suturing it to surrounding soft tissues or by using temporary transcutaneous pullout sutures. Screw fixation of the implant to the skeleton has several benefits. It prevents any movement of the implant and assures application of the implant to the surface of the bone (Figure 3-11). Because each facial skeleton has a unique and varying surface topography, a nonconforming implant will leave gaps between the implants and the skeleton. Screw fixation also allows for final contouring of the implant in position. This final contouring is particularly important where the implant interfaces with the skeleton. Any step-off between the implant and the skeleton will be palpable and possibly visible in thin patients.

Technique

Areas for Augmentation. The mid and lower face are the areas most often altered with implants. In the midface, implants are specifically designed to augment the malar, paranasal, and infraorbital rim areas. In the lower face, each of the anatomic areas of the mandible—the mentum, body, angle, and ramus are amenable to augmentation with alloplastic materials.

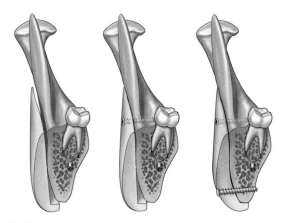

● **FIGURE 3-11.** Screw fixation applies the implant to the skeleton and obliterates the gaps. (Gaps are equivalent to an increase in augmentation.) (Left) Coronal view shows discrepancy in contour between anterior surface of mandible and posterior surface of implant resulting in gaps. (Center) The upper screw is in place and has fixed and immobilized the implant to the skeleton. (Right) The lower screw has been place. The posterior surface of the implant is now congruent with the anterior surface of the mandible.

Malar. Patients who seek malar augmentation may have midface hypoplasia or normal anatomy and usually seek greater prominence of their middle malar prominence.[38]

Paranasal. A relative deficiency in lower midface projection may be congenital or may be acquired, particularly after cleft surgery and trauma. Patients with satisfactory occlusion and midface concavity can have their aesthetic desires satisfied with skeletal augmentation. Implantation of alloplastic material in the paranasal area can simulate the visual effect of LeFort I advancement.[39]

Infraorbital Rim. Augmentation of this area is useful for patients with severe deficiencies of the midface and infraorbital rim area that result in excessively prominent eyes. Infraorbital rim augmentation can effectively reverse the "negative" vector of midface hypoplasia.[40]

Most often, infraorbital rim augmentation is combined with a subperiosteal midface lift which elevates the midface soft tissues on its new infrastructure (Figure 3-12).

Chin. The projection of the chin should be interpreted in the context of the surrounding facial features,

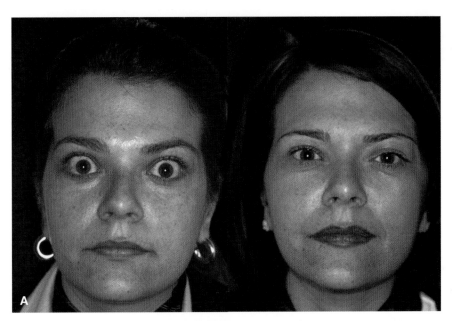

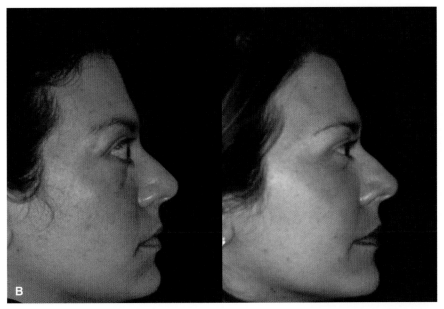
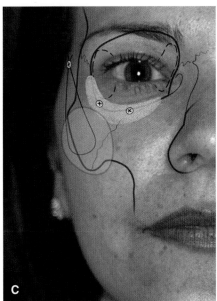

● **FIGURE 3-12.** A 30-year-old woman with Graves disease underwent medial and lateral orbital decompression with preservation of the lateral orbital rim. Globe-rim relations were further improved by augmenting the infraorbital rim, elevating the midface soft tissue and performing lateral canthopexy. (A) Preoperative and postoperative frontal. (B) Preoperative and postoperative lateral. (C) Diagrammatic representation of procedure.

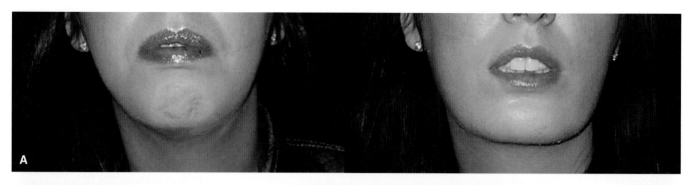

A

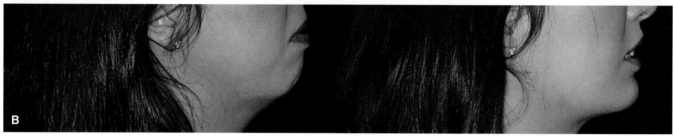

B

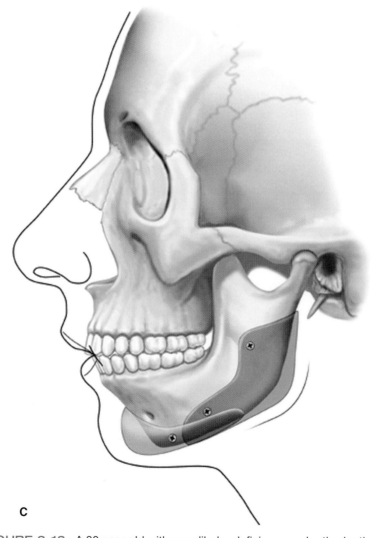

C

● **FIGURE 3-13.** A 30-year-old with mandibular deficiency and orthodontically corrected occlusion underwent chin and mandibular augmentation with alloplastic implants. (A) Pre- and postoperative frontal. (B) Pre- and postoperative lateral. (C) Artist's rendition of surgery.

including the projection of the nose, the relationship to the lips, and the depth of the labiomental sulcus. There is a consensus among surgeons that the ideal profile portrays a convex face with the upper lip projecting incisions approximately 2 mm beyond the lower lip and the lower lip projecting approximately 2 mm beyond the chin.[41]

Early implant designs augmented the mentum only and often created a stuck-on appearance, as a result of failure of the lateral aspect of the implant to merge with the anterior aspect of the mandibular body. "Extended" chin implants have tapered lateral extensions that enable the chin implant to better merge with more lateral mandibular contours.[42,43] I prefer a two-piece chin implant.[44] A two-piece implant allows the inferior border of the implant to follow the inferior border of the mandible. This is usually not possible with a one-piece chin implant.

Ramus and Body

Patients with skeletal mandibular deficiency who have had their malocclusion treated with orthodontics alone are left with mandibular skeletal deficiencies that may be displeasing. The skeletal anatomy associated with mandibular deficiency that can be camouflaged with implants include the obtuse mandibular angle with steep mandibular plane and decreased vertical and transverse ramus dimensions (Figure 3-13). The addition of an extended chin implant will camouflage the poorly projecting chin.[45]

Many patients perceive a wider lower face with a well-defined mandibular border as an enhancement to their appearance. Patients in this treatment group often present with a desire to emulate the appearance of models, actors, and actresses who have a defined, angular lower face. This patient group benefits from implants designed to augment the ramus and posterior body of the mandible.

Implants Used to Camouflage Soft Tissue Depressions

The implants discussed in this section are designed to increase the surface projection of the facial skeleton. Some surgeons have used implants placed on the facial skeleton to disguise overlying soft tissue volume inadequacy, usually caused by involutional changes brought on by age. These include the submalar, prejowl, and tear trough implants. Augmentation of the skeleton to compensate for a soft tissue deficiency should be extremely conservative. Skeletal augmentation does not give the same visual effect as the soft tissue augmentation. Similarly, soft tissue augmentation beyond 1 or 2 mm provides a different visual effect than skeletal enlargement. For example, a chin point augmented with fat to increase projection by 5 mm reads as a fatty chin pad, not as a more projecting chin.

Complications. There is no scientific data to document the complication rate related to facial skeletal augmentation. Prospective studies that control for surgical technique, implant site, patient selection, and follow-up time do not exist. Because all the biomaterials commonly used for facial skeletal augmentation are biocompatible, complications are usually technique related—improper implant size, contour, or placement. Infections are unusual when implants are placed through cutaneous incisions. When infection occurs, the most reliable treatment is implant removal.

● SUMMARY

Augmentation or replacement of nonload-bearing portions of the facial skeleton with alloplastic materials provides powerful means to restore or improve facial appearance. Virtually any area of the facial skeleton can be reconstructed. Requisites for success include implants of appropriate size and shape, adequate soft tissue cover, and careful subperiosteal dissection during exposure and implant placement.

REFERENCES

1. Rubin JP, Yaremchuk MJ. Complications and toxicities of implantable biomaterials used in facial reconstructive and aesthetic surgery: A comprehensive review of the literature. *Plast Reconstr Surg.* 1997;100:1336.

2. Klawitter JJ, Bagwell JG, Weinstein AM, Sauer BW. An evaluation of bone growth into porous high density polyethylene. *J Biomed Mater Res.* 1976;10:311.

3. Spector M, Flemming WW, Sauer BW. Early tissue infiltrates in porous polyethylene implants into bone: A scanning electron microscope study. *J Biomed Mater Res.* 1975;9:537.

4. Spector M, Harmon SL, Kreutuer A. Characteristics of tissue ingrowth into Proplast and porous polyethylene implants in bone. *J Biomed Mater Res.* 1979;13:677.

5. Berghaus A, Mulch G, Handrock M. Porous polyethylene and Proplast: Their behavior in a bony bed. *Arch Otorhinolaryngol.* 1984;240:1165.

6. Maas CS, Merwin GE, Wilson J, et al. Comparison of biomaterials for facial bone augmentation. *Arch Otolaryngol of Head Neck Surg.* 1990;116:551.

7. Eppley BL. Alloplastic implantation. *Plast Reconstr Surg.* 1999;104:1761.

8. Eppley BL, Sadove AM, German RZ. Evaluation of HTR polymer as a craniomaxillofacial graft material. *Plast Reconstr Surg.* 1990;86:1085.

9. Chiroff R, White E, Weber J. Tissue ingrowth of Replamineform implants. *J Biomed Mater Res.* 1975;6:29.

10. Gosain AK, Song L, Riordan P, et al. Part I: a 1-year study of osteoinduction in hydroxyapatite-derived biomaterials in an adult sheep model. *Plast Reconstr Surg.* 2002;109:619.

11. Gosain AK. Biomaterials for reconstruction of the cranial vault. *Plast Reconstr Surg.* 2005;116:663.

12. Holmes R, Halger H. Porous hydroxyapatite as a bone graft substitute in cranial reconstruction: A histometric study. *Plast Reconstr Surg.* 1988;81:662.

13. Fiala TGS, Paige KT, Davis TL, et al. Comparison of artifact from craniomaxillofacial internal fixation devices: Magnetic resonance imaging. *Plast Reconstr Surg.* 1994;93:725.

14. Saxe AW, Doppman JL, Brennan MF. Use of titanium surgical clips to avoid artifacts seen on computed tomography. *Arch Surg.* 1982;117:978.

15. Fiala TGS, Novelline RA, Yaremchuk MJ. Comparison of CT imaging artifacts from craniomaxillofacial internal fixation devices. *Plast Reconstr Surg.* 1993;92:1227.

16. Wehmoller MW, Eufinge H, Kruse D, Massberg W. CAD by processing of computed tomography data and CAM of individually designed prostheses. *Int J Oral Maxillofac Surg.* 1995;24:90.

17. Eufinger H, Wehmoller MW, Machtens E, et al. Reconstruction of craniofacial bone defects with individual alloplastic implants based on CAD/CAM manipulated CT data. *J Craniomaxillofac Surg.* 1995;23:175.

18. Eppley BL, Kilgore M, Coleman JJ. Cranial reconstruction with computer generated hard-tissue replacement patient-matched implants: Indications surgical techniques and long-term follow-up. *Plast Reconstr Surg.* 2002;109:864.

19. Ledezma CJ, Hoh BL, Carter BS, et al. Successful use of custom stereolithographic-designed high-density porous polyethylene cranioplasty implants to correct cranial defects after neurosurgical procedures. Submitted to the *Journal of Neurosurgery*.

20. Taub PJ, Rudkin GH, Clearihue WJ, Miller TA. Prefabricated alloplastic implants for cranial defects. *Plast Reconstr Surg.* 2003;111:1232.

21. Manson PN, Crawley WA, Hoopes JE. Frontal cranioplasty: risk factors and choice of cranial vault reconstructive material. *Plast Reconstr Surg.* 1986;77:888.

22. Hammon WM, Kempe LG. Methyl methacrylate cranioplasty: 13 years experience with 417 patients. *Acta Neurochir.* 1971;25:69.

23. Rish BL, Dillon JD, Meirowsky AM, et al. Cranioplasty: a review of 1030 cases of penetrating head injury. *Neurosurgery.* 1979;4:381.

24. Stelnicki EJ, Ousterhout DK. Prevention of thermal tissue injury induced by the application of polymethylmethacrylate to the calvarium. *J Craniofac Surg.* 1996;7:192.

25. Constantino PD, Friedman CD, Jones K, et al. Experimental hydroxyapatite cement cranioplasty. *Plast Reconstr Surg.* 1992;90:174.

26. Burstein FD, Cohen SR, Hudgins R, et al. The use of hydroxyapatite cement in secondary craniofacial reconstruction. *Plast Reconstr Surg.* 1999;104:1270.

27. Constantino PD, Friedman CD, Jones K, et al. Hydroxyapatite cement: I Basic chemistry and histologic properties. *Arch Otolaryngol Head Neck Surg.* 1991;117:379.

28. Friedman CD, Costantino PD, Jones K, et al. Hydroxyapatite cement. II. Obliteration and reconstruction of the cat frontal sinus. *Arch Otolaryngol Head Neck Surg.* 1991;117:385.

29. Moreira-Gonzalez A, Zins J. The use of hydroxyapatite bone cement in the repair of large full thickness cranial defects: a caution. Presented at: American Association of Plastic Surgeons, 84th Annual Meeting; Scottsdale, AZ; 2005.

30. Matic D, Phillips JH. A contraindication for the use of hydroxyapatite cement in the pediatric population. *Plast Reconstr Surg.* 2002;110:1.

31. Bite U, Jackson IT, Forbes GS, et al. Orbital measurements in enophthalmos using three dimensional CT imaging. *Plast Reconstr Surg.* 1985;75:502.

32. Manson PN, Clifford CM, Su CT, et al. Mechanisms of global support and post-traumatic enophthalmos. I. The anatomy of the ligament sling and its relation to intramuscular cone orbital fat. *Plast Reconstr Surg.* 1985;77:193.

33. Manson PN, Grivas A, Rosenbaum A, et al. Studies on enophthalmos. II. The measurement of orbital injuries and their treatment by quantitative computed tomography. *Plast Reconstr Surg.* 1985;77:201.

34. Tessier P. Inferior orbitotomy. A new approach to the orbital floor. *Clin Plast Surg.* 1982;9:569.

35. Glassman RD, Manson PN, Vanderkolk CA, et al. Rigid fixation of internal orbital fractures. *Plast Reconstr Surg.* 1990;86:1103.

36. Rubin PAD, Shore JW, Yaremchuk MJ. Complex orbital fracture repair using rigid fixation of the internal orbital skeleton. *Ophthalmology.* 1992;99:553.

37. Yaremchuk MJ, Manson PN. Reconstruction of the internal orbit using rigid fixation techniques. In: Yaremchuk MJ, Gruss JS, Manson PN, eds. *Rigid Fixation of the Craniomaxillofacial Skeleton.* Boston, MA: Butterworth-Heinemann; 1992.

38. Whitaker LA. Aesthetic augmentation of the malar midface structures. *Plast Reconstr Surg.* 1987;80:337.

39. Yaremchuk MJ, Israeli D. Paranasal implants for correction of midface concavity. *Plast Reconstr Surg.* 1998;102:51.

40. Yaremchuk MJ. Infraorbital rim augmentation. *Plast Reconstr Surg.* 2001;107:1585.

41. McCarthy JG, Ruff JG. The chin. *Clin Plast Surg.* 1988;15:125.

42. Flowers RS. Alloplastic augmentation of the anterior mandible. *Clin Plast Surg.* 1991;18:137.

43. Terino EO. Facial contouring with alloplastic implants. *Facial Plast Surg Clin North Am.* 1999;7:55.

44. Yaremchuk MJ. Improving aesthetic outcomes after alloplastic chin augmentation. *Plast Reconst Surg.* 2003;112:1422.

45. Yaremchuk MJ. Mandibular augmentation. *Plast Reconstr Surg.* 2000;106:697.

chapter 4

Reconstructive Transplantation: Evolution, Experience, Emerging Insights

Vijay S. Gorantla, MD, PhD / *W.P. Andrew Lee, MD* / *Joseph E. Losee, MD*

● INTRODUCTION

Reconstructive transplantation is among the newest of transplant areas and combines the time-tested techniques of reconstructive microsurgery with the immunologic principles of transplant surgery. It involves the transplantation of composite tissues, including skin, muscle, mucosa, ligament, tendon, nerve, blood vessel, bone, joint and cartilage, bone marrow, and lymph nodes.[1] The overall goal of reconstructive transplantation is to improve the quality of the life of patients with significant tissue defects.

There is currently no national database or registry in the civilian population regarding the millions of individuals each year who sustain trauma or tumor extirpation or undergo complex reconstruction for other congenital or acquired tissue defects or deficits. It is reasonable to estimate that management of these disfiguring, disabling, and debilitating tissue injuries/losses costs the US health care system tens of millions of dollars each year. For example, current surgical procedures after major trauma are limited by available tissues for reconstruction, morbidity from extensive surgery, prolonged rehabilitation, and costs of multiple surgeries. For such complex injuries, reconstructive transplantation of composite grafts can achieve near-perfect restoration of tissue defects with improved functional and aesthetic outcomes and avoidance of multiple surgeries.

Despite the obvious advantages offered by reconstructive transplantation, one factor has hampered its widespread application. This is the need for long-term immunosuppressive therapy to maintain the allograft. The risks posed by antirejection drugs are considered by many to be justified in lifesaving procedures such as solid organ transplants in patients with terminal organ failure. However, such risks are considered to be too high a price to pay for life-enhancing (nonlifesaving) transplants such as hand or face composite grafts.

Reconstructive transplantation has now been performed successfully at more than a dozen centers worldwide[2] and at seven centers in the United States.[3] During the past decade, more than 100 reconstructive transplant procedures have been performed around the world, including 70 hand and 18 facial transplants, with encouraging outcomes. The growth has been slow, largely due to initial skepticism of the immunological feasibility[4] and currently for concern for the life-long risks of immunosuppression.[5] There have been a few deaths and graft failures secondary to complications, noncompliance, or chronic rejection. Yet, the proof of concept of these procedures has been established with favorable intermediate and long-term success.[6,7] There have been growing efforts in the United States and the rest of the world toward wider application of reconstructive transplantation, and many centers are establishing vascularized composite allograft programs. Thus, the outlook for reconstructive transplantation seems promising, but long-term predictions on outcomes are not yet possible.

This chapter is organized into three sections focusing on the past, present, and future of this groundbreaking specialty.

● EVOLUTION OF RECONSTRUCTIVE TRANSPLANTATION

History

The earliest reports of tissue and organ transplantation, including that of the heart, date to between the second centuries BCE and CE in China.[8] Restoration of mutilating injuries of the nose and ear with pedicled autografts from the forehead, neck, and cheek are discussed in the *Sušruta Samhita*.[9–11] This treatise, written by the Indian surgeon Sušruta who lived around 480 BCE, describes in detail the techniques of rhinoplasty. Although this was the first credible account of reconstructive transplantion, mythology credits the patron saints Cosmos and Damian with performing the first limb allotransplantation about 870 years later.[12–15] Per the legend, around the year 348, they transplanted the right leg of a dead Moor onto a patient after amputating his gangrenous leg. Similar legend is also depicted in a fifteenth century fresco in the St. Julius Basilica in Milan, showing St. Julius replanting the amputated thumb of a man.[16] In the sixteenth century, the Italian surgeon from Bologna, Gaspare Tagliacozzi, described a method of nasal and aural alloreconstruction in his book *De curtorum chirurigia per insitionem* (*On the Surgery of Mutilation by Grafting*).[17–19] He used skin from the inner aspect of the arm from a slave to reconstruct the nose of a wealthy patient who injured it during a sword fight. Unsubstantiated reports indicate that the reconstructed nose allegedly survived for 3 years after which the donor flap was rejected. In his book, Tagliacozzi concludes that allografts are possible, but the binding of tissues to one another for a sufficient length of time was prevented by a "force and power." This was possibly the earliest reference to immunologic phenomenon of allograft rejection, as we now know it.

During the next three centuries, the focus of organ transplantation was technical and led to advancements in antisepsis, anesthesia, hemostasis, and organ preservation. However, the most important challenge to replacing tissues or transferring a body part from one person to another lay in graft revascularization. Alexis Carrell in 1902 described the surgical technique of vascular anastomosis, thus laying the foundation for conventional vascular surgery.[20–22] However, he failed to achieve permanent graft acceptance. Carrell attributed this "organ failure" to vascular complications because he had no knowledge of the process of rejection.

The problem of rejection began to be realized clinically in the twentieth century when allografting became the model for research. In 1900, Karl Landsteiner and C. Philip Miller were the first to recognize that humans could be grouped according to the presence of agglutinins in their sera. They eventually discovered ABO, Rh, and other red cell antigens and laid the foundation for histocompatibility testing.[23] In 1924, Emile Holman recognized that a single donor's skin graft rejected more rapidly on the second application.[24] This observation was eventually referred to as the second set phenomenon and, as a result, some believed allografting to be a useless and fruitless endeavor. Meanwhile, other scientists were studying the biologic aspects of transplantation. In 1932 and 1937, the first attempts at skin grafting were performed between identical twins.[25,26] In 1937, Peter Alfred Gorer discovered the first histocompatibility antigen in humans[27] and established the concept of "self vs nonself" after realizing that antigens on tissue cells are genetically determined and capable of eliciting foreign graft destruction. In 1943, Peter Brian Medawar, a young zoologist in Britain, had made the historic discovery rejection.[28] Investigating skin grafting in rabbits, he differentiated between immune responses to homografting and autografting. He also made the observations that skin grafts from a family member were better tolerated than those from an unrelated donor, and those skin grafts from an identical twin were better tolerated than from other family members. Medawar subsequently described the basic characteristics of the immune response—recognition, destruction, and memory.

In 1944, Richard Hall described the technical aspects of cadaveric upper extremity transplantation, including the need for surgical team expertise with organ preservation, bone fixation, and microsurgery as well as availability of appropriate facilities, but there was no mention of rejection.[29] Ironically, Hall had no knowledge of the work of Landsteiner, Gorer, or Medawar.

Following Medawar's groundbreaking findings in skin grafting,[30] other significant breakthroughs led to the foundations of modern organ and reconstructive transplantation. These include the discovery of leukocyte blood groups in humans by Jean Dausset in 1952.[31] Dausset recognized that individuals who had received multiple blood transfusions had leukoagglutinins in their sera, whereas those who had received few or no transfusions had no isoagglutinins in their sera. This important distinction led to the accurate conclusion that alloantibodies, as well as autoantibodies, exist, and it paved the way for discovery of the human leukocyte antigen (HLA) locus in humans. In the 1950s, Simonson and Mitchison observed that acute rejection was not mediated by antibodies but by lymphocytes.[32,33]

Building on Holman's preliminary work, Medawar in collaboration with Thomas Gibson, a plastic surgeon, is credited with establishing the first reliable animal model for the second set response.[34] However, attempts at skin allotransplantation were repeatedly unsuccessful, leading investigators to other areas of transplantation. In a landmark procedure, another plastic surgeon, Joseph Murray, in association with his colleagues Merrill and Hartwell, performed the first kidney transplant between identical twins in 1954.[35–39] Following this, in 1959, the first successful composite tissue allograft was performed by yet another plastic surgeon, Erle Peacock who transplanted a digital flexor tendon mechanism en bloc.[40,41] Indeed, it was Peacock who coined the term "composite tissue allograft" to differentiate these transplants that were composed of modules of multiple tissues unlike solid organs.

It was not until the 1960s and 1970s, though, that disparity at the major histocompatibility complex (MHC) was recognized as a genetic basis for rejection. In 1964, Paul Terasaki[42] developed the microlymphocytotoxicity test to detect preformed circulating cytotoxic antibodies in recipients. In the same year, Roberto Gilbert Elizalde performed the first hand transplantation in Guayaquil, Ecuador.[43,44] However, Gilbert did not have insight into the immunology of skin-containing grafts, such as hand transplants, as well as access to effective pharmacologic immunosuppression. The combination of prednisone and azathioprine could not prevent acute rejection of the transplanted hand in 14 days that had to be re-amputated. This bold and pioneering attempt at hand transplantation underscored the need to understand the immunology of composite grafts as well as improve immunosuppressive strategies to prevent or treat acute rejection.

Immunosuppression

It is only the knowledge gained from landmark discoveries in the past century that facilitated the manipulation or suppression of the immune response, allowing successful prolongation of graft survival. After Medawar's demonstration that rejection was an immunologic event, the next logical question was: Why not prevent this phenomenon by suppressing the immune system? The innovation of induced immunosuppression in the setting of transplantation is credited to John Loutit, who in the 1950s experimented with total body irradiation in rodents undergoing skin grafting.[45] In 1958, this form of immunosuppression was applied to humans by Murray in Boston and Hamburger in Paris.[38,46,47] Graft survival improved, but was still dismal because these drugs acted indiscriminately and were associated with severe organ-specific and systemic adverse effects.

Success was rare until the era of pharmacologic immunosuppression. The introduction and application of the antimetabolite 6-mercaptopurine by Schwartz and Dameshek and Zukoski and Calne dramatically changed the course of early attempts at organ transplantation.[48–50] Wider clinical use came with the development of a precursor drug, azathioprine (Imuran) by Hitchings and Elion.[51] It was Murray and Calne who first used it clinically in 1962.[52,53] Since 1962, all transplantation of organs and tissues between unrelated individuals has been performed under pharmacologic immunosuppression. The last third of the twentieth century witnessed the realization of liver, heart, lung, pancreas, and small bowel allotransplantation as drug protocols were fine-tuned.[54]

The 1960s and 1970s saw the advent of polyclonal antibody technology, followed by cyclosporine and monoclonal antibodies during the 1980s. Cyclosporine dramatically changed the science and the practice of transplantation by increasing dramatically allograft survival, which made it possible for widespread clinical application of extrarenal transplantation.[55–57] The FDA approved cyclosporine A for use in the United States in 1983. The calcineurin inhibitor tacrolimus (FK 506) was discovered in 1987,[58] clinical trials were conducted in 1989,[59] and FDA approval came in 1994. Tacrolimus led to dramatic improvements in solid organ transplantation,[60–63] allowing highly immunogenic grafts such as the small bowel to be transplanted.[64–66] The success of the calcineurin inhibitors cyclosporine A and tacrolimus made them the cornerstone drugs of the modern era of transplantation.[54] The 1990s saw the introduction of novel drugs such as the antimetabolite mycophenolate mofetil[67] (approved by the FDA in 1995) and rapamycin[68] (sirolimus, discovered in 1976 but FDA approved only in 1999). Combining these drugs with a calcineurin inhibitor[69–73] significantly reduced acute rejection and improved solid organ graft survival with a reduction in adverse effects.

Current immunosuppressive regimens are a far cry from the rudimentary combination of prednisone and azathioprine used in the 1960s. But things are changing with the realization that these advances are tempered by drug toxicities, leading to considerable morbidity and even mortality. The use of calcineurin inhibitors, the dominant paradigm for the past two decades, is being challenged as a result of the long-term effects of these agents on allografts. Investigators and clinicians alike are also looking to avoid corticosteroids that have been the mainstay of immunosuppressive regimens, and to minimize global immunosuppression after transplantation.

Immunology

Plastic surgeons have been intimately involved in the evolution of organ transplantation. Although Gibson, Peacock, and Murray made equally significant contributions, it was Murray who earned the coveted recognition of being the first and only plastic surgeon to date to receive the Nobel Prize in Medicine.[74]

However, as a specialty, our understanding of the immunologic behavior of allografts lagged behind technical developments in surgery. Much knowledge concerning the immunologic aspects of reconstructive transplantation has been gained from studies in small and large animal models.

Vascularized composite tissue allografts (CTAs), such as hand or face transplants, differ from solid organ transplants in several important aspects:[75] (1) CTAs are composed of tissues derived from multiple germ lines such as ectoderm, endoderm, and mesoderm such as skin, muscle, blood vessels, nerve, fat, cartilage, bone, and bone marrow; (2) the functional allograft is easily and grossly visible for inspection by the patient and clinical management team; and (3) for the most part, CTAs are not strictly life-sustaining.

Transplantation of multiple tissue constructs such as CTAs is associated with a quantitatively graded recipient immune response to individual graft components.

Traditionally, skin has been considered the most immunologically difficult allograft to transplant. This impression has been verified experimentally. Skin, subcutaneous tissue, muscle, bone, nerve, and blood vessels have been evaluated for their intrinsic and relative antigenicities.[76] Skin is the most immunogenic component, and it usually triggers and is the target of acute rejection.[77] Following skin, muscle, bone, cartilage, and nerve predictably induce a relatively lower immune response in that order.

Skin is the largest organ and is both a physical and immunologic barrier.[78,79] Due to its exposure to the environment, the skin, like the small bowel and lung, has a robust and effective local immune system, called the skin immune system, which contributes to its heightened antigenicity.[80,81] Langerhans cells are immature dendritic cells that are the primary dermal antigen presenting cells. They are extremely efficient at initiating innate responses to trigger sensitization and priming of naïve host T cells to attack the graft. Langerhans cells make up 2% to 4% of epidermal cells. Keratinocytes make up 90% of epidermal cells and play an accessory role in initiating or supporting cell mediated immune responses. Apart from Langerhans cells, skin also has other types of dendritic cells such as dermal dendritic cells.[82] These dendritic cells, due to their migratory capability, can carry antigenic information from skin to secondary lymphoid organs and present to lymphocytes for priming and stimulation.[83,84] Human skin also has tissue specific minor antigens that may contribute to its antigenicity.[85] These are similar to antigens such as Skn and embryonic prealbumin 1, which are potent contributors to skin antigenicity in murine models and swine models.[86,87]

Skin antigenicity correlates with clinical findings in reconstructive transplants. It initially shows the first signs of rejection and is associated with maximal cellular infiltrate in established rejection.[88,89] Experimentally, it has been possible to induce tolerance toward all tissues of a CTA except the skin (split tolerance).[90] More powerful conventional/standard immunosuppression regimens have successfully treated skin rejection and prolonged CTA graft survival; but, like other allografts, in most cases, standard baseline immunosuppression is still unable to prevent long-term skin rejection/deterioration. Although other tissues are less antigenic, rejection of even one component of a CTA could result in graft dysfunction or compromise.

The gross visibility and accessibility of CTAs, such as reconstructive transplants, enables direct visual inspection with comparison to nonallograft tissues for routine clinical evaluation, directed biopsy, and topical therapy. This potentially enables more localized therapy, and possibly, reduced systemic exposure to standard immunosuppressive medications, lessening side effects for recipients, who for the most part, are healthy.[91]

Reconstructive transplants differ from all other solid organ grafts in regard to bone marrow content. No other solid organ graft carries an intact vascularized bone/bone marrow environment/component. Liver grafts do possess significant hematopoietic potential and intestinal grafts carry a heavy mature lymphocyte burden due to the presence of the gut-associated lymphoid tissue, but neither contains functional bone marrow. Both of these organs have produced cases of graft-versus-host disease (GVHD) in transplant recipients and with both organs fatal cases of GVHD have been reported.[92,93] When bone marrow or hematopoietic stem cells are transplanted for treatment of malignancy, GVHD is quite commonly seen and is frequently a severe, life-threatening disease. Composite tissue grafts containing bone marrow and lymph node components carry the potential for producing GVHD, but no episodes have been reported to date in clinical reconstructive transplantation. The unique presence of vascularized bone marrow within its intact microenvironment facilitates the implementation of tolerogenic or immunomodulatory strategies in reconstructive transplantation unlike in any other solid organ.

Another major difference between solid organ grafts and reconstructive transplants is the relative level of exposure to the environment. Lung and intestine transplants are exceptional in that they are constantly exposed to environmental factors and both have proven to be highly prone to bacterial, viral, or fungal infections.[94,95] These infections have compromised the survival of both of these grafts and appear to significantly limit success rate in these transplants. It was thought that reconstructive transplants would be subject to infections as well due to constant environmental exposure, especially if the integrity of the skin component was compromised by graft rejection and/or injury. Fortunately, this has not been the case. No reconstructive transplants performed to date have reported any serious infection in the graft itself. Some infections have been reported in the recipients but these have most often been the infections encountered in all immunosuppressed patients, eg, cytomegalovirus (CMV) infection. Although the recipients of reconstructive transplants are immunosuppressed and are subject to the opportunistic infections frequently encountered in all transplant populations, environmental exposure does not appear to increase the incidence of infection in these grafts.

● EXPERIENCE WITH RECONSTRUCTIVE TRANSPLANTATION

Program Establishment and Organization

Implementing a reconstructive transplant program poses tremendous challenges. Solid organ transplantation is a time-tested procedure and is now standard of care. Reconstructive transplantation on the other hand is an emerging specialty that is the amalgamation of the scientific principles of reconstructive surgery and the concepts of organ transplantation. Thus for any reconstructive transplant program to be successful, it must be collaboration between a multidisciplinary team comprised among others of a core group of hand and transplant surgeons (Figure 4-1). Such a joint effort can overcome the challenges that are inherent in a complex therapeutic option that integrates multiple specialties during the planning,

Team composition and expertise

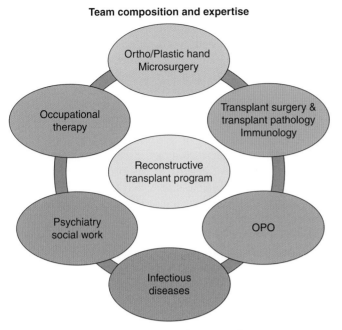

● **FIGURE 4-1.** The reconstructive transplant multidisciplinary team.

personnel, procedural and post-transplant phases. The core team is composed of a team leader, scientific director, and program coordinator who orchestrate the complex transplant logistics in conjunction with the surgical team and the ancillary team (Figure 4-2).

The key steps in the planning and preparation for a reconstructive transplant program are institutional/organizational support, completion of an exhaustive fiscal analysis, organizational or extramural fiscal assurance or strategies for such support, completion of regulatory review and approval, provision for study compliance and oversight, evaluation of infrastructure, facilities and resources, presence of a multidisciplinary team with appropriate expertise, agreement on a protocol for transplant, and organ procurement organization (OPO) support and collaboration.[96,97]

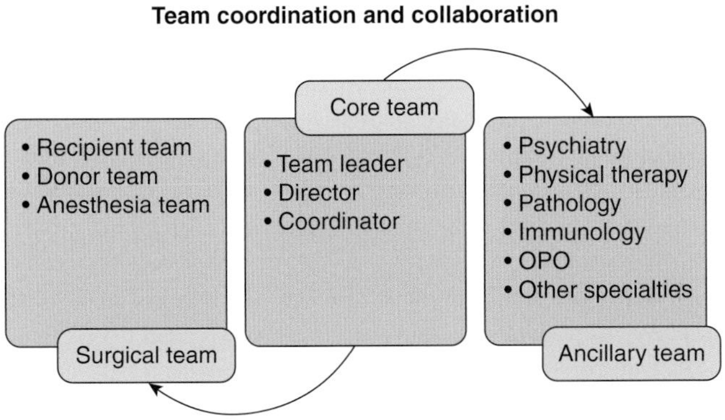

Team coordination and collaboration

- Recipient team
- Donor team
- Anesthesia team

Core team
- Team leader
- Director
- Coordinator

Surgical team

- Psychiatry
- Physical therapy
- Pathology
- Immunology
- OPO
- Other specialties

Ancillary team

● **FIGURE 4-2.** Team coordination and collaboration.

Institutional review board or ethics board review ensures a thorough informed consent process, sound research design with data monitoring, qualified investigators/researchers, favorable risk/benefit analysis, and equitable selection of subjects. The consent process must be

- Comprehensive—includes research procedure, purpose, risks, benefits, alternatives, etc
- Customized—functions of intelligence, rationality, maturity, and language skills; presentation of information must be adapted to the patient's capacity
- Voluntary—requires conditions free of coercion and undue influence

Study compliance or oversight is usually accomplished by an independent data safety monitoring board composed of specialists, statisticians, ethicists, and psychologists.

It is very important to obtain the support of the local/regional OPO for the program. The roles of the OPO relate but are not limited to facilitation of donor screening, evaluation, and selection, donor family education and consent, graft procurement/acquisition/allocation, and donor transportation logistics.

Lastly, given that reconstructive transplant procedures are emerging, innovative, and novel, they are high profile and media intensive in nature. Thus, public relations are an important consideration for every program.

This is important for timing and coordination of press releases, protection of donor identity and patient confidentiality, and announcement of positive or negative outcomes. The media services in the institution can help with website design and planning, distribution of study material, press releases, preparing team members for briefings and video and photographic coverage, and archival of procedures.

Patient and Procedural Considerations

Proper screening evaluation, selection, and management of donors and potential recipients are very important for successful outcomes in reconstructive transplantation. Decades of experience with solid organs have allowed us to establish criteria for donor and recipient selection. In a novel field like reconstructive transplantation, parameters for inclusion and exclusion of donors and recipients have not yet been conclusively defined nor standardized and such criteria as well as technical considerations vary by type of transplant, eg, hand, face, etc.[98,99]

Most of the criteria used for donor selection are similar to that in organ transplantation. These include histocompatibility testing for tissue matching and blood cross-matching (cross-match negative). The ideal patient is a donor who is a nonsmoker in good health with no history of drug abuse or trauma to the graft to be procured, and whose age matches as closely as possible with the recipient. Specifically, the transplant donor is selected after matching for sex, color, tone of skin, age, and comparable phenotypic characteristics of the recipient. Figure 4-3 shows a donor hand graft following retrieval. Absolute contraindications

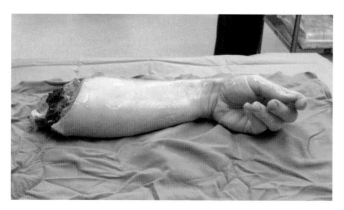

● **FIGURE 4-3.** Donor hand graft after harvest, before transplantation.

are history of previous malignancy, viral hepatitis (B or C), or viral infections such as HIV. The presence of seropositivity for CMV or Epstein-Barr virus (EBV) is not a contraindication for donor selection; however, antiviral prophylaxis is indicated in CMV seronegative recipients receiving transplants from such donors.

Recipients younger than 18 years of age are not considered to be adults, and, therefore, there are issues of informed consent in an experimental procedure. Furthermore, pediatric patients are more likely to develop immunosuppressive-related complications, such as post-transplant lymphoproliferative disease, than adults.[100] Recipients over the age of 65 are usually not considered by programs because of increased immunosuppression-related complications, limited years of potential gain from the transplant, and decreased nerve regeneration. Medical screening of recipients includes a complete medical history and physical examination; routine laboratory studies; blood typing and cross-matching; HLA typing; testing for panel-reactive antibodies; and serology for EBV, CMV, HIV, and viral hepatitis. Other tests include radiography, Panorex imaging, angiography (to exclude abnormal vascular patterns), ultrasound, electromyography, nerve conduction velocity, MRI, and functional MRI as relevant. Reconstructive transplantation, unlike organ transplantation, is usually limited to healthy patients. A patient who is in renal, cardiac, pulmonary, or hepatic failure is excluded whether previously transplanted with solid organs or not.

A thorough assessment of body image adaptation, including the psychological meaning of the transplant to the candidate, the psychological impact of the disfigurement or defect on identity and relationships, coping/adjustment to the injury, motivation for transplantation, anticipated comfort with the transplant, prosthetic use and phantom-limb sensation (in hand transplants) is performed in all candidates.[101] Evaluation of the total family support system is also important. The apparent ideal candidate without family support is not an ideal candidate. These patients will be dependent on a positive family structure, certainly within the first 6 months if not for the life of the transplant. A family support system that does not encourage

strict adherence to the rigorous postoperative regimen will fail. This rigorous regimen includes physical therapy, timely compliance with medications, repeated medical assessments, and avoiding certain activities and substances that may increase the risk of immunosuppressive-related complications. The degree of expectations concerning the transplant outcome and the recognition of the experimental/investigational nature of these procedures are also estimated. Finally, the level of personality strength, including coping skills and regression, are assessed. An additional objective perspective regarding the pros and cons of the particular transplantation is provided (independent of the transplant team) to the recipient through a "patient advocate" who is a respected peer from the home community of the recipient. It is beyond the scope of this chapter to elucidate how this delicate decision is made. Psychological criteria are used to evaluate the competency of recipients to comply with the rigorous pre- and post-transplant rehabilitation program or drug regimens for the rest of their lives.

Programs must cover or ensure coverage of lifelong costs of immunosuppressive medications and other expenses related to post-transplant management of recipients, including complications. Some programs may exclude patients without insurance and/or financial security during the selection process. It has been argued that enrolling patients on the premise of paying for all postoperative medications and management of complications raises the issue of moral hazard related to monetary enticement for transplantation.

Protocol Related Aspects

The current immunosuppressive protocols applied to reconstructive transplantation are extrapolated from regimens used in solid organ transplantation. The overall amount of immunosuppression required to ensure graft survival is comparable with that used in renal transplantation. Such conventional immunosuppression has resulted in patient and graft survival that is 100% at 1 year after upper extremity transplantation and 87% after face transplantation.[101] The majority of transplant patients received either polyclonal (antithymocyte globulins) or monoclonal (alemtuzumab, basiliximab) antibody preparations as induction therapy followed by high-dose, triple-drug combination for maintenance therapy, including tacrolimus, mycophenolate mofetil, and steroids, although the doses and trough levels of each drug differed between some centers. Such regimens have proved sufficient to prevent early immunologic graft loss but were not able to prevent acute rejection. Some programs follow steroid avoidance regimens while others rely on monotherapy immunosuppression. Successful reversal of acute rejection episodes has been achieved using topical clobetasol or tacrolimus ointment with or without short-term bolus steroid doses.[102,103]

Acute rejection is a T cell and/or antibody-mediated attack of the transplant by the recipient's immune system resulting in damage and ultimately loss of the graft. The skin has been demonstrated to be the prime target of rejection and monitoring of the skin by inspection is therefore considered most important for monitoring. Protocol graft skin or mucosal biopsies must be routinely performed until the first year plus whenever clinically indicated (visible signs of rejection such as a maculopapular rash). Biopsy samples may be analyzed by means of histology and immunohistochemistry (staining for CD3, CD4, CD8, CD20, and CD68) for quantification and characterization of cellular infiltrates. Scoring for severity of acute rejection is accomplished using established standard grading criteria, such as the Banff classification.[104,105] Important clinical characteristics of acute rejection include edema, erythema, escharification, and necrosis. Biopsies must also be examined for evidence of chronic rejection, including intimal hyperplasia and subintimal foamy histiocytes in the vessels of the skin or muscle and tissue fibrosis.

Recipient and donor cells must be typed pretransplant for HLA.[106,107] Additional DNA samples from recipient/donor must be stored for future typing for *MICA* (MHC class I chain A related) genes in those patients in whom anti-MICA antibody is detected. All sera should be screened by antihuman globulin-enhanced complement-dependent cytotoxicity assays, by enzyme-linked immunosorbent assay (to identify immunoglobulin G anti-HLA class I– and class II–specific antibodies independently), and by Luminex (allows for the identification of anti-MICA antibodies, as well as ascertainment of their donor specificity). The MICA and MICB antigens are expressed on the surface of endothelial cells and epithelial cells and elicit a strong antibody response in recipients of solid organ transplants. Cell-mediated immunity may be measured by the ImmuKnow assay that detects adenosine triphosphate (ATP) synthesis in CD4 cells. Immune responses are reported in ng/mL of ATP and categorized as strong (>525), moderate (226–524), or low (<225). The desirable target zone for all transplant recipients is 280 ng/mL ATP with a 96% negative predictive value for rejection or infection. An outline of the procedures and protocols used in reconstructive transplantation are listed in Figure 4-4.

Procedures | Protocols

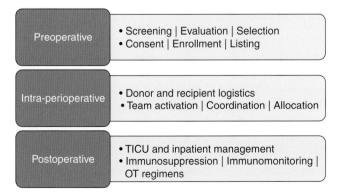

● **FIGURE 4-4.** Procedures and protocols used in reconstructive transplantation.

World Experience

Over the past two decades, reconstructive transplantation has emerged as a new field, with hand, face, and other transplants being performed around the world at multiple centers.[1,91] The overall world experience counts 70 hands transplanted in 50 recipients and 15 face transplants. Good functional results have been achieved with excellent patient satisfaction, acceptably low morbidity, and no mortality.[7]

The first American patient has the longest surviving hand transplant 13 years after surgery.[6] There have been exceptions to this encouraging record. These include the first French patient[108] and the discouraging Chinese experience.[109] Bilateral hand transplants performed in conjunction with face transplants were lost to complications in two cases in Amiens, France and Boston. One patient in Louisville, Kentucky lost his graft to chronic rejection.[110] In some of the above-mentioned cases, transplanted hands were amputated more than 2 years after transplantation. These cases have shown that the operation is fully reversible. More importantly, re-amputation provided an opportunity to observe the evolution of untreated acute rejection in the event of noncompliance, treatment withdrawal, and early chronic rejection.

Since 2005, 15 facial transplantations have been performed in five different centers in three countries. Four teams have reported their outcomes in separate publications. Overall, long-term function of facial grafts has been reported in seven cases with good sensory and motor recovery. Functionality reported in patients included lip and dental occlusion, phonation, olfaction, gustation, mastication, and endobuccal pressure. Sensory return was also seen in the majority of patients with recovery of protective, fine touch, vibratory, and temperature sensation.

● EMERGING INSIGHTS

Chronic Rejection

Unlike acute rejection, we are as yet unclear regarding the magnitude of risk for chronic rejection or how it manifests in reconstructive transplants, but there is enough experience with animal models and other solid organs that manifestations can be reasonably and accurately predicted.

In solid organ transplantation, both immunologic and nonimmunologic factors play roles in chronic rejection pathogenesis (Table 4-1).[111] Immunologic risk factors, are by far, the more important for all allografts. Include are the frequency, severity and temporal onset of acute rejection, greater HLA mismatch, panel reactive antibody status of recipient, racial mismatch between donor/recipient (eg, Caucasian donor into non-Caucasian recipient); sex mismatching (female donor to male recipient and vice versa); and CMV seromismatch (CMV + donor to CMV − recipient), listed largely in order of influence.

TABLE 4-1. Chronic Rejection Factors

Immunologic	Non-Immunologic
Timing of AR (late vs early)	Older donor
Severe, repetitive, humoral AR	Donor atherosclerosis
Greater HLA mismatch	Cadaver donor
Higher PRA of recipient	Prolonged cold ischemia
CMV + Donor to CMV − Recipient	Hypertension, DM, Obesity, High cholesterol
Steroid resistant AR	Unstable donor
Antidonor antibodies + C4D	Non-compliance

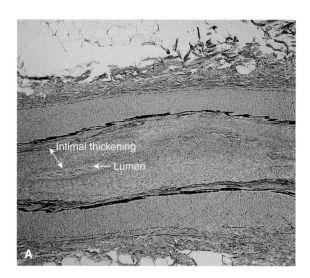

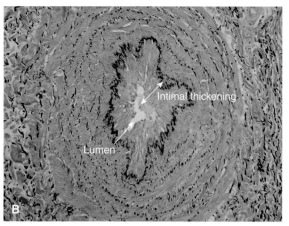

● **FIGURE 4-5.** Chronic rejection leading to progressive ischemia.

Data from almost every form of solid organ transplantation have indicated decreased graft survival in the face of CMV infection.[112] CMV infection has a far greater effect on the allograft than on native organs, increasing the risk of both acute rejection and chronic rejection.[113] This is engendered by cytokines, chemokines, and growth factors.

Chronic rejection may begin weeks to months after transplantation, especially if there are many high-grade acute rejection episodes. In kidney transplants, late, severe, or persistent acute rejection episodes occurring more than 1 year after transplantation are particularly strong and consistent predictors of chronic rejection.[114] The acute rejection may be predominantly cellular or antibody mediated. Antibody-mediated rejection has a considerably worse prognosis than acute cellular rejection.[115] Thus, in kidney transplants, severe, late-onset acute rejection with a significant humoral component may be more predictive of chronic rejection. However, such a correlation may not be totally valid in other organ transplants. For example, in liver transplants, early, mild acute rejection and late episodes of acute rejection are usually not associated with later chronic rejection.[116]

Late-onset acute rejection may be seen in inadequately immunosuppressed or noncompliant patients.[117] Medication noncompliance accounts for one third of late-graft losses and is an important factor contributing to chronic rejection. Though the exact determinants are unclear, some factors associated with noncompliance include inadequate physician–patient relationship, long duration after transplant surgery, multiple immunosuppressive medications, nontolerance of medications, missed clinic visits, and poor transplant outcomes.[118]

Common histopathologic features of chronic rejection in solid organs include (a) patchy organized (lymphoid neogenesis) interstitial inflammation; (b) patchy interstitial fibrosis and associated parenchymal atrophy; (c) graft vascular disease, which primarily manifests as concentric fibrointimal hyperplasia of arteries; (d) destruction of epithelial-lined conduits; and (e) destruction and atrophy of organ-associated lymphoid tissue and lymphatics.[119]

Hand transplant recipients, to date, have been monitored for chronic rejection by clinical and functional exams, skin biopsies, digital subtraction angiography, and standard vascular imaging. The Louisville team has reported[110] the loss of the transplant in their fourth patient to ischemia secondary to progressive Campath 1H confirmed on histopathology (Figure 4-5). Conventional testing failed to reveal any evidence of chronic rejection but deep tissue biopsies were positive for Campath 1H in all of their other patients (Dr. Warren Breidenbach, personal communication). The team concluded that the incidence and severity of Campath 1H correlated with cellular and humoral parameters as well as the immunosuppression load. This is the first conclusive report of chronic rejection–related findings in clinical reconstructive transplantation. There is also a similar report of Campath 1H leading to loss of CTA wherein chronic allograft vasculopathy was seen in vascularized knee transplantation.[120] Within 5 years, 100% of the grafts were lost. Histopathology confirmation of the cases revealed "diffuse concentric fibrous intimal thickening and occlusion of graft vessels." The authors agree that the "lack of adequate tools for monitoring graft rejection might have allowed multiple untreated episodes of acute rejection, triggering myointimal proliferation and occlusion of graft vessels" and that "adequate tools for monitoring need to be developed." It seems clear that these extremities were lost secondary to Campath 1H, and this must be considered a possible chronic rejection. The inability of conventional techniques to monitor and diagnose Campath 1H as the primary predictor of chronic rejection is concerning and has implications for long-term outcomes after reconstructive transplantation.

At this point, we do not conclusively know if factors that play a role in genesis of chronic rejection in solid organs also mediate the phenomenon in reconstructive transplantation, but the expectation is that the pathophysiology will be similar. With prolonged survival of reconstructive transplants beyond 10 years, we will inevitably see more grafts develop signs of chronic rejection or succumb to chronic rejection. We will then be able to better define, diagnose, and grade this condition. Meanwhile, we are limited to minimizing the known risk factors (from solid organ experience) that may contribute to a postulated increase of chronic rejection in reconstructive transplants and also invest collective scientific intellect into identifying novel diagnostic tools and therapeutic strategies to monitor and possibly treat chronic rejection.

Cortical Reorganization

A unique phenomenon observed after reconstructive transplantation of the hand or face is the reassignment of portions of the recipient's brain in the sensorimotor cortex to control the graft. This is called "re-organization" or "plasticity" of the brain. Both the hand and face are contiguously represented in the homunculus. For example, previous studies have demonstrated that changes

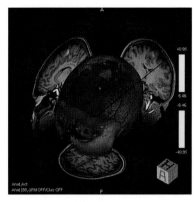

● **FIGURE 4-6.** Functional MRI demonstrating neural integration of the transplanted limb into the premotor cortex.

in cortical organization of the homunculus occur after amputation. However, the impact of limb transplantation on spatial reorganization of the motor cortex is just now being revealed.[121,122] After a hand is amputated or the face is subjected to devastating injury, the area of the brain that was receiving signals from the hand or face is gradually lost and is taken over by other functions. However, after a hand or face transplant, that area of the brain can reestablish its original function, and the signals from the new hand or face go back to the area of brain that was used to control the original area. Such neural integration of the transplant into the premotor cortex has been demonstrated using functional magnetic resonance imaging (Figure 4-6), diffusion tractography, or magnetoencephalography studies. This phenomenon has not been reported after organ transplantation. Figure 4-7 shows high-definition fiber tracking imaging before and after transplantation demonstrating reintegration of nerve fiber inputs to the sensory motor cortex.

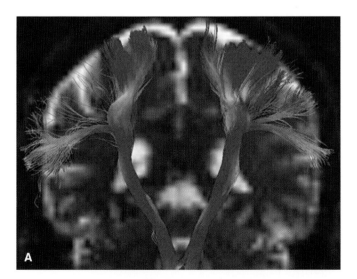
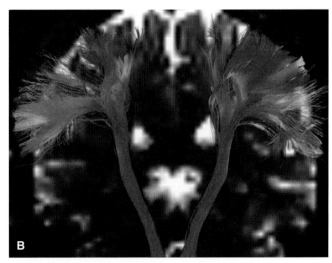

● **FIGURE 4-7.** High-definition imaging of neural fiber inputs into the sensory cortex: (A) pre-transplant; (B) post-transplant.

Strategies for Reduction or Elimination of Immunosuppression

Despite the excellent results thus far, the full potential and clinical applicability of reconstructive transplantation has not yet been realized because of the hazards associated with the long-term use of immunosuppressive drugs. Modern research into mechanisms of immune tolerance offers the promise of reprogramming the immune system, so as to harness the body's natural tolerance mechanisms in the service of graft acceptance. This would allow the minimization of immunosuppressive treatment and offers the prospect of eventually weaning transplant recipients off their drugs.

Fifty years ago, Medawar and colleagues demonstrated transplantation tolerance elicited by infusion of foreign marrow into a newborn mouse.[123] This was the first demonstration of acquired immunological tolerance, and as such, offered a challenge for achieving transplantation tolerance as a clinical goal in an immunologically mature adult—a goal yet to be realized as a routine procedure. Medawar's experiment was used as evidence to support the clonal selection theory and the notion that self-tolerance arises from purging of self-reactive lymphocytes from the immune repertoire. Later studies demonstrated that marrow infusions provided a source of stem cells able to establish a state of mixed (both recipient and donor) blood chimerism. This would guarantee a permanent source of donor antigen to ensure continuous purging of alloreactive lymphocytes, so setting the stage for current concepts of inducing tolerance therapeutically.

Tolerance can be defined as the indefinite acceptance of the grafted tissue after only a short course of immunomodulatory treatment. These findings have galvanized efforts to achieve tolerance in the clinic, although this is proving a formidable task. The goal of achieving clinical tolerance "up front" is enormously challenging, given the genetic heterogeneity of donor/recipient combinations and prior priming of the immune system to environmental antigens, which cross-react with those of the donor organ.[124] Furthermore, continuing improvements with immunosuppressive drugs that produce good medium-term outcomes make it difficult to introduce new "tolerance" protocols that risk loss of the transplanted organ. The emerging compromise has been to aim at harnessing tolerance mechanisms as a means of minimizing the dose and number of drugs administered.[125]

Some of the strategies for immunosuppression minimization or allograft tolerance include approaches using donor bone marrow transplantation or inducing peritransplant depletion of recipient T cells. The mixed chimerism model involves induction of allograft tolerance by establishing long-term mixed chimerism, a state in which both donor and recipient hematopoietic cells coexist after engraftment.[126] One of the lymphocyte depletion approaches includes the use of Campath 1H, which is an antibody that binds to the CD52 receptor,

critical for T cell function in humans. Campath 1H leads to depletion of T cells, B cells, and monocytes, but spares bone marrow stem cells. Early trials with Campath 1H in renal transplants demonstrated that allograft survival could be prolonged but with low doses of maintenance immunosuppression.[127] Campath 1H induction has been implemented in a few hand transplant programs with successful reduction of maintenance immunosuppression. Such a state of tolerance is called "prope tolerance" or "tolerance lite."[125]

Over the past five decades, more than 50 different methods of tolerance induction have succeeded in small or large animal models. Yet tolerance protocols have not widely replaced immunosuppression in clinical organ or reconstructive transplantation. The reason for this is straight forward. Many of the tolerance protocols are too risky for clinical application. In other protocols, the risks remain unknown. Therapies designed to reprogram the immune system toward better self-regulation will require biomarkers for monitoring rejection, tolerance, and undesired toxicity. These will in time provide surrogate measures of efficacy, so as to bypass the need for protracted clinical trials. Simplicity and clinical utility dictate that such diagnostic aids should be aimed at readily available tissue biopsies and body fluids.[128]

The momentum for harnessing tolerance processes is now unstoppable. At this stage, we really do not know how far we can go on the route to reprogramming the immune system. At some point, we will need to take stock and decide whether the patient's interests can best be served by maintaining them on a safe dose of drugs; or whether we aim for complete tolerance with the possibility that some stochastic event may disturb that process and so jeopardize the transplanted organ. Perhaps the compromise will be that of aiming for tolerance by weaning patients off their minimal drug regimens.

Reconstructive transplantation has introduced exciting new possibilities with procedures that offer new hope that was not available to patients just a few years ago. The important goals of reconstructive transplantation are to promote patient and public education; increase awareness of these procedures as treatment options with quality of life restoration as justification; and education of referring physicians, case managers, and patient advocacy groups and coalition with professional societies. Current technology is clearly sufficient to allow for successful transplantation and maintenance of these complex grafts, but controversy continues over the ethics of these procedures. Potentially endangering the life of a patient with immunosuppression in order to maintain what is often referred to as a quality of life graft continues to provoke debate. Advancements in immunosuppressive therapy, particularly in the induction of transplant tolerance, will reduce and possibly eliminate the controversy and open a window of opportunity for many patients deserving of such reconstruction.

REFERENCES

1. Shores JT, Brandacher G, Schneeberger S, et al. Composite tissue allotransplantation: hand transplantation and beyond. *J Am Acad Orthop Surg.* 2010;18(3):127–131.

2. Petruzzo P, Lanzetta M, Dubernard JM, et al. The international registry on hand and composite tissue transplantation. *Transplantation.* 2008;86:487–492.

3. Jones JW, Gruber SA, Barker JH, Breidenbach WC. Successful hand transplantation. One-year follow-up. Louisville Hand Transplant Team. *N Engl J Med.* 2000; 343:468–473.

4. Lanzetta M, Nolli R, Borgonovo A, et al. Hand transplantation: ethics, immunosuppression and indications. *J Hand Surg Br.* 2001;26:511–516.

5. Pollard MS. Hand transplantation–risks of immunosuppression. *J Hand Surg Br.* 2001;26:517.

6. Breidenbach WC, Gonzales NR, Kaufman CL, et al. Outcomes of the first 2 American hand transplants at 8 and 6 years posttransplant. *J Hand Surg Am.* 2008;33(7):1039–1047.

7. Petruzzo P, Lanzetta M, Dubernard JM, et al. The International Registry on Hand and Composite Tissue Transplantation. *Transplantation.* 2010;90(12):1590–1594.

8. Veith I, trans. *Huang Ti Nei Ching Su Wen. The Yellow Emperor's Classic of Internal Medicine.* Baltimore, MD: Williams & Wilkins Co; 1949.

9. Bhishagratna KC. An English translation of the Sushruta Samhita, based on original Sanskrit text. Calcutta: 1907.

10. Hoernlé AFR. *Studies in the Medicine of Ancient India.* Oxford, UK: Clarendon Press; 1907.

11. Hoernlé AFR. *Archaelogical Survey of India.* Calcutta 22, 1893.

12. Da Varagine J. *Leggenda Aurea.* Florence, Italy: Libreria Editrice Fiorentina 648; 1952.

13. Kahan BD. Cosmas and Damian revisited. *Transplant Proc.* 1983;15(4 suppl1-2):2211–2216.

14. Danilevicius Z. Cosmas and Damian: The patron saints of medicine in art. *JAMA.* 1967;201:1021–1025.

15. E Rinaldi. The first homoplastic limb transplant according to the legend of saint Cosmas and saint Damian. *Ital J Orthop Traumatol.* 1987;13(3):393–406.

16. Converse JM, Casson PR. The historical background of transplantation. In: Rapaport FT, Dausset J, eds. *Human Transplantation.* New York: Grune & Stratton; 1968.

17. Tagliacozzi G. *De curtorum chirurgia per insitionem.* Venice, Italy. University of Milan Library, 1597.

18. Tagliacozzi G. *De curtorum chirurgia*, Lib. I, Reiner G (ed.). Berloni: Chaps 12,18 (and passim), 1831.

19. Gnudi M. The sympathetic slave. In: *The life and times of Gaspare Tagliacozzi.* Los Angeles, CA: Zeitlin and Ver Brugge; 1976:285–286.

20. Carrel A. La technique operatoire des anastomoses vasculaires et la transplantation des visceres. *Lyon Med.* 1902;99:859.

21. Carrel A. The surgery of blood vessels. *Bull Johns Hopkins Hosp.* 1907;18:18.

22. Carrel A. Results of the transplantation of blood vessels, organs and limbs. *JAMA.* 1908;51:1662.

23. Landsteiner K. Cell antigens and individual specificity. *J Immunol.* 1928;15:589–600.

24. Flye MW. History of transplantation. In: Flye MW, ed. *Principles of Organ Transplantation.* Philadelphia, PA: WB Saunders Co; 1989.

25. Padgett EC. The full-thickness skin graft in the correction of soft tissue deformities. *JAMA.* 1932;98:18.

26. Brown JB. Homografting of skin: with report of success in identical twins. *Surgery.* 1937;1:558.

27. Gorer PA, Schütze H. Genetical studies on immunity in mice: II. Correlation between antibody formation and resistance. *J Hyg (Lond).* 1938;38(6):647–662.

28. Medawar PB. The behavior and fate of skin autografts and skin homografts in rabbits. *J Anat.* 1944;78:176.

29. Hall RH. Whole upper extremity transplant for human being: General plans of procedure and operative technique. *Ann Surg.* 1944;120:12.

30. Gibson T, Medawar PB. The fate of skin homografts in man. *J Anat.* 1943;77:299.

31. Dausset J. Iso-leuco-anticorps. *Acta Haematol.* 1958;20: 156–166.

32. Simonson M, Buemann J, Gammeltaft A. Biological incompatibility in kidney transplantation in dogs. I. Experimental and morphological investigations. *Acta Pathol Microbiol Scand.* 1953;32:1–35.

33. Mitchison NA. Graft rejection, the histocompatibility complex and the Langerhans' cell. Clin Exp Dermatol. 1979;4(4):489–493.

34. Medawar P. A second study of the behavior and fate of skin homografts in rabbits. (A report to the War Wounds Committee of the Medical Research Council). *J Anat.* 1945;69:157–176.

35. Harrison JH, Merrill JP, Murray JE. Renal homotransplantation in identical twins. *Surg Forum.* 1955;6:432–436.

36. Merrill JP, Murray JE, Harrison JH, Guild WR. Successful homotransplantation of the human kidney between identical twins. *JAMA.* 1956;160(4):277–282.

37. Merrill JP, Murray JE, Harrison JH, et al. Successful homotransplantation of the kidney between non-identical twins. *N Engl J Med.* 1960;262:1251–1260.

38. Murray JE, Merrill JP, Dammin GJ, et al. Kidney transplantation in modified recipients. *Ann Surg.* 1962;156: 337–355.

39. Murray JE, Merrill JP, Harrison JH, et al. Prolonged survival of human-kidney homografts by immunosuppressive drug therapy. *N Engl J Med.* 1963;268:1315–1323.

40. Peacock EE Jr. Some problems in flexor tendon healing, *Surgery.* 1959;45:415–423.

41. Peacock EE Jr. Restoration of finger flexion with homologous composite tissue tendon grafts of the digital flexor mechanism in human beings. *Trans Bull.* 1960;7: 418–421.

42. Terasaki PI, McClelland JD. Microdroplet assay of human serum cytotoxins. *Nature*. 1964;204:998–1000.

43. Anonymous. Historic cadaver-to-man hand transplant. *Med World News*. March 13, 1964.

44. Anonymous. Helping hand. *Time*. March 6, 1964.

45. Barnes DW, Ford CE, Ilbery PL, et al. Tissue transplantation in the radiation chimera. *J Cell Physiol Suppl*. 1957;50 (suppl 1):123–138.

46. Hamburger J, Vaysse J, Crosnier J, et al. Transplantation of a kidney between non-monozygotic twins after irradiation of the receiver: good function at the fourth month. *Press Med*. 1959;67:1771.

47. Hamburger J, Vaysse J, Crosnier J, et al. Renal homotransplantations in man after radiation of the recipient. *Am J Med*. 1962;32:854.

48. Schwartz R, Dameshek W. The effects of 6-mercaptopurine on homograft reactions. *J Clin Invest*. 1960;39:952–958.

49. Calne RY. The rejection of renal homografts: inhibition in dogs by 6-mercaptopurine. *Lancet*. 1960;1:417–418.

50. Zukoski CF, Lee HM, Hume DM. The prolongation of functional survival of canine renal homografts by 6-mercaptopurine. *Surg Forum*. 1960;11:470–472.

51. Hitchings GH. Chemotherapy and comparative biochemistry: G. H. A. Clowes memorial lecture [review]. *Cancer Res*. 1969;29(11):1895–903.

52. Murray JE, Merrill JP, Harrison JH, et al. Prolonged survival of human-kidney homografts by immunosuppressive drug therapy. *N Engl J Med*. 1963;268:1315.

53. Calne RY. The initial study of the immunosuppressive effects of 6-mercaptopurine and azathioprine in organ transplantation and a few words on cyclosporin A. *World J Surg*. 1982;6(5):637–640.

54. Gorantla VS, Barker JH, Jones JW Jr, et al. Immunosuppressive agents in transplantation: mechanisms of action and current anti-rejection strategies. *Microsurgery*. 2000;20(8):420.

55. Dreyfuss M, Harri E, Hofmann H, et al. Cyclosporin A and C; new metabolites from Trichoderma polysporum. Rifai. *Eur J Appl Microbiol*. 1976;3:125.

56. Borel JF, Feurer C, Gubler HU, et al. Biological effects of cyclosporine A; a new antilymphocyte agent. *Agents Actions*. 1976;6:468.

57. Calne RY, White DJG, Thiru S, et al. Cyclosporine A in patients receiving renal allografts from cadaver donors. *Lancet*. 1978;2:1323.

58. Goto T, Kino T, Hatanaka H, et al. Discovery of FK-506, a novel immunosuppressant isolated from Streptomyces tsukubaensis. *Transplant Proc*. 1987;19:4.

59. Starzl TE, Todo S, Fung JJ, et al. FK 506 for human liver, kidney and pancreas transplantation. *Lancet*. 1989;2:1000.

60. Fung JJ, Todo S, Jain A, et al. Conversion of liver allograft recipients with cyclosporine related complications from cyclosporine to FK 506. *Transplant Proc*. 1990;22:6.

61. Armitage JM, Kormos RL, Griffith BP, et al. The clinical trial of FK 506 as primary and rescue immunosuppression in cardiac transplantation. *Transplant Proc*. 1991;23:1149.

62. Todo S, Fung JJ, Starzl TE, et al. Liver, kidney and thoracic organ transplantation under FK 506. *Ann Surg*. 1990;212:295.

63. Starzl TE, Fung JJ, Jordan M, et al. Kidney transplantation under FK 506. *JAMA*. 1990;264:63.

64. Starzl TE, Abu Elmagd K, Tzakis A, et al. Selected topics on FK 506: With special reference to rescue extrahepatic whole organ grafts, transplantation of "forbidden organs," side effects, mechanisms, and practical pharmacokinetics. *Transplant Proc*. 1991;23:914.

65. Todo S, Tzakis AG, Abou Elmagd K, et al. Intestinal transplantation in composite visceral grafts or alone. *Ann Surg*. 1992;216:223.

66. Todo S, Tzakis AG, Abou Elmagd K, et al. Cadaveric small bowel and small bowel-liver transplantation in humans. *Transplantation*. 1992;53:369.

67. Allison AC, Eugui EM. Immunosuppressive and other effects of mycophenolic acid and an ester prodrug, mycophenolate mofetil. *Immunol Rev*. 1993;136:5.

68. Vezina C, Kudelski A, Sehgal SN. Rapamycin (AY-22989), a new anti-fungal antibiotic: Taxonomy of the producing streptomycete and isolation of the active principle. *J Antibiot (Tokyo)*. 1975;28:721.

69. Halloran P, Mathew T, Tomlanovich S, et al. Mycophenolate mofetil in renal allograft recipients: a pooled efficacy analysis of three randomized, double blind clinical studies in prevention of rejection. The International Mycophenolate Mofetil Renal Transplant Study Groups. *Transplantation*. 1997;63:39.

70. McAlister VC, Gao Z, Peltekian K, et al. Sirolimus-tacrolimus combination immunosuppression. *Lancet*. 2000;355:376.

71. Kahan BD, Podbielski J, Napoli KL, et al. Immunosuppressive effects and safety of sirolimus/cyclosporine combination regimen for renal transplantation. *Transplantation*. 1998;66:1040.

72. Shapiro JAM, Lakey JRT, Ryan EA, et al. Islet transplantation in seven patients with type-1 diabetes mellitus using a glucocorticoid free immunosuppressive regimen. *N Engl J Med*. 2000;343:230.

73. Burnet FM. The new approach to immunology. *N Engl J Med*. 1961;264:24.

74. Murray JE. Nobel Prize lecture: the first successful transplants in man. http://www.stanford.edu/dept/HPS/transplant/html/murray.

75. Gorantla V, Maldonado C, Frank J, Barker JH. Composite tissue allotransplantation (CTA): current status and future insights. *Eur J Trauma*. 2001;27(6):267–274.

76. Lee WP, Yaremchuk MJ, Pan YC, et al. Relative antigenicity of components of a vascularized limb allograft. *Plast Reconstr Surg*. 1991;87(3):401–411.

77. Bos JD. The skin as an organ of immunity. *Clin Exp Immunol*. 1997;107(suppl 1):3–5.

78. Swann G. The skin is the body's largest organ. *J Vis Commun Med*. 2010;33(4):148–149.

79. Jensen JM, Proksch E. The skin's barrier. *Ital Dermatol Venereol*. 2009;144(6):689–700.

80. Bos JD, Luiten RM. Skin immune system. *Cancer Treat Res.* 2009;146:45–62.

81. Bos JD, Zonneveld I, Das PK, et al. The skin immune system (SIS): distribution and immunophenotype of lymphocyte subpopulations in normal human skin. *J Invest Dermatol.* 1987;88(5):569–573.

82. Steinman RM. The dendritic cell system and its role in immunogenicity. *Annu Rev Immunol.* 1991;9:271–296.

83. Nestle FO, Di Meglio P, Qin JZ, Nickoloff BJ. Skin immune sentinels in health and disease. *Nat Rev Immunol.* 2009;9(10):679–691.

84. Roediger B, Ng LG, Smith AL, et al. Visualizing dendritic cell migration within the skin. *Histochem Cell Biol.* 2008;130(6):1131–1146.

85. Aoki T, Fujinami T. Demonstration of tissue-specific soluble antigens in human skin by immunodiffusion. *J Immunol.* 1967;98(1):39–45.

86. Steinmuller D, Wakely E, Landas SK. Evidence that epidermal alloantigen Epa-1 is an immunogen for murine heart as well as skin allograft rejection. *Transplantation.* 1991;51(2):459–463.

87. Fuchimoto Y, Gleit ZL, Huang CA, et al. Skin-specific alloantigens in miniature swine. *Transplantation.* 2001;72(1):122–126.

88. Kanitakis J, Jullien D, Petruzzo P, et al. Clinicopathologic features of graft rejection of the first human hand allograft. *Transplantation.* 2003;76(4):688–693.

89. Cendales LC, Kirk AD, Moresi JM, et al. Composite tissue allotransplantation: classification of clinical acute skin rejection. *Transplantation.* 2006;81(3):418–422.

90. Mathes DW, Randolph MA, Solari MG, et al. Split tolerance to a composite tissue allograft in a swine model. *Transplantation.* 2003;75(1):25–31.

91. Brandacher G, Gorantla VS, Lee WP. Hand allotransplantation. *Semin Plast Surg.* 2010;24(1):11–17.

92. Deeg HJ, Storb R. Graft-versus-host disease: pathophysiological and clinical aspects. *Annu Rev Med.* 1984;35:11–24.

93. Zhang Y, Ruiz P. Solid organ transplant-associated acute graft-versus-host disease. *Arch Pathol Lab Med.* 2010;134(8):1220–1224.

94. Sims KD, Blumberg EA. Common infections in the lung transplant recipient. *Clin Chest Med.* 2011;32(2):327–341.

95. Mao Q, Li YS, Li JS. The current status of multivisceral transplantation. *Hepatobiliary Pancreat Dis Int.* 2009;8(4):345–350.

96. Amirlak B, Gonzalez R, Gorantla V, et al. Creating a hand transplant program. *Clin Plast Surg.* 2007;34(2):279–289.

97. Gordon CR, Siemionow M. Requirements for the development of a hand transplantation program. *Ann Plast Surg.* 2009;63(3):262–273.

98. Hollenbeck ST, Erdmann D, Levin LS. Current indications for hand and face allotransplantation. *Transplant Proc.* 2009;41(2):495–498.

99. Kvernmo HD, Gorantla VS, Gonzalez RN, Breidenbach WC 3rd. Hand transplantation. A future clinical option? *Acta Orthop.* 2005;76(1):14–27.

100. Younes BS, McDiarmid SV, Martin MG, et al. The effect of immunosuppression on posttransplant lymphoproliferative disease in pediatric liver transplant patients. *Transplantation.* 2000;70(1):94.

101. Klapheke M, Marcell C, Taliaferro G, Creamer B. Psychiatric assessment of candidates for hand transplantation. *Microsurgery.* 2000;20:453.

102. Kanitakis J, Jullien D, Petruzzo P, et al. Immunohistologic studies of the skin of human hand allografts: Our experience with two patients. *Transplant Proc.* 2001;33:1722.

103. Schneeberger S, Gorantla VS, van Riet RP, et al. Atypical acute rejection after hand transplantation. *Am J Transplant.* 2008;8(3):688–696.

104. Cendales LC, Kanitakis J, Schneeberger S, et al. The Banff 2007 working classification of skin-containing composite tissue allograft pathology. *Am J Transplant.* 2008;8(7):1396–1400.

105. Cendales LC, Kirk AD, Moresi JM, et al. Composite tissue allotransplantation: classification of clinical acute skin rejection [Erratum in: *Transplantation.* 2006;81(3):422.]. *Transplantation.* 2006;81(3):418–422.

106. Zeevi A. Immunomonitoring after human limb allotransplantation. *Transplant Proc.* 1998;30:2711.

107. Ting A, Terasaki PI. Lymphocyte-dependent antibody cross-matching for transplant patients. *Lancet.* 1975;1:304–306.

108. Kanitakis J, Jullien D, Petruzzo P, et al. Clinicopathologic features of graft rejection of the first human hand allograft. *Transplantation.* 2003;76(4):688–693.

109. Pei G.Long term follow up of hand allografts. *J Reconst Microsurg.* 2004;1(21):Part II.

110. Kaufman C. Vasculopathy in vascularized composite allotransplantation. Presented at: the 10th IHCTAS Meeting; April 7-10; Atlanta, Georgia.

111. Demetris AJ, Murase N, Lee RG, et al. Chronic rejection. A general overview of histopathology and pathophysiology with emphasis on liver, heart and intestinal allografts. *Ann Transplant.* 1997;2(2):27–44.

112. Rubin RH. Impact of cytomegalovirus infection on organ transplant recipients. *Rev Infect Dis.* 1990;12(S7):S754.

113. Rubin R. Infection in organ transplant recipients. In: Rubin RH, Young LS, eds. *Clinical Approach to Infection in the Compromised Host.* 3rd ed. New York and London: Plenum Medical Book Company; 1994:629.

114. Matas A. Chronic rejection in renal transplant recipients–risk factors and correlates. *Clin Transpl.* 1994;8(3):332.

115. Michaels PJ, Fishbein MC, Colvin RB. Humoral rejection of human organ transplants. *Springer Semin Immunopathol.* 2003;25(2):119.

116. Junge G, Tullius SG, Klitzing V. The influence of late acute rejection episodes on long-term graft outcome after liver transplantation. *Transplant Proc.* 2005;37(4):1716.

117. Baines LS, Joseph JT, Jindal RM. Compliance and late acute rejection after kidney transplantation: a psychomedical perspective. *Clin Transplant.* 2002;16:69.

118. Chapman JR. Compliance: the patient, the doctor, and the medication? *Transplantation.* 2004;77(5):782.

119. Demetris AJ, Murase N, Starzl TE, Fung JJ. Pathology of chronic rejection: an overview of common findings and observations about pathogenic mechanisms and possible prevention. *Graft*. 1998;1(2):52–59.

120. Diefenbeck M, Nerlich A, Schneeberger S, et al. Allograft vasculopathy after allogeneic vascularized knee transplantation. *Transpl Int*. 2011;24(1):e1–e5.

121. Giraux P, Sirigu A, Schneider F, et al. Cortical reorganization in motor cortex after graft of both hands. *Nat Neurosci*. 2001;4(7):691.

122. Frey SH, Bogdanov S, Smith JC, et al. Chronically deafferented sensory cortex recovers a grossly typical organization after allogenic hand transplantation. *Curr Biol*. 2008;18(19):1530–1534.

123. Billingham RE, Brent L, Medawar PB. Actively acquired tolerance of foreign cells. 1953. *Transplantation*. 2003; 76(10):1409–1412.

124. Adams AB, Pearson TC, Larsen CP. Heterologous immunity: an overlooked barrier to tolerance. *Immunol Rev*. 2003;196:147–160.

125. Calne R, Friend P, Moffatt S, et al. Prope tolerance, perioperative campath 1H, and low-dose cyclosporin monotherapy in renal allograft recipients. *Lancet*. 1998;351(9117): 1701–1702.

126. Prabhune KA, Gorantla VS, Maldonado C, et al. Mixed allogeneic chimerism and tolerance to composite tissue allografts. *Microsurgery*. 2000;20:441.

127. Calne R, Moffatt SD, Friend PJ, et al. Campath 1H allows low-dose cyclosporine monotherapy in 31 cadaveric renal allograft recipients. *Transplantation*. 1999;68(10):1613.

128. Li B, Hartono C, Ding R, et al. Noninvasive diagnosis of renal-allograft rejection by measurement of messenger RNA for perforin and granzyme B in urine. *N Engl J Med*. 2001;344(13):947–954.

chapter 5

Negative Pressure Wound Therapy

Mark B. Schoemann, MD / *Christopher Lentz, MD, FACS, FCCM*

● HISTORY AND DEVELOPMENT

Negative pressure wound therapy (NPWT) is a relatively recent development in the history of wound care. This innovative approach uses a closed system that applies negative pressure to a wound, thereby promoting formation of granulation tissue and maintaining a moist, wound-healing environment. The use of NPWT has rapidly gained acceptance into the armamentarium of the plastic surgeon, as a growing body of research has demonstrated its benefits and successful outcomes. Multiple animal studies and clinical trials have not only supported its use in plastic surgery but across other fields. Papers on NPWT have been published in almost all surgical specialty journals, but the best represented are general surgery, orthopedics, urology, and trauma.

The concept of using negative pressure to treat surgical wounds was first described in 1952, although it took approximately another 50 years before NPWT came into its own as an accepted wound treatment modality. Raffl, in his 1952 article, described the placement of closed suction drains under postmastectomy skin flaps. The drains were connected to continuous negative pressure in order to maintain flap adherence to the abdominal wall and to remove serous fluid. Two years later, Silvis et al., applied these principles of negative pressure to patients who had undergone radical neck dissections. The authors felt an external pressure dressing to the neck was ineffective; therefore, closed suction drains were placed under the dissection flaps and removed in 72 hours. They concluded, "continuous suction has marked advantages over pressure dressings."

Forty years later, Nakayama and Soeda described the use of a negative pressure dressing to affix a split-thickness skin graft to the dorsum of the hand. A fine silastic mesh was placed over the skin graft, on top of which a closed suction drain and two clear adhesive drapes were placed to seal the system. The authors concluded that their "vacuum package" dressing was superior to a conventional bolster dressing over a skin graft because it provided constant uniform pressure over an uneven wound surface.

Throughout the 1990s, development of a negative pressure dressing system gained momentum as plastic surgeons pioneered the next great advancement in wound care. Argenta and Morykwas from the Bowman Gray School of Medicine of Wake Forest University in North Carolina pioneered the development of a universal negative pressure dressing system through extensive basic science research and numerous clinical trials. In 1995, the FDA approved the marketing of the Vacuum Assisted Closure (V.A.C.) device in the United States. As a large body of research accumulated showing the efficacy of the V.A.C., the FDA expanded its clinical indications in 2000.

● SCIENCE AND PHYSIOLOGY

Many studies have elucidated the basic science principles that make NPWT an effective modality for treatment of acute and chronic wounds. The studies were performed using the V.A.C. device, the only commercially available NPWT system, and showed it to stimulate wound healing by several physiologic mechanisms. NPWT improves wound healing by maintaining a moist environment, removing edema fluid, decreasing bacterial colonization, and augmenting local blood flow.[1] On the cellular level, subatmospheric pressures cause deformation of individual cells, which promotes proliferation in the wound microenvironment. Ultimately, blood flow levels are augmented with the use of subatmospheric pressure leading to increased granulation tissue and improved wound healing.

Animal studies in swine have shown that blood flow increases fourfold in wounds with the use of negative pressure dressings. These studies were performed with laser Doppler flow needle probes placed into the subcutaneous tissue of wounds covered with a NPWT dressing. A peak blood flow of four times baseline was seen with subatmospheric pressures of 125 mm Hg. Increasing the amount of negative pressure to values greater than 400 mm Hg, however, did not enhance but rather decreased blood flow. Local blood flow also declined to baseline when subatmospheric pressure was turned off for 5 to 7 minutes. It is believed that the application of continuous negative pressure to a wound removes sufficient interstitial edema to decompress small blood vessels and increase local flow.

In addition to increasing local blood flow, NPWT has been shown to increase the rate of granulation tissue formation in a healing wound. The V.A.C. dressing and saline moistened gauze were placed in wounds on the backs of swine and compared. Subatmospheric pressure applied continuously at 125 mm Hg resulted in a 63% increase in granulation tissue volume when compared with saline gauze dressing. Mechanical forces that are applied to cells cause them to proliferate and divide. Plastic surgeons have long used tissue expanders and the Ilizarov technique to exploit this property of cells. Subatmospheric pressures exert micromechanical forces to the exterior of the cell, which are then transmitted to the intracellular cytoskeleton causing the release of intracellular second messengers that promote cellular proliferation. The V.A.C. device can exert tissue strain from approximately 5% to 20%, which is the range of stretch necessary to induce cellular proliferation and increase formation of granulation tissue. The pores of the NPWT foam, which range in size from 400 to 600 μm, draw up tissue from the superficial surface of the wound and are responsible for exerting cellular stretch and microdeformation, leading to cellular proliferation.[2]

Infection of a wound with significant number of bacteria ($>10^5$ organisms/gram tissue) severely interferes with the normal wound healing process. Application of subatmospheric pressure to a wound with a clinically significant number of bacteria improves clearance. Initial animal studies examining pig wounds inoculated with 10^8 organisms of either *Staphylococcus aureus* or *Staphylococcus epidermidis* had decreased bacterial counts after application of NPWT. By day 4, there was a statistically significant drop in bacterial counts to less than 10^5 in the group treated with NPWT vs wounds not treated with NPWT. Wongworawat et al. showed that application of NPWT using the V.A.C. in wounds with positive cultures was extremely effective. They noted an average reduction of 43% in wound size at 10 days in patients with culture-positive abscesses that were debrided, irrigated, and treated with NPWT. However, one study that quantified bacterial loads in wounds treated with saline moist gauze and NPWT found no major difference between treatment arms. While overall bacterial load was similar in the saline moist gauze and NPWT treatment groups, NPWT was shown to significantly decrease nonfermenting gram-negative bacilli ($P<0.05$) and increase *S aureus* ($P<0.05$).

PATIENT EVALUATION AND SELECTION

In 1995, the FDA approved the first NPWT device known as the V.A.C. for the general treatment of nonhealing chronic wounds. The indications for V.A.C. use were later expanded in 2000 to include acute, traumatic, and dehisced wounds in addition to ulcers of the diabetic and pressure variety. Indications at this time now include treatment of wounds containing flaps and grafts. Use of NPWT in each of these clinical situations is discussed later in the chapter.

Contraindications to use of NPWT are presence of malignancy in the wound, untreated osteomyelitis, nonenteric and unexplored fistulas, and presence of necrotic tissue with eschar. Although mechanical stretch causes proliferation of normal cells, its effect on malignant cells that already have a propensity to proliferate is unknown. Therefore NPWT is not recommended in a wound with known malignancy. NPWT can be placed in wounds that are the result of an oncologic resection, provided that all gross tumor is removed. NPWT should not be used in wounds with active osteomyelitis. Osteomyelitis requires debridement of devitalized tissue and appropriate systemic antibiotic treatment prior to initiation of NPWT. Use of NPWT on devitalized or necrotic tissue in general will be futile as the NPWT can only enhance wound healing of viable tissue. Additionally, application of the polyurethane sponge used in NPWT directly over exposed vessels is contraindicated, as there is the possibility that subatmospheric pressure might compromise vessel wall integrity. It is imperative to place fascia or tissue as a protective layer over vessels if NPWT is to be placed in close proximity. However, there have been several case reports of V.A.C. placement directly over exposed femoral bypass grafts for the treatment of groin infections after lower extremity vascular bypass surgery. A nonadherent dressing was interposed between the V.A.C. sponge and the exposed vessels; no complications were reported with this approach.

Although the use of anticoagulation is not a contraindication to application of a V.A.C. dressing, precaution should be used in these situations. Exsanguination of an anticoagulated patient from a V.A.C. dressing is not possible. The V.A.C. canister, which is typically 250 to 500 mL, will turn off when completely full, alarming patient care staff; or, alternatively, the tubing will become occluded with coagulated blood first. There have been several reports that NPWT in fully anticoagulated patients can lead to complications, mainly occlusion of the suction tubing with coagulated blood, which renders the treatment ineffective. In these cases, discontinuation of NPWT is recommended and institution of a more conventional mode of wound dressing be utilized.

● PATIENT PREPARATION

The first step to ensure successful outcomes with NPWT is to prepare the wound bed for application of a subatmospheric dressing. Devitalized and necrotic tissue must be debrided adequately from the wound. As mentioned earlier, NPWT is only able to augment the healing of viable tissue, therefore, any necrotic tissue must be removed before placement of the foam. Irrigation of the wound with normal saline or a pulse irrigator with or without antibiotic solution may be required in contaminated wounds. Achieving adequate hemostasis is imperative, as removal of copious amounts of blood from the wound can lead to occlusion of the suction tubing.

Once the wound has been adequately debrided and adequate hemostasis achieved, the NPWT foam dressing is then placed into the wound. Three types of foam dressing are currently marketed to be used with the V.A.C. system: a black polyurethane foam, a white polyvinyl alcohol foam, and a silver impregnated foam dressing. The black polyurethane foam dressing (pore size 400–600 μm) is the traditional foam dressing that can be used in a variety of wounds. The smaller pore size of the newer polyvinyl alcohol foam (pore size 60–270 μm) is designed to prevent the ingrowth of granulation tissue into the foam, which is beneficial when dressing skin grafts and painful wounds with NPWT. Placement of a layer of nonadherent gauze, such as Xeroform or Adaptic, which is readily available in the operating room, between a skin graft and the black polyurethane foam can prevent ingrowth of granulation tissue. GranuFoam Silver, the most recently introduced foam dressing, is impregnated with silver, which provides a continuous release of antimicrobial silver ions that interfere with the electron transport chain of a wide spectrum of bacteria. Randomized trials comparing the bacterial clearance of the silver impregnated foam to the traditional black polyurethane foam have not yet been performed.

Following the appropriate selection of the foam dressing, it must be cut to suitable dimensions for placement in the wound. Heavy mayo scissors are adequate in the operating room to cut through the 1-inch thick foam. When placing a NPWT foam dressing in a superficial wound of large surface area, we recommend cutting the 1-inch thick foam dressing into two, half-inch thick, pieces. The foam dressing should cover the entire wound base, sides, and undermined areas and should fit easily into the wound without the need for packing it forcibly. The foam should not be placed in direct contact with native epidermis at the edges of the wound. Multiple pieces of foam should be in direct contact, so that subatmospheric pressure is distributed evenly throughout the wound. A surgical stapler can be used to keep multiple pieces of foam in continuity. Placing a foam dressing in a wound with irregular contour can be difficult. In wounds encompassing the partial circumference of the

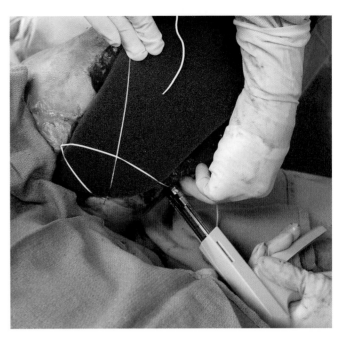

● **FIGURE 5-1.** Placing the NPWT foam dressing in wounds with irregular contour or convex shape can be problematic. To secure the foam dressing, vessel loops are secured at the edges of the wound with a stapler and then interlaced over the top of it. The surgeon is then able to apply the occlusive dressing with both hands unconstrained.

leg or arm, we secure the foam dressing in place with vessel loops. The vessel loops are secured to the edges of the wound with a stapler and then crisscrossed over the foam and then eventually tied down (Figure 5-1). This allows manipulation of the extremity while placing the occlusive drape without dislodgement of the foam.

After the foam dressing has been appropriately sized and placed into the wound, the occlusive dressing is then applied. For the occlusive dressing to maintain adequate seal, the periwound area must be clean and dry. Generous application of Mastisol, Tincture of Benzoin, or Cavilon No Sting Barrier Film to the periwound skin is recommended. Once the skin preparation has had time to adequately dry, the occlusive dressing is placed over the foam dressing with a 3 to 5 cm border of overlap around the wound. The wound drape comes supplied in 25 cm × 35 cm sheets in the package. We have found that trying to place such large sheets over irregularly shaped wounds and joints to be cumbersome. Cutting the occlusive wound drapes into approximately 10 cm wide strips allows easier application; however, each strip should overlap the previous one by approximately 2 cm (Figure 5-2A). More complex wounds with irregular contours, such as those encountered in the groin and across joints, should be dressed with even thinner strips of the occlusive dressing (Figure 5-2B). Wounds with copious effluent can also pose problems of maintaining adequate periwound seal with the occlusive dressing. Often times, wound effluent will pool in the dependent portion of the wound. The occlusive drape should be applied here last.

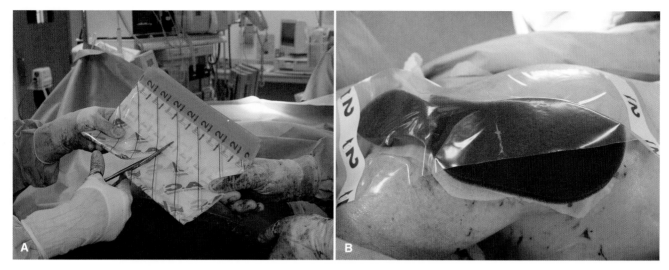

● **FIGURE 5-2.** (A) Application of the occlusive dressing is made easier by cutting it lengthwise into approximately 10 cm wide strips. (B) Wounds with more irregular contour require thinner strips of occlusive dressing. Subsequent strips should be laid down with 3 to 4 cm of overlap.

With the nondependant portions dressed first, the suction tubing can be attached and connected to standard operating room suction tubing. This maneuver will reduce wound effluent and pooling in the dependent portion, allowing placement of the occlusive drape to a drier area.

With the foam placed into the wound and occlusive dressing applied, the last step to successful NPWT is placement of suction tubing. Older V.A.C. units came with a noncollapsible suction tubing that was to be placed into the foam dressing directly and then covered with occlusive dressing. Suction tubing could not be placed over bony prominences or weight bearing areas, as there was the possibility of soft tissue breakdown. Newer V.A.C. devices come with a noncollapsible suction tubing terminating with a circle of self-contained occlusive drape called the TRAC pad. A small, 1 cm cut is made through the occlusive dressing that is covering the foam and the TRAC pad is simply placed over it. Either type of tubing is then connected to a V.A.C. device and the desired amount of subatmospheric pressure established. When NPWT is applied to two different anatomic sites, a Y connector can be used to connect two pieces of suction tubing to one V.A.C. device. If two sites are in close proximity, a bridge can be formed to extend the subatmospheric pressure from the primary NPWT site to a nearby secondary site. This can be accomplished by placing a section of arterial line tubing or nasogastric suction tubing, both of which are non-compressible, between the sites and covering with occlusive dressing (Figure 5-3). Alternatively, a bridge can be formed by placing a piece of NPWT foam between two sites provided the native skin underneath the bridge is protected with either Xeroform gauze or DuoDERM (Figure 5-4).

Two of the most common problems encountered with NPWT are the presence of an air leak from the occlusive wound drape and occlusion of the suction tubing. When the V.A.C. device alarms that an air leak has been detected,

it is crucial to handle this problem in a timely manner. An inadequate seal will result in loss of a moist wound environment and potential wound desiccation on account of a continuous air current over the wound surface. The first maneuver is to check the suction tubing and ensure that it has not been disconnected from the V.A.C. device or is kinked. If the tubing appears to be intact, then the leak is likely from disruption of the periwound occlusive dressing. An additional piece of occlusive wound drape can be placed over the initial dressing in order to obtain adequate sealing. The occlusive drape supplied with the V.A.C. device should be used, as Tegaderm or Opsite are porous and will not be able to sustain an adequate seal at

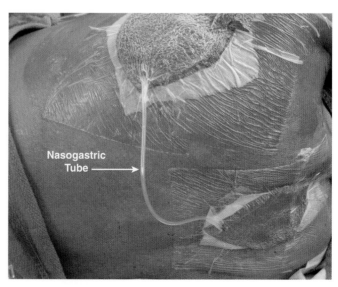

● **FIGURE 5-3.** Two wounds in proximity that have been treated with NPWT can be connected with noncompressible tubing, such as arterial line tubing or in this case a nasogastric tube.

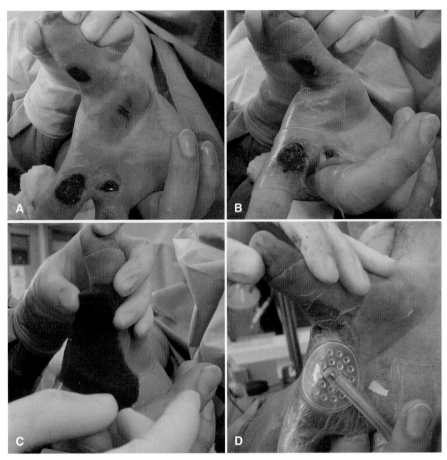

● **FIGURE 5-4.** (A) A young man presents with partial-thickness injuries of the hand after grabbing a hot metal pipe. His wounds have been debrided and prepared for NPWT application. (B) DuoDERM is placed around both wounds in order to protect the native epidermis and to allow the placement of one large foam dressing instead of two smaller foam dressings. (C) Large foam dressing is placed over DuoDERM and both wounds. (D) NPWT applied to both wounds simultaneously.

subatmospheric pressures. If placement of multiple pieces of occlusive dressing does not solve the problem, then the initial occlusive dressing should be taken down and a new one applied with thorough skin prep. Occlusion of the suction tubing can occur commonly in wounds that produce a thick effluent. Placement of a new piece of suction tubing onto the foam dressing will remedy this problem.

● **TECHNIQUES**

Perioperative Use of Negative Pressure Dressings on Skin Grafts

Skin grafting with full-thickness and partial-thickness grafts is an integral tool in the plastic surgeon's reconstructive armamentarium. In order for a skin graft to survive, it must have sufficient contact with the recipient bed and shear forces minimized. A bolster dressing, consisting of cotton fluff secured with interlacing sutures, is commonly used to accomplish this. In small, flat, well-granulated beds with minimal motion, these types of dressings are adequate. However, in larger recipient beds

subjected to excessive shear force, graft survival can be severely compromised. Recognizing that bolster dressings apply variable pressure and can conceal a developing hematoma, Nakayama et al., were the first to describe the use of NPWT to secure split-thickness skin grafts in 1990. They noted NPWT to be superior to conventional bolster and pressure bandages. NPWT provides constant uniform pressure over the entire area of the skin graft, as well as on irregular surfaces and recipient beds subjected to excessive motion (Figure 5-5).

As the use of the V.A.C. became more widespread in the 1990s and its indication were broadened, use of NPWT as a perioperative dressing for skin grafts, instead of the traditional bolster dressing, became more widespread. Early case reports in the literature described successful skin grafting with NPWT in even the most difficult anatomic locations, including the perineum and axilla. Soon after, Schneider, Morykwas, and Argenta reported using the V.A.C. to secure split-thickness skin graft to recipient beds in over 100 patients.[3] They noted complete graft take in all but two patients who incidentally had chronic wounds that were grossly contaminated. A retrospective

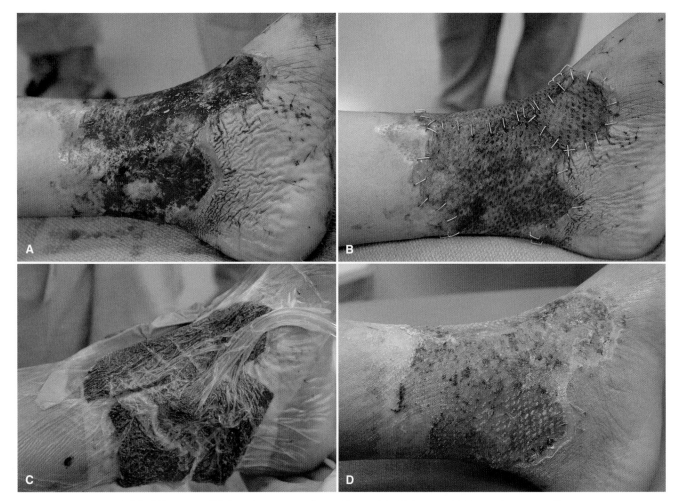

● **FIGURE 5-5.** (A) A patient presenting with partial-thickness skin loss after the cuff of his pants caught on fire. (B) Skin grafts have been applied after the wound bed was adequately debrided of nonviable tissue. (C) Ankle after NPWT has been applied. (D) Skin graft 3 weeks after removal of NPWT.

review of 61 patients requiring split-thickness skin grafts for acute traumatic and thermal injury burns demonstrated that the V.A.C. was superior to bolster dressings. Patients receiving traditional bolster dressings had less graft take (89%) and required more repeat skin grafts (19%) when compared to the V.A.C. group which had a take rate of 96% and required repeat grafting in 3%.[4] With the ability to conform to irregular contours, NPWT has expanded the possibilities of skin grafting and broadens the plastic surgeon's ability to place skin grafts in difficult locations.

In order to use NPWT as a perioperative skin graft dressing successfully, one must first adhere to the basic plastic surgery principles of skin grafting. The recipient bed must be prepared in the usual manner with adequate debridement of necrotic and nonviable tissue along with adequate hemostasis. Once this is achieved, the skin graft is placed onto the recipient bed and its edges trimmed. We secure the skin graft to the edge of the wound with surgical staples. A protective layer must be placed between the skin graft and the polyurethane foam dressing in order to prevent ingrowth of the skin graft into the foam and eventual graft disruption when the foam is removed. Either Xeroform gauze or Adaptic is sufficient to prevent ingrowth. With the skin graft and protective layer down, the foam dressing is cut to size, placed onto the wound, and covered with the occlusive adhesive dressing. Suction tubing is connected and set to continuous negative pressure of 125 mm Hg.

The NPWT dressing should be left in place for 5 full days; others have reported securing skin grafts with NPWT for 3 days. Postoperatively the patient is able to move around without fear of disrupting the skin graft. When the NPWT dressing is ready to be removed after 5 days, it must be removed slowly, layer by layer, in order to avoid unintentionally harming the graft. Removal of the NPWT dressing can sometimes be painful and provoke feelings of anxiety for the patient and, therefore, premedication with analgesics in selected patients is reasonable. Staples from the edges of the wound are carefully removed. Routine postoperative care of the skin graft ensues.

Treatment of Pressure Ulcers and Chronic Wounds

Pressure ulcers result when sustained pressure hinders blood flow to vulnerable areas of the body, mainly the dependent portions: buttocks, hips, and heels. With localized ischemia, the structural integrity of the soft tissue begins to deteriorate leading to a progression from partial-thickness skin loss to full-thickness skin loss and then destruction of underlying subcutaneous fat, fascia, and bone. These wounds pose a particular challenge to the plastic surgeon, as healing is often impaired secondary to local factors (infection, pressure, and edema) and by systemic factors (diabetes mellitus, peripheral vascular disease, and malnutrition). Combined, these factors hinder the timely and orderly progression of wound healing, ultimately leading to a chronic wound.

Both studies and case reports have confirmed NPWT as a useful adjunct in the treatment of these complex and difficult wounds. Recently, Isago and colleagues showed that application of NPWT in 10 patients with pressure ulcers (five sacral, three trochanteric, and two ischial) penetrating the deep fascia and involving bone, resulted in a 55% reduction in wound area and 61% reduction in wound depth. Wounds were small enough to heal by secondary intention in three patients, while the other seven required operative intervention for definitive closure. Joseph et al. randomized 24 patients with 36 chronic wounds (79% pressure ulcers) to receive either saline wet-to-moist dressing changes or NPWT with the V.A.C. device. Wound volume at 6 weeks was reduced 78% in the NPWT group vs 30% in the standard saline dressing group ($P=0.038$). Histologically, 64% of wounds treated with NPWT exhibited granulation tissue, while 81% of the standard saline dressing group showed evidence of inflammation and fibrosis.

The etiology of pressure ulcers is multifactorial and therefore requires a multidisciplinary approach involving physicians from plastic surgery, orthopedic surgery, internal medicine, as well as nutritionists and nurses. Before the wound is evaluated, local and systemic factors inhibiting wound healing should be identified. The wound is then examined and classified according to the National Pressure Ulcer Advisory Panel as stage I, II, III, or IV pressure ulcer. NPWT is not an appropriate treatment modality for stages I and II pressure ulcers; however, patients with stages III and IV may be candidates. If the ulcer is amenable to closure with a surgical procedure and the patient is a good surgical candidate, then surgical intervention is recommended. If the wound can be closed surgically but the medical and nutritional status of the patient does not permit going to the operating room, NPWT can be initiated while patient health status is optimized. The wound should be debrided of necrotic tissue and exudate prior to initiation of NPWT. With dressing changes every 48 to 72 hours, the wound is re-evaluated at the end of 2 weeks and surgical intervention is pursued if the patient's condition has been optimized. Otherwise, NPWT is continued for an additional 2 weeks and the patient re-evaluated for surgery. For patients with stage III or IV pressure ulcers who will not be surgical candidates because of medical comorbidities, NPWT can be initiated as a primary treatment modality in an attempt to close the wound by secondary intention. This is providing that there are no patient characteristics that would make NPWT an unfavorable option, such as inability to adhere to a treatment protocol of consistently offloading pressure, intolerable pain with dressing changes, and bleeding disorders/platelet dysfunction. Wound characteristics that would make NPWT a poor option in nonsurgical candidates include inadequate vascular supply, desiccation and fibrosis, and inability to maintain a seal due to hyperhidrosis and incontinence.

Sternal Wound Infections

Approximately 650,000 open heart operations are performed every year and, although mediastinitis and sternal wound infections are rare, they harbor significant morbidity and mortality. Pooled data from retrospective studies has shown the prevalence of mediastinitis and deep sternal wound infections to be 1.2% with an average mortality of 20%. Plastic surgeons are often consulted to manage and treat these challenging wounds. There has been an evolution in the treatment of sternal wound infections since the introduction of the median sternotomy by Julian in 1957. In the past, aggressive debridement followed by wet-to-dry dressing changes and antibiotic irrigation with catheters was the norm. Once the wound had contracted sufficiently, definitive closure could be accomplished with flaps. Recently, the use of NPWT has been shown to be efficacious as a primary treatment modality, or a bridge to sternal wound reconstruction.

Initial case reports of using NPWT for sternal wounds showed it to be a promising technique to eliminate the need for wet-to-dry dressing changes and bridge the patient to definitive closure. Song and colleagues performed a retrospective review of 35 consecutive patients treated for sternal wound complications. After surgical debridement, 18 patients were treated with traditional wet-to-dry dressing changes twice a day while 17 patients were treated with NPWT using the V.A.C. device. In comparison to the traditional dressing group, the V.A.C. therapy group had a shorter interval between debridement and flap closure (6.2 days vs 8.5 days), significantly less mean dressing changes (3 vs 17; $P<0.05$), and required less soft tissue flaps per patient (0.9 vs 1.5; $P<0.05$). Two years later, Song reported the largest series of patients treated with NPWT for sternal wound complications. Of the 103 patients who had NPWT after surgical debridement, 68% eventually underwent open reduction internal fixation with and without flap closure while 32% had no definitive operation. Of the patients who had no definitive closure, 18 patients died secondary to their disease process, and 15 closed by secondary intention. The authors therefore concluded that NPWT could be used as a first-line treatment modality for sternal wound reconstruction in select patients, avoiding local flaps.[5]

As with all wounds, adequate debridement of necrotic soft tissue and bone is essential for successful outcomes with NPWT. In the operating room, all grossly infected soft tissue and osteomyelitis should be thoroughly debrided and irrigated. Once debrided, a NPWT foam dressing is placed into the wound with adequate contact with remaining bone and soft tissue structures in the wound. In some cases, extensive sternal bone debridement may leave exposed epicardium. This presents a particular problem as the porous black polyurethane foam can become adherent when placed directly over the heart. Some have reported that petrolatum-coated gauze or Xeroform gauze placed between the heart and the NPWT foam results in adherence of the gauze to the epicardium. Harlan reported good results using a thin (0.01 inch thick) sheet of silicone placed between the epicardium and the NPWT foam and reported no adherence problems. The NPWT dressing should be changed every 24 to 48 hours, depending on the original level of gross infection. Adequate analgesia should be administered with each dressing change. Disconnecting the suction tubing and instilling sterile saline through the tube and saturating the foam can loosen it and make dressing changes less painful. Duration of NPWT is based on clinical judgment. For large chest wounds in which NPWT is used as a bridge for flap reconstruction, there should be sufficient granulation tissue and no evidence of necrotic or infected tissue in the wound. For superficial wounds with localized areas of infection, placement of a NPWT dressing after debridement may be all that is needed for closure by secondary intention.

Complex Orthopedic Wounds

Orthopedic wounds with exposed bone, tendon, rods, or plates present particular reconstructive problems because these wounds are subject to malunion, infection, and can be devoid of soft tissue, especially after high-energy trauma. In the past, plastic surgeons often performed technically challenging and complex free flap coverage of these lower extremity wounds. NPWT has been tested in the realm of acute and chronic orthopedic wounds and has proven to be useful as a bridge to local soft tissue transfer, avoiding the need for free flaps, and in select patients, a primary treatment modality. In large open wounds, NPWT can be applied after debridement, converting the open wound to a contained closed wound. With removal of edema fluid and an increase in local blood flow, these large open wounds can be stabilized and enriched with healthy granulation tissue in anticipation for soft tissue transfer. Small areas of exposed bone, tendon, and orthopedic hardware can be treated with NPWT and then closed primarily or covered with a split-thickness skin graft, avoiding the need for complex reconstruction.

Recognizing the positive impact of NPWT in other types of wounds, DeFranzo and Argenta investigated the efficacy of using the V.A.C. device in orthopedic wounds.[6] Their series consisted of 75 patients, of which 49 had orthopedic wounds secondary to acute trauma and 26 had wounds due to postsurgical dehiscence, infection, or failed flap coverage. After adequate operative debridement, a V.A.C. dressing was applied and changed every 48 hours. Definitive wound closure was achieved in 95% of the patients, of which 77% were skin grafted, 16% closed primarily, and 6% had reconstruction with local musculocutaneous or fasciocutaneous flaps. No patients enrolled in the study required free flap coverage. Parrett and colleagues also noted a decreased trend in free flap coverage of open tibia-fibula fractures when they retrospectively evaluated 290 consecutive patients over a 12-year period. The decrease in free flap coverage coincided with the introduction of NPWT technology and thus free tissue transfer dropped from 42% to 11% over a 12-year period. Herscovici et al. utilized NPWT on 26 wounds with soft tissue defects that were the result of high-energy trauma and noted that 57% were closed primarily or with skin grafts avoiding free tissue transfer. While the use of NPWT does not eliminate the need for free tissue transfer, it allows less invasive and complex surgical techniques to be employed for adequate coverage.

In the management of complex orthopedic wounds, and all other types of wounds treated with NPWT, initial debridement in the operating room is paramount. All necrotic soft tissue and nonviable bone must be aggressively debrided for NPWT to be successful. Placing NPWT over large areas of exposed orthopedic hardware is advisable as a temporary measure to better control the wound and prepare it for muscle coverage or split-thickness skin graft if granulation tissue is sufficient. Smaller areas of exposed hardware can be treated with NPWT and soft tissue closed primarily after acceptable contraction of wound skin edges. Independent of wound size, any hardware that is covered with a NPWT dressing must be fixed in solid healthy bone. Plate and screw exposure time should be limited before initiation of NPWT, preferably less than 72 hours.

Dermal Substitutes

In addition to increasing the rate of skin graft take on irregularly contoured wounds, NPWT has been shown to improve incorporation of the dermal template Integra. Integra is a bilaminar sheet consisting of a collagen/glycosamine matrix and a protective silicone covering. In wounds requiring full-thickness coverage, an Integra sheet is placed onto the wound and secured at the wound edges, much like a skin graft. After 2 to 4 weeks, the dermal template becomes fully integrated into the wound bed and the protective silicone layer can be removed. An ultrathin (<0.0005 inch) split-thickness skin graft is then placed over the neodermis. Use of this technique can improve the cosmesis and function of a reconstruction and can avoid full-thickness skin graft donor sites. Placement of Integra with subsequent split-thickness skin grafting allows full-thickness coverage with only minimal cost to the patient, using a split-thickness skin graft donor site.

Preliminary studies with Integra reported excellent take rates of 95% to 100% although other researchers and clinicians were not able to reproduce such results, especially in difficult to graft areas. Use of NPWT as a bolster to secure Integra can decrease incorporation time to approximately 1 week with excellent take rates upward of 95%. Thus, a two-stage approach consisting of resurfacing with Integra followed by skin grafting can be reduced from 2 to 4 weeks to approximately 11 to 12 days. Furthermore, it is reported that NPWT can facilitate incorporation of Integra over bone and tendon, which can then be skin grafted, obviating the need for complex rotational or free flaps.

Miscellaneous Applications

In addition to the aforementioned applications, NPWT has been used in a variety of clinical situations by taking advantage of its ability to maintain a moist wound environment, increase local blood flow, and increase granulation tissue. There are many case reports in the literature about new and innovative applications of NPWT.

Full-thickness skin loss of the scalp with exposed bone due to burns, trauma, and oncologic resections present a reconstructive challenge to the plastic surgeon. These wounds were often treated in the past with multiple-staged procedures with local or free flaps. Recognizing the utility of NPWT for securing skin grafts, Molnar and colleagues reported four cases of successfully skin grafting exposed skull with NPWT in a single operation. The outer table of the skull was burred down to the diploic space and split-thickness skin grafts were secured at the periphery with suture. A V.A.C. device was placed over the skin graft with an intervening layer of Adaptic and removed in 4 days. Graft taken using this approach was 99% amongst the four patients. Thus, NPWT is a useful adjunct to treating wounds with exposed skull in a single operation, averting the need for more complex flap coverage.

Skin defects of the penile shaft that occur with burns, trauma, necrotizing soft tissue infections, or oncologic resections, while uncommon, are difficult reconstructive problems. Resurfacing the irregular contour of the male genitalia with split-thickness skin grafts using conventional bolsters is problematic because the skin grafts are subjected to considerable shear forces when the patient moves. Several case reports in the literature point to NPWT as an ideal method of securing a split-thickness skin graft for penile reconstruction. In one case report, NPWT was applied circumferentially to resurface the penile shaft in three patients with Fornier gangrene and one patient after oncologic resection. NPWT was maintained for 72 hours with reports of good graft take. Others have reported similar outcomes but described placing sterile wooden tongue blades longitudinally in the V.A.C. sponge to maintain the penis in a linear orientation.

● FUTURE DIRECTIONS

Although application of NPWT stimulates a fourfold increase in blood flow in open wound beds, its effect on closed wounds and intact skin have only recently been elucidated. Timmers et al. applied NPWT to the intact forearm skin of 10 volunteers and measured cutaneous blood flow with noninvasive laser Doppler probes in response to varying degrees of negative pressure. At 300 mm Hg of negative pressure, cutaneous blood flow increased 5.6-fold over baseline with the polyurethane foam dressing ($P=0.009$) and 2.9-fold over baseline with the polyvinyl alcohol foam dressing ($P=0.063$).[7] The clinical significance of these findings is currently unknown but the concept of increasing cutaneous blood flow with NPWT could be beneficial in preventing skin loss in myocutaneous flaps and other superficial wounds with diminished blood supply.

Wound instillation therapy is a recent development in the evolution of NPWT that allows the delivery of different therapeutic solutions to the wound bed, allowing the physician to manipulate the wound milieu as deemed appropriate. The V.A.C. Instill system was designed to improve wound healing in particularly difficult wounds with chronic or acute infections. It is composed of the standard V.A.C. dressing along with an additional piece of tubing to allow for infusion of solutions into the foam dressing. Subatmospheric pressure is stopped by the V.A.C. Instill machine, fluid delivered via the second tube by positive pressure, and then subatmospheric pressure resumed after a predetermined length of time. Solutions that can be instilled include topical cleansers, anesthetics, antibiotics, antiseptics, and antifungals. Research evaluating the efficacy of instillation NPWT with the aforementioned instillation therapies along with enzymatic and proteolytic agents is continuing. Clinical studies will help uncover which solutions are best suited for a particular clinical situation and what the ideal cycling of instillation and NPWT is. As wound healing research progresses on the molecular level, it is possible that instillation NPWT will someday permit the delivery of cytokines and growth factors, allowing the plastic surgeon fundamental control of the wound healing process.

The advent of NPWT over the past 10 years has triggered a paradigm shift in the way that plastic surgeons treat wounds. Although initially used for the treatment for chronic nonhealing wounds, the creativity of surgeons across all surgical subspecialties has brought about an ever-expanding list of NPWT applications. NPWT has thus modified the reconstructive ladder by allowing placement of skin grafts in previously inhospitable recipient beds, decreasing the time needed for dermal template incorporation, and avoiding the use of complex free tissue flaps. It is likely that in the ensuing years, the ingenuity of surgeons will expand the list of indications for NPWT. However, it is essential that large prospective trials be performed evaluating the effectiveness of these new applications as they emerge.

REFERENCES

1. Morykwas MJ, Argenta LC, Shelton-Brown EI, McGuirt W. Vacuum-assisted closure: a new method for wound control and treatment: animal studies and basic foundation. *Ann Plastic Surg.* 1997;38(6):553–562.

2. Saxena V, Hwang CW, Huang S, et al. Vacuum-assisted closure: microdeformations of wounds and cell proliferation. *Plast Reconstr Surg.* 2004;114(5):1086–1096; discussion 1097–1098.

3. Schneider AM, Morykwas MJ, Argenta LC. A new and reliable method of securing skin grafts to the difficult recipient bed. *Plast Reconstr Surg.* 1998;102(4):1195–1198.

4. Scherer LA, Shiver S, Chang M, et al. The vacuum assisted closure device: a method of securing skin grafts and improving graft survival. *Arch Surg.* 2002;137(8):930–933; discussion 933–934.

5. Agarwal JP, Ogilvie M, Wu LC, et al. Vacuum-assisted closure for sternal wounds: a first-line therapeutic management approach. *Plast Reconstr Surg.* 2005;116(4):1035–1040; discussion 1041–1043.

6. DeFranzo AJ, Argenta LC, Marks MW, et al. The use of vacuum-assisted closure therapy for the treatment of lower-extremity wounds with exposed bone. *Plast Reconstr Surg.* 2001;108(5):1184–1191.

7. Timmers MS, Le Cessie S, Banwell P, Jukema GN. The effects of varying degrees of pressure delivered by negative-pressure wound therapy on skin perfusion. *Ann Plastic Surg.* 2005;55(6):665–671.

chapter 6

Anesthesia for Plastic Surgery

Meredith S. Collins, MD / Sameer Bashey, MD / Laurence M. Hausman, MD

● INTRODUCTION

According to the American Board of Plastic Surgeons, more than 11 million cosmetic procedures are performed annually in the United States.[1] With the continued increase in the number and complexity of plastic surgical procedures performed each year, careful clinical decision making for the safe and effective administration of anesthesia for these patients is imperative. Many plastic surgical procedures are performed not only in hospitals and free-standing ambulatory surgery centers but also in the office-based setting. This shift in surgical venues has served to reinforce the need to consider all factors impinging on patient safety.

Furthermore, patients are discharged home soon after the completion of their surgical procedure without an overnight or extended stay.[2] It is for these reasons that the anesthetic technique is as vital as the procedure itself. The technique in which the various anesthetic agents are used may impact the quality and quantity of recovery time. Moreover, the anesthetic technique may contribute not only to patient safety, but also to the overall success of nearly every cosmetic procedure.

● PATIENT EVALUATION AND SELECTION

An anesthetic complication during cosmetic surgery is rare in part because of the rigorous screening process a patient undergoes prior to any elective procedure. The patient should be medically optimized before receiving any type of anesthetic ranging from local anesthesia alone through minimal, moderate, or deep sedation and general anesthesia. The American Society of Anesthesiologists (ASA) has defined these depths of sedation along an anesthetic continuum.[3] In preparing a patient for surgery, it is useful to use the ASA Physical Status (ASA PS) score to help determine his or her risk from anesthesia. Within this scoring system, a patient's physical condition is classified into one of six categories:[4]

ASA PS I—Completely healthy
ASA PS II—Mild controlled illness or disease with no interference to patient's daily life
ASA PS III—Illness or disease of more than two organ systems
ASA PS IV—Uncontrolled illness or disease, which is a constant threat to life
ASA PS V—Expected to die within 24 hours with or without surgery
ASA PS VI—Organ donor

Most would agree that a class I or II patient is a suitable candidate for an elective, outpatient procedure, while a class III patient would most likely need additional assessment before being considered suitable for outpatient procedures and may even be better operated upon in an inpatient setting. In addition to a thorough history and physical exam, laboratory screenings are often required. Commonly ordered tests include hemoglobin and hematocrit, electrolytes, blood glucose, urinalysis, an EKG, and a chest x-ray. All laboratory studies should be ordered based on the patient's comorbidities. Routine laboratory screenings should be considered a thing of the past. The only routine screening that should be considered is that any menstruating woman should have a negative urine pregnancy test within 24 hours of the procedure. An EKG for patients older than 50 years of age may also be a helpful screen. A specific preoperative visit with an anesthesiologist is not routinely required because the primary care physician should be able to furnish all of the above information.

PATIENT PREPARATION

All patients should be instructed to abstain from solid food 8 hours prior to surgery and clear liquids 2 hours before surgery. The history of this recommendation likely comes from a report published in 1946 by Mendelson, who noted a high incidence of pulmonary aspiration in obstetric patients undergoing general anesthesia. More recently, the American Society of Anesthesiologists Task Force on Preoperative Fasting published a concrete recommendation.[5] They require a minimum fasting period for clear liquids of 2 hours and a minimum of 6 hours for milk or a light meal. This fasting period should be extended to 8 hours for patients who have ingested any meal containing fried or fatty foods. Since it is easiest and safest to adopt a single, preoperative fasting rule prior to elective surgery, 8 hours is the most appropriate because it covers all foods and liquids. In most healthy adults undergoing elective cosmetic surgery the following morning, there is minimal inconvenience from an overnight fast.

In addition to urging a patient to get plenty of rest the night before the procedure, the surgeon may consider prescribing a medication that provides somnolence and a small degree of anxiolysis. It is common for patients to feel anxiety and apprehension before surgery. A preoperative benzodiazepine is a suitable choice because of its ability to provide both somnolence and anxiolysis. In fact, many plastic surgeons treat preoperative anxiety prophylactically. Specific benzodiazepines such as alprazolam (Xanax) or lorazepam (Ativan) can be prescribed to patients 1 to 3 days prior to the procedure in doses of 0.25 to 0.50 mg three times daily and 2 to 4 mg twice daily, respectively.[6] Additionally, clonidine, an alpha-2 agonist given in doses of 0.1 to 0.2 mg orally the morning of surgery, has been shown to be dually beneficial by decreasing blood pressure and hence decreasing operative blood loss, and providing a degree of sedation.[7] Informed consent for the surgical procedure should be obtained in advance of the surgery, and many anesthesiologists do not feel that a small dose of a preoperative anxiolytic will interfere with the patient's ability to be adequately consented for an anesthetic. Ultimately, the perioperative course of a calm, relaxed patient will more than likely be much smoother than that of an irritable and anxious patient.[8]

TECHNIQUE

Preparation

Upon the patient's arrival to the surgical suite on the morning of surgery, both the anesthesiologist and plastic surgeon should confirm that no interval changes have occurred in the patient's medical condition. If a significant change in the patient's health status occurs immediately prior to the operation, the entire procedure may need to be delayed. Ostensibly, the paramount concern is patient safety.

After assuring that all the required paperwork and consent forms are in order, the patient may be brought into the operating room. Prior to the induction of anesthesia, an intravenous line is inserted for administration of medications. Intraoperative monitoring is mandated by ASA and includes continuous EKG monitoring, noninvasive blood pressure measurements at least every 5 minutes, a pulse oximeter for measuring oxygen saturation, an end tidal carbon dioxide monitor, and the availability of a temperature probe. Compression boots should be placed on the calves prior to the induction of general anesthesia as it has been shown to prevent the incidence of deep vein thrombosis in patients.[9] A bladder catheter is generally advisable for cases longer than 4 hours to safely manage fluid resuscitation, or to keep the bladder decompressed for abdominal procedures. For procedures that go beyond the expected time, a catheter can be placed temporarily in the operating room or postoperative care unit.

Positioning the patient on the operating room table should take into consideration the risk of permanent nerve injury from continuous pressure. The patient's position must allow the anesthesiologist to have adequate access to the airway in case there is a problem with ventilation. If the patient's face is in the operative field and a problem arises, the airway should be addressed expeditiously at the temporary expense of sterility before continuing with the procedure. Finally, the length and placement of all cords of both electrical devices as well as patient monitoring systems must be taken into account. They should be arranged in a fashion that is safe and do not cause distractions during the surgery.

It is important to note that the temperature of the operating room is a vital consideration when planning a surgical procedure. Due to the vasodilatory nature and the direct inhibition of the hypothalamus caused by many anesthetic agents, all patients are susceptible to hypothermia or loss of body heat during surgery. This may result in platelet dysfunction and bleeding, enzymatic inactivity, cardiac dysfunction, or postoperative shivering.[10] Hence, the ambient temperature of the operating room should be kept at a temperature that minimizes body heat loss and a warming blanket be used for longer procedures as well as warming of all intravenous fluids. While hypothermia is probably not a likely occurrence in short cases, a warming blanket is relatively inexpensive compared with other adjunctive devices.

Both patients and surgeons are interested to know what role music has in the operating room. In fact, much has been documented about the use of music before, during, and after surgical procedures. A recent study found that patients undergoing a regional anesthetic who listened to music preoperatively and intraoperatively were calmer and less preoccupied with their surgical procedure than were their counterparts.[11] Furthermore, a similar study reported a measurable difference in heart and respiratory rates, as well as blood pressures between patients undergoing ambulatory surgery who listened to music compared with those who did not.[12] Additional studies sought to determine the effect of music not just on patients, but on the entire operating room, including the staff and the surgeons. Not surprisingly, the studies showed that listening to music allayed preoperative anxiety in patients and neither improved nor hindered the concentration of the surgeons performing the procedures.[13] Thus, while helping patients moderate their anxiety, the use of music in the operating suite seems to be simply a matter of personal preference and precedent.

Local Anesthesia

Most patients associate surgery with general anesthesia but other forms of anesthesia exist along the spectrum of choices for intraoperative sedation/analgesia and can be effectively used for such procedures. The choice of anesthetic technique for plastic surgery varies based on the discretion of the anesthesiologist, the surgeon, and the procedure. Local anesthesia is useful when the procedure is relatively short and is addressing a small, localized area of the body.

Local anesthetics are typically injected with a small-bore needle (23–25 gauge), in the skin and subcutaneous tissues in the area of the planned procedure. The two classes of local anesthetics that are commonly used, amino-esters (procaine, benzocaine) and amino-amides (lidocaine, bupivicaine), are weak bases that share a similar mechanism of action. Both types provide regional anesthesia by inhibiting nerve conduction via prevention of the depolarizing sodium influx into surrounding sensory nerves with varying duration of action, depending on the chosen anesthetic. Potency of local anesthetics is directly correlated to the lipid solubility of the medication.

Local anesthetics are often combined with epinephrine, which provides several benefits related to regional vasoconstriction, including improved hemostasis in the area of infiltration, and increased duration of action of the anesthetic medication. The vasoconstriction effects of epinephrine are apparent several minutes after injection.[14]

Selection of a local anesthetic is based on the pharmacokinetics and pharmacodynamics of each drug as well as the surgical needs. A combination of local anesthetics is usually chosen to ensure optimal anesthetic timing for the procedure. Also, by combining local anesthetics, one can use less of each drug and limit the possibility of toxicity. Use of a fast-acting anesthetic with a short duration of action, such as lidocaine (onset 1–2 min, duration 1–4 h), with a slower-acting agent with an extended duration, such as bupivicaine (onset 5 min, duration 2–8 h), is a common practice.[12] Additionally, sodium bicarbonate may be added to the solution to both hasten the onset of action of the local anesthetic and decrease the pain associated with the infiltration of the medication into the tissues.[15]

Local anesthetics are not without risk and should be dosed appropriately according to the weight of the patient. The maximum dose of lidocaine is 5 mg/kg patient weight, and 7 mg/kg patient weight when combined with epinephrine. Allergy to local anesthetics is rare, and is more common with the ester-type anesthetics. Practitioners should be aware of the systemic toxicities associated with local anesthetics and how to treat them, should these complications

arise. A common cause of local anesthetic toxicity is inadvertent intravascular injection of the medication. Signs of toxicity may be limited to relatively harmless symptoms, including circumoral numbness, restlessness, and tinnitus, but may progress to more serious conditions, including seizures, hypotension, myotonia, respiratory failure, cardiac arrhythmias, myocardial depression, and coma. Treatment of these symptoms includes benzodiazepines for control of seizures, endotracheal intubation for respiratory failure, epinephrine with calcium channel blocking agents for cardiac arrhythmias, or in cases involving bupivicaine, a 20% Intralipid infusion for cardiovascular collapse.[13] Further up to date information and directions for the use of Intralipid can always be found on the website www.LipidRescue.squarespace.com.[14]

Local anesthetics are useful for providing regional anesthesia, and may prove to be especially helpful in the setting of a small office-based procedure. Eliminating the need for sedation or general anesthesia has both safety and economic benefits. This technique puts the patient at less risk from sedation, reduces the cost of the procedure, and reduces the time required to complete the surgery. However, all practitioners should be cautious when using these medications and bear in mind the potentially dangerous side effects that can occur with both inadvertent intravascular injections or exceeding the therapeutic dosages.

Monitored Anesthetic Care

The technique of monitored anesthesia care (MAC) uses a combination of local anesthesia, intravenous analgesia, and sedative medications. Although MAC does not correlate with any specific depth of anesthesia (rather it refers to sedation administered by a professional anesthesia practitioner), it usually refers to a depth of sedation with a "minimally depressed level of consciousness that retains the patient's ability to maintain an airway independently and continuously and to respond to physical stimuli and verbal commands."[16,17] This level of sedation will provide for a patient that is sedated and will not have any keen sense of environmental awareness. However, unlike in general anesthesia where unconsciousness is induced and spontaneous respiration is depressed, patients will continue to breathe on their own.

Monitored anesthetic care has been shown to be effective and safe in large study populations.[18-20] Typically, a combination of two or more medication types is used to achieve the desired level of sedation and analgesia. Commonly used agents include rapid acting drugs such as fentanyl, midazolam, and propofol.[21,22]

As previously mentioned, anesthetic depth is a continuum and thus the administration of high dosages of sedative medications will cause the patient to ultimately lose protective airways reflexes and move into a state of general anesthesia. In some instances, this will require securing the airway, and in others it may require assistance in maintaining a patent airway while decreasing the dose of the anesthetic agents to allow the patient to regain spontaneous respiration. For this reason, monitored anesthesia care has all of the same perioperative requirements as general anesthesia. Patients should be screened preoperatively, vigilantly monitored intraoperatively according to ASA standards, and meet the same discharge criteria. Emergence from monitored anesthesia care will be discussed below.

General Anesthesia

"General anesthesia is defined as a controlled state of unconsciousness accompanied by a loss of protective airway reflexes [in addition to] the inability to maintain a patent airway the patient will be unresponsive to verbal commands."[23] With this type of anesthesia, the patient may require respiratory or cardiovascular support. The insertion of an endotracheal tube after induction will allow control of ventilation. Throughout the surgical procedure, the patient is closely monitored to note any changes in physiologic status (eg, oxygen saturation, blood pressure, heart rate and rhythm, breathing rate and rhythm, and temperature). General anesthesia can be divided into three phases: induction (when the patient loses consciousness), maintenance (when unconsciousness is maintained during the procedure), and emergence (when the patient regains consciousness).

Induction

Understandably, a smooth induction with minimal hypertension and tachycardia is desirable for cosmetic anesthesia. Prior to induction, the anesthesiologist should consider a number of premedications. Midazolam, a short-acting benzodiazepine, can produce sedative-hypnotic effects or can even induce anesthesia at very high doses. It is also characterized by its ability to cause amnesia, hypnosis, and the relaxation of muscles with relative celerity. In fact, the onset of sedation following intravenous administration of midazolam is usually within 1 to 3 minutes, though there is some degree of patient variability. Intravenous midazolam will depress the ventilatory response to carbon dioxide stimulation, which may already be impaired in patients with chronic obstructive pulmonary disease. In young, healthy patients, intravenous sedation with midazolam alone in small doses does not appear to adversely affect respiration. As far as cardiac sensitivity is concerned, the use of midazolam is associated with decreases in mean arterial pressure, cardiac output, stroke volume, and systemic vascular resistance. Consequently, *midazolam is relatively contraindicated in patients with acute pulmonary insufficiency or severe chronic obstructive pulmonary disease.* Nevertheless, studies have reported that the administration of certain barbiturate and benzodiazepine drugs by an anesthesiologist preoperatively may "reduce the overall anesthetic requirements [of the procedure itself], thereby improving recovery time [later]."[24]

Postoperative nausea and vomiting (PONV) is a major concern with any anesthetic procedure. Preoperative antiemetics should be used to prevent PONV following the use of numerous anesthetic agents, including narcotics and nitrous oxide. Many anesthesiologist avoid narcotics altogether to minimize the incidence of PONV. Alternative analgesics include local anesthetics, ketamine, and ketorolac. Others still advocate the use of narcotics for painful procedures and utilize a variety of available antiemetics to minimize PONV. Granisetron (0.2–1 mg IV) and ondansetron (1–4 mg IV) are serotonin antagonists that reduce the autonomic neuro-activity in the vomiting center of the brain. Dexamethasone (4–10 mg IV), a steroid, and scopolamine, a tropane alkaloid, both may be used to resolve dizziness and nausea. Fosaprepitant dimeglumine, a newer antiemetic, is increasingly being used.[25,26] Multimodal therapy using several antiemetics is advisable for patients with a high risk for PONV. These patients would include young women, nonsmokers, those with a history of PONV or car sickness, and patients undergoing breast, gynecologic, or laparoscopic surgery.[27]

Various drugs can be used to induce general anesthesia. One commonly used induction agent is propofol, a short-acting intravenous drug used in adult and pediatric patients. It may also be used during the procedure for the maintenance of anesthesia. Side effects include hypotension and apnea following induction, as well as pain on injection, which can be ameliorated by pretreatment with intravenous lidocaine.[28] Propofol is often used for cosmetic procedures because it is associated with reduced PONV and can even be used as an antiemetic. Thiopental is another induction agent. Thiopental is a barbiturate that affects fine motor skills and is notorious for producing a heavy "hangover" effect and significant PONV.[29] Midazolam and ketamine can also be used for induction, although they are associated with a longer recovery time postoperatively. Ketamine, a phencyclidine derivative, is an anesthetic agent approved for human and veterinary use, whose popularity in the outpatient arena has increased over the past several years.[30] Its effects include analgesia and sedation with minimal to no respiratory depression. However, hallucinations, hypertension, increased intracranial pressure and salivation have limited its appeal. It has been used successfully with propofol and midazolam for cosmetic procedures since it may be used without the need for endotracheal intubation, supplemental oxygen, or narcotics.[31]

Airway Protection

General anesthesia requires control of the patient's airway. The drugs used to induce unconsciousness are often associated with muscle weakness, and the loss of many autonomic reflexes, including the ventilatory response to carbon dioxide and hypoxia.[32] Thus, patients under general anesthesia often require mechanical ventilation. Adequate airway control may be achieved either with a traditional endotracheal tube (ETT) that passes beyond the vocal cords or with a laryngeal mask airway (LMA) that is inflated above the vocal cords at the laryngeal aperture. As with all considerations in cosmetic surgery, the means of securing the airway depends on the procedure being performed.

For procedures that do not involve frequent head turning, the LMA provides a safe alternative to the ETT since it does not risk vocal cord injury and has less of an incidence of postoperative laryngeal irritation and "bucking on the tube."[33] However, since the LMA does not occlude the trachea, patients at high risk for aspiration should still use a traditional ETT.

The device itself may be secured to the face in various ways. For procedures not involving the face, adhesive tape is most often used to secure the tube to the maxilla. For facial procedures, the tube may be prepped into the field or covered with sterile plastic or stockinet to maintain sterility. Of paramount importance is that the surgeon and anesthesiologist weigh surgical exposure versus sterility and always respect the need for emergent visualization of the numerous connections within the patient's anesthetic breathing circuit should problems with ventilation arise. Because surgical preparation of the face often dislodges the tape holding the tube, it may be advisable to place a suture around the tube and then around the teeth in the midline. Of course, this is impractical in patients with dental restoration, such as a bridge or an implant.

Following the induction of general anesthesia, the anesthesiologist must vigilantly monitor changes in the patient's cardiovascular status, including alterations in oxygen saturation, blood pressure, heart rate and rhythm, respiratory rate, and temperature, while continuously administrating anesthetics for the duration of the operation. To accomplish this, the anesthesiologist carefully administers a combination of drugs while closely assuring that the patient's heart rate and blood pressure are well controlled.

A constant stable blood pressure in the low-normal range for the duration of the cosmetic procedure is desirable to minimize blood loss and bleeding into the tissues that contributes to prolonged postoperative ecchymosis and edema. More severe consequences of prolonged hypertension include cardio-pulmonary-hepatic congestion or anasarca, and possibly even heart or renal failure. If the blood pressure drops too low, the patient will not adequately perfuse vital organs and can develop circulatory collapse.

The choice of drugs used to maintain anesthesia is also important to minimize PONV and allow for a rapid recovery process. Nitrous oxide has been historically used as an inhalational agent, in conjunction with other volatile or intravenous anesthetics, to maintain anesthesia. Nitrous oxide reduces the need for higher concentrations of these other volatile inhalational agents. It is, however, associated with PONV and should be limited to concentrations under 50%.[34]

Isoflurane is one of a number of volatile inhalation agents commonly used for maintenance of anesthesia. Desflurane is shorter-acting member of this class of drugs and may be more suitable for plastic and ambulatory surgery. Its quick recovery time results from a higher vapor pressure. However, desflurane often causes postoperative respiratory irritation and coughing largely due to its pungent smell. Sevoflurane is better tolerated than desflurane since it lacks a characteristic odor. As a result of the lower solubility of these newer volatile agents, cognitive functions return to baseline more rapidly when compared with inhaled isoflurane.

Continuous intravenous anesthetics are commonly employed in cosmetic surgery. Propofol, remifentanil, dexmedetomidine, and ketamine are among the most commonly used. Propofol was discussed earlier as a drug of choice for induction, but can also be used as a continuous infusion (75–150 μg/kg/min) to maintain anesthesia. Remifentanil may be used just prior to induction to suppress the autonomic responses to intubation and during maintenance to suppress other autonomic responses to surgical stimuli. Because it is also an ultra short-acting narcotic, it is ideal for the end of the procedure since it is a potent cough suppressant. However, as with all narcotics, it can cause PONV.[35] It must also be appreciated that since remifentanil is so short acting, it will not produce any significant postoperative analgesia. Last, ketamine, like propofol, can be used for both induction and maintenance, though it is often associated with an increase in blood pressure and salivation, as well as bad hallucinations. The dysphoria associated with ketamine can be ameliorated with the concomitant use of midazolam and propofol. Fortunately, ketamine is not associated with PONV.

Emergence

Emergence should be a well-planned event. The ideal emergence from anesthesia following cosmetic surgery would not be associated with an increase in blood pressure or heart rate, there would be no "bucking on the tube" from irritation of the trachea by the endotracheal tube, and no respiratory complications.[36] While the concentration of inhalational and intravenous anesthetics are lowered to allow the patient to regain consciousness, additional medications are administered to restore muscle strength to allow the patient to breathe spontaneously and to permit extubation. Maneuvers that are particularly stimulating, such as nasogastric decompression or suctioning, are done while the patient is still deeply sedated to prevent hypertension. Gagging at the conclusion of any procedure is undesirable because it raises blood pressure and may trigger subcutaneous bleeding. The prevention of nausea and vomiting is important to minimize fluctuations in blood pressure. Patients should be reminded as they emerge from anesthesia that they may have blurred vision due to the ointment and should be prevented from attempting to rub their eyes.

General Anesthesia Compared with Monitored Anesthesia Care

Each of the aforementioned anesthetic techniques has both advantages and disadvantages, thus the selection of one method over the other truly depends on the nature of the surgical procedure and the comfort level of the anesthesiologist and surgeon alike.

For shorter, less complicated procedures, either method of general or monitored care may be used. For difficult and time-consuming procedures, general anesthesia is often more appropriate. In the monitored anesthesia care model, the patient drifts in and out of consciousness during the procedure and may become more anxious, irritable, and emotional than patients undergoing general anesthesia.[37] PONV, however, may be reduced.

It should be noted that the administration of both types of anesthesia in an ambulatory setting are safe. Largely due to the meticulous preoperative screening and technological advancements in anesthesia, morbidity and mortality resulting from outpatient anesthesia are rare.[38] A recent study reported no significant differences between either form of anesthetic technique employed as it relates to patient recovery time, sensitivity to pain, and safety.[39] A joint study conducted by Yale University and the State University of New York at Stony Brook evaluated the safety of outpatient anesthesia for plastic surgery procedures on the face. The study reported no deaths or severe complications among the 1200 cases retrospectively reviewed.[40]

Patients undergoing cosmetic surgery are generally well informed regarding the nature of the procedure and the reputation of their surgeon, but overlook the importance of the anesthetic technique needed to effectively perform the procedure. A successful cosmetic procedure involves both a skilled plastic surgeon and a knowledgeable anesthesiologist. Cosmetic surgeons realize the importance of this and often choose to work with one or more select anesthesiologists with whom they have developed a rapport and a tacit understanding of what is needed before, during, and after surgery.

COMPLICATIONS

After the induction of general anesthesia, every effort should be made to protect the patient's eyes and cornea specifically from inadvertent injury. Closed eyes must always remain closed during surgery, especially procedures on the face. With the various surgical instruments being passed between the nurse and surgeon, accidents may occur. To minimize the risk of corneal abrasion, a gentle ophthalmologic lubricant, with or without antibiotic placed in the lower fornix of each eye at the start of the procedure, may be helpful. Sterile tapes are also recommended to keep the eyelids closed if possible.[41] Ointment is not easily washed from the eye, so that unlike tape that may come loose during the procedure, ointment tends to remain for the duration.

Episodes of prolonged, excessive hypertension under anesthesia can cause congestion in the heart, lungs, and liver, leading to anasarca and possibly organ failure. Conversely, if the blood pressure drops too low, the patient will not adequately perfuse vital organs and can develop circulatory collapse. Keeping the blood pressure constant at a level that ensures adequate perfusion without the aforementioned complications cannot be overemphasized.

As noted, PONV is a major concern with any anesthetic procedure. Strategies to prevent or minimize PONV include the use of preoperative antiemetics and the avoidance of narcotics in lieu of alternative analgesics such as local anesthetics and ketorolac. Available antiemetics include the serotonin antagonists granisetron and ondansetron, the steroid dexamethasone (4–10 mg IV), the alkaloid scopolamine, and fosaprepitant, as well as combination therapy.

OUTCOMES

Anesthetic care does not end once the endotracheal tube has been removed and the patient is restored to consciousness. Patients must be closely monitored postoperatively for signs and symptoms of hypoxia, hypertension, pain, PONV, and even unconsciousness. This is an important part of the continuum of anesthesia care. A patient may be discharged once an assessment of home readiness test is conducted.[38] In this evaluation, patients are closely observed to ensure that their vital signs are stable, to make sure they are environmentally aware, and to make sure they can walk without falling or becoming excessively dizzy. Patients are also evaluated for pain, PONV, and bleeding at the surgical site. Most delays in discharge are due to pain, PONV, hypotension, and dizziness upon ambulating.[38] All patients require analgesia postoperatively, and some may require stronger medications than acetaminophen or NSAID-type drugs as part of their postoperative regimen.

REFERENCES

1. 2000/2005/2006 National Plastic Surgery Statistics. American Society of Plastic Surgeons. http://www.plasticsurgery.org.

2. Zukowski ML, Ash K, Klink B, et al. Breast Reduction under intravenous sedation: A review of 50 cases. *Plast Reconstr Surg.* 1997;99(1):256.

3. American Society of Anesthesiologists. Continuum of Depth of Sedation: Definition of General Anesthesia and Levels of Sedation/Analgesia. 21 Oct. 2009. http://www.asahq.org/For-Members/Standards-Guidelines-and-Statements.aspx; 2009.

4. ASA Physical Status Classification System. American Society of Anesthesiologists. http://www.asahq.org/clinical/physicalstatus.htm.

5. Practice guidelines for preoperative fasting and the use of pharmacologic agents to reduce the risk of pulmonary aspiration: application to healthy patients undergoing elective procedures: a report by the American Society of Anesthesiologist Task Force on Preoperative Fasting. *Anesthesiology.* 1999;90(3):896.

6. Rankin MK, Borah G. Anxiety disorders in plastic surgery. *Plast Reconstr Surg.* 2004;113(7):2199.

7. Taittonen M, Kirvelä O, Aantaa R, Kanto J. Cardiovascular and metabolic responses to clonidine and midazolam premedication. http://eresources.library.mssm.edu:2060/pubmed/9088819. *Eur J Anaesthesiol.* 1997;14(2):190–196.

8. Pearson S, Maddern GJ, Fitridge R. The role of pre-operative state-anxiety in the determination of intra-operative neuroendocrine responses and recovery. http://eresources.library.mssm.edu:2060/pubmed/15969856. *Br J Health Psychol.* 2005;10(Pt 2):299–310.

9. Okuda Y, Kitajima T, Egawa H, et al. A combination of heparin and an intermittent pneumatic compression device may be more effective to prevent deep-vein thrombosis in the lower extremities after laparoscopic cholecystectomy. *Surg Endosc.* 2002;5:781.

10. Rundgren M, Engström M. A thromboelastometric evaluation of the effects of hypothermia on the coagulation system. *Anesth Analg.* 2008;107(5):1465.

11. Eisenman A, Cohen B. Music therapy for patients undergoing regional anesthesia. *AORN J.* 1995;62(6):947.

12. Augustin P, Hains AA. Effect of music on ambulatory surgery patients' preoperative anxiety. *AORN J.* 1996;63(4): 750,753–758.

13. Sármány J, Kálmán R, Staud D, Salacz G. Role of the music in the operating theatre." *Orv Hetil.* 2006;147(20):931.

14. Liu SS, Lin Y. Local anesthetics. In: Barash PG, Cullen BF, Stoelting RK, et al., eds. *Clinical Anesthesia.* Philadelphia, PA: Lippincott Williams & Wilkins; 2009:541.

15. Palmon SC, Lloyd AT, Kirsch JR. The effect of needle gauge and lidocaine pH on pain during intradermal injection. *Anesth Analg.* 1998;86(2):379.

16. Stevens MH, White PF. Monitored anesthesia care. In: Miller RD, ed. *Miller's Anesthesia.* 4th ed. Philadelphia, PA: Churchill Livingstone; 1994:1465–1480 [Chapter 44].

17. Task Force on Sedation and Analgesia by Non-Anesthesiologists. Practice guidelines for sedation and analgesia by non-anesthesiologists: An updated report by the American Society of Anesthesiologists Task Force of Sedation and Analgesia by Non-Anesthesiologists. *Anesthesiology.* 2002;4:1004.

18. Bitar G, Mullis W, Jacobs W, et al. Safety and efficacy of office based surgery with monitored anesthesia care/sedation in 4778 consecutive plastic surgery procedures. *Plast Reconstr Surg.* 2003;111:150.

19. Kryger ZB, Fine NA, Mustoe TA, et al. The outcome of abdominoplasty performed under conscious sedation: six-year experience in 153 consecutive cases. *Plast Reconstr Surg.* 2004;113:1807.

20. Marcus JR, Tyrone JW, Few JW, et al. Optimization of conscious sedation in plastic surgery. *Plast Reconstr Surg.* 1999;104(5):1338.

21. Cinella G, Meola S, Portincasa A, et al. Sedation analgesia during office-based plastic surgery procedures: comparison of two opioid regimens. *Plast Reconstr Surg.* 2007; 119(7):2263.

22. Yoon HD, Yoon ES, Dhang ES, et al. Low-dose propofol infusion for sedation during local anesthesia. *Plast Reconstr Surg.* 2002;109:956.

23. Nique TA. Ambulatory office general anesthesia. In: Nique TA, Tu HK, eds. *Anesthesia for Facial Plastic Surgery.* New York: Thieme Medical Publishers; 1993.

24. Reves JG, Glass PSA, Lubarsky DA. Nonbarbiturate intravenous anesthetics. In: Miller RD, ed. *Miller's Anesthesia.* 4th ed. Philadelphia, PA: Churchill Livingstone; 1994: 247–290 [Chapter 11].

25. Kolodzie K, Apfel CC. Nausea and vomiting after office-based anesthesia. *Curr Opin Anaesthesiol.* 2009;22(4): 532.

26. Gray H. Aprepitant for postoperative nausea and vomiting. *Anaesth Intensive Care.* 2009;37(1):135.

27. Gan, TJ Meyer TA, Apfel CC, et al. Society for Ambulatory Anesthesia guidelines for the management of postoperative nausea and vomiting. *Anesth Analg.* 2007;105(6):1615.

28. Piper SN, Röhm KD, Papsdorf M, et al. Dolasetron reduces pain on injection of propofol [German]. *Anasthesiol Intensivmed Notfallmed Schmerzther.* 2002;37(9):528.

29. Fragen RJ, Avram MJ. Barbiturates. In: Miller RD, ed. *Miller's Anesthesia.* 4th ed. Philadelphia, PA: Churchill Livingstone; 1994:229–246 [Chapter 10].

30. Friedberg BL. Facial laser resurfacing with the propofol-ketamine technique: room air, spontaneous ventilation (RASV) anesthesia. *Dermatol Surg.* 1999;25(7):569.

31. Friedberg BK. Propofol-ketamine technique: dissociative anesthesia for office surgery (a five year review of 1,264 cases). *Aesthetic Plast Surg.* 1999;23:70.

32. Knill RL, Clement JL. Variable effects of anesthetics on the ventilatory response to hypoxia in man. *Can Anaesth Soc J.* 1982;29:93.

33. Cork, RC, Depa MC, Standen JR. Prospective comparison of use of the laryngeal mask airway an endotracheal tube during ambulatory anesthesia. *Anesth Analg.* 1994;79:719.

34. Moffitt EA, Sethna DH, Gary RJ, et al. Nitrous oxide added to halothane reduces coronary flow and myocardial oxygen consumption in patients with coronary disease. *Can Anaesth Soc J.* 1983;30:5.

35. Egan TD, Lemmens HJ, Fiset P, et al. The pharmacokinetics of the new short-acting opiod remifentanil (G197084B) in healthy adult male volunteers. *Anesthesiology.* 1993; 79(5):881.

36. Koga K, Asai T, Vaughan RS, Latto IP. Respiratory complications associated with tracheal extubation. Timing of tracheal extubation and use of the laryngeal mask airway during emergence from anesthesia. *Anaesthesia.* 1998; 53(6):540.

37. Boskovski, N. Regional anesthesia. In: Nique TA, Tu HK, eds. *Anesthesia for Facial Plastic Surgery.* New York: Thieme Medical Publishers; 1993.

38. Ostman PL, White PF. Outpatient anesthesia. In: Miller RD, ed. *Miller's Anesthesia.* 4th ed. Philadelphia, PA: Churchill Livingstone; 1994:2213–2246 [Chapter 69].

39. Hasen KV, Samartzis D, Casas LA, Mustoe TA. An outcome study comparing intravenous sedation with midazolam/fentanyl (conscious sedation) versus propofol infusion (deep sedation) for aesthetic surgery. *Plast Reconstr Surg.* 2003;112(6):1683.

40. Gordon NA, Koch ME. Duration of anesthesia as an indicator of morbidity and mortality in office-based facial plastic surgery. *Arch Facial Plast Surg.* 2006;8:47

41. Orlin SE, Kurata FK, Krupin T, et al. Ocular lubricants and corneal injury during anesthesia. *Anesth Analg.* 1989; 3:384.

chapter 7

Malignant Skin Lesions

Wesley N. Sivak, MD, PhD / *Roee E. Rubinstein, MD* / *Howard D. Edington, MD, MBA*

● PATIENT EVALUATION AND SELECTION

The initial evaluation of any cutaneous lesion must include an assessment of a patient's risk factors for malignancy. Lifetime sun exposure should be estimated through a detailed patient history. Determination of a patient's Fitzpatrick skin type (Table 7-1) is a useful method of stratifying patients based on their sunburn and tanning history, and patients with type I and II skin are at significantly higher risk of developing cutaneous malignancies.[1] Likewise, a personal or family history of skin cancer dramatically increases an individual's risk, and should be considered and documented.[2]

Once an individual's personal and family histories have been considered, the natural history of any lesion in question should be explored in further detail. The American Cancer Society's "ABCD" criteria are useful for assessing potential malignancies (*a*symetry, *b*order irregularity, *c*olor variegation, *d*iameter >6 mm). Any change in size, shape, or color of a previously stable pigmented lesion warrants close observation or preferably biopsy. New pigmented lesions appearing in older patients are highly suspicious, as most benign acquired nevi have developed by age 40 years. Bleeding, scaling, and ulceration are concerning signs often associated with invasion. The clinical diagnosis is confirmed with appropriate biopsy. If the diagnosis of melanoma is entertained, the biopsy must be full thickness to allow accurate measurement of the thickness of the primary (Breslow depth in mm) which has prognostic importance and directs appropriate treatment. An incisional or excisional biopsy is appropriate, whereas a shave biopsy is to be avoided.

Melanoma

Melanoma is currently the sixth most frequently diagnosed cancer in the United States. Although the National Cancer Institute recognizes nonmelanoma skin cancer as the most common cancer in the United States the overall mortality from melanoma is three times higher than from all other cutaneous malignancies combined.[3] Melanoma tends to occur on body surfaces that receive at least occasional sun exposure. Exposures and behaviors in childhood and early adulthood are particularly critical in determining lifelong risk of melanoma. The disease mostly affects Caucasians, with rates substantially lower in Asian and Hispanic populations; melanoma is rare among black persons.

There is strong evidence for the importance of intense, intermittent sun exposure vs cumulative exposure in the etiology of melanoma.[4] The size, type, and number of nevomelanocytic nevi on the skin have been consistently associated with melanoma risk to a greater degree than any direct measure of sun exposure.[5] Atypical nevi are thought to be both markers of elevated risk and melanoma precursors; however, as many as half of all melanomas arise in individuals who are unaffected by these lesions. A small percentage (3%–5%) of lesions appear to occur in individuals with inherited risk.[6] Primary cutaneous melanomas have been classified into four subtypes based on growth pattern with each having distinct phenotypic and histological features. While these features define and distinguish the melanoma subtypes, the key unifying element is that tumor thickness is an important prognostic factor for all melanomas. This again underscores the importance of an early diagnosis

Superficial Spreading Melanoma (SSM). The most common type of cutaneous melanoma, accounting for 70% of all cases diagnosed, most commonly occurs on the legs and back in women, and on the upper back in men (though it can occur in any location) . The peak incidence of SSM is in the fourth and fifth decades, earlier than other melanoma subtypes. SSM may initially present as a deeply pigmented asymmetric macule or slightly raised plaque, and may appear as a new lesion or as a focal darkening

TABLE 7-1. Fitzpatrick's Classification of Sun-reactive Skin Types

Skin Type	Skin Color	Characteristics
I	White; very fair; red or blond hair; blue eyes; freckles	Always burns, never tans
II	White; fair; red or blond hair; blue, hazel, or green eyes	Usually burns, tans with difficulty
III	Cream white; fair with any eye or hair color; very common	Sometimes burns, gradually tans
IV	Brown; typical Mediterranean Caucasian skin	Rarely burns, tans with ease
V	Dark brown; Middle Eastern skin types	Rarely burns, tans easily
VI	Black	Never burns, tans easily

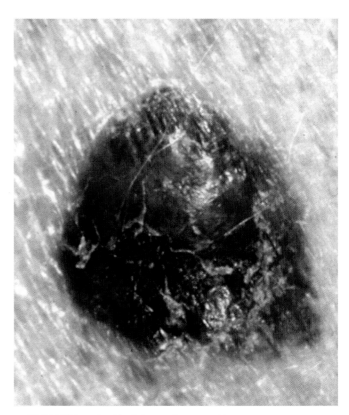

● FIGURE 7-2. Nodular melanoma: Homogenous pigmentation and nodular appearance.

within an existing nevus (Figure 7-1). SSM is the variant of melanoma most likely to arise within or in continuity with a preexisting melanocytic nevus. During the radial growth phase, which may last months to years, it usually develops asymmetry and border irregularities that may raise suspicion in the patient or physician. Color variegation is characteristic of SSM, and hypopigmented areas of regression may be evident. If left undetected or untreated, the lesion transitions into a vertical growth phase, heralded by papular or nodular changes within the lesion, and the melanoma can become deeply invasive. It is often at this stage that the patient may bring the lesion to the attention of the physician. Biopsy is imperative.

Nodular Melanoma (NM). The second most common form of melanoma, with a frequency of 15% to 30% of all

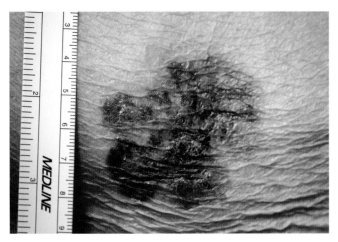

● FIGURE 7-1. Superficial spreading melanoma: Elements of the ABCD criteria are evident. Initial management requires excisional or incisional biopsy.

cases diagnosed, favors individuals in their fifth and sixth decades, and may arise within existing nevi or de novo. NM exhibits rapid expansion and progression without an identifiable radial growth phase, and may be deeply invasive at the time of initial diagnosis. Clinically, NM presents as an enlarging papule, nodule, or pedunculated lesion, often with a history of bleeding, and may measure 1 to 2 cm in diameter. Distinct from other types of melanoma, NM often lacks color variegation, appearing typically as a uniform dark blue-black, steel gray, blue-red, or amelanotic nodule, with or without superficial ulceration (Figure 7-2). The amelanotic melanoma may appear clinically innocuous and is readily misdiagnosed or overlooked. The differential diagnosis includes hemangioma, pyogenic granuloma, blue nevus, and pigmented basal cell carcinoma. Nodular melanomas are highly aggressive and the diagnosis must be considered in any rapidly growing cutaneous nodule.

Lentigo Maligna Melanoma (LMM). Lentigo maligna melanoma rises from an in situ (intraepidermal) precursor (Figure 7-3A,B). In situ melanomas have not yet invaded the basement membrane (Figure 7-3B); have a very low metastatic potential; and should be excised with 5 mm margins. Lentigo maligna (LM) comprises 4% to 10% of all melanomas. LM presents as a macule or patch with variegated brown-black pigmentation in a sun-exposed area (Figure 7-4) The differential diagnosis includes solar lentigo and seborrheic keratosis, as well as pigmented actinic keratosis. LM lesions undergo a slow, progressive

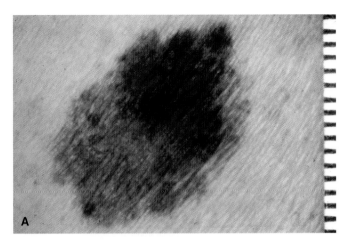
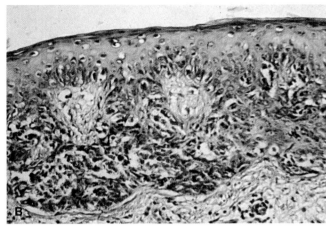

● FIGURE 7-3. (A) In situ melanoma: Clinical appearance. (B) In situ melanoma: Pathology confirms intraepithelial location without invasion.

enlargement during a prolonged radial growth phase, often over many years, but can progress rapidly once the vertical growth phase is initiated. Vertical growth into the dermis and development of invasive LMM are often heralded by intralesional dark papules and/or indurated nodules (Figure 7-4). The margins of LM and LMM often extend well beyond the clinical area of pigmentation, and surrounding skin is often actinically damaged, making histologic evaluation difficult. LMM, when compared to other melanoma types, has the lowest propensity for metastasis and the best prognosis. Despite this, the lifetime risk of invasive melanomatous change is estimated at 30% to 50% and surgical excision of LM is recommended.[7]

Acral Lentiginous Melanoma (ALM). Acral lentiginous melanoma is relatively rare, accounting for 2% to 8% of melanomas diagnosed. ALM is the most common form of melanoma in dark-skinned individuals, representing 70% of melanomas in blacks and up to 46% in Asians.

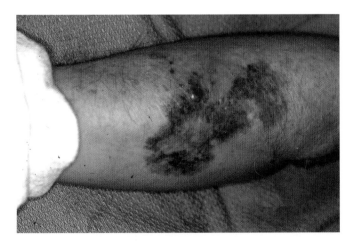

● FIGURE 7-4. Lentigo maligna melanoma: This lesion involves an extremity. The bulk of this lesion is in situ disease. Note the nodular component representing invasive changes and note also depigmented areas of regression.

Its incidence peaks in the seventh decade of life, and it is usually diagnosed late due to delayed presentation. These lesions involve the plantar or palmar skin and may occur in the subungual location. They are often misdiagnosed as fungal infections and biopsy is frequently delayed for up to a year at which point the disease is often in an advanced stage with no realistic hope for cure—again, emphasizing the need for a high index of suspicion and low threshold for biopsy. Subungual lesions require removal of the nail for accurate biopsy (Figure 7-5A,B)

Nonmelanoma Skin Cancer

Nonmelanoma skin cancer (NMSC) is the most commonly diagnosed malignancy in the United States, accounting for 33% to 50% of all newly diagnosed cancers each year. More than 1 million new cases are diagnosed in the United States and 3 million in the world every year. Basal cell carcinoma (BCC) (75%) and squamous cell carcinoma (SCC) (20%) account for the vast majority of NMSC (>95%). Because of their slow growth and negligible risk for metastasis, the mortality associated with these cancers is low; however, they cause considerable functional and cosmetic deformity.

A number of genetic disorders exist that are characterized by an increased incidence of NMSC. Xeroderma pigmentosum is a rare autosomal recessive disorder (prevalence 1:250,000) characterized by a defect in the normal detection and repair mechanism of the UV-induced DNA damage.

Nevoid basal cell syndrome (or Gorlin syndrome) is a multisystemic disorder characterized by the occurrence of multiple BCC often in the hundreds, odontogenic cysts of the jaw, calcification of the falx cerebri, pitting in the palms and soles, and various skeletal abnormalities (bifid ribs, brachymetacarpalism, broad nasal root, and overdeveloped supraorbital rim). BCCs usually develop between the second and third decade and distant metastasis is rare. Other genetic syndromes that predispose to skin carcinoma include

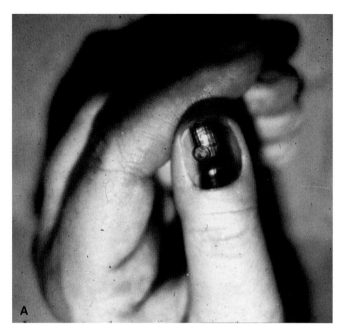
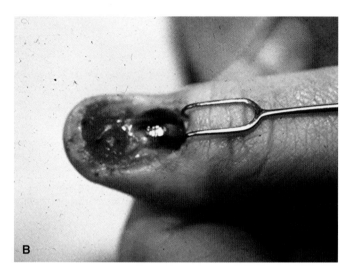

● FIGURE 7-5. (A) Subungual melanoma: Note pigmentation of the nail which is consistent with a diagnosis of acral lentiginous melanoma. A biopsy through the nail performed elsewhere failed to confirm the diagnosis. (B) Subungual melanoma: Correct confirmatory biopsy requires removal of the nail. The lesion involving the more proximal nailbed germinal matrix is apparent.

albinism (increased risk of SCC), porokeratosis (13% chance of SCC formation), and epidermodysplasia verruciformis.

A number of skin lesions are also associated with the development of NMSC, and understanding the associated risk of malignant degeneration facilitates management of the patient. Actinic keratosis is the most common premalignant lesion, as it develops in 16% of North American Caucasians during their lifetime. The transformation rate to SCC ranges between 10% and 13%. Nevus sebaceous of Jadassohn is a well-circumscribed, raised, yellowish plaque that is present at birth on the scalp and face; degeneration into BCC is seen in 5% to 10% of cases. The cutaneous horn is a hard keratotic growth that is taller than its base, and the incidence of an underlying squamous cell carcinoma is thought to be about 10%. Specific deficiencies of cell-mediated immunity are also correlated with the development of BCC and SCC. Advanced and or extensive NMSCs are associated with low T cell levels and apparent tumor anergy. Patients receiving chronic immunosuppressive therapy have a 50% risk of developing SCC within 20 years of transplantation; 30% of such cancers are considered highly aggressive.

Basal Cell Carcinoma. BCC is the most common malignancy among whites, and its incidence shows clear geographic variation reflecting the likelihood of significant sun exposure. Among Caucasians in North America, the incidence has increased at more than 10% a year, leading to a lifetime risk of 30% of developing BCC. Patients with BCC have an increased risk of developing a second BCC of the skin (35% at 3 years, 50% at 5 years), which increases with number of previous skin cancers, solar damage, and skin sensitivity. Histologic type correlates with malignant potential and recurrence and suggests wider clinical margins of resection.

Nodular BCC. The most common BCC subtype (50%–55%), it presents as a small solitary nodule or papule on the surface of the skin of the face with a shiny, pearly, translucent appearance and often small or large telangiectatic vessels traversing throughout. The nodule is round or oval, and the depth is usually similar to the width. Over time, the clinical picture may be dominated by central ulceration surrounded by a rolled pearly border and bleeding, thus masking the nodularity ("rodent ulcer"). Although most are red or flesh colored, they may show variable amounts of pigmentation mimicking or even masking underlying melanoma.

Superficial BCC. The second most common BCC type (10%) presents as an erythematous, flaking lesion usually containing superficial ulcerations or crusting. The borders are usually round or oval, although they may be irregular. The lesions tend to occur mostly in the trunk. They are indolent and may be confused with a variety of benign disorders, including psoriasis, eczematous dermatitis, and Bowen disease (in situ SCC; see below). Excision may be incomplete because the tumor may extend beyond the clinical margin or because the margin may be obscured by erythema from associated inflammation. Typically, the tumor is confined to the epidermis, and growth is more radial than vertical.

Morpheaform (Sclerosing) BCC. A rare (2%–5%) but aggressive variant that presents as a tan, white, or yellowish atrophic plaque with ill-defined borders leading to difficulty in diagnosis and late presentation. Inflammatory induration is almost always present. The extent of the tumor is usually not apparent on clinical examination, and the surgical specimen frequently has involved margins. The growth pattern is primarily radial, and ulceration remains infrequent.

Pigmented BCC. A rare subtype (6%) that may be confused with melanoma. The pigment is melanin and can render the lesion a variety of colors ranging from tan to black.

Squamous Cell Carcinoma. SCC is the second most common skin cancer after BCC and usually is preceded by sun damage, leukoplakia, actinic keratoses, or radiation damage. Varying degrees of keratinocyte dysplasia identifies SCC; keratin pearls and intercellular bridging are seen on histologic examination. The grade of the tumor is determined by the degree of cellular differentiation, with high-grade tumors marked by increased cellular atypia and loss of keratinization. SCC typically presents as a painless, erythematous, poorly defined lesion with elevated borders; they may resemble an actinic keratosis. Compared with BCC, these tumors are more aggressive and nodal metastases occur at greater frequency.

SCC can be associated with long-standing wounds, irritation, or inflammation. Long-standing wounds have a 2% risk of harboring an SCC. Originally described in the setting of burn wounds (Marjolin ulcer), malignant degeneration may occur in any chronic wound, including venous stasis ulcers, decubitus ulcers, hidradenitis, and chronic osteomyelitis. Wound or scar-associated SCC is generally more aggressive than its UV-induced counterpart and metastasizes more frequently (20%–30%). The overall prognosis for patients with metastatic disease is dismal. Of patients with squamous cell carcinoma, 30% will develop an additional SCC after 5 years and more than 50% will develop an additional nonmelanoma skin cancer. For SCC, the differential includes squamous cell carcinoma, keratoacanthoma, eczema and atopic dermatitis, contact dermatitis, psoriasis, pseudoepitheliomatous hyperplasia, bowenoid papulosis, and seborrheic dermatitis.

Bowen's Disease. A SCC in situ with epidermal and follicular involvement. Only 10% of cases become locally invasive; the rest remain localized for long periods.

Verrucous Carcinoma. A well-differentiated variant of SCC so named due to its wart-like appearance. Local invasion is common. Underlying bone involvement may occur; however, metastases are rare. Involvement of the palmar and plantar skin is common.

Merkel Cell Carcinoma. Merkel cell carcinoma (MCC) an uncommon but highly aggressive primary malignant tumor of the skin. It is often classified as a neuroendocrine tumor and the pathologic diagnosis may be difficult. MCC is a rare tumor; therefore, limited prospective, statistically significant data are available to verify or validity of any prognostic features or treatment outcomes. Treatment generally includes wide local excision with consideration for sentinel node mapping and biopsy. Staging includes a metastatic imaging evaluation. Referral to medical and radiation oncology for discussion about adjuvant thereapy is appropriate. Several large reviews document the development of local recurrence in 25% to 33% of all cases of MCC, regional disease in 25% of all cases, and distant metastatic disease in 33% of cases. The overall 5-year survival rates range from 30% to 64%. MCC usually presents after the sixth decade as a solitary nodule on a sun-exposed area (up to 75% in the head and neck area).

Dermatofibrosarcoma Protuberans (DFSP). Dermatofibrosarcoma protuberans is a rare fibrohistiocytic sarcoma that manifests clinically as a distinctive, raised, hard lesion that begins as a plaque or small nodule. Most patients are 20 to 40 years old. DFPS is uncommon, low-grade sarcoma and the incidence rate of 0.8 cases/million-persons/year. The local recurrence rate for DFSP in studies ranges from 0% to 60%, whereas the rate of development of regional or distant metastatic disease is only 1% and 4% to 5%, respectively. Tumor characteristics include long, irregular, subclinical extensions. Delayed reconstruction may be advisable pending confirmation of clear margins. The treatment is wide local excision. The tumor has a propensity for subclinical deep invasion, and deep resection is appropriate.

● PATIENT PREPARATION

Patient preparation begins preoperatively with counseling regarding the need for complete tumor removal in order to gain local control of disease. Cosmetic concerns must be factored into the surgical plan, but they should not limit the degree of resection required to obtain clear and adequate surgical margins. Patients should be prepared for the possibility of positive margins and the need for re-excision. Perhaps, more importantly, the surgeon should also be prepared, and a complex postablative reconstruction should be staged if there is any concern about resection margins. Realistic goals and expectations must be set and thoroughly explained to the patient. The indications for staging should be discussed, especially the potential role for sentinel node mapping and biopsy in patients having melanoma or Merkel cell carcinoma. Imaging studies for patients at risk for metastatic disease should be ordered and reviewed. The results may obviously impact the anticipated surgical plans in the event that metastatic disease is evident. General anesthesia is appropriate for larger procedures, but many resections can be performed with only local. Patients should be positioned to allow access to the entire tumor area and any potential flap donor sites needed for reconstruction. Sterile technique is vital, as the potential for infection remains high. Essential equipment will vary, depending on the surgeon and procedure. In general, electrocautery and bolster dressing supplies should be available for all excisions.

● SURGICAL TREATMENTS

Management of Melanoma

Currently, surgery is the only acceptable therapy for primary melanoma. Surgical resection of the primary involves an en bloc resection with a surrounding margin of normal skin and underlying soft tissue. The need for wide margins was recognized by Handley in 1907, who recognized that growth of the primary was discontinuous and that narrow margins of resection while seeming complete would fail to remove the subclinical spread along dermal lymphatics and result in local recurrence. [8] The exact margins of resection remain a subject of much debate and consensus recommendations exist (Table 7-2). [9] Attempts to move toward thinner margins in the context of clinical trials are met with an increasing risk of local recurrence. Unfortunately, local recurrence portends a poor prognosis. The goals of surgical treatment are to provide local disease control for all patients, even when the risk of systemic spread is high, and to achieve a high cure in patients with early stage disease. Surgical practice calls for these goals to be met without compromise, but also with consideration of functional impairment and cosmetic disfigurement Understanding the relationship between surgical margins, local recurrences, regional failures, and survival has motivated a standardization of surgical melanoma care and, while the consensus margin recommendations are not sacrosanct, they still bear medicolegal importance and should be modified only if there are significant functional or cosmetic concerns. In addition to the radial surgical margins, questions regarding the depth of excision have been addressed. It is currently accepted that the excision need not include the underlying fascia but should extend down to but not including the muscle fascia. Patients having subungual melanoma (acral lentiginous type) are managed with distal amputation of the involved digit (usually at the distal interphalangeal level).

Mohs micrographic surgery, a technique primarily used by dermatologists, employs intraoperative margin assessment to map the histologic extent of a malignant lesion, allowing excision with a minimal surgical margin and maximizing preservation of uninvolved tissue. The efficacy of this approach is well established for the management of basal cell and squamous cell carcinoma (see below); however, no prospective randomized clinical trials comparing Mohs techniques and standard surgical excisions have been undertaken to date, and this technique is not considered standard of care for the management of primary melanoma. Evaluation and management of regional lymphatic involvement of melanoma is essential for both cancer staging and patient survival. Once there is regional spread of melanoma, prognostic factors related to the primary lesion (Breslow thickness, ulceration, histology, site, number of mitoses) contribute very little to the overall prognostic outlook. The status of the sentinel node is the single most important prognostic factor for a patient having melanoma. [10] Nodal metastases alone decrease 5-year survival by roughly 40%. The sentinel lymph node (SLN) is defined as the first node (or nodes), within the chain or network of nodes comprising the lymphatic basin, to receive drainage form the primary tumor. The SLN is therefore at highest risk of developing melanoma metastases. The histology of the SLN accurately reflects the histology of the entire of the basin. It was recognized only fairly recently (mid 1990s) that lymphatic drainage is dynamic and unpredictable. The correct preoperative identification of the sentinel node and by definition the appropriate nodal basin requires a lymphoscintigram usually performed with Tc 99m–labeled sulfur colloid (Figure 7-6). The sentinel node mapping and biopsy procedure is best performed at the time of definitive surgical management of the primary. Lymphoscintigraphy is obtained prior to surgery, usually several hours preoperatively. The primary site is injected intradermally with vital blue dye (Isosulfan Blue seems to be best) (Figure 7-7). An intradermal injection is critical, and a subcutaneous injection may identify

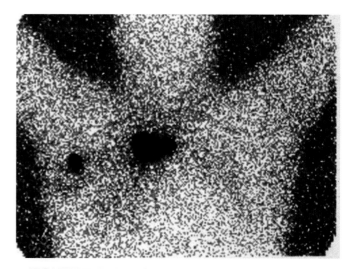

● **FIGURE 7-6.** Lymphoscintigram: The study demonstrates the unilateral axillary drainage pattern of a midline melanoma of the back. Drainage patterns of midline lesions are highly variable and lymphoscintigraphy is a necessary component of the sentinel node mapping procedure.

TABLE 7-2. Recommended Margins of Excision for Melanoma

Thickness	Excision Margins
In situ	5 mm
<1 mm	1 cm
>1 mm	2 cm
>4 mm	2 cm at least

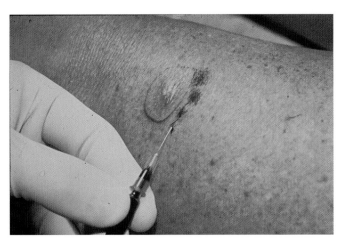

● **FIGURE 7-7.** Intradermal injection: Vital blue dye (Isosulfan Blue) is injected into the primary site (primary removed as an excisional biopsy) in preparation for operative identification of the sentinel node.

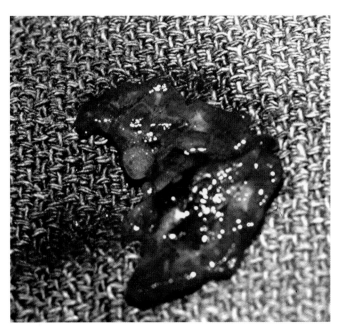

● **FIGURE 7-9.** Sentinel node: The sentinel node containing blue dye and radiocolloid is removed and submitted for pathological assessment.

the wrong node. The draining nodal basin is explored using the blue dye as well as a handheld gamma probe (Figure 7-8). The combination of both the blue dye and the radiocolloid increase both the accuracy and ease of the procedure. The sentinel node(s) are removed and submitted for pathological review (Figure 7-9). The pathological review should include multiple-step sections and the use of immunohistochemistry, both of which increase the accuracy of the subsequent staging. The exact indications for sentinel node mapping and biopsy remain a source of controversy; however, it is generally accepted that patients having a primary lesion of Breslow depth 1 to 4 mm are appropriate candidates. Patients with thin lesions (<1 mm) having additional poor prognostic signs such as ulceration or Clark's level IV are at higher risk for having nodal disease and therefore reasonably staged with sentinel node mapping and biopsy.

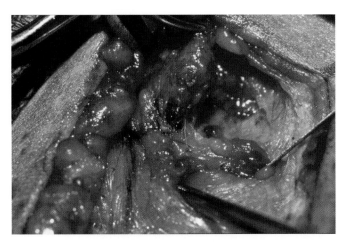

● **FIGURE 7-8.** Intraoperative sentinel node identification. Lymphatics containing blue dye and identifying the sentinel node are apparent.

Management of Nonmelanoma Skin Cancer

Nonmelanoma skin cancers include Merkel cell carcinoma, for which wide excision with margins comparable to the recommendations for melanoma as above. Sentinel node mapping and biopsy is evolving as an appropriate staging procedure for MCC. DFSP tumors should also be widely excised to fascia. Nodal disease is uncommon and therefore sentinel node biopsy (SNB) is not usually performed.

Treatment options for squamous cell and basal cell carcinomas include surgical excision, curettage and electrodessication, cryosurgery, fractionated radiotherapy, topical chemotherapy or immunotherapy (5-fluorouracil, imiquimod), carbon dioxide laser, photodynamic therapy, intralesional interferon, and retinoids. Laser treatment offers theoretical advantages for certain patients, such as those taking anticoagulants. However, primary excision remains the most common treatment for BCC and SCC. Cure rates can approach 99% when surgical margins are negative. Recurrent NMSC is difficult to manage having only a 50% cure rate. Mohs micrographic surgery is a reasonable option for the management of the recurrent BCC. When planning the excision, the size of the tumor, the clinical type, grade, depth of invasion, the location, the ramifications of local recurrence, and patient factors (age, general health, aesthetic considerations, etc) should be taken into consideration.

The appropriate margin of resection for BCC is not set in stone; rather, the surgeon must balance the risk of recurrence with loss of function or diminished cosmesis. Excision with 5-mm margins has been recommended by numerous authors as a general guideline, although large lesions may require wider margins because

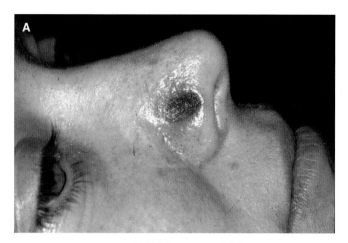
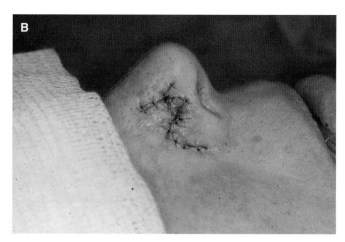

● FIGURE 7-10. (A) Postablative defect: A typical postablative defect following surgical removal of a basal cell carcinoma. Definitive reconstruction in this case was staged to allow confirmation of clear margins. (B) Flap reconstruction: The postablative defect is readily reconstructed with a banner-type transposition flap.

margin positivity and recurrence rates increase with size. Excisions of recurrent BCC are challenging because of the high failure rates. Recurrence rates are highest in the head and neck, especially the nose, and recurrent tumors may be managed with Mohs micrographic surgery. Reconstruction of the postablative defect may require the use of local skin flaps as described in Chapter 2 (Figure 7-10A,B).

Definitive surgical margins for the management of SCC are also unclear and dependent on tumor and host characteristics. For lesions smaller than 2 cm, a 4-mm margin is likely adequate; whereas lesions larger than 2 cm may be better managed with a 1-cm margin. The size of the margins may be modified depending on the differentiation, size, and the invasion of surrounding structures. Some authors advocate wider margins (3.5 cm margin for a >3 cm tumor) to achieve a 95% cure rate. For high-risk SCC, the margin should be 6 mm and the excision should be into the subcutaneous fat. Early re-excision is recommended in the event of positive resection margins. SNB is not usually performed, although may be justified in cases where subclinical disease is likely based on either patient or lesion risk factors.

Management of Nodal Disease. Patients having documented nodal disease are managed with completion lymphadenectomy and/or radiotherapy and should be evaluated by medical oncology for adjuvant systemic therapy.

● POSTABLATIVE RECONSTRUCTION

Ideally, the resection is planned as an ellipse with the long axis pointing toward the draining nodal basin or coincident with lines of relaxed skin tension (cosmesis). The smaller defects are closed primarily over a suction drain as needed. Despite current evidence-based guidelines reflecting a

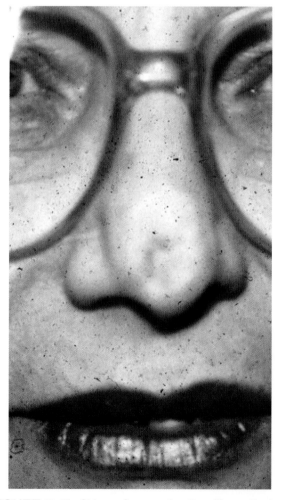

● FIGURE 7-11. Skin graft reconstruction: The patient underwent skin graft reconstruction of a postablative (basal cell carcinoma excision) nasal defect elsewhere. The contour deformity is apparent. While this approach is reasonable and appropriate, a better cosmetic result may be obtained with a local flap reconstruction.

trend toward conservatism, surgical excision often results in a defect that cannot be closed primarily. As noted above, if there is doubt that the primary has been resected with clear margins, definitive reconstruction should be staged pending pathologic confirmation of clear margins. Care should be taken to avoid any cross-contamination between the ablative fields and flap or skin graft donor sites, as cutaneous malignancies can be transplanted. Primary closure is often complicated after resections involving the distal extremities, face, and scalp. For these defects, either split- or full-thickness skin grafts are reasonable options for coverage. The shortcomings of skin grafting include suboptimal cosmetic results, donor site morbidity, and the necessity for patient immobilization postoperatively (Figure 7-11). Local flaps, when appropriate and feasible, offer superior cosmetic results and earlier patient mobility. In our experience, use of the versatile rhomboid flap, or rotation flaps have been valuable when primary closure is not feasible or cosmetically acceptable (see Chapter 2). Rarely, more sophisticated reconstructive techniques such as pedicled flaps or free flaps may be required. Flap closure of melanoma excision defects is not associated with increased local recurrence rates.

● COMPLICATIONS

Wound complications following primary resection occur with a frequency that is related to the size and location of the defect and include infections, dehiscence and hematoma, or seroma formation. Seroma formation may be expected with a 30% incidence after SNB. Management options include aspiration and formal incision and drainage. Local-regional recurrences may occur with an incidence that is proportional to the thickness of the primary but may also reflect inadequate management of the primary lesion. Recurrences are managed with re-excision usually with the more conservative 1-cm margin.

● OUTCOMES ASSESSMENT

Staging for Melanoma

The staging of melanoma is important to practitioners, as it provides a precise nomenclature for description of lesions based on prognosis, a reliable system of patient stratification in terms of risk of metastasis and survival rates, and a consistent tool for judicious clinical decision making. It is likewise important to researchers, as it permits fair

TABLE 7-3. TNM Staging Categories for Melanoma

T Classification	Thickness (mm)	Ulceration Status/Mitoses
Tis	N/A	N/A
T1	≤1.00	a: Without ulceration and mitosis $< 1/mm^2$
		b: With ulceration and mitosis $\geq 1/mm^2$
T2	1.01–2.00	a: Without ulceration
		b: With ulceration
T3	2.01–4.00	a: Without ulceration
		b: With ulceration
T4	>4.00	a: Without ulceration
		b: With ulceration
N Classification	**No. of Metastatic Nodes**	**Nodal Metastatic Burden**
N0	0	N/A
N1	1	a: Micrometastasis
		b: Macrometastasis
N2	2–3	a: Micrometastasis
		b: Macrometastasis
		c: In transit metastases/satellites without metastatic nodes
N3	4+ metastatic nodes, or matted nodes, or in transit metastases/satellites with metastatic nodes	
M Classification	**Site**	**Serum LDH**
M0	No distant metastases	N/A
M1a	Distant skin, subcutaneous, or nodal metastases	Normal
M1b	Lung metastases	Normal
M1c	All other visceral metastases	Normal
	Any distant metastases	Elevated

LDH, lactate dehydrogenase; M, metastasis; N/A, not available; N, nodes; T, tumor.
Micrometastases are detected after sentinel lymph node biopsy.

TABLE 7-4. Anatomic Stage Groupings for Melanoma

	Clinical Staging				Pathologic Staging		
	T	*N*	*M*		*T*	*N*	*M*
0	Tis	N0	M0	0	Tis	N0	M0
IA	T1a	N0	M0	IA	T1a	N0	M0
IB	T1b	N0	M0	IB	T1b	N0	M0
	T2a	N0	M0		T2a	N0	M0
IIA	T2b	N0	M0	IIA	T2b	N0	M0
	T3a	N0	M0		T3a	N0	M0
IIB	T3b	N0	M0	IIB	T3b	N0	M0
	T4a	N0	M0		T4a	N0	M0
IIC	T4b	N0	M0	IIC	T4b	N0	M0
III	Any T	N>N0	M0	IIIA	T1-4a	N1a	M0
					T1-4a	N2b	M0
				IIIB	T1-4b	N1a	M0
					T1-4b	N2a	M0
					T1-4a	N1b	M0
					T1-4a	N2b	M0
					T1-4a	N2c	M0
				IIC	T1-4b	N1b	M0
					T1-4b	N2b	M0
					T1-4b	N2c	M0
					Any T	N3	M0
IV	Any T	Any N	M1	IV	Any T	Any N	M1

M, metastasis; N, nodes; T, tumor.

comparison of different treatment regimens and simplifies inclusion criteria for clinical trials. The staging of cutaneous melanoma has undergone many changes and modifications over the years based on ongoing research aimed at determining the relationship between gross and histopathologic characteristics and clinical behavior of the disease. Late in 2009, a multidisciplinary Melanoma Staging Committee of the American Joint Committee on Cancer met to revise the existing system of TNM classification and staging to reflect the expanding understanding of the disease[11] (Tables 7-3 and 7-4). Important changes include: (1) mitotic rate is now a criterion for defining T1b melanomas; (2) in patients with distant metastases, the site of metastases and LDH level define the M category; (3) all patients with microscopic metastases are now classified as stage III. In short, melanoma staging is based on anatomic compartmentalization and categorizes patients with localized melanoma into stages I/II, those with regional skin, subcutaneous or nodal metastases to stage III, and those with distant metastases to stage IV.

REFERENCES

1. Mihm MC Jr, Sober AJ. Melanoma before and after Thomas B. Fitzpatrick. *J Invest Dermatol.* 2004;122:32–33.

2. Ford D, Bliss JM, Swerdlow AJ, et al. Risk of cutaneous melanoma associated with a family history of the disease. The International Melanoma Analysis Group (IMAGE). *Int J Cancer.* 1995;62:377–381.

3. Weinstock MA. Death from skin cancer among the elderly: epidemiological patterns. *Arch Dermatol.* 1997;133:1207–1209.

4. Elwood JM, Jopson J. Melanoma and sun exposure: an overview of published studies. *Int J Cancer.* 1997;73:198–203.

5. Tucker MA, Halpern A, Holly EA, et al. Clinically recognized dysplastic nevi. A central risk factor for cutaneous melanoma. *JAMA.* 1997;277:1439–1444.

6. Ford D, Bliss JM, Swerdlow AJ, et al. A. Risk of cutaneous melanoma associated with a family history of the disease. The International Melanoma Analysis Group (IMAGE). *Int J Cancer.* 1995;62:377–381.

7. Carucci JA. Treatment of lentigo maligna. *Cutis.* 2001;67:389–392.

8. Handley WS. The pathology of melanotic growths in relation to their operative treatment. *Lancet.* 1907;1:927–933.

9. Lens MB, Nathan P, Bataille V. Excision margins for primary cutaneous melanoma. *Arch Surg.* 2007;142(9):885–891.

10. Gershenwald JE, Thompson W, Mansfield PF, et al. Multi-institutional melanoma lymphatic mapping experience: the prognostic value of sentinel lymph node status in 612 stage I or II melanoma patients. *J Clin Oncol.* 1999;17:976–983.

11. Balch CM, Gershenwald JE, Soong S, et al. Final version of 2009 AJCC melanoma staging and classification. *J Clin Oncol.* 2009;27(36):6199–6206.

chapter 8

Vascular Malformations

David W. Low, MD / *M. Renee Jespersen, MD*

● INTRODUCTION

Hemangiomas are the most common vascular anomaly of infancy, occurring in 10% of full-term infants, but parents can be largely reassured that all hemangiomas will pass from a proliferative to an involutional phase, and up to 70% of hemangiomas will not require any specific interventional therapy. Chapter 9 addresses treatment options for problematic hemangiomas.

Vascular malformations represent the remaining anomalies, and it is important to distinguish these conditions from hemangiomas, as the clinical course and treatment options can be significantly different. Unlike hemangiomas, the vast majority of vascular malformations do not have the ability to involute. Medicolegal situations can arise if parents are advised to wait for slow regression that, in fact, will never occur. Some conditions such as port wine stains warrant immediate therapy beginning in infancy. This chapter will address the most common vascular anomalies and outline their clinical characteristics, diagnostic studies, and treatment options.

● PATIENT EVALUATION AND SELECTION

Vascular Malformations— General Considerations

Vascular malformations represent structurally abnormal vessels, predominantly due to abnormal in utero development, but also influenced by actinic, hormonal, or gravitational influence. Any type of vessel can be involved, and the malformations are classified by the type or types of vessels involved. These include:

Capillary vascular malformations (port wine stains)
Venous malformations (including blue rubber bleb nevus syndrome and glomus tumors)
Lymphatic malformations

Venolymphatic malformations
Arterial and arteriovenous malformations
Capillary, venous, and lymphatic malformations (Klippel-Trenaunay syndrome)
Capillary and arteriovenous malformations (Parkes-Weber syndrome)

Small collections of abnormal dermal vessels have historically been given descriptive names, some of which are not entirely accurate but have persisted through widespread usage:

Pyogenic granulomas (lobular capillary hemangiomas)
Adenoma sebaceum (angiofibromas)
Broken blood vessels (telangiectasias)
Spider angiomas
Spider veins
Cherry angiomas

Many of these conditions are also treated by dermatologists, and it is useful to develop a good working relationship with these specialists, as they are the major referral source of patients with vascular conditions needing surgical intervention.

Nonsurgical Therapy for Vascular Malformations

Some vascular malformations are best treated by nonsurgical methods. Decongestive massage and compression wrapping by rehabilitation medicine specialists, compression garments, and compression pumps are often the treatment of choice for lower extremity malformations characterized by venous engorgement and lymphedema.

Sclerotherapy by an interventional radiologist is an extremely useful option for many venous, lymphatic, and venolymphatic malformations. This will often avoid the need for surgical excision, or at least decrease the risk of intraoperative bleeding. Sclerosing agents such as absolute alcohol, doxycycline, sodium tetradecyl sulfate (Sotradecol) injected under fluoroscopic or ultrasonic guidance can be used for subcutaneous or deeper subfascial and intramuscular malformations. Plastics surgeons may also perform sclerotherapy for superficial dermal vessels using agents, such as hypertonic saline, sodium sotradecyl sulfate, or recently FDA-approved polidocanol (Asclera). 30-gauge needles, 1 cc syringes, loupe magnification, and a steady hand are recommended for successful cannulation of extremely tiny vessels. Post-treatment compression with dental rolls or cotton balls and support stockings will facilitate obliteration of spider and even (nonsaphenous) varicose veins without the need for stripping and ligation.

Steroids and beta-blockers have no role in the treatment of congenital vascular malformations, in contrast to hemangiomas. Steroids and beta-blockers suppress endothelial proliferation associated with hemangioma growth, but have no ability to limit vascular dilatation and hypertrophy associated with vascular malformations.

● PATIENT PREPARATION

Laser Considerations

Lasers that target either oxyhemoglobin or water may be useful in the palliative and occasionally curative treatment of many vascular malformations. Although the continuous beam Argon laser (blue-green light, 488 and 515 nm) was the first clinically useful laser for treating vascular conditions, currently the pulsed yellow dye laser is the most commonly used laser for a wide variety of dermal vascular malformations. The organic rhodamine dye initially emitted a pure yellow 577 nm wavelength, but succeeding generations of pulsed dye lasers have increased the wavelength to 585 nm and currently 595 nm to achieve deeper dermal penetration (Perfecta Vbeam). High-energy, short duration pulses of light tend to cause vascular disruption and purpura rather than coagulation, and limit heat injury to the vessels themselves. By respecting the "thermal relaxation time" of the vessels, pulsed lasers destroy vessels with minimal damage to the surrounding dermis, a process described as "selective photothermolysis."

Continuous beam lasers that travel through fiberoptic cables, such as the KTP and Nd:YAG lasers (Laserscope) can achieve deeper coagulation through largely non-specific heat transfer. These lasers may be more likely to leave cutaneous scars, but may be more useful for bulky, engorged vascular lesions such as venous malformations and cherry angiomas. The fibers can also be passed percutaneously through large gauge hypodermic needles or transmucosally to avoid excessive superficial thermal damage (Figure 8-1). Endovenous laser ablation is growing in popularity as an alternative to venous stripping and ligation for varicose veins, and it can also be used to treat other venous malformations.

Carbon dioxide laser light is absorbed by water, making them appropriate for vaporization or coagulation of a

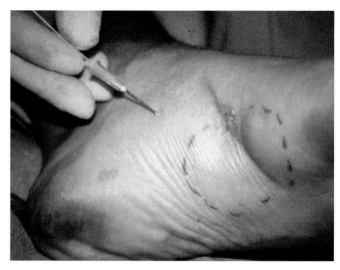

● FIGURE 8-1. Percutaneous deep laser photocoagulation using a KTP laser fiber and a hypodermic needle avoids excessive heat damage to the epidermis.

variety of superficial vascular lesions such as lymphatic vesicles, angiokeratomas (crusted venolymphatic skin lesions), and angiofibromas (commonly called adenoma sebaceum, a misnomer).

● SURGICAL TREATMENT OF VASCULAR MALFORMATIONS

Capillary Vascular Malformations

Capillary vascular malformation, commonly called port wine stains, occur in 3 out of 1000 babies and can appear anywhere on the body, but those on the face are obviously the most distressing to parents. Often following a roughly dermatomal distribution, capillary vascular malformation that include the V1 distribution of the head may also involve ocular structures and the leptomeninges (Sturge-Weber syndrome) (Figure 8-2). These patients should be routinely monitored for glaucoma, and parents should be aware of the potential for seizures.

Pulsed yellow dye laser therapy is the treatment of choice for capillary vascular malformations. Treatment can begin in infancy, and depending upon the location of the malformation, the discomfort of the laser pulses can be reduced by a cryogen spray coupled to the laser handpiece, local anesthetic cream, field block local anesthetic injection (uncommon), or a general anesthetic (particularly for facial port wine stains that involve the periorbital area). Parents should be aware that although most capillary vascular malformations will lighten with laser therapy, virtually none will completely disappear. Also, lasers characteristically leave purpuric spots for about 2 weeks, followed by slow lightening of the vascular pigmentation over 2 to 3 months. Most patients receive six to eight treatments until a plateau in improvement is reached. Residual pigmentation is presumably due to deep dermal vessels that cannot be reached by the laser light. The neck and

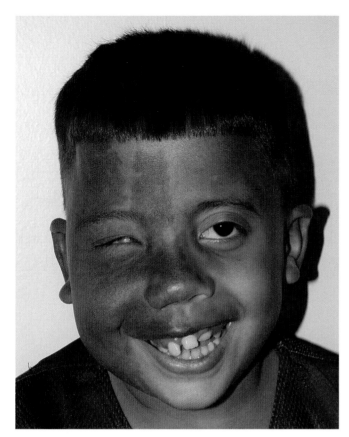

● **FIGURE 8-2.** Capillary vascular malformations involving the V1 distribution require monitoring for glaucoma and seizure activity, clinical features of Sturge-Weber syndrome. This patient has a prosthetic right eye.

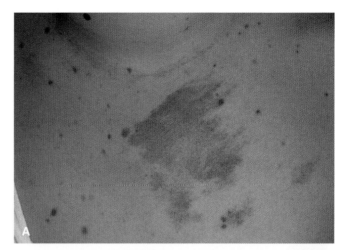

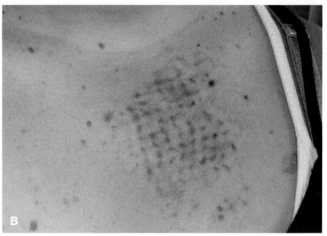

● **FIGURE 8-3.** (A, B) Port wine stains of the neck and chest respond extremely well to pulsed yellow dye laser therapy. Significant lightening is apparent after just one laser treatment. Additional treatments may be given every 2 to 3 months until no further lightening is observed.

chest areas often lighten remarkably, the face lightens to a variable degree, and hands and feet often show minimal improvement (Figure 8-3).

The goal of laser therapy is to lighten the vascular pigmentation as much as possible and also to try to avoid hypertrophy of the capillaries and venules, which can lead to deeper purple pigmentation, a raised nodular texture, and sometimes significant soft tissue hypertrophy and distortion. Pediatric patients who have reached a plateau in improvement may exhibit an increase in vascular pigmentation during their teenage and adult years due to ongoing hypertrophy of the residual dermal vessels. Laser therapy may again be effective in reducing the vascular engorgement.

Macular stains, often called "stork bite" or "angel's kiss," are pale pink patches that present in the midline glabella and forehead and at the nape of the neck. Unlike port wine stains, they have the inexplicable ability to fade spontaneously over the first year of life, and therefore initial treatment is conservative. Persistent macular stains virtually disappear with 1 or 2 pulsed yellow dye laser treatments, suggesting that these malformations are extremely superficial and easily obliterated by the laser light. Port wine stains, in addition, may develop problematic bleeding nodules and even pyogenic granulomas (lobular capillary

hemangiomas) that usually are best treated by direct surgical excision.

Mid and lower facial capillary malformations (V2, V3 distribution) may also create significant lip and cheek hypertrophy. Lasers are not effective in retarding or reducing this bulk, and surgical removal of full-thickness vertical wedges and transverse ellipses of vermilion and skin are usually needed for adequate palliation (Figure 8-4). Temporary placement of noncrushing vascular clamps along the commissures will help to reduce bleeding. Aggressive debulking is analogous to surgical removal of a lip cancer, and it may be necessary to remove one third to one half of the lip to achieve adequate reduction (Figure 8-5). Overcorrection may be desirable, as the residual involved tissue will have a tendency to undergo additional hypertrophy.

Venous Malformations

Venous malformations range from small venous lakes to extensive networks of dilated veins. They may be present at birth or appear throughout life. They may be submucosal,

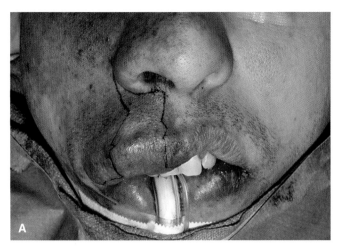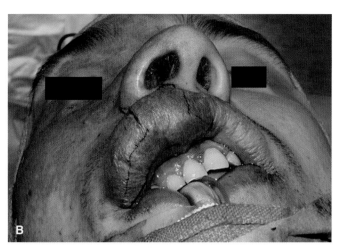

● **FIGURE 8-4.** (A, B) Upper lip hypertrophy associated with capillary vascular malformations requires debulking in three dimensions to improve symmetry.

intradermal, subcutaneous, intramuscular, intra-articular, intracranial, and intra-abdominal. Most venous malformation dilate slowly over time. In addition to progressive contour deformities, patients may develop palpable phleboliths, painful thromboses, hematoma or hemarthrosis formation from vascular rupture, and aching pain from the mass effect on local nerves. It is important to recognize that patients with venous and venolymphatic disorders are at risk for disseminated intravascular coagulopathy, deep venous thrombosis, and pulmonary emboli. Evaluation by a hematologist for elevated D-dimers and low fibrinogen may indicate the need for lifetime anticoagulation.

Depending on location, venous malformations may be followed conservatively, controlled with compression garments and elevation, and treated with NSAID agents for thromboses. Most hematomas can also be followed conservatively, as they will usually resolve slowly without requiring aspiration or drainage.

Persistently problematic venous malformations may be candidates for intralesional sclerotherapy by an interventional radiologist (multiple treatments are usually necessary for optimal results, and patients should be advised that treatments are usually palliative rather than curative), laser photocoagulation, or surgical debulking.

Well-circumscribed malformations can sometimes be cured by excision. *Blue rubber bleb nevus syndrome* involves acquired scattered venous malformations rather than melanocytic nevi. These hereditary malformations can occur anywhere, including along the gastrointestinal tract, in which case severe anemia and heme-positive stools may warrant exploratory laparotomy and bowel resection. Discrete subcutaneous lesions can sometimes be completely removed by surgical excision (Figure 8-6), but new lesions commonly occur.

Lasers have a useful role in the treatment of venous malformations of the head, particularly those involving the lips and oral cavity. Continuous wave lasers, which tend to nonselectively coagulate vessels and surrounding

tissue, are generally well tolerated by the vermilion and oral mucosa. The KTP laser, 532 nm green wavelength, targets oxyhemoglobin and travels through a glass fiber. Superficial venous lakes can be coagulated using a defocused beam. Deeper penetration can be achieved by compressing the lesion with a glass slide and allowing the light to pass through the glass. Intralesional deep coagulation can be achieve by passing the fiber through the mucosa at a point slightly remote from the malformation and using a combination of palpation and transillumination to gauge the location of the fiber tip. The fiber can be passed through a hypodermic needle if one is entering the vermilion or intact skin, or the fiber tip can be placed directly against the mucosa, and a quick burst of laser energy will create a small hole through which the fiber is directed. This technique is highly operator dependent, and care must be taken to avoid excessive heat destruction or improper placement of the buried fiber tip. Endovascular laser ablation using ultrasound to document the treatment endpoint is a more accurate way to achieve the therapeutic goal.

Often, a combination of sclerotherapy and surgical debulking is necessary for extensive venous malformations of the face and oral cavity. Bleeding can be excessive, occasionally necessitating surgical abandonment. Tongue debulking can be facilitated by the placement of vascular clamps at the base of the tongue (Figure 8-7).

Glomus tumors, also known as glomangiomas and glomulovenous malformations appear as solitary or disseminated bluish purple clusters resembling the venous malformations of blue rubber bleb nevus syndrome.[1] Composed of glomus cells (perivascular cells of the glomus body, which controls arteriovenous shunting in the dermis and contributes to temperature regulation), they may present as exquisitely sensitive subungual nodules, or as mildly tender dermal and subdermal nodules elsewhere. The disseminated form is transmitted as an autosomal dominant condition. Laser and sclerotherapy have

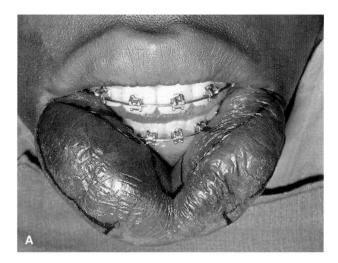
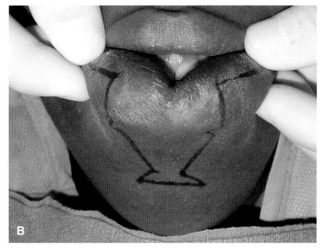
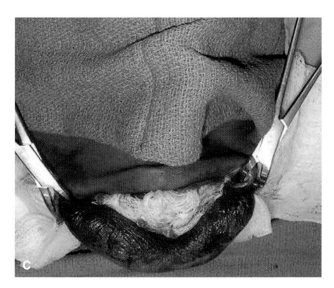
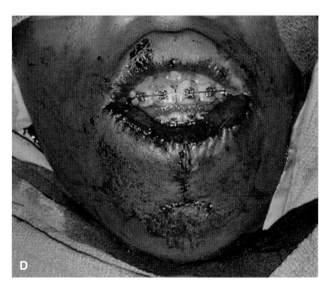

● FIGURE 8-5. (A–D) Massive lower lip hypertrophy associated with a capillary vascular malformation of the lower face. Aggressive debulking may require wide wedge resections. Temporary placement of vascular clamps will decrease intraoperative bleeding.

been described as treatment options, but direct excision is usually the treatment of choice. A minimal margin is needed, as malignant glomangiosarcomas are extremely rare. Microscopic analysis will confirm the presence of glomus cells, distinguishing them from small venous malformations (Figure 8-8).

Varicose veins of the extremities, whether congenital or acquired, may be candidates for sclerotherapy, intravenous laser coagulation, surgical ligation and division/excision, or a combination of the above. Preoperative assessment should confirm the presence of a normal venous drainage system, as removal of the abnormal system is contraindicated if it is the only source of vascular outflow. Additionally, sclerotherapy may be less effective or contraindicated if the abnormal veins connect directly to large normal veins, as it will be difficult to keep the sclerosant from flowing proximally. Combined venous ligation and division combined with sclerotherapy in such situations may produce outstanding results (Figure 8-9).

Lymphatic and Venolymphatic Malformations

Lymphatic malformations are among the most difficult to treat due to their extensive distribution and tendency to microscopically extend into normal appearing tissues, often making complete removal impossible or undesirable. Since veins and lymphatics travel together, it is common to have malformations that involve both structures, and many lymphatic cysts also contain blood from adjacent veins. Lymphatic malformations are present at birth but not always clinically apparent. Time and gravity may lead to progressive lymphatic engorgement that was not obvious in early childhood.

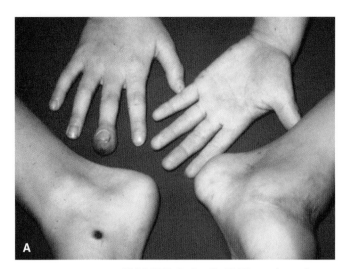
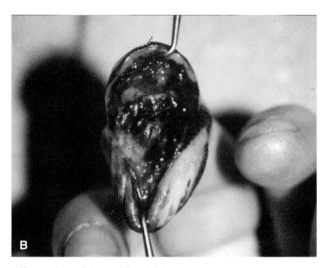

● **FIGURE 8-6.** (A, B) Disseminated venous malformations (blue rubber bleb nevus syndrome) involving all four extremities. These can be directly excised if they become symptomatic, as in the case of this long fingertip malformation. Large malformations may be better candidates for sclerotherapy.

Although the location and age of presentation have led to various names such as cystic hygromas for congenital cervicofacial lymphatic malformations, Milroy disease for congenital lymphedema of the extremities present at birth,[2] Meigs disease (lymphedema praecox) for lymphedema presenting after birth and up to age 35 years, and lymphedema tarda for lymphedema presenting after age 35 years; in fact, one can think of each of these conditions as a form of lymphatic malformation with varying degrees of severity.

Lymphatic malformations become problematic because of their tendency to undergo increasing soft tissue distortion as individual lymphatic cysts enlarge, but also because dermal lymphatic vesicles have a tendency to rupture and bleed. Cellulitis is a common problem requiring periodic

antibiotic suppression. Hypertrophy of the involved area, including osseous overgrowth, complicates attempts at debulking surgery. Recurrent episodes of cellulitis and inflammation make dissection difficult as tissue planes are obliterated and vital structures such as nerves are difficult to identify and preserve. Cervicofacial lymphatic malformations can be life-threatening because of the risk of airway obstruction, and a tracheostomy may be necessary for airway management.

MRI scans are useful to document the extent of a lymphatic malformation and also distinguish macro from microcystic disease. Large lymphatic cysts may shrink significantly with intralesional sclerotherapy, and the morbidity of surgical debulking can often be avoided with the aid

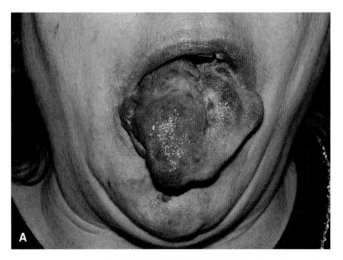
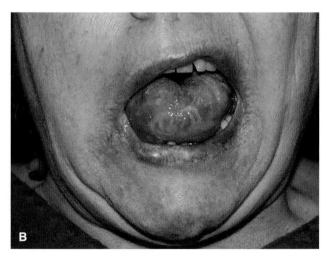

● **FIGURE 8-7.** (A, B) Massive tongue hypertrophy associated with venous malformations of the oral cavity can be safely debulked, resulting in significant improvement in tongue mobility and oral airway obstruction.

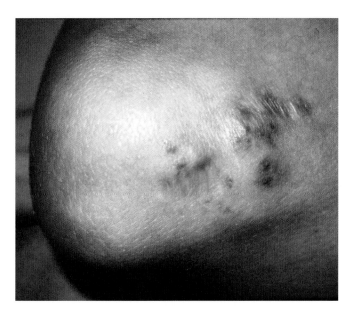

● **FIGURE 8-8.** Glomus tumors appear as clusters of dark bluish nodules in the dermis and subcutaneous tissues. Surgical removal is indicated for those that are symptomatically tender.

of a skilled interventional radiologist. Alcohol and doxycycline are commonly used in the United States; whereas in Japan, a streptococcal protein derivative OK-432 is an effective sclerosant that still awaits FDA approval.

Surgical debulking involves dissection and removal of large discrete lymphatic cysts or empiric debulking of excessive lymphatic tissue characterized by countless small cysts (Figure 8-10). It is important to remind patients that reoccurrence is common and the degree of improvement is often disappointingly small and often temporary. It is not uncommon to spend hours of tedious dissection on a cervicofacial lymphatic malformation, only to have postoperative edema obscure the postoperative result, complicated by a facial nerve injury. Compression garments and wraps, where applicable, may prolong the beneficial effect of surgical debulking.

Carbon dioxide laser vaporization of ulcerated cutaneous lymphatic vesicles may offer palliative relief from constant lymphatic drainage, as the fibrosis caused by the laser may help to cap the leaking lymphatic vessels. If the vesicles contain heme, the KTP laser may offer similar palliation as the blood in the vesicles absorbs the laser energy.

Klippel-Trenaunay Syndrome

The combination of a patchy capillary vascular malformation (port wine stain), an underlying venolymphatic malformation, and (usually) hypertrophy of the involved area is characteristic of Klippel-Trenaunay syndrome (Figure 8-11). In the lower extremity, a prominent lateral varicose vein may be evident, a persistent lateral vein that normally obliterates in utero. Dermal lymphatic

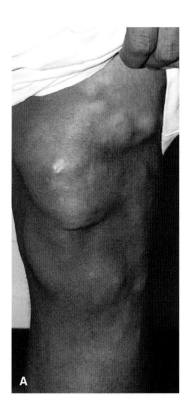
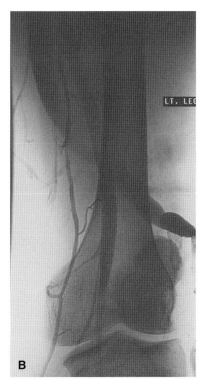
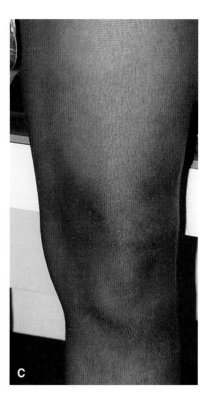

● **FIGURE 8-9.** (A–C) Congenital venous malformation of the thigh and knee. A diagnostic venogram shows massively dilated veins. Surgical ligation and division of the draining vein adjacent to its junction with the femoral vein, followed by ultrasound-guided sclerotherapy, produced outstanding results.

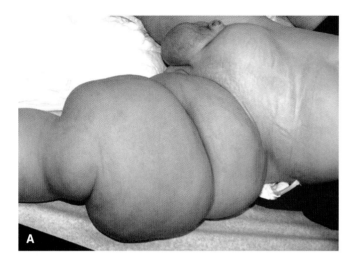

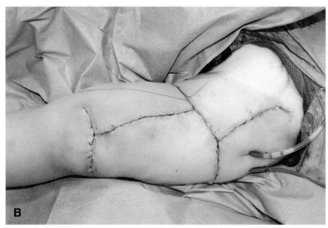

● **FIGURE 8-10.** (A, B) Congenital lymphatic malformation of the left leg. Aggressive debulking results in a significant contour improvement, but the treatment is only palliative, and a compression stocking is recommended to control recurrent edema and tissue hypertrophy.

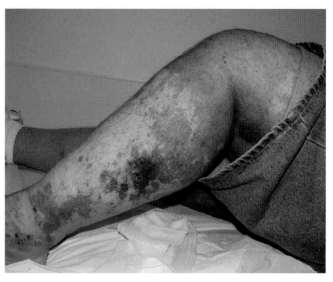

● **FIGURE 8-11.** Klippel-Trenaunay syndrome is characterized by a patchy port wine stain with an underlying venolymphatic malformation and hypertrophy of the involved region. When the leg is involved, a persistent lateral varicose vein is often present, which may cause problematic bleeding.

involvement often creates problematic crusting lesions within the area of capillary malformation (angiokeratomas). Patients complain of ulcerated angiokeratomas that cause troublesome bleeding, which is actually heme-colored lymphatic drainage that clots poorly. The KTP laser may be useful for palliative photocoagulation, directed through a glass slide to control bleeding. Alternatively, direct excision and suture closure will also control these annoying cutaneous vascular lesions.

Compression garments, particularly when the lower extremity is involved, are the treatment of choice. Surgical debulking and sclerotherapy can usually be avoided if compression stockings are used on a consistent basis. Most patients with Klippel-Trenaunay syndrome are poor surgical candidates, given the extensive distribution of the malformation. Occasionally, limited involvement can be surgically debulked, but microscopic peripheral involvement makes cure unlikely.

Hypertrophy of the lower extremity may also manifest itself as excessive limb length, and periodic plane films of the femur and tibia are used to document exact limb length. A shoe lift for the shorter leg may be prescribed by a pediatric orthopedic surgeon, and destruction of the growth plate (epiphysiodesis) may be indicated when the longer leg reaches predicted adult size.

Arteriovenous Malformations

Arteriovenous malformations are usually congenital, but acquired arteriovenous shunting can occur as the result of penetrating injuries and central line placement. These high-pressure, high-flow malformations can occur anywhere, and they are potentially dangerous as they progressively expand, particularly during puberty.

Clinical characteristics include a pulsatile mass with increased warmth, sometimes with an audible bruit. An arteriovenous malformation (AVM) may have an overlying capillary vascular malformation (Parkes-Weber syndrome). An MRI/MRA scan with contrast will provide the most information to formulate a treatment plan.

Complete surgical excision represents the best chance for cure, and preoperative embolization by an interventional radiologist on the day prior to surgery can limit surgical blood loss as well as provide a useful roadmap to aid surgical dissection (Figure 8-12). By staying just peripheral to the malformation, the surgeon can operate in normal tissues and avoid excessive bleeding. Feeding arterial branches outlined on the MRA scan or arteriogram can be sequentially ligated and divided. Extensive resections may require flap reconstruction or skin grafting to achieve closure.

Palliative, highly selective embolization by an interventional radiologist may be done periodically for facial AVM that are not problematic enough to warrant extensive extirpative and reconstructive surgery. Patients must

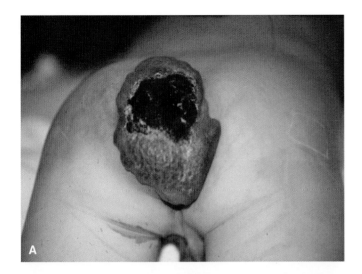

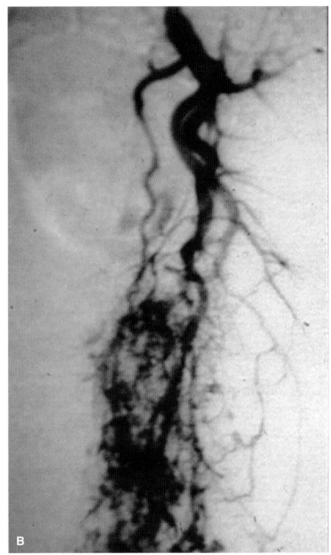

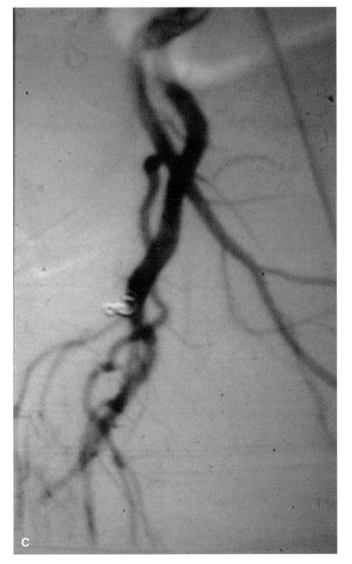

● FIGURE 8-12. (A–C) Arteriovenous malformations of the buttocks supplied by the middle sacral and internal iliac arteries. Preoperative embolization reduced intraoperative bleeding and provided a vascular roadmap to assist with surgical planning and complete excision.

understand that these procedures are not intended to be curative, but may decrease much of the flow, bulk, and discomfort associated with these malformations. The procedure avoids embolization of the external carotid artery itself, as this would only encourage collateral flow from the internal carotid or contralateral carotid system, making future embolization technically impossible or prohibitively dangerous.

Pyogenic Granulomas

Pyogenic granulomas are a true misnomer, being neither pyogenic nor granulomatous. They are more accurately termed lobular capillary hemangiomas, benign dermal vascular tumors that may arise from minor skin trauma. They can occur at any age, and are often seen in pregnant women, suggesting a hormonal component in their pathophysiology.

They present as shiny red papules with a fragile epidermal cover that ulcerates easily. Bleeding can be frighteningly excessive, and many patients present with silver nitrate stains and bandages (souvenirs of the local emergency room).

Surgical excision provides definitive treatment and a biopsy specimen, but at the cost of a surgical scar. Tangential excision followed by either KTP laser or electrocautery coagulation of the residual dermal proliferative vessels provides a biopsy specimen and often no perceptible scar (Figure 8-13). Complete destruction by electrocautery or laser without a biopsy may be curative, but it is medicolegally risky because it fails to provide a confirmatory pathology report.

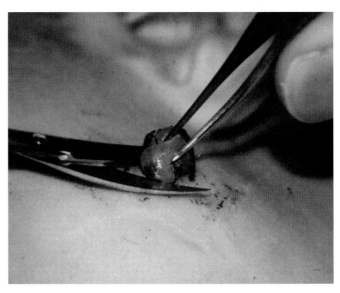

● **FIGURE 8-13.** Pyogenic granuloma of the cheek. Tangential biopsy followed by laser or electrocautery of the base has a high success rate and a scar that may be superior to excision and suture closure.

Angiofibromas

Patients with tuberous sclerosis develop erythematous papular lesions in a prominent butterfly distribution on the face, but also on the chin and alar regions. Historically called "adenoma sebaceum," they are neither adenomatous nor sebaceous and are instead fibrovascular nodules that are more accurately called angiofibromas. Although the pulsed yellow dye laser has been recommended for the hypervascular erythema, most patients and their parents are more concerned with the nodular skin irregularity. The carbon dioxide laser is very effective in vaporizing these lesions, using a slightly defocused 1 mm spot and 1 to 3 watts of power (Figure 8-14). Patients should expect about 2 weeks of crusting until each spot re-epithelializes. The treatments are palliative and completely smooth skin is an unrealistic expectation, but the degree of improvement can be dramatic. Recurrent angiofibromas can be periodically retreated.

Telangiectasias, Spider Angiomas, Cherry Angiomas, and Spider Veins

All of these vascular malformations are characterized by dilated dermal vessels that are readily apparent to the

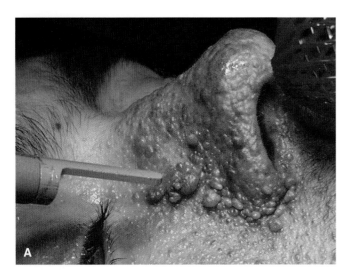

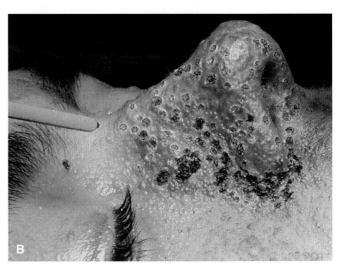

● **FIGURE 8-14.** (A, B) Angiofibromas associated with tuberous sclerosis can be easily vaporized with minimal bleeding using a carbon dioxide laser. Laser safety precautions include the use of protective scleral shields and a plume evacuator.

naked eye. Telangiectasias are often called "broken blood vessels" because they undulate at different depths within the dermis. Although the vessels are continuous, only the superficial segments are easily visualized. Spider angiomas have a central feeding arteriole that arborizes into many peripheral branches, similar to a tree trunk and its branches. They blanch with digital pressure, then fill readily from the central feeder out to the periphery when pressure is released. Cherry angiomas are dilated superficial dermal vessels that appear as papular red spots. Spider veins consist of small dilated dermal vessels that can appear on the nose, face, and legs.

Laser is a popular modality to treat all of these conditions, and there are a wide variety of vascular lesion lasers that are potentially effective. Pulsed yellow dye lasers rapidly cover large areas, and circular handpieces are generally preferred for discrete spots like cherry or spider angiomas, while the elliptical 3 × 10 mm handpiece is appropriate for tracing spider veins. Continuous wave lasers require meticulous yet rapid tracing of tiny spider veins, with care being taken to avoid prolonged energy delivery to any given spot to minimize the risk of burn injury. The patient should be aware of the need for multiple treatment sessions for best results, and realize that it is not possible to remove every spider vein and telangiectasia. On the other hand, spider angiomas and small cherry angiomas are commonly obliterated with a single laser treatment. Continuous wave lasers such as the KTP laser may be more effective than pulsed lasers in obliterating cherry angiomas as the heat penetrates throughout the vascular cluster.

Large spider veins, particularly on the nose and legs may be refractory to multiple laser treatments, and greater success may be achieved with either sclerotherapy, or the combination of sclerotherapy followed immediately by laser photocoagulation for a synergistic vascular insult.

Intense pulsed light may be effective for both small telangiectasias as well as benign melanocytic pigmentation, depending on the filters used to target oxyhemoglobin and melanin.

● COMPLICATIONS OF TREATMENT OF VASCULAR MALFORMATIONS

Laser therapy is basically selective thermal delivery to the abnormal vessels to cause intentional rupture or coagulation. Nonselective photothermolysis can occur with excessive energy delivered to the tissues. Blisters, ulceration, crusting, and scarring can occur when the energy density, the pulse duration, or the laser power setting is too high.

Sclerotherapy can cause cutaneous ulceration and tissue necrosis if the sclerosant is erroneously injected extravascularly, or if the sclerosant extravasates into the soft tissues. In addition to skin necrosis, muscle and nerve injury can occur, and depending on the type of sclerosant this may be permanent. More importantly, excessive intravascular injection can cause hemodynamic complications and death. Airway compromise from postsclerotherapy edema may require prolonged intubation when treating oropharyngeal venous and lymphatic malformations.

Embolization of the feeding arteries to treat AVMs can cause undesirable distal ischemia of unintended targets, particular when treating the extremities. When treating head and neck AVMs, the risk of potential stroke must be discussed with the patient.

Excessive bleeding during debulking procedures, especially with high-flow arteriovenous malformations or large venous or venolymphatic malformations, may warrant the use of a cell saver, and blood and plasma transfusions may be required. Patients should be advised of the potential need to abort the debulking procedure if life-threatening hemorrhage occurs.

Patients with large venous or venolymphatic malformations may have ongoing clotting issues (disseminated intravascular coagulation) which put them at risk for deep venous thrombosis and pulmonary embolism. Surgery and sclerotherapy may result in life-threatening thrombosis and embolism. Patients should be evaluated by a hematologist prior to their procedures, which may warrant lifetime anticoagulation therapy. Placement of a vena cava filter is not a guarantee against pulmonary embolism in the setting of venous malformations which may present atypical vascular anatomy that allows clots to bypass the filter.

REFERENCES

1. Meyerle JH. Dermatological manifestations of glomus tumors. http://www.emedicine.com/derm/topic167.htm. Updated Sept 17, 2010.

2. Kiel RJ. Milroy disease. http://www.emedicine.com/med/topic1482.htm. Updated June 21, 2006. Accessed August 30, 2006.

SUGGESTED READING

Arneja JS, Gosain AK. Vascular malformations. *Plast Reconstr Surg.* 2008;121(4):195e–206e. Huang JT, Liang MG. Vascular malformations. *Pediatr Clin North Am.* 2010;57(5): 1091–1110.

Marler JJ, Mulliken JB. Current management of hemangiomas and vascular malformations. *Clin Plast Surg.* 2005;32(1): 99–116.

chapter 9

Hemangiomas

David W. Low, MD / Richard L. Agag, MA, MD

● INTRODUCTION

Hemangiomas are the most common benign tumor of infancy, occurring in 10% of full-term babies and up to 25% of premature babies. Although hemangiomas can occur anywhere, the majority occur in the head and neck region, raising cosmetic as well as functional concerns. Whereas historically pediatricians involved plastics surgeons in the care of patients with persistent deformity in late childhood, nowadays with widespread access to the Internet and hemangioma support groups, parents are seeking early plastic surgical consultation and surgical solutions to this common vascular anomaly.

Natural History

Typical hemangiomas are not present at birth, but appear during the first few weeks of life. Dermal hemangiomas appear as bright red strawberry patches that gradually protrude above the surface of the skin. Subcutaneous hemangiomas are also composed of proliferating capillaries but appear blue in pigmentation due to their deeper location. Many hemangiomas have both a subcutaneous and dermal component (Figure 9-1). Hemangiomas may also occur in solid organs such as the parotid gland and liver. Large facial hemangiomas may be part of a constellations of anomalies designated by the mnemonic PHACES (**p**osterior cranial fossa abnormalities, **h**emangiomas, **a**rterial abnormalities, **c**oarctation of the aorta and other cardiac anomalies, **e**ye abnormalities, and **s**ternal clefting). Midline back hemangiomas may be associated with a tethered spinal cord.

Proliferation typically occurs over the first 6 to 12 months, followed by slow regression over many years. Regression is characterized by a change in pigmentation as the bright strawberry color gives way to grayish white, and the hemangioma becomes less engorged and decreases in size. Pediatricians tend to advise parents that most hemangiomas will disappear by age 5 years, but only 50% of patients will have completely regressed by that time (70% of hemangiomas fully regress by age 7 years). Although all hemangiomas will show regression, 30% will leave significant residual deformity in the form of redundant skin and excess fatty bulk that may warrant plastic surgical intervention. More importantly, cosmetically important areas, such as the eyelids, nose, lips, and cheek, seem to have a much higher risk of leaving significant deformity, creating not only great concern amongst parents, but also the potential for litigation if parents feel an alternative management strategy might have resulted in less deformity.

Nonsurgical Therapy for Hemangiomas

Pediatric plastic surgeons are in a unique position to become the primary treating physicians for young infants with proliferating hemangiomas, as they can offer the entire spectrum of treatment options. In many cases first-line therapy is medical rather than surgical, and consists of systemic or intralesional steroid therapy. Steroid therapy may significantly decrease the degree of residual deformity, and although it may not remove the need for later reconstructive surgery, it may simplify the complexity of the surgical procedure and increase the chance for a successful outcome.

Oral prednisolone is commonly used for airway or vision-threatening hemangiomas, but it is also widely used for potentially disfiguring hemangiomas of the face. Nasal and lip hemangiomas routinely leave permanent deformity and most parents readily opt for steroid suppression to limit the degree of deformity. Orapred is commonly prescribed as it is reportedly the most palatable and more concentrated than other oral preparations. The starting dose is 2 to 4 mg/kg/d, usually mixed with the morning bottle. Most patients will show obvious signs of regression

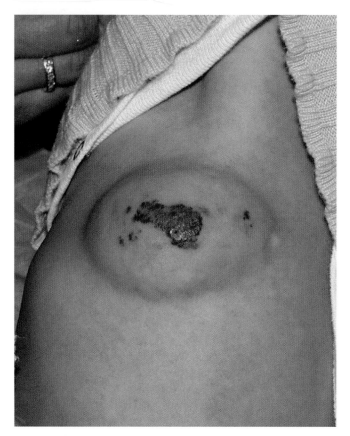

● FIGURE 9-1. Typical compound hemangioma with both a central dermal and a subcutaneous component.

as-needed basis is certainly easier than daily oral administration, but there is no evidence that it avoids systemic side effects. Injection is unlikely to distribute the medication uniformly within the tumor, and it is not appropriate for large hemangiomas.

Recent Medical Advances

Propranolol, used as a non-selective, beta-adrenergic receptor blocker in young children with cardiologic indications, was observed serendipitously to have dramatic effects on the growth of hemangiomas. Due to the variable response rates of systemic corticosteroid therapy (range 30%–60%) and side effects, excitement has grown over this new therapy. After the sentinel case report, multiple case reports and then a larger follow-up report by the initial authors has shown much promise; however, much of the details still need to be worked out. In this follow-up study, because of the potential side effects, the children were admitted into the hospital for a 24-hour period and the drug was administered 2 mg/kg/d divided over two to three doses. The responses to the drug were remarkable (Figure 9-2). Included in these 32 patients were 13 infants who had shown no response or at best stabilization of the lesion after treatment with systemic corticosteroids. Within 24 hours of treatment of propranolol, therapeutic effects were seen, including change in color and softening of the lesions.

Yet another case report showed treatment of a multicentric airway hemangioma with rapid regression and resolution of symptoms. This subset of children often suffer from symptoms such as stridor, breathing difficulties, feeding difficulties, respiratory distress, barking cough, hoarseness, and acute airway obstruction. The patient in this case suffered from biphasic stridor, which improved over the course of 10 days after administration of propranolol. Reduction in bulk and improved subglottic stenosis was confirmed by repeat laryngotracheobronchoscopy 1 week after initiation of the drug.

However, use of propranolol does not come without risk, although seemingly less than that of corticosteroids. FDA labeling indicates that safety and effectiveness of propranolol have not been established in pediatric patients. The most common hemodynamic side effects are bradycardia and hypotension. Hypoglycemia is also another reported side effect. There is also a subset of patients that are at risk for high-output cardiac failure. These include patients with posterior fossa brain malformations, cardiac abnormalities, and suspected PHACES (segmental facial hemangioma) to name a few. These patients require a careful premedication screening and clearance.

Little is known about how propranolol directly affects hemangiomas; however, there is data on the mechanism of action of the drug to which these effects can be attributed. Specifically, how propranolol interferes with endothelial cells, vascular tone, angiogenesis, and apoptosis. Early effects (brightening of the hemangioma surface within 1–3 days)

within a week. Although steroid tapering schedules vary by physician, it is usually easiest for parents to taper the dose every 1 to 2 weeks in easily measured increments. Parents should be advised that infants may require steroid therapy for many months, and at lower steroid dosages rebound growth may necessitate a temporary increase in dose and a more gradual taper. Side effects commonly include a change in appetite, increased irritability, gastrointestinal upset, cushingoid facies, and a plateau in growth, all of which are temporary and reversible. Hypertension may necessitate a more rapid taper or the addition of antihypertensive therapy. Live, attenuated virus vaccinations (measles, mumps, rubella, and chicken pox) should be withheld until steroid therapy has been discontinued for a month.

To decrease the risk of gastrointestinal upset associated with steroid therapy, Zantac liquid is administered orally 3 mg/kg/d until steroids are discontinued.

The ophthalmologic literature supports the potential benefit of triamcinolone (Kenalog-40) as an intralesional injection for periorbital hemangiomas. The risk of potential embolization of the steroid suspension to the retinal artery with subsequent blindness suggests that steroid injection in this area be limited to ophthalmologists and oculoplastic surgeons. However, small discrete hemangiomas in other parts of the face or body can be carefully injected by plastic surgeons. Intralesional injection on a monthly

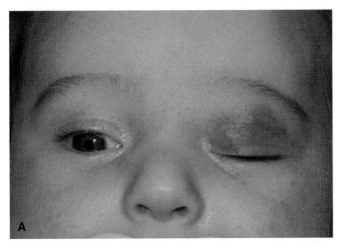 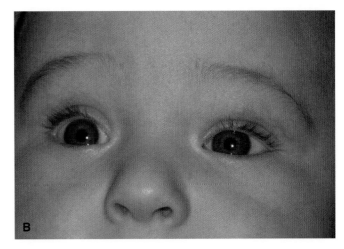

● FIGURE 9-2. Patient at 3 months of age with a left eyelid hemangioma. Improvement after 1 months of propranolol treatment. (*Photographs courtesy of Albert Yan, MD, Department of Dermatology, Children's Hospital of Philadelphia.*)

are attributed to vasoconstriction due to decrease nitrous oxide release. Intermediate effects are due to blocking of pre-angiogenic signals (vascular endothelial growth factor, basic fibroblast growth factor, matrix metalloproteinases 2/9), which result in arrest of growth. Long-term effects are the result of apoptosis in proliferating cells, which results in tumor regression.

We have developed a protocol at the Children's Hospital of Philadelphia which included contributions from multiple specialties. Our relative contraindications to propranolol include history of hypersensitivity to beta-blocker therapy, ischemic intracranial anomalies, structural cardiac abnormalities, decrease cardiac output, and active hypoglycemia or reactive airway disease. Patients with these conditions require a more extensive workup including a cardiology consult. We do not routinely consult cardiology before initiation of propranolol unless contraindications to the therapy are elucidated after history, physical examination, and electrocardiogram. Parents need to be made aware of the off-label nature of treatment during the consent process. The patient is admitted to the ICU setting or inpatient hospital floor based on risk stratification. Baseline vitals are taken and then propranolol treatment is initiated at 0.5 mg/kg/d divided in three doses. Blood glucose levels measurements are taken 1 hour after each of the first two doses. Day 2 and day 3 of hospital admission include increasing the dosage to 1 mg/kg/d to 2 mg/kg/d with continued monitoring of blood glucose levels, blood pressure, and heart rate. If suboptimal results are obtained, doses may be escalated to 3 to 5 mg/kg/d in 0.5 to 1 mg/kg/d increments. After target dose has been achieved, heart rate and blood pressure monitoring is recommended weekly or biweekly in an ambulatory setting. Anticipation is that the propranolol therapy may be necessary for approximately 3 to 6 months, or until the child is 6 to 12 months of age.

● SURGICAL TREATMENT OF HEMANGIOMAS

Patient Evaluation and Selection

The vast majority of hemangiomas do not require urgent surgical intervention during the proliferative phase and never come to the attention of a plastic surgeon until pediatricians and pediatric dermatologists refer those with inadequate involution for debulking and scar revision. However, if life-threatening subglottic hemangiomas with airway obstruction and periorbital hemangiomas with visual obstruction respond poorly to steroid suppression, they may require urgent debulking surgery, usually by otolaryngologists and oculoplastic surgeons, respectively. Intrahepatic hemangiomas associated with high-output cardiac failure may require selective embolization by an interventional radiologist if steroid therapy is ineffective.

Urgent plastic surgical intervention may be needed for ulcerated hemangiomas that have eroded into an artery large enough to cause significant hemorrhage, periorbital hemangiomas that are causing visual obstruction and decreased visual acuity, large lip hemangiomas that are interfering with feeding, and occasionally, ulcerated hemangiomas of the lips and perineum that are causing excruciating pain.

Elective plastic surgical intervention is appropriate for hemangiomas that are destined to leave significant residual deformity in the form of redundant skin, fibrofatty bulk, significant dermal fibrosis, scarring alopecia of the scalp, distortion of involved facial features, and potential functional problems anywhere on the body (Figure 9-3).

Patient Preparation

Timing. While it is technically feasible to operate on any patient with a significant hemangioma as soon as they

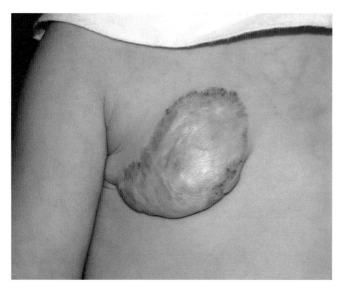

● FIGURE 9-3. Involuted chest hemangioma that has left residual fibrofatty tissue and redundant skin. Excision is indicated since the anticipated contour benefit outweighs the anticipated surgical scar.

present for consultation, one should take into consideration how far along the course of its natural history the hemangioma has progressed. Although it is a continuum, one can semi-arbitrarily divide the clinical course into multiple phases:

1. Proliferative phase—the hemangioma is still actively growing without any signs of regression.
2. Early involutional phase—the hemangioma shows signs of pigmentary lightening and reduced turgor, suggested a diminution in blood flow, but still fills readily after compression.
3. Mid involutional phase—the hemangioma still has some flow, fills slowly after compression, and much of its vascular pigmentation is gone.
4. Late involutional phase or completely involuted—the flow has essentially stopped, leaving stable fibrofatty tissue and redundant skin without any expectation of further improvement.
5. RICH—*r*apidly *i*nvoluting *c*ongenital *h*emangiomas
6. NICH—*n*on*i*nvoluting *c*ongenital *h*emangiomas

Proliferative Phase. Hemangiomas in the very early proliferative phase are candidates for conservative observation, laser, or steroids, but surgical excision is rarely indicated as one cannot predict the growth of the hemangioma and excision will always leave a scar. Additionally, many hemangiomas proliferate over an extensive area and removal of a small nidus will not reliably prevent peripheral growth.

Biopsy of an atypical hemangioma is indicated in the proliferative phase to rule out a more aggressive vascular tumor such as a kaposiform hemangioendothelioma or vascular malignancy, or a soft tissue malignancy. Kaposiform hemangioendotheliomas tend to feel harder than hemangiomas and are associated with thrombocytopenia (Kasabach-Merritt syndrome).

Hemangiomas that are well into their proliferative phase and are causing significant disfigurement and parental anxiety must be carefully evaluated, and the risks and benefits of early excision must be thoroughly weighed.

Ulcerated hemangiomas with significant hemorrhage may be urgently controlled with a hemostatic suture. Excruciatingly painful ulcers can be palliated with 2% lidocaine jelly. Ulcerated hemangiomas always leave a cutaneous scar, and therefore small problematic hemangiomas can be excised, and parents will readily accept the surgical scar in exchange for peace of mind.

Early Involutional Phase. Hemangiomas that have stopped growing will take years to naturally regress, and parents' eagerness to resolve the problem as soon as possible must be weighed against the risks of general anesthesia, the increased risk of perioperative bleeding, and the chance that the permanent surgical scar will be more disfiguring than natural involution. A linear central cheek scar may be far more noticeable than a flat patch of atrophic skin, and the overly aggressive plastic surgeon may be doing his young patient a lifelong disservice by operating too early. Pedunculated hemangiomas will almost certainly leave excessive skin and soft tissue, and can be considered for early excision. Hemangiomas that are too large to be completely excised in a single stage may be better left to a later year when the risk of hemorrhage and wound dehiscence is lower.

Mid-Involutional Phase. The majority of hemangioma excisions take place during this period, when it is obvious that the hemangioma is not going to regress satisfactorily, and the risk of intraoperative hemorrhage is lower as the blood flow has decreased. If the procedure can be done without the risk of needing a transfusion and with minimal risk of injury to local vital structures, then there is no need to make the parents wait for complete involution.

Late or Complete Involutional Phase. These patients usually have excess skin and/or bulky fibrofatty tissue and few residual vessels. Therefore, it is much easier to estimate how much tissue to excise or leave behind, and ancillary procedures such as liposuction or tissue expansion can be planned without risk of excessive bleeding.

RICH—Rapidly Involuting Congenital Hemangiomas. A small subset of hemangiomas appear to demonstrate in utero growth and accelerated regression during the first year of life. Rapid involution may be associated with problematic ulceration and central tissue necrosis. Treatment should be individualized and the timing of surgical intervention can follow the same guidelines as for typical hemangiomas.

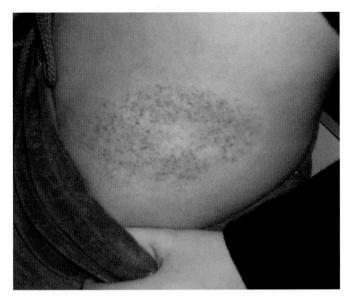

● FIGURE 9-4. NICH—noninvoluting congenital hemangioma. These hemangiomas show no tendency to regress and are characterized by bluish pigmentation and small cutaneous ectatic vessels. Surgical excision is curative.

NICH—Noninvoluting Congenital Hemangiomas. Another subset of hemangiomas that do not follow the expected course of typical hemangiomas show no tendency to involute. They often have the clinical appearance of bluish subcutaneous masses with small cutaneous telangiectasias and increased warmth to palpation (Figure 9-4). Elective excision is curative.

Laser Considerations

A variety of vascular lesion lasers that target oxyhemoglobin may be useful in treating hemangiomas, predominantly in the early proliferative or the late involutional phases. The laser energy is absorbed by dermal blood vessels, resulting in either rupture or coagulation, depending on whether the laser delivers pulses or a continuous beam of light.

Pulsed Yellow Dye Lasers. The current fourth generation yellow dye laser (Perfecta Vbeam) has a wavelength of 595 nm, handpieces that range from 5 to 12 mm, adjustable power density and pulse duration, and a cryogen spray that decreases the discomfort of the laser pulse and provides a protective coolant effect that decreases the risk of epidermal damage. Initially developed for the treatment of port wine stains, this laser has applicability for early proliferating hemangiomas, ulcerated hemangiomas, and involuted hemangiomas with persistent ectatic vessels. The laser light penetrates no more than 1 to 2 mm into the dermis; therefore, it is most effective for flat dermal hemangiomas. It may completely abort small hemangiomas, significantly shrink larger hemangiomas, and decrease the pain of ulcerated hemangiomas.

Parents should be advised that hemangiomas may show rebound growth after 2 to 4 weeks, and a series of treatments may be needed until permanent involution occurs. The manufacturer supplies a cookbook recipe of suggested treatment parameters. The practitioner should be aware that overly aggressive laser treatment can actually cause ulceration and scarring; therefore, conservative power settings may be preferable during the initial laser session.

Residual vascular pigmentation in the form of telangiectasias and spider veins following complete involution may respond to a series of pulsed yellow dye laser treatments (Figure 9-5). Sclerotherapy for larger residual vessels can be combined with laser treatment for a synergistic benefit. Intravascular sclerosis followed immediately by laser photocoagulation may significantly obliterate persistent vessels.

KTP and Nd:YAG Lasers. Continuous beam lasers such as the Nd:YAG laser (1064 nm) and the KTP laser (532 nm) (Laserscope) offer deeper penetration and vascular coagulation, but risk cutaneous scarring from nonspecific heat delivery to the tissues. Although fiberoptic insertion into the hemangioma has been described for deep coagulation, the amount of energy delivery is difficult to quantify and the technique is heavily operator dependent.

General Techniques

The vast majority of hemangiomas are excised like nevi, the circular or oval wound converted into an elliptical (spindle) shape to avoid excessive dog ears at the ends of the linear closure. Although the orientation of the ellipse is readily apparent for most hemangiomas, areas like the glabella are often unpredictable, and it is preferable to excise these hemangioma as a circle and then manipulate the wound margins to determine the best direction of closure.

Hemangiomas with both a central dermal and a larger subcutaneous component can be debulked by incising around the border of the dermal portion and then using this opening to remove the deeper portion, analogous to a skin-sparing mastectomy.

It is not always desirable to remove the entire hemangioma, particularly when the dermal part extends into cosmetically important areas or complete excision will leave a soft tissue deficiency. Bipolar cautery may be extremely useful when it is necessary to debulk a hemangioma with active vessels.

Fully involuted hemangiomas with subcutaneous bulk and minimal residual circulation are often amenable to suction-assisted lipectomy when skin excision is not necessary.

Although circular excision followed by purse-string closure has been advocated to try to minimize the size of the surgical scar, the prolonged pleating and potential need for a second stage excision have made this approach less attractive to most surgeons.

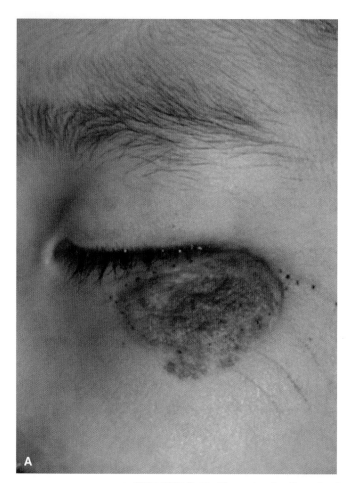 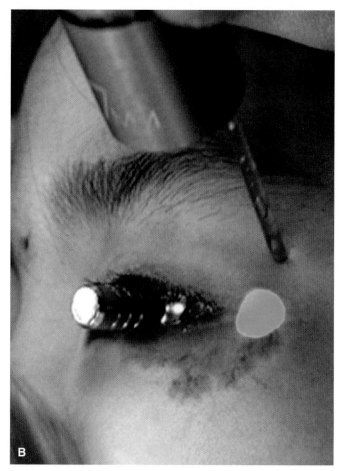

● **FIGURE 9-5.** The pulsed yellow dye laser can remove residual hemangioma vessels in situations where complete excision is contraindicated. An ellipse of redundant hemangioma is initially excised, orienting the scar along the natural wrinkle lines, followed at a later date by Vbeam photocoagulation.

Region-specific Techniques

Periorbital. Similar to cosmetic blepharoplasty, redundant upper or lower eyelid skin with subcutaneous bulk can be excised using elliptical incisions, with care being taken to avoid excessive skin excision. Extensive brow hemangiomas may lead to scarring alopecia and loss of eyebrow hair, or expanded skin with distorted brows and inadequate hair density. Micrografting or scalp strip grafts can be used to reconstruct missing eyebrows. Micropigmentation may be preferable to hair transplantation to restore eyebrow contour if one is unwilling to deal with the constant trimming needed for transplanted scalp hair.

Significant upper eyelid scarring may benefit from a large full-thickness skin graft applied to the entire aesthetic unit. A graft of sufficient size and excellent color match can be prefabricated by tissue expanding the post-auricular donor site.

More complicated deformities of the lids such as true ptosis or missing tissue are beyond the scope of this chapter and may be better left to the expertise of ophthalmologists and oculoplastic surgeons.

Nasal. Nasal hemangiomas may occur anywhere along the nose and can create significant permanent deformities of the nasal ala, alar base, nasal tip, nasal dorsum, radix, and paranasal regions. Nasal tip hemangiomas commonly act as tissue expanders that create redundant tip skin, splay the alar cartilage, and leave behind bulky fat—the "Cyrano deformity." Steroid therapy may significantly reduce the severity of the deformity and is highly recommended to facilitate later reconstruction. It may be exceedingly difficult to normalize the appearance of tip hemangiomas that have created marked skin redundancy and dermal scarring. Most parents are anxious to have the nasal tip debulked prior to complete involution, so usually the procedure requires cutting through active bleeding vessels.

The basic strategy in nasal tip reconstruction involves removal of redundant skin, removal of excess hemangioma or redundant subcutaneous tissue, and centralization of the alar domes. Although a wide variety of patterns exist, a particularly useful technique is analogous to an open rhinoplasty approach, except that the rim incisions are externally placed to permit removal of redundant skin (Figure 9-6). The hemangioma is left attached to

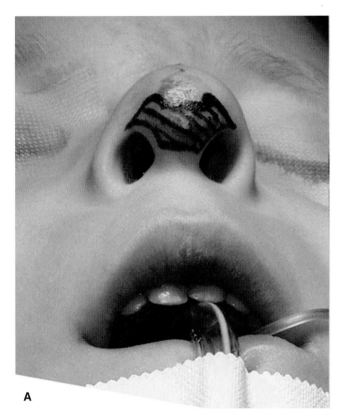 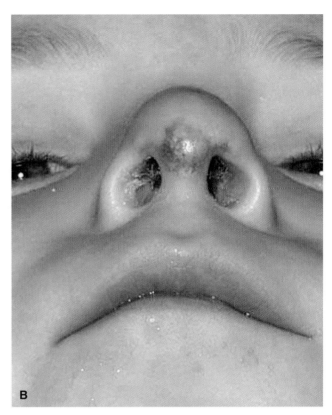

● **FIGURE 9-6.** Modified, open rhinoplasty approach to nasal tip hemangiomas. This provides excellent exposure of the tip cartilage for centralization of the domes, facilitates judicious tip debulking and excision of redundant skin, and leaves a favorable scar.

the overlying skin as the alar domes and lateral crura are exposed. Clear monofilament suture is used to centralize the domes. Excess hemangioma tissue is excised but it is essential to leave some attached to the overlying dermis for future subcutaneous padding. Aggressive removal and combined with ongoing hemangioma regression can leave thin atrophic skin with inadequate subcutaneous tissue. Lastly redundant skin is excised, leaving a scar in the naturally shaded underside of the nose.

If there is minimal excess skin, the hemangioma can be debulked through internal nasal incisions, or via small crescent-shaped nasal rim incisions (Figure 9-7). Again, it is important to avoid excessive debulking that may leave long-term contour deficiency.

Lip. Lip hemangiomas rarely regress satisfactorily, and therefore the presence of a lip hemangioma is a relative indication for steroid therapy. Many lip hemangiomas are transmural, extending from the vermilion or dermis, through the orbicularis, to just beneath the mucosa. Vermilion involvement frequently leads to ulceration and subsequent scarring. Despite some improvement with regression, the majority of patients are left with excess bulk and significant distortion. The vermilion border is often involved and obliterated by the expanding hemangioma.

The approach to upper lip hemangiomas involves many of the principles of cleft lip repair. Debulking procedures create an iatrogenic cleft deformity, and accurate preoperative marking are essential to identify key anatomic landmarks and determine the amount of tissue that needs to be removed. Fully regressed hemangiomas that have left excessive but stable soft tissue are easier to gauge than hemangiomas in mid-involution, in which case the surgeon must allow for some additional loss of volume through natural regression. Furthermore suture lines are at risk for partial dehiscence and delayed healing if one is approximating skin edges involved with hemangioma-infiltrated dermis.

Cupid's bow marking are made as best as possible, and if the hemangioma is unilateral, the uninvolved side is used as a template. Unlike a cleft lip, the involved side is too large, and therefore the philtral column and lip height need to be shortened by removing triangular wedges of tissue. Commonly a full thickness vertical wedge of upper lip is removed to decrease the width of the involved side, followed by a multilayered closure (Figure 9-8).

Hemangiomas involving only the vermilion may be excised with vertically oriented ellipses, leaving scars that mimic natural lip creases. A T-shaped closure, with the crossbar hidden inside the transition to wet mucosa may

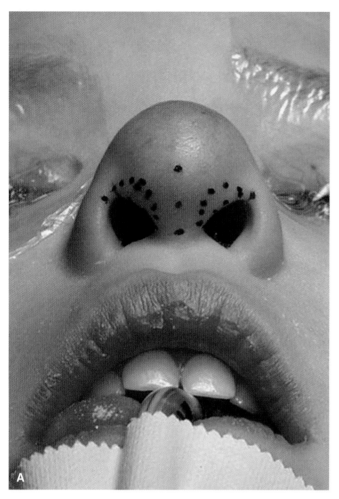
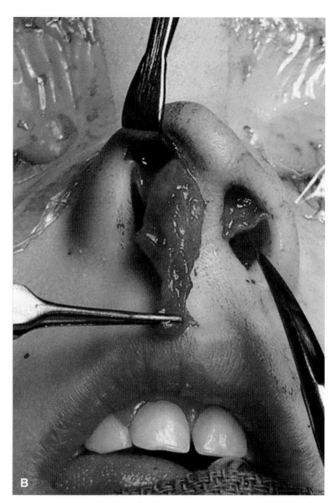

● **FIGURE 9-7.** Similar to a bilateral cleft nasal repair, hemangiomas with limited skin redundancy can be debulked using crescent-shaped rim incisions. The splayed tip cartilage can then be sutured together to improve tip projection.

be useful for larger hemangiomas with excessive vermilion. Hemangiomas along the free vermilion margin can be excised with a horizontally oriented ellipse, to completely hide the surgical scar.

Lower lip hemangiomas may also require wedge excisions to shorten excessively wide lips. Alternatively, a transverse ellipse is useful for hemangiomas that cross the vermilion border, strategically placing the mucosa/skin suture line along the obliterated vermilion border.

Ear. Significant ear distortion and redundant skin can result from periauricular hemangiomas, but it is important to realize that hemangiomas in this area often regress remarkably, leaving only atrophic skin. It may be advisable to wait until mid to late involution to avoid overcorrection and deficient soft tissue bulk, particularly with the lobule. Staged excision may be useful to palliate a severe deformity, postponing the final stage until after complete involution. A protruding or lop ear deformity from a bulky

postauricular hemangioma may warrant early excision and conservative splinting to prevent a permanent deformity.

Cheek/Parotid. Cheek hemangiomas may occur in the dermis and/or subcutaneous layer only, or they may commonly involve the parotid gland. Bilateral parotid involvement is usually an indication for steroid suppression to avoid external ear canal obstruction and hearing problems. Hemangiomas with both a dermal and a subcutaneous component will often leave a patch of atrophic scar or redundant skin and subcutaneous fat, and therefore the use of systemic or intralesional steroids may be justified. Purely subcutaneous or intraparotid hemangiomas of small to moderate size, without a skin component, may regress completely with excellent cosmetic results. Conservative observation is recommended and a surgical scar can usually be avoided.

Large parotid or subcutaneous hemangiomas may act as tissue expanders and create redundant skin. The potential

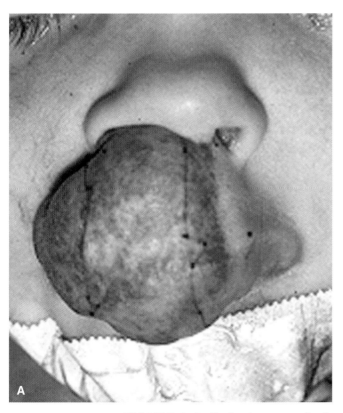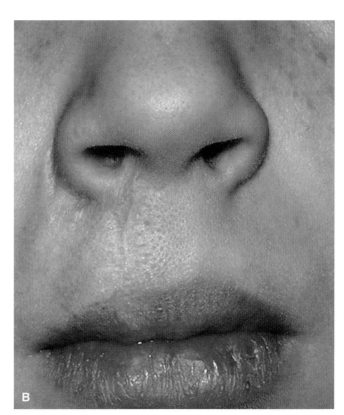

● **FIGURE 9-8.** Redundant upper lip tissue often requires a full-thickness wedge excision. The closure pattern is analogous to a cleft lip repair, with strategic cuts designed to reestablish symmetry.

benefit of steroid suppression should be weighed against the risks of steroid therapy. Often a unilateral facelift approach can address the problem of redundant cheek skin, but only if the skin envelope exceeds the expected volume of the growing face.

Medially and centrally located cheek hemangiomas can be excised at the expense of obvious linear scars. Parents and patients may be advised to postpone surgery until it is certain that the hemangioma is going to leave a contour deformity that is more noticeable than the surgical scar. Trying to strategically place the scar along the nasolabial fold may be useful for medially located hemangiomas. Large, relatively flat cheek hemangiomas with textural irregularities may be better candidates for laser skin resurfacing or dermabrasion than surgical excision. If excision is felt to be the best option, staged excision may be preferable to a single procedure that may result in excessive scar widening due to a tight closure.

Tissue expansion may be useful to replace large areas of dermal scar, particularly in children with extensive cervico-facial hemangiomas (Figure 9-9). The technique is similar to burn scar reconstruction. Pre-expanded rotation flaps may offer more creative options than direct excision. As with tissue expansion for burns or giant congenital nevi, all the risks and benefits of tissue expanders must be discussed with the parents.

● **COMPLICATIONS: AVOIDANCE AND MANAGEMENT**

The greatest controversy in the surgical treatment of hemangiomas relates to the timing of the procedure. Small hemangiomas can be safely removed at any age with minimal risk of bleeding, but judgment must be exercised to decide which hemangiomas may spontaneously resolve without needing excision. Larger hemangiomas may risk perioperative hemorrhage, nerve injury, and wound healing complications, particularly in the case of large facial hemangiomas that cannot be completely excised. Overly anxious parents and overconfident surgeons may be doing their young patients a disservice by operating too early. Over-resection may result in soft tissue deficiency. Hemangiomas of the breast should generally be followed conservatively in girls to avoid injury to the developing breast bud.

From a medicolegal standpoint, parents must be advised of all treatment options, whether they be medical or surgical, and unrealistic expectations must be discouraged. Facial hemangiomas commonly leave permanent deformities despite the best efforts of treating pediatricians, dermatologists, and surgeons, and parents should never be admonished or led to believe they did not offer their children the standard of care.

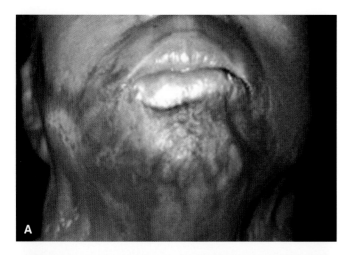

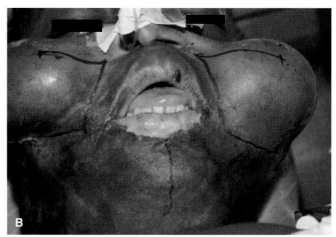

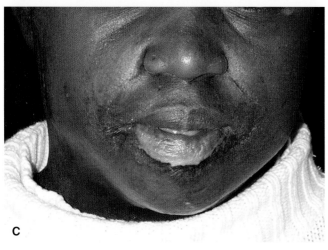

● **FIGURE 9-9.** Extensive cervico-facial scarring from a large ulcerated hemangioma. Bilateral cheek expanders provide good quality skin flaps for lower facial skin replacement.

SUGGESTED READING

Frieden IJ, Haggstrom A, Drolet BA, et al. Infantile hemangiomas: current knowledge, future directions: proceedings of a research workshop on infantile hemangiomas. *Pediatr Dermatol.* 2005; 22(5):383–406.

Lawley LP, Siegfried E, Todd JL. Propranolol treatment for hemangioma of infancy: risks and recommendations. *Pediatr Dermatol.* 2009;26(5):610–614.

Marler JJ, Mulliken JB. Current management of hemangiomas and vascular malformations. *Clin Plast Surg.* 2005;32(1): 99–116.

Sans V, Dumas de la Roque E, Berge J, et al. Propranolol for severe infantile hemangiomas: follow-up report. *Pediatrics.* 2009;124:e423–e431.

chapter 10

Burn Reconstruction

Brian M. Parrett, MD / Julian J. Pribaz, MD

PATIENT EVALUATION AND SELECTION

The goal of burn reconstruction is restoration of function and appearance. Reconstruction is aimed at the correction of tissue deficiency and deformity manifested as contractures, hypertrophic scarring, or exposed structures.

A single patient will often have multiple needs and their chief complaints and deformities should be analyzed, noting damaged tissue as well as unburned tissue. Functional reconstruction is the priority followed by aesthetic reconstruction. Procedures should be divided into urgent, essential, or desired. Urgent procedures include eyelid contracture release and coverage of exposed bone or tendons. Essential procedures restore function. Desirable procedures improve appearance. In general, nonurgent reconstruction should be delayed for more than 1 year to allow scar maturation and maximization of conservative management.

If the patient can tolerate a procedure medically and emotionally, there are few, if any, contraindications to burn reconstruction. Reconstruction should continue until the patient is satisfied or the surgeon has no procedures left to offer that can improve the patient's appearance or function.

PATIENT PREPARATION

Patient preparation begins with the prioritization of reconstructive needs. A set of carefully planned procedures, often occurring over many years, should be developed; proper sequence is important—don't "burn bridges." Planning should involve all burn team members, patients, and their families. Realistic goals and expectations must be explained to the patient.

General anesthesia is appropriate for most procedures. Donor sites should be identified and rationed prior to the procedure. Patients should be positioned to allow access to the burnt areas and donor sites. Sterile technique is essential as the potential for infection is high.

Essential equipment will vary depending on the procedure. Generally, a dermatome, electrocautery, bolster dressing supplies, and splinting devices should be available.

SURGICAL TREATMENTS

Reconstructive Ladder

Surgical treatments are aimed at scar revision, contracture release and coverage of exposed structures. The reconstructive ladder, considering the simplest procedure to achieve the desired result before using more complex alternatives, guides burn reconstruction.[1] It is not uncommon to utilize every modality of the ladder in the reconstruction of multiple deformities in a single patient.

Direct Closure. Excision of a burn scar followed by primary closure is the first option in scar revision. One should orient scars parallel to relaxed skin tension lines and approximate the dermis properly.

Z-plasty. Z-plasty lengthens the line of contracture (Figure 10-1). In a simple z-plasty, three lines of equal length are made with the central limb on the line of tension. The angles between the central and lateral lines should be less than 90 degrees and equal to each other. The resulting two triangular flaps are mobilized and transposed. The flap bases will then lie along the line formerly occupied by the central limb, resulting in a gain of length along the scar. The greater the angle between the central and lateral lines, the greater the length gain, but the more difficult the transposition. Within these limits, a variety of z-plastys are possible (Figure 10-1).

Skin Grafts. Scar and contracture incisional or excisional release with skin autograft coverage is the mainstay of burn reconstruction. The release should penetrate through the burn scar to the normal tissue underneath. An incision can

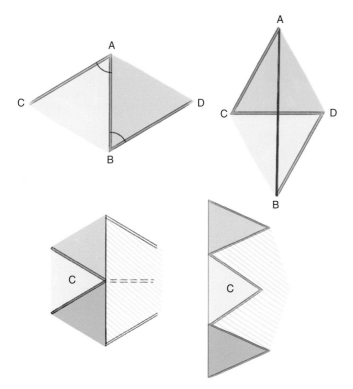

● **FIGURE 10-1.** (Upper Row) A simple z-plasty is designed with diagonal lines *(AC* and *BD)* drawn at 60-degree angles to the central limb, which is along the scar band *(AB)*. The triangular flaps and the surrounding skin are undermined. The flaps are transposed and the length of the wound *(red line)* is increased. (Lower Row) A 5-flap z-plasty places two opposing z-plastys along the same band, such that they are mirror images. This results in a central flap *(C)*, which inserts additional tissue into the band. The flaps of the z-plastys are transposed and the central flap advanced in a Y-V fashion, providing a gain in length.

often release a contracture, whereas a full excision of a scar may leave a better aesthetic result.

Donor sites should be of similar texture, thickness, and color to the recipient site. The nearer the donor site to the recipient, the better the match. Recipient site hemostasis is essential. Full-thickness skin grafts (FTSG) are preferred as they are less likely to contract and resemble normal skin better than split-thickness skin grafts (STSG). However, STSG, preferably at least 0.016 inches in thickness in adult patients, are less limited by donor site availability and work well in most situations. STSG may be applied as sheet or mesh grafts harvested with a dermatome, but mesh grafts generally have poorer aesthetic results. The graft should be secured with chromic gut sutures or staples and a bolster placed to immobilize the graft. A vacuum-assisted closure device (eg, V.A.C.) can also be used as a bolster at a pressure of 100 mm Hg. The bolster is usually removed after 4 to 5 days for a STSG and longer after a FTSG, reflecting the longer time for graft revascularization.

Tissue Expansion and Flaps. Tissue expanders are implanted into a nearby subcutaneous tissue pocket 1 cm larger than expander, and inflated with saline over several weeks, thus expanding the skin peripheral to the scar. The length of the expander should be at least the length of the defect to be covered and should result in an expanded dome 2.5 to 3.0 times the width of the defect. The expanded skin is then used as a FTSG, a regional advancement flap or a free flap.

Local and free flaps are useful in select difficult wounds, including extensive neck contractures, flexural contractures, and areas of exposed bone, tendon, or joints. Generally, local flaps are the first option followed by free flaps. Thin fasciocutaneous flaps are preferable in the head, neck, and hand while musculocutaneous flaps are often needed in the lower extremity. Most flaps will require future debulking for thinning.

Prefabrication and prelamination expand the flap options in burn reconstruction and are utilized when conventional flaps are not feasible.[2] Prefabrication involves the implantation of a vascular pedicle into a new territory followed by a period of maturation of 6 to 8 weeks and then flap transfer based on the new pedicle. Flaps may be prefabricated at a distant site by transferring a vascular pedicle to a more superficial location with a goal to create thin flaps; the flap is then transferred as a free flap in a second operation. Alternatively, flaps can be prefabricated near the recipient site to match color and texture by the local or free transfer of a vascular pedicle. The flap is then rotated into the defect. This is especially useful for facial reconstruction using the neck, scalp, supraclavicular and retroauricular skin. Pretransfer expansion of free and prefabricated flaps is useful as it expands and thins donor skin, often allowing primary closure of the donor site.

Head and Neck Burn Reconstruction

Excision and grafting is required in acute deep partial thickness or full thickness facial burns and post-burn facial scar reconstruction.[3] Excisions should be performed as aesthetic units (Figure 10-2) and grafts placed with seams at the unit boundaries.[4] FTSGs are preferable, but unmeshed thick STSGs may be used and should be 0.018 to 0.021 inches thick in adults and 0.008 to 0.012 inches thick in children. For best color match, grafts and flaps are preferably harvested from nearby donor sites, above the nipple line, including the neck, post- and preauricular area, and supraclavicular area. Bolster dressings are applied to provide compression to enhance graft take and prevent hematomas.

The following are common cervicofacial burn deformities and reconstruction approaches.[1-3,5]

Eyelid Contractures. Perform ectropion release in a timely fashion to prevent any exposure keratopathy. Make releasing incisions 2 mm from the ciliary margin and extend lateral to the lateral canthus and medial to the medial canthus. Avoid injury to the orbicularis oculi muscle and do not violate the supratarsal fold in the upper eyelid. Apply a FTSG for the upper lid, which may be harvested from

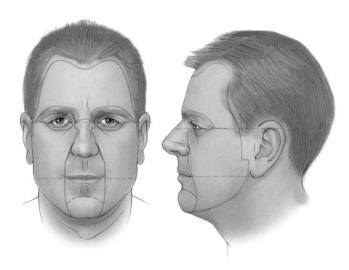

● **FIGURE 10-2.** Face reconstruction proceeds according to the aesthetic units of the face shown in the image.

the contralateral upper lid or retroauricular area. A FTSG is used for the lower lid, harvested from the retroauricular area. Apply grafts with the eyelids pulled by traction sutures and fix with bolsters. Perform upper and lower lids as separate procedures.

Perioral Contractures. Perioral contractures are best treated once the scars have matured. However, microstomia causing diminished oral opening should be treated early. A release of the oral commissure contracture can be performed with a transverse skin incision with a T or Y lateral extension followed by an intraoral mucosal advancement flap.

For upper lip ectropion, an incisional release is made along both nasolabial folds and the base of the nose. The lip should fall back into its normal position and a FTSG is applied. Reconstruction of the philtrum is best performed with a composite cartilage and skin graft from the triangular fossa of the ear. An everted lower lip release should proceed with an incision at the vermilion scar junction and must be released fully so that all of the teeth are covered. The underlying scar, especially from the labiomental crease, can often be used as a local turnover flap to augment the chin and help accentuate the labiomental crease. A FTSG is then placed to cover the entire subunit (Figure 10-3). Chin implants can help reestablish chin projection in select cases.

Mustache and beard reconstruction can be performed with a pedicled or free scalp flap based on the superficial temporal artery. Another option is a prefabricated flap in the hair-bearing scalp region with second-stage pedicle transfer to the mustache and beard area.

Cheek Contractures and Hypertrophic Scarring. Cheek contractures and scarring are treated by excision of the entire cheek aesthetic unit. The defect is then closed with a thick STSG, FTSG, or flap. Flap reconstruction involves tissue expansion of the neck skin, which is then advanced to the cheek area. Additionally, neck skin can be prefabricated, tissue expanded, and then advanced to the cheek defect. Care must be taken to avoid lower eyelid traction that can cause ectropion.

Nasal Scarring and Deformities. The nose is very commonly involved in facial burn injuries, with subtotal or total loss of the tip being the most common injury. For complex defects, use the subunit principles detailed by Burget and Menick[6] and replace each layer to provide nasal lining, skeletal support, and skin coverage. Nasal lining can be obtained from local turn-in flaps or mucosal bipedicle or septal flaps. Nasal support is provided by cartilage grafts. Skin coverage is best obtained with a midline forehead flap using the subunit principles.

For smaller defects in the upper two thirds of the nose a FTSG may be used. Alar deformities may be reconstructed with nasolabial flaps after scar release and attention to adequate nasal lining and support. Full release of an alar contracture is performed with a curved incision in the region of the alar crease extending medially to the nasal tip.

Nostril stenosis is corrected with z-plasty in minor stenosis and with excisional or incisional release in more significant stenosis. A FTSG is sewn into the defect and a nostril stent placed. Otherwise, an inferiorly based nasolabial flap is elevated and transferred to the defect.

If most of the nose is destroyed, total nasal reconstruction is the procedure of choice. This can be performed with a forehead flap but, if unavailable, a radial forearm free flap or dorsalis pedis free flap may be used. A classical Tagliacozzi flap is rarely indicated today.

Scalp Defects and Alopecia. Small scalp defects (<3 cm) are corrected with scar excision and primary closure. Medium-sized defects can be covered with local flaps from the temporal, parietal, or occipital scalp based on the superficial temporal artery. Use a Doppler to map the vessel territory, perform wide undermining and scoring of the galea, then flap transposition.

Alopecia reconstruction should be delayed until wounds are healed. Tissue expanders can reconstruct burnt areas of up to 50% of the scalp. Expanders are placed in the subgaleal plane of the hair-bearing scalp and expanded weekly for 2 to 4 months. The scar is then excised and the expanded tissue is advanced or rotated to fill the defect. For extensive areas of alopecia, multiple-staged expansion procedures are used (Figure 10-4).

Cranial bone exposure requires a local scalp flap or a free flap. A classical method of covering a small area of exposed bone is Millard's crane principle in which a scalp flap is rotated into the defect and allowed to mature for 3 weeks.[1] The flap is raised and returned to its donor site, leaving tissue over the calvarium. The scalp wound is then grafted. Larger areas of exposed bone often require free flap coverage with musculocutaneous flaps, such as latissimus dorsi flap, or fasciocutaneous flaps, such as the parascapular or radial forearm flap. Later tissue expansion of the remaining hair-bearing skin can be used with gradual excision of the

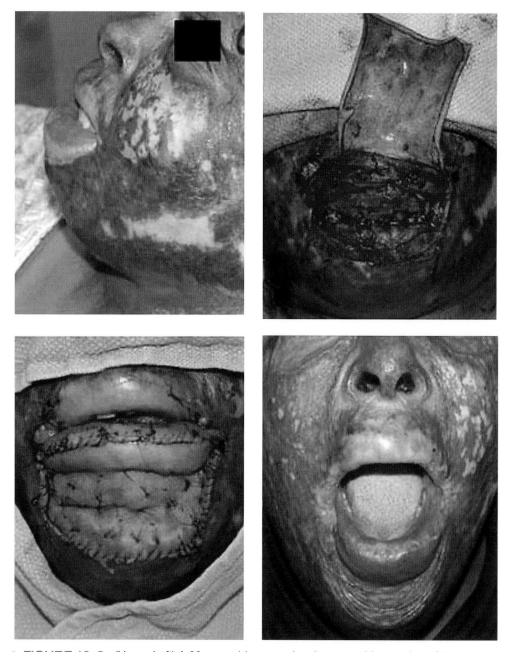

● FIGURE 10-3. (Upper Left) A 28-year-old woman has hypertrophic scarring of lower lip complex causing lip eversion. (Upper Right) The scar is excised as an entire aesthetic unit. (Lower Left) An FTSG is placed with seams at the unit boundaries. (Lower Right) One year later, there is proper mouth opening and no lip eversion.

non-hair bearing flap. Residual non-hair bearing areas can be treated with punch hair grafts.

Forehead Scarring. Forehead scars should be excised and small defects closed primarily. If less than half of the forehead is involved, tissue expanders may be placed under the frontalis muscle and then flaps advanced for coverage. If a majority of the forehead is involved, excise the entire aesthetic unit from the eyebrows to hairline and the outer canthi bilaterally (Figure 10-2). Resurface with a thick STSG or FTSG that is oriented transversely and placed

symmetrically. Exposed bone requires free tissue transfer, most often with a parascapular or radial forearm flap.

Eyebrow Deficit. Eyebrows can be reconstructed with a composite hair-bearing temporal scalp graft. Using a pattern mimicking the opposite eyebrow, extend the incision through the galea, trim excess fat and galea and insert into the recipient site. This gives a thin, less dense eyebrow, ideal for women. Hair growth can be unpredictable and may need to be supplemented with micro- and mini-grafting.

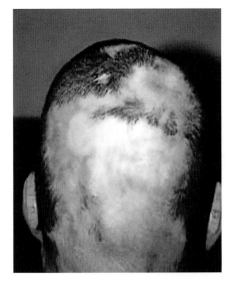 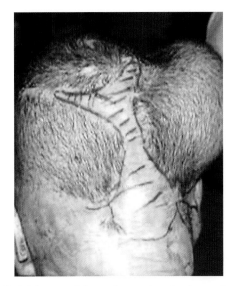 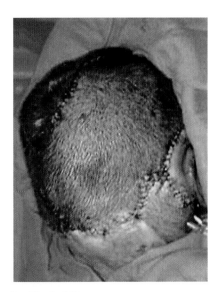

● **FIGURE 10-4.** (Left) A 30-year-old man has extensive burn alopecia. (Center) He had serial expansions and excisions and is shown with an occipital scalp expander after 3 months of expansion. The region of scar alopecia is marked for excision. (Right) The expanded hair-bearing skin is then rotated into the defect.

A temporal scalp flap based on the superficial temporal artery may be used for men to give a fuller, wider eyebrow, but hair growth can be excessive requiring frequent trimming. To perform this flap, Doppler the branches, outline the pedicle, and raise a wide strip of superficial temporalis fascia with overlying scalp of the ipsilateral scalp. Tunnel the flap subcutaneously to the eyebrow.

For partial eyebrow loss, micro- and mini-grafting with occipital scalp hair can be performed. In expert hands, this may in fact be the preferred method of eyebrow reconstruction.

Neck Contractures. Neck contractures should be released early. Z-plasty or local flaps work well in isolated contractures of one third or less of the anterior neck with unburned skin on each side of the contracture. If one third to two thirds of the neck is involved and the adjacent skin is unburnt, tissue expanders can be expanded above the platysma, allowing local flaps to be advanced after scar excision. If more than two thirds of the neck is involved, incisional release or preferentially complete excision of the scar should be performed, including the platysma muscle if involved in the scar. The resulting defect can be covered with a thick STSG, which should be long, wide, harvested as a sheet, and placed in a hammock-like fashion, extending well beyond the scar on each lateral aspect of the neck. Alternatively, flap coverage may be performed. Pre-expanded, pedicle flaps from the infraclavicular area, the deltoid area and the trapezius area have been described. Free tissue transfer employing a parascapular flap, prefabricated thigh flap, or groin flap may be performed (Figure 10-5). Flaps tend to be bulky and need future debulking to decrease blunting of cervicomental angle. Grafts require postoperative splinting and compression.

Upper Extremity and Hand Burn Reconstruction

Extremity contractures are released from proximal to distal. Linear contractures are corrected with z-plastys, and broader contractures with release and skin grafting or flap closure. Joint contractures are released with an incision in line with the axis of rotation. The extent should be judged on improvement in joint mobility. Stabilize bone and joints in position of function; postreconstructive splinting is crucial.

Hand reconstruction is performed under tourniquet control. Proceed with incisional release of contractures at each joint level and excisional release of hypertrophic scars. Resurface hands with thin and pliable tissue. FTSGs are preferred but thick STSGs may be used. If STSGs are used, sheet grafts or 1 to 1.5 meshed grafts should be placed followed by a compressive dressing. Sheet grafts have a better aesthetic outcome and are preferred if there are adequate donor sites.

Pedicle and free flaps are important in upper extremity reconstruction. Local or regional fasciocutaneous flaps, even using previously burnt or grafted arm skin, are reliable for burn coverage as the fascia and vessels are usually spared.[7]

The most common upper extremity deformities and their reconstruction are reviewed.[1,8]

Exposed Bone/Joints/Tendons. The proximal interphalangeal (PIP) joint is the most commonly exposed joint. The joint may be stabilized with an axial Kirschner wire (K-wire), multiple moist dressing changes performed and skin grafting performed when sufficient granulation tissue develops. In small areas of the fingers, local flaps may be

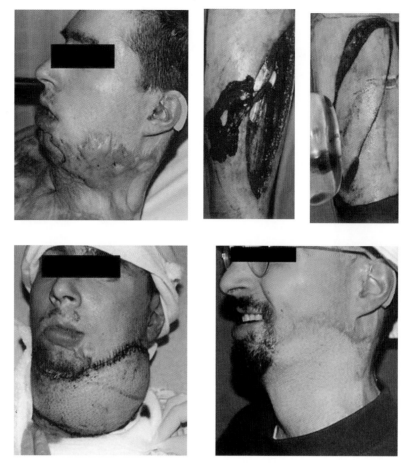

● **FIGURE 10-5.** (Upper Left) A 30-year-old male has extensive neck contractures. (Upper Center) A prefabricated thigh flap is designed. The descending branches of the lateral femoral circumflex vessels and a small amount of attached muscle and fascia are transferred superficially over a tissue expander. (Upper Right) After 8 weeks of maturation, a Doppler exam is performed and a thin flap is raised based on the implanted pedicle. (Lower Left) After excision of the contracture, the prefabricated free flap is transferred to the neck. (Lower Right) The patient is shown 3 years later after debulking.

performed with proximally or distally based fasciocutaneous flaps based on the digital or metacarpal arteries. Cross-finger flaps can also be used for dorsal or volar coverage.

More extensive bone exposure in the hand and arm requires acute coverage with flaps. Groin or abdominal flaps are the "workhorse" flaps and require 2 to 3 weeks of immobilization (Figure 10-6). Local flaps for the wrist and hand include the proximally based digital or first metacarpal flap or the distally based reverse radial, reverse ulnar, or reverse posterior interosseous flaps (Figure 10-7). Otherwise, a free tissue transfer is required using the radial forearm (opposite arm and covers entire dorsum of hand and digits), dorsalis pedis (sensate if includes superficial peroneal cutaneous nerve), temporoparietal fascia (covered with a STSG), or scapular or lateral arm flaps.

Axillary Adduction Contractures. Solitary scar bands in the axilla are released with z-plasty. If only the axillary folds are involved, an incisional release, followed by closure with a thick STSG, can be performed. If the contractures involve

the axillary folds and the axillary dome, one can perform an incisional release involving the entire axis of rotation of the shoulder. A pedicled parascapular flap, island scapular flap or pedicled latissimus flap is then rotated into the defect (Figure 10-8). Postoperatively, abduction splints are applied, especially if skin grafts are used.

Elbow Contractures. Elbow contractures are incisionally released and resurfaced with a thick STSG. When the release results in exposed bone or when there is olecranon ulceration, several flaps are available for closure, the most common being the reverse lateral arm flap (Figure 10-9). Other local flaps that may be used include the proximally based radial, ulnar, or posterior interosseous flaps. The elbow is splinted in extension with a volar splint.

Dorsal Hand Contractures and Hypertrophic Scarring. Linear contractures with adequate lateral tissue laxity are corrected with z-plastys. Otherwise, an incisional release is made proximal to metacarpophalangeal (MCP) joints. If

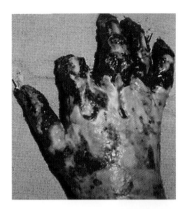
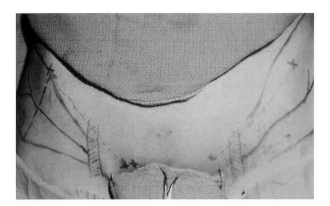
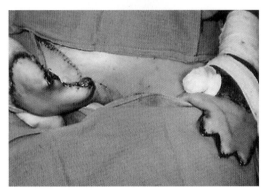
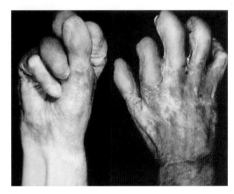

● **FIGURE 10-6.** (Upper Left) A 53-year-old man with bilateral hand burns with exposed bone and tendons shown in the right hand. (Upper Right) Groin flaps are centered over the superficial circumflex iliac arteries, which are traced laterally by Doppler past the anterior superior iliac spine. (Lower Left) The flaps are inset into the hand defects with direct donor site closure and tubing of the attached pedicle. The pedicle is divided 2 to 3 weeks later. (Lower Right) The right hand is shown 1 year later after debulking to create web spaces.

the entire dorsal surface is involved, release extends from the medial to lateral joint axis. The release should result in a resistance-free complete range of motion of the MCP joints. The defect is closed with an FTSG, and the hand is splinted in the intrinsic-plus safe position. Alternatively, postgrafting stabilization in a full-flex hand position with flexion at the distal interphalangeal and PIP and MCP joints may be useful.[1] Extensive dorsal scarring should be excised completely, grafted, and splinted.

Digital Flexion Contractures. Digital flexion contractures are treated with z-plasty if linear (Figure 10-10) or, if broader, with a transverse incision and a FTSG or local flap. Fixed or immobile joints may need release of periarticular structures, including the volar plate, collateral ligaments, or joint capsule. The flap option of choice for reconstruction is the local side-finger fasciocutaneous flap, based on the digital and metacarpal vessels, and can be proximally or distally based. Cross-finger flaps can also be used. When

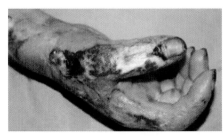
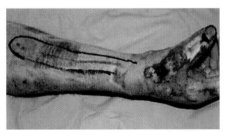
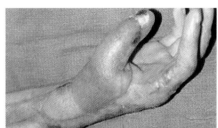

● **FIGURE 10-7.** (Left) There is extensor tendon exposure of the thumb after a burn injury. (Center) A distally based reverse radial artery flap is marked for reconstruction. (Right) The result is shown 6 months later.

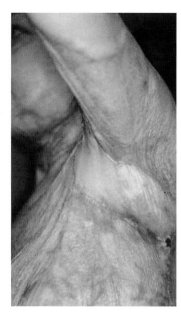
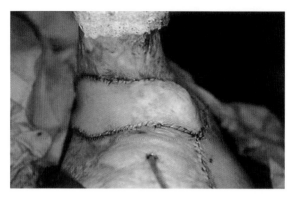
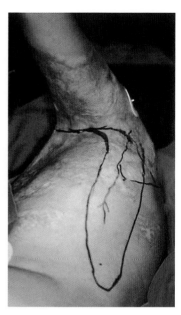

● **FIGURE 10-8.** (Left) A 52-year-old woman has dense axillary contractures and is marked for a pedicled parascapular flap. (Center) The contracture is incisionally released and the flap is rotated into the defect. (Right) One year later, she has improved shoulder abduction.

using arterialized side-finger flaps, a Doppler exam is performed to ensure patency of both digital arteries, and the flap is raised with the artery in the flap. Fingers are splinted in the extended position.

Web Contractures and Syndactyly. Web contractures manifest as dorsal hooding over the web space or syndactyly. Dorsal hooding is corrected with z-plastys or incisional release with a FTSG. Syndactyly is corrected with web space release and web reconstruction with a dorsal pedicle flap. The classic dorsal flap is proximally based and extends from the MCP joint up to two thirds the length of the proximal phalanx. The subcutaneous fat, fascia, and dorsal metacarpal vessels are included in the flap. The flap is inset with a 45-degree incline in the dorsal-to-volar direction, with the distal edge ending at the midshaft of the proximal phalanx. The flap should provide a wide web space, and residual defects on the separated fingers are covered with an FTSG. Postoperatively, compression gloves with web space conformers are worn.

First web space contractures cause thumb adduction and are released with a five or four flap z-plasty (Figure 10-10). Alternatively, after release, the defect may be covered with a thick STSG, FTSG, or a local flap. Postoperative splinting keeps the thumb in extension.

Boutonniere Deformity. Boutonniere deformity at the PIP joint is common and reconstruction of the central extensor tendon slip and cutaneous coverage with a local flap can be pursued. However, if the deformity is complicated and the joint is stiff, the repair may be performed with fusion of the PIP joint at a 25- to 50-degree angle, increasing toward the more ulnar digits.

Breast Burn Reconstruction

Chest contractures can restrict breast enlargement during puberty, causing asymmetry and displacing the nipple areolar complex. Reconstruction is performed when normal breast growth is affected. Nipple-areola reconstruction is delayed until breast mound reconstruction is complete. Use the opposite unburned breast as a model for reconstruction.[9]

Breast Contractures. Contracture release is obtained by incision or excision of the restricting burn scar. Care must be taken to not disturb the breast bud in young girls, as this can lead to severe breast hypoplasia. A wide release of the inframammary fold is performed down to the muscle fascia. Occasionally, release will require incisions superior to the breast mound, around the areola, or between the breasts. STSG are applied to the defect and bolsters placed. Occasionally, the entire breast bud is destroyed and needs to be reconstructed with a regional musculocutaneous flap such as a latissimus dorsi flap with a tissue expander or a transverse rectus abdominus myocutaneous flap. Balancing procedures are often required on the opposite breast.

Nipple-Areola Deformities. For a malpositioned nipple-areola complex, the scar is released and the nipple-areola complex advanced as a flap into a better, more symmetrical

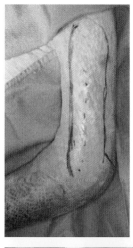
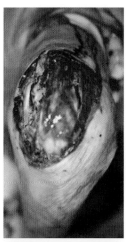
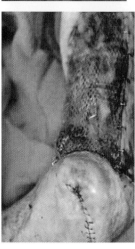
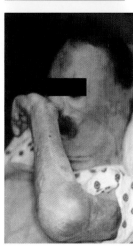

● FIGURE 10-9. (Upper Left) A 45-year-old man has a burn contracture of his elbow limiting flexion. He is marked for a distally based reverse lateral arm fasciocutaneous flap using previously grafted skin. (Upper Right) The contracture is excised resulting in exposed joint and bone. (Lower Left) A lateral arm flap is rotated into the defect. (Lower Right) He has appropriate elbow flexion and wound coverage 1 year later.

position. An STSG may be needed in the resulting defect. If the nipple is lost, it will require reconstruction as after mastectomy, using a C-V flap or a skate flap. For nipple reconstruction on a grafted breast, tent up a circle of skin and place a tight FTSG around the base. Composite grafts, such as postauricular cartilage or toe pulp, can also be used to construct a nipple. It is best to make the nipple larger than the opposite side, allowing for long-term flattening. The areola is reconstructed with an FTSG taken from the opposite breast areola with an outer "donut" technique or taken from hairless groin skin. Alternatively, the areola may simply be tattooed once the nipple reconstruction has healed.

Perineum Burn Reconstruction

Scar contracture is common after perineal burns. Surgical reconstruction of the external genitalia is complex, and often requires multiple specialized procedures.

Perineal Contractures. Isolated perineal scar bands are released with multiple z-plastys with the patient placed in the lithotomy position. More diffuse scars require incisional or excisional releases followed by the placement of meshed STSG, which are more pliable and better fit the perineal contour. Local flaps from the perineal area or medial thigh can also be used.

Lower Extremity Burn Reconstruction

Meshed STSGs are the mainstay of treatment in the lower extremity. However, narrow scar bands can be divided and lengthened with z-plastys. Immobilization is needed post-reconstruction, with the long-term use of postoperative splinting.

Fourth-degree Burns. Exposed tendon or bone requires flap closure. The gastrocnemius and soleus muscle flaps can be used for knee or proximal tibial defects. Common free flaps used for exposed tibia include the rectus abdominus, latissimus dorsi, or parascapular flap. Small ankle and foot defects can be closed with a broad array of local flaps. The abductor hallucis, abductor digiti minimi, and extensor digitorum brevis muscle flaps can cover small proximal dorsal defects. The abductor hallucis, abductor digiti minimi, and flexor digitorum brevis muscle flaps can cover malleolar and weight-bearing heel defects. The lateral calcaneal artery flap is useful for heel and Achilles tendon defects. The dorsalis pedis artery fasciocutaneous or myofascial flap with an STSG can reconstruct ankle defects and, when used in a reverse fashion, distal foot defects.

Extensive exposed foot structures require free flap coverage. This can be accomplished with a radial forearm or temporoparietal fascia flap to the dorsal foot. For plantar defects, a muscle flap, such as the latissimus dorsi, gracilis, or rectus abdominus flap, or a fasciocutaneous flap, such as the tensor fascia lata flap, can be used.

The V.A.C. device and tibial burr holes are options in patients who cannot undergo flap closure. The V.A.C. is placed at 125 mm Hg and changed every 2 to 3 days. If the wound contracts and granulates enough, it can be closed with delayed primary closure or grafting. Tibial burr holes may help expedite granulation tissue formation by burring through the outer table of bone. Dressing changes or the V.A.C. should follow this. If these interventions fail or result in a poorly functional leg, amputation may be the best option. Attempts should be made to maintain as much limb length as possible.

Foot Contractures. Dorsal foot contractures or hypertrophic scarring are released with excision of the scar tissue and coverage with a STSG. Plantar contractures can be incisionally released and an STSG placed under a bolster. Postoperative immobilization is necessary and may require K-wire fixation. With extensive and severe contractures, free flap transfer may be required.

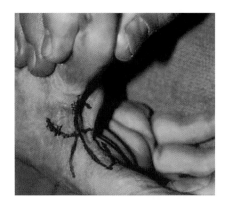
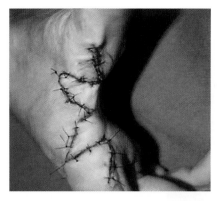
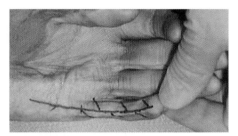
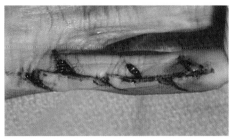
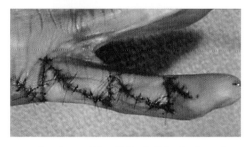

● **FIGURE 10-10.** (Upper Left) A long linear contracture of the fifth digit is designed with multiple z-plastys in series along the contracture. (Upper Center and Right) The flaps are incised and transposed with successful lengthening of the contracture. (Lower Left) A 5-flap z-plasty is designed over a first web space contracture. (Lower Right) Flap transposition lengthens the web space.

Popliteal Flexion Contractures. Popliteal contractures require incisional release, avoiding injury to the underlying neurovascular structures of the popliteal fossa. The defect is closed with an STSG or a flap if there are exposed vessels or tendons. If adjacent tissue is viable, a transposition flap can be created adjacent to the defect with the length of the flap equal to the length of the scar release and rotated into the defect. Postoperative immobilization in knee extension is required.

● COMPLICATIONS

The most common adverse outcomes of burn reconstruction are infection, failed grafting and recurrent scarring. Strict sterile technique is necessary. Tissue expanders are prone to infection and should only be used in healed wounds and removed at any sign of infection. Expansion works best in the head, neck, and torso; but overall have high complication rates due to infection and expander extrusion or exposure.

The final functional results of grafts are largely determined by postoperative care, including compression garments, facemasks, and extremity splints. Grafts should be immobilized and compressed with bolster dressings. After bolster removal, the grafts should be protected for an extended period of time.

Customized pressure garments should be applied as soon as possible after wound healing and continued for at least 6 months to control scar maturation and minimize hypertrophic scarring. Compression and splinting for the face is important for several months after grafting and is achieved with custom fit pressure garments or masks. Splints should be applied to extremities as well as the neck. Occupational or physical therapy programs should be initiated to maintain mobilization and prevent contractures after reconstruction. Postoperative contractures will reoccur if physical therapy and joint splinting are not pursued.

● OUTCOMES ASSESSMENT

Successful outcomes are dependent on forming a realistic long-term reconstructive plan that involves the patient, surgeon, therapists, and other health care providers. Psychological response to burn scars or contractures is a main factor in influencing the functional rehabilitation and psychological state of burn patients. Thus, reconstruction of these deformities can have a profound impact on the psychological well-being of patients, allowing future social reintegration and improvement in function.

REFERENCES

1. Herndon DN. *Total Burn Care.* London: Saunders; 2002.

2. Pribaz JJ, Fine N, Orgill DP. Flap prefabrication in the head and neck: a 10-year experience. *Plast Reconstr Surg.* 1999; 103:808.

3. Klein MB, Moore ML, Costa B, et al. Primer on the management of face burns at the University of Washington. *J Burn Care Rehabil.* 2005;26:6.

4. Gonzalez-Ulloa M. Restoration of the face covering by means of selected skin in regional aesthetic units. *Br J Plast Surg.* 1956;9:212.

5. Achauer BM. Reconstructing the burned face. *Clin Plast Surg* 1992;19:623.

6. Burget GC, Menick F. The subunit principle in nasal reconstruction. *Plast Reconstr Surg.* 1985;76:239.

7. Pribaz JJ, Pelham FR. Use of previously burned skin in local fasciocutaneous flaps for upper extremity reconstruction. *Ann Plast Surg.* 1994;33:272.

8. Smith MA, Munster AM, Spence RJ. Burns of the hand and upper limb–a review. *Burns.* 1998;24:493.

9. MacLennan SE, Wells MD, Neale HW. Reconstruction of the burned breast. *Clin Plast Surg.* 2000;27:113.

chapter 11

Head and Neck Embryology

Geoffrey H. Sperber, BDS, MSc, PhD, FICD

● INTRODUCTION

The significance of head and neck embryology to surgical practice is based on a required understanding of the underlying developmental phenomena leading to normal craniofacial morphology. This, in turn, provides insights into how maldevelopment leads to dysmorphology that the clinician is called upon to analyze, treat, and prognosticate its occurrence. The essence of treating any malady is to fully understand its etiology and eliminate the causative factors. The emergence of molecular genetics and advances in gene identification aided by the imaging capabilities of electron, scanning, transmission, fluorescence, and confocal laser microscopy, together with immunohistochemistry, polymerase chain reaction (PCR) technology, and stem cell and experimental cloning have revolutionized our capabilities for investigating developmental events. Molecular diagnostics have begun to revolutionize medicine. Identification of biomarkers allows the characterization of the molecular basis of dysmorphology and possible therapeutic intervention. Understanding these technologies is changing embryology from a descriptive science into a predictive science, with the potential for control of its mechanisms.[1]

The craniofacial complex, subserving the elements of the sensory organs of sight, hearing, olfaction, and taste, while providing a muscularized masticatory apparatus and a bony protective braincase is a composite of numerous disparate evolutionary components melded into an essential functioning appendage to the body. This complexity of diverse purposes contained in the head is reflected in its complicated embryology.

The emerging fields of regenerative medicine and potential stem cell therapy are rooted in an understanding of the mechanisms of embryogenesis and developmental differentiation of the initial unicellular totipotential zygote resulting from the union of the male and female gametes. Furthermore, the prenatal imaging capabilities of embryoscopy, fetoscopy, and ultrasonography have accelerated gestational development into the field of concern to the clinician. Chorionic villus sampling and amniocentesis provide advance information on the chromosomal and genetic status of the developing fetus and any possible abnormalities, thus allowing for possible therapeutic intervention.

● EARLY EMBRYOLOGY

Embryogenesis is a series of cascading events transforming the coded instructions contained in the genome of the conceptus into proteins, tissues, and organs in an ordered manner (Figure 11-1).[2] The instructions of regulatory genes and signaling factors shape an indeterminate mass of cells into complex morphologies. The combination of molecular biology with classical embryology results in the production of an unfolding embryo turning into a fetus at 8 weeks postconception and ultimately into an infant (Figure 11-2).

The embryonic disk that develops from cellular differentiation consists of the primary germ layers, ectoderm, endoderm, and mesoderm, all of which contribute to the craniofacial structures. The intermediate mesodermal germ layer is deficient in two locations in the trilaminar disk—at the prechordal plate cranially and at the cloacal plate caudally—demarcating the sites of the future entrance and exit of the gut (Figure 11-3). The persistent contact of ectoderm and endoderm at these two locations determines the dissolution of these two plates, which are denoted as the oropharyngeal and cloacal membranes, respectively, and perforate at the mouth and anus. The oropharyngeal membrane sinks into a central depression, the stomodeum, around which the future face is built.

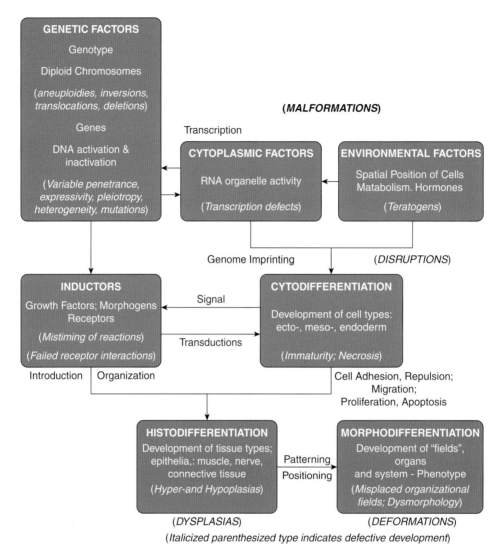

● FIGURE 11-1. Schema of embryogenesis. (*Reprinted from Sperber GH. Embryology of the head and neck. In: English GM, ed. Otolaryngology. Philadelphia: JB Lippincott; 1990:1–36.*)

● **NEURAL CREST TISSUE (ECTOMESENCHYME)**

The neural crest is a pluripotent cell population derived from the crests of the neural folds that form the neural tube and brain. During neural tube closure (failure of which leads to neural tube defects), induction by differential tissue interactions produces an epithelial-mesenchymal transformation resulting in ectomesenchyme that gives rise to a diverse variety of tissues (Table 11-1). Migration, proliferation, and differentiation of neural crest cells provide the prominences of the embryonic face and neck.[3] The segmental pattern of migrating neural crest is foreshadowed by hindbrain neuromeres, termed rhombomeres, that are determined by the *HOX* genes (Figure 11-4). It is the brain underlying the future face that is a key component of cephalogenesis.[4]

Deficiencies in neural crest migration, proliferation, or differentiation account for a wide range of craniofacial malformations, the neurocristopathies, manifested in a variety of syndromes. Abnormalities in form or function of

neural crest cells range from von Recklinghausen neurofibromatosis through acoustic neuroma (neurofibroma) to DiGeorge and Klein-Waardenburg syndromes.

● **CRANIOFACIAL DEVELOPMENT**

Most of the skeletal and connective tissues of the face and pharyngeal arch apparatus are dependent on neural crest tissue migrating as ectomesenchyme into the ventral regions of the future skull, face, and neck (Figure 11-5).[5,6] Any defect in the quantity and quality of migrating ectomesenchyme manifests itself in nearly every congenital anomaly observed clinically, ranging from major holoprosencephaly to the most minor clefts of the lips and dimples in the cheeks.[7–11]

During the critical days 21 to 31 of development, the central stomodeum is surrounded by five facial prominences formed by underlying neural crest migration and proliferation displaying selective regional characteristics.

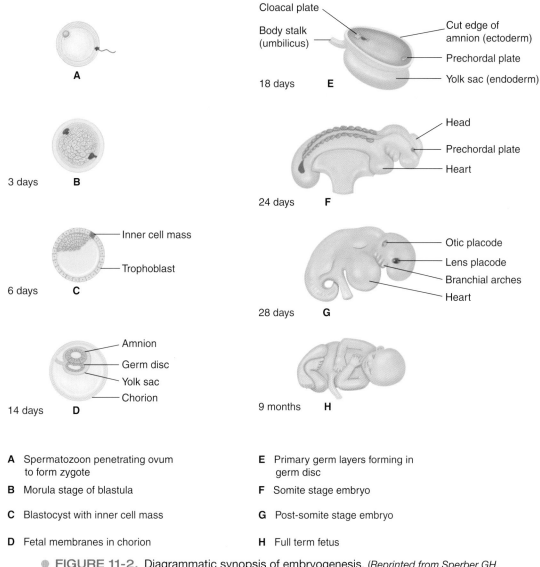

A Spermatozoon penetrating ovum to form zygote

B Morula stage of blastula

C Blastocyst with inner cell mass

D Fetal membranes in chorion

E Primary germ layers forming in germ disc

F Somite stage embryo

G Post-somite stage embryo

H Full term fetus

● **FIGURE 11-2.** Diagrammatic synopsis of embryogenesis. (*Reprinted from Sperber GH. Embryology of the head and neck. In: English GM, ed. Otolaryngology. Philadelphia: JB Lippincott; 1990:1–36.*)

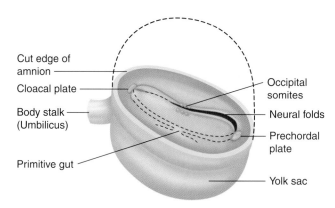

● **FIGURE 11-3.** Diagram of 21-day-old embryonic disk elevating neural folds, encompassed by fetal membranes. (*Reprinted from Sperber GH. Embryology of the head and neck. In: English GM, ed. Otolaryngology. Philadelphia: JB Lippincott; 1990:1–36.*)

Ectomesenchyme from the mesencephalic region contributes to the leptomeninges and the frontal and nasal bones, whereas the parietal bones are derived from mesoderm. The interaction at the boundaries between these dissimilar cell populations may be influential in growth control, potentially accounting for craniosynostotic syndromes.

Neural crest cells around the midbrain form part of the trigeminal, facial, glossopharyngeal, vestibulcochlear, and vagal nerve ganglia, joined by neuroblasts from the maxillomandibular placodes. Lateral evaginations of the forebrain, the optic vesicles, induce lens placodes in the surface ectoderm, around which neural crest cells migrate to form the scleral and choroid optic coats and the facial frontonasal prominence innervated by the ophthalmic division of the trigeminal nerve. More caudally located migrating neural crest cells encounter pharyngeal endoderm, with which they interact to form the five pharyngeal arches. Springing from the first pharyngeal arches

TABLE 11-1. Derivatives of Neural Crest Cells

Connective Tissues
Ectomesenchyme of facial prominences and pharyngeal
   arches
Bones and cartilages of facial and visceral skeleton
   (basicranial and pharyngeal arch cartilages); portions
   of ear ossicles
Dermis of face and ventral aspect of neck
Stroma of salivary, thymus, thyroid, parathyroid and
   pituitary glands
Corneal mesenchyme
Sclera and choroid optic coats
Blood vessel walls (excepting endothelium); aortic arch
   arteries
Dental papilla (dentin); portion of periodontal ligament;
   cementum

Muscle Tissues
Ciliary muscles
Connective tissues, sheaths of pharyngeal
   arch muscles (masticatory, facial, ossicular,
   faucial, laryngeal) combined with mesodermal
   components

Nervous Tissues
Supporting tissues
Leptomeninges of prosencephalon and part of
   mesencephalon
Glia
Schwann sheath cells

Sensory ganglia
Bipolar neurons of vestibular and cochlear ganglia of
   vestibulocochlear nerve
Autonomic ganglia
Spinal dorsal root ganglia
Sensory ganglia (in part) of trigeminal, facial
   (geniculate), glossopharyngeal (otic and superior)
   and vagal (jugular) nerves

Autonomic nervous system
Sympathetic ganglia and plexuses
Parasympathetic ganglia (ciliary, ethmoid,
   sphenopalatine, submandibular, enteric
   system)

Endocrine Tissues
Enteric ganglia
Adenohypophysis mesenchyme
Adrenomedullary cells and adrenergic
   paraganglia: chromaffin cells
   (phaeochromocytes)
Calcitonin (C) cells—thyroid gland (ultimobranchial
   body)
Carotid body
Part of pineal body

Pigment Cells
Melanocytes in all tissues; melanophores of iris

bilaterally are the maxillary and mandibular prominences (innervated by the respective branches of the trigeminal nerve); these prominences form the superolateral and inferior boundaries to the wide stomodeal chamber. The median superior boundary is the frontonasal prominence (Figure 11-6). On the inferolateral corners of the frontonasal prominence there develop bilateral nasal placodes, precursors of olfactory epithelium. The nasal placodes sink into the face to form the nasal pits that become the anterior nares consequent to the elevation of the horseshoe-shaped medial and lateral nasal prominences. The posterior aspect of each nasal pit is initially separated from the oral cavity by the oronasal (bucconasal) membrane, which disintegrates by the end of the fifth week to form the posterior choanae.

Elevation of the lateral nasal prominences creates the alae of the nose. Defects of the medial nasal prominences may produce arhinia, or a bifid nose, or contribute to clefts of the upper lip. The medial tip of the maxillary prominences that contribute to the upper lip makes contact with the medial nasal prominence separated by an intervening epithelial "nasal fin" that normally degenerates, allowing mesenchymal merging. Persistence of the nasal fin contributes to clefting of the upper lip and anterior palate.[12]

Clefting of the upper lip is one of the most frequent of all congenital anomalies; its unilateral occurrence (usually on the left) varies among different racial groupings, indicating its inherited character: it is highest in incidence in Mongoloid peoples, intermediate in frequency among whites and least in blacks, varying from 1:500 to 1:2000 births. The degree of clefting varies enormously; the anomaly is rarely median, indicative of a major holoprosencephaly syndrome. Lip clefts may be coincidentally associated with cleft palate, which is inherited separately. The lower lip is rarely defective but, if so, it is clefted in the midline (Figure 11-7).

● THE MOUTH

The primitive wide stomodeal aperture is reduced by migrating mesenchyme fusing the maxillary and mandibular prominences to form the commissures of the definitive mouth. Inadequate fusion results in macrostomia (uni- or bilateral), a form of facial clefting, while excessive fusion produces microstomia or astomia (Figure 11-7).

The initial shallow depression of the stomodeum becomes the familiarly deep oral cavity by forward growth of the surrounding facial prominences. The stomodeum becomes the common oronasopharyngeal chamber and entrance to the gut by disintegration of the dividing oropharyngeal membrane, providing continuity between the mouth and pharynx. Rare persistence of the membrane results in oropharyngeal atresia.

The foregut, extending from the oropharyngeal membrane gives rise to the esophagus and the laryngotracheal groove, generating the larynx and trachea (Figure 11-8).[13]

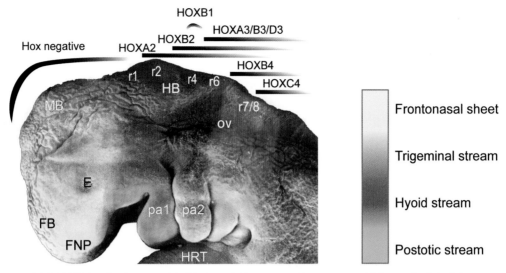

● **FIGURE 11-4.** A stage 15, 33-day-old human embryo upon which are depicted the neural crest streams emanating from the rhombomeres (r1-r8), influenced by *HOX* gene expression patterns. FNP, frontonasal prominence; FB, forebrain; E, eye; MB, midbrain; HB, hindbrain; OV, otic vesicle; HRT, heart; pa 1, pa 2, pharyngeal arches. (*Modified from Hinrichsen KV. Human-Embryologie. Berlin: Springer-Verlag; 1990.*)

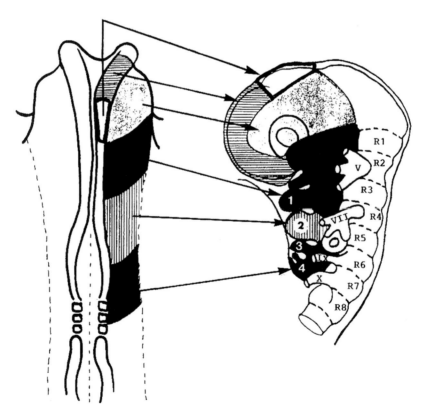

● **FIGURE 11-5.** Schematic depiction of the fate map of neural crest tissue segments (*left*) and their facial and pharyngeal arch destinations. R1-R8, rhombomeres; 1-4, pharyngeal arches; v, vii, ix, x, cranial nerves. (*Reprinted from Sperber GH. Embryology of the head and neck. In: English GM, ed. Otolaryngology. Philadelphia: JB Lippincott; 1990:1–36.*)

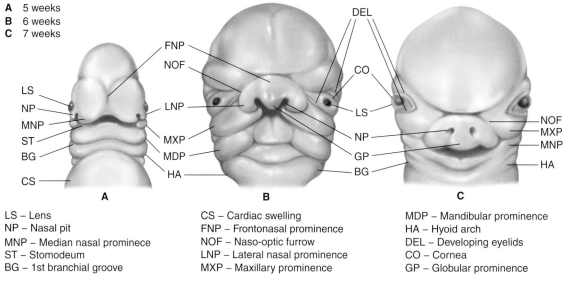

A 5 weeks
B 6 weeks
C 7 weeks

LS – Lens
NP – Nasal pit
MNP – Median nasal prominece
ST – Stomodeum
BG – 1st branchial groove

CS – Cardiac swelling
FNP – Frontonasal prominence
NOF – Naso-optic furrow
LNP – Lateral nasal prominence
MXP – Maxillary prominence

MDP – Mandibular prominence
HA – Hyoid arch
DEL – Developing eyelids
CO – Cornea
GP – Globular prominence

● **FIGURE 11-6.** Schematic depiction of facial formation at 4, 5, 6, and 7 weeks postconception. (*Reprinted from Sperber GH. Embryology of the head and neck. In: English GM, ed. Otolaryngology. Philadelphia: JB Lippincott; 1990:1–36.*)

● THE PHARYNGEAL ARCHES

Ventrally migrating neural crest cells surround mesodermal cores containing the six aortic arches to form the pharyngeal arches (Figure 11-9). Only five pairs of arches are discernible, however, since the fifth is extremely transitory. The arches are separated by ectodermal grooves externally and endodermal pharyngeal pouches internally.

Common to the initial arches are a central cartilage rod, surrounded by mesoderm accompanied by a nerve along the aortic arch artery. The fates of the archetypal elements in each of the pharyngeal arches are outlined in Table 11-2. The consequences of maldevelopment of the derivatives of the pharyngeal system are listed in Table 11-3.[14,15]

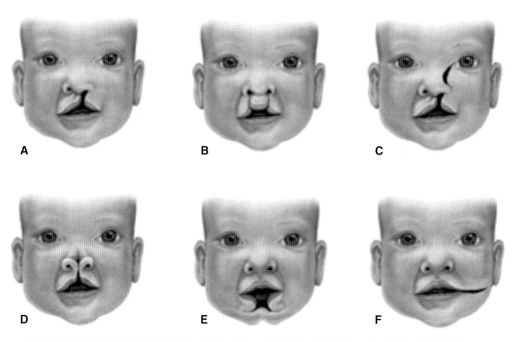

● **FIGURE 11-7.** Orofacial clefts: (A) unilateral cleft lip; (B) bilateral cleft lip; (C) oblique facial cleft; (D) median cleft lip and nasal defect; (E) median mandibular cleft; (F) unilateral macrostomia.

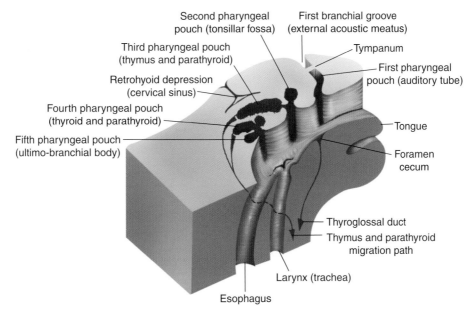

● **FIGURE 11-8.** Schematic depiction of pharyngeal pouch derivatives and their migration paths. (*Reprinted from Sperber GH. Embryology of the head and neck. In: English GM, ed. Otolaryngology. Philadelphia: JB Lippincott; 1990:1–36.*)

● **THE PALATE**

Three elements make up the secondary definitive palate: the two lateral palatal shelves projecting into the stomodeum from the maxillary prominences and the anterior midline primary palate derived from the frontonasal prominence. These elements are initially widely separated owing to the advancing edges of the lateral shelves being deflected vertically on either side of the tongue that occupies most of the stomodeal chamber. Concomitantly, the cartilaginous nasal septum descends from the roof of the stomodeum (Figure 11-10).[16]

Consequent to expansion of the stomodeum and mouth opening, the tongue withdraws from between the palatal shelves, allowing their elevation into the horizontal plane, enabling them to contact each other in the midline, with the primary palate anteriorly and with the vertical nasal septum superiorly. Thereby is the single chamber stomodeum converted into a three-chambered oronasal orifice—the two nasal fossae and the mouth.

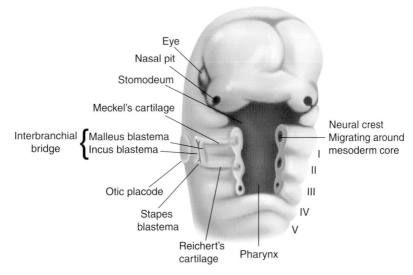

● **FIGURE 11-9.** Diagramatic sectioned view of facial and pharyngeal arch development. (*Reprinted from Sperber GH. Embryology of the head and neck. In: English GM, ed. Otolaryngology. Philadelphia: JB Lippincott; 1990:1–36.*)

TABLE 11-2. Derivatives of the Pharyngeal System

Pharyngeal Arch	Ectodermal Groove	Endodermal Pouch	Skeleton	Viscera	Artery	Muscles	Motor Nerve	Sensory Nerve
1st Mandibular	Ext. acoustic meatus; Ear hillocks; Pinna	Auditory tube; Middle ear tympanum	Meckel's cartilage; malleus; incus (mandible template)	Body of tongue	Ext. carotid artery; Maxillary artery	Masticatory Muscles; Tensor tympani; Mylohyoid, tensor palati; Ant. digastric	Mand. Div. V. Trigeminal	V Lingual nerve
2nd Hyoid	Disappears	Tonsillar fossa	Stapes, styloid process; sup hyoid body	Midtongue; Thyroid gland anlage; Tonsil	Stapedial artery (disappears)	Facial, stapedius, stylohyoid, post. digastric	VII Facial	VII Chorda tympani
3rd	Disappears	Inf. parathyroid 3; Thymus	Inf. hyoid body, grt. cornu hyoid	Root of tongue; Fauces; Epiglottis; Thymus; Carotid body; Inf. Parathyroid 3	Int. carotid artery	Stylopharyngeus	IX Glossopharyngeal	IX Glossopharyngeal
4th	Disappears	Sup. parathyroid 4	Thyroid & laryngeal cartilages	Pharynx; epiglottis; Sup. Parathyroid 4	Aorta (L); Subclavian (R)	Pharyngeal constrictors; Levator palatini; Palatoglossus; Palatopharyngeus; Cricothyroid	X Superior laryngeal nerve Vagus	X Auricular N. to ext. acoustic meatus
6th	Disappears	Telopharyngeal (Ultimobranchial) body (cyst); Calcitonin "C" cells	Cricoid, Arytenoid, Corniculate cartilages	Larynx	Pulmonary arteries; Ductus arteriosus	Laryngeal muscles; Pharyngeal constrictors	X Inferior laryngeal nerve Vagus	X Vagus
Postbranchial region; Somites 4; Occipital somites			Tracheal cartilages; SCLEROTOMES Basioccipital bone			Trapezius; Sternomastoid; MYOTOMIC MUSCLE; Intrinsic tongue muscles; Extrinsic tongue muscles (Styloglossus, Hyoglossus, Genioglossus); Extrinsic ocular muscles	XI Spinal accessory; XII Hypoglossal; III. Oculomotor, IV. Trochlear, VI. Abducens; Spinal nerves, C1, C2	
Prechordal somites; Upper cervical somites			Nasal capsule; Nasal septum; Cervical vertebrae			Geniohyoid; Infrahyoid muscles		

TABLE 11-3. Possible Anomalies of the Pharyngeal System

Arch	Ectodermal Groove	Endodermal Pouch	Skeleton	Artery	Muscles	Nerve
1st Mandibular	Aplasia, atresia, stenosis, duplication of ext. acoustic meatus	Diverticulum of auditory tube; aplasia, atresia, stenosis of tube	Aplasia/dysplasia of malleus, incus, mandible	Hypoplastic/absent ext. carotid & maxillary arteries	Deficient masticatory/facial muscles	Absent mand. nerve
2nd Hyoid	Cervical (Branchial) cleft, sinus, cyst, fistula	Tonsillar sinus, pharyngeal fistula	Aplasia/dysplasia of stapes, styloid process	Persistent stapedial artery	Deficient facial, stapedial muscles	Deficient facial, chorda tympani N.
3rd	Cervical cleft, sinus, cyst, fistula	Cervical thymus; thymic cyst; aplasia parathyroid 3; aplasia thymus (DiGeorge anomaly)	Defective hyoid bone	Hypoplastic/absent int. carotid artery		Deficient glossopharyngeal nerve
4th	Cervical cleft, sinus, cyst, fistula	Fistula/sinus from pyriform sinus; aplasia parathyroid 4	Congenital laryngeal stenosis, cleft, atresia (Fraser syndrome)	Double aortae; aortic interruption; right aorta	Deficient faucial muscles	Deficient vagus nerve
6th		Aplasia of calcitonin "C" cells (DiGeorge anomaly)		Aortico-pulmonary septation anomalies (DiGeorge anomaly)		

Palatoschisis

Clefting of the palate is a consequence of failure of any one of the complex embryological interactions necessary for intact palate formation. Palatal shelf developmental defects can be categorized as (1) failure of shelf formation; (2) fusion of palatal shelf(ves) with the tongue or mandible; (3) failure of shelf(ves) elevation; (4) failure of shelves to contact each other; and (5) persistence of the midline medial edge epithelium that normally transforms into mesenchyme or disintegrates (apoptosis).[17]

All degrees of clefting may occur, ranging from nondysfunctional submucous clefts to the major incapacitating cleft lip and palate (cheilouranoschisis) (Figure 11-11). The consequences of palatal clefting are multifarious, ranging from oronasal food regurgitation, speech impediments, dental malocclusion, facial growth retardation, and social isolation.

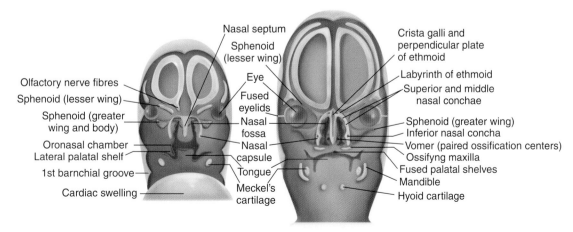

● **FIGURE 11-10.** Coronal sections of head at 7 weeks (A); 12 weeks (B) revealing nasal capsule and palate development. (*Reprinted from Sperber GH. Embryology of the head and neck. In: English GM, ed. Otolaryngology. Philadelphia: JB Lippincott; 1990:1–36.*)

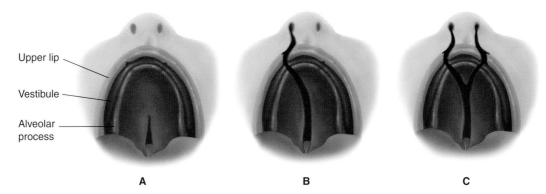

Upper lip

Vestibule

Alveolar
process

A   B   C

● **FIGURE 11-11.** Cleft palate variations: (A) bifid uvula; (B) unilateral cleft palate and lip; (C) bilateral cleft palate and lip. (*Reprinted from Sperber GH. Embryology of the head and neck. In: English GM, ed. Otolaryngology. Philadelphia: JB Lippincott; 1990:1–36.*)

● THE SKULL

The neurocranium encapsulating the brain is divided developmentally into the vault or calvaria, of membranous bone origin, and the cranial base of endochondral bone formation. Herein lies the discrepancy of embryopathological distinctions of calvarial and basicranial developmental lesions (Figure 11-12).

The viscerocranium, composed of the face and orognathic apparatus, is derived from the facial prominences, previously described, and the pharyngeal arches. Ossification of these components, either intramembranously or endochondrally follows a genetically determined timetable, commencing at 8 weeks postconception at various ossification centers that coalesce to constitute the osseous components of the skull. The intervening sutures are of enormous significance in determining skull size and shape, and are the source of clinical syndromes of skeletal dysplasias.

The calvaria is surgically significant for its brain protective function and its reflection of the morphology of the underlying brain. Microcephaly, hydrocephaly, and macrocephaly

are revealed by the calvarial contour created by the frontal, parietal-occipital, and temporal bones. Patency of the sutures between these bones is critical for brain expansion during fetal development and subsequent infancy. Skull growth results from a combination of (1) bone remodeling (deposition and resorption), (2) bone apposition at sutures and synchondroses, and (3) transposition and displacement of enlarged and remodeled bones. Premature synchondrosal fusion in the basicranium, prior to adolescence, will lead to a foreshortened chondrocranium (brachycephaly) that usually causes calvarial expansion and bulging frontal bossing. Premature fusion of the calvarial sutures, converting syndesmoses into synostoses results in distorted skull shapes characterizing craniosynostotic syndromes (Apert, Crouzon) or isolated sutural fusions.[18–21]

● THE MASTICATORY APPARATUS

Development of the masticatory apparatus comprises the jaws, temporomandibular joint, teeth, and masticatory musculature derives from the first pharyngeal

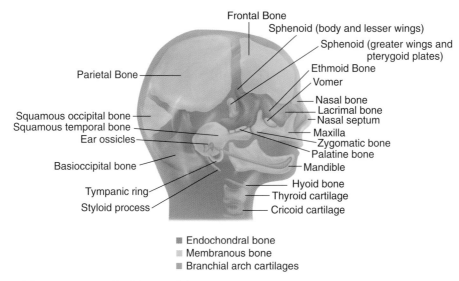

Frontal Bone
Sphenoid (body and lesser wings)
Sphenoid (greater wings and pterygoid plates)
Ethmoid Bone
Vomer
Nasal bone
Lacrimal bone
Nasal septum
Maxilla
Zygomatic bone
Palatine bone
Mandible
Hyoid bone
Thyroid cartilage
Cricoid cartilage

Parietal Bone

Squamous occipital bone
Squamous temporal bone
Ear ossicles

Basioccipital bone

Tympanic ring
Styloid process

■ Endochondral bone
■ Membranous bone
■ Branchial arch cartilages

● **FIGURE 11-12.** Skull bone origins. (*Reprinted from Sperber GH. Embryology of the head and neck. In: English GM, ed. Otolaryngology. Philadelphia: JB Lippincott; 1990:1–36.*)

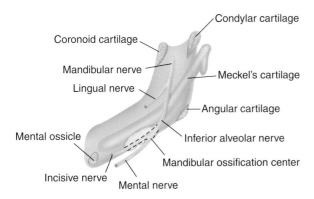

● **FIGURE 11-13.** Cartilages and membranous ossification center of fetal mandible (*lateral view, left half*). (*Reprinted from Sperber GH. Embryology of the head and neck. In: English GM, ed. Otolaryngology. Philadelphia: JB Lippincott; 1990:1–36.*)

arch.[22] Maxillary and palate development are previously described. The primary template of the mandible, Meckel's cartilage, is the skeleton of the first pharyngeal arch, to which are added secondary accessory cartilages, for the head of the condyle and coronoid process (Figure 11-13).

Aplasia of the mandible (agnathia) and the hyoid bone (first and second arch syndrome) is a rare lethal condition with multiple defects of the orbit and maxilla, reflecting deficiencies of neural crest tissue migration to these areas of the face and neck. Mandibular hypoplasia leads to micrognathia, characteristic of Pierre Robin sequence, the cri du chat (cat cry) syndrome, mandibulofacial dysostosis (Treacher Collins syndrome), progeria, Down syndrome (trisomy 21), oculomandibulodyscephaly (Hallermann-Streiff syndrome), and Turner syndrome (XO).

● **THE TEMPOROMANDIBULAR JOINT**

This complex double joint is secondary to the primary jaw joint in utero between the malleus and incus formed in Meckel's cartilage between weeks 8 and 23. The definitive temporomandibular joint develops as upper and lower cavities arise in the mesenchyme between the condylar cartilage and the temporal fossa, leaving a meniscus between the bones, creating a double joint (Figure 11-14).[23,24] Since the condylar cartilage acts uniquely as both an articular and growth cartilage, damage to the cartilage by trauma, infection, or any of the arthritides impacts mandibular growth, leading to unilateral or bilateral micrognathia. Conversely, continued growth past adolescence accounts for prognathism in acromegalics.

● **DENTITION**

Dental development is enormously complex, incurring interactions between ectoderm (forming enamel) neural crest ectomesenchyme (forming dentin, pulp and cementum), and mesoderm (forming portion of the periodontal ligament). The genetics of odontogenesis has expanded prodigiously into a specialty invoking the whole of the embryonic, fetal, infant, adolescent, and adult stages of life. The prolonged chronology of odontogenesis makes teeth the most protracted developing set of organs in the body, exposing them to the greatest extent of possible maldevelopment. This life-long duration of dental dysmorphology, ranging from anodontia, and supernumeraries to malocclusion requires the specialty of dentistry to devote to its stomato-odontognathological requirements.[25] Full details of odontogenesis are available in Sperber et al.[7]

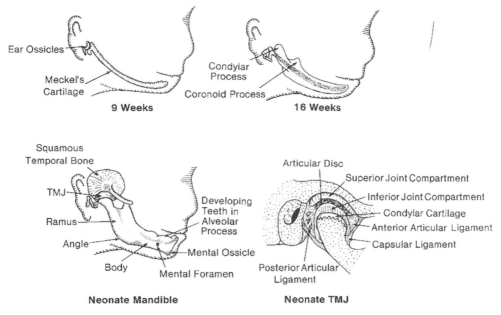

● **FIGURE 11-14.** Development of the mandible and temporomandibular joint.
(*Reprinted from Sperber GH. Embryology of the head and neck. In: English GM, ed. Otolaryngology. Philadelphia: JB Lippincott; 1990:1–36.*)

● CONCLUSION

These synoptic insights into embryogenesis and development provide the clinician with better comprehension of the origin of the maladies they are called upon to remedy and allow for insightful treatment planning to achieve normality of function and performance. The multiferous syndromes of the head and neck are rooted in deviations of development that require etiological diagnosis before surgical remediation.[26] Evaluation of congenital facial anomalies is enhanced by computer tomography (CT) scanning and magnetic resonance imaging (MRI) in conjunction with maldevelopmental insights to appropriately manage rehabilitational surgical interventions.[27]

● ACKNOWLEDGMENTS

Grateful thanks are accorded to Joanne Lafrance for her meticulous word processing skills.

REFERENCES

1. Scheller EL, Krebsbach PH. Gene therapy: design and prospects for craniofacial regeneration. *J Dent Res.* 2009;88:585.

2. Korshunova Y, Tidewell R, Veile R, et al. Gene expression profiles of human craniofacial development [poster]. COGENE. Updated February 14, 2003. http://hg.wustl.edu/cogene. Accessed February 2, 2010.

3. Cordero DR, Brugmann S, Chu Y, et al. Cranial neural crest cells on the move: their roles in craniofacial development. *Am J Med Genet A.* 2011;155:270.

4. Le Douarin NM, Brito JM, Creuzet S. Role of the neural crest in face and brain development. *Brain Res Rev.* 2007;55:237.

5. Chai Y, Maxson RE Jr. Recent advances in craniofacial morphogenesis. *Dev Dyn.* 2006;235:2353.

6. Helms JA, Cordero D, Tapadia MD. New insights into craniofacial morphogenesis [erratum *Development.* 2005; 132(12):2929]. *Development.* 2005;132:851.

7. Sperber GH, Sperber SM, Guttmann GD. *Craniofacial Embryogenetics and Development.* 2nd ed. Shelton, CT: PMPH-USA; 2010.

8. Brugmann SA, Tapadia MD, Helms JA. The molecular origins of species-specific facial pattern. *Curr Top Dev Biol.* 2006;73:1.

9. Francis-West P. Craniofacial development: making headway [editorial]. *Dev Dyn.* 2006;235:1151.

10. Radlanski RJ, Renz H. Genes, forces and forms: mechanical aspects of prenatal craniofacial development. *Dev Dyn.* 2006;235:1219.

11. Tapadia MD, Cordero DR, Helms JA. It's all in your head: new insights into craniofacial development and deformation. *J Anat.* 2005;207:461.

12. Song L, Li Y, Wang K, et al. Lrp6-mediated canonical Wnt signaling is required for lip formation and fusion. *Development.* 2009;136:3161.

13. Ioannides AS, Massa V, Ferraro E, et al. Foregut separation and trachea-oesophageal malformations: the role of tracheal outgrowth, dorso-ventral patterning and programmed cell death. *Dev Biol.* 2010;337:351.

14. Passos-Bueno MR, Ornelas CC, Fanganiello RD. Syndromes of the first and second pharyngeal arches: a review. *Am J Med Genet A.* 2009;149A:1853.

15. Johnson JM, Moonis G, Green GE, Carmody R, Burbank HN. Syndromes of the first and second branchial arches, Part 2: Syndromes. *Am J Neurorad.* 2011;32:230.

16. Bush JO, Jiang R. Palatogenesis: morphogenetic and molecular mechanisms of secondary palate development. *Development* 2012;139:231.

17. Sperber GH, Sperber SM. Embryology of orofacial clefting. In: Losee JE, Kirschner RE, eds. *Comprehensive Cleft Care.* 2nd ed. New York: McGraw-Hill Medical; 2009:3.

18. Connerney J, Andreeva V, Leshem Y, et al. Twist1 homodimers enhance FGF responsiveness of the cranial sutures and promote suture closure. *Dev Biol.* 2008;318:323.

19. Opperman LA, Gakunga PT, Carlson DS. Genetic factors influencing morphogenesis and growth of sutures and synchondroses in the craniofacial complex. *Semin Orthod.* 2005;11:199.

20. Rice DP. *Craniofacial Sutures: Development, Disease and Treatment. Frontiers of Oral Biology.* Vol 12. Basel, Switzerland: Karger AG; 2008.

21. Roybal PG, Wu NL, Sun J, et al. Inactivation of Msx1 and Msx2 in neural crest reveals an unexpected role in suppressing heterotypic bone formation in the head. *Dev Biol.* 2010;343:28.

22. Eames BF, Schneider RA. The genesis of cartilage size and shape during development and evolution. *Development.* 2008;135:3947.

23. Gu S, Wei N, Yu L, et al. Shox2-deficiency leads to dysplasia and ankylosis of the temporomandibular joint in mice. *Mech Dev.* 2008;125:729.

24. Wang Y, Liu C, Rohr J, et al. Tissue interaction is required for glenoid fossa development during temporomandibular joint formation. *Dev Dyn.* 2011;240:2466.

25. Fleming PS, Xavier GM, DiBiase AT, et al. Revisiting the supernumerary: the epidemiological and molecular basis of extra teeth. *Brit Dent J.* 2010;208:25.

26. Hennekam RCM, Allanson J. *Gorlin's Syndromes of the Head and Neck.* 5th ed. New York: Oxford University Press; 2010.

27. Baxter JG, Shroff M. Congenital midface abnormalities. *Neuroimag Clin N Am.* 2011;21:563.

SUGGESTED WEBSITES

Embryo Images Normal and Abnormal Mammalian Development. http://www.med.unc.edu/embryo_images

Virtual Human Embryo Project. http://virtualhumanembryo.lsuhsc.edu/

chapter 12

Cleft Lip Repair

William Y. Hoffman, MD

● PATIENT EVALUATION

Cleft lips occur in a wide range of phenotypes, from a minimal notch to complete cleft lip and palate (Figure 12-1). The lip is formed in the sixth week of gestation by the fusion of the frontonasal process and the maxillary processes. The frontonasal process gives rise to the nose and the central lip (the prolabium) and the premaxilla back to the incisive foramen (the primary palate). The fusion of the maxillary processes with the central lip is stabilized by migration of mesenchymal tissue, which is derived from the neural crest. The stabilization of neural crest by folate is well documented and contributes to the decrease in cleft occurrence with administration of perinatal folate. Although the remainder of the palate unites at a later point in fetal development, cleft lip and palate frequently occur together. Approximately one fourth of clefts are of the lip only, one fourth of the palate only, and one half of the cleft lip and palate.

Classification may be done with simple description: the most minimal cleft is described as microform or forme fruste, incomplete clefts with intact nasal sill may be described in terms of the percentage of the lip involved, while complete clefts involve the nasal sill and floor. The extent of involvement of the alveolus should be documented as well as the palate. Kernahan formulated a diagrammatic system to standardize these descriptions (Figure 12-2).

Approximately 30% of clefts occur in association with a known genetic syndrome. We are only beginning to understand the expression of specific genes in relation to the formation of clefts. Almost all syndromes present with a right-sided cleft, although left-sided clefts represent about two thirds of unilateral clefts. The presence of a right-sided cleft should prompt heightened surveillance for possible syndromic involvement.

Some syndromes are more common and should be recognizable by the practitioner. Relatively common is Van Der Woude syndrome, which is manifested by clefts in association with lip "pits," which in fact are sinus tracts of the minor salivary glands. This syndrome, as with many, is autosomal dominant but has variable phenotypic expression, from submucous cleft palate through complete bilateral cleft lip and palate. It is associated with the interferon regulatory factor 6 (*IRF6*) gene, also found in popliteal pterygium syndrome.

Inheritance of nonsyndromic clefts is not typically Mendelian; if an otherwise unaffected family has a child with a cleft, there is a 2% to 5% chance that another child will be affected. If two children are affected, the chances for a third child is 9%; if a parent and a child are affected, the chances for another child rise to 15%.

In general, there are few contraindications to cleft lip repair. While the presence of a syndrome, particularly one with significant developmental delay, may mitigate against cleft palate repair because of airway concerns, these concerns are not as significant regarding the lip. In bilateral lip repairs the very short columella may result in a relatively restricted nasal airway, but the use of nasal stents postoperatively will help both in lengthening of the columella and in maintaining patency of the nasal airway.

● PATIENT PREPARATION

The classic mnemonic for cleft lip surgery is the "rule of 10s"—the child should be 10 weeks old, weigh 10 pounds, and have a hemoglobin level above 10 g/mL. These are still useful criteria but it is important to remember that they are based on an evaluation of the general well-being of the infant. Ten to 12 weeks is the average age where the other goals can be met. The hemoglobin is perhaps the

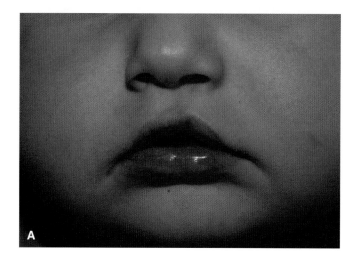

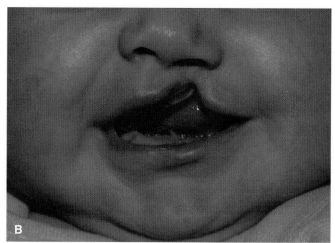

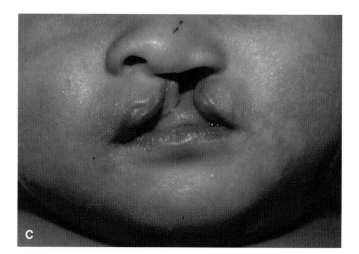

FIGURE 12-1. (A) Microform of cleft lip (forme fruste). (B) Incomplete unilateral cleft lip. (C) Complete unilateral cleft lip.

least important of the three, as fetal hemoglobin begins to disappear at birth to be replaced by adult hemoglobin, resulting in a nadir at about 6 to 8 weeks of age. However, the expected blood loss for a lip repair should be negligible

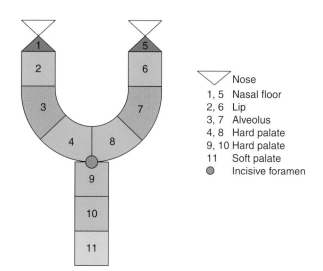

FIGURE 12-2. Kernahan system for classification of clefts.

Nose
1, 5 Nasal floor
2, 6 Lip
3, 7 Alveolus
4, 8 Hard palate
9, 10 Hard palate
11 Soft palate
⬤ Incisive foramen

and a hemoglobin level of 8 or 9 may be acceptable if the child is otherwise fine.

The child's weight is a general reflection of adequate nutritional intake. If there is a cleft palate in association with the cleft lip, the child will not be able to suck adequately for breastfeeding and requires specialized feeding appliances. Inadequate intake, gastroesophageal reflux, and increased effort of breathing all may contribute to poor weight gain, and these must be investigated thoroughly prior to surgery.

Lastly, if there is a complete cleft through the lip and alveolus (and generally the palate as well) the child must be prepared for surgery by controlling the position of the maxillary segments. Reduction of the gap in a unilateral cleft and, even more importantly, controlling the position of the premaxilla in a bilateral cleft are important factors in preoperative preparation which make the surgery both more facile as well as producing better results.

There are multiple means of manipulation of the alveolar segments and the premaxilla. Latham originally described alveolar molding plates as pin-fixed appliances; these have largely been supplanted by denture-like plates that are maintained with denture adhesive. These can be fashioned by orthodontists or pediatric dentists; creating

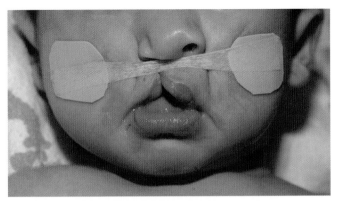

● **FIGURE 12-3.** Taping the cleft segments can be an effective and readily available means of narrowing the cleft prior to surgical closure.

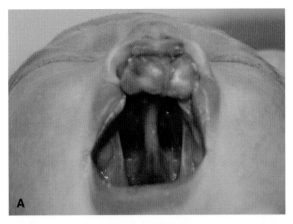

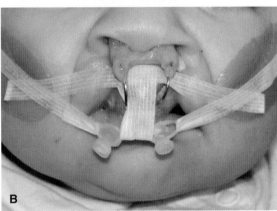

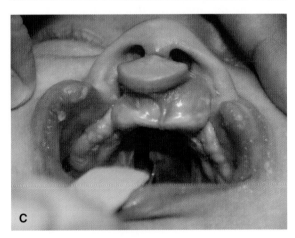

● **FIGURE 12-4.** (A) Bilateral cleft lip and palate with marked anterior displacement of premaxilla. (B) Nasoalveolar molding device shown in place. (C) Premaxilla shown in good position in relation to the lateral segments. Note the improvement in nasal contour as well.

space on one side and adding material on the other can gradually move the alveolus. The addition of prongs to stretch out the abnormal nostril(s) has given rise to the popular acronym NAM (nasal alveolar molding). These devices generally require weekly visits to the orthodontist and may require 3 to 4 months to accomplish. Treatment must be started early as the segments are much more mobile in the neonate.

In unilateral clefts, taping with gentle compression will significantly narrow the gap between the alveolar segments (Figure 12-3). While this is a reasonable and inexpensive alternative to NAM in the unilateral cleft, in the bilateral cleft it is difficult to move the premaxilla in a predictable fashion and NAM is preferable, if available (Figure 12-4).

Performing an operation on a 3-month-old child is a significant undertaking, even when the surgery is essentially superficial. Pediatric anesthesiologists should be administering anesthesia. Standard monitoring is sufficient (blood pressure, pulse oximetry), and the use of an oral Ring–Adair–Elwin (RAE) endotracheal tube is recommended, as this can be secured to the chin without distortion of the upper lip or commissures. Occlusive plastic sheets are placed over the eyes for protection and to allow antiseptic preparation of the entire face. Betadine is used for prepping as chlorhexidine is contraindicated for facial preparation.

The oral RAE tube is useful for positioning; by turning the patient 90 or even 180 degrees, the surgeon has access to the entire face and the endotracheal tube is still directed toward the ventilator and the anesthetist.

The lip repair should be marked with a fine-tipped marking pen. The author's preference is for brilliant green dye, which is alcohol based and produces a fine line with a cut, cotton-tipped applicator, even on mucosa. The mucocutaneous junction is tattooed with the dye as well. This is critical for repairing the white roll during the closure, as the mucosal blanching that occurs from epinephrine may make this line obscure during the surgery. Once this is completed, the lip is injected with lidocaine 0.5% and

epinephrine 1:200,000; 1 cc/kg can be safely administered, although generally no more than 3 to 4 cc is required.

● **TECHNIQUES**

Unilateral Cleft Lip Repair

In all unilateral cleft lip repairs, the goal is to lengthen the cleft side to achieve a symmetrical appearance of the

Cupid's bow. In the first half of the twentieth century, recognition that a straight-line repair would inevitably contract and shorten led to breaking up of the scar, initially with quadrilateral repairs and later with the triangular lip repair (also known as the Tennison repair, later modified by Randall), which is still popular today. In essence, the triangular lip repair is a z-plasty placed just above the vermilion border; as with any z-plasty, length is obtained at the expense of width. The triangular lip repair creates excellent length but because the area just above the white roll is the tightest, the lip appears somewhat flat on lateral view. In addition, lip revision may be more difficult due to the geometric closure.

The rotation advancement repair, also known as the Millard repair after the initial description, addresses many of these issues, by moving the z-plasty to just below the nasal sill (Figure 12-5). This places the tightest area of closure at the top of the lip rather than the bottom, and creates a more natural appearing lip with normal pout. The scar follows the natural line of the philtral column on the side of the cleft, contributing to the more normal appearance. The introduction of a small z-plasty above the white roll can reduce scar contraction but does not break up the philtrum significantly.

The rotation flap is designed by first establishing the high point of Cupid's bow on the medial segment. This is established by first marking the high point on the intact side, then the midline. Note that the midline is not usually obvious and that the gradually curving prolabium can often be marked correctly in a number of locations. A narrow prolabium is much more normal in appearance

and moving the midpoint and high point further medially reduces the amount that the lip needs to be rotated for symmetry. The most common error is to have the high point too far lateral, resulting in a scar that is too far lateral, a prolabium that is too wide and a lip that is too short on the repaired side.

Once the high point is established, the rotation flap is designed from that point upwards, curving up to the junction of the lip with the columella. The cutaneous portion that is lateral to the rotation flap becomes the "c" flap, which will be used to lengthen the columella. The same line is continued down into the mucosa, creating the medial mucosal flap that will be used for lining the vestibule. Note that in an incomplete cleft, the medial and lateral mucosal flaps are basically trimmed near the vestibule to permit suturing of the lateral lip flap.

The key to designing the advancement flap is again the determination of the point that will be closed at the white roll. The height of the lip is again the critical factor; the point on the advancement flap is established by measuring the normal side with calipers from the high point to the nasal sill, then measuring the same length on the advancement flap (Figure 12-6). The advancement flap is drawn with a line along the mucocutaneous junction, taking care not to include any mucosa in the skin portion of the flap,

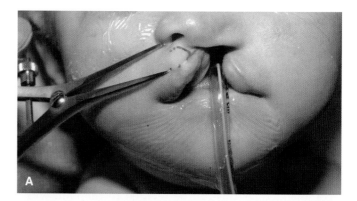

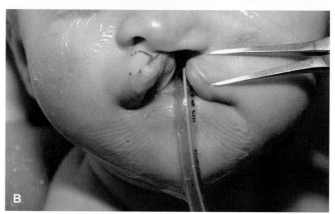

● **FIGURE 12-6.** (A) Measuring the height of the lip on the non-cleft side. (B) Transfer of the measurement from the normal side to the cleft side. This determines the location of the advancement flap on the cleft lateral segment.

● **FIGURE 12-5.** Typical markings for a rotation advancement repair. Note the small triangular flap of dry mucosa on the lateral segment which will be used to augment dry mucosa on the medial side.

as this will result in a permanently pink scar (this is true for the c flap as well). The upper part of the advancement flap is cut just below the nasal sill but does not continue around the alar base, where the scar is more obvious. The mucosal flap on this side is a little more complex, leaving a small triangular flap of dry mucosa on the lateral lip element to insert into the central portion of the lip, where the dry mucosa is almost always deficient. The lateral mucosal flap is taken from the remaining medial mucosa.

The incisions on both sides are made just through the dermis, as the orbicularis muscle is quite superficial. On both sides, the orbicularis must be dissected circumferentially from skin and mucosa. Medially, the dissection should be limited to the midpoint of the philtrum to preserve any central depression that exists. On both sides the muscle must be released from the abnormal attachments to the nose; medially from the columella, laterally from the nasal sill and alar base. The lateral dissection should not be carried any farther than is necessary to complete the circumferential release of the muscle.

Once the flaps are all completely dissected, the nose is addressed by separating the nasal skin from the alar cartilage using small tenotomy scissors. This dissection is carried out over the opposite alar dome and onto the nasal dorsum, creating a space for rotation of the cleft side alar cartilage up and medial, partially correcting the nasal deformity. Sutures are placed at the end of the procedure, either through an internal method or over external bolsters to hold the alar cartilage in the new position.

Adequate release of the lateral lip is crucial to obtaining a tension-free repair. The lateral vestibular incision permits release of the lip and muscle as a unit, with dissection above the periosteum of the maxilla (some surgeons have proposed a subperiosteal dissection but in general it is felt that this may interfere with subsequent maxillary growth). The nose is released along the piriform aperture laterally to allow the nasal ala to be brought into a symmetrical position with the opposite side. This creates a lateral mucosal defect in the nasal sidewall, which is closed with the lateral mucosal flap. The medial mucosal flap is turned over to line the vestibule and the floor of the nose. The alar base is anchored to the columella with an absorbable suture, which brings the columella into the midline and should attempt to position the ala symmetrically with the opposite side. This is generally an "air knot," where the surgeon ties it while watching the symmetry from above the patient.

Closure of the lip repair follows that of the nose and starts along the lateral maxillary vestibule, as this is difficult to see later. The orbicularis oris muscle is repaired with two or three absorbable mattress sutures. In general, the medial muscle must be rotated somewhat inferiorly to achieve proper alignment of the two lip segments. A good muscle repair is critical to avoid tension on the skin closure, and is associated with more normal lip growth in the future. The majority of the muscle repair is near the lower part of the lip to achieve appropriate fullness and contour. There have been techniques described to separate specific muscle

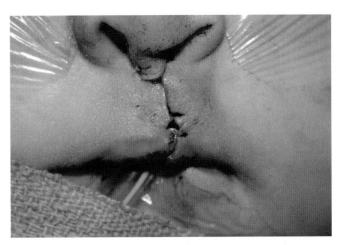

● **FIGURE 12-7.** Noordhoff triangular flap is a z-plasty just above the mucocutaneous junction which can increase length of the lip repair slightly as well as decreasing scar contracture.

components to place in different sites, but the author has found this technically difficult and unnecessary.

The lip skin is closed with 6-0 fast-absorbing catgut sutures; these are dissolved in a matter of days, obviating the need for suture removal and avoiding cross-hatching. If the lip repair appears at all short at the time of repair, Noordhoff triangular lip flap (really a small, 1–1.5 mm z-plasty above the white roll) is an excellent means of obtaining a little extra length and reducing scar contracture (Figure 12-7). The mucosa is closed with particular attention to the "red line," the junction between the wet and dry mucosa. In most unilateral clefts the dry mucosa is deficient on the medial side, and an incision at the red line will allow insertion of the dry mucosa that was preserved with the lateral lip element at the outset, improving the amount of dry mucosa and ensuring alignment of the two types; retention of wet mucosa in the external lip repair can be quite obvious and will mar an otherwise good effort. If there is any tension on the wet mucosa, a z-plasty is placed near the vestibule to avoid notching.

The nasal correction is completed at the conclusion of the lip repair. With the McComb technique, two bolster sutures are placed. The first goes through the lateral portion of the dome and is brought out through the dorsum of the nose on the contralateral side. This should bring the alar cartilage up to a slightly overcorrected position; the second suture anchors the lateral crus at the point where it is most prominent in the nasal sidewall. The sutures used are 4-0 monofilament, and are tied over red rubber bolsters. The internal bolsters have silk sutures attached as well, which makes removal in clinic (time: less than 1 week) very straightforward.

Bilateral Cleft Lip Repair

The bilateral cleft lip presents a number of additional challenges compared with the unilateral situation. First, as noted above, the premaxilla can be almost at 90 degrees to the plane of the lip in a complete bilateral cleft, and considerable effort should be devoted to repositioning the premaxilla prior to surgery. It is critical to the final outcome that there be minimal tension on the lip repair and also that the orbicularis muscle from the two lateral segments be brought together across the premaxilla in the midline, and both of these require that the premaxilla be brought back more in line with the lateral segments. Although taping or elastics have been used with reasonable success, alveolar molding plates are an excellent choice, as these can also control the position of the lateral segments, which tend to collapse behind the premaxilla. If these efforts are unsuccessful, either due to absence of resources or family compliance, a last alternative is use of the vomer osteotomy at the time of surgery. This requires a small longitudinal incision along the vomer behind the premaxilla, and removal of about 4 to 5 mm of bone from the vomer with a small rongeur. The premaxilla then rotates back, usually into contact with the lateral segments. This maneuver has been associated anecdotally with decreased maxillary growth but there are no good long-term studies documenting growth in this situation.

The second challenge is the short columella. This is due to multiple factors: there is separation of the alar cartilages with interposed fibrofatty tissue, but there is also a true lack of length of the columella as well. Various proposals for correction of the columella fall into three primary categories: preoperative lengthening with the addition of prongs to the NAM device; intraoperative suturing and internal rotation of the alar cartilages; and later procedures such as forked flaps or V-Y advancements to lengthen the columella, usually at about age 4 to 5 years. All of these have some shortcomings: NAM may provide inadequate length despite some definite improvement; suturing of the alar cartilages may rotate the tip upward as in any rhinoplasty, adding to the already foreshortened nose; later procedure produce scars and may not produce adequate length as well. Virtually all patients with unilateral or bilateral clefts require rhinoplasty in their teens.

Lastly, while subtle, there is minimal or no dry mucosa in the prolabium. The design of the lateral lip incisions, which is otherwise similar to the Millar repair above, must have a step-cut with preservation of the dry mucosa to be repaired in the midline beneath the prolabium. This author preserves 1 to 2 mm of existing dry mucosa with the prolabium; others remove all mucosa and suture the lateral mucosa to the prolabial skin.

With an appreciation of these issues, one can then design the bilateral cleft lip repair. The central tenet is that the prolabium must be narrowed to about 4 to 5 mm; the central lip always becomes wider and a prolabium of 15 mm or more in an adolescent is an obvious stigma of the bilateral cleft even with good scars (Figure 12-8). The length of the prolabium determines the length of the cutaneous lip repair; there is not really any method of increasing this length at the time of the initial repair. The central

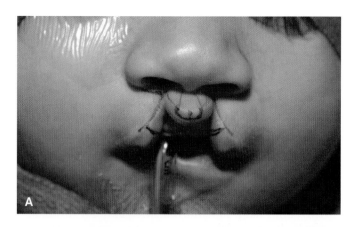

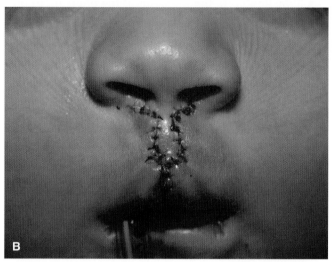

● **FIGURE 12-8.** (A) Markings for a bilateral lip repair. Note the narrow prolabium and the step-cut on the lateral segment to preserve additional dry mucosa. (B) Bilateral cleft lip repair completed. Note the alignment of the dry mucosa in the midline below the prolabium, and absence of whistle deformity.

lip is hinged on the columella, and this is the source of blood supply. The additional skin on either side of the prolabium can be preserved as "forked flaps" to be inset under the nasal sill on each side and used later for columellar lengthening. The lateral lip element is tailored to fit the length of the prolabium. The two alar bases are sutured to each other, which may exaggerate the short columella in more severe cases.

The nose may be addressed at the time of lip repair. Mulliken was an early proponent of suturing the alar domes together to obtain additional columellar length. Initially this was done through a midline incision in the tip of the nose, but this has now evolved to a procedure done through bilateral rim incisions with excision of excess overhanging skin at the alar margin. Cutting proposes doing a modified open rhinoplasty by elevating the medial crura of the alar cartilages together with the prolabium and the columella. This is done to preserve blood supply to the prolabium, but requires a retrograde dissection of the nasal tip in order to suture the tip cartilages together. Both of these techniques show very nice improvement in the columella but in lateral views the tip is often rotated cephalad.

Gingivoperiosteoplasty

Gingivoperiosteoplasty (GPP) refers to the creation of subperiosteal flaps at the cleft margin to close the alveolar cleft. Skoog described this many years ago, and Delaire later proposed more extensive subperiosteal dissection of the lateral lip element. It is well documented that these repairs will result in bone bridging the alveolar gap in a majority of cases, but it is also widely held that extensive undermining of the periosteum may create maxillary growth deficiency. Cutting and Grayson have popularized GPP after NAM in both unilateral and bilateral clefts but have emphasized that this should only be done if there is perfect alignment of the alveolar segments with a minimal gap (1–2 mm at most). Orthodontists are divided about the benefit of this procedure, as it may be more difficult to manipulate the alveolar segments if there is bony continuity.

● COMPLICATIONS

Complications of lip repair are quite rare, as there is excellent blood supply; infections and dehiscence occur in well under 1% of patients. While not specifically a complication, hypertrophic scarring can occur commonly, particularly in darker complexions. This is often seen at about 3 to 6 weeks following surgery and usually resolves without specific treatment. Taping and massage may be beneficial. With hypertrophic scarring the lip usually becomes somewhat shorter along the line of repair, but in general the length returns as the scar diminishes and softens (this may take as long as a year).

● OUTCOMES

It is rare that a critical plastic surgeon would not see something to "touch up" in any cleft lip repair. The goal should be to minimize such interventions, as repeated revisions will remove some normal tissue with each procedure and will inevitably result in a lip that is tight. Unless there is a severe problem, the earliest revision should be considered is in preschool, around age 5 years. Better still, if possible revision should be delayed until orthodontic treatment is completed, so that the fullness of the lip can be evaluated appropriately. As children mature they should be involved in the discussion of any revision; there is a surprising range of opinions among the patients.

Nasal deformity is almost always addressed in early to mid teens. Most unilateral cleft patients have septal deviation into the side of the cleft and usually have deviation of the bony pyramid to the opposite side. A septorhinoplasty allows correction of the breathing issues and harvesting of septal cartilage to use as graft material for any residual tip asymmetry. An inverted U osteotomy allows the bony pyramid to be shifted as a unit back into the midline.

● CONCLUSION

Cleft lip is best treated by a team approach, and consistent good results are now the expectation rather than the exception. It is often the small details that make a large difference in the final outcome.

SUGGESTED READING

Losee JF, Kirschner RE, eds. *Comprehensive Cleft Care*. New York: McGraw-Hill; 2008. An excellent text that is encyclopedic in its coverage of cleft lip and palate with multiple techniques reviewed.

Millard R. *Cleft Craft*. New York: Little Brown; 1976–1980. Out of print but well worth the effort as a review of many techniques and the evolution of the rotation advancement repair.

chapter 13

Cleft Palate

Peter J. Taub, MD, FACS, FAAP / Joseph E. Losee, MD, FACS, FAAP

● INTRODUCTION

A palatal cleft represents one of the more commonly recognized congenital anomalies (Figure 13-1). Anatomically, the palate separates the oral and nasal cavities from the lip to the uvula. It is divided at the incisive foramen into the primary palate anteriorly and the secondary palate posteriorly. More commonly, however, the palate is described as being composed of hard and soft portions, from the alveolar ridge to the uvula. The soft portion is also referred to as the velum.

The teeth develop within the maxilla and erupt into the softer inferior alveolar bone. The central and lateral incisors develop within the midline premaxillary portion of the palate, separate from the canines, premolars, and molars. The premaxilla eventually fuses with the two lateral elements, each of which houses the remaining complement of teeth. Typical clefts occur in the region of the lateral incisor and canine, either of which may or may not be present.[1]

Among ethnic groups, the incidence of clefting is highest in Native Americans, followed by Caucasians, Asians, and African Americans. Clefts of the lip, with or without a palatal cleft, are now thought of as a separate entity from isolated clefts of the palate. The two differ significantly in terms of their epidemiologic profiles. The incidence of clefts of the lip with or without a cleft palate is approximately 1 in 700 live births, while that of isolated clefts of the palate is closer to 1 in 2000 live births. The isolated variety is also more commonly seen in females, while clefts of the lip with or without a cleft palate are more commonly seen in males.

● PATIENT SELECTION

At the time of consultation, a thorough history and physical examination should note any family history of relatives with clefting or congenital anomalies and any prenatal problems that might be related to development of the cleft. The sequellae of an open palate include difficulty with feeding and maintaining adequate nutrition, collection of fluid in the middle ear possibly leading to hearing loss, abnormal speech production and language development, and distortion of facial growth.

Palatal clefts are generally described in terms of their uni- or bilaterality, their completeness, and the specific structures that are affected. The lip may or may not be involved and the alveolar ridge may or may not be part of the cleft. A rare combination may include a cleft of the lip, with an intervening intact alveolus, and a cleft palate. The simplest form of a cleft palate is a bifid uvula, which occurs in roughly 2% of the population and may go undetected. The bifid uvula, however, may be a clue to the presence of an underlying submucous cleft palate. Here, the oral and nasal mucosal surfaces are intact, but the levator veli palatini muscle fibers are divergent. This may present in older children without a prior diagnosis of an overt cleft palate. Patients are referred with speech concerns despite a period of therapy that has failed to provide adequate results. The specific findings that might accompany a patient's hypernasal speech include a bifid uvula, a notch of the posterior nasal spine, and a "zona pellucida" or clear area in the middle of the soft palate.

A cleft palate may be seen in infants as part of a syndrome encompassing other craniofacial anomalies, such as Apert syndrome, Stickler syndrome, Treacher Collins syndrome, Van Der Woude syndrome, and velocardiofacial syndrome. In patients with Pierre Robin sequence (Figure 13-2), the cleft is usually in the secondary (or soft) palate. Here, it arises as a result of the associated micrognathia and inability of the tongue to remain out of the way of the descending palatal shelves which normally fuse in the midline before birth. In such patients, prone positioning, tongue-lip adhesion, tracheostomy, or

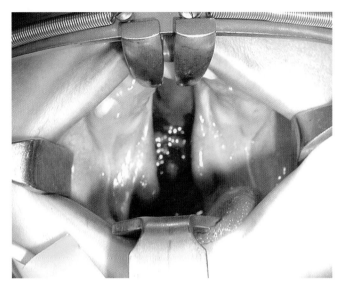

● **FIGURE 13-1.** Intraoperative photograph of an infant with a near complete cleft of the hard and soft palate.

early distraction of the mandible may be required before closure of the palate in order to stabilize the infant's airway.

Adults who present with an unrepaired cleft of the hard and/or soft palate are likely to have greater speech concerns than are younger patients. Adults often develop significant errors of articulation as a means of compensation for the cleft. Depending on their access to health care, some patients may or may not have had years of speech therapy in an attempt to overcome the physiologic problem of palatal incompetence. While closure is important to improve resonance and oral hygiene, it is usually difficult to achieve near-normal speech quality in older patients.

● **PATIENT PREPARATION**

In developed countries, the diagnosis of a cleft palate may be made as early as 12 weeks into pregnancy by a skilled ultrasonographer (Figure 13-3). In such cases, it is helpful for the parents to visit with a multidisciplinary team of clinicians to discuss the nature of the problem and management strategies in advance of the birth. More often, however, a cleft palate is diagnosed at birth as a defect "in the roof of the mouth."

Early problems related to a cleft palate include difficulty in maintaining nutrition, especially with breastfeeding, and regurgitation. Most infants do better with head-up positioning and the use of specially designed nipples that facilitate intake of milk or formula by diminishing resistance to flow or creating force to push fluid from the bottle in the presence of a weak suck.

The timing of cleft lip closure is related more to the social implications than to the functional problems. Infants with an open lip and an intact palate usually feed with minimal difficulty. Palatal clefts, on the other hand, require closure to improve oral and nasal hygiene and allow for the development of intelligible speech with normal resonance. As such, cleft lip repair is generally performed at about 3 months of age, a time chosen due to the relative safety of general anesthesia in an infant.

Prior to formal lip repair, consideration for presurgical, nasoalveolar molding of the palatal arches should be entertained. In some children, especially those with either a complete unilateral or bilateral cleft of the lip and palate, distortion of the palatal arch is present. This may make lip repair problematic due to the tension required to approximate the cleft margins. Nasoalveolar molding, using either passive or active appliances, may dramatically realign the palatal components so that the lip may be repaired under minimal tension, the nasal contour may

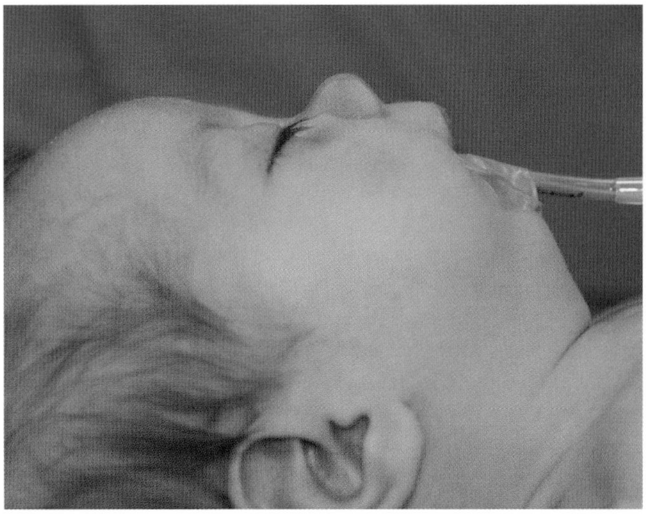

● **FIGURE 13-2.** Photograph of an infant with Pierre Robin sequence demonstrating the micrognathia which contributes to the formation of a palatal cleft.

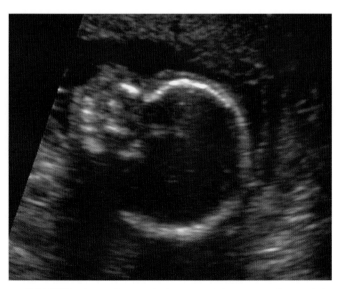

● **FIGURE 13-3.** Prenatal ultrasound demonstrating a cleft of the palate.

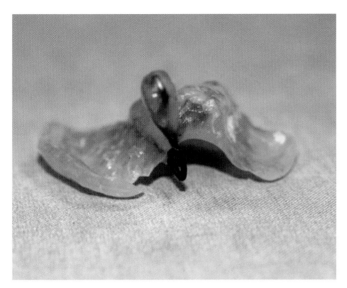

● **FIGURE 13-4.** Appliance fabricated from a palatal impression for use in presurgical nasoalveolar molding.

be improved, and possibly the alveolar mucosa closed at the time of lip repair to avert bone grafting in the future (gingivoperiosteoplasty).

Nasoalveolar molding requires obtaining an impression of the palate as soon as possible—often within the first few days of life—from which an appliance may be fabricated (Figure 13-4). Frequent follow-up visits are necessary over the ensuing weeks to ensure correct and adequate movement of the arches in anticipation of cleft lip, and eventually palate repair. Modifications include attachment of a nasal bulb to facilitate recontouring of the alar rim.

Prior to the advent of nasoalveolar molding, a wide cleft lip was closed in stages. An adhesion procedure was performed first using soft tissues from the margins of the cleft that were not to be used for the later formal repair. After allowing the tension from the closure to mold the palatal arches, the lip was then repaired at a second setting using standard techniques described elsewhere. The adhesion facilitates not only lip repair but also the later palatal closure.

The timing of palatal repair is controversial and varies from center to center. It is widely accepted that repair before 18 months of age minimizes problems related to speech and language development while not causing drastic effects on midfacial growth.[2] Early palate closure creates normal anatomy for the development of proper speech development but may interfere with midfacial growth. Several studies, looking at cephalometric data in patients who underwent early palatal repair, however, failed to demonstrate a difference in midfacial growth.[3,4] Later repair, although ideal to minimize scar formation during growth, leads to errors of articulation that become more difficult to reverse as the child gets older.

Some surgeons have advocated repair of the palate in stages. The soft palate, which is more intimately involved

with speech production, is repaired as early as 3 to 4 months of age, often at the time of lip repair. This is followed by later repair of the hard palate, delayed either months or years to minimize the detrimental affects on facial growth.[5] A palatal obturator may be used in the interim to seal off the oral cavity. Long-term evaluation, however, has failed to support any benefit of this approach on normal speech development.[6,7]

Many patients with a submucous cleft palate do not require surgical intervention and it is assumed that a large percentage go undiagnosed. Studies of patients with a known submucous cleft palate have demonstrated that many require no treatment at all.[8] Studies for a suspected diagnosis of a submucous cleft palate include nasopharyngoscopy and/or videofluoroscopy. The former involves passage of a small-caliber endoscope through the nose into the nasopharynx while the patient is awake. For this reason, younger children may not tolerate the procedure as well as older ones and the study may need to be deferred until the child is more cooperative. The camera is positioned above the soft palate and is able to visualize closure of the velum during phonation (Figure 13-5). In the patient with a suspected cleft palate, ridging of the lateral palatal elements may be indicative of incomplete muscle union in the midline. The soft palate may then fail to contact the posterior pharyngeal wall at the level of Passavant ridge opposite the second cervical vertebra during phonation. Videofluoroscopy provides similar information but does so by imaging the nasopharynx with radiography. It provides detailed information about the movement of the velum with speech. However, a fluoroscopic image provides only a single, cross-sectional view of the palate, usually in the sagittal plane. It is not possible to record multiple planes simultaneously and therefore cannot ascertain whether adequate velopharyngeal closure is possible.

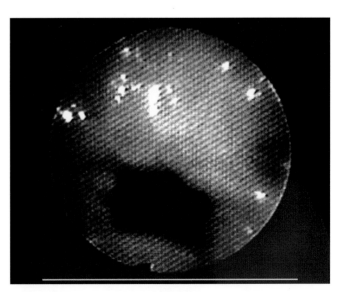

● **FIGURE 13-5.** Nasoendoscopic image of the velum and posterior wall of the pharynx demonstrating incomplete closure with phonation.

● TECHNIQUE

Palate repair is performed under general anesthesia with the patient in a supine position. The head and neck may be slightly extended and a shoulder roll placed across the upper back to improve exposure. Following intubation, a mouth prop is placed to adequately visualize the palate. The tongue blade has a groove for the endotracheal tube and the proper size should be chosen so as to hold the tongue out of the way in the midline yet not press on the posterior pharynx. The attached cheek retractors should sit just anterior to the mandibular rami. A moistened throat pack is placed in the pharynx to minimize blood loss into the stomach. A dilute epinephrine and anesthetic solution is injected into the lateral palatal shelves for hemostasis and the face and mouth prop are prepped in the usual sterile fashion. Care is taken to avoid ocular injury with lubricant and tape. Antibiotics may be given preoperatively and continued postoperatively at the surgeon's discretion.

Reconstruction of the hard palate begins with elevation of the lateral mucoperiosteum using a scalpel and periosteal elevator. The flaps are freed from the underlying palatal bone and advanced towards the midline for closure. Adequate mobilization requires careful dissection posteriorly around the vascular pedicle. The von Langenbeck repair leaves the anteriormost portions of the hard palate shelves attached to the alveolar ridge creating two bipedicle flaps that are then approximated in the midline (Figure 13-6).[9] For the more common complete cleft, the Veau-Wardill-Kilner repair creates two axial-pattern peninsular flaps based on the greater palatine artery and vein. These flaps are similarly approximated in the midline. They may also be fixed back to the premaxilla or hard palate anteriorly (Figure 13-7). In both instances, the resultant lateral defects may be packed with a gelatin material or left open to heal spontaneously in several weeks.

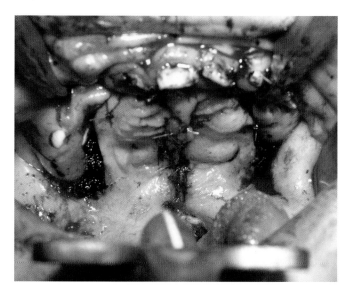

● **FIGURE 13-7.** Completed intraoperative view of Veau-Wardill-Kilner repair for closure of the palate.

The two basic options to address closure of the cleft of the soft palate include a straight-line repair or one that employs double-opposing z-plasty flaps. The straight-line repair involves dissection of the soft palate into its component parts: oral mucosa, palatal muscle, and nasal mucosa. The muscular components are invariably misdirected, inserting along the posterior edge of the hard palate. They are detached and redirected to the midline.

Repair begins with closure of the thin nasal mucosa anteriorly. This may not always be possible due to the size of the defect and the limited potential for mobilization of the lateral nasal mucosal edges. Flaps of mucosa from the midline vomer bone may be recruited to separately close each posterior nasal cavity. The use of vomerine mucosa during infancy has been questioned due to its possible adverse effects on facial growth.[10] Posterior to the vomer, the lateral mucosa does not always reach the midline without tension. In the past, one solution was to divide the nasal mucosa superior to the hard palate via the nose and allow it to advance posteriorly to close this potential defect. Recently, acellular dermis has been used to reconstruct this area; however, further investigation needs to clarify whether the addition of nonautogenous tissue is detrimental to palate repair.

The posterior soft palate normally contains the musculature that acts to elevate and pull the palate posteriorly, thus sealing off the nasal cavity from the pharynx. Six muscles have some attachment to the palate and all serve slightly different functions. These include the tensor veli palatine, the levator veli palatini, the palatoglossus, the palatopharyngeus, the superior constrictor, and the uvulus. In most cases of cleft palate, the tensor muscles, which normally originate laterally and insert in the midline, aberrantly insert along the posterior edge of the hard palate.[11] The abnormal muscle position also prevents adequate regulation of air and fluid flow through the distal Eustachian

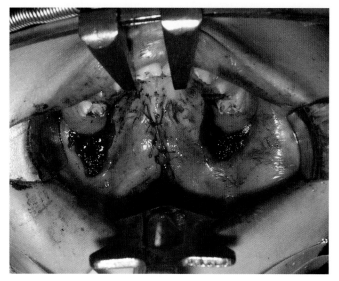

● **FIGURE 13-6.** Completed intraoperative view of von Langenbeck repair for closure of the palate.

tube predisposing to fluid buildup in the middle ear. Re-approximation of the muscle in the midline (intravelar veloplasty) following closure of the nasal mucosa serves to restore the normal anatomy of the palatal musculature.

Finally, the oral mucosa is closed in the midline. Controlled medial pressure on the soft tissues by a blunt instrument laterally within the Space of Ernst may assist in further mobilizing the soft tissues, minimizing tension across the repair, and thus diminishing the incidence of fistula formation. The greatest area of tension is often at the junction between the hard and soft palates. It is here that fistulae may develop and need to be addressed separately.

Fracture of the hamular process of the maxilla—the small bony protruberance around which the tensor veli palatini muscle runs—has been proposed as an adjunctive technique. It was suggested to improve medial displacement of the lateral tissues and minimize midline tension along the repair. Fracture of the hamulus appears to have neither obvious benefit nor detrimental effect on closure and its continued use is questionable in cleft palate surgery.[12]

Furlow devised the double-opposing z-plasty as an alternative technique for closure of the soft palate.[13] The objective is to realign the muscles while lengthening the palate, which may be inherently short and further shortened with postoperative scarring. Opposing z-plasty flaps are elevated on either side of the defect, one anteriorly based and the other posteriorly based. On the posteriorly based side (usually the patient's left for a right-handed surgeon), the flap contains oral mucosa and muscle separate from nasal mucosa. The nasal mucosa is cut as an opposing anteriorly based flap. On the contralateral side of the defect, an anteriorly based flap of oral mucosa is elevated off the muscle and nasal mucosa. The muscle and nasal mucosa are kept together and cut as an opposing posteriorly based flap. The flaps are rotated and the nasal mucosa is re-approximated followed by the oral mucosa (Figure 13-8). The muscles naturally realign in the midline and the length of the palate is increased.

The most important reported benefit of the double-opposing z-plasty technique is the improved speech results.[14] The dynamic lengthening of the palate is achieved by using the principles of the z-plasty in combination with the rearrangement of the muscle fibers. The disadvantages include the need for adequate mobilization of the flaps, since length is usually gained at the expense of width, and the more extensive suture lines which may be sites of fistualization. The Furlow palatoplasty has also been advocated as a conversion procedure in those patients who have previously undergone straight-line palate repair with an intravelar veloplasty and less than optimal speech results. It is felt that incomplete release and transposition of the muscles fail to produce optimal speech results. At the time of repeat palatoplasty some patients are also noted to have scarring of the muscles back down to the posterior edge of the hard palate, which compromises postoperative function.[15]

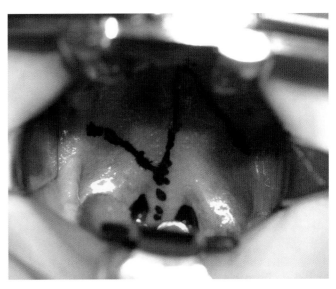

● FIGURE 13-8. Intraoperative view of the markings for a double-opposing z-plasty to repair a submucous cleft palate.

The most anterior portion of the palate, the alveolar ridge, is often closed separately. The oronasal fistula in the region of the cleft is usually small and, despite problems with regurgitation, has little impact on speech production. Reconstruction in this area requires bone graft to create a stable palatal arch, provide bone into which the erupting teeth may anchor, support the alar base of the nose, and provide a base for prosthetic dental restoration.

Closure of the alveolus has been described at various times during the management of a cleft palate. Some authors advocate mucosal closure at the time of initial lip repair (gingivoperiosteoplasty), noting that the bony defect may then heal without the need for later grafting.[16] Others advocate early bone grafting, about the time of palatal repair at around 1 year of age.[17] Others prefer to delay grafting anywhere between 2 to 12 years of age.[18] A better gauge for timing repair may be based on dental eruption. In this scheme, suggested times for alveolar grafting include (1) prior to eruption of the permanent incisor, (2) after eruption of the incisor but before eruption of the cleft side canine, and (3) after eruption of the cleft side canine. Details of the technique are beyond the scope of this chapter and are discussed elsewhere.

● **COMPLICATIONS**

The two significant early complications of cleft palate repair are bleeding and airway compromise. Bleeding following cleft palate repair is rare if care is taken to protect the greater palatine artery and control blood loss intraoperatively. Infiltration of local anesthetic with dilute lidocaine and epinephrine is useful prior to beginning the procedure and intraoperatively the blood pressure should be carefully monitored and controlled. Once the palate is closed, gentle compression over the bone may be useful prior to emergence from anesthesia.

Postoperative airway compromise in the obligate nose breather may result from edema and blood present in an already small nasopharynx. It may also result from swelling due to compression beneath the Dingman mouth gag and subsequent edema of the tongue. As a precaution, many surgeons place a suture through the tip of the tongue at the completion of the repair to assist in pulling the tongue forward in the event of airway compromise. In small children, the tongue may be difficult to grasp in an emergent setting, making the suture potentially lifesaving. It is easily removed on the first postoperative day with no adverse sequellae.

More common complications related to palatal closure are those related to wound healing problems. Dehiscence and fistula formation may be minimized by closing the medial palatal margins under as minimal tension as possible. To achieve this, wide lateral undermining is required. The surgeon, however, must be cognizant of the location of the pedicle to maximize dissection of the surrounding soft tissues while avoiding vascular injury.

The mucosal repair needs to be watertight since the incision lines are continuously bathed by saliva and mucus from the time the palate is closed. Furthermore, oral feedings need to be restarted in the postoperative period to maintain adequate nutrition. To combat the difficulty in creating a watertight seal, several authors have advocated the use of tissue sealants in cleft palate repair.[19] Cyanoacrylate adhesive may be instilled beneath the mucoperiosteal flaps to fix the flaps in place and minimize dead space or placed as a topical sealant. It has yet to be shown whether such maneuvers minimize the risk of fistula formation.

Often, some amount of tension is placed across the repair and a fistula forms at the point of maximal tension (Figure 13-9). Fistulae as small as 5 mm^2 may interfere with speech production.[20] Rates of formation vary among published series, but is approximately 5% to 10% (and higher for patients older than 2 years). Secondary closure

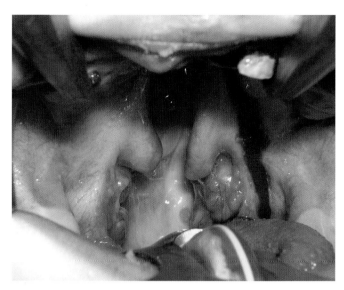

FIGURE 13-10. Photograph of the nasopharynx demonstrating purulent fluid arising from the unseen Eustachian tube.

of a palatal fistula is difficult due to the scarring that is present at the margins of the defect. Alloplastic material (acellular dermis), local flaps (adjacent palate), or distant flaps (tongue flap), may be used to cover the defect and better results are obtained with a two-layer closure.

Wound dehiscence may result from infection at the time of repair. Generally, the palate tolerates the normal colonization of bacterial flora within the oral cavity and does not become infected. In the oral cavity, common flora include staphylococcal and streptococcal species, as well as *Enterobacter*, *Neisseria*, *Bordetella*, and *Corynebacterium*. However, children with clefts often have fluid in the middle ear which may harbor more virulent organisms and act as a source of contamination (Figure 13-10). Since repair is considered elective, deferring surgery until after any infection has subsided is often prudent.

OUTCOMES ASSESSMENTS

Following successful cleft palate closure, the major parameter to observe is the patient's speech development and language production. Children born with a cleft palate are at risk for speech and language problems related to velopharyngeal insufficiency. Reports of insufficiency range from 7% to 30%. Frequently, adjunctive speech therapy is needed to correct errors of articulation that develop as a compensatory mechanism. Despite advances in the surgical management of cleft palate, preschoolers continue to require speech therapy as an integral component of their global care.

Speech impairments specific to velopharyngeal incompetence affect those sounds that require pressure in the oral cavity, either anteriorly or posteriorly. These include the sibilant consonants soft g, /s/, /z/, /ch/, /sh/, and /zh, and the intraoral pressure consonants /b/, /d/, hard g,

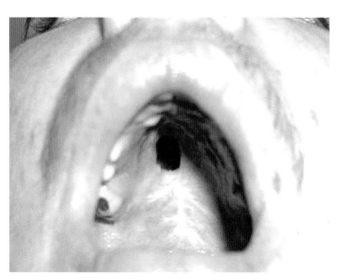

FIGURE 13-9. Chronic fistula of the hard palate.

/k/, /p/, and /t/. Such problems have been shown to be more prevalent in patients with a complete cleft of the hard and soft palate or those with associated congenital anomalies.[21]

Technique and surgeon skill may each play a role in the ultimate success of cleft palate repair. Longitudinal closure with an intravelar veloplasty was compared with Furlow palatoplasty in nonsyndromic cleft palate patients operated upon by a single surgeon.[22] Patients who had undergone straight-line closure had a 34% higher incidence of hoarseness, nasal air escape, and hypernasality at 3 years of age than those who underwent Furlow palatoplasty. No difference was noted in the rate of fistula formation. In a separate study, nonsyndromic patients with an incomplete cleft palate demonstrated a higher rate of adequate velopharyngeal function following Furlow palatoplasty as opposed to von Langenbeck palatoplasty.[23] The Furlow technique was also noted to have fewer complications and the results of velopharyngeal function translated to improved results in speech and language production.

Midfacial growth is also a concern following repair of the palate. It is thought that the production of scar tissue near the growth centers of the face interferes with normal skeletal development. This finding has been noted since the early 1900s when Gilles and Fry observed posterior displacement and narrowing of the maxillary arch in patients who underwent early hard palate repair. Similarly, Ortiz-Monasterio et al.,[24] among others,[25] noted excellent jaw relationships in adult patients who did not undergo timely palate closure. As a result, surgical protocols were developed that closed only the soft palate at an early stage while the hard palate was obturated with a prosthesis until facial growth was complete.[26] The belief was that closure of the more pliable soft palate had less of an effect on facial growth than did closure of the hard palate. It should be noted however that other studies have failed to show an adverse affect on facial growth by repair of the palate.[27] To date, prospective, well-controlled studies are still lacking to establish the long-term effect of hard palate repair on facial growth. Creation of such a study would likely be unethical in light of the speech concerns that would develop in the control group of patients with portions of their cleft left unrepaired.

Currently, modern interventions for patients with a cleft palate result in a good outcome in terms of speech development and facial appearance with a low risk of complication. Management should be directed by a team of clinicians with experience in treating children with clefts of the lip and palate. Continuing long-term evaluations are equally important to analyze the choices that are made with respect to the timing and techniques of cleft palate repair.

REFERENCES

1. Vichi M, Franchi L. Eruption anomalies of the maxillary permanent cuspids in children with cleft lip and/or palate. *J Clin Pediatr Dent.* 1996;20:149.

2. Witzel MA, Salyer KE, Ross RB. Delayed hard palate closure: The philosophy revisited. *Cleft Palate J.* 1994;21:263.

3. Randall P, LaRossa DD, Fakhraee SM, et al. Cleft palate closure at 3 to 7 months of age: A preliminary report. *Plast Reconstr Surg.* 1983;712:624.

4. Semb G. A study of facial growth in patients with unilateral cleft lip and palate treated by the Oslo Cleft Lip and Palate Team. *Cleft Palate Craniofac J.* 1991;28:1.

5. Schweckendiek H. Zur Frage der Fruh-und Spat-operationen der angeborenen Lippen-Kiefer-Gaumen-Spalten (mit Demonstrationen). *Z Laryng Rhin Oto.* 1951;30:51.

6. Schweckendiek W. Primar veloplasty: Long-term results without maxillary deformity. A twenty-five year report. *Cleft Palate J.* 1978;15:268.

7. Bardach J, Morris HL, Olin WH. Late results of primary veloplasty: The Marburg Project. *Plast Reconstr Surg.* 1984;73:207.

8. McWilliams BJ. Submucous clefts of the palate: How likely are they to be symptomatic? *Cleft Palate Craniofac J.* 1991;28:247.

9. Trier WC. Primary palatoplasty. *Clin Plast Surg.* 1985;12:659.

10. Friede H, Johanson B. Adolescent facial morphology of early bone grafted cleft lip and palate patients. *Scand J Plast Reconstr Surg Hand Surg.* 1982;14:41.

11. Braithwaite G, Maurice DG. Importance of levator veli palatine muscle in cleft palate closure. *Br J Plast Surg.* 1968;21:60.

12. Kane AA, Lo LJ, Yen BD, et al. The effect of hamulus fracture on the outcome of palatoplasty: a preliminary report of a prospective, alternating study. *Cleft Palate Craniofac J.* 2000;37:506.

13. Furlow LT. Cleft palate repair by double opposing Z-plasty. *Plast Reconstr Surg.* 1986;78:724.

14. Gunther E, Wisser JR, Cohen MA, Brown AS. Palatoplasty: Furlow's double-reversing Z-plasty versus intravelar veloplasty. *Cleft Palate Craniofac J.* 1998;35;546.

15. Noorchashm N, Dudas JR, Ford M, et al. Conversion Furolw palatoplasty. *Ann Plast Surg.* 2006;56:505.

16. Santiago PE, Grayson BH, Cutting CB, et al. Reduced need for alveolar bone grafting by presurgical orthopedics and primary gingivoperiosteoplasty. *Cleft Palate Craniofac J.* 1998;35:175.

17. Dado DV, Rosenstein SW, Alder ME, Kernahan DA. Long-term assessment of early alveolar bone grafts using three-dimensional computer-assisted tomography: a pilot study. *Plast Reconstr Surg.* 1997;99:1840.

18. Cohen M, Polley JW, Figueroa AA. Secondary (intermediate) alveolar bone grafting. *Clin Plast Surg.* 1993;20:691.

19. Turkaslan T, Ozcan H, Dayicioglu D, Ozsoy Z. Use of adhesives in cleft palate surgery: A new flap fixation technique. *J Craniofac Surg.* 2005;16:719.

20. Witt PD, D'Antonio LL. Velopharyngeal insufficiency and secondary palatal management: A new look at an old problem. *Clin Plast Surg.* 1993;20:707.

21. Persson C, Elander A, Lohmander-Agerskov A, Söderpalm E. Speech outcomes in isolated cleft palate: impact of cleft extent and additional malformations. *Cleft Palate Craniofac J.* 2002;39:397.

22. Gunther E, Wisser JR, Cohen MA, Brown AS. Palatoplasty: Furlow's double reversing Z-plasty versus intravelar veloplasty. *Cleft Palate Craniofac J.* 1998;35:546.

23. Yu CC, Chen PK, Chen YR. Comparison of speech results after Furlow palatoplasty and von Langenbeck palatoplasty in incomplete cleft of the secondary palate. *Chang Gung Med J.* 2001;24:628.

24. Ortiz-Monasterio F, Serrano Reveil A, Valderrama M, Cruz R. Cephalometric measurements on adult patients with nonoperated cleft palates. *Plast Reconstr Surg.* 1959;24:53.

25. Mestre JC, De Jesus J, Subtelny JD. Unoperated oral clefts at maturation. *Angle Orthodon.* 1960;30:78.

26. Schweckendiek W. Primary veloplasty: long-term results without maxillary deformity. A twenty-five year report. *Cleft Palate J.* 1984;15:268.

27. David DJ, Anderson PJ, Schnitt DE, et al. From birth to maturity: a group of patients who have completed their protocol management. Part II. Isolated cleft palate. *Plast Reconstr Surg.* 2006;117:515.

chapter 14

Secondary Deformities of the Cleft Lip, Palate, and Nose

Jamal M. Bullocks, MD, FACS / *Samuel Stal, MD*

● INTRODUCTION

Secondary deformities of the cleft patient are inevitable. Despite timely and appropriate care, the intrinsic congenital insult confers overwhelming forces on the anatomical structures associated with the cleft. Throughout the lifetime of the patient, theses forces are not overcome, conversely growing with the patient causing continual deformation and challenges to repair efforts.

Once of controversy was the chronological age at which clefts were repaired. Arguments for delayed repair touted the benefits of improved structural outcomes leading to fewer secondary deformities. However, it is without a doubt that early primary repair of the cleft lip and palate produce significant improvements in speech and subsequent cognitive and language development. Additionally, the social and psychological advantages have proven to be innumerable. Therefore, early primary repair of the cleft lip and palate is now the standard despite its potential negative effects on the growth of the maxilla and subsequent secondary deformities.[1]

At the root of secondary deformities of the cleft lip, palate, and nose is the deformed maxilla. The maxilla is hypoplastic, and retruded with outward rotation of the cleft elements. With regard to the bilateral cleft, there is inherent premaxillary instability. These structural anomalies results in a midface configuration that defies the ability to harmoniously reconstruct the soft tissues of this region. The soft tissues are displaced by the cleft and are aberrantly inserted in the bony cleft margin which effectively tethers these structures. Lastly, the associated soft tissue structures are themselves hypoplastic and deformed during development, making primary repair difficult.

The secondary deformities of the cleft patient are not only the result of this overwhelming congenital disposition, but are also influenced by the other factors. Of greatest importance is the overall health and associated comorbidities of the patient. Functional primary repairs of the lip and palate are plagued when there is a strong history of morbidity in the upper airway. Chronic coughing, gagging, and infections delay wound healing after primary repair and predispose the patient to failure and to the development of secondary deformities. The type and technique of the primary repair will also influence the development of secondary deformities. This aspect is a direct correlation of the cleft surgeons judgment and ability, which is the most controllable variable in this equation.

The evaluation and treatment of secondary deformities of the cleft lip, nose and palate requires an astute appreciation of the evolution of the cleft. Secondary deformities are predictable; the presenting embryologic insult dictates the development of deformities despite repair. Finally, because of the three-dimensional configuration of the lip, nose, and palate along the cleft, it is appreciated that these deformities do not occur in isolation. Properly timed concomitant repair of all defects will increase the ability to restore anatomic congruity and ultimately minimize the need for additional secondary procedures.

● SECONDARY DEFORMITIES OF THE CLEFT LIP

Secondary deformities of the lip after primary repair are a spectrum of anomalies that range from superficial scar abnormalities to full-thickness derangement of the skin, muscle, and mucosa. Evaluation of the lip involves careful assessment of the mucosa, vermilion, orientation of the orbicularis, symmetry of the philtral complex, and examination of the lip scar with special attention to the alignment of the white roll. Normally, in the adult, the philtrum is 17 mm in length with the philtral columns diverging from the collumela and ending at the peaks of the Cupid's bow.[2] At the superior aspect of the philtrum, the columns are 6 to 9 mm apart, while at the base are 8 to 12 mm apart.[2] In the young patient, these measurements are appreciably smaller but similar in proportion. Ideally there should also be an uninterrupted white roll with a smooth transition of the contiguous lip skin and vermilion mucosa. The orbicularis muscle is oriented circumferential to the vermilion without bulges or tethering to either the lip skin or mucosa. Additionally important to the lip anatomy, is the anterior projection of the upper lip compared with the lower. When the patient is relaxed the upper lip projects 2 to 3 mm anterior to the lower lip.[1]

The most frequent secondary anomalies after primary repair include vermilion deficiency contributing to the "whistle" deformity, lip skin excess (long lip), lip skin deficiency (short lip), orbicularis disorientation, and vermilion misalignment.[3] Although these secondary deformities are seen after both unilateral and bilateral repair, patients with bilateral cleft lip are predisposed to another subset of secondary deformities. In patients with bilateral cleft lip, secondary deformities are either a problem of relative excess or deficiency. At the time of primary repair, the integrity of the prolabium as well as the surgical plan controls the ability to create a symmetric philtrum with the proportions described above. In a situation in which there is adequate prolabial substance, errors in planning contribute to a lip that will ultimately be wide. The philtrum is in excess of tissue, appearing wide without the discrepancy in the collumelar and base distances of the philtral columns. When there is a relative deficiency of prolabial tissue a short retracted philtrum will result despite adequate technique during primary repair.[4] The so-called "tight lip" results from horizontal deficiency of the philtrum.[1] These aberrations of the philtral skin also occur in the mucosa, conferring either a deficiency or excess of vermilion. Lastly, both unilateral and bilateral cleft patients are susceptible to abnormalities associated with the scars from the primary repair. The scar may be hypertrophic, widened, or abnormally contracted, thereby distorting the symmetry of the repair.

Modalities for preventing secondary cleft lip deformities stem from appropriate presurgical treatment, choice of operative technique, and meticulous attention to detail during operative repair. Over the past two decades, the advent of presurgical orthopedics has improved our ability to perform primary repair on patients with very wide clefts.[5,6] An intraoral appliance is fixed to the maxilla along the cleft margins. The maxillary segments are then actively or passively aligned into a more normal anatomic relationship. Presurgical orthopedics is initiated early in the postnatal period in order to shorten the distance between the cleft margins so that primary repair can be performed at

3 months of age.[5–7] The surgical technique for lip repair should address the full height of the lip extending into the nasal sill, as well as the orbicularis muscle. The tension should be placed on the upper third of the repair as in the Millard rotation advancement. At the time of primary repair every effort should be made to free all the soft tissues completely from the cleft in order to create a tension-free repair. It is also at this point where there is the best chance to align the white roll and vermilion to prevent subsequent deformities that are more difficult to correct secondarily.

Secondary deformities of the cleft lip, once identified, should be addressed when there has been adequate development of the soft tissue to allow easy manipulation. Once the wounds of the primary repair have healed, an integral growth period is allowed for maturation of the lip elements. This will establish an appropriate consistency of soft tissue and accurately define the deformity to increase the likelihood of success with secondary repair. Repair of secondary cleft lip deformities should then be approached in one operation with as many procedures necessary.[1]

Cleft Lip Scar Abnormalities

The scar of the secondary cleft lip deformity represents abnormalities of superficial and deep components of the lip, including the skin, vermilion, and underlying orbicularis muscle. Isolated superficial scar abnormalities along the skin portion of the repair are in the form of hypertrophy, contracture, notching, and tethering of the vermilion (Figure 14-1). Deformities in the postoperative period may not be present until the onset of scar maturation, at which time the intrinsic characteristics of wound healing predispose the incisions to the development of such deformities. In the early postoperative period, these abnormal scars should be treated conservatively. The parents are instructed to constantly massage the scars with the application of coca butter, vitamin E, or Mederma.[1]

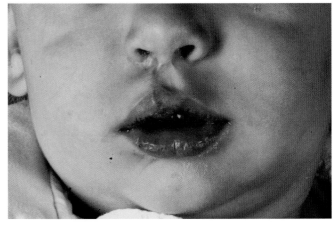

● **FIGURE 14-1.** The spectrum of secondary cleft lip deformities: malalignment of the white roll, vermilion excess with notching, long lip deformity, and hypertrophic scarring.

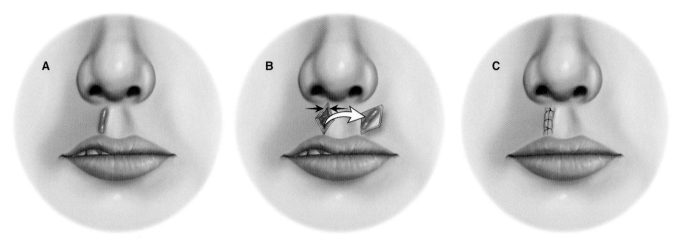

● FIGURE 14-2. Diamond-shaped excision of philtral scars are suitable for minor superficial scar revisions, and are particularly useful in increasing the scar length and reducing vermilion height.

Scars that are refractory to conservative therapy are readdressed with more aggressive, invasive treatment at an interval of 12 months after primary repair. After at least 1 year, the scar has been given ample opportunity to mature, at which point revision should be considered. The elevated scar may be treated simply with corticosteroid injection or dermabrasion. However, these therapies are less effective on widened scars as compared with raised scars. Surgical revision of abnormal scars entails elliptical or diamond-shaped excision of the scar with linear re-approximation (Figure 14-2). If notching of the vermilion is a problem this reorientation will serve to lengthen the scar and relieve minor problems. Often, full-thickness excision is required with re-approximation of the orbicularis, when muscular derangement is encountered on evaluation. As painful as it is to the family, aggressive revisions are sometimes warranted.

Malalignment of the Vermilion

Continuity of the white roll is often the most judged component of the lip repair (Figure 14-3A,B). Inaccurate alignment of the vermilion at the time of primary repair is the culprit, causing lack of color continuity along the skin and vermilion border. Discrepancies of as small as 2 mm are noticeable at conversational distances.[1,3,8] Surgical correction is the only remedy (Figure 14-4). The vermilion should be used to reconstruct the vermilion step-off instead of mucosa with tissue rearrangement opposing like-with-like tissue. Z-plasty rearrangement is efficacious in reorienting the skin vermilion step-off. This is accomplished with the z-plasty designed along the vertical component of the step off with horizontal extensions at 45 degrees. Transposition of the two skin flaps creates a smooth continuous white roll without distortion of other components of the lip.

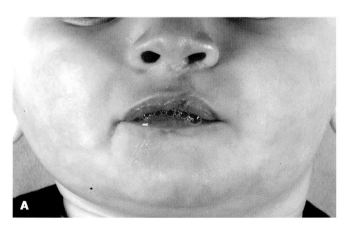
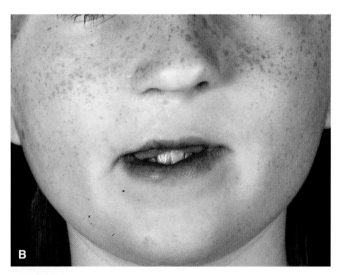

● FIGURE 14-3. Alignment of the white roll is a major component of determining success in primary cleft lip repair. (A) Poor alignment of less than 3 mm is obvious at conversational distances. (B) Proper alignment includes reconstruction of the Cupid's bow.

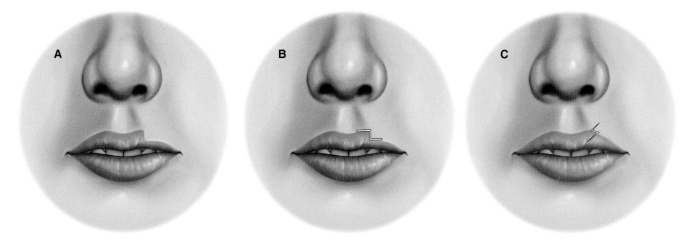

● **FIGURE 14-4.** Malalignment of the white roll corrected with superficial z-plasty rearrangement.

When elevation of the vermilion at the site of repair occurs (Figure 14-5), this may be due to varying severity of deformity. This includes superficial scar contracture causing shortening of the involved philtral column or muscular malalignment tethering the skin superiorly toward the cleft. In minor superficial cases, conservative therapy with scar massage is instituted. If there is persistent deformity 12 months after primary repair, the scar margins are excised along the length of the philtrum across the white roll into the vermilion in a diamond shaped (Figure 14-2). Closure is then preceded in a pants-over-vest fashion to maintain fullness along the margin (Figure 14-6).[8] Full-thickness deformities representing malalignment of the orbicularis result from inadequate rotation of the lateral lip elements at the time of primary repair.[8-10] This deformity can only be corrected by disassembling the reconstruction and re-rotating the lip elements with careful re-approximation of the orbicularis.

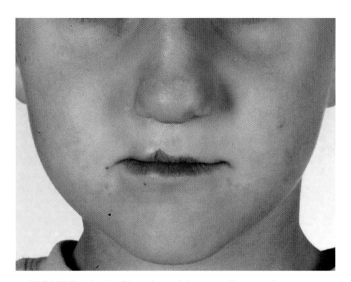

● **FIGURE 14-5.** Elevation of the vermilion produces notching of the scar margin.

Orbicularis Oris Deformities

The importance of orbicularis continuity cannot be overstated. Proper restoration of orbicularis orientation not only improves the appearance and function of the lip but also provides a stable base for correction of cleft palate and nasal deformities. Prevention of secondary muscle deformity is most effectively accomplished with proper primary repair. The deformed muscle inserts vertically along the cleft margin and the alar base. The initial reconstruction should involve complete release of the muscular attachments to the cleft followed by direct approximation of both the superficial and deep layers of the orbicularis. Restoring continuity during primary repair additionally provides a driving force for shaping the premaxilla and palatal shelves. Therefore, orbicularis deformities have a profound effect on the lip, palate, and nose as well as the subsequent prognosis of the repair of these structures.

Orbicularis diastasis is evident by the presence of bulging along the incision of the cleft repair. This is particularly evident with attempted animation. Once secondary orbicularis deformities are identified, repair should be performed by completely releasing the scar and resorting continuity of the muscle. After the scar is opened the orbicularis is separated from the skin and mucosa in subdermal and submucosal planes, respectively. The muscle is then rotated form its vertical position to a more anatomical horizontal position. In the unilateral cleft, the muscle is re-approximated to the contralateral orbicularis without distortion of the philtrum. In bilateral cleft deformity, the muscle is reoriented horizontally and attached to the lateral aspect of the prolabial skin.

Vermilion Deficiency

Vermilion deficiencies occur in unilateral and bilateral cleft patients in different forms. In unilateral deformity, deficiency of the vermilion on the medial lip element is a common problem. This causes an apparent fullness on the

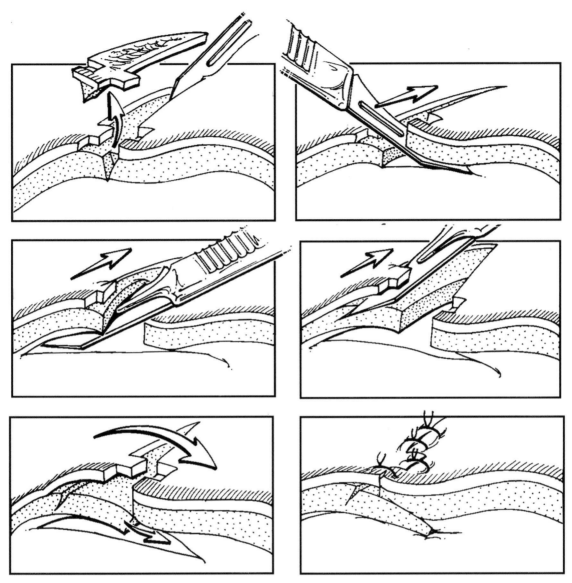

● FIGURE 14-6. Pants-over-vest closure prevents scar depression and adds bulk to maintain fullness along the scar.

vermilion of the lateral lip element, the "whistle" deformity or vermilion notch. In addition to the deficiency of the vermilion in the bilateral cleft lip patient, there is also appreciable shortening of the philtrum. The philtrum is usually normal in height in the unilateral cleft patient, making techniques for repair quite different in these two patient populations.

Mild to moderate deficiencies of the vermilion may be simply camouflaged with fillers. Traditionally, dermal fat grafts and injectable autologous fa, has served this purpose.[11] More recently, a variety of nonautologous fillers have been described, including bovine collagen, acellular dermal matrix, and hyaluronic acid. Fillers represent the least invasive technique for correcting minor deformities and are particularly useful when there is not overwhelming scar contracture along the lip repair. In the severely scarred lip, there will be considerable difficulty generating enough force to overcome the tissue forces and

appropriately disperse the implanted material. Variable absorption of theses fillers may mandate repeat or multiple applications to sustain their structural effect.[11]

More significant deficiencies of the vermilion require local tissue rearrangement to properly address the deformity. The most common configuration in the unilateral cleft lip patient is vermilion deficiency medial adjacent to vermilion excess laterally along the scar. Repair involves first resecting the entire scar, then the excess lateral vermilion is redistributed to the medial deformity. This can be easiest accomplished with a simple z-plasty along the upper border of the vermilion without disturbing the white roll (Figure 14-7). If distortion of the remaining lip element, particularly along the white roll, is predicted with redistribution of the lateral lip vermilion, tissue may be recruited by V-Y advancement of the mucosa to replace the deficient vermilion.[12]

Vermilion deficiencies in bilateral cleft secondary deformities respond less favorably to fillers and local tissue

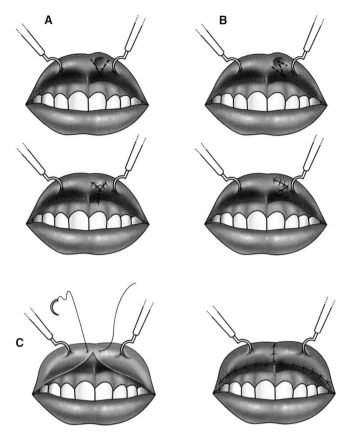

● **FIGURE 14-7.** Recruitment of the local vermilion into an area of vermilion deficiency may be accomplished by varying techniques: (A) local V-Y advancement; (B) z-plasty; (C) V-Y advancement of the labial vermilion.

rearrangement, unless these defects are minor. Due to the concomitant philtral deficit, favorable results are better obtained with lower to upper lip switch procedures, such as an Abbe flap (Figure 14-8). The Abbe flap helps correct projection discrepancies between the upper and lower lips, in which the lower lip excess is transferred to the upper lip deficiency. Although lip switch procedures are reliable procedures for correcting vermilion and philtral deficiencies, in patients with reasonable dimensions, these flaps should be considered second line to scar revision and local tissue rearrangement.

● CUPID'S BOW: SECONDARY DEFORMITIES

The caudal portion of the philtrum represents a complex and aesthetically intricate structure, the Cupid's bow. Secondary scar and mucosal deformities distort the philtral tubercle and the slight peak of the vermilion at the base of the philtral column. These deformities are a variety of abnormalities of vermilion discrepancy, ranging from notching (Figure 14-5) to complete absence of Cupid's bow. For patients with vertical deficiency lateral to the cleft and subsequent loss of alignment of the white roll at the peak of the bow, simple triangular skin excision and

superior advancement of the vermilion will treat this problem effectively (Figure 14-2). In cases of smaller step-offs, z-plasty reorientation of the white roll as described earlier may suffice. When performing these techniques that advance the vermilion, care is taken not to rotate the inside "wet" vermilion to the dry external surface. Although, these techniques of skin excision and vermilion advancement are effective, the associated scarring of the wounds may induce an artificial appearance to the lip. Therefore, in these instances, particularly in patients with abnormal scarring after primary repair, the repair should be taken down to repeat rotation advancement of the lateral lip.

When the Cupid's bow portion of the vermilion is totally absent, as is frequently the case in bilateral cleft lip deformities, then reconstruction with a Abbe flap should be considered to provide adequate vermilion and vermilion ridge to reshape the Cupid's bow on the cleft side. In certain instances, the vermilion portion of the Cupid's bow may be correctly aligned but have poor superior projection. In these cases, elevation of the white roll is performed with tissue fillers (hyaluronic acid or autologous fat) to accentuate the peak of the Cupid's bow. When there is vermilion deficiency, the vermilion portion of the Cupid's bow can be similarly augmented with dermal fat grafts or injectable fillers with a modest degree of overcorrection at the time of implantation.

The Short Lip

In unilateral cleft lip deformity, the short lip refers to positioning of the lateral lip elements at a deficient vertical height with respect to the medial lip elements and is usually accompanied by asymmetry of Cupid's bow.[8] The short lip is often noted to be 3 to 4 mm shorter in length as compared with the normal lip.[1,3] This secondary deformity is usually the result of scar contracture, but also results from inadequate rotation and advancement at the time of primary repair.[1,3,8] The most effective way of correcting this deformity is by releasing the scar completely and performing rotation and advancement of the lateral elements similar to the technique described by Millard for primary repair.[13] During secondary rotation and advancement, attention to additional downward positioning is paramount. If a rotation and advancement repair was performed as the initial repair, then a full-thickness z-plasty, including the muscle and mucosa, can also be effective. Minor length discrepancies can be treated with superficial diamond-shaped skin excision and closure to lengthen the scar.

The short lip is also occasionally secondary to vermilion and labial mucosa deficiencies.[1,3,8] In these instances, correction with z-plasty and V-Y mucosal advancement is not adequate, as it is the case with vermilion length discrepancies alone. There is an additional tissue requirement that can be addressed with a dermal fat graft or lateral buccal fat. This type of deformity is more commonly seen in bilateral secondary cleft lip deformities and is also amenable to Abbe flap reconstruction when the shortness is both in

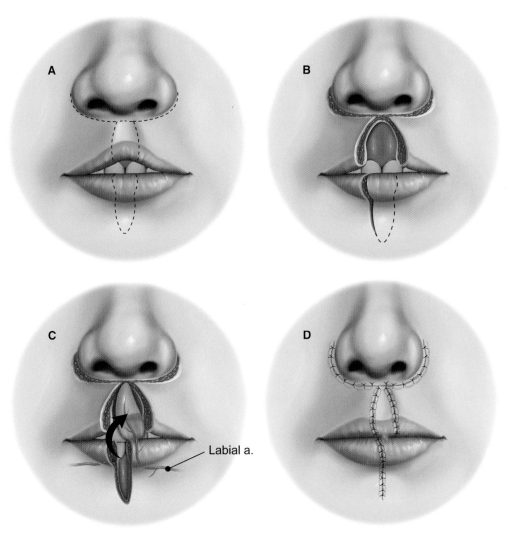

● **FIGURE 14-8.** (A–D) Lip switch procedure (Abbe flap), based on the inferior labial artery. Transfer of a central lower lip segment to augment the central upper lip and reconstruction of the vermilion.

the lateral and vertical dimension. The Abbe flap provides composite tissue to replace the vertical skin and mucosa deficiency.[14]

The Long Lip

In long lip deformity, the lateral lip elements are inferiorly positioned compared with the medial lip elements. This occurs more commonly after unilateral compared with bilateral cleft lip repair. The Tennison triangular flap repair of the cleft lip often resulted in the long lip.[15] This is due to the inadequately addressed upper third of the lip during primary repair. With the increasing utilization of the rotation advancement technique being performed for primary repair of the cleft lip, this secondary deformity is seen in less frequently.

Correction of long lip deformity requires opening the entire lip from the base of the nose to the vermilion. The skin, muscle, and musocal elements are re-approximated

from the bottom up. The associated dog ear is incorporated into the nasal sill and alar base. The excess tissue is then excised along the lateral alar base. Although it is tempting to perform a lesser simple excision of the tissue below the alar base and pexy, the elongated lip to the piriform aperture, this technique is doomed to failure. The overwhelming forces of gravity and underlying musculature will pull down on the base of the ala on the cleft side, making the lower border on the cleft side appear long.

The Tight Lip

The tight lip represents tissue deficiency in the horizontal plane after primary lip repair.[8] This deformity is more commonly seen after bilateral cleft lip repair.[8] The width of the cleft and the degree of prolabial protrusion predisposes to the formation of this secondary deformity after primary repair. After primary repair, the prolabium remains short

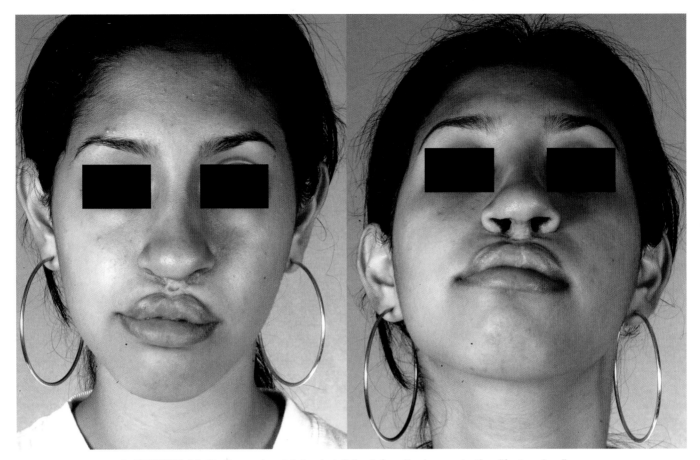

● **FIGURE 14-9.** Secondary bilateral cleft lip deformity demonstrating "festooning," philthral deficiency, and long lateral lip elements.

compared with the lateral lip elements (Figure 14-9). This is an example in which the initial congenital insult is difficult to overcome secondary to the relative paucity of tissue available for primary repair. With the advent of presurgical orthopedics which attempts to decrease the cleft distance before primary repair, hopefully this deformity will be seen less frequently.

In order to correct the problem of upper lip deficiency, tissue must be recruited into this region. Historically, this has been done most successfully with a lip switch procedure (ie, Abbe flap).[16] The Abbe flap will reduce the tightness of the upper lip and reduce the projection discrepancy of the lower lip.[14,16] In addition to providing skin and vermilion to the upper lip, an Abbe flap will also provide addition muscle, which has been shown to improve orbicularis function.[14] Technically, the flap should always be placed centrally to replace the philtral portion of the lip regardless of where the upper lip deficiency exists. If there is relative lateral deficiency contributing to a tight lip deformity, the flap is again placed centrally in order to provide symmetry of the upper lip, lateral elements are rotated and advanced to restore orbicularis continuity. Depending on the vermilion deficit that is present in the upper lip, the flap can be designed with either V- or M-shaped donor excision to recreate the upper lip tubercle or Cupid's bow region.[16]

The Wide Lip

Contrary to the tight lip, the wide lip represents horizontal excess of the upper lip. This deformity again more commonly occurs after bilateral cleft lip repair. This secondary deformity is the result of both technical design errors during initial repair and mechanical forces stretching the dimensions of the repair.[1,3] At the time of initial lip repair in the 3-month-old infant, the philtral width should be designed to be approximately 6 mm.[1,3] Additionally, during primary repair, the orbicularis muscle must be firmly attached to itself across the midline. If the muscle fails to unite with the prolabium, the orbicularis will pull either side of the lateral lip elements away for the prolabium widening this region over time. If this is the instance, there will be concomitant hypertrophy and excess fullness of the lateral lip.

To correct the wide lip deformity, there must be reduction of the wide prolabium in conjunction with correction of the orbicularis. A new philtrum is designed after excision of the excess philtral tissue. The orbicularis is redirected into a horizontal position and firmly affixed to the prolabium. If possible, depending on the adequacy of tissue in the philtrum, an attempt should be made to reconstitute the orbicularis across the cleft. Orbicularis reconstitution is easily performed in patients with wide unilateral cleft deformities. Finally, it is equally important to design the new philtrum smaller than the final desired size to anticipate the inevitable stretching that occurs during healing.

● CLEFT PALATE: SECONDARY DEFORMITIES

Secondary deformities of the cleft palate represent a complex conglomeration of soft tissue and bony structural abnormalities that results in both cosmetic and functional abnormalities. The misaligned palatal shelves and the hypoplastic maxilla are the culprits of these secondary deformities. Despite timely primary repair of the palate, the predisposing structural aberrations decrease the chance for an acceptable primary repair. The cleft palate can be either V or U shaped with aberrant insertion of the palatal soft tissues into the cleft margins, particularly the tenor veli palatine muscle which serve to elevate the palate and close the communication between the nose and mouth during speech and deglutination (Figure 14-10). The relative distance of the palatal shelves and the length of the palatal diastasis will predict the occurrence of secondary deformities. For instance, a wide, complete cleft of the palate that requires multiple procedures to close will inevitably develop secondary deformities after primary repair.

Confounding the development of secondary palatal deformities is the negative effect the primary repair has on growth of the maxilla. Inhibition of maxillary growth is believed to result from the transient devascularization of the palate that occurs in most techniques used for palatoplasty. Delaying the primary repair to allow the

maxillary elements to become more robust may minimize the development of secondary deformities. However, delay in primary palate repair is not an option because of the overwhelming negative effect it has on speech, language, and cognitive development.[1] Therefore, early repair of the cleft palate is the rule and secondary deformities are inevitable. Understanding the management of these deformities is essential knowledge for a cleft surgeon.

The palate is embryologically separated into primary and secondary components by the incisive foramen. The premaxillary segment forms from the fusion of the medial nasal process, a derivative of the frontal nasal process and the lateral maxillary elements. The premaxillary segment will form the midportion of the lip and house the alveolar segment of bone containing the incisors. Failure of fusion of this structure produces a cleft of the primary palate. It is important to recognize that the primary cleft is a three-dimensional structure that extends from the nose to the anterior alveolar segment (Figure 14-10). The resultant secondary deformities of the primary cleft palate are in the form of oronasal fistulas, anterior alveolar fistulas, and a varying array of dentolalveolar aberrations.

Posterior to the incisive foramen is the secondary palate. The secondary palate forms from the fusion of the palatine shelves and mesenchymal infiltration across the cleft margins. There can be complete or incomplete formation along the length of the cleft. Repair of the secondary palate is designed not only for coverage of the defect but more importantly to reorient the deranged levator veli palatini muscle. Secondary deformities of the secondary palate present with varying degrees of palatal fistulae and velopharyngeal incompetence.

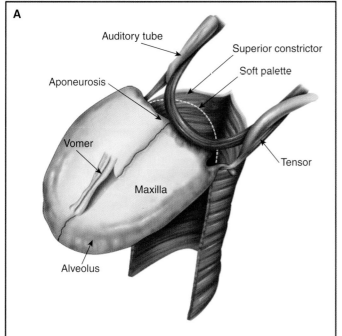
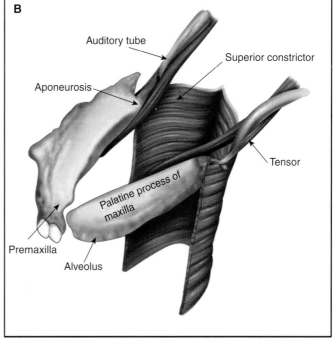

● **FIGURE 14-10.** (A) Normal compared to (B) a cleft morphology of the palate and the pharyngeal musculature.

Generally, fistulae are the most common defects of the hard palate after repair. Anterior to the alveolar ridge, the defect is termed an oronasal fistula and posterior it is termed a palatal fistula.[17] The majority of fistulae are small and present with regurgitation of food and liquid through the nose. Speech is rarely affected by small fistulae; however, larger defects can cause variable degrees of hypernasality. Fistulae also result from orthodontic treatment, specifically after rapid expansion of the dental arches. Most commonly, fistulae occur at the junction of the primary and secondary palate followed by the hard palate alone. There is an increased incidence of fistula formation with increasing severity in the cleft. Of all fistulae, 61% occur after repair of bilateral deformities of the lip and palate, 26% after unilateral deformities of the lip and palate, and 15% after isolated palatal defects.[18,19]

Repair of Oronasal Fistulae

Oronasal fistulae most frequently represent a residual cleft in the maxillary alveolus that was not closed at the time of primary palatoplasty and is not a true fistula. If the fistula is small and without functional significance, closure may occur spontaneously with growth; therefore, intervention should be delayed. Small symptomatic fistulae anterior to the alveolar arch can be closed by primary gingivoperiosteoplasty at the time of lip repair.[8,20] This technique may eliminate or minimize the need for bone grafting. Placement of bone into the oronasal fistula serves to provide a matrix into which the teeth can erupt, as well as to stabilize the maxillary arch to allow proper alignment of the maxillary teeth. Closure of the oronasal fistula with bone grafting is performed between 6 and 12 years of age during the period of mixed dentition.[21–23]

As a general rule, fistulae should be closed by re-approximating the oral and nasal layers separate from one another. Most fistulae are closed with local tissues within which the bone graft is contained (Figure 14-11). Frequently, a turn-over flap can be employed to close the nasal layer after which cancellous bone is packed into the recesses of the cleft and covered with a shield of cortical bone, if available. The iliac bone, harvested from the posterior surface of the crest, is easily procured and is a plentiful source for grafting. Palatal, buccal, or labial flaps are then used to close the oral layer (Figure 14-12).

Palatal Fistulae

Palatal fistulae vary in size and location and have a high recurrence rate. Repair of palatal fistulae involve rearrangement of local tissues to close the defect in a double-layered fashion. Large or recalcitrant fistula may require the use of regional oral flaps or free flaps for closure. Small palatal fistulae can be closed in two layers, using one turnover flap from the palatal side to close the nasal mucosa and a second large palatal flap to close the oral mucosa (Figure 14-13). The nasal mucosa can also be closed in a purse-string fashion if the fistula is small and the adjacent tissue is supple

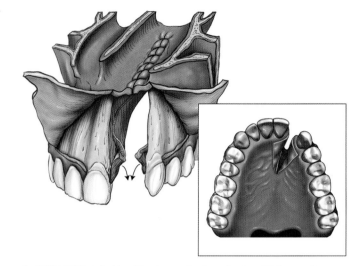

● **FIGURE 14-11.** Gingivoperiosteoplasty utilizing soft tissue flaps from the cleft margin to close the floor (oral mucosa) and the roof (nasal floor) of an oronasal fistula. (*From Kelly P, Taylor T, Hollier L, Stal S. Alveolar bone grafting. In: McCarthy JG, Galiano RD, Boutros SG, eds. Current Therapy in Plastic Surgery. Philadelphia: Saunders Elsevier; 2006.*)

and mobile. The oral mucosa flaps should be designed large enough to compensate for their scarred and inelastic quality. The design can be a unipedicle or a bipedicle flap and be performed unilaterally or bilaterally (Figure 14-14). These flaps often mimic those used in primary palatoplasty.

If there is a relative paucity of reliable adjacent tissue or the fistula is large, consideration should be given to recruiting tissue from regional sources. Large anterior defects can be closed using buccal mucosa flaps. A portion of the buccal sulcus is tunneled through the nasal fossa onto the defect in the hard palate, which provides single-layer closure of the nasal mucosa. The oral mucosa is then closed using large palatal flaps. Fistulae in the posterior palate, particularly the soft palate, can be closed either primarily or with pharyngeal flaps, depending on the amount of tension. Pharyngeal flaps provide fresh vascular tissue to close the defect and obturate the nasophayngeal aperture, which is of particular benefit in patients with velopharyngeal incompetence.

For large recurrent defects, other regional flaps from the tongue and the buccal mucosa are employed when previous attempts at repair have failed. The tongue flap described by Guerrerosantos and Altamirano[24] (Figure 14-15) mobilizes a superficial portion of the tongue based on a posterior pedicle. At a second procedure 3 weeks later, the flap is then divided and inset. A larger portion of the lateral buccal mucosa may be transferred to cover the entire oral palate based on the facial artery (Figure 14-16).[25,26] The facial artery myomucosal flap transfers a portion of buccinator and lateral buccal mucosa based either antegrade off the facial artery or retrograde off the buccal branch of the maxillary artery.[25–27]

Crippling fistulae that have failed repeated closure attempts may require free tissue transfer. Reserved as

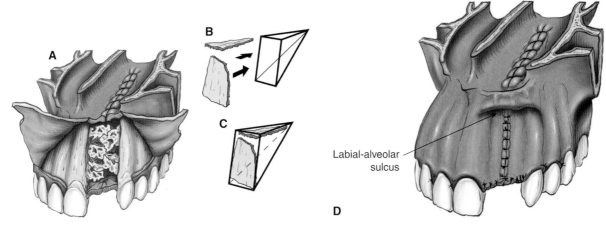

Labial-alveolar sulcus

● FIGURE 14-12. (A) Oronasal cleft after cancellous bone grafting. (B, C) Cortical bone fragments are utilized to strut the nasal and alveolar margin reducing tension on the flap closure. (D) The final closure of the oronasal defect. (*From Kelly P, Taylor T, Hollier L, Stal S. Alveolar bone grafting. In: McCarthy JG, Galiano RD, Boutros SG, eds. Current Therapy in Plastic Surgery. Philadelphia: Saunders Elsevier; 2006.*)

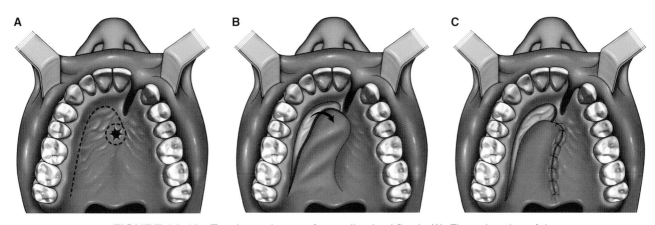

● FIGURE 14-13. Two-layer closure of a small palatal fistula (A). First, elevation of the fistula margin and turnover closure of the nasal mucosa (B). Second, rotation of a large oral mucosa flap (unipedicle) over the nasal closure (C).

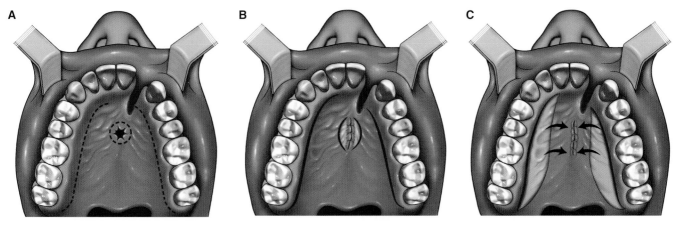

● FIGURE 14-14. Two-layer closure of a palatal fistula (A). The nasal mucosa is closed (B) and bipedicle oral mucosa flaps are advanced over the defect (C).

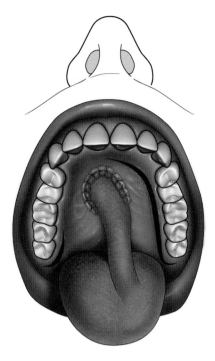

● **FIGURE 14-15.** Regional flaps for closure of recalcitrant palatal fistulae. The tongue flap described by Guerrerosantos and Altamirano.[24]

the last option, the radial forearm free flap has been used to close resistant large defects. This thin fasciocutaneous flap provides composite tissue to reconstruct both the oral and nasal linings. The flap is superior to other thin facsiocutaneous flap due to its long pedicle that can reach a variety of recipient vessels in the neck. The use of acelluar dermal matrix has recently been advocated for closure of palatal fistulae.[28,29] The alloderm essentially serves as a scaffold for the migration of granulation tissue from the surrounding vascularized structures that eventually differentiates into dermis. Alloderm can provide a layer of tissue in cases where reconstruction of only one layer is possible (Figure 14-17). Lastly, a prosthesis can be fabricated to obturate the fistula and should be considered when multiple attempts at closure have proven to be futile.[8] The prosthesis can serve multiple functions, including closure of the fistula, camouflage of the missing teeth, and improved velopharygeal competence when a posterior extension is included.

● MAXILLARY GROWTH DISTURBANCE

As mentioned previously, the mandatory early repair of the cleft palate has a negative effect on maxillary growth. This exacerbates the abnormal development of the already deformed maxilla.[30] The result is the development of a hypoplastic maxilla that causes noticeable cosmetic deficiencies and abnormal occlussal relationships.[30] The extent

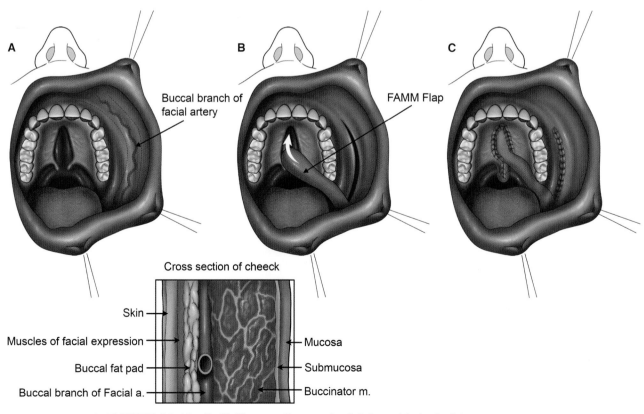

Buccal branch of facial artery

FAMM Flap

Cross section of cheeck

Skin
Muscles of facial expression
Buccal fat pad
Buccal branch of Facial a.

Mucosa
Submucosa
Buccinator m.

● **FIGURE 14-16.** (A–C) Closure of large palatal defect with the facial artery myomucosal (FAMM) flap.

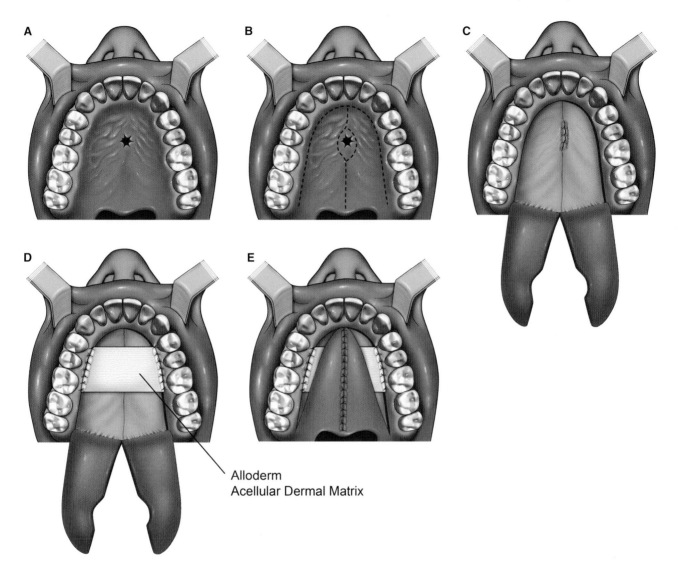

● FIGURE 14-17. Three-layer closure of palatal fistulae using acellular dermal matrix. (A) Fistula. (B) Incisions for oral mucosa flap. (C) Elevation of bilateral peninsular flaps around the fistula based on the greater palatine arteries. (D) Placement of the acelluar matrix. (E) Final three-layer closure.

of the maxillary hypoplasia is secondary to the timing of the primary repair, the extent of the defect (with bilateral defects being more injurious than unilateral defects), and the amount of secondary scarring. The maxilla is also narrow, causing crowding, crossbite, and apertognathia. Occlussal abnormalities frequently require orthodontic intervention. Maxillary expansion may also be required to achieve adequate width to accommodate permanent dentition.

In the majority of cases, the maxillary hypoplasia is localized to the base of the nose on the cleft side. Orthodontic correction of the occlusal abnormalities along with bone grafting of the cleft will provide adequate contour to the lip and base of the nose.[31] In wide cleft deformities, the lateral maxillary arch may collapse and not be amenable to orthodontic treatment. In these instances, a transverse unilateral osteotomy through the maxillary sinus

is created on the cleft side.[31] This allows mobilization of the collapsed arch segment inferiorly and buccally into occlusion. Subsequent maxillary defects are bone grafted and the reconstruction is immobilized for 6 weeks using intermaxillary fixation. An additional secondary effect of maxillary hypoplasia is an apparent maxillary retrusion and class II malocclusion. This is corrected by performing a transverse maxillary osteotomy (LeFort I osteotomy). The mobilized maxillary segment is then moved anterior and inferior to correct the retrusion and vertical height deficiency. Again, bone grafting may be required to fill any gap and to stabilize the malar-maxillary complex. This technique is often needed to restore facial contour and proper occlusion with the mandibular dentition. Generally, maxillary osteotimies are performed in the late teens after the completion of maxillary and mandibular growth.[8]

● CLEFT NASAL DEFORMITY

The cleft nasal deformity is influenced greatly by the extent of the cleft deformity and the result and technique used for primary lip repair and palate repair. The lip and nose share a common deficiency in soft tissue and the abnormal insertion of the orbicularis muscle pulls and widens the nasal deformity. At the base of the cleft nasal deformity, there is a hypoplastic nasal spine that opposes adequate projection. There is also a negative effect caused by the displacement of the weaker, lower lateral cartilage. The lateral crus is displaced outward, further flattening the tip-defining point. The cleft nose is deviated with a resultant tilting of the nasal bones and deflection of the septum. The vomer is crooked and often displaced off the vomerine crest. If inadequately addressed at the time of lip repair, the collumella is shortened secondary to a deficiency of skin and nasal lining. In the complete bilateral cleft, support for the nasal tip is deficient on both sides, causing retro-positioning of the entire tip complex and producing a broad flat bulbous tip with no projection.

Overall, the most apparent distortion of the cleft nose is the obvious abnormalities of the lower lateral cartilages (Figure 14-18). The flattened, laterally displaced lateral cartilages do not form the acute angle at the genu necessary for proper tip definition, leading to inadequate tip projection. Poor tip projection is secondary to the weak, malformed lower lateral cartilage and the lowered angle of septum (Figure 14-19). Maintenance of projection of the tip can only be accomplished with proper support of the lower lateral cartilage.

Beginning in the neonatal period, nasoalveolar molding is used to remodel the lower lateral cartilage.[1,32–34] During this period the cartilage has a remarkable ability to be reshaped

due to the high levels of circulating estrogens.[35,36] Using a nasal extension to the passive palatal presurgical devices and appliance is placed to shape the nose in the first months of life. The appliance elevates the lower lateral cartilage and stretches the nasal lining (Figure 14-20). Nasoaveolar molding is the first step in a series of procedures in early childhood that helps increase the prognosis of definitive rhinoplasty when the patient is of appropriate age. In the first year of life, the cleft lip-nose patient will have a number of procedures to correct the lip deformity. It is advantageous to perform additional molding techniques on the lower lateral cartilage. At the time of lip repair, the lower lateral cartilage is freed from the overlying skin; the lower lateral cartilage is then suspended to the dermis in the desired position (Figure 14-21). These dermal suspension sutures serve to define the apex of the alae and reposition the skin and mucosal envelope opening the nasal aperture.

While minor procedures may be performed in early childhood, formal septorhinoplasty to correct the residual sequellae of the cleft nasal deformity is best deferred until growth of the nose is complete. This age is approximately 11 to 12 years in girls and 13 to 14 years in boys.[32] In early adolescence, patients are likely to be mature enough to consider septorhinoplasty. The goals of the procedure are focused on correcting the nasal bones and septal deviation and resorting tip support. However, before reshaping of the tip is to occur, the alar base is addressed. The poorly projected tip is based on a hypoplastic maxilla. Consideration for augmentation of the piriform should be made using a bone graft, diced cartilage, or hydroxyapatite. The augmentation is performed using an intraoral incision and the material is secured in a subperiosteal location below the cleft side of the alae. In patients, with maxillary retrusion contributing not only to poor alar base support but also

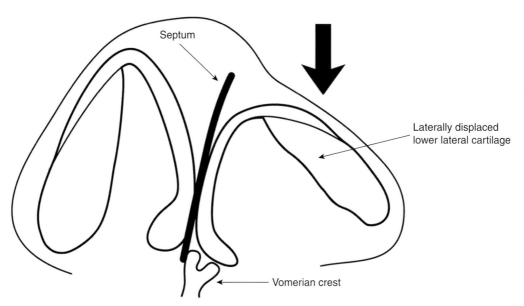

● **FIGURE 14-18.** Characterization of the cleft nasal deformity. Lateral and inferiorly displacement of the lower lateral cartilage, septal deviation, and rotation of the vomerian crest secondary to deforming forces of the cleft (*down arrow*).

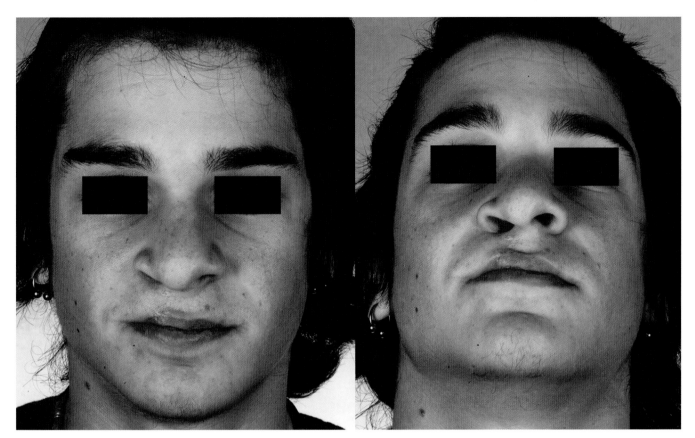

● **FIGURE 14-19.** Cleft nose deformity, illustrating poor tip projection and definition secondary to the weak, flattened, laterally displaced lower lateral cartilages and the lowered angle of the septum.

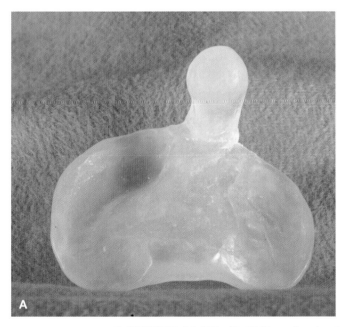
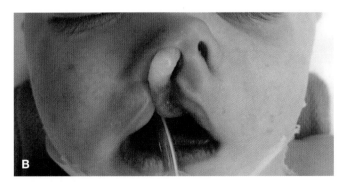

● **FIGURE 14-20.** (A, B) Nasoalveolar device applied in the neonatal period elevates the lower lateral cartilage and stretches the nasal lining as the first step in a series of procedures in early childhood that helps increase the prognosis of definitive rhinoplasty when the patient is of appropriate age.

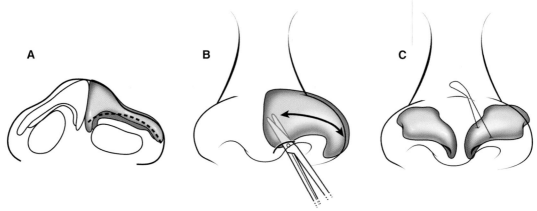

● **FIGURE 14-21.** Lower lateral cartilage dermal suspension. (A) Vestibular infra cartilaginous nasal incision. (B) Dissection and exposure of the lower lateral cartilage. (C) Suture placement through the cartilage then skin and brought through the same site and tied in the nasal vestibule.

to functional malocclusion, a LeFort I osteotomy with advancement should ideally be performed before definitive rhinoplasty.[8]

Definitive rhinoplasty is best performed through an open approach to carefully analyze and directly address the lower lateral cartilages. The soft tissues are completely released and the support structures are visualized.[37] The septum is dissected and associated anomalies corrected. At this point, septal cartilage can be harvested for later use as either a columellar strut, an alar batten graft, or a spreader graft. Generous attention is given to reshaping the lower lateral cartilages. Symmetry to the lower lateral cartilages is created using intradomal and interdomal suture techniques (Figure 14-22).[38] The tip may also need additional support in the form of a columelar strut, which also serves as scaffold for equalizing the domes. Tip projection may require additional augmentation with a separate graft. To correct any deviation of the nasal

bones, osteotomy and repositioning can be performed.[37,38] Definitive septoplasty is performed to correct deviations and alterations of the septum on the vomerian crest.

In the bilateral cleft lip nasal deformity, the collumella is deficient, the nostrils are obliquely oriented and the alar base is widened. Correction requires advancement from either the bilateral nasal sill or the lateral aspect of the philtrum for lengthening (Figure 14-23). The columella is also wide with loss of the central waist. The columella can be reshaped by direct excision or narrowing with plication sutures placed between the medial crura. The bilateral cleft lip deformity includes bilateral flaring of the lower lateral cartilages, causing abnormally elongated and enlarged nostrils. The elongated appearance is secondary to overall poor projection, and is repaired by recreating the middle crura and supporting the tip with a columellar strut. A widened alar base is corrected with caudal lateral crus spanning sutures.[38]

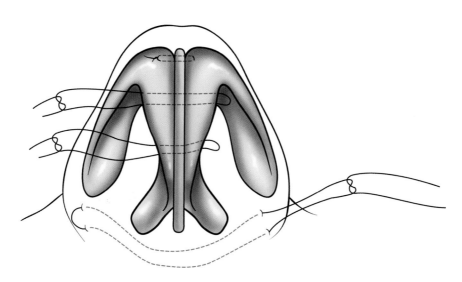

● **FIGURE 14-22.** Suture techniques for the correction of tip and alar base deformities in cleft rhinoplasty.

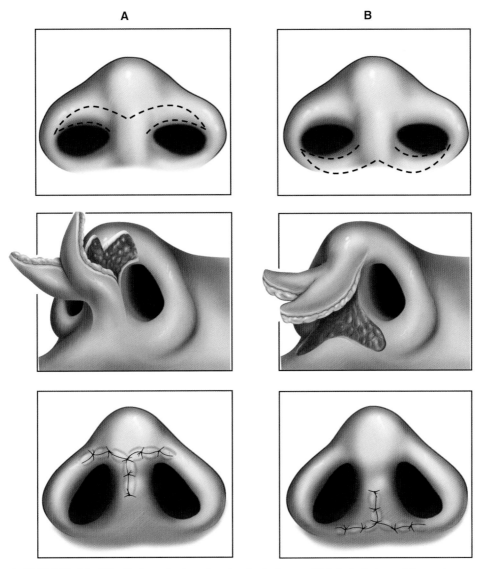

FIGURE 14-23. Collumelar lengthening techniques. (A) Inferiorly based flap using the superior vestibular tissue and (B) superiorly based flap rotating the soft tissue of the nasal sill.

CONCLUSION

Secondary deformities of the cleft lip, palate, and nose are multiple. They have multiple etiologies, with inherent congenital deformation and subsequent primary repair being the two most influential. Presurgical orthopedics can have a profound beneficial effect in preventing these deformities and improving outcome of primary repair. Once a diagnosis is established, multiple procedures may be required to correct the deformity. In planning reconstruction, careful attention should be placed on the hypolastic maxilla and the insertion of the soft tissues into the margins of the cleft. The timing of repair is dictated by requirements for function and growth.

REFERENCES

1. Stal S, Hollier LH. Secondary deformities of the cleft lip, nose, and palate. In: Mathes SJ, ed. *Plastic Surgery.* 2nd ed. Philadelphia: WB Saunders; 2005:339–363.

2. McCarthy JG, Cutting CB. Secondary deformities of cleft lip and palate. In: Georgiade GS, Riefkohl R, Levin LS, eds. *Georgiade: Plastic, Maxillofacial, and Reconstructive Surgery.* 3rd ed. Baltimore, MD: Williams & Wilkins; 1997: 247–257.

3. Stal S, Hollier LH. Correction of secondary cleft lip deformities. *Plast Reconstr Surg.* 2002;109(5):1672–1681.

4. Mulliken JB, Wu JK, Padwa BL. Repair of bilateral cleft lip: review, revisions, and reflections. *J Craniofac Surg.* 2003;14(5):609–620.

5. Georgiade NG, Latham RA. Maxillary arch alignment in the bilateral cleft lip and palate infant, using the pinned coaxial screw appliance. *Plast Reconstr Surg.* 1975;56(1):52–60.

6. Latham R, Qusy R, Georgiade N. An extraorally activated expansion appliance for cleft palate infants. *Cleft Palate J.* 1976;13:252–261.

7. Grayson BH, Santiago PE, Brecht LE, et al. Long term effects of nasoalveolar molding in infants with cleft lip and palate. *Cleft Palate Craniofac J.* 1999;36:486–498.

8. Stal S, Spira M. Secondary reconstructive procedures for patients with clefts. In: Sursin D, Georiade NG, eds. *Pediatric Plastic Surgery.* St. Louis, MO: CV Mosby; 1984: 352–378.

9. Jackson IT, Fasching MC. Secondary deformities of cleft lip, nose, and cleft palate. In: McCarthy JG, ed. *Plastic and Reconstructive Surgery.* Vol. 4. Philadelphia: WB Saunders; 1990.

10. Cohen M. Secondary correction of the nasal deformity associated with cleft lip. In: Cohen M, ed. *Mastery of Plastic and Reconstructive Surgery.* New York: Little, Brown, and Company; 1994:702–719.

11. Coleman SR. Facial recontouring with lipostructure. *Clin Plast Surg.* 1997;24:347–367.

12. Kapetansky DI. Double pendulum flaps for whistling deformities in bilateral cleft lips. *Plast Reconstr Surg.* 1971; 47:321–323.

13. Millard DR Jr. *The Unilateral Deformity.* Boston, MA: Little, Brown & Co; 1976. *Cleft Craft: the Evolution of its Surgery; Vol 1.*

14. Jackson IT, Soutar DS. The sandwich Abbe flap in secondary cleft lip deformities. *Plast Reconstr Surg.* 1980;66:38–45.

15. Stal S, Klebuc M, Taylor T, et al. Algorithms for the treatment of cleft lip and plate. *Clin Plast Surg.* 1998;25(4):493–507.

16. Abbe R. A new plastic operation for the relief of deformity due to double harelip. *Med Rec.* 1898;53:477–478.

17. Oneal RM. Oronasal fistulas. In: Grabb WC, Rosenstein SW, Brock KR, eds. *Cleft Lip and Palate.* New York: Little, Brown, and Company; 1971.

18. Schultz RC. Management and timing of cleft palate fistula repair. *Plast Recontr Surg.* 1986;78:739.

19. Schultz RC. Cleft palate fistula repair. Improved results by the addition of bone. *J Craniomaxillofac Surg.* 1989;17:34.

20. Randall P. Discussion of "Management and timing of cleft palate fistula repair" by RC Schultz. *Plast Reconstr Surg.* 1986;78:746.

21. Abyholm FE, Bergland O, Semb G. Secondary bone grafting or alveolar clefts. *Scand J Plast Reconstr Surg.* 1981;15:127.

22. Jackson IT, Vandervord JG, McLennan JG, et al. Bone grafting of the secondary cleft lip and palate deformity. *Br J Plast Surg.* 1982;35:345.

23. El Deeb M, Messer LB, Lehnert MW, et al. Canine eruption into grafted bone in maxillary alveolar cleft defects. *Cleft Palate J.* 1982;19:9.

24. Guerrerosantos J, Altamirano JT. The use of lingual flaps in repair of fistulas of the hard palate. *Plast Reconstr Surg.* 1966;38:123–128.

25. Ashtiani AK, Emami SA, Rasti M. Closure of complicated palatal fistula with facial artery musculomucosal flap. *Plast Reconstr Surg.* 2005;116(2):381–386.

26. Nakakita N, Maeda K, Ando S, et al. Use of a buccal musculomucosal flap to close palatal fistulae after cleft palate repair. *Br J Plast Surg.* 1990;43(4):452–456.

27. Joshi A, Rajendraprasad JS, Shetty K. Reconstruction of intraoral defects using facial artery musculomucosal flap. *Br J Plast Surg.* 2005;58(8):1061–1066.

28. Steele MH, Seagle MB. Palatal fistula repair using acellular dermal matrix: the University of Florida experience. *Ann Plast Surg.* 2006;56(1):50–53.

29. Clark JM, Saffold SH, Israel JM. Decellularized dermal grafting in cleft palate repair. *Arch Facial Plast Surg.* 2003;5(1): 40–44.

30. Smahel Z, Mullerova Z. Effects of primary periosteoplasty and facial growth in unilateral cleft lip and palate: 10 year follow-up. *Cleft Palate J.* 1988;20:356.

31. Vargervik K. Growth characteristics of the premaxilla and orthodontic treatment principles in bilateral cleft lip and palate. *Cleft Palate J.* 1983;20(4):289–302.

32. Stal S, Hollier L. Correction of secondary deformities of the cleft lip nose. *Plast Reconstr Surg.* 2002;109(4):1386–1392.

33. Tan S, Abramson D, MacDonald D, et al. Molding therapy for infants with deformational auricular anomalies. *Ann Plast Surg.* 1997;3:263–268.

34. Cutting C, Grayson B, Brecht L. Presurgical columella elongation with one-stage repair of the bilateral cleft lip and nose. Proceedings of the American Cleft Palate-Craniofacial Association. 1995;52:58.

35. Brown F, Colen L, Addante R, et al. Correction of congenital auricular deformities by splinting in the neoneonatal period. *Pediatrics.* 1986;78:406–411.

36. Matsuo K, Hayashi R, Kiyono M, et al. Nonsurgical correction of congenital auricular deformities. *Clin Plast Surg.* 1993;17:333–395.

37. Stal S, Hollier LH. Correction of secondary deformities of the cleft lip nose. *Plast Reconstr Surg.* 2002;109(4): 1386–1392.

38. Van Beek AL, Hatfield AS, Schnepf E. Cleft rhinoplasty. *Plast Reconstr Surg.* 2004;114:57e.

chapter 15

Velopharyngeal Insufficiency

Rachel A. Ruotolo, MD / Richard E. Kirschner, MD, FACS, FAAP

● INTRODUCTION

Normal speech depends on the functional and structural integrity of the velopharynx. This complex and dynamic structure allows for uncoupling of the oral and nasal cavities during speech. Dysfunction of the velopharyngeal valve (velopharyngeal dysfunction, or VPD) may result in hypernasality, nasal air emission, and compensatory articulation errors, all of which may impair speech intelligibility and lead to social stigmatization. The goal of surgical intervention is to restore velopharyngeal competence while avoiding the complications of upper airway obstruction. Successful surgical management of VPD requires careful preoperative assessment and individualization of treatment. Optimization of surgical outcome is critically dependent on a thorough analysis of each patient's history, structural anatomy, and velopharyngeal dynamics. This analysis is best performed with close interdisciplinary collaboration of the surgeon, the speech pathologist, and the other members of the cleft-craniofacial team.

The velopharyngeal port is composed of several striated muscles that play a role in velopharyngeal valving. These include the superior pharyngeal constrictor, the musculus uvulae, and, most importantly, the levator veli palatini. If these muscles are structurally abnormal, as in cleft palate, or if their function is impaired, the oral and nasal cavities may not be adequately uncoupled during sound production. The cranial base likewise contributes to the overall configuration of the velopharyngeal port. If the cranial base angle is abnormally obtuse, the resulting increase in pharyngeal depth may lead to velopharyngeal disproportion and, consequently, to valvular dysfunction. The procedures most often employed for the physical management of VPD are the Furlow palatoplasty, the sphincter palatoplasty, and the posterior pharyngeal flap (PPF). Each of these techniques will be discussed below.

● PATIENT EVALUATION AND SELECTION

Patient Evaluation

Patients with known or suspected VPD are best evaluated by an interdisciplinary team of specialists. A comprehensive history, physical examination, and speech and language evaluation, including appropriate instrumental measures and imaging studies, are essential to the evaluation of patients with VPD.

The elicited history should focus on patient/family concerns with speech; pregnancy and birth history; primary medical/genetic diagnoses (eg, cleft palate, syndromes, cardiac defects, neuromuscular disease, etc); family history of cleft lip/palate or VPD; feeding or swallowing difficulties; hearing loss or ear disease; snoring or symptoms of obstructive sleep apnea (OSA); surgical history, including prior cleft palate repair, pharyngoplasty, tonsillectomy, or adenoidectomy; hearing loss, developmental delays, or learning disabilities; and history of speech therapy. A history of snoring or other signs of upper airway obstruction should alert the physician to obtain a preoperative polysomnogram. Each patient should undergo direct craniofacial and intraoral examination, focusing on craniofacial symmetry, oral/facial movement and symmetry, dentition and occlusion, structural integrity of the palate (eg, fistulae or clefts), signs of submucous cleft palate, including bifid uvula, zona pellucida, and notching of the posterior hard palate, velar length and elevation during phonation, and tonsil size and symmetry.

As noted above, the size of the tonsils and adenoids should also be evaluated and documented. Rarely, enlarged tonsils or an enlarged, irregular adenoid pad can cause dysfunction of the velopharyngeal valve. In such instances, patients may benefit from tonsillectomy or adenoidectomy alone. Conversely, adenoidectomy may result in VPD in predisposed patients, such as those with submucosal cleft

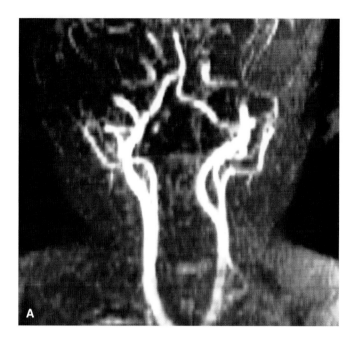

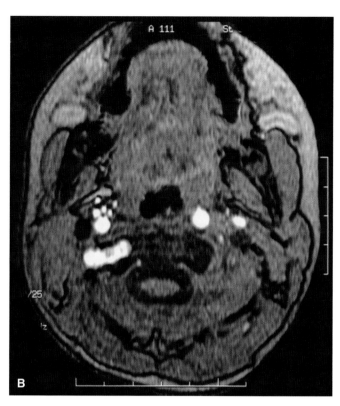

● **FIGURE 15-1.** Preoperative magnetic resonance angiogram (MRA) showing medially deviated left carotid artery in coronal section (A) and axial section (B).

palate or velopharyngeal disproportion (as in patients with 22q11.2 deletion syndrome). In such patients, adenoidectomy should be avoided. Patients with 22q11.2 deletion syndrome often have associated anomalies of the great vessels, including medially deviated carotid arteries (Figure 15-1), and such patients should undergo preoperative MRI evaluation for anatomic documentation and to guide surgical management.[1-4] If PPF surgery is performed in a patient with medial carotid deviation, the base of the flap can be skewed in order to avoid vascular injury.[5,6]

It is important to obtain information about any prior surgical procedures (eg, Furlow palatoplasty, adenoidectomy, PPF) and elucidate the timing of any changes in the patient's speech. Each patient should be evaluated by a speech pathologist familiar with cleft speech disorders. Perceptual speech assessment remains the gold standard in the diagnosis of VPD. The components of a standard speech evaluation for the assessment of velopharyngeal closure for speech should include an assessment of resonance, nasal emission, voice, and articulation. When clinical speech evaluation suggests the presence of VPD, instrumental assessment of speech and velopharyngeal closure may be useful as an adjunct to perceptual judgments. Instrumental measures can provide confirmation of perceptual judgments and further evidence of the need for intervention, as well as allow for objective pre- and post-treatment measurements. The most popular clinical tools for indirect instrumental evaluation include acoustic assessment of nasality and aerodynamic testing.

Imaging of the velopharynx is critical for making the most appropriate treatment decision, as optimization of surgical outcome is critically dependent on tailoring

the surgical procedure to each patient's velopharyngeal anatomy and function. In addition, imaging provides for assessment of the adjacent structures of the upper airway, which could impact treatment planning, such as the tonsils and adenoid pad. Objective assessment of the velopharyngeal valve is conducted using multiview videofluoroscopy (Figure 15-2) and/or nasopharyngoscopy (Figure 15-3). With either technique, the velopharyngeal closure pattern, contribution of lateral pharyngeal wall motion, gap size, and site of attempted velar closure on the posterior pharyngeal wall should be noted and documented.

Procedure Selection

Following thorough assessment, the proper surgical procedure for management of VPD may be determined to be one of three surgical procedures: Furlow double-opposing z-palatoplasty, PPF, or sphincter pharyngoplasty. Leonard Furlow first described the double-opposing z-plasty technique for the treatment of cleft palate.[7] This technique allows for anatomic reorientation of sagittally oriented levator veli palatini fibers, and at the same time reduces the potential for velar shortening that can occur with a longitudinal scar. A patient with a submucous cleft and small gap VPD will benefit from levator repositioning and velar lengthening and thus represents the ideal candidate for Furlow palatoplasty. In contrast, patients with horizontally oriented levator muscles and those who have had prior reconstruction of the levator sling should not be considered candidates for the Furlow technique.

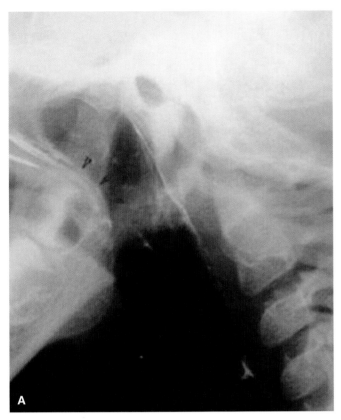
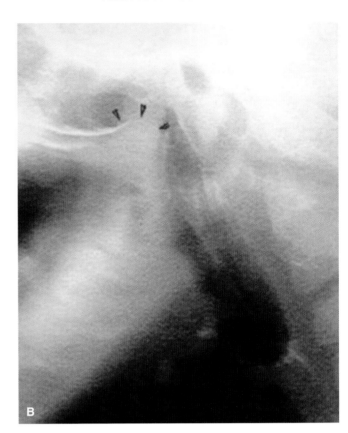

● FIGURE 15-2. Videofluoroscopy during rest (A) and attempted closure, with arrows showing velar bulge (B).

The PPF serves as an obturator to nasopharyngeal air escape. Patients with good lateral wall motion, or sagittal velopharyngeal closure patterns, are ideally suited for management using this technique. In contrast, patients with coronal closure patterns may derive greater benefit from a sphincter pharyngoplasty. Previous surgical intervention must be taken into account, however. For

example, if the patient has had a previous tonsillectomy, the posterior tonsillar pillars may be scarred, making a sphincter pharyngoplasty an unfavorable option. Both PPF surgery and sphincter pharyngoplasty carry some risk of postoperative sleep apnea, thus any history of snoring or airway obstruction warrants a preoperative polysomnogram, and the decision to proceed with

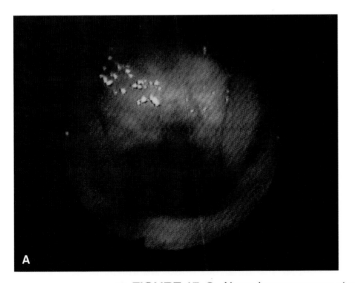
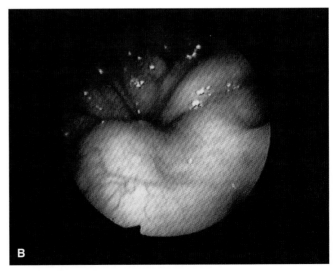

● FIGURE 15-3. Nasopharyngoscopy at rest (A) and with complete closure during speech without evidence of velopharyngeal insufficiency (VPI) (B).

surgical management of VPD must be tempered by the study results.

As noted above, surgical outcomes are critically dependent on individualizing surgical technique. Proper patient evaluation and selection includes both subjective and objective measures, and every aspect of the preoperative evaluation must be weighed in determining the best modality of treatment for each patient.

● PATIENT PREPARATION

Informed Consent

A detailed informed consent must be obtained from the parents preoperatively. Risks of VPD surgery include bleeding, dehiscence, OSA, hyponasal speech, and persistent VPD/hypernasal speech. Patients with preoperative symptoms of airway obstruction are at an increased risk for OSA postoperatively and should be monitored accordingly. Patients with 22q11.2 deletion syndrome and a medially deviated internal carotid artery are at a theoretical increased risk for arterial injury when performing either PPF surgery or sphincter pharyngoplasty, and parents/patients should be made aware of this increased risk preoperatively.

Anesthesia

General anesthesia is standard in surgical correction of VPD. Pediatric anesthesiologists familiar with treating patients with complicated airways should be available, especially when patients have a history of preoperative airway obstruction, Pierre Robin sequence, or syndromic diagnoses.

Equipment and Positioning

The patient is positioned supine on the operating table with the neck slightly extended. Exception to this should be made in patients who have cervical spine abnormalities that predispose to cervical instability. In such cases, hyperextension of the neck should be avoided. A Dingman mouth gag is placed to allow for a reliable, unobstructed view of the palate and velopharynx. Once adequate visualization of the operating field is achieved, the operation can proceed with efficiency.

● TECHNIQUE

Furlow Double-Opposing Z-Palatoplasty (Figure 15-4)

This technique involves the creation of mirror image z-plastys on the nasal and oral sides of the velum; the central limb is placed along the palatal midline. On the oral side, the posteriorly based triangular flap is composed of muscle and mucosa. The deep plane of dissection is the nasal submucosa. The tip of the flap is placed at the junction of the hard and soft palate, and its most posterior extent is placed the hamulus. Once the oral myomucosal flap is elevated, the anteriorly based nasal mucosa flap can be created. This flap extends from the base of the uvula medially toward the hamulus laterally. On the contralateral side, the anteriorly based flap is an oral mucosal flap, while the posteriorly based flap is a nasal myomucosal flap. In essence, the oral and nasal z-plastys are mirror images of one another. It is important to note that proper design of the z-plastys is based on the palatal anatomy and not on a predetermined geometric pattern. The palatal aponeurosis must be freed completely from the posterior hard palate in order for the posteriorly based flaps to be properly rotated and the levator fibers to be properly retrodisplaced. The palate is then closed in two layers: the nasal flaps are transposed and sutured, followed by the oral flaps.

Sphincter Pharyngoplasty (Figure 15-5)

The most widely used technique today is a variation of the technique first described by Hynes.[8-10] The posterior tonsillar pillars, made up of the palatopharyngeus muscles and overlying mucosa, are dissected and elevated as superiorly based flaps. These flaps are rotated 90 degrees and inset into the posterior pharynx. The level of flap inset should be at the level of attempted velopharyngeal closure, as determined by preoperative imaging. Of note, the superior-most extent of flap inset may be limited by the inferior portion of the adenoid pad. If the level of attempted velar closure is determined to be above this level, preoperative adenoidectomy is advised, thereby allowing for inset of the pharyngoplasty at the proper level of the posterior pharyngeal wall. Once both flaps are inset, their respective donor sites are closed.

Posterior Pharyngeal Flap (Figure 15-6)

PPF width (and, conversely, lateral port size) is determined preoperatively, based on velopharyngeal imaging studies. Flap width should be tailored to gap size and to the extent of lateral pharyngeal wall motion. The base of the flap should be designed at the level of attempted velar contact with the posterior pharyngeal wall. This flap may be superiorly or inferiorly based, although the former is the technique most often utilized. Flap length is determined as that necessary for proper inset, depending on the specific technique used. The posterior pharyngeal mucosa and underlying superior pharyngeal constrictor are divided to the prevertebral fascia. The flap is then elevated to its base in this avascular plane. The distal end of the flap is sutured into the soft palate, which may be split in a sagittal or in a horizontal ("fish mouth") orientation. In general, a wider, shorter flap has less of a tendency to tube on itself, resulting in less narrowing of the flap postoperatively. The undersurface of narrower flaps, in contrast, should be lined by nasal mucosal flaps based on the posterior velum in order to prevent such tubing. The donor site in the posterior pharynx may be closed primarily or left open to remucosalize secondarily.

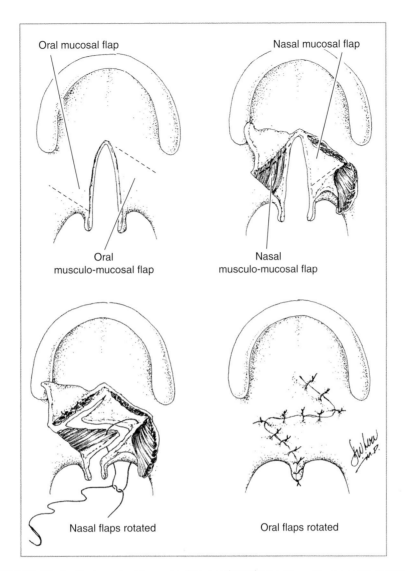

Oral mucosal flap

Nasal mucosal flap

Oral
musculo-mucosal flap

Nasal
musculo-mucosal flap

Nasal flaps rotated

Oral flaps rotated

● **FIGURE 15-4.** Furlow double-opposing z-palatoplasty. (*From Kirschner RE. Palatal anomalies in 22q11.2 deletion syndrome. In: Murphy K, Scambler P, eds. Velo-Cardio-Facial Syndrome: Understanding Microdeletion Disorders. Cambridge; New York: Cambridge University Press; 2005.*)

● COMPLICATIONS

In general, complications are infrequent following any of the above surgical techniques and include bleeding, dehiscence, oronasal fistula, nasal airway obstruction, and sleep apnea. The incidence of each of these complications varies significantly depending upon the technique used.

Furlow Palatoplasty

Postoperative complications specific to the double-opposing z-plasty technique include bleeding, oronasal fistula, and nasal airway obstruction. Bleeding can often be avoided simply by meticulous attention to hemostasis. Although some have reported a relatively high incidence of oronasal fistula formation following use of the Furlow technique for repair of cleft palate, the incidence of fistula formation following its use for management of VPD has

not been reported but can be presumed to be quite low. Risk factors for fistula formation include previous cleft surgery, comorbid conditions, and, most importantly, tension on the repair. Finally, although airway obstruction can occur following Furlow palatoplasty, it is less frequent and usually transient, when compared to PPF surgery.[11,12] It is important to monitor the respiratory status of all patients postoperatively, particularly those with a prior history of upper airway obstruction.

Sphincter Pharyngoplasty

Bleeding, flap dehiscence, nasal airway obstruction, and OSA have all been reported following sphincter pharyngoplasty. In cases where VPD was noted to persist postoperatively, partial or total flap dehiscence was most often cited as the etiologic factor.[13] Sphincter pharyngoplasty has often been as "dynamic" or "physiologic." Whereas dynamism of

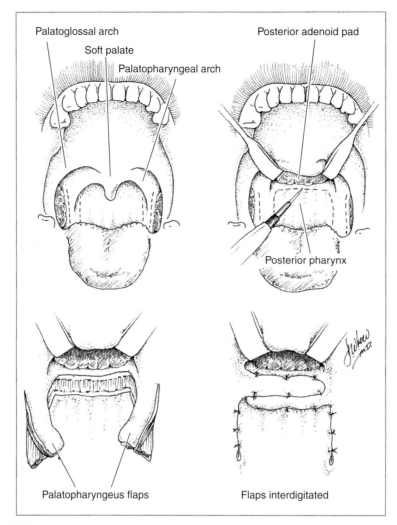

● **FIGURE 15-5.** Sphincter pharyngoplasty. (*From Kirschner RE. Palatal anomalies in 22q11.2 deletion syndrome. In: Murphy K, Scambler P, eds. Velo-Cardio-Facial Syndrome: Understanding Microdeletion Disorders. Cambridge; New York: Cambridge University Press; 2005.*)

sphincter pharyngoplasty is not a constant finding, reduction in velopharyngeal port size is assured.[14,15] Nasal airway obstruction, which may present as hyponasal speech, nasal airway congestion, or OSA are potential unwanted outcomes, although some have reported that nasal airway obstruction may be less frequent after sphincter pharyngoplasty than after PPF surgery. Patients most at risk are those with comorbid conditions such as tonsillar hyperplasia or a history of Pierre Robin sequence or OSA. When airway obstruction does occur, however, it is most often transient. Persistent upper airway obstruction may often be successfully treated using continuous positive airway pressure (CPAP) at night.[16,17]

Posterior Pharyngeal Flap

The most commonly reported complications of PPF surgery include bleeding, flap dehiscence, and airway obstruction. Rare cases of death have been reported.[18,19] Bleeding often occurs during the first 24 to 48 hours at the open donor site in the posterior pharynx. This risk can be reduced with careful hemostasis, use of electrocautery in flap elevation, and primary closure of the donor site. Many patients show signs upper airway obstruction in the immediate postoperative period, but this often resolves in several days to weeks as edema resolves. Patients at greatest risk for airway complications include those with a history of Pierre Robin sequence, hypotonia (22q11.2 deletion syndrome), and enlarged tonsils. Preoperative or concomitant tonsillectomy is recommended in patients with significant tonsillar hyperplasia. All patients should be monitored with continuous pulse oximetry overnight. Patients with wide flaps should be considered for placement of a temporary nasopharyngeal airway and observation in an intensive care unit.

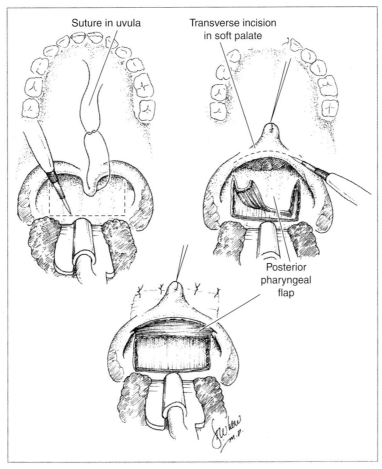

● **FIGURE 15-6.** Posterior pharyngeal flap. (*From Kirschner RE. Palatal anomalies in 22q11.2 deletion syndrome. In: Murphy K, Scambler P, eds. Velo-Cardio-Facial Syndrome: Understanding Microdeletion Disorders. Cambridge; New York: Cambridge University Press; 2005.*)

● OUTCOMES ASSESSMENT

Successful outcome of surgical management of VPD is measured by the effective elimination of hypernasality and nasal air emission while avoiding overcorrection that may lead to hyponasality or sleep apnea. Postoperatively, each patient should undergo formal speech evaluation at 6 months, at 12 months, and then at yearly intervals. In addition, careful monitoring of the upper airway is essential. Patients who demonstrate signs or symptoms of OSA that persist beyond the immediate postoperative period should undergo polysomnographic evaluation. Patients with significant OSA that persists postoperatively may require CPAP therapy or, in some cases, surgical revision. Obstructing PPFs may be narrowed or converted to sphincter pharyngoplasty, based on the results of studies that document a lower incidence of OSA following the latter procedure.[20]

Although hypernasality is successfully reduced or eliminated in the majority of patients who undergo surgery, approximately 10% to 20% of patients will demonstrate persistent hypernasality requiring revisional surgery.[13] All such patient should undergo the same comprehensive evaluation that was performed before the primary procedure. Persistent VPD may be due to fistula, flap dehiscence, scarring and tethering of the flap, poor selection of primary technique, or improperly low placement of the flap or sphincter on the posterior pharyngeal wall. Patients should undergo objective assessment via diagnostic imaging using either nasendoscopy or videofluoroscopy. Revisional surgery for the management of persistent VPD should only be performed in patients with a stable airway and no signs of OSA.

Patients with persistent VPD after Furlow palatoplasty may be managed by PPF or sphincter pharyngoplasty, the selection of which should be based on the findings of postoperative imaging studies. In some patients, persistent VPD after PPF may be found to be secondary to narrowing and/or inferior migration of the flap. If the flap is noted to be too narrow, the flap may be augmented or divided and a new, wider flap created. If the flap is noted to be tethered inferiorly, it can be advanced using a V-Y technique, divided and replaced by a new flap, or taken down and replaced by a sphincter pharyngoplasty. Persistent VPD following sphincter pharyngoplasty is most often managed by re-elevating the flaps and tightening the central port. Close monitoring of speech and airway stability is critically important following secondary surgery. The risk of OSA has not been found to be greater after secondary speech surgery.[13,21]

It is essential to base the operative plan on the preoperative assessment of velopharyngeal motion and closure patterns, both for optimizing speech outcomes and limiting the risk of complications. This is equally important in the setting of primary and revisional surgery. Because the nature of VPD varies from patient to patient, reliably successful outcomes depend on careful execution of the surgical technique as well as diagnostic precision and selection of technique.

REFERENCES

1. D'Antonio LL, Marsh JL. Abnormal carotid arteries in the velocardiofacial syndrome. *Plast Reconstr Surg.* 1987;80:471.

2. MacKenzie-Stepner K, Witzel MA, Stringer DA, et al. Abnormal carotid arteries in the velocardiofacial syndrome: a report of three cases. *Plast Reconstr Surg.* 1987;80:347.

3. Mitnick RJ, Bello JA, Golding-Kushner KJ, et al. The use of magnetic resonance angiography prior to pharyngeal flap surgery in patients with velocardiofacial syndrome. *Plast Reconstr Surg.* 1996;97:908.

4. Ross DA, Witzel MA, Armstrong DC, et al. Is pharyngoplasty a risk in velocardiofacial syndrome? An assessment of medially displaced carotid arteries. *Plast Reconstr Surg.* 1996;98:1182.

5. Tatum SA 3rd, Chang J, Havkin N, et al. Pharyngeal flap and the internal carotid in velocardiofacial syndrome. *Arch Facial Plast Surg.* 2002;4:73.

6. Witt PD, Miller DC, Marsh JL, et al. Limited value of preoperative cervical vascular imaging in patients with velocardiofacial syndrome. *Plast Reconstr Surg.* 1998;101:1184.

7. Furlow LT Jr. Cleft palate repair: preliminary report on lengthening and muscle transposition by z-plasty. Southeastern Society of Plastic and Reconstructive Surgery. Boca Raton, FL; 1978.

8. Hynes W. Pharyngoplasty by muscle transplantation. *Br J Plast Surg.* 1950;3:128.

9. Hynes W. The results of pharyngoplasty by muscle transplantation in failed "cleft palate" cases, with special reference to the influence of the pharynx on voice production. *Ann R Coll Surg Engl.* 1953;13:17.

10. Hynes W. Observations on pharyngoplasty. *Br J Plast Surg.* 1967;20:244.

11. Liao YF, Noordhoff MS, Huang CS, et al. Comparison of obstructive sleep apnea syndrome in children with cleft palate following Furlow palatoplasty or pharyngeal flap for velopharyngeal insufficiency. *Cleft Palate Craniofac J.* 2004;41:152.

12. Liao YF, Yun C, Huang CS, et al. Longitudinal follow-up of obstructive sleep apnea following Furlow palatoplasty in children with cleft palate: a preliminary report. *Cleft Palate Craniofac J.* 2003;40:269.

13. Witt PD, Myckatyn, T, Marsh JL. Salvaging the failed pharyngoplasty: intervention outcome. *Cleft Palate Craniofac J.* 1998;35:447.

14. Witt PD, Marsh JL, Arlis H, et al. Quantification of dynamic velopharyngeal port excursion following sphincter pharyngoplasty. *Plast Reconstr Surg.* 1998;101:1205.

15. Kawamoto HK Jr. Pharyngoplasty revisited and revised. In: Jurkiewicz MJ, Culbertson JH Jr, eds. *Operative Techniques in Plastic and Reconstructive Surgery.* Philadelphia: W.B. Saunders; 1995:239.

16. Witt PD, Marsh JL, Muntz HR, et al. Acute obstructive sleep apnea as a complication of sphincter pharyngoplasty. *Cleft Palate Craniofac J.* 1996;33:183.

17. Saint Raymond C, Bettega G, Deschaux C, et al. Sphincter pharyngoplasty as a treatment of velopharyngeal incompetence in young people: a prospective evaluation of effects on sleep structure and sleep respiratory disturbances. *Chest.* 2004;125:864.

18. Hofer SO, Dhar BK, Robinson PH, et al. A 10-year review of perioperative complications in pharyngeal flap surgery. *Plast Reconstr Surg.* 2002;110:1393.

19. Valnicek SM, Zuker RM, Halpern LM, et al. Perioperative complications of superior pharyngeal flap surgery in children. *Plast Reconstr Surg.* 1994;93:954.

20. Pensler JM, Reich DS. A comparison of speech results after the pharyngeal flap and the dynamic sphincteroplasty procedures. *Ann Plast Surg.* 1991;26:441.

21. Barone CM, Shprintzen RJ, Strauch B, et al. Pharyngeal flap revisions: flap elevation from a scarred posterior pharynx. *Plast Reconstr Surg.* 1994;93:279.

chapter 16

Craniosynostosis

Mitchel Seruya, MD / Stephen B. Baker, MD, DDS, FACS / Jeffrey Weinzweig, MD, FACS

● PATIENT EVALUATION AND SELECTION

Craniosynostosis is defined as the premature closure of a cranial suture which causes abnormal calvarial growth. Virchow's law states that skull growth is arrested in the direction perpendicular to the fused suture and expanded at the sites of unaffected sutures, leading to characteristic calvarial deformations.[1] This condition can be classified into simple (single suture) versus complex (multiple sutures) and nonsyndromic versus syndromic subtypes (Tables 16-1 and 16-2).

Preoperative assessment for craniosynostosis includes a detailed medical history, physical examination, and radiographic imaging. Medical history should elicit skull irregularities, associated syndromes, family history of calvarial deformities, and symptoms of intracranial hypertension (headache/vomiting, developmental changes, irritability, and oculomotor paresis). Physical examination should evaluate for characteristic calvarial shapes and asymmetries, premature closure of the anterior fontanelle (normally open until 8–12 months of age), perisutural ridging, and signs of intracranial hypertension (papilledema, supraorbital retrusion, severe towering [turricephaly], and severe frontal/occipital bossing). Head circumferences, cranial indices, and anthropometric measurements should be documented.

Radiological investigation may be necessary to corroborate the diagnosis and/or rule out any associated intracranial abnormalities. Computed tomography (CT) remains the most sensitive barometer of bony fusion and may provide evidence for elevated intracranial pressure, as noted by erosion of the inner calvarial table ("copper-beaten" appearance also referred to as "thumb printing") (Figure 16-1). CT imaging and MRI are also helpful in evaluating the underlying brain for structural or functional abnormalities, including hydrocephalus, holoprosencephaly, cortical dysplasias, and Chiari malformations.

Surgical intervention is indicated in craniosynostosis both for the correction of calvarial contour deformities and the prevention of psychosocial dysfunction, intracranial hypertension, and/or mental retardation. Studies have shown that the presence of intracranial hypertension is dependent on the number of affected sutures, ranging from approximately 14% for single-suture synostosis to approximately 47% in multisuture synostosis.[2-3] Sutural release in simple craniosynostosis has been advised due to the concerns regarding increased intracranial pressure as well as the mild but significant developmental delay in the aging child. Patients with complex synostoses present with increased severity of physical and neurological symptoms; therefore, surgical intervention is even more imperative.

● PATIENT PREPARATION

Preoperative considerations include the optimal type and timing of surgical correction for craniosynostosis. A broad range of surgical options exist in the armamentarium of contemporary craniofacial surgical reconstruction, all with the primary objective of releasing the affected suture(s) to permit normalization of skull growth in the setting of accelerated cerebral growth. An open craniofacial approach remains the mainstay of therapy, relying on wide scalp dissection, extensive calvarial osteotomies, and skull reconfiguration that is individually tailored to each cranial vault deformity.[4] To address concerns regarding incision length, operative blood loss, and length of stay for open craniofacial procedures, minimally invasive techniques have been proposed. These techniques include endoscopic sutural release,[5] spring-assisted cranioplasty,[6] and distraction osteogenesis.[7]

The optimal surgical age has been a source of contention, given its differential effects on intraoperative hemodynamics, postoperative cranial growth, and subsequent mental

TABLE 16-1. Classification of Craniosynostosis

Affected Suture	Phenotypic Presentation
Sagittal	Dolichocephaly, scaphocephaly
Coronal (unilateral)	Anterior plagiocephaly
Coronal (bilateral)	Brachycephaly
Metopic	Trigonocephaly
Lambdoid	Posterior plagiocephaly
Multiple sutures	Cloverleaf (Kleeblattschädel), acrocephaly, oxycephaly

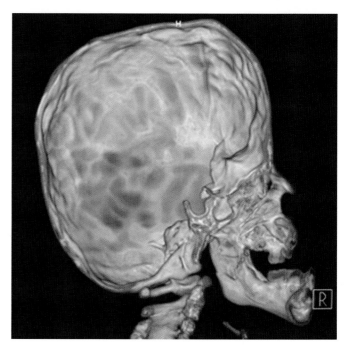

● **FIGURE 16-1.** CT findings of elevated intracranial pressure. This sagittal CT image demonstrates the classic "copper-beaten" appearance, also referred to as "thumb printing," resulting from increased intracranial pressure.

development. While the literature is inconclusive regarding the appropriate timing for correction of craniosynostosis, the majority of craniofacial surgeons operate between 3 and 12 months of age. Surgical age is also dependent on the type of surgical approach employed. Minimally invasive techniques, which rely on dynamic cranial vault alteration during rapid calvarial growth, are generally performed at an earlier age than open surgical correction.

Given the senior authors' extensive experience with open craniofacial reconstruction for craniosynostosis, surgical considerations, operative steps, and outcomes shall be described for this type of surgical approach in the accompanying sections. In preparation for open craniosynostosis surgery, measures for ensuring adequate blood resuscitation should be undertaken. These include obtaining a blood type and cross, autologous blood donation, and/or allogenic blood direct donation from a family member. Parents should be instructed that open craniosynostosis surgery is performed under general anesthesia. For most types of open craniosynostosis surgeries, patients are placed in the supine position to facilitate calvarial exposure. However, if the posterior vault is being addressed, as in a lambdoidal synostosis or some sagittal synostoses, the patient is ideally placed in the prone position. In the prone position, care must be taken to ensure adequate protection of the globes, facilitated by bilateral tarsorrhaphies and periorbital cushioning.

A plating system is used by most surgeons to maintain the proper position of the osteotomized bone segments after they have been placed in the desired position. Historically, titanium was used but fell out of favor when it was noted that the plates translocated with continued

calvarial growth. Resorbable plates eliminate the problems associated with translocation. They maintain strength across the osteotomy long enough for the bone to heal but are resorbed by the body after several years. Most surgeons today employ some type of resorbable fixation for cranial vault remodeling.

● **TECHNIQUE**

Metopic Synostosis (Trigonocephaly)

Metopic synostosis is marked by a variable degree of phenotypic severity, ranging from mild ridging to the formation of a triangular shaped head (trigonocephaly) or prominent "keel" forehead with or without hypotelorism. Although an endocranial ridge is not commonly seen in patients with metopic synostosis, an endocranial notch can be observed on axial CT images and is virtually diagnostic of premature suture fusion. Weinzweig termed this radiographic finding

TABLE 16-2. Craniofacial Dysostosis Syndromes

Syndrome	Involved Suture	Morphological Presentation
Crouzon	Coronal, sagittal	Midface hypoplasia, shallow orbits, proptosis, hypertelorism
Apert	Coronal, sagittal, lambdoid	Midface hypoplasia, shallow orbits, proptosis, hypertelorism, *symmetrical syndactyly of hands and feet*, choanal atresia, ventriculomegaly, genitourinary/cardiovascular anomalies
Pfeiffer	Coronal, sagittal	Midface hypoplasia, proptosis, hypertelorism, *broad great toe/thumb*

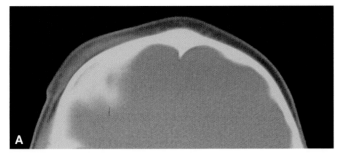 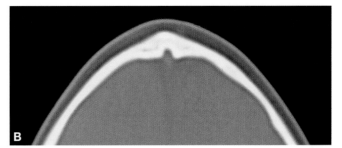

● **FIGURE 16-2.** The metopic notch. Axial CT images demonstrate the endocranial bony spur associated with normal metopic suture fusion (A), and the Ω (omega)-shaped *metopic notch* (B). Moderate ectocranial ridging is also appreciated in this patient.

the *metopic notch*, a morphologic abnormality that is seen in 93% of synostotic patients (Figure 16-2).[8] A metopic notch is not seen in *any* nonsynostotic patients and, therefore, can be used to diagnose metopic synostosis even *after* the period physiologic suture closure. This notch represents the anatomic site of attachment of the falx, a dural reflection off the crista galli with basicranial origins, and suggests a role for the cranial base in metopic suture fusion.

Whereas a metopic notch describes the endocranial finding on axial CT images in patients with metopic synostosis, a corresponding three-dimensional groove is found on the endocranial surface of the actual skull that extends from the nasion to the anterior fontanelle in these patients. Weinzweig termed this clinical finding the *metopic groove*, an anatomic abnormality that can reliably be found in patients with metopic synostosis (Figure 16-3).

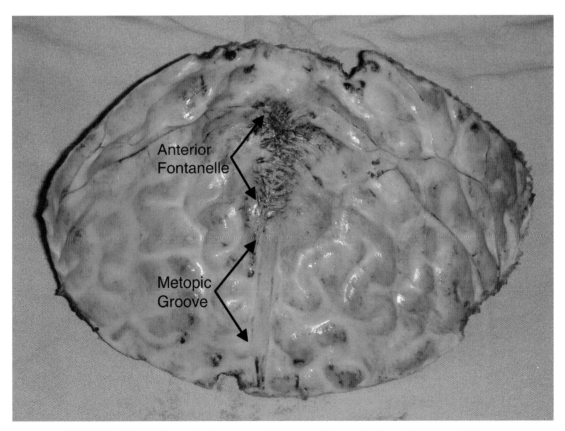

● **FIGURE 16-3.** The metopic groove. Intraoperative evaluation of the inner table of the anterior cranial vault of a previously untreated 9-year-old child with metopic and bicoronal synostosis and Crouzon syndrome demonstrates a *metopic groove*. While Crouzon syndrome is commonly associated with bicoronal synostosis, this child demonstrated both a metopic notch and metopic groove, pathognomonic findings consistent with metopic synostosis. The metopic groove typically extends from the nasion to the anterior fontanelle. Note the severe depressions of the inner table of the skull indicating increased intracranial pressure in this older child.

In general, the goals of surgery are the normalization of the forehead with reconstitution of a normal supraorbital rim when necessary. Individuals presenting solely with a prominent midline keel may be best served by simple contouring of the frontal bone or by removal of the frontal bone flap followed by reconfiguration. Conversely, patients with significant trigonocephaly and hypotelorism will require a fronto-orbital reconstruction, recontouring the frontal bone, and laterally expanding the orbits, often with cranial bone graft placed in the midline of the frontal bandeau at the level of the nasion.

The essentials of fronto-orbital reconstruction involve a standard "stealth" (zig-zag) coronal incision, providing for adequate exposure of the fronto-orbital region while minimizing any postoperative scar. Perioperative antibiotics and steroids are given prior to the start of surgery. The incision is infiltrated with 0.25% lidocaine and 1:400,000 parts epinephrine to minimize intraoperative bleeding. The frontal and temporal regions are dissected in the subgaleal plane and care is taken to preserve the periosteum on the surface of the bone, which helps minimize blood loss and may be used to stabilize osteotomized bony segments. The dissection is taken down to the level of the periorbital tissues, with caution taken to avoid any injury to the underlying globes. Following exposure of the frontal and orbital regions, the frontal bone is removed, providing access to the intracranial compartment. The supraorbital rim is then removed in one piece to facilitate reconstruction of the previously triangular-shaped supraorbital bar. Care is taken to remove sufficient bone in the region of the sphenoid bone to allow for growth at the midface and orbits. If the orbits require correction of hypotelorism, it will be necessary to displace the lateral walls of the orbit as well as to split the midline and interpose a calvarial bone graft. Reconfiguration of the supraorbital bar often requires a midline osteotomy to facilitate a flattened forehead with additional partial-thickness bone cuts at the lateral (pterional) angle to promote normalization of the lateral supraorbital angle. The supraorbital reconfiguration is maintained by the utilization of intervening bone grafts as well as resorbable hardware. Following placement of the supraorbital bar as a foundation, the frontal bone is reconstructed using the remaining portions of bone. It is often possible to reverse the original frontal bone flap (posterior portion is now in an anterior position) to obtain an adequate width and contour with the new frontal bone flap. It is important to provide adequate enhancement at the pterional region to avoid long-term supratemporal hollowing or recession.

Sagittal Synostosis (Scaphocephaly, Dolichocephaly)

Children with sagittal synostosis will present with a narrow, elongated skull (*dolichocephaly*, long headedness; *scaphocephaly*, boat shaped). Depending on the region of greatest premature fusion of the sagittal suture, the child may manifest frontal or occipital bossing, or a combination of both.

The treatment for sagittal synostosis remains controversial, with surgical approaches ranging from minimal removal of the involved suture and bone to extensive total calvarectomy and reconfiguration. Simple synostectomy or simple strip craniectomy is safe and well tolerated, providing adequate cosmetic results in select patients with mild deformities. This procedure, however, has several disadvantages stemming from the fact that it strictly addresses the fused suture and not the compensatory changes in skull shape. It also leaves a large unprotected area over the vertex of the skull, an area with a high rate of restenosis and renewed growth restriction.

An extended synostectomy provides immediate restoration of normal skull contour by shortening the anteroposterior dimension, expanding the biparietal dimension, and addressing the frontal and occipital prominences. Amongst extended synostectomy techniques, the pi procedure has become a widely utilized approach for older infants (3–12 months of age) with scaphocephaly. The essential steps involve removal of bone along both sides of the sagittal suture as well as over the coronal suture, in the design of the Greek letter pi (Π). Cranial bone overlying the sagittal sinus is left intact to minimize bleeding. Drill holes are placed in the adjacent osteotomized bone flaps, allowing for placement of an absorbable suture that helps narrow the anteroposterior dimension while expanding the biparietal length.

Staged or partial vault remodeling procedures also work well in indicated patients. In some cases, the majority of the deformity occurs anteriorly or posteriorly. In these cases, vault remodeling may be limited to the most involved area (posterior vs anterior) of the cranium. In properly selected cases, this approach is less morbid and produces excellent results.

To address older infants beyond the period of maximal cerebral growth (>12–18 months of age), as well as those children with significant frontal or occipital prominence, procedures with more aggressive craniectomies and reconstruction must be undertaken.[9] Total calvarectomy and reconstruction in the setting of severe or late presentation scaphocephaly has been proposed to offer superior cosmetic results with a minimal increase in morbidity. This may be accomplished by removal of the frontal, occipital, and both parietal bones. Subsequently, reconfiguration is carried out and aimed at providing a shortened anteroposterior dimension in addition to a widened biparietal diameter. The use of rigid fixation is indispensable in these cases, providing greater three-dimensional conformational stability and decreased intraoperative time, bleeding, and postoperative infection.

Coronal Synostosis (Anterior Plagiocephaly/Brachycephaly)

Patients with unicoronal synostosis present with anterior, or frontal, plagiocephaly whereas those with bilateral coronal involvement demonstrate brachycephaly. Phenotypic features of anterior plagiocephaly include ipsilateral perisutural ridging, forehead flattening, and orbital recession, coupled with contralateral compensatory frontal bossing. Facial deformities are also common, including nasal root displacement toward the ipsilateral side, anterior displacement of the ipsilateral ear, increased orbital aperture, and chin deviation toward the contralateral side. Pathognomonic radiographic findings diagnostic of unicoronal synostosis include elevation of the ipsilateral orbit which is seen secondary to superior displacement of the greater wing of the sphenoid, also known as the "harlequin" deformity (Figure 16-4A–C). Phenotypic features of brachycephaly include forehead retrusion and flattening, frontal towering, and biparietal widening. The nasal dorsum can be low and hypertelorism may be present.

Surgical intervention in unicoronal and bicoronal synostoses aims to correct both the frontal and orbital asymmetries. With the current understanding that unilateral coronal synostosis presents with bilateral dysmorphic changes,

bilateral correction is now believed to be the optimum approach. For anterior plagiocephaly, a bilateral fronto-orbital advancement procedure is employed for expansion of the affected forehead and orbit with concomitant recession of the contralateral orbit (Figure 16-4D–I). Excellent symmetry can be achieved in this manner (Figure 16-4J,K). Bilateral fronto-orbital advancement also serves in the correction of bicoronal synostosis.

The bilateral fronto-orbital advancement reconstruction (FOAR) involves the release of both coronal sutures while providing bilateral frontal and orbital correction (Figure 16-5). A standard coronal skin incision is made. A bifrontal bone flap is removed typically in one piece, leaving a 1–2 cm wide supraorbital bandeau. Extending the osteotomy posterior to the coronal suture will often provide adequate width and a satisfactory new frontal reconstruction when this bone flap segment is inverted. The sphenoid wing is osteotomized and the coronal sutures are

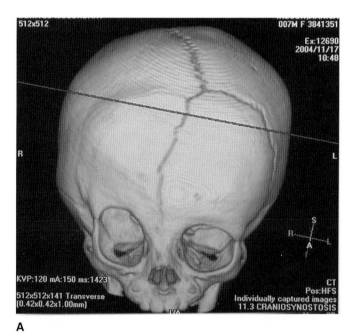

A

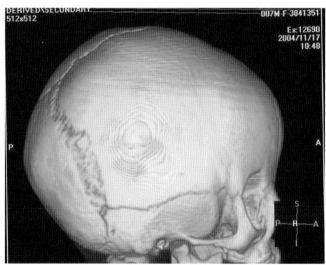

B

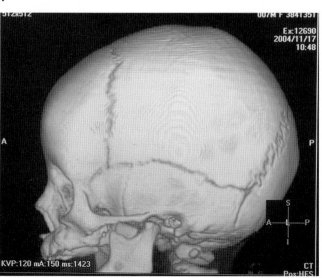

C

● FIGURE 16-4. Bilateral fronto-orbital reconstruction for unicoronal synostosis. Three-dimensional CT scans demonstrate right coronal synostosis and a harlequin deformity (A, B), and a normal, patent contralateral coronal suture (C).

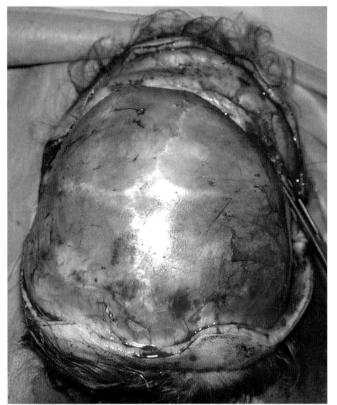

D

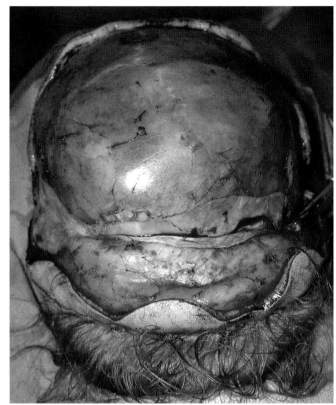

E

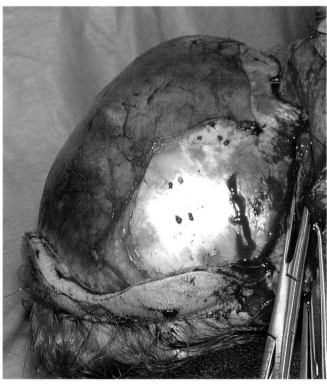

F

● FIGURE 16-4. (*continued*) Intraoperative exposure demonstrates right coronal synostosis, ipsilateral frontal flattening, and contralateral frontal bossing (D–F).

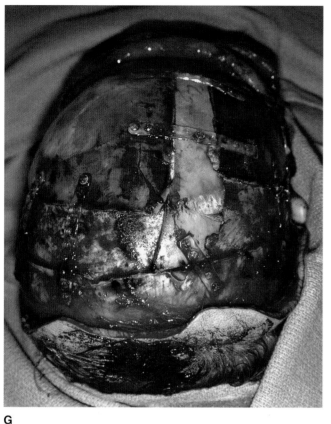

G

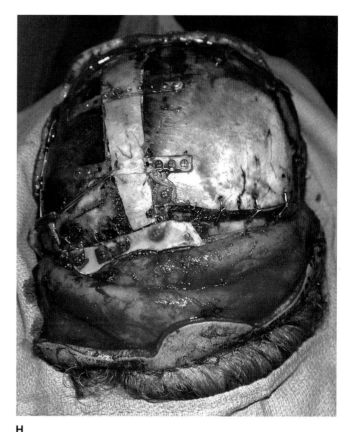

H

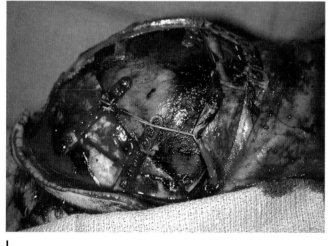

I

● FIGURE 16-4. (*continued*) Bilateral fronto-orbital advancement is performed for expansion of the affected frontal bone and orbit with concomitant recession of the contralateral orbit. Fixation is performed using resorbable plates and screws (G–I).

opened to the level of the skull base, serving to prevent continued growth restriction and resultant postoperative hollowing of the pterional regions. Caution must be exercised when performing the osteotomy across the sphenoid wing on the affected side, as its superior displacement may cause technical difficulty upon frontal bone flap removal and lead to dural laceration if caution is not exercised. After removal of the frontal bone flap, the orbital bandeau is freed with osteotomies performed across the lateral orbit at the frontozygomatic suture, the orbital roof, and the nasion just above the nasofrontal suture. Care is taken to protect the underlying brain as well as orbital contents with judicious placement of retractors. The bandeau is then reconfigured using partial osteotomies at the midline

while using absorbable hardware on the interior surface to maintain the newly contoured shape. The newly configured supraorbital bar is replaced, its lateral aspects and midline fixed to the calvarial foundation with resorbable fixation for improved healing and postoperative maintenance of the surgical construct. It is frequently necessary to overcorrect the expansion of the affected side by 5% to 10% while also providing a convex shape at the lateral border for a satisfactory reconstruction. Often, the unaffected orbit is mildly set back to correct for preoperative compensatory overgrowth. The frontal bone flap is then attached to the supraorbital bar, taking care to match it to the previously overcorrected (5%–10%) orbital bandeau on the affected side. Remaining portions of bone are fixed

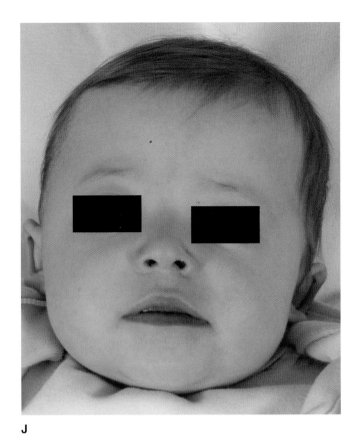

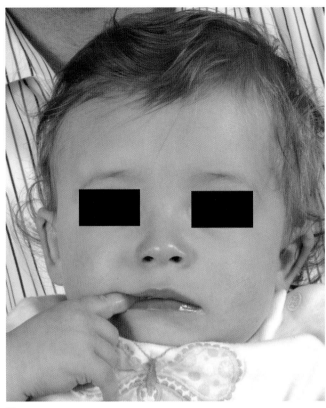

J

K

● **FIGURE 16-4.** (*continued*) Preoperative (J) and postoperative (K) photographs demonstrate correction of the orbital and frontal bone asymmetries. Note the increased aperture of the right eye in the preoperative photo and subsequent correction.

with absorbable plates or suture, and closure is performed in a routine fashion with placement of subgaleal drains.

Lambdoid Synostosis and Posterior Deformational Plagiocephaly

Posterior plagiocephaly due to lambdoid suture synostosis is rare, with the majority of observed posterior plagiocephaly secondary to positional molding. Understanding the phenotypic differences between lambdoid synostosis and posterior deformational plagiocephaly is critical toward making the appropriate diagnosis and designing the proper course of treatment. Children with lambdoid synostosis characteristically have a trapezoid-shaped head in association with posterior displacement of the ipsilateral ear, contralateral occipital bossing, and frequent ridging of the affected lambdoid suture. In contrast, posterior deformational plagiocephaly is marked by a parallelogram-shaped head, anterior displacement of the ipsilateral ear, and ipsilateral frontal bossing in the absence of palpable ridging along the lambdoid sutures.

Infants with true lambdoid synostosis may benefit from a variety of surgical approaches, aiming to release the affected suture(s) and normalize the posterior calvarial vault contour. Options include simple synostectomy, unilateral reconfiguration of the affected occipital region, and bilateral occipital reconstruction with or without the use

of an occipital bandeau. The majority of lambdoid surgical candidates have significant parietal and frontal compensatory changes in addition to their occipital deformation; therefore, they are best served by a more extended calvarectomy and reconstruction.

For an extended calvarial reconfiguration, the globes are protected with bilateral tarsorrhaphies and patients are placed in a prone position. Perioperative antibiotics and steroids are administered. Intraoperative bleeding is minimized with the use of local anesthetic mixed with epinephrine as well as controlled hypotensive anesthesia. A coronal incision is then undertaken followed by subgaleal dissection to expose the occipitoparietal regions. Both parietal bone flaps are subsequently removed with osteotomies taken posterior to the coronal and anterior to the lambdoid sutures. A midline strip of bone is then left to protect the underlying sagittal sinus. After removal of the parietal bone flaps, dissection is carried out at the level of the lambdoid suture under direct visualization, taking great caution at the level of the transverse, sagittal and sigmoid sinuses. Osteotomies are brought to within 1 cm on either side of the midline, with the final cut made after the underlying dura and sinus have been clearly dissected free under direct visualization. Inadvertent entry into the sinus, particularly at the region of the asterion, may lead to significant blood loss over a short period and constitutes the greatest risk encountered with this approach.

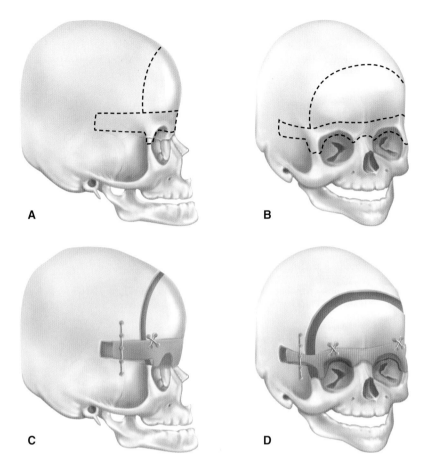

● **FIGURE 16-5.** Bilateral FOAR for bicoronal synostosis. The FOAR procedure involves release of both coronal sutures while providing bilateral frontal and orbital correction. A bifrontal bone flap is removed, typically as a single segment, leaving a 1–2 cm wide supraorbital bandeau. A tongue-and-groove osteotomy of the bandeau facilitates advancement and fixation (A, B). Fixation of the frontal bone to the supraorbital bar is then performed (C, D).

Nevertheless, with appropriate care and meticulous dissection, this complication may be avoided in the majority of individuals. The removed calvarial plates are reconfigured to provide adequate reshaping of the occipital contour and stabilized with resorbable hardware, deliberately leaving open the region of the prior lambdoid suture. Subgaleal drains are then placed and closure is carried out in routine fashion.

Treatment of posterior deformational plagiocephaly is a function of both the age and severity at presentation. When presenting before the age of 6 months, therapy consists of positional modifications combined with physiotherapy in the case of constrained neck movements or asymmetric neurological development. In cases of no improvement or progression of the deformity despite repositioning after 2 to 3 months, cranial orthotic (helmet) therapy is indicated.

● **COMPLICATIONS**

Perioperative morbidity may include wound infection, dural laceration, superficial brain injury, cerebrospinal fluid leak, encephalocele formation, subgaleal hematoma, and ocular injury. Intraoperative blood loss and transfusion requirements, leading to hemodynamic instability, constitute great dangers to the patient and should never be underestimated. It is imperative to accurately gauge the extent of blood loss and match accordingly with packed red blood cells. Other serious perioperative complications consist of ischemic brain injury, venous air embolism, epidural and subdural hemorrhage, and severe transfusion reactions.

Long-term postoperative concerns include recurrent calvarial deformities, cranial bone defects that fail to fill in over time, and hardware-related problems. Depending on the extent of morphologic asymmetry, intracranial hypertension, and developmental delay, recurrent calvarial deformities may require a minor or major reoperation. Defects larger than 2 cm in patients older than 18 to 24 months will often persist and may need eventual correction with split calvarial bone graft or bone substitute. Persistent hardware may also be problematic, particularly in patients in whom resorbable hardware was used. It is not uncommon for the polylactic/polyglycolic constructs to remain in place for 12 to 18 months before eventual resorption. In rare individuals, sterile abscesses may develop at sites of hardware resorption and subsequently require exploration for debridement. Postoperative mortality rates are low and continue to decline with technological advancements and experience.

● OUTCOMES ASSESSMENT

Based on outcomes data on open craniosynostosis surgery, estimated blood loss spans 25% to 500% of estimated blood volume (EBV), transfusion requirement range from 25% to 500% of EBV, complication rates are between 6.8% and 23.3%, and mortality rates center around 0% to 1.1%. Hospital length of stay is typically between 4 and 7 days, with longer admissions for complex synostoses. Reoperation rates range from 7.2% to 23.3% and are indeed higher for complex synostoses.

Outcome studies have also demonstrated that conservative therapy is beneficial in the reduction of calvarial deformities secondary to positional molding. Postural changes and helmet therapy are most effective between 4 and 12 months of age, during the period of rapid brain growth. Approximately 95% of infants can be expected to have satisfactory cosmetic improvement with conservative management. Counterpositioning with or without physiotherapy or helmet therapy may reduce skull deformity, with better results noted with increasing compliance.

REFERENCES

1. Virchow R. Uber den Cretinismus, namentlich in Franken und uber pathologische Schadelformen. *Verh Phys Med Ges (Wurzburg).* 1851;2:230–271.

2. Renier D, Sainte-Rose C, Marchac D, Hirsch JF. Intracranial pressure in craniostenosis. *J Neurosurg.* 1982;57(3):370–377.

3. Thompson DN, Harkness W, Jones B, Gonsalez S, Andar U, Hayward R. Subdural intracranial pressure monitoring in craniosynostosis: its role in surgical management. *Childs Nerv Syst.* 1995;11(5):269–275.

4. Whitaker LA, Munro IR, Salyer KE, Jackson IT, Ortiz-Monasterio F, Marchac D. Combined report of problems and complications in 793 craniofacial operations. *Plast Reconstr Surg.* 1979;64(2):198–203.

5. Jimenez DF, Barone CM, Cartwright CC, Baker L. Early management of craniosynostosis using endoscopic-assisted strip craniectomies and cranial orthotic molding therapy. *Pediatrics.* 2002;110(1 Pt 1):97–104.

6. Lauritzen CG, Davis C, Ivarsson A, Sanger C, Hewitt TD. The evolving role of springs in craniofacial surgery: the first 100 clinical cases. *Plast Reconstr Surg.* 2008;121(2):545–554.

7. Akai T, Iizuka H, Kawakami S. Treatment of craniosynostosis by distraction osteogenesis. *Pediatr Neurosurg.* 2006;42(5):288–292.

8. Weinzweig J, Kirschner R, Farley A, et al. Metopic synostosis: defining the temporal sequence of normal suture fusion and differentiating it from synostosis on the basis of computed tomography images. *Plast Reconstr Surg.* 2003;112:1211–1218.

9. Weinzweig J, Baker SB, Whitaker LA, Sutton LN, Bartlett SP. Delayed cranial vault reconstruction for sagittal synostosis in older children: an algorithm for tailoring the reconstructive approach to the craniofacial deformity. *Plast Reconstr Surg.* 2002;110(2):397–408.

chapter 17

Hemifacial Microsomia

Fernando Molina, MD

● INTRODUCTION

The term hemifacial microsomia (HFM) syndrome refers to a spectrum of congenital anomalies development and growth of craniofacial structures derived from the first and second branchial arches. The malformations include microtia and facial asymmetry secondary to hypoplasia of structures such as the mandible, temporal bone, lateral parts of the face, and the cranium. The syndrome can vary in severity from almost unnoticeable to severely disfiguring, and in some cases it may be associated with malformations in other regions of the anatomy. Bilaterality occurs in 15% to 30% of cases and may also present with asymmetrical involvement.

The most commonly used term, hemifacial microsomia, was popularized by Gorlin and Pindborg.[1] Other terms that have been used include otomandibular dysostosis, first and second branchial arch syndrome, and auriculo-branchiogenic dysplasia.[2] If the deformity includes orbital dystopia and skull asymmetries, then it is referred to as craniofacial microsomia. In any case, associated craniofacial anomalies may include macrostomia, micrognathia, cleft lip (with or without cleft palate), preauricular skin tags or pits, and ocular dermoid cysts (Figure 17-1A,B). The occurrence of epibulbar dermoid cysts with this pattern of anomaly, especially when accompanied by vertebral anomalies, has been designated Goldenhar syndrome.[3]

● EPIDEMIOLOGY

The incidence of HFM has not been established, although it is known to be the second most common group of birth defects after cleft lip and palate.[4] It occurs more commonly on the right side. Because half of all cases of microtia occur in association with syndromes, in particular HFM, some authors concluded that microtia should be considered a microform of HFM.[5] Other investigators support this view.

A family history of HFM, auricular anomalies, or hearing loss was associated with a greater risk of HFM. A positive familial association of approximately 50% has been observed in large series, and patterns of both autosomal dominant and autosomal recessive inheritance have been described.

● PATHOGENESIS

The clinical signs spectrum seen in HFM arises when the normal developmental processes in the first and second branchial arches are disrupted. Under normal circumstances, the first branchial arch forms Meckel cartilage, which further develops into the mandible, the muscles of mastication, a major portion of the malleus, and the incus. The second branchial arch forms Reichert cartilage, which further develops into the hyoid bone, the styloid process, and the muscles of facial expression. A major portion of the stapes is also derived from this cartilage.

In 1973, Poswillo[6] was able to induce phenocopies of HFM by administering triazines to mice and thalidomide to monkeys. Drugs induced hematomas in the region of the stapedial artery. Secondary tissue necrosis caused by the ischemia had produced similar facial anomalies in the animals. As major was the hemorrhage, more severe is the syndrome and for these reasons we can explain the broad spectrum of abnormalities that can be seen. Retinoic acids produce anomalies in the axial skeleton and craniofacial region, as well as in the cardiovascular and central nervous systems, similar to those seen in HFM.[7,8]

● PATIENT EVALUATION AND SELECTION

Classification

The most effective classification should be universally acceptable to allow clinicians and investigators to

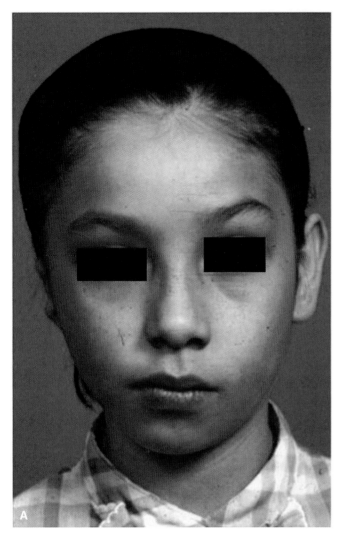
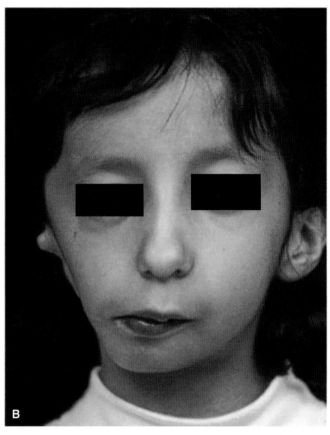

● **FIGURE 17-1.** (A) A 7-year-old girl with right hemifacial microsomia. Facial asymmetry, microtia, soft tissue deficiency, and chin deviation to the affected side are the typical signs. (B) A 6-year-old girl with Goldenhar syndrome. Ocular dermoid cysts and vertebral anomalies are characteristic clinical features together with the facial asymmetry.

communicate data unambiguously, and should also help in treatment planning and prognosis. The earliest classification by Pruzansky[9] and Murray et al.[10] focused on the mandibular deformity into four grades:

Grade I—hypoplasia affects only the gonial angle

Grade II-A—the angle and the ascending ramus are affected

Grade II-B—hypoplasia is a more severe affecting angle, ascending ramus with a flat and rudimentary condyle

Grade III—Complete absence of the ramus and condyle

The OMENS classification is an acronym that means *o*rbit, *m*andible, *e*ar, *n*erve, and *s*oft tissue.[11] Later revised to OMENS-Plus,[12] it further differentiated between the mandible and orbit skeletal components, and distinguished between facial nerve involvement and soft tissue

involvement. The expansion of OMENS to indicate the presence of extracranial anomalies by adding "plus" to the classification creates a more complete system.

Clinical Presentation

Mandibular hypoplasia and microtia remains the hallmarks of this deformity. The more affected mandibular structure is the ascending ramus. In the severe cases, the lack of bone at the mandible secondarily affects the growth of the ipsilateral maxilla and orbit. Approximately 15% of patients have orbital involvement. In the affected side, the orbit is lower when compared with the orbit on the opposite side. Microtia is the most common auricular malformation and frequently is situated in a very low position. Middle ear anomalies are also observed. Seventh nerve involvement is present in less than half of the patient; the more affected is the marginal branch with unilateral lip palsy. The second is the frontal branch and the patients are unable to elevate the eyebrow.

Whereas a soft tissue deficiency is present in most patients, the masticatory muscles are affected in different degrees. Usually there is no relationship between the bone hypoplasia and the muscles involvement. However, in grade III HFM, the masticatory group of muscles are severely affected and in many cases absent.

Other commonly associated anomalies include macrostomia, preauricular ear tags, palatal deviation, epibulbar dermoids, vertebral and long bone anomalies, and rib anomalies. Palatal deviation is usually the result of muscular palsy and hypoplasia and is not related to any cranial nerve weakness.

● PATIENT PREPARATION

The objective in the treatment of the patients with HFM is to obtain facial symmetry and to correct the functional alterations. Children must be seen regularly by a craniofacial team consisting of a craniofacial surgeon, an orthodontist team, a geneticist, a speech pathologist, an audiologist, an otolaryngologist, an ophthalmologist, and a social worker. This will ensure a more thorough assessment of the underlying problem and better treatment planning.

Frequent ear examinations and hearing tests are recommended to identify and treat ear infections and/or hearing loss. Microtia is usually associated with a 50 to 55 dB hearing loss on the affected side.

Velopharyngeal insufficiency is present in up to one third of children with HFM, and speech evaluation should be recommended.

Patients should first be clinically examined with the intention of providing a quantitative and qualitative assessment protocol for determining soft and hard tissue components of the facial deformity.

In patients with facial asymmetry, with the use of a compensatory head posture corrected, the clinician subjectively assesses the level of the asymmetry. One should note forehead, orbital, zygoma, and external ear position and relationships by viewing the patient frontally. The quality and thickness of the cheek soft tissue should also be observed. Additional anthropometric measurements must be made, the distance between the lateral canthus to the buccal commissure and from a central point of the inferior orbital rim to the buccal commissure are recorded before and after distraction. The position and contour of the chin (pogonion), as well as the inferior border and angle of the mandible (gonion), are likewise recorded.

The intraoral examination documents the status of the occlusion: the occlusal plane/cant, molar relationship, and presence of crossbites. Evaluation of the temporomandibular joint is routinely performed: mandibular excursions, including maximum interincisal opening, and lateral movements are documented.

Preoperatively, lateral and posteroanterior cephalometric studies are done. Panorex views are used to compare both sides of the mandible and to locate the tooth buds

and dental nerve, in order to avoid their injury during surgery. In the first cases, the superimposing method of Björk and Skieller[13] was used to obtain a mandibular growth prediction to assess the ideal dimension of the mandible and to reproduce the rotational movements (anterior and posterior) that it performed during growth. 3D-CT offers refinement in anatomic and morphologic mapping to aid in the diagnosis, treatment planning, and postsurgical control in the long term of patients.

● TECHNIQUE

Macrostomia and preauricular skin tags are the most obvious deformities that may need to be addressed early in life. Untreated macrostomia may cause feeding difficulties because of the incompetence of the mouth. Not infrequently, preauricular tags have cartilage remnants extending into the deeper subcutaneous tissue, and to avoid depression deformity of the scar, it is important that the cartilage remnants be completely removed using blunt dissection with the deeper layers approximated. For repair of macrostomia, the distance from midline to the oral commissure on the noncleft side is measured and used as a reference for the future oral commissure on the cleft side. Frequently there is a distinct demarcation at the site of macrostomia, and this usually coincides with the other side. Revisions may be necessary, although one may be able to minimize the risk associated with revision by reconstructing an oral commissure 1 to 2 mm close to the midline to compensate for laxity. Incision at the mucocutaneous junction exposes the underlying muscle in the cleft, which is then properly repaired. A z-plasty at the mucosal commissure is included to recreate the crease of the mouth. In the skin, the surgeon should avoid the presence of z-plasty since the final result is always anesthetics.

It may be possible to excise epibulbar dermoid cysts with minimal scarring of the cornea. Children with these cysts should be referred to an experienced ophthalmologist for management to avoid secondary symblepharon. Auricular reconstruction is usually performed after the age of 9 years. Using costochondral graft to fabricate a cartilage framework, the ear reconstruction is achieved. Six months later the new ear is separated from the cranium using a skin graft. There after, surgical refinements are done to obtain a satisfactory final ear. Mandibular distraction may be considered before reconstruction of a low-set microtia in an attempt to position the reconstructed ear in a symmetrical location.

Velopharyngeal insufficiency is very seldom observed. If a patient requires a treatment related to palatal muscle hypoplasia, it should be performed on the basis of nasoendoscopic findings. Upper airway compromise resulting from severe mandibular micrognathia in bilateral HFM may require consideration of bilateral mandibular distraction or the need for tracheostomy early in life.

The mandibular hypoplasia is treated with distraction osteogenesis to achieve simultaneous skeletal and soft tissue correction with minimal surgery. The technique has only recently become popular in the craniofacial skeleton and present a treatment modality with unique properties that offer a superior clinical and functional results not only by augmenting the craniofacial skeleton but also the overlying soft tissue.[14-17] The bones of the craniofacial skeleton are membranous in embryologic origin. As such, they are of a relatively smaller dimension, have a much richer blood supply, and are more accessible to surgical manipulation due to wide subperiosteal dissection.

Under general anesthesia and a dilute solution of xylocaine and epinephrine is injected over the oblique line and buccal surface of the ramus. A 3-cm incision is made on the lateral vestibule oral mucosa. Subperiosteal dissection is performed exposing the gonial angle and the neighboring area of the ascending ramus. This maneuver is simple and provides an excellent exposure of the bone hypoplasia area. The site of the planned external corticotomy and pin placement is marked with gentian violet, avoiding the mental nerve and tooth buds. This step is critical since the selection of the pin hole sites dictate the vector of distraction.

The corticotomy is not just external, but rather is an external and extended corticotomy that attempts to preserve the nerve, the intramedullary vascularity, and the tooth buds. It should be done with a side-cutting burr. The osteotomy begins at the retromolar angle, cutting along the medial and lateral buttresses and extending through the lateral aspect of the mandibular angle, including the entire cortex down to the cancellous layer. Along the inferior aspect, the corticotomy is extended widely around the angle where the bone is quite thick (Figure 17-2). Only

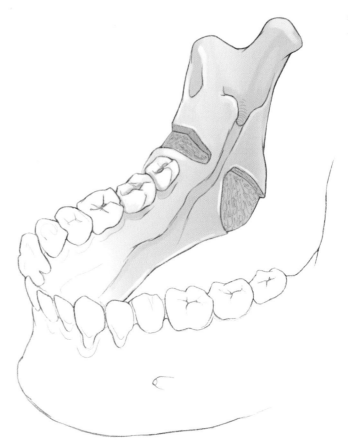

● FIGURE 17-3. The diagram shows the remaining 6 to 8 mm of the internal cortical layer protecting the neurovascular bundle. Different zones of bone resistance are encountered, minor at the angle but major resistance at the alveolar ridge, that will be elongated differently under a perpendicular distraction vector. The remaining lingual cortex eventually will be disrupted by the distraction forces. This fact usually occurs during the second week of the distraction period.

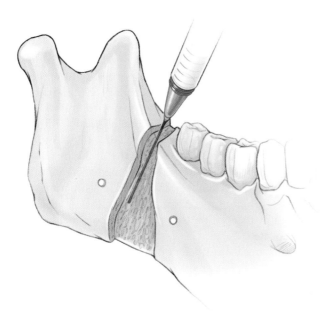

● FIGURE 17-2. Diagram showing the external and extended corticotomy. The cortical bone is widely cut from the retromolar triangle to the mandibular angle exposing the cancellous bone. Two points has been selected to introduce the pins through the full thickness of the mandible.

6 to 8 mm of the internal cortical layer is preserved to protect the nerve and artery (Figure 17-3). In fact, with this external extended corticotomy, different zones of bone resistance are encountered, less at the angle and more at the alveolar ridge, which will be elongated differently with a perpendicular distraction vector to achieve multidimensional mandibular lengthening (Figure 17-4A,B). In fact, this technique will produce bone lengthening with simultaneous bone remodeling. Increases in the vertical height of the ramus and the new bone formation at the mandibular angle allow clockwise mandibular rotational growth movements. During the consolidation period, the patient is allowed use of the mandible to eat, talk, etc. and the masticatory muscles work on the regenerate bone to modify the mandibular morphology. The bigonial distance is increased in the vertical dimension of the coronoid process and also in the musculature. All of the changes explain the role of the functional matrix on mandibular distraction osteogenesis and it is clearly observed when the neurovascular bundle and intramedullary vascularity are preserved.

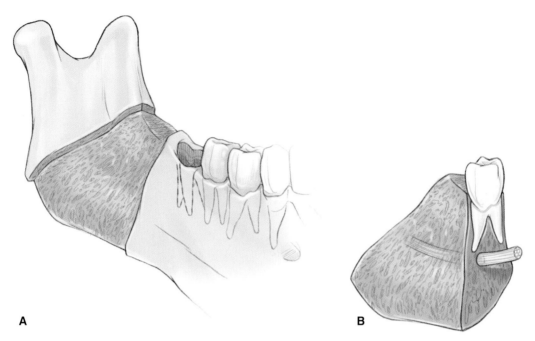

A

B

● **FIGURE 17-4.** (A) Bone elongation and remodeling should be achieved at the gonion and the ascending ramus in the hypoplastic hemifacial microsomia mandible. If the bone elongation area does not recreate the normal mandible anatomy, major occlusion problems will occur and facial asymmetry will remain. (B) The diagram shows the multidimensional new bone formation area at the mandible after the proper use of distraction vectors. Neurovascular components and tooth buds always should be preserved.

Vectors of Distraction

The position of the pins placement will determine the vector of distraction. This is different in each patient according to the grade of mandibular hypoplasia (Figure 17-5). In patients with grade I HFM, the corticotomy extends obliquely from the posterior edge of the hypoplastic gonial angle to the retromolar angle in the alveolar ridge. The pins must be placed perpendicular to the corticotomy to obtain an oblique vector of distraction that produces greater bone elongation in the angle and less in the alveolar ridge.

In patients with grade II-A HFM, the distraction process must remodel and elongate the angle and the initial portion of the ascending ramus. For this reason, the corticotomy is placed obliquely at the junction of the angle and ramus and the pins must be inserted in an intermediate position between a vertical and oblique distraction vector.

In patients with grade II-B HFM, the corticotomy is placed horizontally at the base of the ascending ramus and the pins must follow a vertical distraction vector in order to obtain more elongation in the hypoplastic ascending ramus.

The Semirigid External Devices

Two pins, from 2.0 to 3.5 mm in diameter (age depending), are introduced percutaneously through the whole thickness of the mandible (bicortical), 3 to 5 mm in front and behind the corticotomy. The diamond tip design of the pins makes it unnecessary to drill a hole before its introduction in the bone. Care must be taken to position the pins parallel to each other and facilitate their fixation to the distraction device and one must avoid injuries in the unerupted dental follicles.

The mucosa is closed with a fine absorbable suture and the distraction device is applied. The device is made of two hollow plates with a central perforation to allow the entrance of the mandibular pins. The two plates are joined by another stainless steel screw running free in one of them and transversing the whole length of the plate at the other, so when it is turned the distance between the plates is increased or decreased (Figure 17-6A,B). The steel resistance of the distractor device is softer than the pins; this produces a flexible device that can bend under the masticatory muscle action and externally reflects the shape of the elongated bone area.

● THE POSTOPERATIVE PERIOD

Elongation is commenced on the fifth postoperative day (latency period) at a rate of approximately 1 mm per day (rhythm). It is done by the parents with minimal discomfort to the patient. In the event that the patient is resistant to turning the distractors, an age-appropriate dose of acetaminophen may be given 20 minutes prior to turning. The elongation is usually completed in 3 to 4 weeks (distraction period), and the device is left in place for an additional 6 to

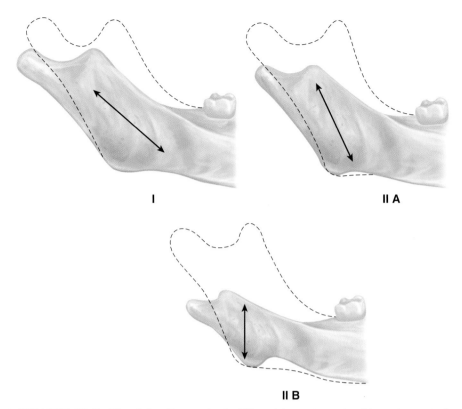

● **FIGURE 17-5.** The distraction vector is different in each grade of bony hypoplasia. The mark in the mandibular angle shows the different vectors. Notice the oblique vector in the grade I and the vertical vector in grade II-B.

8 weeks (consolidation period) until radiological evidence of new cortical bone formation is found. At that time, the screws are easily removed under sedation.

Measurements of the distance between the pins and soft tissue structures (external canthus-buccal commissure and the inferior orbital rim-buccal commissure) are recorded weekly. Dental casts and follow-up plain radiographs are taken at the end of the distraction period and 6 to 8 weeks later to assess osteogenesis at the site of the corticotomy, as well as noting any occlusal changes. The progress of distraction is monitored by documenting changes in the relationships of the maxillary and mandibular occlusion and the position or level of the occlusal plane, oral commissure, and chin position.

In general, the results following mandibular distraction have been highly satisfactory.

● **COMPLICATIONS**

Mandibular distraction has been a benign process for patients. Morbidity is limited to the presence of skin scars slightly enlarged by the distraction which have evolved satisfactorily over time and no revisions have been necessary. To minimize the length of the scar, the cheek skin is pinched between the thumb and the index finger before introducing the second pin to allow for stretching. The second complication presented in this series is the use of an inadequate distraction vector which will produce bone

elongation, but misses the opportunity of bone remodeling and the production of occlusal disasters in the vast majority of the cases.

Regarding the temporomandibular joint, no symptoms of functional disruption have been noted from follow-up radiographic studies. It has been observed in unidirectional cases that the condylar head becomes more upright and increased in size and volume. Also, on account of the multidimensional bone remodeling in the gonial angle, the condyle, which is initially laterally displaced, moves into a medial and more anatomically correct position that resembles the contralateral side. This change in condylar morphology occurs during the consolidation period. The contralateral unexpended condyle maintained its size and shape and did not show evidence of deformational changes.

● **OUTCOMES ASSESSMENT**

In patients with grade I HFM, lengthening varies from 12 to 18 mm (mean 16 mm). Dental occlusion remains stable without development of a posterior open bite. No active functional orthodontic appliances have been required. The aesthetic results were excellent with restoration of facial symmetry by descent of the buccal commissure to match the contralateral side and leveling of the menton in the midline. Long-term follow-up has shown stable clinical and occlusal results (Figure 17-7A–F).

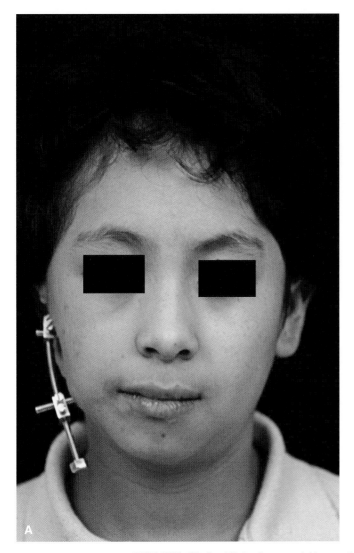
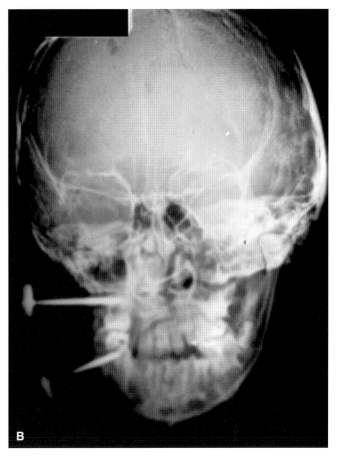

● **FIGURE 17-6.** (A) An 8-year-old boy using an unidirectional external device. This is made of two hollow plates with a central perforation to allow the entrance of the mandibular pins. When it is activated, the distance between the plates is increased or decreased. The resistance of the distractor device is softer than the pins; this produces a flexible device that can bend under the masticatory muscle action and externally reflects the shape of the elongated bone area. (B) Posteroanterior cephalogram showing the mandibular changes during bone elongation.

In grade II-A HFM, mandibular elongation has ranged from 14 to 22 mm (mean 19 mm). The dental occlusion is disrupted, creating a contralateral crossbite and a posterior open bite of 1 to 3 mm in half of the patients treated. Posterior bite blocks, worn on the mandibular dentition and dynamic orthodontic appliances are used to maintain the space in order to allow the vertical growth of the constricted maxillae into the open bite. In the following 2 to 3 months, the bite block is serially reduced in size to allow the entire maxillary occlusal plane to become level and maintain the elongation and occlusion (Figure 17-8A–F). In patients younger than 4 years of age, the maxillary teeth quickly fill the space and the above orthodontic maneuver is often not necessary. The aesthetic results are excellent

with restoration of facial symmetry and horizontalization of the chin and the buccal commissure.

The group of patients with grade II-B HFM characteristically have a stable but incorrect dental occlusion with marked deviation of the mandibular midline teeth to the affected side. During the vertical distraction of the mandibular ramus, bite blocks are required to maintain the posterior open bite and are gradually reduced to allow vertical maxillary growth. Dynamic orthodontic appliances are also used in all patients at an early stage. After the distraction, the initial occlusion is reproduced in the opposite direction on the contralateral side as a result of overcorrection. The maxilla has to be expanded to correct the crossbite with a classical palatal expansion device. The aesthetic

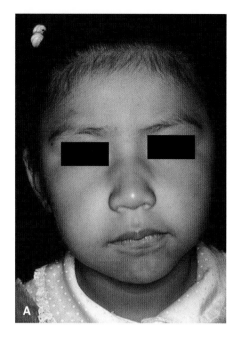
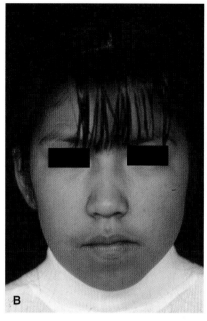
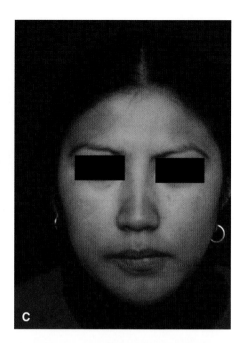
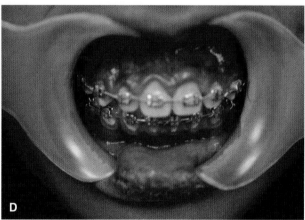
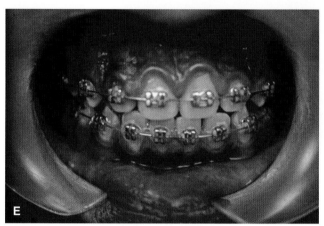
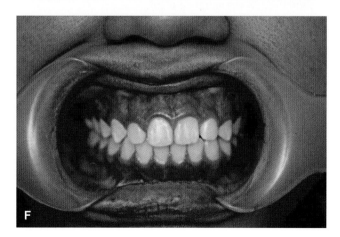

● FIGURE 17-7. (A) Preoperative frontal view of a 5-year-old girl with hemifacial microsomia grade I. Despite the minimal mandibular hypoplasia, a notorious facial asymmetry is observed. (B) Postoperative view after a mandibular elongation of 16 mm. Facial symmetry has been recovered. (C) Long-term control at age 17 years. Facial symmetry is stable and the soft tissue changes remain. (D) Preoperative dental occlusion. Notice the inferior incisors midline deviation to the affected side. (E) Postdistraction dental occlusion. Maxillary transversal expansion, the use of posterior bite blocks and myofunctional intraoral devices are the most common orthodontics maneuvers to achieve occlusal stability. (F) The occlusion at age 17 years.

improvement and the restoration of symmetry have also been impressive in these patients (Figure 17-9A–D).

An important benefit of bone distraction is the simultaneous expansion of the soft tissues of the face (skin, muscles, fascia, vessels, and nerves). In fact, we were surprised to see the rapid descent of the buccal commissure to a normal position, the horizontalization of the chin, the increase in the distance between the buccal commissure and the external canthus-inferior orbital rim, and the remarkable improvement in facial symmetry in all the

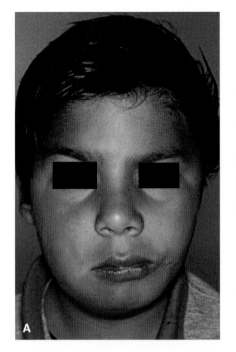
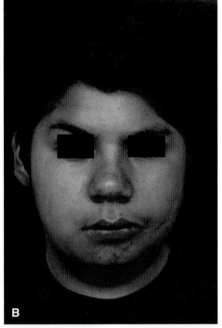
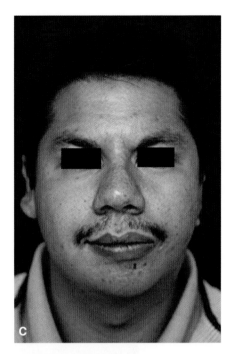
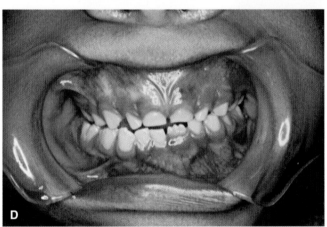
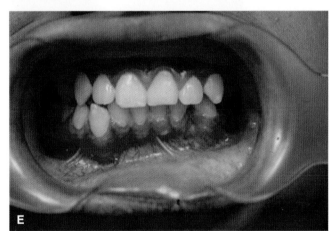
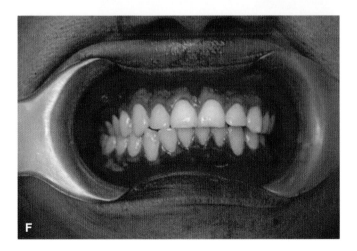

● FIGURE 17-8. (A) Preoperative view of a 6-year-old boy with left hemifacial microsomia. The macrostomia was repaired at age 8 months. (B) Postdistraction view at age 9 years. Notice the level of both oral commissures. To improve the left cheek soft tissue deficiency, a dermal fat graft has been added. Also a macrostomia scar revision has been performed. (C) Postdistraction frontal view control at age 20 years. Clinical stability of facial symmetry is maintained. (D) Preoperative occlusal view. (E) Postdistraction occlusal view showing a horizontal occlusal plane and a good relationship between superior and inferior teeth. (F) Long-term occlusal view at age 20 years.

unilateral cases. The secondary expansive effect on the soft tissues and muscles is also reflected in the fact that there is minimal, if any, evidence of clinical relapse; in contrast to the dental-skeletal relapse observed following traditional orthognathic advancements procedures to reconstruct the ramus in HFM patients.

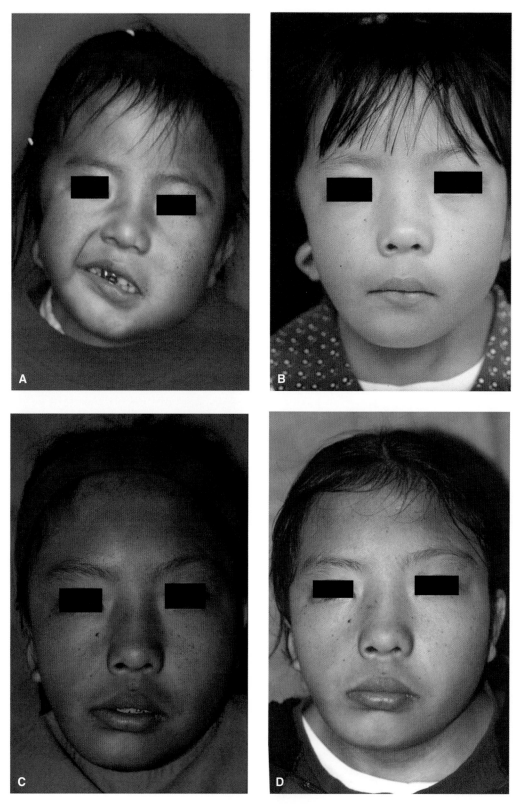

● **FIGURE 17-9.** (A) Preoperative view of a 3-year-old girl presenting with hemifacial microsomia grade II-B. A severe facial asymmetry and inferior lip palsy is observed. (B) Postdistraction view showing the obtained facial symmetry after a mandible elongation of 38 mm of the right ascending ramus. (C) Long-term control at age 11 years. Notice the slight chin deviation to the affected side. (D) Long-term control at age 16 years. Bone changes at the mandible and at soft tissue remain stable. For a final perfect facial symmetry an asymmetrical menton osteotomy will be added.

Minimal to moderate soft tissue deficiencies may not require treatment until after puberty, at which time fat aspirated from the lower abdomen or thighs may be used for soft tissue augmentation. Large soft tissue defects may require transfer of dermal fat grafts. More volume should be added around the mandible angle. Since secondary fat reabsorption has been shown to approach 40%, usually observed after the dermal fat graft insertion, two to three sessions of fat injection should be necessary to obtain a final aesthetic contour of the cheek and a very good facial symmetry.

REFERENCES

1. Gorlin RJ, Pindborg JJ, Cohen MM Jr. *Syndromes of the Head and Neck*. New York: McGraw-Hill; 1976:546–552.

2. Mellor DH, Richardson JE, Douglas DM. Goldernhar's syndrome: oculo-auriculo-vertebral dysplasia. *Arch Dis Child*. 1973;48:537–541.

3. Goldernhar M. Associations malformatives-fistula auris congenial et ses relations avec la dysostose mandibulo-faciale [French]. *J Genet Hum*. 1952;1:243–282.

4. David DJ, Mahatumarat C, Cooter RD. Hemifacial microsomia: a multisystem classification. *Plast Reconstr Surg*. 1987;80(4):525–535.

5. Kaye CI, Rollnick BR, Hauck WW, Martin AO, Richtsmeier JT, Nagatoshi K. Microtia and associated anomalies: statistical analysis. *Am J Med Genet*. 1989:34(4):574–578.

6. Poswillo D. The pathogenesis of the first and second branchial arch syndrome. *Oral Surg Oral Med Oral Pathol*. 1973;35:302–328.

7. Lammer EJ, Chen DT, Hoar RM, et al. Retinoic acid embriopathy. *N Engl J Med*. 1985;313(2):837–841.

8. Sulik KK, Johnston MC, Smiley SJ, Speight HS, Jarvis BE. Mandibulofacial dysostosis (Treacher Collins syndrome): a new proposal for its pathogenesis. *Am J Med Genet*. 1987;27(2):359–372.

9. Pruzansky S. Not all dwarfed mandibles are alike. *Birth Defects*. 1969;1:120.

10. Murray JE, Mulliken JB, Kaban LB, Belfer M. Twenty-year experience in maxillocraniofacial surgery: An evaluation of early surgery on growth, function and body image. *Ann Surg*. 1979;190(3):320.

11. Vento AR, LaBrie RA, Mulliken JB. The O.M.E.N.S. classification of hemifacial microsomia. *Cleft and Palate Craniofac J*. 1991;28(1):68–71.

12. Horgan JE, Padwa BL, LaBrie RA, Mulliken JB. OMENS-plus: analysis of craniofacial and extracranial anomalies in hemifacial microsomia. *Cleft Palate Craniofac J*. 1995;32(5): 405–412.

13. Björk A, Skieller V. Normal and abnormal growth of the mandible. A synthesis of longitudinal cephalometric implant studies over a period of 25 years. *Eur J Orthod*. 1983;5: 1–46.

14. McCarthy JG, Schreider J, Karp N, Thorne CH, Grayson BH. Lengthening the human mandible by gradual distraction. *Plast Reconstr Surg*. 1992;89(1):1–8.

15. McCormick SU, Grayson BH, McCarthy JG, Staffenberg D. Effect of mandibular distraction on the temporomandibular joint. Part 2, Clinical study. *J Craniofac Surg*. 1995; 6:364–367.

16. Molina F, Ortiz Monasterio F. Extended indications for mandibular distraction: unilateral, bilateral and bidirectional. In: Ortiz Monasterio F, ed. *Craniofacial Surgery 5*. Bologna, Italy: Monduzzi Editore; 1993.

17. Molina F, Ortiz Monasterio F. Mandibular elongation and remodeling by distraction: A farewell to major osteotomies. *Plast Reconstr Surg*. 1995;96(4):825–840; discussion 841–842.

chapter 18

Craniofacial Clefts

Jeffrey A. Fearon, MD, FACS, FAAP

● PATIENT EVALUATION AND SELECTION

Facial clefting is the most common facial birth defect, yet craniofacial clefts are one of the least frequently seen craniofacial anomalies. What constitutes a craniofacial cleft? Basically, all facial clefts, aside from the commonly seen cleft lip and palate, comprise the spectrum of craniofacial clefts. These clefts may occur unilaterally or bilaterally, and just about anywhere on the face. Clefting can be barely discernible, limited just to the soft tissues as a forme fruste, or may involve the deeper underlying bone. Some clefts may affect the bone primarily and have only minimal overlying soft tissue involvement. Adding to the confusion as to what exactly constitutes a craniofacial cleft has been the previous inclusion by some authors of facial hyperplasias, hypoplasias, and aplasias.

Epidemiology

Determining the true incidence of craniofacial clefts remains a daunting challenge, and the inclusion of syndromes such as hemifacial microsomia and Treacher Collins within the craniofacial clefting spectrum has further muddied these waters. Moreover, clefts may present with a wide phenotypic variability with some clefts going unrecognized for years. Kawamoto estimated that the incidence for craniofacial clefts is somewhere between 1.4 and 4.9:100,000 births.[1] Another way of calculating the incidence of these rare anomalies is to consider their proportion to the more commonly seen cleft lip and palate. Cleft lip and palate is often quoted as occurring as frequently as 1:550 births (varying with family history, race, socioeconomic status, etc). At the Craniofacial Center in Dallas, excluding the hyper- and hypoplasias (eg, frontonasal dysplasia, Treacher Collins, hemifacial microsomia), craniofacial clefts comprise about 10% of all facial clefts treated. The Australian Craniofacial Unit has reported a similar proportion of treated craniofacial clefts to cleft lip and palate of about 9%.[2] These proportions

suggest an incidence for the rare craniofacial clefts as common as 1:5500 births. However, it is likely that this estimate is significantly influenced by the nature of referral patterns to major craniofacial centers (complicated clefts being more likely to be referred, and simple cleft lip and palate less likely to be referred), and that the true incidence of craniofacial clefts is actually much lower. Ortiz Monasterio et al. reviewed their cleft experience in Mexico City and noted that during the same time period they had treated 174 craniofacial clefts and 5412 cleft lip and palates (a ratio of 1:31, yielding an incidence of >1:17,000 births).[3] Finally, the Texas Birth Registry, from 1996 to 2003 reported 36 cases of facial clefts for 2,419,928 births for an incidence of 1.5:100,000 births. Suffice it to say, craniofacial clefts are exceedingly uncommon.

Etiology

The most commonly cited theory explaining the anomalous embryological development resulting in a cleft lip implicates a failure of mesodermal penetration. During the first 2 months of fetal development, supporting mesodermal tissue migrates underneath an intact facial ectodermal layer. Failure of this migration results in an overlying ectodermal loss, resulting in a cleft. Much of the craniofacial skeleton is believed to originate from migrating neural crest cells. Facial skeletal hypoplasia results by interrupting neural crest cell migration in the chick embryo, supporting the theory that craniofacial clefts might arise from an inhibition of normal migration, or cell death, during embryogenesis. Also, a correlation between limb ring constrictions and craniofacial clefting has been noted, and craniofacial clefts have also been artificially induced in an in utero animal model using a suture constriction band technique. Finally, craniofacial clefts also may occur in conjunction with midline encephaloceles, raising the question: Which came first? Currently, given the wide variability in

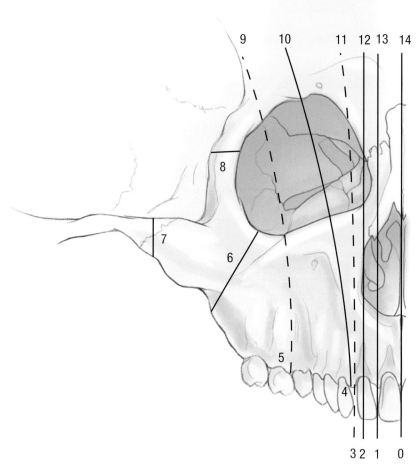

● FIGURE 18-1. The Tessier Classification for Rare Craniofacial Clefts.

the presentation of rare craniofacial clefts, their etiology appears to be multifactorial.

Classification

A number of classifications for craniofacial clefts had been proposed prior to Tessier's landmark publication describing a new schema that was based on his own considerable personal experience.[4] His classification assigns a specific number to each craniofacial cleft, depending on the anatomic location (Figure 18-1), and partially relies on a horizontal axis through the center of the orbits. The first cleft is designated #0, and describes a vertical cleft occurring in the maxillary midline (and central upper lip) up to the midorbital horizontal line. A midline craniofacial cleft arising above this horizontal line is given a separate number, #14. A full-length midline cleft, extending both above and below the orbital horizontal, is designated as a #0-14 cleft (however, the bony hyperplasia associated with frontonasal dysplasia has also been considered a #0-14 "cleft"). As the location of the lower clefts shifts laterally, a higher number is assigned. A single number is used to describe each cleft, unless the cleft crosses the

midorbital horizontal line, at which point a second number is added. For continuous clefts, extending above and below the orbital horizontal, their combined numbers will add up to 14. For example: a #1 cleft below the orbit becomes a #13 above the orbit, similarly a #2 below becomes a #12 above, etc. The vertical facial clefts (becoming more oblique as they occur lateral to the midline) include #0-14, #1-13, #2-12, #3-11, #4-10, and #5-9. However, clefts do not always occur in a continuous line. Tessier opined that the facial clefts falling medial to the infraorbital foramen (#0-14 through #4-10) are more likely to present with overlying soft tissue deficiencies, and those falling lateral to the infraorbital nerve are more likely to have significant bony clefting (others have questioned this relationship). Tessier also observed that clefts affecting the bony skeleton did not necessarily imply the absence of principle neurovascular structures, and that clefts of the soft tissues and bone do not always coincide. The lateral facial clefts, assigned the numbers, #6, #7, and #8, are used to describe Treacher Collins syndrome, as well as auriculo-oculo-vertebral spectrum anomalies, including hemifacial microsomia and the Goldenhar variant (with and without true bony clefting). An isolated lateral facial cleft, extending through the soft tissues of the oral commissure is designated a #7 cleft (as is a vertical cleft of the zygomatic arch). Finally, a separate number, #30, was used by Tessier to describe a cleft occurring through the midline of the lower lip and mandible. A number of years ago I had the occasion to ask Tessier why he had assigned the #30 to the lower lip, instead of #15, or even a #-14? He replied: "I simply wanted a very different number." Detractors of Tessier's classification note that it does not take embryological development into account, while supporters point out that most craniofacial clefts do not occur along lines that correspond to the fusion planes for the various facial processes. One aspect of the Tessier classification, which has somewhat obscured exactly what constitutes a rare craniofacial cleft, is the broad net that has been cast over multiple different conditions. Telorbitism, with intervening bony hyperplasia, has been considered a #14 cleft. The bony and soft tissue hypoplasias associated with milder Treacher Collins and hemifacial microsomia fall under the lateral facial "clefts" #6, #7, and #8. Should the hyperplasias, hypoplasias, and aplasias all be included under the moniker "cleft"? Moreover, how

necessary is it to differentiate between clefts that arise in such close anatomic proximity, and does the treatment of craniofacial clefts differ sufficiently to require a classification that includes 16 different clefts, with multiple possible combinations? Published reviews that include all craniofacial clefts tend to be protean in length. Finally, few physicians are able to classify craniofacial clefts, or conjure up a visualization of a cleft when given a descriptive number, without first consulting a diagram. Instead of attempting to split facial clefts along fairly minutely spaced anatomic locations, which are not always germane to treatment paradigms, clefts can be classified more regionally based on variations in surgical planning.[5] Using the aforementioned criteria, it is possible to categorize all craniofacial clefts, using a *surgical classification*, into one of four primary types (Figure 18-2):

- Type I, midline facial clefts (#0-14, and #30)
- Type II, paramedian facial clefts (#1-13, #2-12)
- Type III, orbital facial clefts (#3-11, #4-10, #5-9)
- Type IV, lateral facial clefts (#6, #7, and #8, excluding hypoplasias)

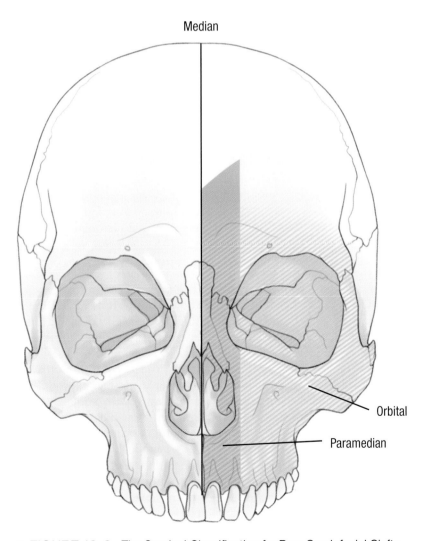

Median

Orbital

Paramedian

● **FIGURE 18-2.** The Surgical Classification for Rare Craniofacial Clefts.

Each cleft type could be further subclassified as frontal, maxillary, or mandibular, if necessary. This simplified classification system would enable surgeons to quickly describe an observed cleft, have a basic treatment paradigm applicable to each location, and permit others to easily understand the location of the cleft.

● PATIENT PREPARATION

Infants born with craniofacial clefts require an expeditious initial evaluation. The common reflexive action is to order a CT scan, but almost all preliminary decision making is based on factors identifiable on physical examination; in fact, arguments can be made for delaying a CT scan evaluation, not only because the results of this test almost never impact treatment decisions in the newborn, but also because of concerns, which some have raised concerning radiation exposure on the growing brain in the first few years of life. Furthermore, bone grafting of clefts is typically not indicated in infancy, unless the cranial vault is involved. Therefore, a physical examination remains the primary evaluation for the majority of rare craniofacial clefts presenting during infancy, and a surprising amount of information can be ascertained by a thorough examination. However, in older children a 3D CT scan may provide invaluable insight into the extent of underlying skeletal defects, providing considerable assistance in the planning of the surgical reconstruction.[6]

Type I, Midline Facial Clefts

In midline craniofacial clefts, an absence of bone running vertically down the central forehead almost always results in an encephalocele. A "widow's peak," or V-shaped midline frontal projection of hair, may be a marker for an underlying bony cleft. A careful evaluation of vision, and interpupillary distance is important (ie, Is vision stereoscopic?). Patency of the nares may be determined simply by placing an unraveled cotton swab under each naris in order to ascertain air movement. The palate should be carefully evaluated for clefting; the presence of a soft tissue mass herniating through a split palate is a basal encephalocele until proven otherwise. Often, palatal clefting will be accompanied by a central upswing of the horizontal occlusal plane. An MRI evaluation is very useful for the midline craniofacial clefts, in order to evaluate brain parenchymal for possible midline defects, as well as to determine the presence and extent of a basal encephalocele. An endocrine workup can also be of great benefit for the midline facial clefts in order to evaluate basic pituitary and hypothalamic function.

The midline clefts, arising below the mouth, may or not involve the underlying mandible (which can be easily assessed by physical examination). The tongue is evaluated for clefts and ankyloglossia, and the neck is extended to look for fibrotic contractures. Although these clefts may extend down into the sternum, treatment of the chest is typically never required. Up to 10% of these rare clefts may be associated with congenital heart anomalies.

Type II, Paramedian Facial Clefts

Clefts occurring lateral to the midline, but sparing the majority of the orbit, are most likely to affect the frontal bone, hemi-nose, and maxilla. These clefts may be as simple as a notch in the alar rim, or can result in heminasal agenesis or a lateral proboscis. Often the nasolacrimal drainage system is compromised. The patency of the ipsilateral naris, if in doubt, should again be determined with a cotton swab as described above.

Type III, Orbital Facial Clefts

The majority of oblique clefts involve the orbit; therefore, evaluation of the globe for exposure is of paramount importance. Often, clefts involving the orbit may affect eyelid coverage, which can quickly lead to an exposure injury of the globe. The oblique clefts may be associated with a normal globe, a hypoplastic globe (microphthalmia), or complete anophthalmia. Intraoral examination of the alveolus and palate are performed, and palpation can provide clues to underlying bony clefts of the maxilla, as well as the supraorbit. The lateral oblique clefts may rarely involve maxillary-mandibular fusion, which can be easily ascertained by examining jaw opening for extent and symmetry.

Type IV, Lateral Facial Clefts

The lateral facial clefts primarily involve the oral commissure and adjacent soft tissues. An assessment can be made of the size of the hemi-mandible, ascending ramus, and temporomandibular joint on the affected side by clinical examination. Observing the chin point in relation to the midfacial plane, and palpating the ascending ramus, may provide clues to the size of the lower jaw. Rocking the body of the mandible on each side allows comparison of the joint spaces, and can assist in determining if the temporal mandibular joints are fully formed.

● TECHNIQUE

The primary goals of surgery vary significantly with both the type of cleft as well as the age of the patient, permitting few generalizations. In the newborn, the adage often attributed to Pichler, "first the bone, then the soft tissue," should be ignored for the exact opposite is typically the more prudent course. Soft tissue coverage is first considered in order to protect exposed structures, such as the globe, and to assist with feeding if the cleft extends intraorally. As children grow older, and the facial skeleton matures, bony osteotomies and grafting are considered. These osteotomies include, but are not limited to, facial bipartitions for the midline clefts, bone grafting of alveolar clefts prior to dental eruption, and cranial bone graft reconstruction of maxillary defects. The volume of bone graft necessary to correct the cleft defects is easy to underestimate and may be surprisingly large. The following descriptions provide general principles and treatment approaches, depending on the anatomic location of the cleft.

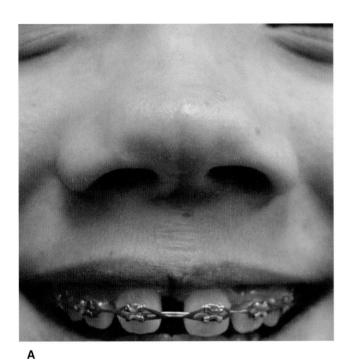

A

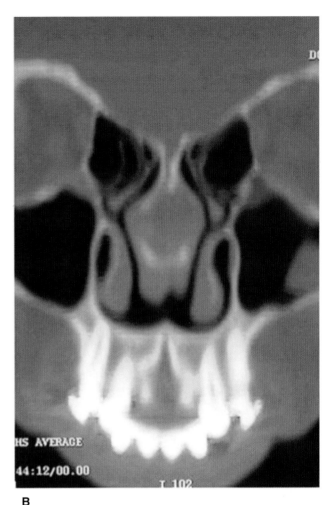

B

● FIGURE 18-3. (A, B) Patients with a "simple" bifid nose need to be evaluated for a possible encephalocele, such as in this patient, which splits the nasal septum.

Type I, Midline Facial Clefts

The surgical treatment of midline facial clefts can be extremely challenging, even for the most experienced craniofacial surgeons. Exceptions to the aforementioned admonishment to avoid early bony reconstructive surgery would include the midline clefts that involve the frontal bone. For these cases, early bone grafting prior to a year of age not only reconstructs the skull and protects the brain, but it is also facilitated by the ability of the dura to regenerate bone, which eliminates the need to reconstruct the donor site. The focus of the surgery for clefts that include frontal bone defects is the correction of the encephalocele. In the absence of a frontal bone defect and corresponding encephalocele, it is best to avoid the correction of any associated hypertelorism during infancy because these early procedures always need to be repeated and any small achievable gains are rarely sufficient to justify the risks. An additional caveat to this reproach might be cases of extreme telorbitism, with impairment of stereoscopic vision; for these individuals, the risks and benefits of early hypertelorism corrections must be carefully balanced. In older children, it is better to undercorrect than overcorrect telorbitism, because mild hypertelorism is generally considered more attractive than mild hypotelorism. It is also prudent to delay, or avoid, the treatment of any intraoral brain herniations in order to avert significant endocrine dysfunction. The author is aware of attempts, at other institutions, to treat basal encephaloceles in children that resulted in complete loss of pituitary function. Reconstruction of the nose may be equally as challenging as an intracranial hypertelorism correction, and may be the crucial step in normalizing facial appearance. These midline nasal reconstructions frequently entail a central skin resection as a component to bringing the hemi-nasal structures together in the midline; however, it is always aesthetically preferable to avoid a nasal scar when possible. For minor central vertical facial clefting, an MRI or CT scan evaluation should be undertaken prior to performing a primary rhinoplasty to rule out an occult encephalocele, which may split the nasal septum (Figure 18-3) potentially leading to dire consequences for the unsuspecting surgeon.

Upper central lip clefts present unique challenges. These midline clefts may include a complete absence of the central lip elements (philtrum and Cupid's bow) that will

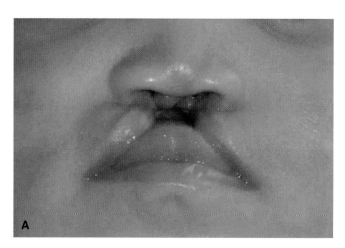
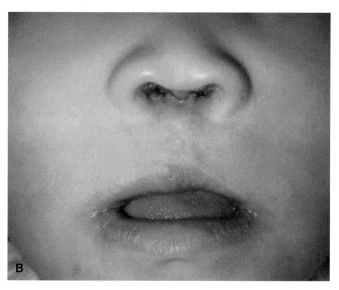

● FIGURE 18-4. (A, B) Treatment of the lower midline facial clefts requires the recruitment of as much local tissue as possible to reconstruct the nasal floor, and lengthening of the anterior abortive columella/septum, to achieve as much nasal height as possible in order to not significantly diminish the nasal airway.

negatively influence postrepair aesthetics. The superior extension of these clefts through the columella requires careful planning, prior to surgical closure, in order to avoid postoperative nasal airway compromise (Figure 18-4). Staged reconstruction with Abbe cross-lip flaps can help to establish normal upper lip dimensions through the creation of a philtrum and central lip tubercle.

The midline lower clefts are usually handled similar to the upper lip clefts. During a primary closure, fibrous union of the lateral mandibular halves may be appreciated. It is best to delay any bony repair until mixed dentition in order to prevent injuring permanent dentition with bone fixation that can damage unerupted tooth follicles.

Type II, Paramedian Facial Clefts

Procedures designed to correct nasal defects, and associated choanal atresia, are best left until a child is about to enter school. Early corrections of choanal atresia have significant failure rates; moreover, there is little truth to the dictum that infants are obligate nasal breathers, as any physician who has treated congenital arhinia can attest. It is probably best to not to even attempt to create a nasal airway for children who have a unilateral functioning nasal airway, as the functional results typically do not justify the surgical efforts.[2] Isolated clefting of the ala can be often addressed with an excision and a z-plasty repair. As the clefts become more extensive, local flaps and full reconstruction with a forehead flap may be required. The general tenet of nasal repair, "replace like with like," should be applied to the treatment of congenital clefts of the nose as well. Nasal repair may be coordinated with palatal repair, when the clefts involve both structures. Reconstruction of the nasolacrimal apparatus is also better delayed until children are bigger, and a larger stent can be used.

Type III, Orbital Facial Clefts

Primary corrections for clefts that involve the orbit are focused on the protection of the globe. Additional consideration is given to reestablishing the oral sphincter, if affected, and providing general soft tissue closure. Orbital clefts typically involve some degree of vertical deficiency, and multiple different repairs have been described using multiple z-plastys, variations on nasolabial flaps, and even rotation flaps. As in any cleft repair, length may be accomplished in one of two ways: wider lateral paring of the cleft with recruitment of tissues medially and laterally, resulting in a straight line scar; or, limited lateral paring of the cleft with the use of z-plastys, or other flaps that recruit tissue laterally and reorient it to increase vertical length. Millard argued, with the presentation of his technique for cleft lip repair, that when flaps are required to provide length, they should used in such a way as to avoid crossing discrete anatomic landmarks. Similar principles should be applied to the treatment of craniofacial clefts, and the author would argue for a restraint in the use of any large facial flaps, whenever possible. If flaps must be used, their design should be kept as small as possible, striving to keep scars along junctions of facial aesthetic units, and tissue discarding should be kept to a minimum.[7] This principle requires greater undermining of the lateral facial mass in closing large clefts. After primary closure is achieved, and early scar contracture has relaxed, the judicious use of carefully placed small z-plastys can be considered. Protection of the globe can be particularly challenging with significant clefting involving the eyelids. Once again, minimizing the use of larger transposition flaps will result in a better aesthetic outcome in the majority of cases. The use of tissue expanders may assist with the closure of extremely wide clefts. Coloboma-type defects can be closed with a small z-plasty, and segmental eyelid

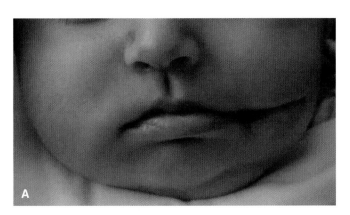 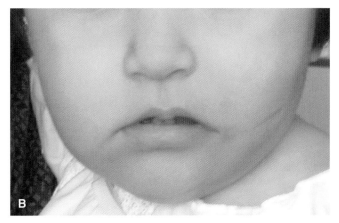

● FIGURE 18-5. (A, B) Lateral facial clefts are best corrected with a straight-line closure, and undercorrection is preferable to overcorrection.

defects can be closed with serial advancement or switch flaps. Once soft tissue closure has been accomplished, secondary cranial bone grafting of the underlying facial skeleton can be considered. Ideally, bone grafting is performed at skeletal maturity (avoiding fixation injuries to unerupted teeth), but any significant aesthetic deformities should be addressed around ages 5 to 7 years, before they lead to any permanent psychosocial issues.

Micro-ophthalmia may best be treated with serial conformers fitted over the globe. Complete anophthalmia may be best treated with orbital expansion. Although the author has used both saline-filled and osmotic orbital expanders; currently, the use of serial static orbital implants is preferred. This involves early placement of an orbital prosthesis, followed by an exchange for a larger prosthesis a few years later. This slower "expansion" needs to be coordinated with a prosthetist, who can serially exchange the appropriate conformers to maintain the sulci for the final eye prosthesis.

Type IV, Lateral Facial Clefts

The key to correcting a lateral facial cleft, or macrostomia, is the repair of the underlying muscle. Multiple variations on the use of w-plastys and z-plastys have been described for repairing the lateral clefts. Macrostomia repairs may be undertaken at any age, but they are typically performed within the first year of life. As with the oblique clefts, the author prefers a straight-line closure, minimizing the use of flaps (Figure 18-5). It is clearly better to undercorrect than to overcorrect these clefts; slight macrostomia is a far more attractive trait than the appearance of an overcorrected macrostomia, which can resemble an electrical burn injury of the oral commissure. Lateral facial clefts may also occur in conjunction with bimaxillary fusion.

● COMPLICATIONS

Very little has been published regarding complications related to rare craniofacial cleft repair, and the discussion of complications is made more problematic by the wide

variety of procedures that are used to repair these clefts. Nevertheless, a failure to achieve a reasonable postoperative appearance may be the most common complication following the treatment of these clefts. As a result of the rarity of such clefts, few surgeons have experience levels that are commensurate with achieving a good result with a minimal risk for complications.

For midline clefts, achieving a satisfactory correction of any associated telorbitism will be more likely in older children, with any procedures performed during infancy or early childhood certain to require subsequent repeat procedures. Infection rates are probably higher in the facial bipartition type procedures than for isolated cranial vault reconstructions that do not breach sinuses. The author is aware of two unpublished cases of panhypopituitarism following surgical procedures performed at other centers intended to treat midline facial clefts by placing bone grafts above palatal defects, which likely resulted in injury to the hypothalamic pituitary axis.

Paramedian clefts are difficult to correct at a young age, and multiple procedures that accomplish little must be considered a complication. It is also extremely unlikely that a permanently patent nasal passage can be satisfactorily accomplished for cases involving congenital atresia.

With orbital facial clefts, unsightly scarring has been reported following the use of large facial z-plastys in treating the oblique facial clefts, emphasizing the need for restraint in using flaps to assist with the closure of facial clefts. In addition, the treatment of congenital anophthalmia with expanders is also prone to potential complications, including expander displacement outside the orbit, expander exposure, and conjunctival scarring. Avoidance of these complications may be possible by instead placing static orbital implants that are serially exchanged two or three times, prior to skeletal maturity.

● OUTCOME ASSESSMENTS

Although the literature is replete with case reports of craniofacial clefts, there are only a few reports describing series of patients with these rare clefts, and none have examined outcomes in any meaningful way. It is reasonable to assume that better outcomes are accomplished in the milder clefts that are treated by the more experienced surgeons.

Whenever possible, patients with the more severe craniofacial clefts should be referred to regional centers with particular expertise with these anomalies.

REFERENCES

1. Kawamoto HK Jr. The kaleidoscopic world of rare craniofacial clefts: order out of chaos (Tessier classification). *Clin Plast Surg.* 1976;3:529.

2. Coady MSE, Moore MH, Wallis K. Amniotic band syndrome: the association between rare craniofacial clefts and limb ring constrictions. *Plast Reconstr Surg.* 1998;101(3): 640.

3. Ortiz Monasterio F, Fuente Del Campo A, Dimopulos A. Nasal clefts. *Ann Plast Surg.* 1987;18(5):377.

4. Tessier P. Anatomical classification of facial, cranio-facial and laterofacial clefts. *J Maxillofac Surg.* 1976;4:69.

5. Fearon JA. Rare craniofacial clefts: a surgical classification. *J Craniofac Surg.* 2008;19:110.

6. David DJ, Moore MH, Cooter RD. Tessier clefts revisited with a third dimension. *Cleft Palate J.* 1989;26:163.

7. Longaker MT, Lipshutz GS, Kawamoto HK. Reconstruction of Tessier no. 4 clefts revisited. *Plast Reconstr Surg.* 1997;99:1501.

chapter 19

Orthognathic Surgery and Cephalometric Analysis

Jesse A. Goldstein, MD / Stephen B. Baker, MD, DDS, FACS

● INTRODUCTION

Orthognathic surgery is the term used to describe surgical movement of the tooth-bearing segments of the maxilla and mandible. Candidates for orthognathic surgery have dentofacial deformities that cannot be adequately treated with orthodontic therapy alone. Children with cleft lip and palate as well as certain craniofacial anomalies are especially prone to develop malocclusion. Indeed, where approximately 2.5% of the general population have occlusal discrepancies that warrant surgical correction, 25% to 30% of patients who undergo surgical correction of cleft lip and palate in infancy will have severe enough midface retrusion to require orthognathic surgery.[1] Maxillary hypoplasia resulting in class III malocclusion is the typical deformity seen in patients with cleft and craniofacial deformities, but class II malocclusion, anterior open bites, occlusal cants, and many other dentofacial deformities can also occur. Regardless of the etiology, patient examination and treatment planning principles remain the same. The goal of orthognathic surgery, therefore, is to establish ideal dental occlusion with the jaws in a position that optimizes facial form and function.

● HISTORY AND PATIENT SELECTION

It is important to obtain a thorough medical, dental, and surgical history from every patient. Systemic diseases such as juvenile rheumatoid arthritis, diabetes, and scleroderma can affect treatment planning. With jaw asymmetries, a history of hyperplasia or hypoplasia from syndromic, traumatic, postsurgical, or neoplastic etiologies affects treatment considerations. Each patient should be questioned regarding symptoms of temporomandibular joint (TMJ)

disease or myofascial pain syndrome. Motivation and realistic expectations are important for an optimal outcome. It is likewise important for patients to have a clear understanding of the procedure, the recovery, and anticipated result. In younger patients, a family discussion in terms they can understand helps to alleviate preoperative anxiety. Orthognathic surgery is a major undertaking, and the patient and family must be appropriately motivated to undergo necessary preoperative and postoperative orthodontic treatment in addition to the surgery itself.

A complete physical examination should be performed on every patient prior to surgery. The frontal facial evaluation begins with the assessment of the vertical facial thirds (trichion to glabella, glabella to subnasale, and subnasale to menton) and the horizontal facial fifths (zygoma to lateral canthus, lateral to medial canthi, and intracanthal segment). The most important factor in assessing the vertical height of the maxilla is the degree of incisor showing while the patient's lips are in repose. Males should show at least 2 to 3 mm, whereas as much as 5 to 6 mm is considered attractive in females. If the patient shows the correct degree of incisor in repose, but shows excessive gingival in full smile, the maxilla should not be impacted. It is more important to have correct incisor show in repose than in full smile. If lip incompetence or mentalis strain is present, it is usually an indicator of vertical maxillary excess.

The inferior orbital rims, malar eminence, and piriform areas are evaluated for the degree of projection. These regions often appear deficient in cleft patients; maxillary advancement is indicated. If they are prominent, posterior repositioning may be necessary. The alar base width should also be assessed prior to surgery since orthognathic surgery may alter this width which, in turn, may accentuate any asymmetries associated with a cleft nasal deformity. Asymmetries of the maxilla and mandible should be documented on physical examination, and the degree of deviation from the facial midline noted.

The profile evaluation focuses on the projection of the forehead, malar region, the maxilla and mandible, the nose, the chin, and the neck. An experienced clinician can usually determine whether the deformity is caused by the maxilla, the mandible, or both simply by looking at the patient. This assessment is made clinically and verified at the time of cephalometric analysis. The intraoral exam should begin with an assessment of oral hygiene and periodontal health. These factors are critical for successful orthodontic treatment and surgery. Any retained deciduous teeth or unerupted adult teeth are noted. The occlusal classification is determined, and the degrees of incisor overlap and overjet are quantified. The surgeon should assess the transverse dimension of the maxilla as prior cleft palate repair will often result in transverse growth restriction. If the mandibular third molars are present, they must be extracted 6 months prior to sagittal split osteotomy. Any missing teeth or periapical pathology should be noted, as should any signs or symptoms of TMJ dysfunction. These issues should be addressed prior to proceeding with orthognathic surgery. The term "dental compensation" is used to describe the tendency of teeth to tilt in a direction that minimizes dental malocclusion. For example, in a patient with an overbite (Angle class II malocclusion), lingual retroclination of the upper incisors and labial proclination of the lower incisors minimize the malocclusion. The opposite occurs in a patient who has dental compensation for an underbite (Angle class III malocclusion). Thus, dental compensation, which is often the result of orthodontic treatment, will mask the true degree of skeletal discrepancy. Precise analysis of the dental compensation is done on the lateral cephalometric radiographs.

If the patient desires surgical correction of the deformity, presurgical orthodontics will upright and decompensate the occlusion, thereby reversing the compensation that has occurred. This has the effect of exaggerating the malocclusion, but it also allows the surgeon to maximize skeletal movements. If the patient is ambivalent or not interested in surgery, mild cases of malocclusion may be treated by further dental compensation, which will camouflage the deformity and restore proper overjet and overlap. The importance of a commitment to surgery prior to orthodontics lies in the fact that dental movements for decompensation and compensation are in opposite directions, so this decision needs to be made prior to orthodontic therapy.[2]

CEPHALOMETRIC AND DENTAL EVALUATION

Identifying the proper patient for orthognathic surgery is a key step to ensure satisfaction and successful outcomes. This includes amassing considerable data beyond a simple history and physical exam and should be coordinated with other members of the care team.

A cephalometric analysis and comparison to normative values can help the surgeon plan the degree of skeletal movement needed to achieve both an optimal occlusion and an optimal aesthetic result. A lateral cephalometric radiograph is performed under reproducible conditions so that serial images can be compared. This film is usually taken at the orthodontist's office using a cephalostat, an apparatus specifically designed for this purpose, and a head frame to maintain consistent head position. It is important to be certain the surgeon can visualize both the bony and soft tissue features in order to facilitate tracing every landmark. Once the normal structures are traced, several planes and angles are determined (Figure 19-1).

The sella-nasion-subspinale (SNA) and sella-nasion-supramentale (SNB) are the two most important angles in determining the positions of the maxilla and mandible relative to each other as well as the cranial base. These angles are determined by drawing lines from sella to nasion to *A point* or *B point*, respectively. By forming an angle with the sella and nasion, this position is referenced to the cranial

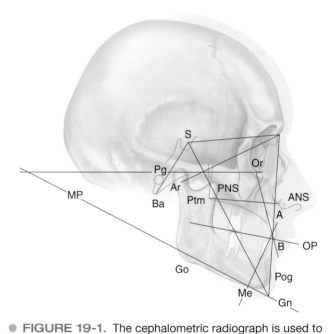

● **FIGURE 19-1.** The cephalometric radiograph is used to identify skeletal landmarks used in determining the lines and angles that reflect facial development. These measurements aid in determining the extent to which each jaw contributes to the dentofacial deformity. (S, sellaturcica, the midpoint of the sellaturcica; N, nasion, the anterior point of the intersection between the nasal and frontal bones; A, *A point*, the innermost point in the depth of the concavity of the maxillary alveolar process; B, *B point*, the innermost point on the contour of the mandible between the incisor tooth and the bony chin; Pg, pogonion, the most anterior point on the contour of the chin; Go, gonion, the most inferior and posterior point at the angle formed by the ramus and body of the mandible; Po, porion, the uppermost lateral point on the roof of the external auditory meatus; Or, orbitale, the lowest point on the inferior margin of the orbit; Gn, gnathion, the center of the inferior contour of the chin; Me, menton, the most inferior point on the mandibular symphysis.)

base. *A point* provides information about the anteroposterior position of the maxilla. If the SNA angle is excessive, the maxilla exhibits an abnormal anterior position relative to the cranium. If SNA is less than normal, the maxilla is posteriorly positioned relative to the cranial base. The same principle applies to the mandible: *B point* is used to relate the mandibular position to the cranial base. The importance of the cranial base as a reference is that it allows the clinician to determine if one or both jaws contribute to a noted deformity. For example, a patient's class III malocclusion (underbite) could develop from several different etiologies: a retrognathic maxilla and a normal mandible as is common in cleft patients, a normal maxilla and a prognathic mandible, a retrognathic mandible and a more severely retrognathic maxilla, or a prognathic maxilla and a more severely prognathic mandible. All of these conditions yield a class III malocclusion, yet each requires a different treatment approach. The surgeon can delineate the true etiology of the deformity by the fact that the maxilla and mandible can be independently related to a stable reference, the cranial base. Next, cephalometric tracings are performed.

Cephalometric tracings give the surgeon an idea of how skeletal movements will affect one another as well as the soft tissue profile. They also allow the surgeon to determine the distances the bones will be moved to achieve the goals of specific procedure. Different tracing methods using acetate paper are used for isolated maxillary, isolated mandibular, or two-jaw surgeries. Much of the traditional hand cephalometric tracing, however, has given way to computer-aided cephalometric analysis which allows the surgeon to electronically position the maxilla and mandible on the cephalogram while recording the soft tissue changes and measuring the degree of repositioning.

Complete dental records, including mounted dental casts, are needed to execute preoperative model surgery and fabricate surgical splints. Casts allow the surgeon to evaluate the occlusion both before and after articulation into proper positions. Analysis of new occlusion gives the clinician an idea of how intensive the presurgical orthodontic treatment plan will be. Casts also allow the clinician to distinguish between absolute and relative transverse maxillary deficiency. Absolute transverse maxillary deficiency presents as a posterior crossbite with the jaws in class I relationship. A relative maxillary transverse deficiency is commonly seen in a patient with a class III malocclusion. A posterior crossbite is observed in this type of patient, raising suspicions of inadequate maxillary width. However, as the maxilla is advanced or the mandible retruded, the crossbite is eliminated. Articulation of the casts into a class I occlusion allows the surgeon to easily distinguish between relative and absolute maxillary constriction.

Using the cephalometric tracings as a guide, the next step is to reproduce the maxillary and/or mandibular movements on articulated dental models. This allows for the fabrication of occlusal splints to be used intraoperatively to guide jaw repositioning in preparation for osteosynthesis. Model surgery begins by obtaining accurate casts of the patient's occlusion. If the surgeon does not have a

dental laboratory, the orthodontist will obtain the casts. The success of the technical portion of orthognathic surgery correlates directly with the accuracy of the model surgery and splint fabrication.

It should be noted that if isolated mandibular surgery is being performed, the casts can be hand articulated into the desired occlusion. The Galetti articulator is a useful tool that allows securing of casts with a screw mount. A universal joint allows the casts to be set in the desired relationship. Surgical splints can then be made from the articulator. If the maximum intercuspal position is the desired postoperative occlusion, a splint is unnecessary. The surgeon can osteotomize the mandible and secure it into its new position using the maximum intercuspal position as a guide to the new position. The surgeon should always verify the desired postoperative occlusion with the othrodontist prior to surgery.

A face bow is a device that is used to accurately relate the maxillary model to the cranium on an articulator. If a maxillary osteotomy is being performed, one set of models should be mounted on an articulator using the face bow. Two other sets of models are used in treatment planning. Next, an Erickson model block is sued to measure the current position of the maxillary central incisors, cuspids, and the mesiobuccal cusp of the first molar. The face bow-mounted maxillary cast is placed on the model block. The maxillary model is then measured to the tenth of a millimeter vertically, anteroposteriorly, and end-on. By having numerical records in three dimensions, the surgeon can reproduce the maxillary cast's exact location, as well as determine a new location. Reference lines are circumferentially inscribed every 5 mm around the maxillary cast mounting. The distances the maxillar will move in anteroposterior, lateral, and vertical directions have been determined from the previous cephalometric exam. These numbers are added or subtracted from the current values measured on the model block to determine the new three-dimensional position of the maxillary cast. The occlusal portion of the maxillary cast is removed from its base using a saw. As much plaster is removed from the cast as is necessary to accommodate the new position of the maxilla. Once the model block verifies the maxilla is in its new position, the cast is secured with sticky wax or plaster to the mounting ring. Now it can be placed on the articulator. At this point, the surgeon has a mounting of the postoperative maxilla related to the preoperative mandible. An acrylic splint is made at this point. This splint is called the intermediate splint and is used in the operating room to index the new position of the maxilla to the preoperative position of the mandible. A second mounting with the casts in the occlusion desired by the orthodontist is used to make a final splint that represents the new position of the mandible to the repositioned maxilla. This is fabricated in a manner similar to the splint for isolated mandibular surgery. If the occlusion is good, intercuspal position can be used to position the mandible without the splint.

Several computer-assisted design (CAD) and computer-aided manufacturing (CAM) programs are commercially available that can assist the surgeon with some or all of the preoperative patient preparation. A CT scan is obtained with the patient wearing a bite jig that correlates natural head position to the 3D CT image of the patient's face. Although conventional helical CT scans with fine cuts through the face are ideal, cone beam CT scans offer a comparable image quality with considerably less cost and radiation exposure (50 μSv compared to 2000 μSv). A cephalometric analysis can then be performed as well as simulated movements of the jaws and chin in any dimension. Once the osteotomy movements are verified by the surgeon, CAD/CAM technology is used to fabricate surgical splints for the patient. If necessary, 3D models of the patient can be made showing the exact proposed movement (Figure 19-2A–E). Some systems can actually "wrap" a 2D digital image around the soft tissue envelope of the 3D CT image, thus replicating a 3D image of the patient's actual face in color.

In our experience, the 3D CT modeling has demonstrated improved accuracy in diagnosis and treatment. The elimination of traditional model surgery saves the surgeon time in patient preparation. Finally, the 3D aspect of this treatment planning approach enhances the surgeons ability to predict how osteotomies may affect soft tissue of the face. These advantages facilitate the ability of the plastic surgeon to provide optimal care for these patients.

● DEVELOPING A TREATMENT PLAN

Once the data are obtained, the surgeon can determine which abnormalities the patient exhibits and the extent to which these features deviate from the norm. The treatment plan is the application of these data to provide the best aesthetic result while establishing a class I occlusion. The goal is not to "treat the numbers" in an attempt to

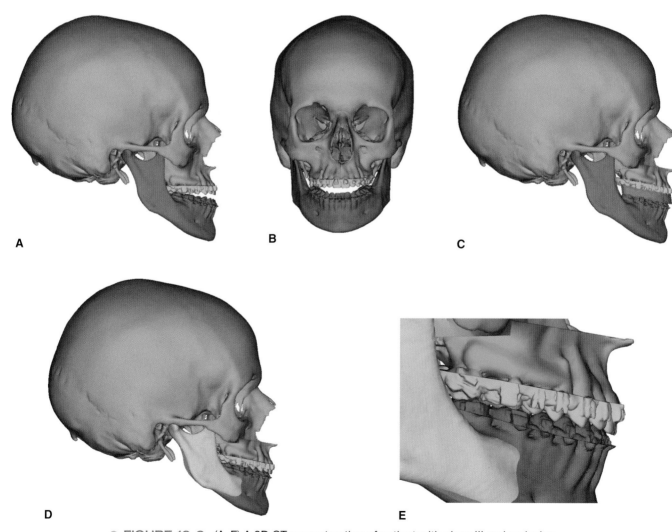

● FIGURE 19-2. (A–E) A 3D CT reconstruction of patient with class III malocclusion and anterior open bite. (A) Lateral preoperative view. (B) Front pre-operative view. (C) Lateral view after LeFort I osteotomy has been simulated with intermediate splint in place. (D) Lateral postoperative view after LeFort I and bilateral sagittal split osteotomies have been simulated with correction of class III malocclusion and anterior open bite. (E) Close-up view of predicted postoperative occlusion.

normalize every patient. The appearance of the soft tissue envelope surrounding the facial skeleton is the most crucial factor in determining the aesthetic success of orthognathic procedures, and the jaws should be positioned so they provide optimal soft tissue support.

Historically, skeletal movements that expanded the soft tissue of the face were less stable, so posterior and superior movements were preferred. Although these movements were more stable, they resulted in contraction of the facial skeleton with the associated soft tissue features of premature aging. Since the introduction of rigid fixation systems, osteotomies that result in skeletal expansion have been achieved with a great degree of predictability. An attempt is made to develop a treatment plan that will expand or maintain the preoperative volume of the face. If a superior or posterior (contraction) movement of one of the jaws is planned, an attempt should be made to neutralize the skeletal contraction with an advancement or inferior movement of the other jaw or the chin. It is important to avoid a net contraction of the facial skeleton, as this may result in a prematurely aged appearance.[3]

As skeletal expansion is increased, soft tissue laxity is reduced and facial creases are softened. These effects increase the definition of the face, creating a more attractive appearance. It has been shown that skeletal expansion is aesthetically pleasing, even if facial disproportion is necessary to achieve the expansion. Women with successful careers as fashion models often exhibit slight degrees of facial disproportion and are considered beautiful. The aesthetic benefits the patient receives by expanding the facial envelope frequently justify the small degree of disproportion necessary to achieve them. Even in young adolescent patients who do not show signs of aging, one must not ignore these principles. A successful surgeon will incorporate these principles into the treatment plan of every patient so that as the patient ages, the signs of aging will be minimized and a youthful appearance will be maintained as long as possible.

A class I occlusion can be achieve with the jaws in a variety of positions. The goal in treatment planning is to use the data from the patient's examination to predict the location of the jaws that will optimize the soft-tissue features of the face. By reducing the emphasis on normal values and increasing the awareness of the soft tissue effects of skeletal movements, preserving skeletal disproportion can often lead to a more favorable result.[7]

● GENERAL PRINCIPLES AND PERTINENT ANATOMY

Several principles have broad application to jaw surgery. Blood loss can be substantial in maxillofacial surgery and even small volumes can have significant clinical implications in the pediatric population. Standard techniques of head elevation, hypotensive anesthesia, blood donation, and administration of erythropoietin are useful adjuncts to reduce blood loss, especially in the younger population. Before incisions are made, an antimicrobial rinse is helpful to minimize the intraoral bacterial count. A topical steroid is applied to the lips to reduce pain and swelling associated

with prolonged retraction. Intravenous steroids may also be useful to reduce postoperative edema.

The occlusion desired may not be the same as maximum intercuspal position. The splint is useful in maintaining the occlusion in the desired location when it does not correspond to maximal intercuspal position. It is easy for the orthodontist to close a posterior open bite, but very difficult to close an anterior open bite with orthodontic treatment. At the end of the case, it is important to have the anterior teeth and the canines in a class I relationship without an open bite.

Guiding elastics are useful postoperatively to control the bite. Class II elastics are placed in a vector to correct a class II relationship (maxillary lug is anterior to the mandibular lug). Class III elastics are applied to correct a class III discrepancy. With rigid fixation, the elastics will not correct malpositioned jaws. They serve only to help the patient adapt to his new occlusion. Minor malocclusions can be corrected with postoperative orthodontic treatment.

Certain skeletal movements are inherently more stable than others. Stable movements include mandibular advancement and superior positioning of the maxilla. Movements with intermediate stability include maxillary impaction combined with mandibular advancement, maxillary advancement combined with mandibular setback, and correction of mandibular asymmetry. The unstable movements include posterior positioning of the mandible and inferior positioning of the maxilla. The least stable movement is transverse expansion of the maxilla. Long-term relapse with rigid fixation has not been demonstrated to be clearly superior to nonrigid fixation in single-jaw surgery. However, in two-jaw surgery, rigid fixation results in less relapse. The judgment of the surgeon will dictate the extent to which the facial skeleton can be expanded without resulting in unacceptable relapse.

The maxilla is associated with the descending palatine artery, the intraorbital nerve, the tooth roots, and the internal maxillary artery. The internal maxillary artery runs about 25 mm from the pterygomaxillary junction, and the descending palatal artery descends into the posteromedial maxillary sinus. The infraorbital nerve exits the intraorbital foramen below the infraorbital rim along the midpupillary line. The maxillary tooth roots extend within the maxilla in a superior direction. The canine has the longest root and is usually visible through the maxillary cortical bone.

The patient who presents with a cleft lip and/or palatal anomaly will have several anatomic differences when compared with an unaffected patient. The maxilla is typically deficient in both the anteroposterior and vertical dimensions. Because the midface retrusion can be significant, it frequently appears that the mandible is prognathic, but it is rare that the mandible demonstrates a true prognathia. It is a relative prognathia secondary to the maxillary deficiency.

● LEFORT I OSTEOTOMY

The first step in any facial osteotomy is satisfactorily securing the nasal endotracheal tube; our preference is a nasal Ring–Adair–Elwin (RAE) endotracheal tube. The vertical

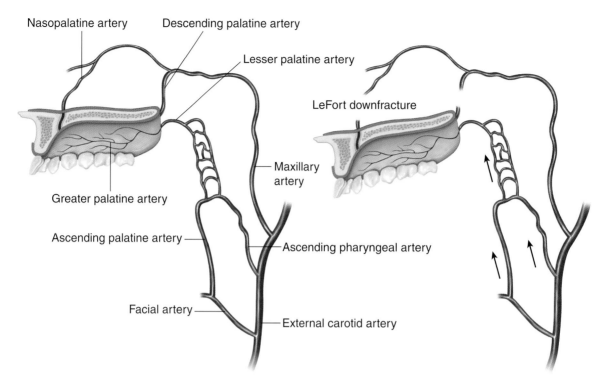

● **FIGURE 19-3.** Blood supply to maxilla before and after LeFort I osteotomy and downfracture. After the nasopalatine and descending palatine arteries are transected, perfusion of the maxillary segment occurs via the lesser palatine artery.

position of the maxilla is recorded by measuring the distance between the medial canthus and the orthodontic arch wire. These vertical measurements are absolutely critical. The maxillary vestibule is injected with epinephrine prior to patient preparation. An incision is made with needle tip electrocautery 5 mm above the mucogingival junction from first molar to first molar. A periosteal elevator is then used to expose the maxilla around the piriform rim and infraorbital nerve. Obwegeser toe-in retractors are held by the assistant at the head of the operating table. As the dissection extends laterally, it is important to remain subperiosteal to avoid exposure of the buccal fat pad. A Woodson elevator is used to initiate reflection of the nasal mucosa, and a periosteal elevator is used to complete the dissection of the nasal floor and lateral nasal wall. A double-balled osteotome is used to release the septum from the maxilla and an uniballed osteotome is used to release the lateral nasal wall. The surgeon can insert a finger on the posterior palate to help feel when the cut is complete. A periosteal elevator is used to protect the nasal mucosa and then a reciprocating saw is used to make a transverse osteotomy from the piriform aperture laterally until the cote descends just posteriorly to the last maxillary molar and drops through the maxillary tuberosity. The cut should be made at least 5 mm above the tooth apices. This distance is determined from preoperative Panorex radiographs. If cuts are complete, the maxilla is downfractured with manual pressure. An alternative is to use Rowe disimpaction forceps. These fit into the piriform aperture and on the palate to provide increased leverage for the downfracture. Pressure

should be applied in a slow steady, controlled fashion, not in a serious of quick movements. If the maxilla is not mobilized with relative ease, the cuts are likely not complete and should be reevaluated. Once the downfracture is complete, a bone hook can be used by the assistant to hold the maxilla down while any remaining bony interferences are removed. The descending palatine arteries will be seen near the posteromedial maxillary sinus. These can be clipped prophylactically without compromising the blood supply to the maxilla (Figure 19-3). The splint is then used to place the maxilla in its proper position in occlusion with the mandible. Mandibulomaxillary fixation (MMF) is then applied with 26-gauge wires around the surgical lugs. The amount the maxilla will be impacted or elongated was determined in the treatment plan. This distance is added or subtracted from the medial canthal-incisor distance to determine the new vertical position of the maxilla. Four 2-mm plates, usually L shaped can be used to secure the maxilla. The MMF is released and occlusion verified prior to closure. If the alar base is wise, an alar cinch can be performed to normalize the width. Lip shortening may also result from closure. A V-Y closure at the central incisor can help alleviate this effect.

In patients who require increased cheek projection, a high LeFort I osteotomy can be performed. This differs in that the transverse osteotomy is made as high as the infraorbital nerve will allow. If further cheek projection is necessary, bode grafts can be added. In the case of inferior or anterior positioning, gaps between the segments greater than 3 mm should be grafted with autogenous bone, cadaveric bone, or block hydroxyapetite. Finally, if simultaneous expansion of the maxilla is necessary, the maxilla can be split into two or more pieces to allow concurrent expansion.

Surgically Assisted Rapid Palatal Expansion

Correction of transverse maxillary constriction are common in patients with repaired cleft palates or those with craniofacial syndromes such as Apert or Cruzon syndrome. Such palatal constriction can be addressed in adolescence with nonsurgical orthodontic appliances. As the sutures begin to close during late adolescence, relapse rates increase. A multiple LeFort I osteotomy can be performed to provide simultaneous maxillary expansion, but the degree of relapse is high. In the young adult, the preferred procedure is the surgically assisted rapid palatal expansion (SARPE) procedure.[8] The orthodontist places a palatal expander prior to the procedure. A LeFort I osteotomy is performed to completely mobilize the maxilla from the upper face. A small osteotome is used to make a thin cut between the roots of the central incisors, and a midline split is completed to the posterior nasal spine. Separation is verified by activating the device. The maxilla is widened until the gingival blanches and then is relaxed several turns to avoid ischemia. The SARPE procedure offers the best stability for maxillary expansion in the young adult and older patient. Transverse deficiencies of the mandible can be corrected with a similar technique, that of distraction osteogenesis (see Chapter 14).

● BILATERAL SAGITTAL SPLIT OSTEOTOMY

The endotracheal tube placement and epinephrine injection are carried out in a similar fashion to the LeFort I osteotomy. The cut is made with electrocautery about 10 mm from the lateral aspect of the molars and extends from the midramus to the region of the second molar. If insufficient tissue is left on the dental side of the incision, closure is more difficult. A periosteal elevator is used to expose the lateral mandible and the anterior coronoid process in a subperiosteal plane. As the coronoid process is exposed, placement of a notched coronoid retractor may facilitate the dissection. A curved Kocher with a chain can be clamped to the coronoid process and the chain secured to the drapes. To optimize blood supply, subperiosteal dissection is limited to those areas required to complete the osteotomy. A J-stripper is used to release the inferior border of the mandible from the attachments of the pterygomasseteric sling. The eternal oblique ridge and inferior border of the mandible should be exposed. The medial aspect of the ramus is also dissected subperiosteally. The mandibular nerve should be identified. A Seldin elevator is inserted medial to the ramus and protecting the nerve. A Lindemann side-cutting burr is used to make a cut on the medial ramus that is parallel to the occlusal plane and extends about two thirds of the distance to the posterior ramus. The cut extends from

medial to lateral until the burr is in the cancellous portion of the ramus. Mandibular body retractors are then placed and a fissure burr or a reciprocating saw is used to make a cut from the midramus down along the external oblique ridge, gently curving to the inferior border of the mandible. The cuts are verified with an osteotome, and then large osteotomes are inserted and rotated to gently separate the segments. The tooth-baring segments are referred to as the distal segment, and the condylar portion as the proximal segment. The inferior alveolar nerve should be identified and found in the distal segment. If part of the nerve is located within the proximal segment, it should gently be released with a small curette. After both osteotomies are complete, the distal segment is placed into occlusion and secured by tightening 26-guage wire loops around the surgical lugs. If a surgical splint is necessary to establish a required occlusion, it is placed between the teeth before MMF wiring. The proximal segments are then gently rotated to ensure they are seated within the glenoid fossa. When each condyle is comfortably seated within the fossa, it is rotated to align the inferior borders of the two segments and secured into position with a clamp. Three lag screws are placed at the superior border of the overlapping segments on each side of the mandible. To ensure that the transbuccal trocar will be placed properly, a hemostat is placed at the proposed screw location and pointed toward the cheek. A small stab incision is made in the skin, and the trocar is placed through the tissue bluntly until the tip enters the oral incision. The trocar is then exchanged for a drill guide, and the 2.0-mm and 1.5-mm drills are used in the lag sequence to make three holes through the overlapping portion of the proximal and distal segments. The screw lengths are measured and the screws inserted. The MMF is released, and the mandible is gently opened and closed to verify the occlusion. If a malocclusion is noted, the most likely etiology is that one or both condyles are not seated properly during application of fixation. The screws should be removed and replaced until the correct occlusion is established. The wounds are irrigated and closed with interrupted 4-0 chromic sutures.

Intraoral Vertical Ramus Osteotomy

A second technique for correcting mandibular prognathism or asymmetry is the intraoral vertical ramus osteotomy. The incision is the same as described above. A subperiosteal dissection is performed from the lateral ramus and a LeVasseur-Merril retractor is used to hold this tissue laterally. An oscillating saw is then used to make a vertical cut from the sigmoid notch to the inferior border of the mandible. The cut must be make posterior to the mandibular foramen on the medial side. The antilingula is a useful landmark. This is an elevation on the lateral mandible that indicates the approximate location of the mandibular foramen. After both sides are complete, the distal segment is moved into occlusion, making sure that the proximal segments remain lateral to the distal segments posteriorly.

Because rigid fixation is difficult to apply, a single wire, or no fixation at all, is used, and the patient remains in MMF for 6 weeks. This osteotomy can be done from an external approach but this incision results in a scar on the neck.

Two-Jaw Surgery

Moving the maxilla and the mandible in one procedure requires osteotomizing both jaws and precisely securing them into position as determined by the treatment plan. If proper treatment planning, model surgery, and splint fabrication are performed, each jaw should be able to be placed into its desired position with precision. The mandibular bony cuts are made first but terminated prior to osteotomy completion. The maxillary osteotomy is made, and the maxilla is placed into its new position using the intermediate splint. The splint is used to wire the teeth into MMF, allowing for indexing the new position of the maxilla to the preoperative (uncorrected) position of the mandible. With the condyles gently seated, the maxillomandibular complex is rotated so that the maxillary incisal edge is at the correct vertical height. The maxilla is plated into position, the MMF is released, and the intermediate splint removed. Next the mandibular osteotomies are completed, and the distal segment of the mandible is placed into the desired occlusion using the final splint. If the teeth are in good occlusion without the splint, the final splint may not be necessary to establish the desired occlusal relationship. Wire loops secure the occlusal relationship and the rigid fixation is completed as previously described.

● GENIOPLASTY

Including a genioplasty in the treatment plan can be a powerful adjunct to mandibular movements, either by offsetting soft tissue collapse with posterior mandibular repositioning or augmenting anterior mandibular movement. When performed asymmetrically, a genioplasty may also correct for minor mandibular asymmetries.

After adequate local anesthetic infiltration, the mucosa is incised from canine to canine with needle tip electrocautery 5 mm below the mucogingival junction. The mentalis is transected, being sure to leave enough muscle cuff to allow for reapproximation during closure. Failure to do so can result in a ptotic soft tissue envelope, or "witch's chin" deformity. Next, the dissection is carried out in a subperiosteal fashion identifying and protecting the mental nerves bilaterally. Using a reciprocating saw, the mandibular midline is gently marked to aid is centric fixation. The transverse osteotomy is made approximately 3 mm below the mental foramina in order to protect the intraosseus course of the mental nerves and the canine tooth roots. The trajectory of the osteotomy can be varied depending on the type of correction required. The mobilized segment is then fixed into the desired position with plates and screws, using the midline mark as a guide. The mentalis is then repaired and the mucosa closed.

Finally, because of lesser segment collapse, the dental midline is often deviated toward the cleft side.

Despite having had alveolar bone grafting performed, many of these patients have deficient or missing bone in the region of the alveolus. Persistent palatal fistulas may be present as well. The lateral incisor is frequently missing in these patients and closure of this space must be taken into consideration at the time of treatment planning. If a large fistula is present in the alveolus, modifications of the LeFort I procedure can be performed to facilitate a tension-free alveolar closure.

The important structures in the mandible that may be injured in the mandibular osteotomy are the mental nerve, the inferior alveolar nerve, and the tooth apices. The third branch of the trigeminal nerve enters the mandibular foramen to become the inferior alveolar nerve. It runs below the tooth roots and exits at the level of the first and second premolars through the mental foramen. The region where it is most medial to the outer cortex is located near the external oblique ridge. This is where the vertical portion of the bilateral sagittal split osteotomy is made because it affords the largest margin of error.

● CLEFT SURGERY

Orthognathic surgery in cleft lip/palate patients is done similar to noncleft patients with the exception of several important modifications that are necessary to maintain blood supply and assist in fistula closure.

In a unilateral cleft lip patient, the standard maxillary incision can be made with little jeopardy to the premaxillary blood supply. Each side of the cleft has an incision made similar to that of the alveolar bone graft incision. This allows for a two-layer closure of the palatal and nasal mucosa. If supplemental bone grafting needs to be done at this time, harvested bone can be placed into the alveolar gap after fixation has been applied. If a wide fistula is present, the surgeon can compress the maxillary segments to reduce the size of the alveolar space. This ensures the soft tissue closure is under minimal tension and the chance of fistula closure is optimized. The canine may now be adjacent to the central incisor, but the restorative dentist can fabricate a prosthetic crown for the canine to make it look like a lateral incisor.

In the bilateral cleft patient, care must be taken not to make the vestibular incision across the premaxilla. The premaxillary blood supply originates from the vomer and the buccal mucosa. Since the vomer will be split, the majority of blood flow to the premaxilla must course from the premaxillary buccal mucosa. A circumvestibular incision that violates this mucosa will severely jeopardize the blood supply of the premaxillary segment. To minimize the risk of complications, the incision is stopped just lateral to the alveolar cleft on each side. One minimizes reflection of the mucosa from the premaxilla in order to preserve the blood supply. The osteotomy of the premaxillary segment is made from a posterior approach just anterior to the incisive foramen. This allows mobilization of the segment without violation of the buccal mucosa. Similar to the unilateral cleft maxilla, residual fistulae and inadequate alveolar bone may be present. If either is identified, it can be corrected by a two-layer mucosal closure and bone graft-ing into the alveolar defect. If large gaps are present that may jeopardize fistula closure, the segments can be com-pressed at the alveolar gaps to reduce tension of the repair. Postoperative orthodontics and prosthetic restorations of the teeth can correct almost any postoperative dental aes-thetic irregularities.

Once the incision is made, the mucosa is reflected in a subperiosteal plane to expose the piriform aperture, the zygomatic buttress, and the posterolateral maxilla. A recip-rocating saw is used to make a high LeFort I osteotomy in most cases. A high LeFort I osteotomy is cut horizontally in a lateral direct line from the piriform aperture to the zygomatic buttress. One takes this line as high as possible while staying at least 5 mm below the inferior orbital fora-men. A vertical cut is now made from the lateral edge of the horizontal cut and taken to an area about 5 mm above the tooth root apices. The lateral nasal walls are cut with a uniball osteotome and mallet. The vomer and septum can be reached through the lateral maxillary osteotomies so the mucosa remains preserved. The pterygomaxillary junc-tion can be separated with a 10-mm curved osteotome or the maxillary tuberosity can be cut posterior to the last molar in the arch. The latter choice makes downfracture easier and results in fewer complications. Downfracture is now completed with either digital pressure or applica-tion of the Rowe disimpaction forceps. If a wide alveo-lar fistula is present, the greater and lesser segments can be compressed at the alveolus. The occlusion that would result from segment compression would be evaluated on the dental casts during preoperative model surgery. Any deficiency of alveolar bone can be corrected with supple-mental bone grafts after application of fixation, and fistulas can be corrected as well.

The surgical splint is then placed orient the new position of the maxilla to the mandible. Twenty 6-gauge wire loops are used to place the patient in maxillomandibular fixa-tion. It is extremely important to make sure the condyles are seated as the maxillomandibular complex is rotated to its new vertical dimension. Generally, cleft patients have vertical maxillary deficiency in addition to the sagittal deficiency. This requires the maxilla to be inferiorly posi-tioned to its new position. If vertical lengthening greater than 5 mm is required, bone grafts are placed between the osteotomy segments to reduce relapse. Rigid fixation is now used to secure the maxilla into its new position. If any instability remains across the maxillary segments, a small plate can be placed across the segments to reduce mobil-ity and maintain the bone graft. Because the osteotomized cleft maxilla results in a multisegment maxilla, the surgical splints are wired in place for 6 to 8 weeks in order to allow for bone healing.

● BASIC APPROACHES TO COMMONLY ENCOUNTERED PROBLEMS

The following paragraphs outline basic treatment approaches to commonly encountered dentofacial defor-mities commonly seen in orthognathic patients.

Skeletal Class II Malocclusion

Class II malocclusion is almost always caused by mandibu-lar retrognathia and is almost always best treated by man-dibular advancement (Figure 19-4). The mandible is small,

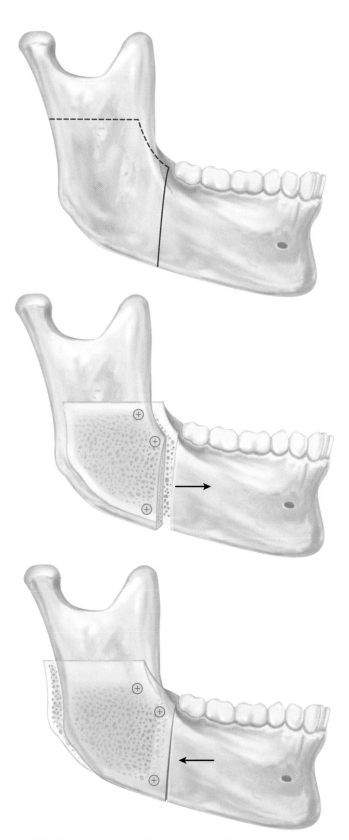

● **FIGURE 19-4.** Mandibular sagittal split osteotomies dem-onstrating mandibular advancement and mandibular setback.

and forward positioning is an expansible movement that enhances facial form. If the maxilla is also slightly deficient or in a normal position, one may consider a bimaxillary advancement to further enhance facial soft tissue definition, especially in more mature patients. If the malocclusion is minimal and there is little preexisting dental compensation, one may choose to have the orthodontist intentionally compensate the dentition to correct the occlusion and avoid surgery. In contrast, if the malocclusion appears minimal but there is dental compensation, the skeletal discrepancy will be more significant after the orthodontist decompensates the dentition, and the patient may be a good surgical candidate.

Skeletal Class III Malocclusion

A class III malocclusion may be treated by advancing the maxilla, posteriorly positioning the mandible, or by combining these procedures. It is important to consider the contributions of the mandible and the chin separately as each may require different treatments to achieve aesthetic goals. If some posterior positioning of the mandible is necessary, one may advance the maxilla to counteract the skeletal contraction produced from posteriorly positioning the mandible. Additionally, the patient may benefit from an advancement genioplasty, counteracting any skeletal contraction occurring from a mandibular setback. As in the class II patient, a minor malocclusion with minimal dental compensation may be corrected with orthodontic treatment alone. In contrast, a minor malocclusion with dental compensation may become a significant malocclusion after dental decompensation, and the patient will be a good surgical candidate.

Maxillary Constriction

Patients can present with a maxilla that is narrow in a transverse dimension. Maxillary constriction may occur as an isolated finding or as one of multiple abnormalities. Up to about age 15 years, the orthodontist can usually expand the maxilla nonsurgically with a palatal expander. If orthopedic expansion cannot be done, the SARPE technique can be performed. If the maxilla requires movement in other dimensions, a two-piece (or multipiece) LeFort I osteotomy can be performed to place the maxilla in its new position while simultaneously achieving transverse expansion (Figure 19-5).

Apertognathia

An anterior open bite is caused by a premature contact of the posterior molars and is commonly seen in patients with syndromic craniosynostoses such as Apert or Crouzon syndrome. The recommended treatment is a posterior impaction of the maxilla. By reducing the vertical height of the posterior maxilla, the mandible can come into occlusion with the remaining mandibular teeth. Posterior maxillary impaction does not necessarily result in incisor impaction; the posterior maxilla is simply rotated clockwise and upward using the incisal tip as the axis of rotation. Therefore, incisor show should not be affected. If a change in incisor show is also desired, the posterior impaction is performed, and then the whole maxilla can be inferiorly positioned or impacted to its new position (Figure 19-6A–C).

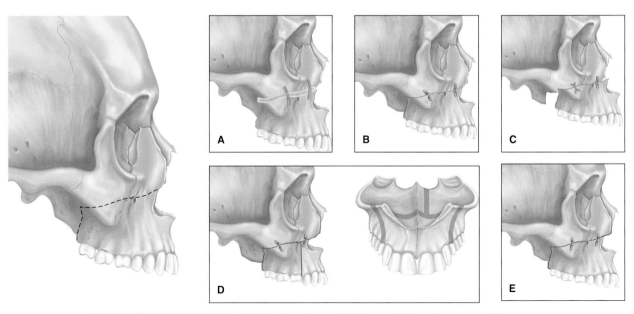

● **FIGURE 19-5.** LeFort I osteotomies demonstrating maxillary advancement, impaction, setback, and multipiece LeFort.

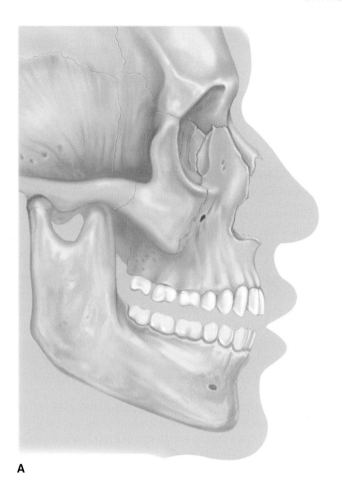

A

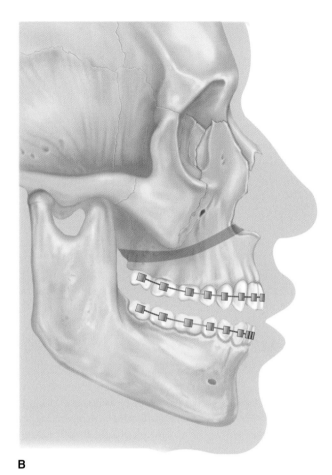

B

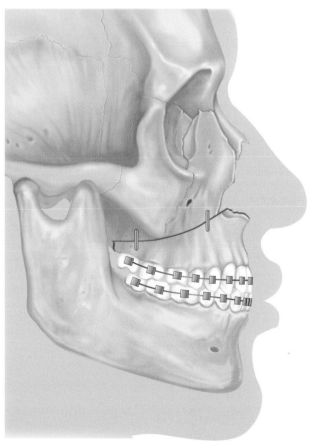

C

● **FIGURE 19-6.** (A) Anterior open bite. (B) The LeFort osteotomy allows posterior impaction of the maxilla and clockwise rotation. (C) Counterclockwise mandibular autorotation closes the anterior open bite.

Vertical Maxillary Excess

Vertical maxillary excess is typically associated with lip incompetence, mentalis strain, and an excessive degree of gingival show (long face syndrome). The treatment approach is to impact the maxilla to achieve the proper incisor show with the lips in repose. Impaction, however, may result in skeletal contraction, so the surgeon must consider anterior repositioning of the jaws to neutralize the associate adverse soft tissue effects. As the maxilla is impacted, the mandible rotates counterclockwise (with respect to a rightward facing patient) to maintain occlusion. This rotation results in anterior positioning of the chin and is called mandibular autorotation. The opposite occurs if the maxilla is moved in an inferior direction. In this case, the chin point rotates in a clockwise direction, resulting in posterior positioning of the chin point. It is important to note that these effects on the cephalometric tracing during treatment planning because a genioplasty may be required to reestablish proper chin position.

Short Lower Face

A short lower face is marked by insufficient incisor show and/or a short distance between subnasale and pogonion. Treatment is aimed at establishing a proper degree of incisor show. The facial skeleton should be expanded to the degree that provides optimal soft tissue esthetics.

As the maxilla is inferiorly positioned, resulting clockwise mandibular rotation leads to a posterior positioning of the chin. The surgeon needs to preoperatively assess the new chin position on the cephalometric prediction tracing to determine if an advancement genioplasty will be necessary to counter the effects of mandibular clockwise rotation.

OUTCOMES, PROGNOSIS, AND COMPLICATIONS

Accurate assessment of orthognathic surgical outcomes is essential to maintaining safe practices, maximizing patient satisfaction, and effectively evaluating an ever-changing field. Indeed, this importance is echoed in the wide range of ways investigators have used to record postoperative results. These include measurement tools such as three-dimensional CT scanning and volumetric analyses to evaluate postoperative changes in bony and soft tissues immediately and over time to questionnaires assessing patient-reported satisfaction scales and quality of life. While there is currently no universally accepted tool to accurately and reliably demonstrate patient outcomes after orthognathic surgery, with reasoned and reasonable expectations on the part of the patient, family and surgeon alike, orthognathic surgery can result in high levels of satisfaction both from a functional and aesthetic level.[4-6]

REFERENCES

1. DeLuke DM, Marchand A, Robles EC, Fox P. Facial growth and the need for orthognathic surgery after cleft palate repair: literature review and report of 28 cases. *J Oral Maxillofac Surg.* 1997;55(7):694–697.

2. Tompach PC, Wheeler JJ, Fridrich KL. Orthodontic considerations in orthognathic surgery. *Int J Adult Orthodon Orthognath Surg.* 1995(10):97–107.

3. Selber JC, Rosen HM. Aesthetics of facial skeletal surgery. *Clin Plast Surg.* 2007;34(3):437–445.

4. Janulewicz J, Costello BJ, Buckley MJ, et al. The effects of Le Fort I osteotomies on velopharyngeal and speech functions in cleft patients. *J Oral Maxillofac Surg.* 2004;62(3):308–314.

5. Posnick JC, Tompson B. Cleft-orthognathic surgery: complications and long-term results. *Plast Reconstr Surg.* 1995;96(2):255–266.

6. Baker SB, Goldstein JA, Seiboth L, Weinzweig J. Posttraumatic maxillomandibular reconstruction: a treatment algorithm for the partially edentulous patient. *J Craniofac Surg.* 2010;21(1):217–221.

7. Proffit WR, Sarver DM. Treatment planning: optimizing benefit to the patient. In: Proffit WR, White RP, Sarver DM, eds. *Contemporary Treatment of Dentofacial Deformity.* St. Louis, MO: Mosby; 2003:213–223.

8. Silverstein K, Quinn PD. Surgically assisted rapid palatal expansion for management of transverse maxillary deficiency. *J Oral Maxillofac Surg.* 1997;55:725–727.

chapter 20

Skull Base Surgery

Stephen P. Beals, MD, FACS, FAAP / *Hahns Y. Kim, MD*

● PATIENT EVALUATION AND SELECTION

Based on the principles established by Tessier more than 40 years ago for the correction of congenital craniofacial anomalies, development of advanced transfacial approaches has made possible the curative resection of many skull base lesions once considered inoperable.[1-8] A six-level classification scheme (Figure 20-1) has been developed to guide the approach based on the location of the tumor.[1,9]

A complete history and physical examination of a patient can provide clues to the location and extent of a tumor. Often, the clinical presentation is vague and nonspecific until the tumor has grown to a large size. The pathophysiology of the specific signs and symptoms may depend on whether the tumor is benign or malignant. With benign tumors, signs frequently result from compression of adjacent tissues. For example, a patient with an angiofibroma may present with nasal obstruction and a patient with fibrous dysplasia may present with proptosis. Signs of malignant tumors are often changes in the function of the tissues due to invasion by the lesion, such as headaches, focal seizures, loss of cranial nerve function, altered facial animation, and visual changes.

Once a thorough understanding of the patient's clinical presentation and deficits related to the tumor is established, further workup should include computed tomography with true coronal cuts as well as magnetic resonance imaging. Angiography may provide added benefit in select patients. Tissue diagnosis through biopsy, when feasible, is always preferred, but surgical resection can proceed with open biopsy and frozen section analysis before full exposure is undertaken or critical structures are sacrificed.

An essential component of evaluating a patient is a multidisciplinary team approach. The skills and training from several surgical disciplines are required to manage the complex needs of a patient with a skull base tumor. A skull base team can establish a centralized center where patients are referred for the treatment of these rare skull base tumors. This allows for adequate volume to maintain a high skill level, to conduct research in order to refine surgical techniques, and to improve outcomes. Specialties involved include the core specialties of neurosurgery, plastic surgery, and head and neck surgery as well as neurology, radiation oncology, endovascular radiology, oncology, ophthalmology, and neurorehabilitation. Coordinated care through a team approach improves communication between physicians, facilitates development of a superior treatment plan, and assists in follow-up and discussions of morbidity and mortality, ultimately giving the patient the best chance for a successful outcome.

● PATIENT PREPARATION

A full discussion of the potential risks and complications associated with the procedure is necessary, as well as ensuring that the expectations of the patient and surgeon are in congruity. The risks of craniotomy include neurologic injury, bleeding, infection, cerebrospinal fluid (CSF) leak. Other possible risks include alteration of orbital adnexal function, such as extraocular muscle imbalance, visual loss, altered globe position, and alteration of blink dynamics, tear production or drainage. There can be loss of olfaction, temporary or permanent change of facial sensation, brow weakness or paralysis, or change in orbital nasal configuration. Soft tissue contour defects can result if temporalis or forehead galeal muscle flaps are used. With extracranial approaches (levels I–III), there can be malocclusion requiring secondary surgery or orthodontic correction or loss of segmental circulation which may result in an oronasal fistula and abnormal speech. In children, there may be loss of secondary tooth buds.

Preparation for patients undergoing a level IV or V approach requires additional workup. The maxillary-mandibular relationship and occlusal relationship need

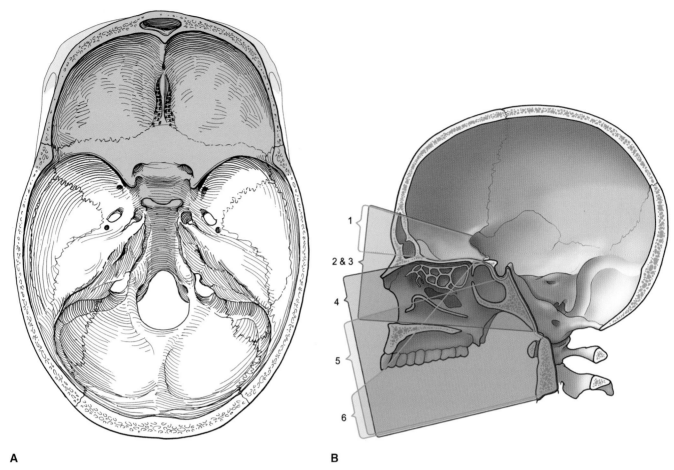

● FIGURE 20-1. (A) Region of tumor sites in the anterior skull base and clivus that can be exposed by direct anterior transfacial routes. (B) Summation of the six levels demonstrating that the anatomical site of the tumor and direction of growth determine the level of the transfacial exposure. (*With permission from Barrow Neurological Institute.*)

to be documented with life-size photographs, dental models, and x-rays, including occlusal views, anteroposterior and lateral cephalometrograms as well as a panoramic of the mandible. A presurgical acrylic splint is fabricated, making sure it is deep enough to allow the two palatal halves to snap into splint, reducing the need for arch bars.

● SURGICAL TECHNIQUE

Classification of Transfacial Approaches

The transfacial approach can be divided into six levels based on the anatomic location of the lesion and the pattern of extension. The kyphotic shape of the skull base is perpendicular to the vertical plane of the face and calls for a more superior approach through the frontonasal region for lesions with anterior extension, while posteriorly located lesions with superior extension would require a more inferior or transmaxillary approach. The surgery can be customized for each patient based on the best angle of approach, combining intracranial and extracranial approaches, if needed.

The upper three approaches (levels I– III) are derived from the supraorbital bar (Figure 20-2). By removing the supraorbital bar, in continuity with the naso-orbital complex, the approach is extended vertically to include the entire midline skull base. Removal of the naso-orbital complex increases the degree of horizontal extension, and an even greater exposure can be obtained by combining levels II and III with a circumferential cribriform plate osteotomy, which allows brain retraction but preserves olfaction. The lower three approaches (levels IV–VI) provide exposure to the skull base through the maxilla. The level IV exposes the entire midline skull base, the level V exposes the lower half, and the level VI exposes the lower third (Figure 20-3).

Intracranial Approaches (Levels I-III)

Patient Positioning. The patient in placed in the supine position and general anesthesia is introduced through an orotracheal tube. The tube can be secured to the lower dentition with a 26-gauge wire to allow for unobstructed access to the surgical field. After monitoring lines and intravenous lines are placed, prophylactic antibiotics are

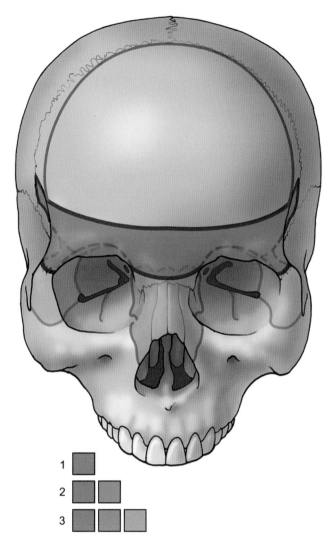

1
2
3

FIGURE 20-2. The three intracranial approaches represent variations of the amount of bone resected with the supraorbital bar. The shaded areas indicated by the numbers 1, 2, and 3 represent the amount of exposure for levels I, II, and II, respectively. (*With permission from Barrow Neurological Institute.*)

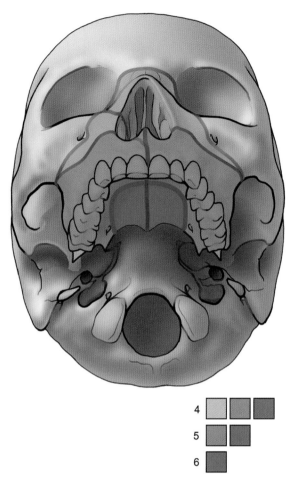

4
5
6

FIGURE 20-3. The extracranial approaches provide increasing exposure as more of the maxilla is removed. The shaded areas indicated by the numbers 4, 5, and 6 represent the amount of exposure for levels IV, V, and VI, respectively. (*With permission from Barrow Neurological Institute.*)

given and a lumbar drain is inserted, if indicated. Rigid three-point fixation is used to position the patient's head, placing the tongs posterior to the ears to allow for a more posterior bicoronal incision. The ISG Frameless Stereotactic Guidance System Wand is attached, and fiduciary reference points are correlated with the MRI and then registered. The patient's face, scalp, and any other anticipated donor sites for reconstruction are prepped and draped. Temporary tarsorrhaphy sutures using 5-0 cardiovascular silk are placed for corneal protection.

Level I—Transfrontal Approach. This approach is indicated for tumors of the anterior cranial fossa and the superior orbital region (Figure 20-4A–C). A bicoronal incision is placed posteriorly (in line with the preauricular

crease) to allow for potential pericranial and frontal galeal flaps of adequate length (Figure 20-5). Dissection is continued until the radix and superior orbits are exposed and the temporalis muscles are reflected. A bifrontal craniotomy is performed and the dura is retracted from the anterior cranial fossa. The supraorbital bar is removed (Figure 20-4C).

After tumor resection, a pericranial flap, cranial autografts, and fibrin glue are used to reconstruct a watertight separation between the nasopharynx and the cranial fossa. The supraorbital bar is fixated with plates and screws.

Level II—Transfrontal Nasal. This approach is indicated for tumors of the anterior cranial fossa, nasopharynx, ethmoidal and sphenoidal sinuses, clivus, and tumors that extend anteriorly or into the superior, medial, and lateral aspects of the orbit (Figure 20-4D–F). A bicoronal incision as in a level I approach is used. Dissection is continued until the radix, nasal bones, nasal process of the

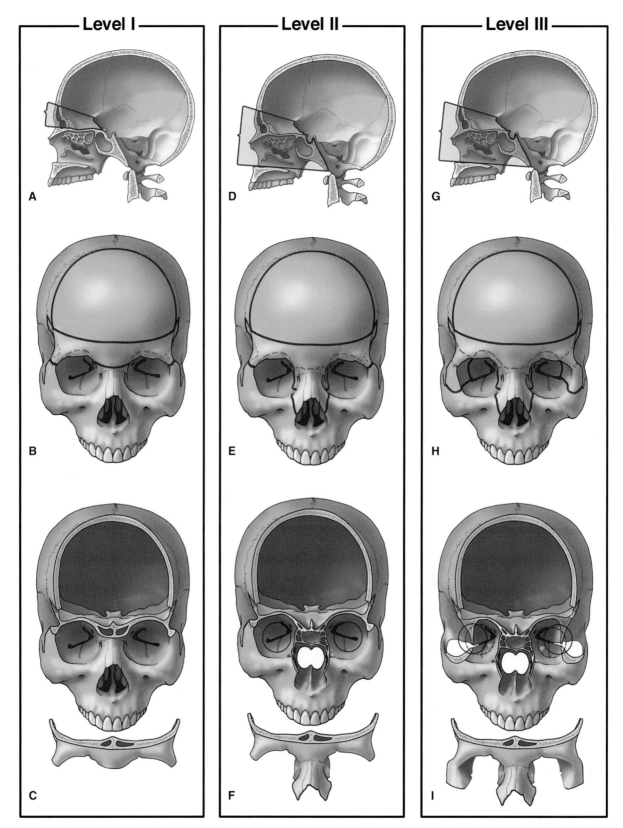

● **FIGURE 20-4.** Composite illustration showing the levels of exposure for the three intracranial approaches and the osteotomies required for each. (A) Level I transfrontal exposure for anterior cranial fossa. (B, C) Level I exposure requires removal of the supraorbital bar. (D) Level II transfrontal nasal exposure for anterior approach to the anterior cranial fossa and clivus. (E, F) Level II exposure requires removal of the frontonasal fragment. (G) Level III transfrontal nasal-orbital exposure for larger lesions of the anterior cranial fossa, nasopharynx, and clivus. This approach is similar to level II, except that it provides a wider exposure by allowing lateral retraction of the globes (see Figure 20-4D). (H, I) Level III exposure requires inclusion of the lateral orbital walls on the frontonasal fragment (frontal nasal-orbital unit). (*With permission from Barrow Neurological Institute.*)

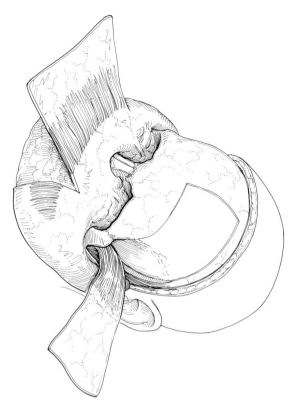

● **FIGURE 20-5.** Frontogaleal and pericranial flaps must be preserved during the initial dissection. (*With permission from Barrow Neurological Institute.*)

maxilla, and the superior orbits are exposed. The periorbita is stripped, taking great care to preserve the nasolacrimal ducts. The medial canthal ligaments are taken down, with a small fragment of bone if desired. The upper lateral nasal cartilages are detached from beneath the caudal margin of the nasal bones, and nasal mucosa dissected off the nasal bones. The temporal muscles are reflected and a bifrontal craniotomy is performed as in a level I approach. The supraorbital bar is removed in continuity with the nasal complex and medial orbital walls to the anterior ethmoid foramen (Figure 20-4F).

Level III—Transfrontal Nasal-Orbital. This approach is indicated for large anterior cranial fossa or nasopharyngeal tumors or for clival tumors with anterior extensions (Figure 20-4G–I). The dissection proceeds as in the level II approach, but when the osteotomies are made, the lateral orbital walls are included with the supraorbital segment from the level of the inferior orbital fissure. A majority of the orbital roof can also be included. This allows for lateral retraction of the globes to allow for greater midline exposure when compared with the level II exposure (Figure 20-4I).

After tumor resection, skull base reconstruction is achieved with a pericranial or temporalis flap and cranial autografts as needed. The upper lateral cartilages are reattached to the nasal bones and transnasal wiring is used to repair the medial canthal ligaments. The frontonasal fragment is secured with rigid fixation.

Cribriform Plate Preservation. When performing a level II or III approach, the integrity of the cribriform plate and olfactory nerves can be preserved when they are not involved with tumor. This is accomplished with a circumferential osteotomy and allows for increased posterior exposure, simplified skull base reconstruction, and reduced risk of CSF leak all while preserving olfaction.[10] After the craniotomy for the level II or III approach is completed, the dura is separated from the anterior cranial fossa as previously described. Osteotomies are performed to remove the frontonasal or the frontonasal-orbital unit, leaving the cribriform plate behind (Figure 20-6). The cribriform plate is osteotomized along its lateral margins into the ethmoidal sinuses. The final cut is made through the planum sphenoidale (Figure 20-6C). While carefully preserving a cuff of nasal mucosa and septum, attached to the inferior side of the plate, the perpendicular plate of the ethmoid is cut, freeing the cribriform plate and allowing retraction with the dura (Figure 20-6D). After resection of the tumor, reattachment of the plate is accomplished with stainless steel wires before reconstruction as described for the intracranial procedures.

Extracranial Approaches (Levels IV through VI)

Patient Positioning. The patient in placed in the supine position and general anesthesia is introduced through an orotracheal tube or a temporary tracheostomy. With orotracheal intubation, the tube can be secured to the lower dentition with a 26-gauge wire. After monitoring lines and intravenous lines are placed, prophylactic antibiotics are given and a lumbar drain is inserted, if indicated. Rigid three-point fixation is used to position the patient's head, placing the tongs posterior to the ears to allow for a more posterior bicoronal incision. The ISG Wand is attached, and fiduciary reference points are correlated with the MRI and then registered. The patient's face, scalp, and any other anticipated donor sites for reconstruction are prepped and draped. Temporary tarsorrhaphy sutures using 5-0 cardiovascular silk are placed for corneal protection. An epinephrine solution is infiltrated into the upper buccal sulcus and mucosa in the anterior maxillary region.

Level IV—Transnasomaxillary. This approach is indicated for large nasopharyngeal and clival tumors that extend in any direction. It provides wide exposure to the entire central skull base region (Figure 20-7A–D). The transnasomaxillary approach is performed through a modified Weber-Ferguson incision. This is continued across the radix and along the opposite subciliary margin of the lower lid (Figure 20-7B). Plates are adapted that will be used for fixation, and then a LeFort II osteotomy is performed. The nasal fragment is divided at the nasal process of the maxilla on one side and at the midline of the palate (Figure 20-7C–D). The nasal soft tissue remains intact and is retracted with the fragment.

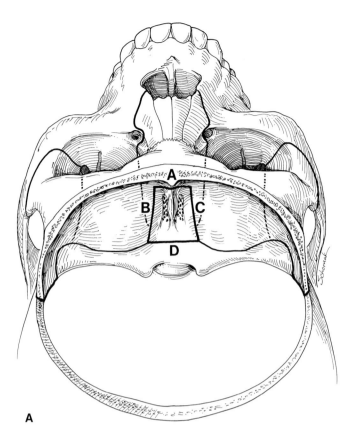

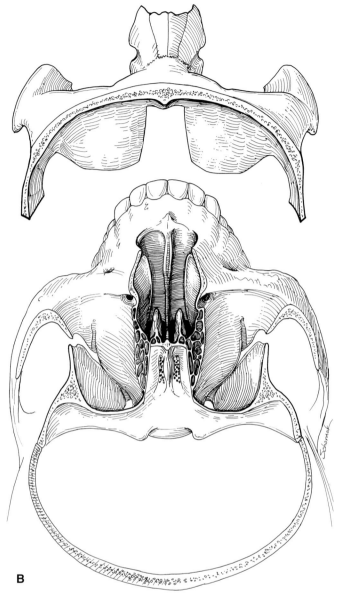

● **FIGURE 20-6.** (A) Anterior cranial fossa demonstrating the initial circumferential cribriform plate osteotomies. (**A**) anterior osteotomy; (**B**, **C**) parasagittal osteotomy; (**D**) posterior osteotomy through the planum sphenoidale. The additional lines indicate osteotomy cuts for removal of the fronto-nasal-orbital unit. (B) All osteotomy cuts, except for the posterior cut, are performed to allow removal of the fronto-nasal-orbital unit.

After tumor resection, the skull base defect may require a fat graft or bone graft before mucosal closure. Fibrin glue can then be used to seal the margins and create a watertight closure. Reconstruction then proceeds with the pre-registered plates and an acrylic splint (prepared ahead of time from dental models). The facial incisions are closed precisely to maximize the aesthetic result. The splint is left in place for 7 to 10 days and a liquid diet is recommended for 4 weeks.

Level V—Transmaxillary. This approach is indicated for moderate-sized clival tumors with superior, posterior, and inferior extensions and small to moderate-sized nasopharyngeal tumors (Figure 20-7E–G). An upper labial sulcus incision is used to expose the anterior maxilla. A LeFort I osteotomy is performed after adapting plates for later fixation, and the segment is displaced inferiorly providing adequate exposure. When more exposure is required, a midline palatal split and soft palate division on one side of the uvula is made. The two maxillary fragments can then be rotated laterally to expose the clivus (Figure 20-7G). For additional exposure, the pterygoid plates can be included on the fragments.

After tumor resection, a dermal fat graft or bone graft and fibrin glue are used to reconstruct the skull base defect. The preregistered plates and interdental splints are used to complete the facial reconstruction. The splint is left in place for 7 to 10 days and a liquid diet is recommended for 4 weeks.

Level VI—Transpalatal. This approach is indicated for small tumors of the lower clival and upper cervical

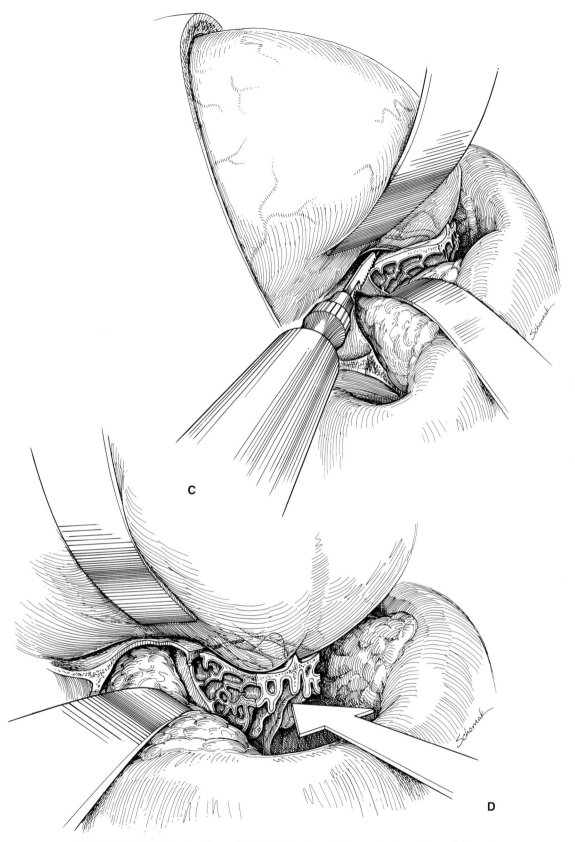

● **FIGURE 20-6.** (*continued*) (C) The final, posterior osteotomy through the planum sphenoidale is performed with appropriate retraction of the frontal lobe dura and paranasal soft tissues. (D) After the trabeculae are divided and a generous cuff of mucosa is left intact, the intact cribriform plate unit is released from the skull base. (*With permission from Barrow Neurological Institute.*)

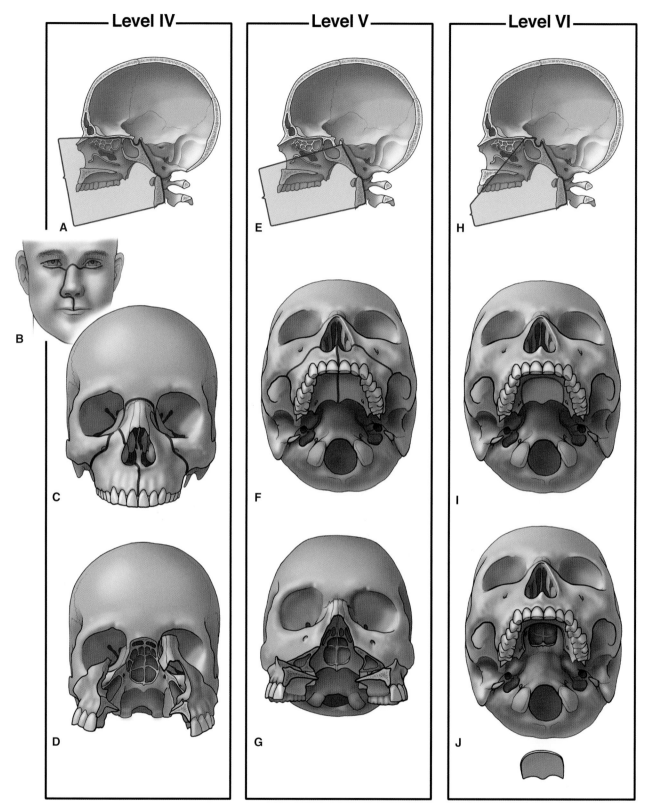

Level IV — Level V — Level VI

● **FIGURE 20-7.** Composite illustration showing the levels of exposure for the three extracranial transfacial approaches and the osteotomies required for each. (A) Level IV transnasomaxillary approach yields a wide exposure of the entire central skull base from the radix to the craniocervical junction. A similar degree of exposure can usually be obtained with a combination of the level III and level V exposures. (B) Skin incisions for the transnasomaxillary approach. (C) Level IV exposure requires a LeFort II osteotomy and then (D) splitting of the maxillary fragment. (E) Level V transmaxillary approach provides exposure of the clivus and nasopharyngeal area. (F) Level V exposure requires a LeFort I osteotomy and (G) splitting of the palate for further exposure. (H) Level VI transpalatal approach provides access to the lower clivus and upper cervical region. Level VI exposure requires an (I) osteotomy and (J) removal of the hard palate. (*With permission from Barrow Neurological Institute.*)

regions (Figure 20-7H–J). An upper labial sulcus incision is made and the nasal floor is exposed. The palatal mucosa is incised in the midline and the soft palate is divided on one side of the uvula. The mucoperiosteal flaps are then elevated, and the hard palate is osteotomized. The septum and nasal groove are separated along the nasal floor, and cuts are made in the lateral nasal wall into the antra with an osteotome. The hard palate is removed and the soft palate is retracted laterally. When more exposure is required, the vomer and perpendicular plate of the ethmoid can be removed with a rongeur.

After tumor resection, a dermal fat graft or bone graft and fibrin glue are used as indicated to reconstruct the skull base defect. The hard palate is then secured with microplates for rigid fixation. The soft tissue is repaired with absorbable sutures.

Combined Surgical Approaches

Any of the transfacial approaches may be combined to provide an overlapping range of exposure for a lesion. The combination of a level II or III and a level V approaches achieves exposure to the entire anterior cranial fossa and midline skull base. When intracranial and extracranial approaches are combined, the intracranial approach is performed first. The tumor is resected from skull base and dural integrity restored. Then the extracranial approach is performed, removing the remaining portion of the tumor. Facial reconstruction is then completed and the incisions closed.

● COMPLICATIONS

The most serious complications that are life-threatening and result in lifelong functional deficits are neurologic. Wide exposure is essential to minimize brain retraction, to allow good visualization for complete tumor resection, and to provide enough space for reconstruction of the dura with a watertight closure. While wide exposure may seem radical, it actually speeds up surgery, thus making it safer. The ISG localizing wand gives greater accuracy in localizing vital structures affected by tumor and allows the resection to be more complete.

Wound complications after skull base surgery are some of the most challenging that plastic surgeons face. The goals of reconstruction are to support the brain, contain CSF, and provide a watertight sealing of the compartment from contamination. Unfortunately, the area is often predisposed to wound healing problems due to prior surgery, irradiation, or dead space. Pericranial flaps and temporalis flaps are the first choice in helping to seal skull base defects. The frontogaleal flap leaves the forehead skin thin, predisposing it to break down, and should be used as a last resort to seal midline defects. The risk of breaking the reconstructive seal with a Valsalva maneuver is present for at least 3 months after surgery, and possibly lifelong. A flimsy reconstructive flap and granulation tissue will not seal the defect effectively and hold up to forces created by a Valsalva maneuver, often resulting in infectious complications. Therefore, an adequate reconstruction is critical.

A CSF leak can doom any skull base reconstruction and can occur despite ideal repair. During the early phase, a lumbar drain is used routinely for 3 to 5 days along with prophylactic antibiotic therapy. If the leak fails to resolve after this time period, localization studies and exploration of the wound is undertaken. Direct repair is preferred for small defects if the adjacent tissues are of good quality. Reinforcement with a fat or muscle graft or a local flap, if available, and fibrin glue is ideal. If the defect is large, or is due to necrosis or flap infection, debridement and secondary reconstruction is performed. Fastidious attention to detail in the reconstruction of the skull base is essential in prevention a CSF leak. Close postoperative surveillance and early intervention are critical to successful management of a postoperative CSF leak.

Malocclusion after level IV and V approaches is usually avoidable with precise technique and adequate preoperative preparation. In patients who undergo a two-piece transmaxillary (level V) approach, a fixation plate or lag screw placed between the two fragments is essential. A plate can be placed on the nasal floor anteriorly or across the anterior nasal spine region. Postoperative intermaxillary fixation is not routinely used. If a postoperative malocclusion occurs and is not correctable with orthodontic treatment, secondary osteotomy at an appropriate time postoperatively is necessary to correct it.

Speech abnormalities can occur not only because of neurologic complications, but also due to a palatal split. Spontaneous improvement is usually noted as the soft palate and nasopharynx heal. Velopharyngeal insufficiency can result secondary to irregularities and concavity of the clival and vertebral junction in the region of the nasopharynx. Speech evaluation with nasoendoscopy can aid in diagnosing the cause.

A palatal fistula can occur after a palatal split and is usually related to surgical technique. Secondary repair may be necessary using palatal flaps to line the nasal and oral sides of the fistula.

Approaches that require an osteotomy near the nasolacrimal duct or require an actual transection of the duct may result in epiphora postoperatively. The surgeon should look for duct disruption during reconstruction and repair and cannulate as indicated. When transection is required, the duct can be repaired over tubes during reconstruction. If postoperative epiphora is persistent, workup is indicated and occasionally a dacryocystorhinostomy is needed.

Orbital volume must be restored to maintain symmetry and globe position. This is accomplished with anatomic reconstruction of the orbital walls. When a large portion of the orbit is removed during resection of the tumor, this reconstruction can prove difficult. If enophthalmos occurs postoperatively, secondary reconstruction of the orbit with autogenous bone grafts is indicated. Strabismus can occur after orbital surgery and may require surgical correction.

● OUTCOMES ASSESSMENT

Although skull base tumors remain challenging and have been associated, in the past, with formidable morbidity and mortality, the emergence of cranial facial disassembly has provided an avenue of safe, wide exposure of this critical region. The past several decades have shown progressively improving survival rates with curative skull base resection. Furthermore, the concomitant evolving techniques and

technology offered by a comprehensive skull base team continues to offer proficient management of such complex cases. There has been some promise that transnasal endoscopic techniques may be successful in managing a subset of patients in a minimally invasive manner.[11] Ultimately, the skull base surgeon can often offer a versatile treatment strategy, and thus the patient can face his or her treatment with confidence.

REFERENCES

1. Beals SP, Joganic EF. Transfacial exposure of anterior cranial fossa and clival tumors. *BNI Q.* 1992;8(4):2–18.

2. Sandor GK, Charles DA, Lawson VG, et al. Transoral approach to the nasopharynx and clivus using the LeFort I osteotomy with midpalatal split. *Int J Maxillofac Surg.* 1990;19(6):352–355.

3. Spetzler RF, Pappas CT. Management of anterior skull base tumors. *Clin Neurosurg.* 1991;37:490–501.

4. Cocke EW Jr, Robertson JH, Robertson JT, et al. The extended maxillotomy and subtotal maxillectomy for excision of skull base tumors. *Arch Otolaryngol Head Neck Surg.* 1990;116:92–104.

5. Brown AM, Lavery KM, Millar BG. The transfacial approach to the postnasal space and retromaxillary structures. *Br J Oral Maxillofacial Surg.* 1991;29:230–236.

6. Weissler MC. Transoral approaches to the skull base. *Ear Nose Throat J.* 1991;70(9):587–592.

7. Osguthorpe JD, Patel S. Craniofacial approaches to tumors of the anterior skull base. *Otolaryngol Clin North Am.* 2001;34(6):1123–1142,ix.

8. Beals SP, Joganic EF. In: Dickman C, Spetzler RF, Sonntag VKH, et al. *Surgery of the Craniovertebral Junction.* New York: Thieme; 1998:395–418.

9. Beals SP, Hamilton MG, Joganic EF, et al. Classification of transfacial approaches in the treatment of tumors of the anterior skull base and clivus. *Plast Surg Forum.* 1993;16:211–213.

10. Spetzler RF, Herman JM, Beals S, et al. Preservation of olfaction in anterior craniofacial approaches. *J Neurosurg.* 1993;79(1):48–51.

11. Solares CA, Ong YK, SNyderman CH. Transnasal endoscopic skull base surgery: what are the limits? *Curr Opin Otolaryngol Head Neck Surg.* 2010;18:1–7.

chapter 21

Overview of Facial Fractures

Alexandre Marchac, MD / *Jeffrey D. Larson, MD* / *Stephen M. Warren, MD*

● INTRODUCTION

In the latter half of the twentieth century, radiologic and implant advancements substantially improved the diagnosis, management, and treatment of facial fractures. In addition, the widespread acceptance of the concept of facial buttresses simplified complex fracture management. The bones of the face are lightened by pneumatic cavities (sinuses) and reinforced by vertical and horizontal pillars (ie, buttresses). These buttresses are linked to the cranial base either directly or indirectly. The buttresses provide support as well as projection for the overlying soft tissues.

The buttress concept does not change the classic anatomy of the face, but the concept is surgically important. Buttresses not only represent areas of bony condensation that conveniently hold screws and plates, but anatomic reduction of fractured buttresses will restore facial contour. Following Paul Mason's work on the structural pillars of the facial skeleton, Gruss and Mackinnon described four paired vertical buttresses in the face: (1) anterior medial or nasomaxillary, (2) anterior lateral or zygomaticomaxillary, (3) posterior or pterygomaxillary buttress, and (4) posterior vertical or mandibular ramus. Anatomic reduction of these vertical buttresses restores facial height. Of note, the posterior vertical maxillary buttress can be ignored if the two anterior maxillary (medial and lateral) and the vertical mandibular buttresses (ramus) are restored. Four paired transverse buttresses maintain facial profile and width to the face: (1) upper transverse maxillary (orbital floor), (2) lower transverse maxillary (palate), (3) upper transverse mandibular, and (4) lower transversal mandibular buttresses. Adequate anatomic reduction of these buttresses restores facial width and provides functional support for the globes and teeth.

● PATIENT EVALUATION

Kelley[1] showed that in a level 1 urban trauma center, the mechanism for facial fractures where largely dominated by assault and interpersonal violence (50%), followed by motor vehicle accidents (28%), gunshot wounds (13%), fall (5%), automobile-pedestrian accidents (3%), contact sports (2%), and stab wounds (2%). Drugs and/or alcohol commonly fuel these traumatic events.

In a conscious patient, the examination begins with a history of the event, with particular attention paid to loss of consciousness, symptoms of intracranial trauma (headache, confusion, etc), medications, and last meal. The examination of the face begins with a general inspection for obvious deformity or asymmetry. All bony surfaces should be palpated: forehead, superior and inferior orbital rims, nasal bones, cheek bones, and borders of the mandible (Figure 21-1). The auditory canals should be evaluated for hemotympanum, which would indicate a skull base fracture. Any face examination must include documentation of vision and extraocular movements; this can be done with a pocket Snellen chart in the awake patient and response to light in the unconscious or sedated patient. The surgeon should also inspect the nose and look for a septal hematoma, which should be incised and drained to prevent septal necrosis. The intraoral area must be examined for step-offs or lacerations, and the examiner must take care to protect his or her hands during this examination, as the unconscious or combative patient may bite down on an examiner's finger (Figure 21-2). Occlusion is to be assessed by asking the patient to clench his teeth and describe any abnormalities. Maxillofacial instability, indicating a possible LeFort injury, is evaluated by manipulating the upper dentition (Figure 21-3). Sensory function

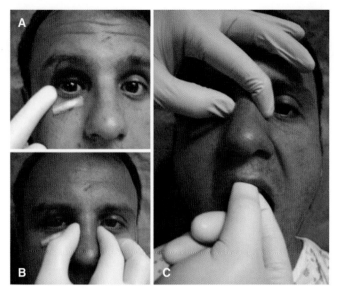

● FIGURE 21-1. Inspection and palpation of patient with facial injuries. (A) Palpation of inferior orbital rim; (B) determining stability of the nasal pyramid; (C) determining stability of the midface.

(cranial nerve V) can be assessed by lightly touching the patient on both sides of the face and assessing for symmetrical sensation. Motor function (cranial nerve VII) is assessed by asking the patient to raise his eyebrows, smile and frown, and observing for symmetry.

Most imaging requirements for diagnosing facial fractures are met by the maxillofacial computed tomography (CT) scan and should be obtained before contacting subspecialty services. Thanks to the technological advances of modern imaging, there is little indication for plain films, although isolated mandible fractures can be adequately imaged by low Townes and panorex x-rays. Nevertheless, panorex requires the patient to sit during the examination, and is commonly unavailable at night.

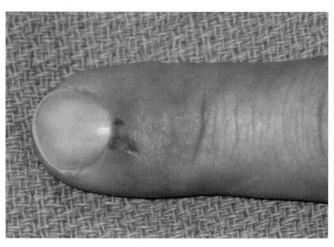

● FIGURE 21-2. Injury sustained during intraoral examination. Note right and left central incision marks on the index finger eponychium.

Computed tomography has become the gold standard for imaging the craniofacial skeleton in facial trauma. Panorex radiograph is useful in diagnosis of mandibular injuries, but it requires a cooperative patient. Two-dimensional CT and three-dimensional reconstructions allow precise diagnosis and valuable tools in preoperative planning.

First developed for dental purposes, cone beam computed tomography (CBCT), where a cone-shaped beam captures a cylindrical volume much faster than conventional slice CT (10–17 s), with a lower radiation exposure, and with less metallic artifacts than CT, yields some very promising applications in facial trauma, including intraoperative imaging.[2] Two-dimensional and three-dimensional CT navigators are now available to the surgeon in the operating room. Software like Osirix, a free, open-source software for navigating in multidimensional, DICOM (Digital Imaging and Communications in Medicine) images, allows

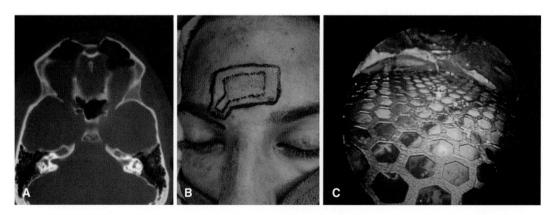

● FIGURE 21-3. Endoscopic treatment of depressed frontal sinus fracture. (A) Axial CT image demonstrating depressed anterior table frontal sinus fracture; (B) dashed inner line marks the borders of the fracture. The solid outer line marks the estimated size of the titanium mesh. Note the right medial eyebrow incision used to allow elevation of the fracture fragments. (C) Endoscopic image of titanium mesh in situ. Note a screw has been placed transcutaneously to affix the fracture fragments to the titanium mesh.

the surgeon to do, on his laptop, most of the complex 3D maneuvers that radiologist perform on desktop computers.[3] Overall, these technological improvements in craniofacial imaging allow better preoperative planning and intraoperative control over the reduction of the bone fragments. This is particularly useful in panfacial "smashed" fractures, when all anchor points have been displaced.

● PATIENT PREPARATION

Treatment of facial fractures should be scheduled in the days following injury (2–3 d) as early as possible. A team approach is necessary in the case of multisystem injuries to coordinate a long facial reconstruction before critical systemic complications occur such as pulmonary, hepatic, or renal dysfunction. Moreover, the surgeon should not wait for the patient's neurologic prognosis to be determined, because doing so often results in untreated fractures and secondary facial deformities. If thoracic or abdominal surgery is required, facial reconstruction can be delayed. Mandibulomaxillary fixation (MMF), however, can easily be combined with chest or abdominal surgery in order to initiate the treatment of panfacial/midfacial injuries to stabilize the fractures and reduce blood loss.

If spine injury has not been ruled out by physical examination and MRI (ligamentous injuries cannot be detected on CT scan), the cervical spine must be immobilized during the operation. Nasotracheal intubation facilitates MMF, but oronasal bleeding can cause fiberoptic intubation to be difficult. Tracheostomy may be necessary for airway protection.

In addition to the initial eye examination, the surgeon should make a careful assessment of the patient's pupil diameter and responsiveness prior to incision. This will allow for comparison at the end of the operation. Preoperative assessment of lower lid laxity and position is important. Patients with lower lid laxity are best treated with a lateral canthopexy and/or Frost stitch to avoid ectropion and sclera show. When operating near the orbit, it is important to document function of the intraocular muscles. Rectus muscle entrapment should be diagnosed by a forced duction test before and after the procedure.

● TREATMENT

Frontal Sinus Fractures

Frontal sinus fractures occur in 5% to 12% of all facial fractures and are associated with 32% of panfacial/maxillary fractures. Of the patients with frontal sinus fractures, 35% present with concomitant orbital fractures, 17% with zygomatic fractures, and 15% with naso-orbitoethmoid (NOE) fractures. Frontal sinus fractures may be considered in four categories: (1) isolated anterior table fractures; (2) combined anterior and posterior table fractures; (3) fractures with nasofrontal duct injury; and (4) isolated posterior table fractures with or without dura mater or brain injury.

Frontal sinus fracture patterns that include the anterior table will induce a contour deformity of the forehead. The subjective degree of comminution, depression, and contour deformity will determine the treatment strategy. Minor injuries may be observed. More modest injuries will require bone fragment elevation. Traditionally, a coronal incision has been used to gain access to the anterior table. Recently, the endoscopic approach has become popular.[4] Isolated anterior wall fractures can be repaired using the endoscope. Small scalp incisions (usually two) are placed 1cm behind the hairline and a third incision is sometimes placed in the medial aspect of the eyebrow (Figure 21-3). Dissecting in a subperiosteal plane, the fracture fragment is repositioned using a threaded fragment manipulator (a long, self-drilling, 2.0-mm screw inserted through a small stab incision on the forehead) or using an elevator inserted through the medial eyebrow incision. The fragment is fixed with a miniplate (titanium or resorbable) and self-tapping screws.[4] If the fracture is severely comminuted, endoscopic reduction and fixation of the outer table is unlikely to succeed and a coronal approach should be used. In unrepaired fractures resulting in a contour deformity of the forehead, Mueller proposes a delayed endoscopic approach (>3 months) to camouflage the defect with hydroxyapatite cement, porous polyethylene custom implants or 0.85-mm porous polyethylene sheets inserted endoscopically.[4] Caution should be exercised against placing alloplastic materials in or around open or potentially communicating sinuses.

The importance of combined anterior/posterior table factures as well as isolated posterior table fractures lies in the presence or absence of concomitant nasofrontal duct and/or dura mater injuries. The drainage to the frontal sinus is provided by ostia which are located bilaterally in the posteromedial aspect of the frontal sinus floor. These ostia drain caudally into the nasal cavity by means of the frontal recess or nasofrontal duct and empty into the middle meatus. Determining whether the nasofrontal ducts have been obstructed by the traumatic event can be difficult. The surgeon should examine CT looking for comminution in the superior portion of the uncinate process (anterior border of the nasofrontal duct), the superior portion of the bulla ethmoidalis (posterior border of the nasofrontal duct), the conchal plate (medial border of the nasofrontal duct), and the suprainfundibular plate (lateral border of the nasofrontal duct). If the nasofrontal ducts appear to be patent, then the anterior/posterior table fracture pattern can be treated as an isolated anterior table fracture (if there is no dural injury). If the nasofrontal ducts appear to be patent, then the isolated posterior table fracture can be observed, unless, again, there is a dural injury.

When the nasofrontal ducts are injured, the surgeon has five options: (1) ablation, (2) exenteration, (3) frontoethmoidectomy, (4) obliteration, or (5) cranialization. When the anterior and posterior tables are comminuted, *ablation* of the frontal sinus can be performed. Ablation (or the Riedel procedure) is the removal of both the anterior and posterior tables of the frontal sinus.[5] While effective, this procedure results in an unacceptable aesthetic result and, therefore, should be reserved for select cases. *Exenteration* is the removal of the anterior table of the frontal sinus.[6] Like the Riedel procedure, exenteration is effective, but it results in an unacceptable aesthetic result.

In 1921, Lynch described an external *frontoethmoidectomy* performed through a relatively small and aesthetically acceptable curvilinear incision located half way between medial canthus and nasal dorsum.[6] The Lynch procedure provided access to the ipsilateral frontal sinus enabling the surgeons to create a frontonasal communication by removing a portion of the nasal septum and nasal floor of the frontal sinus. In the mid-1990s, the Lothrop and modified-Lothrop procedures were introduced. These endonasal procedures enabled the removal of the inferior portion of the interfrontal septum, the superior part of the nasal septum, and the frontal sinus floor to the orbits bilaterally. The lamina papyracea and posterior walls of the frontal sinus remained intact. The endonasal frontoethmoidectomy can restore adequate drainage of the frontal sinus, but does not provide access for reconstruction of a comminuted, depressed anterior table.

Obliteration is the complete removal of frontal sinus mucosa.[7] Typically, this is performed by removing the anterior table, staining the frontal sinus mucosa with methylene blue, and then burring the sinus to remove the mucosa and their podocytic invaginations into the vascular pits of Breschet (Figure 21-4). The nasofrontal ducts are occluded with bone, fat, muscle, fascia, or pericranial tissue, and anterior table is affixed orthotopically with resorbable or titanium miniplates.

When the posterior table is comminuted and the nasofrontal outflow tracts are obstructed, *cranialization* is a simple procedure that allows the removal of the frontal sinus and preservation of the forehead contour (Figure 21-5).[8] After performing an anterior table frontal sinusotomy, the comminuted posterior table is removed, the nasofrontal ducts are occluded with bone, fat, muscle, fascia, or pericranial tissue, and the anterior table is affixed orthotopically with resorbable or titanium miniplates.[9] The space formerly occupied by the frontal sinus is replaced by the anterior expansion of the frontal lobes.

Frontobasal Fractures

Frontobasal fractures result from high-energy trauma. These skull based fractures are commonly found in association with NOE, non-LeFort, and LeFort fractures. Frontobasal fractures can lead to significant neurological morbidity. Manson et al.[10] recently established a frontobasal classification scheme: Type I fractures are isolated linear cranial base fractures; type II fractures are vertical linear fractures of the frontal bone (skull vault) and base; and type III fractures are characterized by comminution of the entire lateral and frontal skull vault and orbital roof. The incidence of cerebrospinal fluid (CSF) fistula and

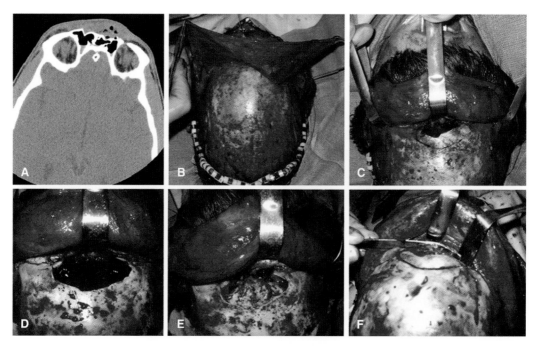

● **FIGURE 21-4.** Obliteration of the frontal sinus. (A) Axial CT image demonstrating anterior table frontal sinus fracture with comminution of the nasofrontal ducts; (B) elevation of a pericranial flap. (C) The perimeter of the anterior table has been marked in blue. (D) The anterior table of the frontal sinus has been removed and the mucosa has been stained with methylene blue. (E) The frontal sinus mucosa has been removed with a bur. (F) The comminuted nasal frontal ducts have been packed with bone; the pericranial flap has been placed in the frontal sinus, and the anterior table has been replaced.

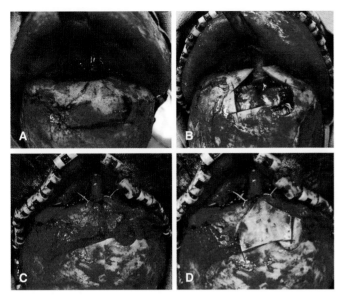

● **FIGURE 21-5.** Cranialization of the frontal sinus.
(A) Perimeter of the frontal sinus outlined in blue. (B) After removal of the anterior table, the comminuted fragments of the posterior table were removed and the dural injury was repaired. (C) Bone was used to occlude the comminuted nasofrontal ducts and pericranial flaps were placed into the space formerly occupied by the frontal sinus. (D) The anterior table was been replaced and the displaced nasal bones have been temporarily wired to the glabella.

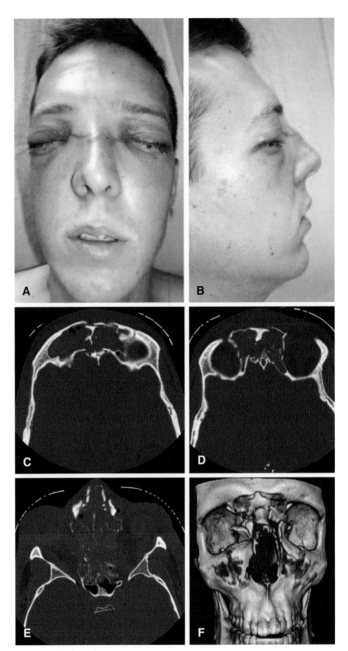

● **FIGURE 21-6.** Patient with naso-orbital-ethmoidal injury. (A) The patient demonstrates telecanthus. (B) The patient demonstrates a collapse nasal dorsum, forehead irregularity, and an obtuse nasolabial angle. (C) Axial CT scan demonstrating anterior and posterior table frontal sinus fractures. Note the nasal bones can be seen in the frontal sinus. (D) Axial CT scan demonstrating medial orbital wall and ethmoid fractures. (E) Axial CT scan demonstrating nasal fractures and lateral displacement of the canthal bearing segments. (F) Three dimensional CT demonstrating NOE fracture.

meningitis, the two most acute deleterious outcomes of frontobasal fractures, relies heavily on the fracture pattern and associated midfacial injury (eg, LeFort II/III and NOE fractures). "Impure" fractures account for half of all frontobasal fractures and for more than two thirds of complications. Half of all types II and III frontobasal fractures have an associated NOE fracture in comparison with only every fourth type I fracture. Naso-orbitoethmoid fractures are more likely to produce a complication than LeFort fractures because of its anatomical relationship to the nasofrontal outflow tract.

Naso-Orbitoethmoid Fractures

Clinically, NOE fractures differ from simple nasal fractures by an apparent telecanthus (increased distance between the internal canthi), globe malposition, and a loss of nasal projection in profile (Figure 21-6). The medial canthal region, the ethmoids and the medial orbital walls are fractured. This corresponds to a disruption of the medial and upper transverse maxillary buttresses. The medial canthal ligament can be avulsed from its osseous insertion, in the region of the lacrymal fossa, causing lateral drifting of the internal canthus and loss of the normal shadow definition of the brow-nose line. The Manson classification of NOE fractures is based on the degree of injury to the medial canthal attachment (Figure 21-7). A type I fracture involves a large bone fragment, displaced only inferiorly at the infraorbital rim and

piriform margin. Type I fractures can commonly be anatomically reduced and plated. A type II fracture involves a comminuted fracture with the medial canthal tendon still attached to a bony fragment. Type II fracture fragments are usually too small to anatomically reduce and plate. These fractures typically require transnasal wiring.

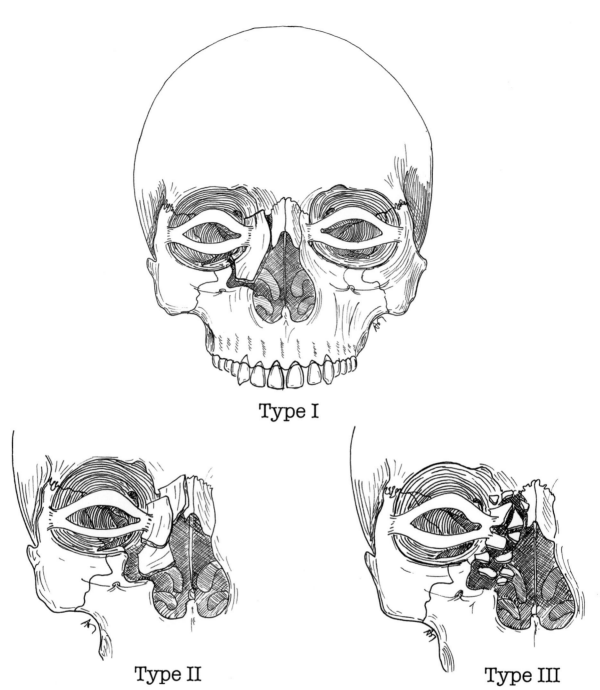

Type I

Type II

Type III

● **FIGURE 21-7.** The classification of NOE fractures is based on the degree of injury to the medial canthal attachment. (A) Type I fracture involves a large bone fragment (open reduction and internal fixation). (B) Type II fracture involves a comminuted fracture with the medial canthal tendon still attached to a bony fragment (transnasal wiring). (C) Type III NOE fractures, the medial canthal ligament is either avulsed from its osseous attachments or the bone fragments are severely comminuted (transnasal wiring). (*Adapted from Markowitz BL, Manson PN, Sargent L, et al. Management of the medial canthal tendon in nasoethmoid orbital fractures: the importance of the central fragment in classification and treatment. Plast Reconstr Surg. 1991;87(5):843–53.*)

In type III NOE fractures, the medial canthal ligament are either avulsed from there osseous attachments or the bone fragments are severely comminuted. Either way, a type III NOE fracture requires transnasal reduction.

In addition to restoring medial canthal position, a patient with an NOE fracture requires reconstruction of his/her nose. Often, the nasal bones can be retrieved from the ethmoid or frontal sinuses, anatomically reduced, and

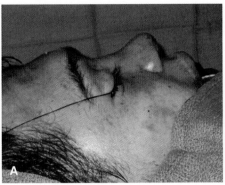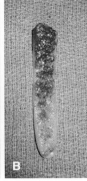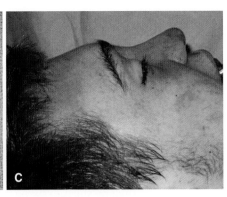

● **FIGURE 21-8.** Cantilever bone graft treatment of a patient with a NOE fracture. (A) After anatomic reduction of the type I NOE fracture fragments, the patient's comminuted nasal bones could not be reconstructed. Note the collapse of the nasal dorsum. (B) A unicortical cranial bone graft was harvested and fashioned to reconstruct the nasal dorsum. (C) After placement of the cantilever bone graft the nasal dorsum has been restored.

plated. When the nasal bones are comminuted, a cantilever bone graft is necessary to rebuild the nasal dorsum. The cantilever bone graft can be harvested from the cranium or rib (Figure 21-8). The bone graft is cantilevered from the inferior aspect of the glabella and tucked under the lower lateral cartilages.

The medial orbital walls must also be reconstructed. The surgeon may choose alloplastic materials or autogenous bone to rebuild the medial orbital walls (see below). While the lacrymal drainage system may be injured in an NOE fracture, the duct is typically not explored. If the canaliculus is lacerated, it may be repaired over a silastic tube.

Orbital Fractures

Orbital fractures alone or in conjunction with other facial skeletal fractures are the second most commonly encountered midfacial fractures (nasal fractures are most common). Orbital floor fractures can cause diplopia, dystopia, and enophthalmos. While orbital apex fractures are rare, patients can suffer superior orbital fissure syndrome or orbital apex syndrome. In such cases, a combined endovascular and intracranial approach may be necessary to treat an injured carotid artery, decompress the optic nerve, and repair the dural injury.

Orbital floor fractures can be approached through a lower lid incision or endoscopically. At least four access routes to the orbital floor pass through the lower lid: (1) the subciliary (composite skin-muscle flap) incision was described by Converse in 1944; (2) the subtarsal (muscle-splitting incision) described by Converse in the 1960s; (3) the transconjunctival incision first described by Bourquet in 1924, but popularized by Converse and Tessier in the 1970s; and finally, (4) the lower eyelid–cheek junction incision.

As a general rule, in acute trauma, subciliary incisions should be avoided because of a higher risk of ectropion.[1]

Nevertheless, if one chooses a subciliary incision, the nonstepped variant (skin-muscle flap) is preferred over the stepped (skin flap with preservation of a orbicularis muscle sling) because of the risk of skin loss in contused eyelids. (In secondary cases, when circulation to the skin may be expected to be near normal, the stepped incision provides less risk of ectropion than the nonstepped incision). The subtarsal approach should be avoided in young patients, where the transcutaneous incision cannot be camouflaged in a natural skin crease.

Many surgeons favor the transconjunctival incision. A lateral canthotomy may be added to increase lid mobilization and exposure. The transconjunctival incision is made 3 to 4 mm above the fornix, to avoid entropion. The transconjunctival approach can either be preseptal or retroseptal. In the later, the orbital fat is exposed and must constantly be reclined. Our preference goes to the preseptal approach, where the periosteum is incised 2 mm below the orbital floor and elevated to expose the orbital floor. Two concomitant procedures are added before skin closure: (1) a lateral canthopexy (if lateral canthotomy was performed) and (2) a cheek resuspension.[11] Regarding the choice of material for the repair, as usual in plastic surgery, repair should be performed following the Gillies principle of replacing like with like. When the skull is readily available (eg, in a complex panfacial fracture, where a coronal incision was necessary), a cortical graft can be harvested from the outer table of the calvaria. Nevertheless, substitutes have been developed, such as polyethylene with incorporated titanium mesh, PSD plaque, Medpor, etc. The surgeon should explain the risk of and benefits of autologous versus alloplastic reconstructions.

The lower eyelid/cheek junction incision is positioned directly over the bony orbital rim. While this approach is faster than other eyelid incisions and is associated with minimal risk of postoperative eyelid malposition, it results in a visible cutaneous scar and can be associated with lower eyelid edema. Consequently, most surgeons avoid this incision except in patients with significant rhytides and minimal concerns of an external scar.

The endoscopic approach can also be used to repair the orbital floor and medial wall fractures. The most accepted approach to the orbital floor goes through the maxillary sinus and visualizes the orbital floor from beneath.[4] An upper sulcus incision followed by a maxillary antrostomy gives adequate exposure to trapdoor fractures and blowout fractures located between the infraorbital nerve and the medial wall of the orbit. The floor is then replaced by a 0.85 mm thick porous polyethylene sheet or by bioresorbable sheets (polydiaxone) or by a titanium mesh.[4]

Orbital fractures rarely entrap the inferior rectus muscle; however, the authors of this chapter would consider the treatment of a trapped inferior rectus muscle analogous to treatment of any other ischemic muscle. That is to say, inferior rectus muscle entrapment in the orbital floor is a surgical emergency.

While rare, orbital floor fractures in children will more commonly entrap the inferior rectus than an orbital floor fracture in an adult. In children, it is hypothesized that the flexible orbital floor fractures and is displaced inferiorly, allowing infraorbital tissue to enter the fracture site. The orbital floor trapdoor then recoils, trapping the inferior rectus. Children with an entrapped inferior rectus muscle will have upward gaze restriction and diplopia. The CT may demonstrate an entrapped inferior rectus muscle, but this is maybe equivocal (Figure 21-9). The surgeon may look for additional signs and symptoms to make the diagnosis. When the inferior rectus muscle is trapped, the ophthalmic division of the trigeminal nerve is stimulated

and, through the reticular formation, it transmits a signal to the vagus nerve, which then carries the efferent impulse to the stomach, producing nausea.[12] Cohen and Garrett studied 29 children with orbital floor fractures and found that one fourth of the children had nausea/vomiting, and half had trapdoor fractures. Seventeen percent of patients had entrapment of the inferior rectus. The positive predictive value of nausea/vomiting with a trapdoor fracture for entrapment was 83.3% ($P=0.002$; Fisher exact test).[12]

Isolated orbital roof fractures are rare in adults, but more common in children. Patients with orbital roof fractures are at risk of retrobulbar hematoma, optic nerve impingement by a bone fragment, and dural tear. The surgeon should rule out superior orbital fissure syndrome and orbital apex syndrome.

Orbitozygomatic Fractures

Clinically, the zygomaticomaxillary complex fracture deformity presents as a loss of cheek projection and enlargement of facial width. The zygoma is commonly referred to as a "tripod," but it actually articulates with four bones (ie, maxilla, frontal bone, temporal bone, and sphenoid) and, therefore, is more correctly referred to as a "tetrapod." Because the zygoma has four sutures and two orthogonal buttresses (ie, the lateral maxillary and the superior transversal maxillary buttresses), a fracture along the zygomaticomaxillary suture may include the inferior orbital foramen. If the zygomaticosphenoid suture and the two buttresses are not anatomically reduced, there will be a rotational deformity that increases the orbital volume.

Most fractures can be treated through eyelid incisions and gingivobuccal sulcus incisions (Figure 21-10). A coronal incision is required only if the infraorbital rim and zygomaticomaxillary (superior transverse) buttresses are so comminuted that adequate alignment requires arch visualization.[1] The gingivobuccal sulcus incision is performed first. Subperiosteal dissection of the medial and lateral maxillary buttresses is carried all the way to the inferior orbital rim, taking care to identify and preserve the inferior orbital nerve (V2). The dissection of the inferior orbital rim extends laterally, revealing the displaced fracture. A first attempt of reduction should be made at this point with a blunt elevator inserted beneath the zygomatic arch. In case of successful reduction, a miniplate (L shape) will usually be sufficient to ensure fixation. If reduction is not optimal, a lower lid incision should be performed to allow visualization of the fracture. If the zygomaticotemporal suture is displaced, a lateral extension of the upper blepharoplasty incision will allow exposure, reduction, and fixation of the fracture (steel wire or 1.0-mm miniplate). This should be done before fixing the inferior orbital rim, to serve as a reference point while still allowing rotational control. Using a Caroll-Girard screw placed in the lateral portion of the zygoma through the lower lid incision or by

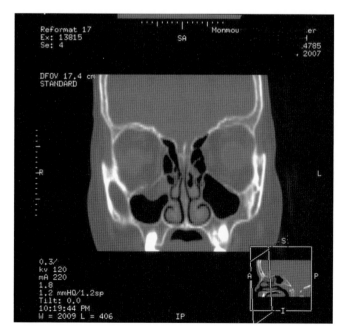

● FIGURE 21-9. CT suspicious of entrapped inferior rectus muscle. This child presented with nausea and vomiting. Altogether, this highly favored entrapment, indicating urgent operation (compartment syndrome).

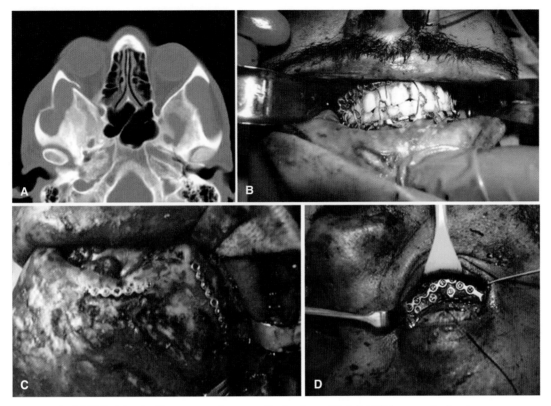

● FIGURE 21-10. Treatment of zygomatic fracture. (A) Axial CT image of a fracture right zygoma. Note zygomatic arch fracture. (B) Maxillomandibular fixation was performed to establish centric occlusion. (C) Titanium miniplate fixation of the zygomatic arch and lateral orbital rim. (D) Inferior orbital rim and orbital floor plates were used.

planting a Ginestet hook in the inferior portion of the zygoma, the inferior orbital rim is then realigned. The lateral orbital wall should be monitored before fixation, to prevent a rotational deformity. Miniplates (1.5 mm) and screws should be placed on the superior aspect of the infraorbital rim rather than on the anterior aspect to avoid palpability. An L miniplate is placed on the lateral maxillary buttress. The orbital floor fracture should then be addressed with a cortical bone graft or an implant (polyethylene with incorporated titanium mesh, PSD plaque, or Medpor).

One should expect an overcorrection of the globe on the operated side at the end of the surgery because of the swelling caused by the trauma and the surgery. If the globes are in identical position at the end of the surgery, enophthalmos will likely occur. The extensive subperiosteal undermining, necessary for the exposure of zygomaticomaxillary fractures, may be a cause of postoperative ptosis of the cheek with traction on the lower lid, therefore causing ectropion.

Cheek resuspension should be performed at the end of the procedure; either by suturing the cheek periosteum to the orbital periosteum on the inferior orbital rim, or by transosseous stitches. The endoscopic approach has not yet gained acceptance in zygomatic arch fractures, because of the difficulty to fix the arch in place with miniplates and the risk of transient frontal nerve palsy.[4]

Nasal Fractures

Nasal fractures are the most common facial fractures. Care should be taken when reducing nasal fractures, because torrential epistaxis and airway obstruction are avoidable complications. Local anesthesia (1:200.000 adrenaline + 0.5% lidocaine) and oxymetazoline gauze are used to control bleeding. A septal hematoma must be diagnosed and drained to avoid septal necrosis and its sequelae, septal perforation, and saddle nose deformity. A deviated septum must be placed back into its original position. A septal Doyle splint and trans septal ("quilting") stitches maintain the septum in place and prevent recurrence of hematoma. The fractures are reduced with a blunt instrument (reversed scalpel handle). In case of greenstick fractures, it is important to complete the fracture. The fragment must be mobilized freely to avoid relapse. In any case, patients must be warned that 50% will require secondary procedure to correct airway obstruction or residual deformity.

Maxillary (LeFort) Fractures

In 1901, René LeFort described patterns of fractures that separated the maxilla from the skull base. LeFort fractures occur when the pterygoid plates are disrupted from the posterior maxilla (pterygomaxillary dysjunction), disrupting the posterior vertical buttress. If the inferior aspects of the medial and lateral maxillary buttresses are fractured at or below the level of the piriform, the maxillary arch (lower transversal maxillary buttress) is set free from the skull base (*LeFort I fracture*). If the inferior lateral maxillary buttress (zygomaticomaxillary suture) and the superior medial maxillary buttress (frontomaxillary suture) are fractured, then the entire maxilla is set free from the skull base (*LeFort II fracture*). If the upper transverse maxillary buttress (zygomatic arch), superior lateral maxillary buttress (frontozygomatic), and superior medial maxillary buttress (maxillofrontal) are fractured, then craniofacial separation has occurred (*LeFort III fracture*). Patients often combine LeFort I, II, and III asymmetric fractures. The hard palate can be fractured sagittally or parasagittally, resulting in a widening of the maxillary arch, causing malocclusion. Sagittal palatal fracture can also explain a unilaterally displaced LeFort fracture.

Treatment of midface fractures should focus on restoration of the patient's baseline dental occlusion and reestablishing the key buttresses of the midface. In severely comminuted fractures, temporary MMF is useful before plating the two bone fragments. Intraoral cortical bone screws are a valid alternative to Erich arch bar and are placed much faster. Nevertheless, the surgeon should be careful not to injure the dental roots while placing the screws. In LeFort I fractures, an intraoral superior sulcus incision provides good visualization of the fracture line. In severely comminuted fractures with bone impaction, corticocancellous bone grafting should be performed immediately to restore maxilla height. Unlike mandibular fractures, muscular tractions are minimal on the maxilla. Therefore, miniplates are sufficient to assure fixation. Resorbable devices are widely used in pediatric craniofacial surgery, but Dorri et al. showed that there is so far no evidence supporting superiority of resorbable material over titanium plates and screws in facial fractures.[13]

In LeFort II fractures, a combination of intraoral superior sulcus incision and lower lid incision is necessary to ensure proper reduction and fixation of the inferior lateral maxillary buttress (zygomaticomaxillary suture) and the superior medial maxillary buttress (frontomaxillary suture). Associated fractures (orbital floor especially) are treated simultaneously by the same incisions. Care must be taken to avoid injury to the lacrymal duct.

In LeFort III fractures, a coronal approach is necessary to expose the root of the nasal pyramid, the zygoma at the zygomaticofrontal suture, the zygomatic arch and the lateral and medial walls of the orbit. The infraorbital rim is explored through a lower eyelid incision, which provides exposure for the medial maxillary buttress fixation. After careful assessment of the dental occlusion, open reduction and internal fixation with microplates and screws is performed. In severely impacted fractures, immediate bone grafting is necessary to restore the height and the width of the face, and especially the nasal dorsum.

Mandible Fractures

Mandible fracture patterns are influenced by the force and direction of impact. For example, Fridrich and associates reported the frequency of mandible fractures in adults according to anatomic location: body (29%), condyle (26%), and angle (25%). Symphyseal fractures accounted for 17% of all mandibular fractures, whereas fractures of the ramus (4%) and coronoid process (1%) occurred less frequently.[14] In automobile accidents, the condylar region was the most common fractured site. In motorcycle accidents, the symphysis was fractured most often. When assault was the cause of injury, the angle was most commonly fractured.[14]

Children have distinctly different fracture patterns than adults. The younger child has more soft tissue cushioning and the mandible tends to be smaller and relatively more protected. Moreover, the force generated in most childhood falls is low. When a child falls, the force of impact tends to be directed at the chin and transmitted to the condylar heads, which sustain a crush-type injury. In Thoren's 1992 study, the condylar region was the most common location of fracture in all pediatric age groups, accounting for 60% of all fractures.[15] In 1993, Posnick et al. reported that most pediatric mandibular fractures occurred at the condyle (55%), followed by the parasymphysial region (27%), then the body (9%), and angle (8%).[16] As the patient ages, the relative incidence of condylar fractures decreases and fractures of the body and angle increase. Patients aged 10 years and older are similar to adults in cause and fracture pattern.

In addition to physical examination, diagnosis of mandible fractures is made radiographically; a panorex and low Townes view (which show the condylar processes) may be sufficient for diagnosis and surgical treatment planning. If a patient has multiple facial fractures, is restrained in a cervical collar, is uncooperative or combative, a maxillofacial CT scan can be obtained. In both adults and children, the surgeon should consider the mandible as a closed "ring"; therefore, if the surgeon identifies a fracture, he or she should look for a second fracture. Multiple mandible fractures has been reported to be as high as 67%.[17]

Successful management of all mandible fractures begins with the restoration of centric occlusion. Under general anesthesia, the mandible is manually manipulated with care taken to look for wear facets and mammelons on the dentition. These occlusal cues will guide the surgeon to reestablishing the patient's preinjury occlusion. Centric occlusion can be maintained by performing MMF (applying arch bars or screws with wires or elastics).

Fractures of the condyle may be successfully managed with MMF and physical therapy alone (Figure 21-11). Functional treatment of condylar fractures includes early mobilization (starting at day 14, when pain has decreased) to restore normal mouth opening (45 mm). Guiding elastic therapy may be used for 6 to 8 weeks. The purpose of functional treatment is to maintain posterior

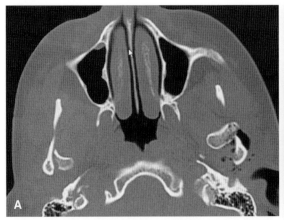 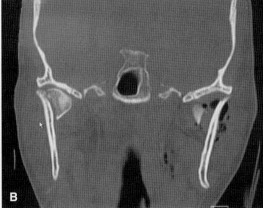

● **FIGURE 21-11.** Condylar fractures. (A) Axial CT image of bilateral condylar fractures. (B) Coronal CT image of bilateral condylar fractures. Note: these fractures were treated with maxilomandibular fixation and early movement.

mandibular height and to intentionally create a pseudo-arthrosis. Indications for open treatment of the condyle include displacement into the middle cranial fossa, pre-existing medical condition precluding MMF (epilepsy, severe mental disorder), inability to obtain occlusion by closed reduction, lateral extracapsular displacement of the condyle, presence of a foreign body, or open fracture with potential for fibrosis.

Subcondylar fractures are often incorrectly treated like condyle fractures. The purpose of condylar fracture treatment is to intentionally create a pseudoarthrosis. The purpose of subcondylar fracture treatment is to heal the fracture in anatomic alignment. While some surgeons use an open approach to subcondylar fractures, we prefer an endoscopic approach because it reduces the risk of facial nerve injury and eliminates preauricular or retromandibular scars (Figure 21-12). After establishing MMF, an intraoral incision is used to expose the fracture. An endoscope is inserted to assist in anatomic reduction of the fracture fragments. A plate is positioned and screws are placed trough cheek stab incisions. MMF is removed at the conclusion of the operation.

Fractures of the body, parasymphysis, and symphysis usually require rigid fixation because the forces exerted on the mandible by the muscles of mastication (eg, temporalis, masseter, medial and lateral pterygoids, and strap muscles) tend to distract the fracture fragments. While favorable fracture patterns do exist in this region and they can be managed with MMF or a soft diet, most surgeons perform open reduction and internal fixation. An intraoral approach is commonly used to treat fractures in these areas. The incision should be made at least 1 cm below the level of the attached gingival (to allow for an adequate cuff of tissue for closure). Care must be taken to avoid the inferior alveolar nerve in the canal and the mental nerve exiting the mental foramen. The inferior alveolar nerve travels in the mandibular canal at the junction of the middle and lower thirds of the mandibular body.[18,19] The mandibular canal terminates by wrapping 4.5 mm beneath the mental foramen and then looping 5.0 mm anteriorly before delivering the mental nerve.[18,19] Fractures in the body, parasymphysis, and symphysis are typically treated with a monocortical "tension band" and a bicortical plate at the lower border.

Fractures of the mandibular angle may be favorable or unfavorable. Favorable fractures may be managed with MMF or a soft diet, but most surgeons perform open reduction and internal fixation. Angle fractures were treated with a tension band and compression plate (similar to body, symphyseal, and parasymphyseal fractures). Alternatively, angle fractures may be treated with a single plate along the external oblique line as described by Khouri and Champy.[20] Exposure and visualization of the fracture line may be difficult for fractures at the angle; in addition to an intraoral approach, a system of cheek retractors and transbuccal trocars may be used to facilitate fixation. Alternatively an extraoral approach may be used, but this exposure increases the risk of facial nerve injury.

The presence of teeth in the fracture line is a point of controversy most relevant in mandibular angle fractures because angle fracture tends to involve the second molar or impacted third molar (when present). Indications for removing a tooth include (1) longitudinal fracture involving the root; (2) dislocation or subluxation of the tooth from its socket; (3) presence of periapical infection; (4) infected fracture line; (5) acute pericoronitis; and (6) inability to achieve anatomy reduction of the mandibular fracture fragments.

● **COMPLICATIONS**

Cerebrospinal Fluid Fistula

Cerebrospinal fluid otorrhea and rhinorrhea are important to detect: clear fluid leakage in facial fractures (upper and midfacial fractures) may indicate a traumatic dural tear, accompanied in 10% to 50% by pneumocephalus.[10]

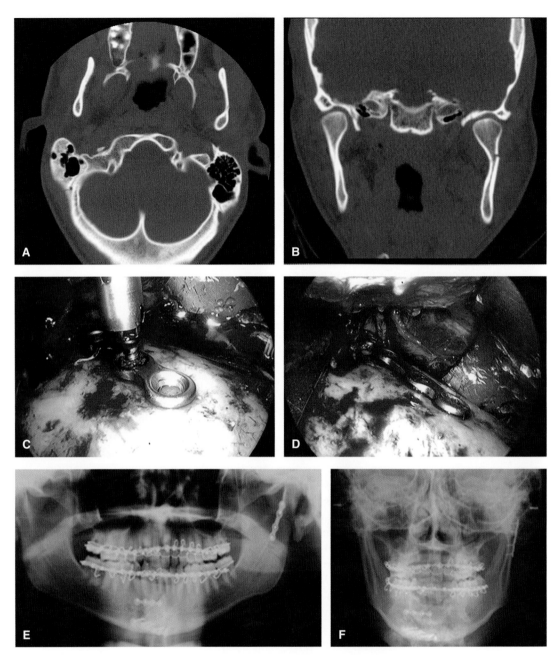

● **FIGURE 21-12.** High subcondylar fracture. (A) Axial CT image of high subcondylar fracture. (B) Coronal CT image of high subcondylar fracture. (C) Endoscopic view of screw placement. (D) Endoscopic view of miniplate fixation. (E) Postoperative panorex demonstrating anatomic reduction of the left subcondylar and right symphyseal fractures. (F) Postoperative posterior-anterior cephalogram demonstrating anatomic reduction of the left subcondylar, right symphyseal fractures, and restoration of posterior mandibular height. Note: maxilomandibular fixation was removed at the conclusion of the operation. The Erich arch bars were left in situ for postoperative guiding elastic therapy.

In case of doubt, especially when it is mixed with blood, the presence of glucose (urinary strip) is an indication of CSF fistula, but has 20% false-positives. Detection of beta-trace protein indicates CSF contamination in oto- and rhinorrhoe with a sensitivity of >90% at a specificity of 100%. It is faster and cheaper than beta-2 transfer-rine.[21] Non–contrast-enhanced, high-resolution CT scans have a specificity of 70% in CSF fistula detections.[10]

Pneumocephalus is often associated with dural fistula. Most CSF fistulae can be observed and 80% will spon-taneously resolve in 1week.[10] In case of isolated CSF leak, the risk of meningitis following 1-week CSF leak is only 3%. Nevertheless, after 2-weeks duration, the risk exceeds 50%.[10] Prophylactic antibiotic therapy should not exceed 24 hours. Prolonged antibiotic therapy does not reduce the rate of meningitis but increases bacterial resistance to antibiotics. Proper surgical wound treatment, dural repair, removal of the mucosa and obliteration of any communication with the contaminated nasal fossa are crucial steps to avoid meningitis.[10] Although its incidence is very low (around 2%), late meningitis (<1 year after trauma) can occur several months after the trauma and patients treated conservatively should be warned and monitored.[10]

Ectropion

Ectropion can be observed postoperatively in 14% of transcutaneous subciliary incision.[1] It results of a combination of factors such as orbicularis oculi muscle traumatic dissection, lateral canthal laxity, and cheek descent following extensive undermining of the soft tissues. The transconjunctival approach should be preferred over the transcutaneous approach when exposing the orbital floor in order to limit injury to the orbicularis oculi. Correction of tarsoligamentous laxity (lateral canthal support with lateral canthopexy)[22] and cheek suspension should be performed at the end of the bony repair. If massive swelling is expected, a temporary tarsorraphy will prevent exposure of the conjunctiva and stretching of the inferior canthal sling. If minimal swelling is expected, a temporary (4–5 d) lower lid suspension preserving sight will provide similar protection.[23]

Entropion of the lower lid is seen as the lashes are turned upward toward the cornea, causing trichiasis.[23] Entropion is consecutive to transconjunctival incision (1.5%), when the scarring or reduction of conjunctiva, subconjunctiva, or internal tarsus results in an inward bowing of the eyelid.[22,23]

Facial Hypoesthesia

Hypoesthesia is a common complication in facial fractures treatment. The three branches of the trigeminal nerve exit the facial skeleton in a reproducible pattern. Traumatic section is less frequent than nerve compression by bone fragments, especially at the maxillary level. Hyposesthesia can also result from excessive traction on a retractor during surgery. Neurapraxia is reversible in a

few weeks, but in case of neurotmesis, either traumatic or surgical, sensory recovery will not occur unless a microsurgical end-to-end suture is performed.

Secondary Displacement (Titanium vs Resorbable Osteosynthesis)

Secondary displacement of the fractures is rare at the upper and midface but can be seen in the mandible, where the powerful mastication muscles apply divergent forces on the fracture lines. Adequate placement of the plates and rigid osteosynthesis material prevents secondary displacement. In the past decade, several resorbable plates and screws have been introduced. Dorri et al.,[13] from the Cochrane Collaboration, a UK public health institute, reviewed the literature looking for randomized controlled trials comparing resorbable versus titanium fixation systems used for facial fractures. After analyzing 53 studies, none were found to be statistically sound and therefore no data were available for analysis. As of today, there is no strong evidence in favor of either fixation system.

● OUTCOMES

In general, the outcome from managing facial fractures should be excellent. Specific measures involve form and function. Patients should have a symmetrical appearance with minimal scarring and no functional concerns. Either observation of minimally displaced fractures or reduction and internal fixation of displaced fractures should yield minimal complications. Understanding the etiology of the notable short-term complications described above and taking appropriate measures to avoid them can minimize their occurrence. Problems arise from internal fixation of poorly reduced fractures. In the periorbital region, this will lead to vertical dystopia and diplopia. In the mandible, it will lead to malocclusion that often puts abnormal wear on the occlusal surface and disproportionate force on the temporomandibular joints. Long-term complications are rare. Occasionally, recurrent inflammation at the site of previously placed hardware warrants removal once the fractures have healed.

REFERENCES

1. Kelley P, Crawford M, Higuera S, Hollier LH. Two hundred ninety-four consecutive facial fractures in an urban trauma center: lessons learned. *Plast Reconstr Surg.* 2005;116(3):42e–49e.

2. Shintaku WH, Venturin JS, Azevedo B, Noujeim M. Applications of cone-beam computed tomography in fractures of the maxillofacial complex. *Dent Traumatol.* 2009;25(4):358–366.

3. Rosset A, Spadola L, Ratib O. Osiri X: an open-source software for navigating in multidimensional DICOM images. *J Digit Imaging.* 2004;17(3):205–216.

4. Mueller R. Endoscopic treatment of facial fractures. *Facial Plast Surg.* 2008;24(1):78–91.

5. Riedel. Schenk Inaug Dissertation. *Jena.* 1898.

6. Lynch RC. The techniques of a radical frontal sinus operation, which has given me the best results. *Laryngoscope.* 1921;31:1–5.

7. Goodale RL, Montgomery WW. Experiences with the osteoplastic anterior wall approach to the frontal sinus; case histories and recommendations. *AMA Arch Otolaryngol.* 1958;68(3):271–283.

8. Donald PJ, Bernstein L. Compound frontal sinus injuries with intracranial penetration. *Laryngoscope*.1978;88(2): 225–232.

9. Rodriguez ED, Stanwix MG, Nam AJ, et al. Twenty-six-year experience treating frontal sinus fractures: a novel algorithm based on anatomical fracture pattern and failure of conventional techniques. *Plast Reconstr Surg*. 2008;122(6): 1850–1866.

10. Manson PN, Stanwix MG, Yaremchuk MJ, et al. Frontobasal fractures: anatomical classification and clinical significance. *Plast Reconstr Surg*. 2009;124(6):2096–2106.

11. Kaufman Y, Stal D, Cole P, Hollier L Jr. Orbitozygomatic fracture management. *Plast Reconstr Surg*. 2008;121(4): 1370–1374.

12. Cohen SM, Garrett CG. Pediatric orbital floor fractures: nausea/vomiting as signs of entrapment. *Otolaryngol Head Neck Surg*. 2003;129(1):43–47.

13. Dorri M, Nasser M, Oliver R. Resorbable versus titanium plates for facial fractures. Cochrane Database of Systematic Reviews. 2009(1):CD007158.

14. Fridrich KL, Pena-Velasco G, Olson RAJ. Changing trends with mandibular fractures: A review of 1067 cases. *J Oral Maxillofac Surg*. 1992;50(6):586–589.

15. Thoren H, Iizuka T, Hallikainen D. Different patterns of mandibular fractures in children. An analysis of 220 fractures in 157 patients. *J Craniomaxillofac Surg*. 1992;20(7): 292–296.

16. Posnick JC, Wells M, Pron GE. Pediatric facial fractures: evolving patterns of treatment. *J Oral Maxillofac Surg*. 1993;51(8):836–844.

17. King RE, Scianna JM, Petruzzelli GJ. Mandible fracture patterns: a suburban trauma center experience. *Am J Otolaryngol*. 2004;25:301–307.

18. Ritter EF, Moelleken BR, Mathes SJ, Ousterhout DK. The course of the inferior alveolar neurovascular canal in relation to sliding genioplasty. *J Craniofac Surg*. 1992;3(1):20–24.

19. Hwang K, Lee WJ, Song YB, Chung IH. Vulnerability of the inferior alveolar nerve and mental nerve during genioplasty: an anatomic study. *J Craniofac Surg*. 2005;16(1):10–14; discussion 14.

20. Khouri M, Champy M. Results of mandibular osteosynthesis with miniaturized screwed plates. Apropos of 800 fractures treated over 10-year period. *Ann Chir Plast Esthet*. 1987;32(3):262–266.

21. Deisenhammer F, Egg R, Giovannoni G, et al. EFNS guidelines on disease-specific CSF investigations. *Eur J Neurol*. 2009;16(6):760–770.

22. Codner MA, Wolfli JN, Anzarut A. Primary transcutaneous lower blepharoplasty with routine lateral canthal support: a comprehensive 10-year review. *Plast Reconstr Surg*. 2008;121(1):241–250.

23. Ridgway EB, Chen C, Lee BT. Acquired entropion associated with the transconjunctival incision for facial fracture management. *J Craniofac Surg*. 2009;20(5):1412–1415.

chapter 22

Orbital Fractures and Deformities

Joshua Fosnot, MD / *Joseph M. Serletti, MD, FACS*

● INTRODUCTION

The orbit is a complex union of multiple bones of the facial skeleton that together provide structure for and house one of the most important sensory organs of the human body: the eye. Although this space provides ample support for normal function and protects against minor trauma, it is prone to fracture in major facial trauma and the resultant deformities can create either an ophthalmologic emergency, poor cosmetic defect, or both. The management of orbital fractures and deformities has advanced significantly owing to an improved understanding of the complex anatomy, traumatic mechanisms, refined imaging, and the advancement of implantable materials for reconstruction. Although facial trauma often is not isolated to the orbit alone, this chapter will focus on the identification and management of the orbital component of facial trauma and resultant deformities; whereas, other chapters will focus on fractures including the naso-orbitoethmoid (NOE), zygomaticomaxillary complex (ZMC), panfacial fractures, and soft tissue injuries.

Orbital Anatomy

A thorough understanding of orbital anatomy is paramount to the overall appreciation of pathologic processes and resultant management of orbital trauma. The bony orbit is composed of the seven separate bones of the membranous facial skeleton. These include the frontal, sphenoid, zygomatic, maxillary, ethmoid, lacrimal, and palatine bones (Figure 22-1). The overall space created by this arrangement is roughly pyramidal in shape, with the base anteriorly and apex posteriorly oriented, respectively. The anterior rim bony margin is fairly dense bone giving the outer edge strength for resistance to fracture. The same is true for the posterior apex, as this area is composed primarily of the cranial floor. The bone of the middle third of the orbit is weak and thin walled by comparison; thus, it is here that the effects of traumatic insult are usually seen. This is particularly true for the inferior wall or floor of the orbit. Composed of the maxilla, the floor separates the orbit from the maxillary sinus. Laterally, the orbit is a bit hardier. Through this wall, made up of the greater wing of the sphenoid and the zygoma, lies the temporal fossa. Also fairly resilient, the superior orbital wall lies under the frontal sinus and anterior cranial fossa and is created by the lesser wing of the sphenoid and the frontal bone. The orbits are separated in the midline by the interorbital space—defined by the nasal cavity and the ethmoid and sphenoid sinuses. The largest portion of the ethmoid, the lamina papyracea, is the weakest portion of the medial wall and is prone to fracture. Also contributing to this wall are the lacrimal bone and portions of the frontal, maxilla, and lesser sphenoid.

The optic nerve passes through the optic foramen at the junction of the sphenoid and ethmoid bones along with the ophthalmic artery. Between the lesser and greater wings of the sphenoid bone lies the superior orbital fissure. Through this cleft pass the motor nerves to the extraocular muscles and the ophthalmic division of the trigeminal nerve. The inferior orbital fissure allows passage of the maxillary division of the trigeminal nerve, the infraorbital artery, zygomatic nerve, autonomic nerve fibers, and branches of the ophthalmic vein (Figure 22-2).

The periorbita (periosteum) lines the orbit and is continuous with the dura of the cranial vault. The soft tissue of the orbit consists of the globe itself, extraocular muscles, lacrimal system, fat, nerves, and vessels. The bulbar fascia (Tenon capsule) surrounds the globe and is interconnected to a series of intermuscular and muscle sheath fascia to ensure that all of the intraorbital contents move in unison. Due to this interconnection, entrapment of even orbital fat may lead to significant visual disturbance.

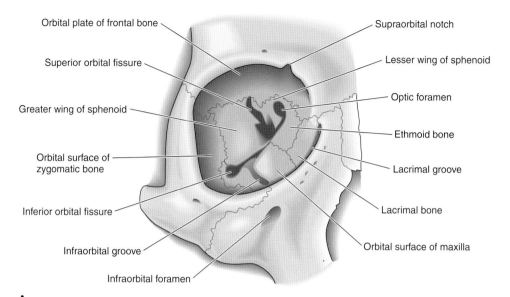

Orbital plate of frontal bone
Superior orbital fissure
Greater wing of sphenoid
Orbital surface of zygomatic bone
Inferior orbital fissure
Infraorbital groove
Infraorbital foramen

Supraorbital notch
Lesser wing of sphenoid
Optic foramen
Ethmoid bone
Lacrimal groove
Lacrimal bone
Orbital surface of maxilla

A

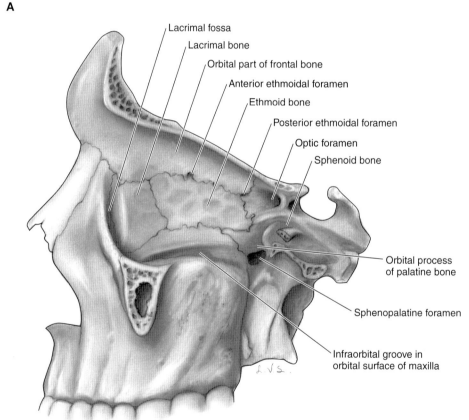

Lacrimal fossa
Lacrimal bone
Orbital part of frontal bone
Anterior ethmoidal foramen
Ethmoid bone
Posterior ethmoidal foramen
Optic foramen
Sphenoid bone

Orbital process of palatine bone
Sphenopalatine foramen
Infraorbital groove in orbital surface of maxilla

B

● FIGURE 22-1. (A) Anterior view of bones of right orbit. (B) Medial view of bony wall of left orbit. (*Reprinted with permission from Riordan-Eva P, Whitcher JP. Vaughan & Asbury's General Ophthalmology. 17th ed. New York: McGraw-Hill; 2008.*)

All of the extraocular muscles, except for the inferior oblique, originate from a common periosteal thickening around the optic nerve called the annulus of Zinn. These muscles work in concert to move the globes in unison. The anterior orbit of course is bounded by the eyelids. The canthal tendons are attached to the maxilla medially and the zygoma laterally.

● **PATIENT EVALUATION**

As previously stated, isolated orbital trauma is quite rare. The impact energy necessary to impart a fracture usually results in additional traumatic injury. This may result in concomitant facial fractures, or trauma throughout the body. As most facial trauma is not life-threatening, it is

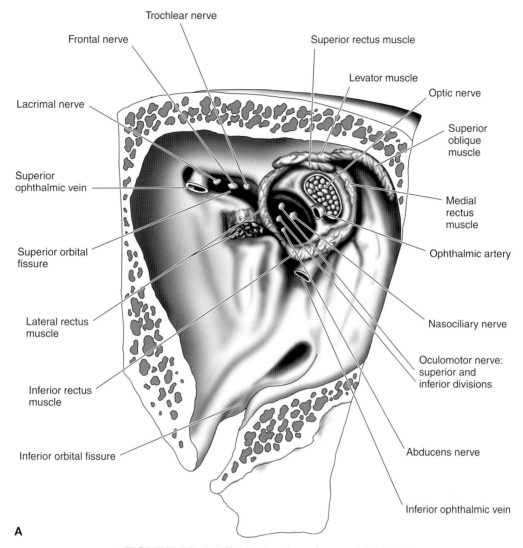

● FIGURE 22-2. (A) Anterior view of apex of right orbit.

important to recognize and treat major injuries first, with proper timing of evaluation and treatment of orbital injury decided through open dialogue with the trauma surgeon.

Orbital trauma is most frequent in the young adult and adolescent male patient population. The most frequent mechanisms of injury are assault and motor vehicle collision. In children, orbital injury is more common in boys who are older in age. The common mechanisms are most frequently related to sports or play. The mechanism of isolated orbital fractures typically involves an object (fist, bat, etc.) compressing the soft tissue and globe in an anterior projection, effectively creating a hydraulic press, which leads to volume expansion and "blow out" of the thin walls of the orbit.

When a patient presents for evaluation, a detailed history and physical are an essential starting point. The mechanistic details are important; however, the most prudent information is related to the visual axis. Patients should be asked about specific changes in vision either immediately after or delayed following traumatic insult. Floaters and flashes may indicate additional pathology such as a retinal

detachment. One should specifically ask about diplopia which may indicate entrapment. Also pertinent however, is the prior ocular/visual history such as use of glasses, history of amblyopia, or prior ocular trauma. If the patient is unconscious or unable to participate, one should take the time to ask family or friends if they are available.

General Exam

The plastic surgeon should be familiar with a basic visual examination, although a formal examination including dilated funduscopic exam is generally warranted by an ophthalmologist as well. Contact lenses should be removed to prevent possible corneal injury. Old photographs are useful for comparison, especially in patients with severe complex facial injuries. The physical examination generally begins with inspection for any obvious trauma and palpation of the periorbital bone and soft tissue. The bony orbital rims are palpated for irregularities or tenderness and this is followed by evaluation of eyelid movement, including proper opening and closure. Exophthalmos (anterior malposition

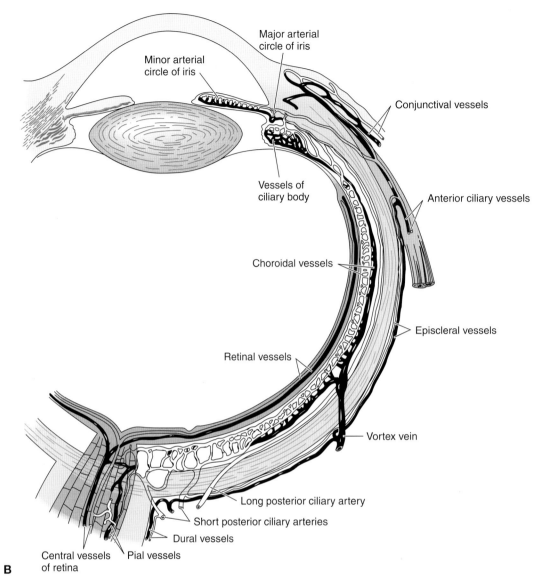

Minor arterial
circle of iris

Major arterial
circle of iris

Conjunctival vessels

Anterior ciliary vessels

Vessels of
ciliary body

Choroidal vessels

Episcleral vessels

Retinal vessels

Vortex vein

Long posterior ciliary artery

Short posterior ciliary arteries

Dural vessels

Central vessels
of retina

Pial vessels

B

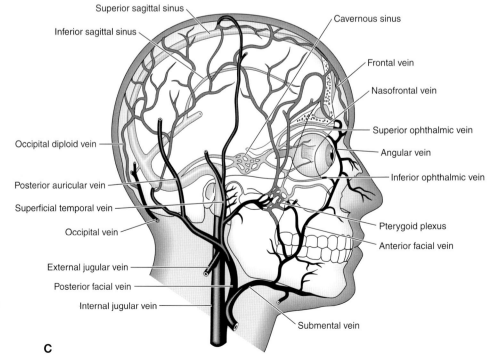

Superior sagittal sinus

Inferior sagittal sinus

Cavernous sinus

Frontal vein

Nasofrontal vein

Occipital diploid vein

Superior ophthalmic vein

Angular vein

Posterior auricular vein

Inferior ophthalmic vein

Superficial temporal vein

Occipital vein

Pterygoid plexus

Anterior facial vein

External jugular vein

Posterior facial vein

Internal jugular vein

Submental vein

C

● FIGURE 22-2. (*continued*)
(B) Vascular supply to the eye. All
arterial branches originate with the
ophthalmic artery. Venous drainage
is through the cavernous sinus and
the pterygoid plexus. (C) Venous
drainage system of the eye.

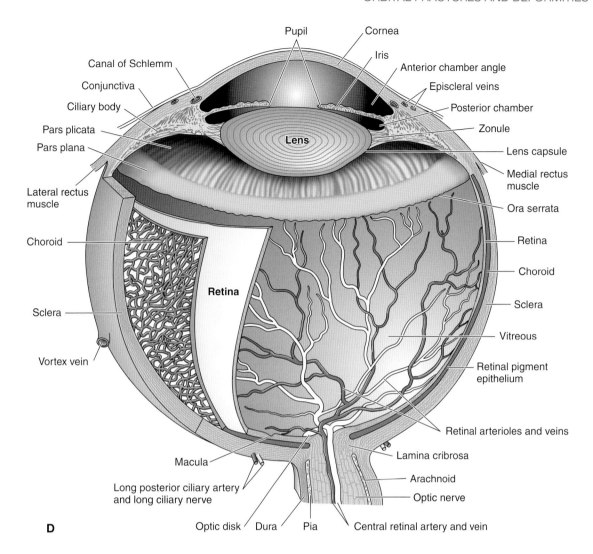

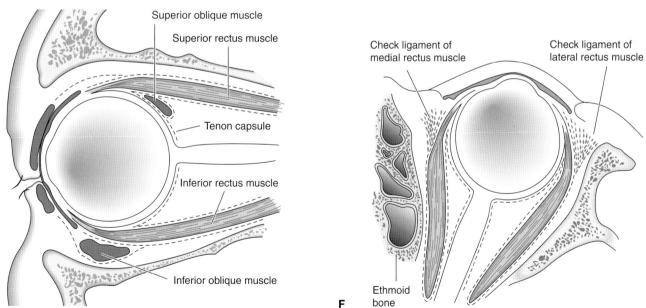

● **FIGURE 22-2.** (*continued*) (D) Internal structures of the human eye. (E) Fascia about muscles and eyeball (Tenon capsule). (F) Check ligaments of medial and lateral rectus muscles, right eye (diagrammatic). (*Reprinted with permission from Riordan-Eva P, Whitcher JP. Vaughan & Asbury's General Ophthalmology. 17th ed. New York: McGraw-Hill; 2008.*)

of the globe) or enophthalmos (posterior malposition of the globe) are best documented by looking down over the patient from above the forehead, or by looking up from below the chin.

Mobility

The patient should be asked to move his eyes in all directions with specific attention to disconjugate gaze or a complaint of diplopia. This can be done quickly by asking the patient to follow the examiner's finger; however, use of a penlight is a more sensitive test for documenting a disconjugate state. If there is concern for a mechanical restriction, a forced duction test may be performed in which the conjunctiva is anesthetized with a topical agent placed into the lower fornix and the globe is manually manipulated by grasping the muscle in question with forceps.

Visual Acuity

The standard approach to documenting visual acuity remains the Snellen eye chart, in which a patient reads characters of varying sizes from a 20-foot distance. In trauma patients, often this test is not possible due to the inability to stand and/or participate. In this case, a Rosenbaum pocket chart may be used in which a patient holds a card at a reading distance. In any test of visual acuity, glasses or contact lenses should be used for examination. Changes in visual acuity are particularly alarming for either nerve or intrinsic structural problems with the visual axis, all of which are ophthalmologic emergencies.

Pupil Exam

The pupil size and shape should be documented at baseline prior to light examination. Anisocoria (asymmetric pupil size) can be normal; however, it is more likely to be an indication of a more sinister process. An abnormally shaped pupil may be indicative of a ruptured globe or displaced lens. The light is next shone in each eye and removed individually. Both eyes should constrict and relax in unison and equally. A relative afferent pupillary defect or Marcus Gunn pupil is present when the eyes constrict equally relative to one another; however, when light is shone in the affected side, the response is less intense bilaterally. This may be indicative of a receptive neurologic defect, vitreal hemorrhage, or retinal injury.

Imaging

While historically, plain x-ray films were obtained to guide diagnosis and treatment, this has largely been replaced by faster and more powerful CT scanning with computer-aided reconstruction and/or modeling. Although plain films may be helpful to screen patients at low risk for fracture in an effort to avoid the radiation dose of a CT, if a CT is to be obtained, plain films can be avoided.

CT scanning is the gold standard for diagnosis and clarification of the extent of orbital injury in trauma. Facial protocol CT scanning with 1 to 3 mm sections in axial acquisition with sagittal and coronal reformatting is standard to evaluate the face thoroughly. CT is very sensitive for picking up fractures and can also clarify soft tissue involvement, hematoma, and entrapment or herniation (Figure 22-3). In fact, studies have shown decent accuracy in predicting eventual enophthalmos through the use of CT imaging and computer modeling.[1]

While ultrasound is incredibly useful for evaluating the extent of injury within the globe itself, its use in diagnosing bony injury is limited. Likewise, MRI can be useful to further characterize soft tissue abnormalities such as tumor; however, its use in trauma is rare due to expense, speed, and availability.

Deformities

The most common fracture from blunt orbital trauma is the inferior wall blowout fracture medial to the groove of the infraortibal nerve with extension onto the inferior portion of the medial orbital wall. In one series, this pattern occurred in roughly 40% of isolated orbital trauma.[2] In this same series, fractures of the orbit involved NOE or ZMC over 50% of the time. Although floor and medial wall fractures are the most common injury patterns, patients may present with lateral wall or roof fractures with resultant deformities.

One clinical deformity common to many orbital fractures is enophthalmos whereby the globe is inferiorly and posteriorly displaced (Figure 22-4). In addition, examination may show pseudoptosis in which the superior eyelid appears to droop with a deepened superior tarsal fold. If enophthalmos is not initially present in the setting of a known fracture, this does not mean it will not develop later. Often, there is concomitant edema and/or hematoma which masks the ability to predict the position of the globe in the future. This may be particularly true in cases where the zygoma is fractured as well. The etiology of enophthalmos has been studied extensively with several different theories; however, it is likely the combined effect of increased orbital bony volume, fat herniation into the maxillary sinus and fat atrophy. All contribute to a globe to orbit volume discrepancy.[3]

In addition to enophthalmos, entrapment is one of the more common conditions resulting from an inferior wall blowout fracture. In this condition, the periorbital fat or extraocular muscles become caught in the fracture line or wall deformity. This tissue is interlaced with a fine network of fascia and as a result may result in tethering and restriction of motion. Due to restriction of motion of the inferior orbital contents, the most common clinical symptom is diplopia in superior gaze. The degree of diplopia is usually proportional to the degree of tissue entrapment and restriction may be further documented with forced duction. It is important to recognize, however, that diplopia can occur with a small nondisplaced fracture as well due to hematoma and edema limiting motion. This type of diplopia is usually temporary and resolves without intervention. Entrapment

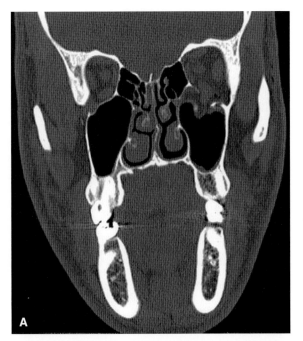

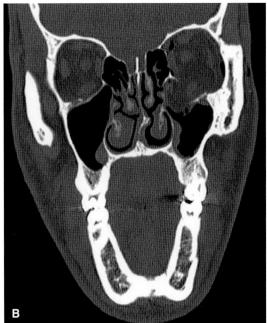

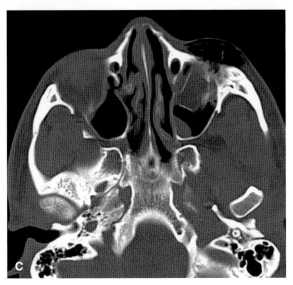

● FIGURE 22-3. This patient was punched in the left eye and presented with a complaint of paraesthesias of the left upper lip extending up to the left eye. (A, B) Two coronal sections of a CT scan of the face showing a left orbital floor blowout fracture with herniation of the orbital contents including the inferior rectus muscle into the maxillary sinus. (C) Axial imaging of the same patient also showing extensive subcutaneous air due to the maxillary sinus involvement.

and resultant diplopia is more common in children owing to more flexible bone. A linear fracture in children snaps back into place leading to a trapdoor with incarcerated contents; whereas, in adults the fracture tends to result in multiple fragments and a frank defect. Due to this trapdoor effect, children without any sign of trauma can present with severe diplopia and oculocardiac reflex symptomatology, the so-called "white-eyed blowout" fracture.

On examination, binocular diplopia must be distinguished from monocular diplopia. The occlusion test is useful for this purpose. Each eye is alternatively covered and the patient is asked to report the presence or absence of diplopia. In diplopia resultant from disconjugate gaze, the patient's symptoms resolve with covering of either eye. The examiner should look at the uncovered eye to determine what corrective measures the eye makes when the contralateral side is occluded. This test

helps differentiate vertical from horizontal diplopia. If the diplopia is present in one eye when the other is covered, this is called monocular diplopia. This may be the result of diffraction errors from corneal or lens pathology or a supratentorial problem.

Orbital Apex Syndrome

Although the vast majority of orbital trauma results in fracture of the middle third of the orbit involving thin bone, occasionally posterior orbital fractures do occur. When this occurs, the fracture typically involves the superior orbital fissure and may include optic nerve injury. The pentad of findings includes loss of vision, ophthalmoplegia, ptosis, pupillary dilation, and anaesthesia of the upper eyelid—together known as orbital apex syndrome. While traditionally this finding was considered permanent obviating the

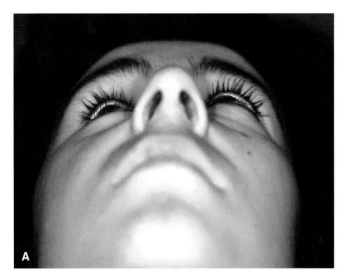 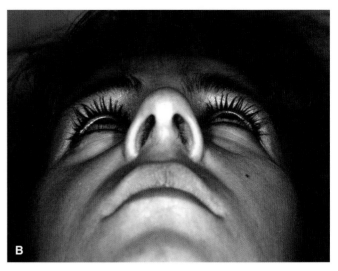

● **FIGURE 22-4.** Preoperative photograph of a patient who had suffered trauma to the right eye resulting in an orbital blowout fracture. (A) This patient suffered from enophthalmos, best seen by looking coronally from below the face. (B) Following surgical repair, the eye is significantly less posteriorly displaced.

need for surgical intervention, the overall approach has changed in recent times and surgery has become more heavily utilized.

● PATIENT PREPARATION

The final common indication for any type of orbital fracture is globe malposition or persistent visual changes such as diplopia. Not all orbital fractures require surgical repair; however, with proper evaluation and dialogue between surgeon and patient, the end results should be predictable through minimally invasive means. Patients with minimal displacement on CT and no or minimal enophthalmos or diplopia on examination do not need immediate surgical intervention and may be followed conservatively. Significant entrapment, enophthalmos of greater than 2 mm, diplopia on primary gaze and fractures occupying more than 50% of the floor are all indications for repair.[4] Although some would argue that conservative management will lead to resolution of diplopia and visual changes, enophthalmos and resultant poor cosmesis rarely, if ever, resolve spontaneously. Thus, patients should be prepared for poor cosmetic outcomes without surgery, even if their vision improves over time.

Timing of orbital floor repair has been a controversial subject historically. The initial thought was that time led to resolution of symptoms and more predictable surgical planes. In recent times, there has been a trend toward early intervention as several studies have shown improved cosmetic results when surgery is offered within at least 2 weeks, if not immediately.[4] Most would agree that immediate surgical repair is indicated in patients with significant diplopia in primary or vertical gaze and those with a persistent oculocardiac reflex (bradycardia, heart block, nausea, vomiting or syncope). In addition, children with a "white

eye" blowout fracture should be operated on immediately. Significant immediate enophthalmos will not improve and warrants immediate repair. Of those patients followed, many eventually need an operation. Those with persistent diplopia, latent enophthalmos or progressive lower eyelid sensory loss all should be operated on by 2 weeks.[5] The 2-week timeline avoids the fibrosis and scarring of waiting for a prolonged period. If there are concomitant injuries such as retinal detachment, hyphema, or severe edema, delayed surgery is still preferred to avoid further injury to the visual axis.

Once a decision has been made to proceed to the operating room, the patient should undergo general anesthesia and be placed in a supine position with the endotracheal tube taped away from the working field. Reversing the direction of the table may be helpful. The patient is prepped and draped and preoperative antibiotics should be administered. Either a corneal protection device or, in some cases depending on approach, transpalpebral suturing may be warranted to protect the cornea.

● TECHNIQUE

Orbital Floor Fracture

For repair of an orbital floor blowout fracture, the two most common incisions are transconjunctival and subciliary. A transoral approach is possible however no longer recommended. Although results are conflicting, most authors report improved outcomes with a transconjunctival approach owing to decreased rates of ectropion and eyelid retraction in the long term.[6] In addition, a transconjunctival incision avoids an external scar on the face. A canthotomy may be necessary to achieve adequate exposure in this approach.

When performing the transconjunctival approach, retraction sutures may be placed opposite one another on the gray line of the eyelid margin and in the depth of the fornix for exposure. Using a low setting on the electrocautery, a curvilinear incision is made blow the level of the tarsus. From here, either a preseptal or postseptal path to the orbital rim may be chosen. The former tends to avoid the fat that lies behind the septum allowing for a less obstructive view. The latter tends to transverse the fat compartment but leaves the attachment of the septum to the rim intact and thereby further minimizes the risk of eyelid retraction and ectropion.

Regardless of the incision, dissection is carried down to the level of the infraorbital rim. Here, an incision is made in the periosteum, allowing for a subperiorbital plane to be developed into the inferior orbit with an elevator (Figure 22-5). With an extensive fracture, the posteriorly directed dissection will lead to easy identification of the fracture and dissection continues until the furthest extent of the fracture is identified. Similarly, the dissection is carried medially and laterally to identify an area around the fracture to support a graft or implant. Commonly, there is a medial component of the fracture necessitating fairly extensive medial dissection. Care should be taken to not injure the infraorbital nerve at this time.

Once completely dissected, a decision is made as to the type of implant needed to span the defect and recreate a new floor. In the past, the calvarial bone graft was the workhorse for this application; however, donor site morbidity has led most surgeons away from this technique. In addition, most of the bone graft is resorbed over time, thus a thick initial graft is necessary to compensate. This leads to initial overcorrection which can be unsatisfactory to the patient. Other autologous options include the conchal or nasal cartilage graft, although these have a tendency to warp and in complex fractures, prevent their use for nasal fracture repair.

As material science has progressed, use of alloplastic material for reconstruction has become more common. Alloplastic options include silastic, nylon, polyethylene, polytetrafluoroethylene, and titanium. When comparing alloplastic materials, no one type has been shown to be

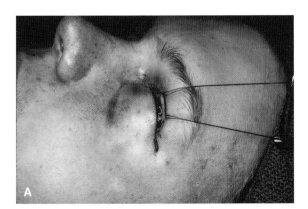

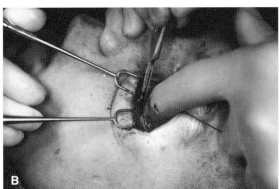

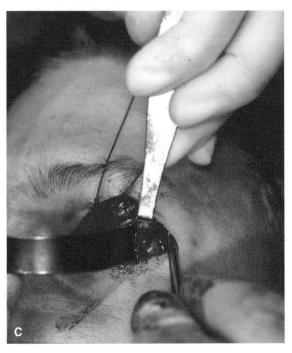

● **FIGURE 22-5.** A subciliary incision allows for adequate exposure of the orbital floor and any traumatic defect in the thin wall of bone. Once exposed, placement of a graft/implant for structure is fairly straightforward.

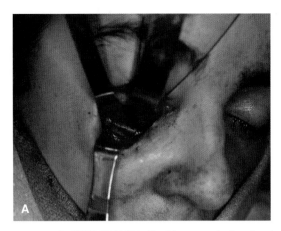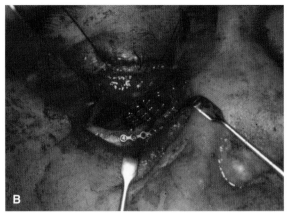

● **FIGURE 22-6.** Placement of an implant is fairly straightforward with adequate access to the inferior orbital rim (A), and performed with fixation of the mesh with titanium screws (B).

superior to another in a prospective trial. The most commonly used implants are Suprafoil (nylon), titanium mesh, and Medpor Titan (titanium embedded polyethylene). They are all fairly easy to use, readily available, and avoid donor site morbidity. Although rare, when infected these implants do unfortunately require explant.

In cases of complex fractures, the horizontal and vertical buttress system of the orbital rim must be stabilized and fixed first (see other chapters for complete description). Only at that time is the implant able to be secured in place. In the case of a titanium implant, this is typically done with a single titanium screw driven into the inferior orbital rim (Figure 22-6). It is crucial that the posterior edge of the fracture is found and spanned with the implant to prevent eventual inferior displacement of the globe or residual hypoglobus. This obviously must be balanced with caution due to the devastating consequence of severing the neurovascular structures entering the orbit from the posterior apex. Once in place, the soft tissue is re-approximated and closed over the implant. This should include the periosteum to help prevent implant migration and fibrosis leading to motility restriction. The surgeon should ensure no ocular limitation of range of motion with forced duction prior to allowing the patient to emerge from anesthesia. If a corneal protection device or transpalpebral suturing were used, these should be removed at this time. Although not performed routinely, repairing the orbital floor through a transconjunctival incision can be performed in standard fashion without closing the wound. The implant is not fixed in place and the incision is not closed primarily. Overall results appear equivalent in small series, with excellent spontaneous wound closure and implant stability.[7]

Medial Orbital Wall

Historically, a coronal incision was used to reach the medial orbit, but this is no longer routinely used. Inferomedial fractures can usually be reached in similar fashion to the technique described above. True medial or superomedial fractures typically require a separate incision. Most authors recommend a transcaruncular or precaruncular incision. Through this incision, exposure is generally acceptable; however, care must be taken not to injure the lacrimal system. In addition, a W-shaped medial canthal skin incision may be used with fairly predictable results. The incision is carried down to the periosteum and the fracture is identified at that time. An implant is used in similar fashion to the floor fracture, although Tisseel glue may be used to affix the implant as there is generally less room for screw fixation.

Orbital Roof

Fractures of the orbital roof are rarely seen in isolation. Most commonly, they involve the orbital rim or frontal sinus and management of this injury pattern will be discussed in another chapter. Nondisplaced roof fractures do not require surgical repair, although an isolated roof fracture resulting in significant proptosis should be fixed surgically. A standard superior blepharoplasty incision allows for the easiest access to the orbital roof. Through this incision, the periosteum is easily identified and able to be lifted in similar fashion to that described above. Care must be taken to avoid injury to the superior oblique muscle and lacrimal gland during this dissection. The fracture may be plated in similar fashion.

Endoscopic Approach

There has been an increasing interest in endoscopic approaches to medial and floor fractures. Through either a transnasal or transmaxillary sinus approach, this technique offers excellent visualization of the fracture. In particular, this technique allows better visualization of the posterior orbit without the need for retraction of the globe.[8]

Authors have advocated either manual reduction of a trapdoor, or insertion of an inflatable balloon in the maxillary sinus which allows for bony healing over a month at which point the balloon is removed. The second branch of the trigeminal nerve is at greater risk of injury. Although a novel approach, not all fractures are amenable to this repair and aside from incision size, there is little if any added outcome benefit.[9]

● COMPLICATIONS

Edema is quite common following orbital trauma and fracture. Steroids have been advocated as a method to decrease edema and some studies have shown faster resolution of diplopia and edema even in those who underwent immediate surgical correction.[10] Standard dosing of dexamethasone does not appear to interfere with wound healing.[11]

Eyelid abnormalities, including hypoaesthesia and ectropion, are common following orbital trauma and subsequent surgical correction. As noted above, this may be less pronounced if a transconjunctival approach is taken; but overall, ectropion may be as high as 12.5%.[6] Transconjunctival approaches are not without risk however, as this does place the patient at risk for entropion. As many as 28% of patients complain of lower eyelid hypoaesthesia likely from infraorbital nerve injury either from the fracture itself or subsequent surgery.[2]

Retrobulbar hematoma is a potential devastating complication of orbital fracture and can occur with or without surgical intervention. The managing physician needs to be immediately aware of any complaint of sudden vision loss, developing proptosis, periocular ecchymosis, or eye pain. Surgical evacuation is mandatory to prevent permanent visual loss.

Given that the sinuses and nasal passages are not sterile and cannot be sterilized in a surgical field, infection is possible. The use of prophylactic antibiotics to prevent this is controversial. No randomized control trials exist to support this practice; however, most surgeons treat patients with a week of broad spectrum antibiotics following surgical repair. Overall infectious risk is roughly 3%.[2] With significant implant infection, the prosthesis needs to be removed; likewise, severe orbital cellulitis is possible, necessitating incision and drainage.

● OUTCOMES

Following orbital trauma, a patient should follow-up with an ophthalmologist for a complete eye exam within 1 week to ensure no changes in vision. Overall, patients tolerate surgical repair well and assuming no other traumatic injury, may return to full function soon after repair (Figure 22-7). Persistent diplopia is particularly meddlesome and should be discussed with the patient preoperatively. The vast

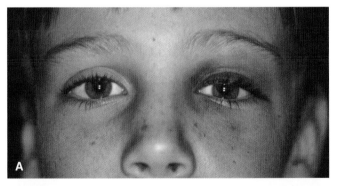
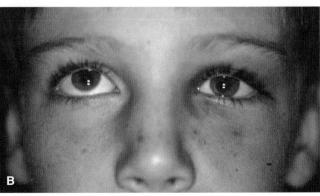
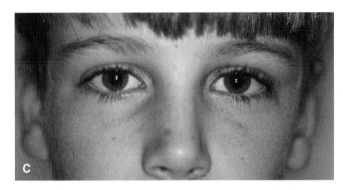
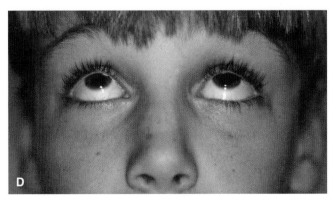

● **FIGURE 22-7.** (A) Preoperative photograph of a young boy with an isolated left orbital floor fracture. Note the significant periorbital edema and ecchymosis associated with hypoglobus and enophthalmos. (B) The patient has significant entrapment causing diplopia in vertical gaze. (C) Postoperative photo of the same patient showing excellent alignment in primary gaze and (D) resolved entrapment.

majority of patients will still complain of diplopia immediately following surgical intervention and up to one third of patients with preexisting diplopia will never be completely asymptomatic.[12] Older patients appear to be at greater risk for persistent diplopia.[13]

One of the primary goals of repair of the orbital blowout fracture is to correct enophthalmos and provide for improved overall aesthetics and facial symmetry. While surgical repair offers a better chance for improved cosmesis, not all patients are corrected satisfactorily. In as much as 2.7% to 7.0% of surgical repairs for enophthalmos, persistent asymmetry will be present in long-term follow-up.[2,13] Not surprisingly, this is more common in patients who have suffered multiple facial fractures.

Although patient satisfaction postoperatively has not been addressed for isolated orbital floor pathology, this has been studied for complex facial fractures, specifically ZMC with orbital floor fracture repair. In this series, 80% of patients were satisfied with their results in the long term. Reasons for dissatisfaction were primarily centered around residual diplopia and enophthalmos.[14]

REFERENCES

1. Ahn HB, Ryu WY, Yoo KW, et al. Prediction of enophthalmos by computer-based volume measurement of orbital fractures in a Korean population. *Ophthal Plast Reconstr Surg.* 2008;24:36–39.

2. Hwang K, You SH, Sohn IA. Analysis of orbital bone fractures: a 12-year study of 391 patients. *J Craniofac Surg.* 2009;20(4):1218–1223.

3. Clauser L, Galiè M, Pagliaro F, Tieghi R. Posttraumatic enophthalmos: etiology, principles of reconstruction, and correction. *J Craniofac Surg.* 2008;19(2):351–359.

4. Liss J, Stefko ST, Chung WL. Orbital surgery: state of the art. *Oral Maxillofac Surg Clin North Am.* 2010;22:59–71.

5. Burnstine MA. Clinical recommendations for repair of isolated orbital floor fractures: An evidence-based analysis. *Ophthalmology.* 2002;109:1207–1210.

6. Ridgway EB, Chen C, Colakoglu S, et al. The incidence of lower eyelid malposition after facial fracture repair: a retrospective study and meta-analysis comparing subtarsal, subciliary, and transconjunctival incisions. *Plast Reconstr Surg.* 2009;124(5):1578–1586.

7. Ho VH, Rowland JP Jr, Linder JS, Fleming JC. Sutureless transconjunctival repair of orbital blowout fractures. *Ophthal Plast Reconstr Surg.* 2004;20:458–460.

8. Farwell DG, Sires BS, Kriet JD, Stanley RB. Endoscopic repair of orbital blowout fractures. *Arch Facial Plast Surg.* 2007;9:427–433.

9. Cheong EC, Chen CT, Chen YR. Endoscopic management of orbital floor fractures. *Facial Plast Surg.* 2009;25:8–16.

10. Flood TR, McManners J, el-Attar A, Moos KF. Randomized prospective study of the influence of steroids on postoperative eye-opening after exploration of the orbital floor. *Br J Oral Maxillofac Surg.* 1999;37:312–315.

11. Thoren H, Snall J, Kormi E, et al. Does perioperative glucocorticosteroid treatment correlate with disturbance in surgical wound healing after treatment of facial fractures? A retrospective study. *J Oral Maxillofac Surg.* 2009;67:1884–1888.

12. Biesman BS, Hornblass A, Lisman R, Kazlas M. Diplopia after surgical repair of orbital floor fractures. *Ophthal Plast Reconstr Surg.* 1996;12:9–16; discussion 17.

13. Hosal BM, Beatty RL. Diplopia and enophthalmos after surgical repair of blowout fracture. *Orbit.* 2002;21:27–33.

14. Folkestad L, Åberg-Bengtsson L, Granström G. Recovery from orbital floor fractures: a prospective study of patients' and doctors' experiences. *Int J Oral Maxillofac Surg.* 2006;35(6):499–505.

chapter 23

Frontal Sinus Fractures

Matthew G. Stanwix, MD / *Eduardo D. Rodriguez, MD, DDS*

● INTRODUCTION

Frontal sinus fractures represent 5% to 15% of all craniomaxillofacial fractures.[1] Improper management leads to devastating and potentially fatal complications due to the proximate relationship of the frontal sinus with the anterior cranial fossa. Concomitant facial fractures along with associated intracranial and bodily injuries confirm the severity of impact required to produce these fractures.

● PATIENT EVALUATION AND SELECTION

Evaluation of the patient by the craniomaxillofacial surgeon begins with a thorough physical examination to assess appearance and contour of the frontal sinus region, presence of a cerebral spinal fluid leak, associated fractures and injuries, and neurological status. Although this initial assessment gives an overall impression of the injury, computed tomography (CT) scans direct patient selection and evaluation. Fine, thin sections in a multidetector CT scanner can provide near-anatomic representation of the fracture pattern. Radiographic evaluation must assess the table(s) involved, presence or displacement or comminution, sidedness (with regard to intersinus septum), and degree of nasofrontal outflow tract injury.

Injury to the nasofrontal outflow tract stands as the cornerstone of treatment; its presence or absence will predict complications in surgical or conservative management.[1,2] Note the use of the term nasofrontal outflow tracts in this chapter, as only 15% or individuals have a true nasofrontal duct, while the majority drains directly into the anterior ethmoidal cells.[1] There are three indicators of nasofrontal outflow tract injury: fracture in the floor of the frontal sinus, anterior table medial wall fracture (anterior ethmoidal cells), and gross outflow tract obstruction (fracture fragments lying in the tract itself) (Figure 23-1). Management of frontal sinus fractures according to the algorithm in

Figure 23-2 shows the importance of nasofrontal outflow tract injury in surgical versus nonsurgical management. Patients who do not have nasofrontal outflow tract injury (no criteria met) can be safely observed with almost no incidence of complications. Although the presence of one or more of these criteria can indicate nasofrontal outflow tract injury, obstruction is the most powerful and important criterion of the three. Obstruction is almost always associated with a more devastating and assiduous injury (Table 23-1), directing surgeons toward prompt and aggressive defunctionalizing surgery (ie, cranialization or obliteration). Those patients with nasofrontal outflow injury, but absence of obstruction, can be either observed or surgically contoured depending on displacement of the fragments.[1]

● PATIENT PREPARATION

Patients encountered in the emergency room or trauma bay frequently have polytrauma that requires a team approach from multiple surgical subspecialties. Serious intracranial, thoracic, or abdominal injuries must be treated with emergent surgery when required. Stabilization of the patient hemodynamically, including proper intracranial pressures, must be met prior to any surgery. Therefore, although prompt and immediate surgical repair of frontal sinus fractures has been shown to decrease complications,[3] ultimately, the timing of the surgery depends on clearance from trauma and/or neurosurgery colleagues.

Frontal sinus fractures with concomitant cranial base injuries (frontobasal fractures) should heighten the craniomaxillofacial surgeon awareness for cerebrospinal leaks. Often, cerebrospinal leaks evade clinical diagnoses, delaying a potentially fatal scenario of subsequent abscess or meningitis. Patients with associated cranial base injuries, especially in the setting of midfacial fractures, must be aggressively worked up for dural fistulae.[3] Beta-2 transferrin detection,

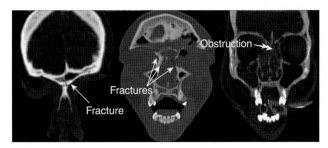

● **FIGURE 23-1.** Computed tomographic diagnosis of nasofrontal outflow tract injury. Fracture of the sinus floor (Left); (Middle) fracture of the medial aspect of anterior table; and (Right) frank obstruction. (*From Rodriguez ED, Stanwix MG, Nam AJ, et al. Twenty-six-year experience treating frontal sinus fractures: a novel algorithm based on anatomical fracture pattern and failure of conventional techniques. Plast Reconstr Surg. 2008;122(6):1852.*)

isotope investigations, intrathecal fluorescein tests, and noncontrast, high-resolution CT scans play a significant role in detecting cerebrospinal leaks. Importantly, the risk of meningitis correlates with duration of dural fistula; thus a team approach of neurosurgical dural laceration repair in coordination with frontal sinus treatment must be pursued without delay. Although many centers use prophylactic antibiotics for cerebrospinal fluid leaks until definitive treatment, evidence-based medicine establishes they should only be administered within the immediate (24 hours) postinjury period; and for those who require dural repair, also limited to the first 24 hours of the perioperative period.[4]

Once the patient is hemodynamically stable for surgical repair, and neurosurgical team is available for dural laceration repair or assistance with exposure, the patient is brought to the operating room. General anesthesia is administered in the supine position with the vertex of the head at the edge of the bed or in a halo device, both arms tucked at the side, and the bed turned 90 degrees for full access. Consent for and preparation of autologous bone graft sites (calvarium, iliac crest, or tibial tuberosity) must always be pursued. Essential equipment for the procedure include a craniomaxillofacial plating set of the surgeons choice (with available mesh plates), power drills and bone burring tips, protected needle-tip cautery set at 18, a head light, liposuction tools if indicated, and osteotomes. Skin preparation with betadine, lubricated corneal eye shields, and strict sterile techniques must fully be implemented.

● **SURGICAL TREATMENTS**

Appropriate surgical management of frontal sinus fractures with outflow tract obstruction relies on defunctionalizing the sinus cavity (removing mucous producing cells by cranialization or obliteration) and proper partitioning of the upper aerodigestive system from the anterior cranial base. If the outflow tract is injured, but patent, then surgery shifts to providing proper contour

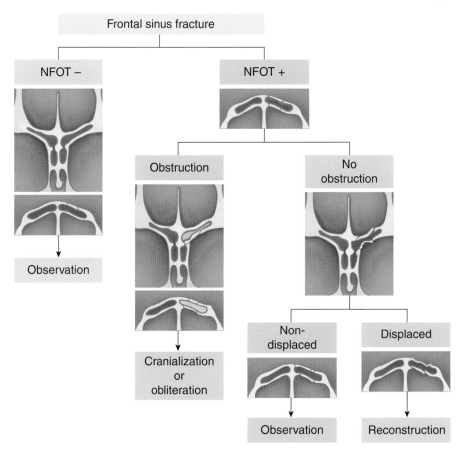

● **FIGURE 23-2.** Frontal sinus fracture treatment algorithm. NFOT, nasofrontal outflow tract. (*Rodriguez ED, Stanwix MG, Nam AJ, et al. Twenty-six-year experience treating frontal sinus fractures: a novel algorithm based on anatomical fracture pattern and failure of conventional techniques. Plast Reconstr Surg. 2008;122(6):1852.*)

TABLE 23-1. Higher Associated Injuries With Outflow Tract Injuries

Injury	NFOT−	NFOT+
Brain	31%	76%
Cerebral spine	7%	14%
Upper extremity fracture	15%	25%
Lower extremity fracture	13%	23%
Pneumothorax	12%	24%
Abdominal	7%	13%
Orbital roof	13%	40%
Orbital wall	7%	13%
Orbital floor	2%	7%
Naso-orbitoethmoid	12%	31%
Zygoma	8%	18%
LeFort	2%	17%
Mandible	3%	5%

NFOT−, nasofrontal outflow tract uninjured. NFOT+, nasofrontal outflow tract injury.

Data from Rodriguez ED, Stanwix MG, Nam AJ, et al. Twenty-six-year experience treating frontal sinus fractures: a novel algorithm based on anatomical fracture pattern and failure of conventional techniques. Plast Reconstr Surg. 2008;122(6):1853.

Treatment of concomitant facial fractures must also be taken into consideration, and proper sequencing pursued.[5] Surgical approach to the frontal sinus area must begin through an inconspicuous bicoronal approach. For reconstruction and contouring alone, very specific instances may arise where a bicoronal approach is not required. Rarely, direct horizontal incisions in the forehead over the fracture fragments may be used in select balding men with thick frontalis rhytids. Additionally, large lacerations or frontal soft tissue loss may be encountered and serve as access for contour alone procedures. Minimally invasive endoscopic techniques seem like a reasonable alternative to large coronal incisions, but utilize foreign bodies (porous polyethylene), have worse contour results, and have higher complication rates.[6] For the overwhelming majority of patients, a bicoronal approach serves as appropriate access for contouring and defunctionalizing surgery, dural laceration repair, and split calvarial bone graft harvesting.

Although the algorithm described thus far in this chapter uses only three surgical techniques (reconstruction, obliteration, and cranialization), there are others currently used which have been found to be inadequate and lead to unacceptably high complication rates (ablation and osteoneogenesis).[1]

Ablation (Exenteration)

Riedel initially described the technique of frontal sinus ablation in 1898, with removal of the frontal bone, supraorbital bandeau, proximal nasal bones, all sinus mucosa, and often the posterior table.[1] This then allows for skin involution against the posterior wall or dura itself. Delayed reconstruction of this severe cosmetic defect at a subsequent surgery is then dangerous and difficult. The only potential indication for the ablation procedure is severe acute infection, where collapse of the dead space and removal

with open-reduction internal fixation, while not pursuing the sinus cavity and its drainage (Figure 23-2). As noted previously, preoperative radiological diagnosis of nasofrontal outflow tract injury, particularly obstruction, fully determines which surgical treatment is indicated (Figure 23-3). Therefore, intraoperative assessment of outflow tract patency through direct outflow tract visualization, probing, or colored fluid investigation (ie, instillation of methylene blue from the sinus to assess drainage inferior to middle meatus) is never required.

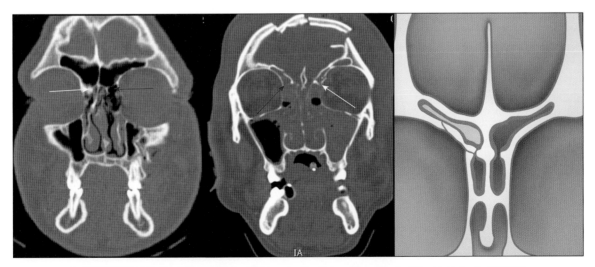

● FIGURE 23-3. Obstruction of the nasofrontal outflow tract. CT scans (Left, Middle) demonstrating a patent outflow tract (red arrows) as well as obstructed outflow tracts (white arrows). On the right is an artist's rendition of outflow tract obstruction.

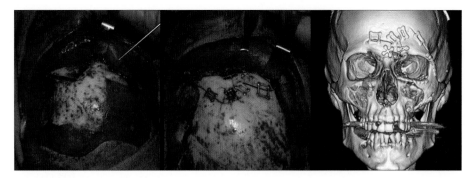

● **FIGURE 23-4.** Open reduction internal fixation of the anterior table. A blunt injury to this patient resulted in an anterior table frontal sinus fracture as well as a concomitant zygomaticomaxillary complex fracture. A bicoronal approach is pursued exposing the fracture segments (Left). Appropriate reduction management by elevating the depressed segments and assuring proper contour is made with various miniplatefixation (Middle). A postoperative CT scan demonstrates proper contour and reduction (Right).

of infected, nonvascularized bone nidus, will protect from mucocele and devastating intracranial infections.

Osteoneogenesis

Much like the other defunctionalizing surgeries that will be discussed below, this procedure strips the mucosa of the sinus cavity, obstructs the nasofrontal outflow tracts, and preserves the empty cavity itself. Spontaneous obliteration then proceeds in a slow, indolent fashion by which scar tissue and bone theoretically fills the empty frontal sinus cavity.

For patients who have displacement or comminution of the anterior table of the frontal sinus, and lack nasofrontal outflow tract obstruction, proper contouring by open reduction internal fixation (reconstruction) is indicated.

Reconstruction

Reconstruction of the anterior table of the frontal sinus begins with a bicoronal scalp incision for exposure. Alopecia can be avoided by making the incision parallel to the hair follicles and meticulous pinpoint hemostasis (thereby avoiding the use of scalp clips). Dissection is then directed with electrocautery in the loose areolar subgaleal plane past the frontal sinus. Preservation of the facial nerve can be guaranteed by sharp dissection deep to the superficial temporal fascia laterally and under the pericranium centrally. At the location of the temporal fat pad, a combination of blunt and sharp dissection is used to protect blood supply to the fat pad (minimizing the risk of temporal hallowing). If one seeks improved lateral supraorbital rim exposure, then extension of the bicoronal flap to the preauricular area at the junction of the tragus and helix is performed. Dissection around the fracture is performed to facilitate reduction of the individual fragments. Careful attention to location and orientation is made before any removal or manipulation. A small hole or removal of a fragment may be needed to create access for instruments to reduce an indented large fracture fragment. Plating is then performed either in situ or on back table. Straight,

box-, T-, L-, or X-shaped 1.3-mm plates can be used to anatomically align the fracture fragments and secure to stable frontal bone (Figure 23-4). Occasionally a 1.3-mm titanium mesh is needed to assist in achieving proper contour in a comminuted section. Cortical bone graft and split calvarial bone grafts are almost never needed, as these are reserved for worse fracture patterns, commonly associated with nasofrontal obstruction.

When sinus defunctionalization and separation of sinonasal communication is required for patients with nasofrontal outflow tract obstruction, cranialization or obliteration is indicated. Although outcome differences are not significant between these techniques, cranialization has several distinct advantages: wide exposure of the injured area allows assessment and repair of dural injury, access to the cranial base for complex frontobasal repair, and elimination of the sinus with its propensity for infection and mucocele formation in a single stage. Although some surgeons advocate combining both of these techniques for one frontal sinus if the intersinus septum is uninjured (cranialize the left, and obliterate the right side), higher complications occur.

Complications of improper fracture management often arise due to inadequate removal of the mucous producing cells, particularly the posterior table. The frontal sinus lining is a tenacious mucoperiosteum that regenerates from residual basilar mucosal cells if simple stripping alone is used. To eliminate the mucosa, the walls must be burred deep to the diploic veins of Breschet, removing all the tails and cells of the mucosa. The fear of the inexperienced surgeon is burring too deep at the posterior table and compromising the dural layer.

Cranialization

Cranialization removes the ducts, posterior sinus wall, and mucosa, and creates a partition between the intracranial and nasal cavities. The area previous occupied by the frontal sinus, in fact, becomes a portion of the intracranial cavity through expansion of the dura and brain after several months. Cranialization often requires the assistance of

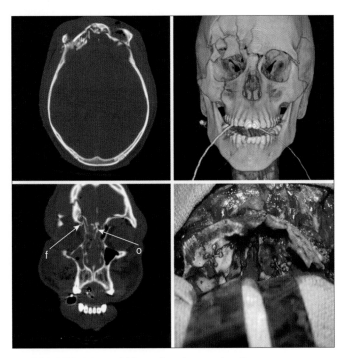

● **FIGURE 23-5.** This patient has a simultaneous anteroposterior displaced fracture seen on the axial cut (Above, *left*) and a three-dimensional reconstruction (Above, *right*) following a motor vehicle accident. The fracture meets all criteria for nasofrontal outflow tract injury: fracture of the medial aspect of the anterior table, sinus floor fracture (*f*), and outflow tract obstruction (*o*) (Below, *left*). (Below, *right*) Photograph obtained intraoperatively with frontal lobe retraction showing comminution and obstruction around the nasofrontal outflow tract. (*Rodriguez ED, Stanwix MG, Nam AJ, et al. Twenty-six-year experience treating frontal sinus fractures: a novel algorithm based on anatomical fracture pattern and failure of conventional techniques. Plast Reconstr Surg. 2008;122(6):1860.*)

a neurosurgery colleague. After bicoronal flaps by the primary team are raised in the standard fashion, the neurosurgeons can proceed with a careful frontal craniotomy to permit frontal lobe retraction for posterior wall visualization (Figure 23-5). Importantly, when raising the coronal incision for a cranialization, care must be made to preserve the pericranium such that one can rotate either a centrally or laterally based pericranium flap. Careful removal of the posterior wall then proceeds by rongeuring larger segments or power-burring techniques. Close attention should be paid to the inferolateral aspect of the posterior table, as the mucosa here is often inadequately eradicated. Meticulous burring of anterior table segments, lateral recesses, and other residual mucosal areas past the foramen of Breschet will eliminate the remaining mucous cells. Attention is then turned to the nasofrontal outflow tracts for definitive separation of the aerodigestive tract from the anterior cranial base. Here the surgeon must fully occlude the nasofrontal outflow tract. Importantly, we use the term "occlude" here to differentiate from the commonly used term "obliterate." "Obliterate" or "obliteration" is a surgical treatment for frontal sinus fractures, and should not be confused with "occlude," when one

seals the nasofrontal outflow tracts. Autologous bone graft can be placed in the nasofrontal outflow tract. Fibrin glue sealant or other modalities may be further implemented to create complete occlusion. The pericranial flap that was preserved during the coronal incision is now rotated down into the aperture of the outflow tracts.

Replacement of the frontal craniotomy segment, covering of the burr hole sites with titanium mesh plates, and frontal contouring is then pursued. Proper reduction of the anterior table by techniques presented above in the "reconstruction" section provides anatomical re-alignment. Titanium mesh may have to be implemented in order to achieve proper frontal contouring. When anterior table defects preclude the use of conventional hardware, split calvarial bone grafts harvested from the parietal lobe are indicated. Prior to final closure of the coronal flap, a suction drain should be placed to eliminate the dead space and prevent seroma formation. Typically, these drains only stay for 2 to 3 days postoperatively. Limitation of postoperative antibiotic therapy to only 24 hours must strictly be adhered to. Importantly, extra vigilance for any cerebral spinal fluid leak in the drain must be monitored as sinonasal communication has been surgically separated precluding typical cerebrospinal fluid rhinorrhea visualization.

Obliteration

Obliteration involves complete removal of the sinus mucosa, burring the sinus walls to eliminate mucosal invaginations, and filling the sinus cavity with fat, muscle, or bone. Exposure of the frontal area follows a typical bicoronal approach identical to cranialization, with specific attention to preserving a pericranial flap. Neurosurgical assistance is not required, as exposure to the contents of the frontal sinus cavity is accessed through comminuted bone segments or removal of an adequate surface area of the anterior table via a reciprocating power saw. Wide exposure is imperative to assure meticulous burring of the posterior and lateral recesses of the bone past the foramen of Breschet. Once all mucosa is stripped, and invaginations burred, occlusion of the nasofrontal outflow tract is performed in an identical manner to that of cranialization. Placement of an obliterating material follows subsequently with the autologous material of choice and then proper frontal vault contouring.

Autogenous materials, including fat, muscle, and bone have been used for decades, but newer alloplastic biomaterials have also been used. Bioactive glass, methylmethacrylate, oxidized regenerated cellulose, and calcium phosphate bone cement harbor intrinsic antibacterial properties and avoid donor site morbidity.[6] However, these potential benefits have not matriculated, and higher complication rates repeatedly are published.[1] Controversy even within autologous materials choices seems to undergo continuous debate. Cancellous bone grafts force the sinus to undergo ossification and provide progenitor cells and integral growth factors, providing an environment suitable for successful obliteration. Fat grafts rely on the viability of damaged bony walls that are poorly vascularized. In fact, over 50% of the fat placed into the cavity is resorbed or atrophies, creating an inadequate obliteration. If the doctrines of careful mucosal removal, proper occlusion of the nasofrontal outflow tracts with bone graft, surgical debridement of mucosal invaginations, and attention to dural integrity are followed, obliteration with cancellous bone graft may be a suitable alternative to cranialization in experienced hands.[7]

COMPLICATIONS

Inadequate treatment of frontal sinus fractures, unlike management of other craniomaxillofacial injuries, leads to severe and potentially fatal injuries. Mucoceles, meningitis, brain abscesses, and death may arise from inadequate partitioning of the upper aerodigestive system from the anterior cranial base and proliferation of unextirpated sinus mucosa. Complications arise in 3% to 10% patients following frontal sinus fracture treatment, but can be minimized by three tenets: meticulous eradication of sinus mucosa, occlusion of the sinonasal communication, and complete elimination of dead space (expanding brain in cranialization or cancellous bone grafting in obliteration).[8]

Complications may be major or minor and arise in the acute post-treatment period (first 6 months) or chronic period. Acutely minor complications proceeding surgery are typical of any procedure: hardware palpability/migration, contour irregularities, wound/skin infections, or skin breakdown. Major acute complications, on the contrary, are serious problems requiring a multiteam approach and intensive care. Meningitis, brain abscesses, and prolonged dural fistula, and death are fortunately rare entities but humble the craniomaxillofacial surgeon.

Late complications arise from inadequate sinus drainage; mucous is continuously produced resulting in pain, mass-like effect, erosion, and ultimately infection. Although early diagnosis seems critical, the propensity of this patient population is to disregard follow-up until clinical manifestations of frontal sinusitis or mucocele formation manifest. Chronic complications have very indolent courses, arising upward from 5 to 20 years after initial management. Surgical intervention is often required to correct complex bone and soft tissue deformities, while eradicating infectious material from the frontobasilar region (Figure 23-6).

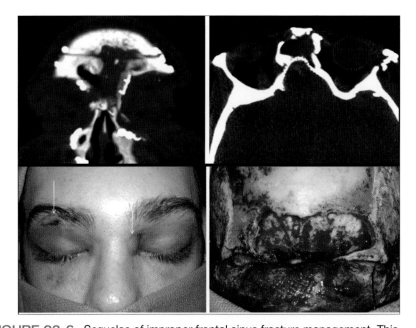

FIGURE 23-6. Sequelae of improper frontal sinus fracture management. This patient underwent management of panfacial fractures after a motor vehicle collision 4 years previously, which included obliteration of the frontal sinus with bone graft. She presented to our clinic with months of progressive frontal pressure, headaches, and throbbing. A mucopyocele formed after inadequate occlusion of the nasofrontal outflow tract (Above, *left*). The direct sinonasal communication seen in the axial cut (Above, *right*) resulted in persistent air and an indolent infection. Images of a 30-year-old patient treated 1 month previously with obliteration of the frontal sinus after sustaining a simultaneous anteroposterior fracture with nasofrontal outflow tract injury (Below, *left, right*). Pus (*arrows*) is expressed from the superior orbital rim and left medial canthus (Below, *left*). Complete removal of previous hardware and anterior table along with extensive burring of the sinus was performed (Below, *right*). (*Above from: Rodriguez ED, Stanwix MG, Nam AJ, et al. Twenty-six-year experience treating frontal sinus fractures: a novel algorithm based on anatomical fracture pattern and failure of conventional techniques. Plast Reconstr Surg. 2008;122(6):1862.Below from: Rodriguez ED, Stanwix MG, Nam AJ, et al. Definitive treatment of persistent frontal sinus infections: elimination of dead space and sinonasal communication. Plast Reconstr Surg. 2009;123(3):962.*)

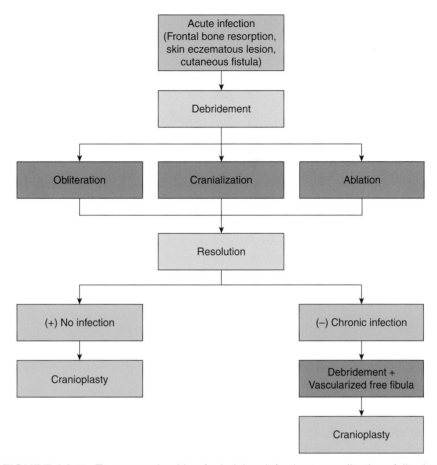

● **FIGURE 23-7.** Treatment algorithm for indolent infectious complications following frontal sinus fractures. (*Rodriguez ED, Stanwix MG, Nam AJ, et al. Definitive treatment of persistent frontal sinus infections: elimination of dead space and sinonasal communication. Plast Reconstr Surg. 2009;123(3):964.*)

Mucoceles as the result of sinus malfunction have an insidious course and are the most frequently encountered long-term complication. Typically, this collection of mucous undergoes recurrent bouts of infection, which is commonly misdiagnosed for frontal sinusitis or chronic headaches by primary care physicians. Initial complaints of frontal pressure or throbbing slowly progress to debilitating periorbital pain, and culminate with central nervous system sequelae. Clinical symptoms of seizures, headaches, photophobia, visual disturbances, and nuchal rigidity may be the only symptoms to push front line clinicians toward proper diagnostic studies. Overall, patients have limitations in activities of daily living, multiple abstained days from work, and a diminished quality of life. Chronicity of the disease, along with recurrent infectious bouts, leads to skin and bony changes.

Eczematous skin changes can be seen along with fistular drainage tracts, and the underlying soft tissue becomes indurated and scarred (Figure 23-6). The bony structure of the anterior table is attenuated and may have smoldering osteomyelitis. Occasionally, the infection will compromise the bone completely, creating a source for intracranial or periorbital extension. The disease perseveres, despite conventional treatment

approaches (antibiotics, endoscopic techniques) due to the duration and extent of bony and soft tissue involvement. Ultimately, treatment requires a combined intracranial-extracranial approach.

Traditionally, initial treatment involves debridement of the infection with hardware and graft removal, and re-obliteration or cranialization (Figure 23-7). Depending on the skin, soft tissue, and bony involvement, single-stage or multiple-stage approaches can be used. Regardless of the treatment pursued, successful management relies on wide local debridement, meticulous reburring of the tables beyond the foramen of Breschet, and removal of infected bone and previous obliteration material. Patients previously obliterated with bone graft or hydroxyapatite may need deeper burring than anticipated because of its osteoinductive capabilities. After completion of debridement, attention must be turned to finalize re-obliteration, cranialization, and reconstruct the anterior table. However, treatment for prolonged infected mucoceles by cranialization or re-obliteration is unsuccessful in over 50% of patients.[8] This is likely due to inadequate debridement, use of nonvascularized or foreign materials in an infected area, poor outflow tract occlusion, or inability to fill all dead space. Previous intracranial manipulation or

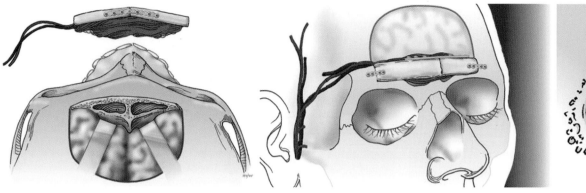

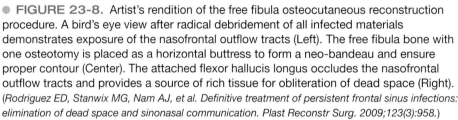

● **FIGURE 23-8.** Artist's rendition of the free fibula osteocutaneous reconstruction procedure. A bird's eye view after radical debridement of all infected materials demonstrates exposure of the nasofrontal outflow tracts (Left). The free fibula bone with one osteotomy is placed as a horizontal buttress to form a neo-bandeau and ensure proper contour (Center). The attached flexor hallucis longus occludes the nasofrontal outflow tracts and provides a source of rich tissue for obliteration of dead space (Right). (*Rodriguez ED, Stanwix MG, Nam AJ, et al. Definitive treatment of persistent frontal sinus infections: elimination of dead space and sinonasal communication. Plast Reconstr Surg. 2009;123(3):958.*)

cranialization forces the dura to scar down and inhibits the expansion of the brain to fill this space. Furthermore, wide local debridement of all infected, necrotic, and non-viable tissues may leave devastating defects that conventional salvage techniques stand inadequate. After salvage techniques fail or extensive defects are encountered, reconstruction commences with assessment and replacement of key missing components along with complete sinonasal separation.

Several donor sites have been used to reconstruct the skin, soft tissue, and bony loss following debridement of persistent frontal sinus infections. Autologous nonvascularized bone grafts such as calvarium, iliac, or ribs have been used to recontour the frontal area. Additionally, alloplastic materials, such as methymethacrylate, titanium mesh, or hydroxyapatite provide for easy on table contouring and avoid donor site morbidity. However, each autogenous or alloplastic materials used are nonvascularized or foreign materials that may predispose an already vulnerable area to re-infection. Nonetheless, each of the above grafts requires a secondary donor site for sinonasal separation by occluding the nasofrontal outflow tracts and a third for soft tissue bulking and dead-space obliteration. Galeal, temporalis muscle, and other local vascularized flaps have donorsite morbidity, and are likely unavailable due to previous surgical attempts or concomitant trauma.

The osteoseptocutaneous-free fibular flap is an ideal choice for single-staged treatment of the infected obliterated frontal sinus as it provides healthy bone and soft tissue (Figure 23-8).[8] The fibular bone recreates the frontal bandeau, and supplies rich vascularity to promote bony union and overcome local infection and osteomyelitis. Additionally, soft tissue and flexor hallucis longus muscle fully separate the anterior cranial base from the aerodigestive system while obliterating all dead space and occluding the nasofrontal outflow tracts (Figure 23-9).

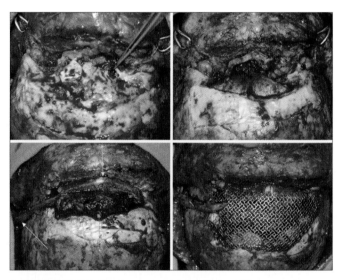

● **FIGURE 23-9.** A mucocele developed 32 years after a Riedel (ablation) procedure. A raised coronal flap displays mucus contamination of the frontal bone and alloplast (Above, *left*). The instrument is pointing to the source of the mucopyocele. After radical debridement and removal of infected methyl methacrylate, the large defect is ready for definitive free tissue reconstruction (Above, *right*). Formal reconstruction of the 9 × 5 cm bony defect, sinonasal separation, and softtissue reconstruction with a one-stage, single osteotomy fibular free flap were performed. The pedicle is anastomosed to the superficial temporal vessels (*white arrow*), the flexor hallucis longus obliterates the sinus and occludes the nasofrontal outflow tract (*blue arrow*), and the fibula forms the frontal neo-bandeau (*yellow arrow*) (Below, *left*). The titanium mesh can now be safely secured to stable, healthy bone for final contour (Below, *right*). (*Rodriguez ED, Stanwix MG, Nam AJ, et al. Definitive treatment of persistent frontal sinus infections: elimination of dead space and sinonasal communication. Plast Reconstr Surg. 2009;123(3):960.*)

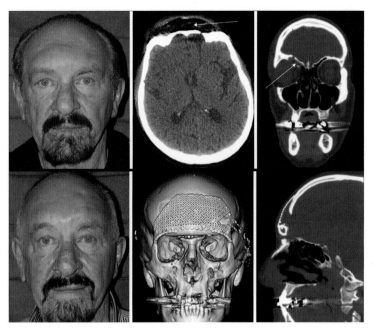

● **FIGURE 23-10.** Photographic and CT depiction of the patient in Figure 23-9. The patient presented with severe cosmetic deformity and diffuse erythema extending over forehead, nasal side walls, and frontal processes of the maxillary bones (Above, *left*). The *white arrows* demonstrate an abundance of undrained mucus found in the frontal sinus on axial (Above, *center*) and coronal views (Above, *right*), along with air (*red arrow*) and slow resorption of the bony posterior wall (*blue arrow*). Three-month postoperative photograph demonstrating resolution of erythema and restoration of contour (Below, *left*). This patient had complete cessation of all preoperative frontal symptoms, allowing for discontinuation of migraine, pain, and other related medications. A CT scan illustrates a neo-bandeau (Below, *center*), along with complete sinonasal separation as noted by the absence of air (Below, *right*). (*Rodriguez ED, Stanwix MG, Nam AJ, et al. Definitive treatment of persistent frontal sinus infections: elimination of dead space and sinonasal communication. Plast Reconstr Surg. 2009;123(3):959–961.*)

Also, careful dissection of the superficial temporal vessels proximally provides for an ideal anastomotic recipient. Radical debridement, meticulous mucosa removal, and obliteration with a free fibula flap achieve all goals of treatment for persistent infectious complications following frontal sinus fractures: a secure horizontal buttress, obliteration of dead space, and occlusion of the nasofrontal outflow tracts (Figure 23-10).

● OUTCOMES ASSESSMENT

Outcomes following sinus fracture treatment must be assessed as two separate entities: acute and chronic. The initial bodily and cranial trauma the patient endures resulting in frontal sinus fracture should make all survivors of the injury fortunate. Acute management, observation or surgical, may potentially lead to devastating and fatal complications. Patients who withstand this hospital course, and subsequently discharged, are usually satisfied with no acute concerns. They may have initial hardware or contour complaints, but fortunately avoided fatal acute complications. Patients should then be followed long term as the indolent and persistent course of late complications may take many years before culminating. Unfortunately, the nature of this patient population is to forego any postoperative care or monitoring and follow-up is often poor. If willing, patients must be indefinitely monitored for signs of infectious chronic complications. Prompt radiological studies must be pursued if any symptom or sign arises. Inadequate or delayed treatment will generate severe multifaceted soft tissue and bony issues that require intracranial-extracranial salvage approaches, or possibly free tissue transfer.

REFERENCES

1. Rodriguez ED, Stanwix MG, Nam AJ, et al. Twenty-six-year experience treating frontal sinus fractures: a novel algorithm based on anatomical fracture pattern and failure of conventional techniques. *Plast Reconstr Surg.* 2008;122(6): 1850–1866.

2. Rohrich RJ, Hollier L. The role of the nasofrontal duct in frontal sinus fracture management. *J Craniomaxillofac Trauma.* 1996;2(4):31–40.

3. Manson PN, Stanwix MG, Yaremchuk MJ, et al. Frontobasal fractures: anatomical classification and clinical significance. *Plast Reconstr Surg.* 2009;124(6):2096–2106.

4. Holloway KL, Smith K. Antibiotic prophylaxis during clean neurosurgery: A large, multicenter study using cefuroxime. *Clin Ther.* 1996;18(1):84–94.

5. Markowitz BL, Manson PN. Panfacial fractures: organization of treatment. *Clin Plast Surg.* 1989;16(1):105–114.

6. Manolidis S, Hollier LH. Management of frontal sinus fractures. *Plast Reconstr Surg.* 2007;120(7 suppl 2):32S–48S.

7. Mickel TJ, Rohrich RJ, Robinson JB Jr. Frontal sinus obliteration: a comparison of fat, muscle, bone, and spontaneous osteoneogenesis in the cat model. *Plast Reconstr Surg.* 1995;95(3):586–592.

8. Rodriguez ED, Stanwix MG, Nam AJ, et al. Definitive treatment of persistent frontal sinus infections: elimination of dead space and sinonasal communication. *Plast Reconstr Surg.* 2009;123(3):957–967.

chapter 24

Nasal Fractures

Ronald E. Hoxworth, MD / Rod J. Rohrich, MD, FACS

● INTRODUCTION

The nose is the most prominent facial feature. The nasal pyramid consists of the paired nasal bones, the frontal process of the maxilla, the paired nasal cartilages (upper lateral and lower lateral), and the nasal septum. The septum is composed of the quadrilateral cartilage anteriorly, the vomer inferiorly, and the perpendicular plate of the ethmoid posteriorly (Figure 24-1). A fracture of the nasal pyramid is the third most common bone fracture in the body and the most common facial fracture, requiring less force than that for any other facial bone.[1–5] The increasing prevalence of this injury presents the plastic surgeon with challenging treatment options. Although nasal fractures are often discussed as minor injuries,[6] the incidence of posttraumatic nasal deformity as reported in the literature is not insignificant (9%–50%). Revision rhinoplasty for traumatic nasal deformity is a difficult procedure; accordingly, guidelines are needed to optimize the management of acute nasal fractures in order to minimize secondary deformities.

The numerous factors that contribute to suboptimal aesthetic and functional results include timing, edema, undetected preexisting nasal deformity, and occult septal deviation/injury. Thus, it is essential for the physician to have a systemic approach or algorithm for acute nasal fracture management that includes a complete evaluation of the nasal deformity (both internal and external) and a precise anatomic reduction under controlled conditions. This algorithmic approach can be used to improve long-term results and to reduce the incidence of posttraumatic nasal deformities.

● PATIENT EVALUATION AND SELECTION

A detailed nasal history and a physical examination are essential to diagnosis and treatment. To begin the assessment, a precise account of the mechanism, including injuring agent, direction of blow, and timing of nasal injury, is recorded. A history of epistaxis (sine qua non for a nasal fracture) indicates a laceration of the involved nasal mucosa.[4] The essential aspects of the nasal history are noted on the nasal fracture datasheet (Figure 24-2). Patients may vary in assessment of preinjury nasal shape; differentiating between new and old nasal deformity is sometimes difficult and must be correlated with patient history and physical findings. To this end, a review of old photographs or a driver's license photo can be very helpful as one third of individuals may have nasal deviation present prior to their injury. Finally, standard seven-view nasal photographs (anteroposterior, right and left laterals, right and left obliques, low and high basals) are taken to complete the nasal history.

The physical examination consists of an integrated systematic approach. During the course of the examination, the physician needs to be aware of the patient's overall status. Quite often the mechanism of injury results in concomitant injuries which may prove more threatening for the patient. As such, the physician must strictly adhere to the ABCs of patient resuscitation prior to conducting any secondary evaluation of nasal injury. Further, cooperation with all members of the team caring for the acutely injured patient is essential. The presence of concomitant life-threatening injuries precludes the need for urgent management of nasal fractures unless there is an associated airway issue involved with the injury.

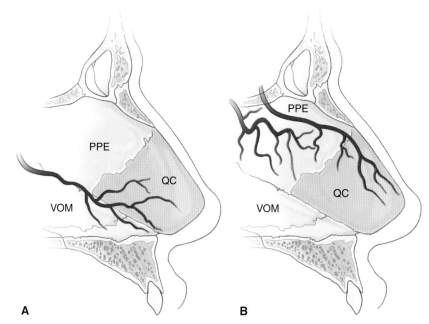

● **FIGURE 24-1.** Sagittal view of the nasal septum, with red and green depicting the most common septal fractures seen with low-velocity (A) and high-velocity (B) injuries. QC, quadrangular cartilage; PPE, perpendicular plate of the ethmoid; Vom, vomer.
(Reprinted with permission from Rohrich RJ, Adams WP Jr. Nasal fracture management: minimizing secondary nasal deformities. Plast Reconstr Surg. 2000;106(2):266–273.)

The external examination includes an inspection for lacerations, wounds, swelling, and deviation. Palpation of the proximal nasal skeleton is done to identify tenderness, crepitus, depression and/ or nasal shortening, and widening of the nasal base. Accurate intercanthal measurements are done to rule out a naso-orbitalethmoid (NOE) fracture, which is especially common in severe, high-velocity frontal or inferior injuries. Next, if present, the fracture type is then defined. Various nasal fracture classifications have been reported in the literature.[7,8] We adopted a practical, clinically applicable nasal fracture classification based on the physical examination as recorded on the nasal fracture datasheet (Figure 24-2). Fractures are graded as simple unilateral (type I) or bilateral (type II), comminuted (type III), and complex with bone and septal disruption (type IV). The most serious fractures (type V) involve associated midfacial or NOE involvement. Edema is graded by the degree of periorbital edema (1+, minimal/no periorbital edema; 2+, moderate periorbital edema; 3+, severe periorbital edema).

A complete assessment of the nasal septum is the single most important step in determining aesthetic and functional outcome in nasal fractures.[4,6] Verwoerd[6] describes the pathogenesis of septal fractures as including three septal zones composed of thicker cartilage-dorsoposterior, basal, and caudal. Conversely, the central caudal portion of the septum is thin. The thicker, posterior septal cartilage provides the primary support for the nasal dorsum. Trauma to the nasal dorsum leads to lesions in the caudal-basal to cephalodorsal supporting cartilage and to horizontal fractures of the thinner central region.[6]

Fry[9,10] presented the progressive distortion of fractured septal cartilage caused by the release of locked internal stresses. Verwoerd[6] and Wexler[11] demonstrated that the septum does not remain straight after manipulation and that the nasal bones tend to unite in the direction of the deviated septum. Accordingly, the septum is the key structure to consider for optimal management of nasal fractures and the prevention of secondary deformities.[12] The extent of septal injury determines the proper technique for septal correction. Renner reported that closed reduction with intranasal splints and packs yielded satisfactory results in most simple septal injuries involving the distal portion of the quadrangular cartilage.[2] Pollock advocated a low threshold for open reduction, with precise septal correction for moderate to severe septal injuries with a complex fracture pattern or an involvement of the perpendicular plate of the ethmoid or vomerine groove.[7] In the absence of a complete evaluation of the entire septum, the mobile anterior portion is reduced, leaving a dislocated, rigid posterior septum that results in late functional deformity after closed reduction.[13] In 1968, Adamson et al. advocated acute submucous resection for severely fractured septums.[14] Eleven years later, Harrison recognized that low horizontal submucous septal resection removing only the quadrangular cartilage-vomerine groove interface was often inadequate because of the overlapping, fractured segment in the perpendicular plate of the ethmoid. To fully address the septal pathology, he recommended an extended low horizontal and posterior vertical submucous resection.[13] Murray et al.[15] also attributed the high rate of postreduction nasal deformity requiring salvage

Nasal Fracture Data Sheet

Name: _____ Date: _____ Age: _____

Mode of Injury: Low Energy   High Energy

Direction: _____ Appearance: _____

Time Since Injury: _____

Associated Injury: Soft Tissue   Facial Fracture

Patient Medical History:

Allergies	_____
Previous Nasal Trauma	_____
Previous Nasal Surgery	_____
Airway Obstruction History	_____
Medications	_____
Pretraumatic Photographs:	Yes No

Physical Examination:

External   Unilateral _____   Bilateral _____   (Width of Nasal Base)
                  Intercanthal Distance   _____
                  Edema   1+   2+   3+
                  Ecchymosis   1+   2+   3+
                  Nasal Bleeding   Right   Left   Bilateral   None

Intranasal   Septal Deviation/Dislocation/Fracture _____
                  Mucosal Status _____
                  Septal Hematoma   Yes   No

Nasal Fracture Classification:
I.   Simple (Unilateral)
II. Simple (Bilateral)
III. Comminuted
     a. Unilateral
     b. Bilateral
     c. Frontal
IV. Complex (Nasal Bone & Septal Disruption)
     a. Associated Septal Hematoma
     b. Associated Open Nasal Laceration
V.   NOE Fracture/Midface Fracture

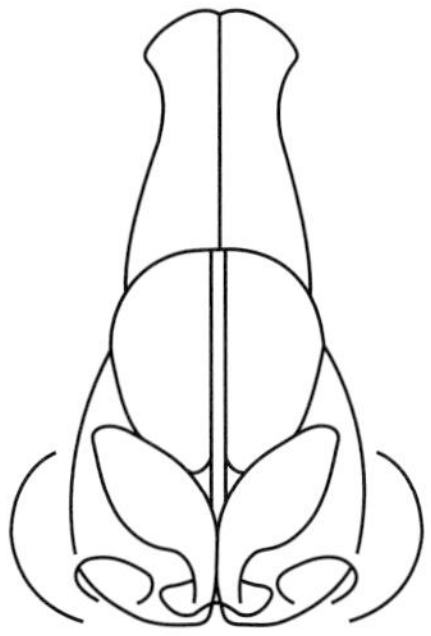

● **FIGURE 24-2.** Nasal fracture datasheet for documenting clinical findings. (*Reprinted with permission from Rohrich RJ, Adams WP Jr. Nasal fracture management: minimizing secondary nasal deformities. Plast Reconstr Surg. 2000;106(2):266–273.*)

septorhinoplasty to an unrecognized septal injury. They found that patients with nasal bones deviated more than half the nasal bridge width had a concomitant, C-shaped fracture of the bony and cartilaginous septum. They also concluded that acute open reduction with submucous septal resection resulted in an improved long-term cosmetic and functional outcome due to the alleviation of overlapped, interlocking fragments of the septum that usually resulted in the secondary nasal bone deformity.

The most common septal fractures in low-velocity injuries occur inferiorly along the vomerine groove as fractures or fracture dislocations.[16] High-velocity injuries or frontal impacts result in more extensive septal fractures through the thin central region of the quadrangular cartilage that extend posteriorly across the interface with the perpendicular plate of the ethmoid and inferiorly

to the vomer (Figure 24-1). Aggressive management of these septal injuries is a major key to the successful management of the nasal fracture.

Plain film radiographs are not necessary for the clinical diagnosis of isolated nasal fractures.[2,17] Approximately half of all patients with nasal fractures will have negative x-ray findings. Logan et al. reported a prospective series evaluating the use of routine x-rays in the diagnosis of nasal fractures, ultimately concluding that they are not cost-effective.[18] However, patients found by x-ray to have displaced nasal fracture are at a higher risk for long-term nasal deformity, thus, anatomic reduction was highly recommended for these individuals. CT scans are likewise not essential for isolated nasal fractures unless there is a suspicion of associated complex facial fractures based on clinical findings or mechanism of injury.

PATIENT PREPARATION

At minimum, the internal examination requires halogen lighting, good suction, a nasal speculum, vasoconstrictive anesthesia, and a 30-degree, 3-mm rigid nasal endoscope of type III or greater. A complete evaluation of the internal structures is performed with particular attention paid to the septum. Specifics of the deformity and evidence of obstruction are recorded on the datasheet. The rigid nasal endoscope is used to fully evaluate the entire septum, especially the posterior bony septum and vomerine regions in types III, IV, and V nasal fractures. A topical anesthesia of 4% lidocaine and oxymetazoline (Afrin) or phenylephrine hydrochloride (Neo-Synephrine) is adequate to perform a full waking examination of the patient. The total septal examination is central to the evaluation of nasal fractures and to the optimization of results; therefore, adequate anesthesia is essential for complete systematic evaluation. After adequate vasoconstriction and topical anesthesia of the nasal mucosa, the diagnostic endonasal procedure can proceed. The patient is seated in an examining chair with the examiner usually sitting or standing to the right side of the patient.

TECHNIQUE

Endoscopic Evaluation

The endoscope is placed in the nasal vestibule and advanced posteriorly under direct vision. This pass of the endoscope is advanced along the floor of the nose, beneath the inferior turbinate. Areas examined include the inferior meatus, turbinates, septum, and the postero-inferior septal junction with the perpendicular plate of the ethmoid. Withdrawal of the scope allows for confirmation of fractures and septal disruption while these areas are re-inspected.

The septal mucosa is inspected for disruptions and evidence of septal fractures. Prompt diagnosis and treatment of septal hematoma are essential to the reduction of fibrosis and subsequent septal distortion, abscess, and complete necrosis with saddle nasal deformity. Wide, dependent drainage followed by careful packing with antibiotic gauze[19] and systemic antibiotic coverage is recommended. Small hematomas are aspirated,[2] followed up closely, and re-aspirated if re-accumulation occurs.

Management of Nasal Fractures

Once a nasal fracture has been diagnosed, the physician needs to consider the proper timing for repair. In the absence of any prevailing injuries or comorbidities, closed reduction should be undertaken within 3 hours of the initial injury. If there is excessive edema due to a delay in treatment, the patient is managed expectantly with head elevation, ice packs, and pain management until the edema resolves in 3 to 5 days. If closed reduction is not accomplished within 5 to 7 days, fibrous union of the fracture may make manipulation difficult. In the case of

a missed diagnosis or unsuccessful reduction in the first 5 to 7 days, it is recommended that an open reduction be planned for 3 to 6 months post injury (Figure 24-3).

Numerous prospective series have been published comparing local versus general anesthesia for the manipulation of nasal fractures.[20–22] In most cases, these studies found local anesthesia to be as clinically effective and less expensive than general anesthesia for closed reduction. Wang et al.[4] stated that most adults with uncomplicated fractures can be treated using either the closed or open technique with topical/local anesthetics and intravenous sedation. Cook et al.[23] found externally infiltrative field anesthesia to the nasal dorsum to be as effective as, and better tolerated than bilateral specific internal blocks of the infraorbital, infratrochlear, and external nasal nerves. This external technique introduces the needle bilaterally at the caudal edge of the nasal bone, midway between the nasal bridge and maxilla.

Brief general anesthesia is recommended for complete nasal fracture reduction,[2,16] on account of its safety, airway control, and unhindered ability to examine, reduce, and manipulate the nose. Local anesthesia with intravenous sedation is used for simple types I and II fractures or at the patient's request. Nasal reductions can be performed in a day-surgery center regardless of the anesthesia type, thereby maximizing the use of superior lighting, nasal fracture/rhinoplasty instruments and enhanced technical assistance available in that setting. This approach yields a more consistent and controlled outcome with less patient discomfort. Pediatric patients, however, routinely undergo nasal manipulation with general anesthesia, as do adults with polytrauma who require the repair of multiple injuries. A topical vasoconstrictive agent (Afrin) and 8 to 10 cc of 1% lidocaine with 1:100,000 epinephrine are always used for nasal hemostasis. The reduction of external nasal bones to their anatomic position is initially accomplished by recreating the fracture; molding the nasal bones with the fingers is the simplest approach.[7,8,24] Impacted nasal bones require instrumentation for reduction and restoration of nasal length, which is the most critical dimension to regain. The Walsham forceps are designed for the reduction of impacted nasal bones,[2,8] whereas the Asch forceps are designed for reduction of the nasal septum, although they may also successfully restore the alignment of impacted nasal bones. Both of these instruments can cause damage to the nasal mucosa; therefore, we prefer using a less traumatic Boies elevator (Figure 24-4). Placing the elevator intranasally and the surgeon's thumb externally over the nasal bones allows appreciation of subtle osseous movements.[2]

The reduction of the fractured nasal septum begins by relocating the displaced base into the vomerine groove (Figure 24-4), a process that may be accomplished with either the Asch forceps or the blunt Boies elevator. If the reduction of the septum is accomplished with this simple technique, it should be reexamined endoscopically or with a nasal speculum and headlight to ensure alignment of posterior elements. The nasal bone reduction should

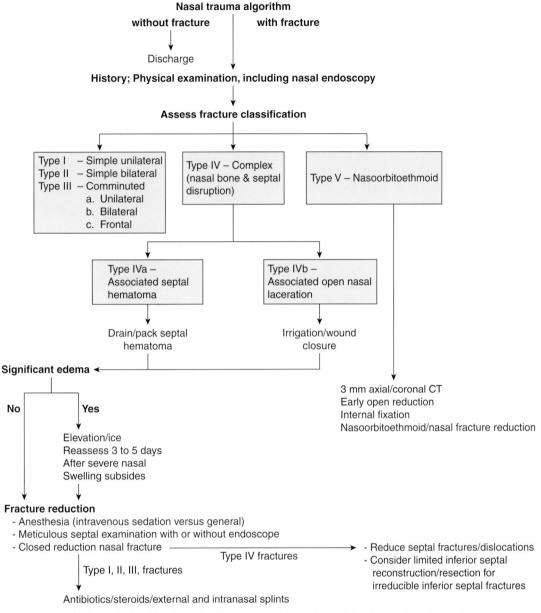

Nasal trauma algorithm

without fracture   with fracture

↓
Discharge

History; Physical examination, including nasal endoscopy

Assess fracture classification

Type I – Simple unilateral
Type II – Simple bilateral
Type III – Comminuted
        a. Unilateral
        b. Bilateral
        c. Frontal

Type IV – Complex
(nasal bone & septal
disruption)

Type V – Nasoorbitoethmoid

Type IVa –
Associated septal
hematoma

Type IVb –
Associated open nasal
laceration

Drain/pack septal
hematoma

Irrigation/wound
closure

Significant edema

No   **Yes**

3 mm axial/coronal CT
Early open reduction
Internal fixation
Nasoorbitoethmoid/nasal fracture reduction

Elevation/ice
Reassess 3 to 5 days
After severe nasal
Swelling subsides

Fracture reduction
  - Anesthesia (intravenous sedation versus general)
  - Meticulous septal examination with or without endoscope
  - Closed reduction nasal fracture ——————→ Type IV fractures ——→ - Reduce septal fractures/dislocations
                                                                          - Consider limited inferior septal
                                                                            reconstruction/resection for
                                                                            irreducible inferior septal fractures
            Type I, II, III, fractures

Antibiotics/steroids/external and intranasal splints

● **FIGURE 24-3.** Algorithm for the management of nasal fractures. (*Reprinted with permission from Rohrich RJ, Adams WP Jr. Nasal fracture management: minimizing secondary nasal deformities. Plast Reconstr Surg. 2000;106(2):266–273.*)

also be reassessed, because shifting may occur during septal manipulation.[7] Comminuted nasal bones may be reduced, followed by dorsal-posterior intranasal packing with gel foam to prevent collapse after reduction.

A nonreducible posteroinferior or anterior septum is considered for acute septal reconstruction, especially in type IV fractures. This has a slightly increased risk of losing traumatized nasal mucosa during undermining with subsequent septal perforation. Nevertheless, given the extremely high rate of posttraumatic nasal deformity secondary to malaligned or occult septal injury, a total anatomic septal reduction and/or reconstruction should be performed if the injury is acute or if the septum is irreducible and posteriorly displaced.

A hemitransfixion or Killian incision is made, and the bilateral inferior mucoperichondrial flaps are developed. Complete visualization of the septum is then able to define the extent of the injury. An inferior and posterior septal reconstruction to dislodge and align the septum and/or to implement septal repositioning may be performed with anterior septal spine figure-of-8 sutures, using 5-0 polydioxanone suture to keep the septum aligned and straight (Figure 24-5). Reduced fractures of the septum are precisely re-approximated using through-and-through, mucosal-septum-mucosal, 4-0 chromic mattress suture (Figure 24-6, Left). Doyle splints are recommended to further stabilize the caudal septum (Figure 24-6, Right). Intranasal and external splints are used for 5 to 7 days,

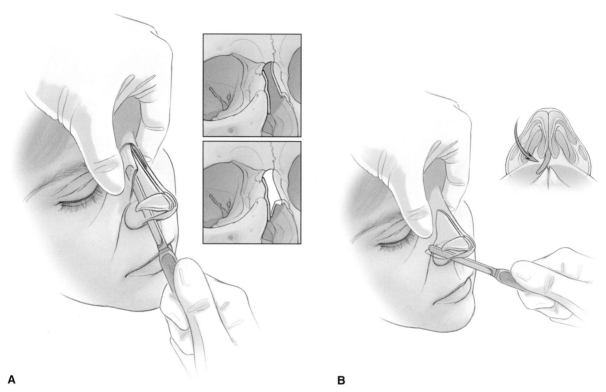

A

B

● **FIGURE 24-4.** (A) Bimanual reduction of a nasal bone fracture using the Boies elevator to minimize nasal mucosa trauma, injury, and bleeding. The inset depicts an anatomic reduction of nasal bones. (B) Relocation of a septal disruption. The inset depicts a septal dislocation out of the vomerine groove, which may be similarly reduced using the Boies elevator. (*Reprinted with permission from Rohrich RJ, Adams WP Jr. Nasal fracture management: minimizing secondary nasal deformities. Plast Reconstr Surg. 2000;106(2):266–273.*)

as are prophylactic antibiotics (Cephalexin) and 3-day steroid-dose packs to reduce postreduction nasal edema.

Clinical Algorithm

A clinical algorithm for acute nasal fracture management was formulated (Figure 24-3) to minimize the incidence of post-traumatic nasal deformity requiring revision septorhinoplasty; however, an algorithm is merely a framework on which to base clinical decisions and does not supplant sound, individualized clinical judgment. Points of emphasis include the following:

1. The diagnosis of an acute nasal fracture is based on a patient's complete history and physical examination, including intranasal examination (± nasal endoscopy), not on radiographic studies.

2. In patients with significant posttraumatic swelling precluding immediate precise reduction, a clinical examination is performed and local measures (eg, ice and elevation) are prescribed, with follow-up in 3 to 5 days. Definitive treatment is instituted 5 to 7 days postinjury, depending on edema resolution in the nose.

3. The septum is the key to nasal fracture management. Using clinical examination and rigid nasal endoscopy, all septal pathology, especially posteriorly, must be identified. Significant septal fractures are directly visualized and limited septal reconstruction/repositioning is considered.

4. This algorithm will yield improved, long-term functional and aesthetic results; however, all patients should be counseled initially regarding the possibility of further nasal procedures.

Previous acute nasal fracture management has been inadequate, with a high incidence of long-term nasal deformity. Primary factors contributing to poor long-term results include acute traumatic edema, unrecognized preexisting nasal deformity, and undetected posteriorly and inferiorly displaced septal fractures. Given these variables, we have devised an algorithm for acute nasal fracture management.

This algorithm was developed and refined during the past 15 years. In the original series of 110 patients,[16] these principles were followed; however, albeit was not possible to stratify these patients with regard to fracture type. The treatment failures were generally those patients with

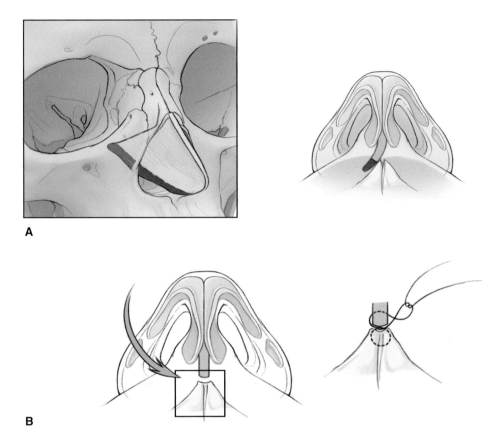

● **FIGURE 24-5.** (A) Submucous resection of an inferior septum. (B) Midline fixation of a dislocated septum using a figure-of-8 suture at the nasal spine. (*Reprinted with permission from Rohrich RJ, Adams WP Jr. Nasal fracture management: minimizing secondary nasal deformities. Plast Reconstr Surg. 2000;106(2):266–273.*)

severe, difficult-to-reduce septal injuries, which emphasizes the importance of the septum. Further detailed data on the type of patients most prone to failure is presently being collected and will further refine the algorithm.

Most reductions are done 3 to 4 days postinjury with appropriate anesthesia in the operating room. Irreducible septal injuries should be treated with limited inferior septal reconstruction in the acute phase to diminish secondary nasal deformity. Using the described algorithm, the need for extensive and difficult posttraumatic revision rhinoplasty should be significantly reduced.

● COMPLICATIONS

Incidence of Post-traumatic Nasal Deformity

In 1947, Maliniac's classic description of the management of acute nasal injuries was published.[25] Since then, there has been considerable debate over the optimal care of acute nasal fractures. Discrepancies in timing, method, and postoperative management are common in the literature.[1–3,7,19,26] The incidence of postreduction nasal deformities requiring subsequent rhinoplasty or septorhinoplasty ranges from 9% to 50%.[16,20,26,27] Several authors[15,20–23,26] report suboptimal results when using simple closed manipulation for acute nasal fractures.

Fry[9,10] and Mayell[28] described unfavorable structural and aesthetic outcomes after nasal fractures. In a study of 29 patients who underwent acute closed nasal fracture reduction, Watson et al. noted a 29% to 50% incidence of secondary nasal deformity.[22] Waldron et al.[20] presented a prospective study of 100 patients comparing local versus general anesthesia for closed reduction. Three months postoperatively, a 14% to 15% incidence of postreduction deformity was found, requiring further surgery. Of those patients with initially identified traumatic septal deviation, 40% to 42% had a significant septal deformity at 3 months that required septorhinoplasty. Cook et al.[21] published a randomized prospective series of 45 patients, again comparing anesthesia for the simple reduction of nasal fractures, resulting in a 14% to 17% incidence of postreduction deformity that required further surgery. Murray and Maran's[26] prospective series of 756 patients treated with simple reduction resulted in a 41% incidence of postreduction deformity. They stated that "When outcome of simple manipulation is assessed objectively the technique has poor success rate; only a proportion of noses are made straight and quite a number left unaltered."[26] Rohrich and Adams[16] presented better outcomes for closed reduction when a systemic approach was employed. Their review of management techniques over an 11-year period involved 110 cases with a 9% (10/110) nasal revision rate. This low

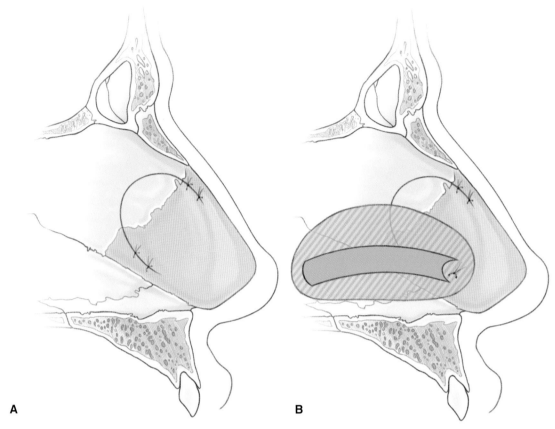

● **FIGURE 24-6.** (A) Stabilization of a septal fracture using through-and-through, 4-0 chromic horizontal mattress sutures. (B) Added septal stabilization using intranasal Doyle splints. (*Reprinted with permission from Rohrich RJ, Adams WP Jr. Nasal fracture management: minimizing secondary nasal deformities. Plast Reconstr Surg. 2000;106(2):266–273.*)

incidence of revision was attributed to complete nasal assessment, use of outpatient controlled general anesthesia, and primary septal reconstruction in cases with severe septal fracture dislocation. The details of the algorithm have been outlined within this chapter (Figure 24-3).

The first step in the treatment of complications is prevention. The authors believe that adoption of a systemic approach to injury may not abolish complications but certainly can minimize the prevalence. It is essential that the physician include the potential for postoperative complications in any preoperative discussion and consent. In the case of nasal fractures, a discussion of the occurrence of secondary deformities requiring further surgical procedures is mandatory.

REFERENCES

1. Haug RH, Prather JL. The closed reduction of nasal fractures: an evaluation of two techniques. *J Oral Maxillofac Surg*. 1991;49(12):1288–1292.

2. Renner GJ. Management of nasal fractures. *Otolaryngol Clin North Am*. 1991;24(1):195–213.

3. Tremolet de Villers Y. Nasal fractures. *J Trauma*. 1975;15(4):319–327.

4. Wang TD, Facer GW, Kern EB. Nasal fractures. In: Gates GA, ed. *Current Therapy in Otolaryngology: Head and Neck Surgery*. Vol. 4. Philadelphia: B. C. Decker; 1990:105–109.

5. Swearington JJ. Tolerances of human face to crash impact. Oklahoma City, OK: Federal Aviation Agency; 1965.

6. Verwoerd CD. Present day treatment of nasal fractures: closed versus open reduction. *Facial Plast Surg*. 1992;8(4):220–223.

7. Pollock RA. Nasal trauma. Pathomechanics and surgical management of acute injuries. *Clin Plast Surg*. 1992;19(1):133–147.

8. Stranc MF, Robertson GA. A classification of injuries of the nasal skeleton. *Ann Plast Surg*. 1979;2(6):468–474.

9. Fry HJ. Interlocked stresses in human nasal septal cartilage. *Br J Plast Surg*. 1966;19(3):276–278.

10. Fry H. Nasal skeletal trauma and the interlocked stresses of the nasal septal cartilage. *Br J Plast Surg*. 1967;20(2):146–158.

11. Wexler MR. Reconstructive surgery of the injured nose. *Otolaryngol Clin North Am.* 1975;8(3):663–677.

12. Gunter JP, Rohrich RJ. Management of the deviated nose. The importance of septal reconstruction. *Clin Plast Surg.* 1988;15(1):43–55.

13. Harrison DH. Nasal injuries: their pathogenesis and treatment. *Br J Plast Surg.* 1979;32(1):57–64.

14. Adamson JE, Horton CE, Crawford HH, Taddeo RJ. Acute submucous resection. *Plast Reconstr Surg.* 1968;42(2):152–154.

15. Murray JA, Maran AG, Mackenzie IJ, Raab G. Open v closed reduction of the fractured nose. *Arch Otolaryngol.* 1984;110(12):797–802.

16. Rohrich RJ, Adams WP Jr. Nasal fracture management: minimizing secondary nasal deformities. *Plast Reconstr Surg.* 2000;106(2):266–273.

17. Humber PR, Horton CE. Trauma to the nose. In: Starks RB, ed. *Plastic Surgery of the Head and Neck.* New York: Churchill Livingstone; 1989.

18. Logan M, O'Driscoll K, Masterson J. The utility of nasal bone radiographs in nasal trauma. *Clin Radiol.* 1994;49(3):192–194.

19. Kurihara K, Kim K. Open reduction and interfragment wire fixation of comminuted nasal fractures. *Ann Plast Surg.* 1990;24(2):179–185.

20. Waldron J, Mitchell DB, Ford G. Reduction of fractured nasal bones; local versus general anaesthesia. *Clin Otolaryngol Allied Sci.* 1989;14(4):357–359.

21. Cook JA, McRae RD, Irving RM, Dowie LN. A randomized comparison of manipulation of the fractured nose under local and general anaesthesia. *Clin Otolaryngol Allied Sci.* 1990;15(4):343–346.

22. Watson DJ, Parker AJ, Slack RW, Griffiths MV. Local versus general anaesthetic in the management of the fractured nose. *Clin Otolaryngol Allied Sci.* 1988;13(6):491–494.

23. Cook JA, Murrant NJ, Evans K, Lavelle RJ. Manipulation of the fractured nose under local anaesthesia. *Clin Otolaryngol Allied Sci.* 1992;17(4):337–340.

24. Dingman RO, Converse JM. The clinical management of facial injuries and fractures of the facial bones. In: Converse JM, ed. *Reconstructive Plastic Surgery.* Vol. 2. Philadelphia: Saunders, 1977.

25. Maliniac JW. *Rhinoplasty and Restoration of Facial Contour: With Specific Reference to Trauma.* Philadelphia: F. A. Davis; 1947:29.

26. Murray JA, Maran AG. The treatment of nasal injuries by manipulation. *J Laryngol Otol.* 1980;94(12):1405–1410.

27. Crowther JA, O'Donoghue GM. The broken nose: does familiarity breed neglect? *Ann R Coll Surg Engl.* 1987;69(6):259–260.

28. Mayell MF. Nasal fractures. Their occurrence, management and some late results. *J R Coll Surg Edinb.* 1973;18(1):31–36.

chapter 25

Midface and Maxillary Fractures

Adam J. Oppenheimer, MD / *Steven R. Buchman, MD, FACS*

● INTRODUCTION

The principles of reconstructive surgery, namely restoration of form and function, have particular importance in traumatic midface reconstruction. Given the density of specialized functional units and highly expressive mimetic tissue, midface fractures can incur significant dysfunction on an individual's way of life. Accordingly, patients sustaining severe midfacial fractures report substantially worse health outcomes and demonstrate poorer occupational productivity than general injury-matched control patients.[1] It is the responsibility of the maxillofacial surgeon not only to prevent short-term morbidity and mortality, but ultimately to restore the patient to their preinjury condition. This chapter keeps this goal in mind, focusing on key reconstructive principles and the avoidance of commonly encountered complications.

While the midface consists of the entire central third of the facial skeleton, this chapter will limit its focus to maxillary fractures and palatal fractures. Those fractures involving the zygoma, naso-orbitoethmoid (NOE) complex, and orbital floor will be discussed elsewhere.

● EPIDEMIOLOGY

Motor vehicle accidents and interpersonal violence account for greater than two thirds of all facial fractures. Alcohol intoxication is frequently cited as an associated and etiological factor. Not surprisingly, facial fractures are intimately related to socioeconomic status and geographic locale. Men are twice as likely to experience facial fractures compared with women, the average age being approximately 33 years.[2]

Associated Injuries

Although facial fractures are rarely a threat to life, those involving the midface are associated with a high proportion of life-threatening injuries. This may be due, in part, to the severity of impact and the degree of force required to sustain this type of fracture. Cerebral trauma, hemorrhagic shock, and airway compromise have all been strongly correlated. Injuries to the cervical spine are reported in approximately 6% of maxillofacial trauma.[3] Stabilization of the cervical spine should be maintained in maxillofacial trauma patients until radiographic and clinical clearance is possible. When traumatic brain injury occurs in concert with facial fractures, patient mortality increases from 5.8% to nearly 17%.[4] Death is also strongly linked to midface fracture. In one study, 84% of patients who died from neurologic injuries had a facial fracture pattern that included the midface.[5] In contrast, isolated mandibular fractures were rarely associated with fatal neurologic complications.

● MIDFACIAL ANATOMY

The anatomy of the maxilla is complex: alternating segments of thick and thin bone are admixed with sinuses and cavities, and neurovascular pathways course throughout. A sound understanding of regional anatomy is therefore crucial to proper midface reconstruction. The maxilla is the keystone of the facial skeleton, establishing the central portion of the midface. The paired maxillary bones define the orbital, nasal, and oral cavities: the so-called functional units.[6] The physiological importance of these units in respiration, mastication, and vision is axiomatic. Reestablishing the functional units of the midface is, therefore, a central goal of posttraumatic midface reconstruction. In addition, several specific anatomic structures deserve additional attention (Figure 25-1). They will be discussed in the context of their relationship to the buttress system.

The Buttresses of the Midface

The maxilla's ability to resist fracture resides in several fortifications of bone: the maxillary buttresses (Figure 25-2).

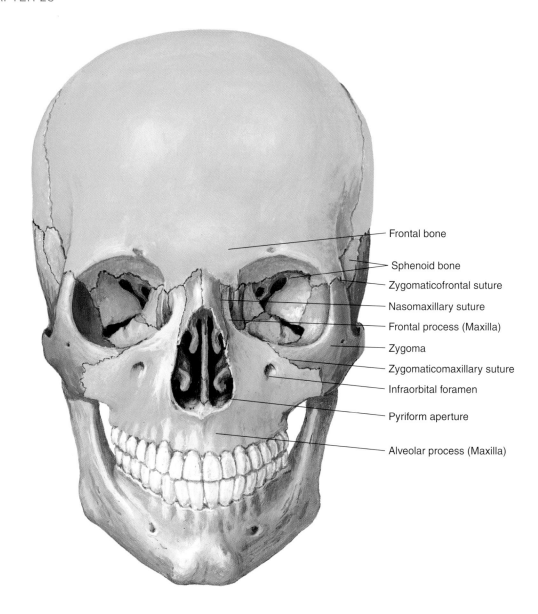

Frontal bone

Sphenoid bone

Zygomaticofrontal suture

Nasomaxillary suture

Frontal process (Maxilla)

Zygoma

Zygomaticomaxillary suture

Infraorbital foramen

Pyriform aperture

Alveolar process (Maxilla)

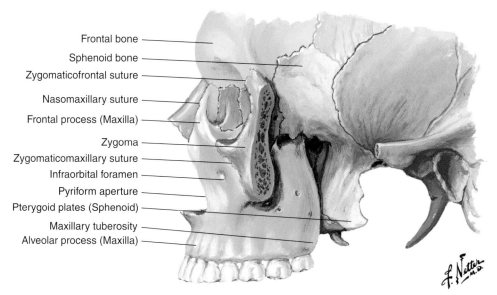

Frontal bone

Sphenoid bone

Zygomaticofrontal suture

Nasomaxillary suture

Frontal process (Maxilla)

Zygoma

Zygomaticomaxillary suture

Infraorbital foramen

Pyriform aperture

Pterygoid plates (Sphenoid)

Maxillary tuberosity

Alveolar process (Maxilla)

● **FIGURE 25-1.** Key anatomical structures in the midface. (*Reprinted with permission from Netter FH, Dalley AF. Atlas of Human Anatomy. 2nd ed. New York: Elsevier; 1997.*)

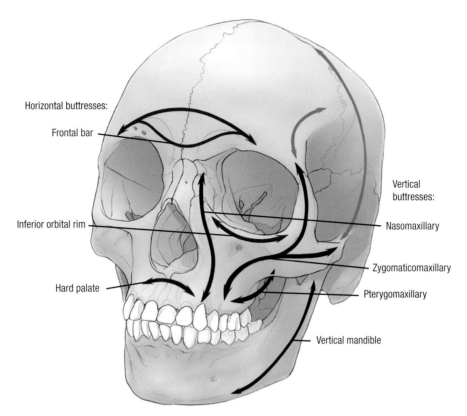

● **FIGURE 25-2.** Midface buttress anatomy. The orange lines (1-4) represent the
vertical buttresses, while the green lines (A-C) represent the horizontal buttresses.
Vertical: (1) nasomaxillary, (2) zygomaticomaxillary, (3) pterygomaxillary. Horizontal:
(B) upper transverse maxillary (inferior orbital rim), (C) lower transverse maxillary
(hard palate). Also shown: (4) the vertical mandibular buttress, and (A) the frontal bar.
*(Reprinted with permission from Mann FA. Imaging of high-energy midfacial trauma: what the
surgeon needs to know. Eur J Radiol. 2003;48:17–32.)*

The buttresses may be likened to the trusses and beams of
a building. In the midface, the buttress system is comprised
of thick confluences of bone that do not transilluminate.
The buttress system provides a framework for dissipating
forces to the cranial base. They are either horizontally or
vertically oriented, each projecting into the sagittal plane.
The midfacial buttresses are a key component in the
reconstruction of the midface as they meet the following
criteria: (1) they are linked to the skull base; (2) they have
sufficient bone to allow stable plate and screw fixation; and
(3) they are accessible through standard surgical incisions.[7]
In contradistinction to the buttresses, the transilluminat-
ing portions of the maxilla (eg, the walls of the maxillary
sinus and laminae paprycea) are particularly susceptible
to fracture, owing to their thin, weak structure. Sufficient
anterior and/or lateral impact to these areas results in fracture, often associated with comminution.

The Vertical Buttresses. The midface is primarily
designed to absorb vertically directed forces, namely, the
forces of occlusion. Finite element analysis has confirmed
that forces indeed flow through these buttresses to the
skull base. Aptly, the vertical buttresses are the strongest
structural components of the midface. There are three
pairs of vertical buttresses in the maxilla. The nasomaxillary buttress is also known as the medial maxillary or nasofrontal buttress. It runs from the anterior alveolar process
cephalad along the border of the piriform aperture and
across the frontal process of the maxilla. After forming the
medial orbital rim, it crosses the nasofrontal junction to
the frontal bone. Its sagittal projection defines the medial
orbital wall. The zygomaticomaxillary buttress or lateral
maxillary buttress originates at the posterior alveolar process and travels cephalad over the body of the zygoma. It
extends superiorly to comprise the lateral orbital rim and
then crosses the zygomaticofrontal suture into the frontal
bone. The pterygomaxillary buttress is also known as the
posterior maxillary buttress. It is unique in that it is not
commonly used in rigid fixation. Nonetheless, fractures
across this buttress—and the pterygoid plates—are the
common thread of all LeFort fractures. This represents the
key point of separation (pterygomaxillary dysjunction)
between the maxilla and the cranial base. The pterygomaxillary buttress joins the pterygoid plates of the sphenoid bone to the posterior maxilla.

The Horizontal Buttresses. When compared with the
vertical buttress system, the horizontal buttresses

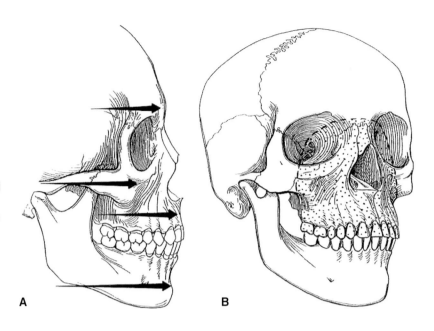

● **FIGURE 25-3.** Buttresses in the sagittal plane. (A) the sagittal extensions of the horizontal buttresses (*black arrows*) are relatively weak. (B) The central midface (*shaded area*) is therefore prone to collapse and deficient projection. (*Reprinted with permission from Manson P. Subunit principles in midface fractures: the importance of sagittal buttresses, soft-tissue reductions, and sequencing treatment of segmental fractures. Plast Reconstr Surg. 1999;103:1287–1307.*)

A　　**B**

are relatively weak, particularly in the sagittal plane (Figure 25-3). Accordingly, the maxilla is highly susceptible to fracture from horizontally directed forces. The upper transverse maxillary buttress runs from the temporal bone to the infraorbital rim via the zygomatic arch. It then travels over the frontal process of the maxilla to the nasal radix, continuing to the contralateral side via a similar path. Throughout its course, the upper transverse maxillary buttress crosses several sutures, which are commonly involved in fracture patterns: the zygomaticotemporal, zygomaticomaxillary, and nasomaxillary. Its sagittal projections are the zygomatic arches laterally and the orbital floors medially. The lower transverse maxillary buttress follows a horseshoe-shaped path along the alveolar process, and includes the hard palate.

The Soft Tissues and Musculature

The facial soft tissue envelope makes a significant contribution to the perception of appearance. Its shape is largely predicated on the underlying skeletal structure. Following injury, internal fibrosis can occur, making subsequent repositioning an onerous and challenging task. Early primary repair of the soft tissues in a layered fashion is advocated, along with tissue resuspension in early fracture reduction. This approach will achieve the best aesthetic result and avoid the long-term consequences of scarring and contraction.

The highly specific facial musculature permits a remarkable diversity of human expression and functionality. The muscles attached to the maxilla include those of facial expression anteriorly, and mastication posteriorly. Standard surgical techniques diffusely elevate, or deglove, the anteriorly located mimetic muscles, potentially disrupting their osseous attachments. Resuspension of the soft tissue envelope should therefore be included as a component of midface fracture repair.

The Neurovasculature

Blood Supply. The dual system of carotid perfusion to the midface permits both tissue viability and resistance to infection following facial injury. A necessary corollary, however, is the coincident possibility of profuse bleeding. The major culprits are the internal maxillary artery, a branch of the external carotid system, and the ethmoidal arteries, branches of the internal carotid system.

Innervation. The maxillary division of the trigeminal nerve (CN V2) provides sensation to the cheek, nasal sidewall and ala, upper lip, and maxillary dentition. The infraorbital nerve, its major branch, exits its named foramen 1 cm below the infraorbital rim in the midpupillary line. This nerve is frequently injured in midface fractures.[8] Paresthesia or anesthesia may be noted in its distribution, depending on the degree of injury. The facial nerve (CN VII) is usually spared in midface fractures. Damage to this nerve is more common in fractures of the cranial base, temporal bone, and mandible.

● PATTERNS OF MIDFACIAL FRACTURE

Rene LeFort, a French orthopedic surgeon, published his classical treatise on facial fractures in 1901.[9] Therein, he described "the great lines of weakness" of the facial skeleton (Figure 25-4). His experimentation on human skulls defined a lexicon for midface fractures that is still widely used more than 100 years later. Although he reported midface fractures with bilateral symmetry, seldom are they seen in pure form. In clinical practice, a myriad of patterns are observed, as the thin bone of the midface is susceptible to multiple fractures that easily collapse. Comminution is the rule, and synchronous injuries to the mandible and the frontal bones are commonplace. In addition, the LeFort classification does not adequately

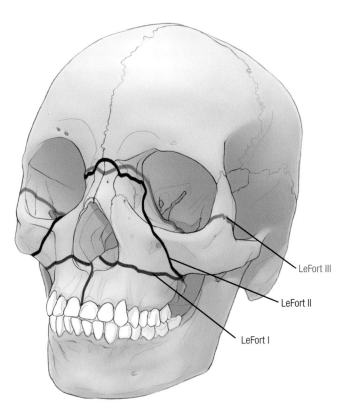

● **FIGURE 25-4.** "The great lines of weakness."
(Reprinted with permission from Mann FA. Imaging of high-energy midfacial trauma: what the surgeon needs to know. Eur J Radiol. 2003;48:17–32.)

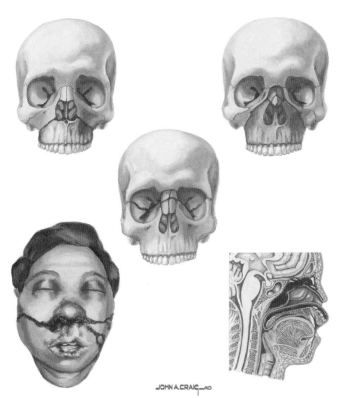

● **FIGURE 25-5.** LeFort fractures. (Upper Left, *blue*) LeFort I. (Upper Right, *orange*) LeFort II. (Center, *green*) LeFort III. (Lower Left) classic "panda facies" appearance. (Lower Right) Edema and hematoma as seen on sagittal section. *(Reprinted with permission from Hansen, J. Netter's Clinical Anatomy. New York: Elsevier; 2006.)*

address palatal fractures or descriptions of coincident bone loss. Regardless, with minimal modification,* LeFort's original classification scheme continues to provide surgeons with a simple, reproducible language for describing midface fractures and their relative points of stability (Figure 25-5).

LeFort I Fractures

Also known as a transverse maxillary fracture, the LeFort I fracture extends across the maxilla in a horizontal fashion above the dental apices. The maxillary sinus is traversed, and the base of the piriform aperture is disrupted. The pterygoid plates are also disrupted (the commonality of all LeFort fractures). A so-called "floating palate" ensues. In essence, the lower transverse maxillary buttress is mobile in relation to the skull.

LeFort II Fractures

The LeFort II fracture assumes a triangular shape and is therefore known as a pyramidal maxillary fracture. The fracture extends through the maxilla across the infraorbital rim and medially to the nasal radix. The orbit is

invariably involved. In this fashion, LeFort II fractures separate and mobilize the midfacial skeleton.

LeFort III Fractures

Most rare of the midfacial fractures, LeFort III fractures occur at the juncture of the cranial and facial skeletons. Apropos, this type of fracture results in craniofacial dysjunction. LeFort III fractures extend into the orbit, and concomitant injury to orbital structures may ensue. The fractures necessarily include a separation of the zygomatic arch. In strictest terms, most LeFort III fractures are actually zygomaticomaxillary complex fractures in combination with LeFort I and/or II fractures (Figure 25-6).

LeFort IV Fractures

Not described in Rene LeFort's original classification, LeFort IV fractures result when the upper midface is fractured in conjunction with the frontal bone. Injury to the NOE complex is nearly ubiquitous with this pattern.

LeFort fractures occur in a relatively predictable frequency, with LeFort II being the most common, followed by LeFort I and LeFort III.[2] Concurrent palatal fractures are observed in approximately 8% of maxillary fractures.

*The numerical designation of fracture levels has since been inverted from LeFort's initial proposal.

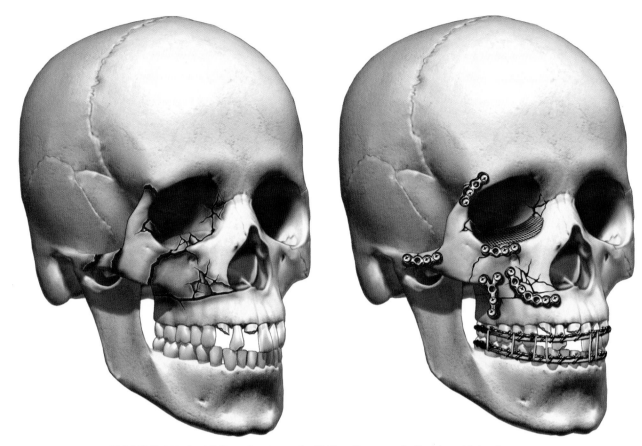

● **FIGURE 25-6.** Midface fractures. (Left) Simultaneous LeFort I and II fractures associated with zygomaticomaxillary complex, zygomatic arch, and orbital floor fractures. (Right) Appearance following reduction and rigid plate fixation. Titanium mesh has been placed in the orbital floor defect and arch bars have been applied. Note the incorrect placement of the L plate, which should be located medially over the nasomaxillary buttress. (*Illustration Copyright © 2006 Nucleus Medical Art. All rights reserved. www.nucleusinc.com.*)

Conversely, palatal fractures are rarely observed in isolation: LeFort I fractures are almost uniformly present. Fractures of the other facial bones (eg, nasal, mandibular) are clinically more common than those of the midface.

Palatal Fractures

Fractures of the palate occur in approximately 8% of all midface fractures.[7] A wide variety of patterns may be observed, based on patient age and nature of injury. Alveolar and para-alveolar fractures cause mobility in an isolated segment of the dentition. They may be misinterpreted as LeFort fractures on bimanual intraoral examination if not carefully delineated.

Sagittal fractures result in a "split palate." The fracture occurs along the intermaxillary and midpalatal sutures. This pattern is commonly seen in children. The palatal suture does not fuse until age 20 to 30 years, allowing for maxillary expansion and growth. For this reason, parasagittal fractures are much more likely in adults. These fractures extend through the piriform aperture anteriorly, and deviate toward the maxillary tuberosity posteriorly.

The transverse palatal fracture is addressed here for completeness sake, as this pattern is rarely observed in clinical practice. The palatal vault is well buttressed sagittally, preventing this type of injury.

Severe palatal fractures may divide the palate obliquely and transversely, comminuting the palate and alveolus. These fractures are extensive, involving combinations of fracture patterns. In summary, the particular pattern of palatal fracture is not as important as the simple recognition of their presence; their management is discussed below.

● ASSESSMENT

Facial trauma is a harbinger of life-threatening injury, indicating the possibility of concomitant injury to the airway, neuroaxis, viscera, and axial skeleton. The potential for unstable hemodynamic phenomena must also be realized. Treatment of these concurrent, systemic injuries should take precedence over maxillofacial reconstruction.

Patients with maxillofacial injuries are often prematurely assigned to the care of subspecialty services. In these cases, it is important that this team reevaluate the patient for the possibility of evolving, life-threatening injury.

Airway

In all trauma settings, adherence to Advanced Trauma Life Support protocol is essential. As such, the initial management of the maxillofacial trauma patient begins with securing the airway. These patients are particularly prone to asphyxia from prolapsed bone and soft tissue, laryngeal fractures, aspiration of dental fragments, and oropharyngeal hemorrhage. While maintaining inline stabilization of the cervical spine, anterior traction on the mandible and direct intraoral examination should be followed by vigorous suctioning to remove blood clot and debris.

A low threshold for intubation should be maintained. In most cases, this can be achieved via orotracheal approach. The endotracheal tube may be wired to the anterior dentition for additional security. Inspection for cerebrospinal fluid (CSF) leakage and consideration of skull base fracture should occur prior to blind insertion of nasogastric tubes or nasal airways. In all facial trauma patients, caution should be used to avoid the inadvertent entry of these devices into the cranial vault through fracture lines. Fiber optic intubation techniques may be implemented for guidance, but careful manual placement is generally sufficient to avoid this complication. The examiner's finger may be placed into the patient's oropharynx to help guide the endotracheal tube inferiorly. If an adequate airway cannot be established through these means, a cricothyroidotomy or tracheostomy should be performed without delay in cases of airway compromise.

Hemorrhage

As previously noted, the blood supply to the maxilla is robust and redundant. Exsanguination and hemorrhagic shock, although rare, may rapidly ensue following severe midface fracture. A thorough knowledge of vascular anatomy permits rapid hemostasis.

The majority of uncontrolled bleeding arises from the internal maxillary artery or its branches. Following the application of direct pressure, persistently bleeding vessels may be carefully ligated. This approach minimizes the damage to adjacent structures, which may result from blind clamping in the field. The superficial temporal and external carotid arteries may be similarly ligated in cases of severe uncontrolled bleeding.

Epistaxis can result from either the anterior or posterior nasal cavity. Anterior bleeding originates from Kiesselbach plexus, which is located on the anterior nasal septum. This vascular confluence is composed of the anterior ethmoidal, sphenopalatine, and superior labial arteries. Anterior epistaxis responds well to topical vasoactive compounds and bilateral, direct, and external pressure to the nasal septum. Posterior bleeding is more difficult to access. It usually arises from Woodruff plexus, which is located on the middle nasal turbinate, and is composed of the posterior nasal, sphenopalatine, and ascending pharyngeal arteries. Layered gauze packing of the nasal floor with bayonet or Debakey forceps is often successful in this context. Tamponade may also be achieved with the introduction and inflation of 30-cc Foley balloon catheters into each nostril. The catheter may be secured at the columella and the balloon released intermittently to avoid pressure necrosis of the nasal septum.

Manual fracture reduction is the definitive management of bleeding and should be employed in a controlled setting as soon as the patient's condition allows. Angiographic embolization, while increasingly facile with interventional techniques, is rarely necessary. The aforementioned means of attaining hemostasis are sufficient in the vast majority of cases.

Physical Examination

A complete maxillofacial examination includes observation for symmetry, palpation for step-off and contour deformities, examination of the visual axis, otoscopy, assessment of the occlusion, and neurological evaluation, including cranial nerve testing.

Midface fractures may present with a combination of ecchymosis, edema, malocclusion, and missing dentition with osseous deformity and mobility. The latter is routinely assessed through bimanual examination. With one hand intraorally on the maxillary alveolus and the other across the midface, a gentle rocking motion will frequently elicit the level(s) of fracture. An overzealous examination, however, may worsen the injury and cause instability where none was previously present.

Prima Non Nocere. An additional stumbling block for the uninitiated examiner is the misinterpretation of a mobile alveolar segment for a complete LeFort fracture. Gently assess the entire midface for mobility. In the maxillofacial trauma patient, malocclusion is assessed through subjective and objective means. Asking the patient, "Does your bite feel normal?" is a highly sensitive way to determine the presence of fracture. The present and pretraumatic status of the occlusion should always be solicited if the patient's clinical condition allows. If there has been a past history of orthodontic treatment, these records should be sought out.

Objectively, the Angle classification of malocclusion is used. In normal occlusion, the mesiobuccal cusp of the first maxillary molar contacts the buccal groove of the first mandibular molar. A class III malocclusion with anterior open bite (ie, negative overbite) is often associated with a LeFort fracture. Inferior maxillary displacement causes an elongated and retruded midface. This "facies equine" results from premature contact of the posterior dentition.

Radiographic Analysis

As noted above, the clinical diagnosis of midface fractures may be complicated by the presence of edema, incomplete fracture, impaction, or a combination of fracture types. Advances in radiographies, particularly in the realm of computed tomography, have greatly enhanced diagnosis and preoperative planning. Plain films are no longer routinely recommended in the evaluation of midface fractures. Far superior in resolution and sensitivity, maxillofacial CT scans have moved to the fore. Sections are generally taken 1.0 to 1.25 mm apart. Coronal reformatting is frequently performed to further delineate fracture lines in alternate planes. Three-dimensional computed tomography permits further analysis of fracture patterns. With this modality, volume and proportionality may be directly assessed.

Particular clues to radiographic diagnosis include the presence of step-off deformities and sinus opacification. Pneumocephalus indicates the possibility of high LeFort fractures with breach of the cranial base. Cerebral edema and diffuse axonal injury may also be appreciated.

Postoperative computed tomography is often eschewed because of its cost and associated radiation exposure. Nonetheless, it is frequently used in the fields of orthopedics and neurosurgery. When used in the reconstructive algorithm, postoperative CT scanning provides a powerful educational tool. It should be considered more strongly in the routine postoperative care of patients with maxillofacial trauma in order to confirm surgical efficacy.

● RECONSTRUCTIVE PRINCIPLES

Historically, multiple treatment modalities have been employed for the stabilization of midface fractures, including external fixation, Kirschner wires, and internal wire suspension. The introduction of rigid plate fixation and its associated benefits has reduced the utility of these earlier forms of repair.[5] It is now generally accepted that rigid osteosynthesis with titanium plating provides the best stability and long-term results. Wide surgical exposure has enabled precise anatomic reduction under direct visualization. In the cases where rigid fixation is difficult to achieve (because of severe comminution or bony instability), more creative solutions must be employed. A thorough understanding and deft skill with mandibulomaxillary fixation (MMF) is a requisite to proficient midfacial fracture management. The judicious use of autogenous bone grafting at the time of injury has yielded additional improvements in bone healing, augmenting the stability and durability of fracture repair. The continued evolution of these techniques has afforded the maxillofacial surgeon the capacity to provide prompt and definitive management in a single-stage operation.[7]

Sequencing

Multiple authors have proposed various methodologies for appropriate sequencing in traumatic midface reconstruction: top-down, bottom-up, inside-out, and vice versa, all have been purported to be ideal. Aptly, Manson states, "The exact order of treatment is not as important as the development of a plan that permits both flexibility and reproducibly accurate positioning."[5] For this to be achieved, a thorough preoperative assessment of the involved facial bone fragments is necessary. This is particularly important in cases of panfacial fracture, which result from concomitant fractures of the mandible, midface, and frontal bones. Midface fractures are generally repaired in the following sequence: arch bar application, fracture exposure, disimpaction and reduction, restoration of occlusion with MMF, rigid fixation, and soft tissue re-suspension and repair. All these techniques are performed with a keen eye to gaining symmetry, restoring projection, and providing a durable and stable repair.

Exposure

The need to widely expose the involved bony buttresses must be balanced against the possibility of iatrogenic soft tissue injury. Accordingly, surgical approaches that maximize exposure and minimize conspicuous scarring are preferred. If significant lacerations are present, these may be used for access; oftentimes, the injury has partially completed the dissection. Based on the location and degree of fracture, several classical approaches to the midfacial skeleton may be used (Figure 25-7).

Gingivobuccal Sulcus. The gingivobuccal sulcus incision is the most commonly used approach to access the midfacial skeleton. It is the least conspicuous incision, and provides exceptional exposure for lower maxillary fractures. Alveolar fractures can also be reduced via this approach. Periosteal elevation permits skeletonization of the fractures while protecting the mimetic muscles and neurovasculature of the soft tissue flap. The naso- and zygomaticomaxillary buttresses are also accessible from this approach, and the infraorbital rim may be reached if the dissection is carried out superiorly. Care should be taken, however, to avoid inadvertent damage to the infraorbital nerve. The gingivobuccal sulcus incision should preserve a 5-mm cuff of tissue on the gingiva and should not be placed at the apex of the sulcus. This technique permits a facile and watertight closure.

Orbital. Transconjuctival, subcilliary, subtarsal, and midlid approaches to the orbit provide the best access to the infraorbital rim component of LeFort II fractures. Each of these approaches has its strengths and weaknesses. The subciliary incision, for example, carries an increased risk of ectropion and scleral show. Extended lateral canthotomy or upper blepharoplasty incisions may be added for access to the zygomaticofrontal suture. Care must be taken to avoid placing incisions within the brow, which can yield a conspicuous and untoward result. Corneal shields are essential when any orbital exposure is attempted.

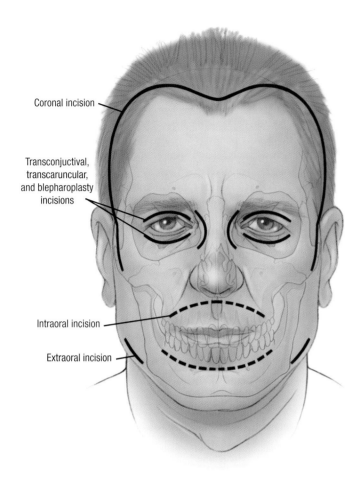

● FIGURE 25-7. Commonly used exposures in midface fracture. (*Reprinted with permission from Mathes S. Plastic Surgery. 2nd ed. Vol 3. New York: Elsevier; 2006.*)

Coronal and Hemicoronal. Wide exposure to the cranial region, upper midface, zygomatic, and nasoethmoid area can be gained through a coronal incision. Such an approach is often indicated when high LeFort fractures with severe comminution are encountered. A "stealth" technique may be used to camouflage the scar. This is performed by making a zig-zag (or sinusoidal) incision, the limbs of which should be approximately 2 cm in length and mutually orthogonal to one another. The incision is carried out from ear to ear (posterior to the ear is better aesthetically) with dissection carried out anteriorly in the subgaleal plane. When the scalp is incised parallel to the hair follicles, the severity of cicatricial alopecia is reduced. Removable surgical clips are applied to the free edge of the flap for hemostasis.

Palalal. Palatal incisions are used if rigid fixation of the hard palate is attempted, which may be considered based on surgeon preference. If utilized, incisions should be kept in the midline or paramedian position to avoid mucosal devascularization. The greater palatine vessels course posterolaterally, adjacent to the maxillary tubercles. Care should also be taken to avoid the nasopalatine

neurovascular bundle as it exits the incisive foramen anteriorly. Access may be achieved through preexisting lacerations, if present.

Anatomic Reduction

For definitive repair of midface fractures, the buttresses must reassume their preinjury alignment. All three dimensions—vertical, horizontal, and sagittal—must be satisfactorily restored. The *sine qua non* of midface fracture repair is anatomic reduction along buttress lines.

Closed reduction techniques are no longer routinely recommended in maxillary fracture management. The use of Rowe or Hayton-Williams disimpaction forceps can create new and undesirable fracture lines that may extend into the orbit or skull base. Nonetheless, when severely impacted fractures are encountered, these instruments may be used in an open and controlled fashion. In general, open techniques provide a safer and more predictable means of reduction. Precise reduction under direct visualization is only possible after adequate exposure and skeletonization of the fracture segments.[7]

Mandibulomaxillary Fixation

MMF is required intraoperatively to restore the preinjury occlusion. Once rigid fixation has been achieved, however, MMF is no longer necessary. Prolonged MMF as a primary treatment strategy has become less commonplace, and is often reserved for situations where true rigid fixation cannot be attained. In these cases, a 2 to 6 week course of MMF may be required. If left in place during the acute phase of hospitalization, it is important to keep wire cutters at the bedside. Should vomiting ensue, MMF must be released to protect the airway and avoid the possibility of aspiration.

After the appropriate fixation period, the wires may be removed and replaced with traction elastics. These can be modified on a weekly basis to make fine adjustments in the occlusion. Frequent observation is suggested during this time period, as "off-axis" forces may disrupt alignment or cause dental extrusion. After several weeks, the elastics may be discontinued, leaving the arch bars in place for an additional "test" week. If centric occlusion has been maintained, the arch bars may be removed. Orthodontic realignment may be required if occlusal restoration is not possible. This strategy, however, should be considered as a last resort.

Splinting may be used as an additional means of stabilization for midfacial fractures. When employed in concert with MMF, splints are particularly efficacious in the fixation of comminuted, unstable, small bone fragments (eg, alveolar fractures). The dentition bearing these fracture segments can also be etched and wired to achieve requisite stability.

Rigid Osteosynthesis

Fractures must be stabilized in three dimensions against both translational and rotational forces.[9] Plates and screws are fixed across adjacent fractures in order to prevent micromovement, thus providing rigid osteosynthesis (Figure 25-6). The most common plating sets used in the maxilla are equipped with 1.5 to 2.0 mm diameter screws. Plates of varying shapes and sizes are part of the surgeon's armamentarium and are used according to the demands of local anatomic topography.

Plates should be placed along the natural lines of force (ie, the buttresses) to permit maximum load bearing.[7] They may be conceptualized as synthetic buttresses, which augment those injured during trauma. At least two screws should be used on either side of the fracture. Interfragmentary wires are a versatile tool that may be used to create an ideal reduction prior to definitive fixation.[7]

Both the amount of bone and degree of comminution largely determine the ability to achieve sufficient fixation. The highest probability of attaining rigid fixation will be realized if the solid bone of the nasomaxillary and zygomaticomaxillary buttresses is used when anchoring screws. It must be reemphasized that other means of stabilization (ie, MMF) should be used for maintaining reduction and fixation if plate deformation or semirigid fixation is present.

Bone Grafting

Bone grafting in maxillofacial injuries was first proposed by Bonanno and Converse,[10] and pioneered by Gruss.[11] The use of interpositional bone grafts along the course of the native vertical buttresses provides functional and structural support to the fractured midface. These grafts enhance bony consolidation and restore facial height. Although not always required, bone grafting to large defects in the anterior maxilla may prevent soft tissue prolapse into the maxillary sinus. Bone grafts are indicated when gaps of 5 mm or wider are found between fracture segments.

Plate and screw fixation or wiring may be used for graft stabilization, but rigid fixation is preferable to attain optimal osteosynthesis.[6] Fracture fragments should be re-used as the primary bone graft source until they are exhausted, thereby limiting donor site morbidity. In severely contaminated wounds, or when tissue covering is inadequate or nonviable, bone grafting is generally contraindicated.

The rib, calvarium, and iliac crest are among the more commonly used donor sites for bone grafting in maxillofacial trauma. The surgeon considers three variables when harvesting bone grafts: (1) bony characteristics; (2) ease of access; and (3) donor site morbidity. Rib grafts, for example, allow for superior contouring, but experience high resorption rates, and carry the risk of pneumothorax during harvest. Calvarial bone, in comparison, is less malleable, but shows decreased resorption over time and is close to the operative field. The risks of dural tears and cerebral injury during harvest, however, must also be considered. The iliac crest provides abundant bone and is easily accessible. The greatest drawback of this site is postoperative pain.

Palatal Reconstruction

The palate, because of its intimate involvement with the occlusion, requires unique reconstructive consideration. The palate is composed of relatively thin bone, making plate and screw fixation a difficult task. Because these small bony fragments are often not amenable to the aforementioned techniques of rigid fixation, adjunctive stabilization methods are often required. While some authors advocate that rigid osteosynthesis be applied to palatal fractures/occlusal splinting is both a viable and effective strategy for their management.

Splinting of palatal fractures provides stability against rotation, creating a point of fixation away from the fracture site. Etched interdental ("buddy") wiring may also be used in this context. Splinting is mandatory in cases of severe palatal comminution.

In order to create an adequate splint, impressions of the dentition must be taken. Dental models are made from these impressions, and then mounted on an articulator. The models are then cut and manipulated in order to restore centric occlusion on the articulator based on facet wear patterns. Once this is established, an acrylic mold, or splint, is created along the restored occlusion. The occlusal splint is then used as a surgical guide. Once the major fracture fragments have been reduced, the splint is then used to facilitate MMF. The rigid osteosynthesis of other maxillary fractures, if present, can then be performed. On release of MMF, the maxillary splint is left in place for approximately 6 weeks.

Soft Tissue Management

The shape of the soft tissue envelope of the face is highly dependent on the underlying skeleton. Upon disruption of the bones of the midface, the overlying soft tissue often suffers concomitant damage resulting in swelling and local response to injury. A thorough understanding of the interactions between the soft tissue and the midfacial fracture is of paramount importance. Remodeling of the soft tissues can occur within 7 to 10 days postinjury, generating problematic contraction and/or tissue atrophy. Internal fibrosis gives the injured tissue "memory," and subsequent repositioning becomes difficult. Therefore, repair of both the bone and soft tissue need to be done in a timely fashion in order to preclude permanent disfigurement. In order to restore a natural appearance, simultaneous soft tissue repair and re-suspension is advised.

The soft tissues should be closed in a standard layered fashion. Re-approximration of muscle and soft tissue also provides bulk over low-profile plates, making step-offs less visible. If this is not performed, soft tissue diastasis may result. The related changes of soft tissue descent (ptosis) result from improper re-suspension of the soft tissues to the underlying skeleton.[7] Periosteal reattachment is required at the malar eminence, infraorbital rim, and medial and lateral canthi. Drill holes may be created at these locations to facilitate re-suspension.

● SPECIAL CONSIDERATIONS

Pediatric facial fractures and panfacial fractures require nuanced management and will be addressed elsewhere in this volume. Several other special considerations merit further discussion here.

The Edentulous Maxilla

The management of the fractured maxilla in the edentulous patient requires special consideration because the occlusion is no longer available as a reconstructive guide.[12] In these patients, the mandibulomaxillary relationship assumes the utmost reconstructive significance. An important corollary is the need to restore the space between the maxilla and the mandible. Adequate intermaxillary space allows for dentures to fit without difficulty.

If the maxilla is not displaced, the fracture may be managed conservatively with a soft diet for 2 to 3 weeks, followed by a gradual reincorporation of dentures. When the maxilla is displaced and the patient's condition is stable, the surgeon should proceed with bony reconstruction. The patient's dentures, or gunning splints, may be used to stabilize MMF and establish the aforementioned requisite intermaxillary height.

Gunshot Wounds

In general, the same principles of midface reconstruction—open reduction, rigid fixation, and early soft-tissue management—are applied to gunshot wounds of the face. After standard resuscitation and stabilization, the management of the patient with a gunshot wound to the face should proceed conservatively: the facial soft tissues should be minimally debrided, and only if clearly devitalized. Packing or loose closure of the skin can be performed between early serial debridements, with a focus on keeping the soft tissues on stretch in preparation for primary closure after bony reconstruction.

The early restoration of the skeletal scaffolding improves facial contour, minimizes soft tissue deformity and decreases the need for extensive reoperation. Therefore, the reconstructive surgeon should employ a low threshold for the use of primary bone grafting.[11]

After the facial skeleton has been adequately restored, external coverage with primary closure, local or free flaps is required.

● COMPLICATIONS

The complications related to midface reconstruction occur on a continuum, beginning at the time of injury. The earliest complications of maxillofacial fracture—airway compromise and uncontrolled hemorrhage—should always be considered prior to further assessment. The following sequelae also deserve attention.

Infection

Although continuous with the sinuses and oropharynx—areas of rich bacterial colonization-maxillary fractures are rarely complicated by infection. This is attributable to the rich blood supply of the face.

Blindness

Blindness is a rare complication of midface fractures, occurring in less than 1% of cases. Blindness at the time of presentation is usually the result of direct optic nerve (CN 2) injury. Postoperative blindness resulting from reduction of facial fractures is exceedingly rare. When observed, it is related to increased pressure in the optic canal. A retro-orbital hematoma is commonly responsible. Steroids are mandated, and a lateral canthotomy is required for decompression. It is important to document visual acuity prior to operative management.

Cerebrospinal Fluid Rhinorrhea

Cerebrospinal fluid leaks may occur with high LeFort injuries when the cribriform plate has been fractured. The diagnosis should be suspected when clear rhinorrhea is observed in the maxillofacial trauma patient. The presence of glucose corroborates the diagnosis, and β-2-transferrin positivity is confirmatory. Meningitis is the feared complication. Nose blowing may cause retrograde bacterial dissemination through the dural defect and should be avoided. Nasal packing is similarly undesirable as it provides a stagnant reservoir for bacterial growth. Prophylactic intravenous antibiotics with good blood–brain barrier penetration (eg, ceftriaxone) should be instituted.

Severely impacted LeFort III and IV fractures, however, may actually "block" a CSF leak. Oftentimes, fracture reduction will restore the flow of CSF and a leak that was not present preoperatively ensues. A high index of suspicion should be gleaned from the fracture pattern on preoperative CT. Early neurosurgical consultation will facilitate their intraoperative availability, if ultimately needed. A lumbar CSF drain may be required in cases of persistent or copious drainage. The majority of cases, however, resolve spontaneously following reduction and fixation.[8]

Nerve Injury

The infraorbital nerve (CN V2) is the most commonly nerve injured in midface fractures.

Paresthesia is frequently related to neuropraxia, resolving over the convalescent period. Unfortunately, permanent sensory disturbance in the cheek, upper lip, and nasal sidewall may also occur. The incidence of this complication was reported as 17% in series of 240 patients. Anosmia (CN I) and ageusia (CN VII, chorda tympani nerve) have also been demonstrated in high LeFort fractures with frequencies up to 20% to 30%. Whether the lesion is related to the fracture itself or proximal brain injury remains unclear.

Soft Tissue Deformities

Soft tissue malpositioning, as previously discussed, may result in descent and deformity. Specifically, canthal dystopia, malar sagging, ectropion, and eclabion may be encountered.

Malocclusion

Malocclusion is a significant deleterious complication that impacts mastication and speech. It can also cause headaches, chronic facial pain, and temporomandibular joint dysfunction. Most commonly, malocclusion is a technical error related to insufficient disimpaction and a poor anatomic reduction of a displaced maxillary fracture. When MMF is performed in these cases, the mandible is forced in centric occlusion (ie, intercuspation of the dentition) at the expense of centric relation (ie, anatomic seating of the mandibular condyle in the glenoid fossa). Upon release of MMF, the condyle translates back into centric relation, but the occlusion is lost. Unfortunately, this error may not be noted until the patient emerges from anesthesia, or worse, when MMF is released several weeks postoperatively. If discovered early, an expeditious return to the operating room for correction is mandated. Otherwise, reoperation with LeFort I advancement is required. This is further evidence for the overall superiority of rigid fixation, which mandates the release of MMF at the end of the case to assess the occlusion before the patient emerges from anesthesia.

Alveolar fractures can cause distinct problems with occlusion in isolated areas. A crossbite (laterognathism) may result if palatal width is not sufficiently restored. This problem is avoided with the proper use of occlusal splints. Close follow-up with dentistry is suggested in this setting, and the reinstitution of MMF may be required.

Malunion and Nonunion

In cases of malunion with partial bony healing, LeFort I osteotomies with repositioning provide a safe and efficient means of secondary repair. Rigid fixation may then be employed without the need for prolonged MMF. Complete nonunion of the maxilla is rarely encountered. When it does occur, the same principles of primary reconstruction apply: the site of nonunion is exposed, the intervening fibrous tissue is resected, and rigid osteosynthesis is then implemented with or without bone grafting.

Symptomatic Hardware

Plates, although inert, are not wholly benign. Common reasons for plate removal include prominence, loosening, pain, infection, and exposure. In cases of symptomatic

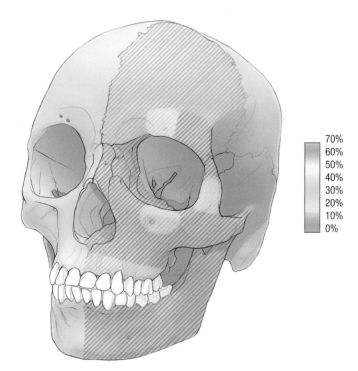

● FIGURE 25-8. The distribution of plate removal in craniomaxillofacial surgery. (*Reprinted with permission from Nagase D. Plate removal in traumatic facial fractures: 13-year practice review. Ann Plast Surg 2005;55:609.*)

hardware, secondary operations are required for their removal, which occurs 12% to 18% of the time.[13] Palatal plates display a similar incidence of symptomatology, with resultant plate removal in approximately 10% of cases. In the midface, plate discomfort is particularly likely with close proximity to the infraorbital foramen and nasal spine (Figure 25-8), and when screws penetrate the tooth roots. Preoperative plain films are useful to document hardware location and provide intraoperative guidance.

The loosening of screws postoperatively may result from osteonecrosis, which can be induced at the time of high-speed drilling. Resident osteoblasts adjacent to the screws die, resulting in bone loss and screw loosening. Cool, constant irrigation during screw placement is recommended to protect against this complication.

● SUMMARY

An early, single-stage repair provides ideal outcomes in traumatic midface reconstruction.

Rigid osteosynthesis is imperative to achieve a stable reduction, and should be universally considered for fracture fixation. Mandibulomaxillary fixation should be used intraoperatively and/or adjunctively in situations where rigid fixation is not possible or less than ideal. These principles allow the maxillofacial surgeon to restore form and function to the facial skeleton, and ultimately return the patient to a meaningful way of life.

REFERENCES

1. Girotto JA, MacKenzie E, Fowler C, et al. Long-term physical impairment and functional outcomes after complex facial fractures. *Plast Reconstr Surg.* 2001;108(2):312–327.

2. Lee R, Robertson S, Manson P. Current epidemiology of facial injuries. *Semin Plast Surg.* 2002;16:283.

3. Tung TC, Tseng WS, Chen CT, et al. Acute life-threatening injuries in facial fracture patients: a review of 1,025 patients. *J Trauma.* 2000;49(3):420–424.

4. Plaisier SR, Punjabi AP, Super OM, et al. The relationship between facial fractures and death from neurologic injury. *J Oral Maxillofac Surg.* 2000;58(7):708–712; discussion 712–713.

5. Manson P, Hoopes J, Su C. Structural pillars of the facial skeleton: an approach to the management of LeFort fractures. *Plast Reconstr Surg.* 1980;66(1):54–62.

6. Rudderman R, Mullen R. Biomechanics of the facial skeleton. *Clin Plast Surg.* 1992;19(1):11–29.

7. Gruss JS, Mackinnon SE. Complex maxillary fractures: role of buttress reconstruction and immediate bone grafts. *Plast Reconstr Surg.* 1986;78(1):9–22.

8. Steidler NE, Cook RM, Reade PC. Residual complications in patients with major middle third facial fractures. *Int J Oral Surg.* 1980;9(4):259–266.

9. LeFort R. Etude experimentale sur les fractures du la machoire superieure. *Riv Chir de Paris.* 1901;23:208.

10. Bonanno PC, Converse JM. Primary bone grafting in management for facial fractures. *N Y State J Med.* 1975;75(5):710–712.

11. Gruss JS, Mackinnon SE, Kassel EE, Cooper PW. The role of primary bone grafting in complex craniomaxillofacial trauma. *Plast Reconstr Surg.* 1985;75(1):17–24.

12. Farmand M, Baumann A. The treatment of the fractured edentulous maxilla. *J Craniomaxillofac Surg.* 1992;20(8):341–344.

13. Orringer JS, Barcelona V, Buchman SR. Reasons for removal of rigid internal fixation devices in craniofacial surgery. *J Craniofac Surg.* 1998;9(1):40–44.

chapter 26

Mandibular Fractures

Jack C. Yu, DMD, MD, MS Ed, FACS / *Ian F. Wilson, MD, MPH*

● INTRODUCTION

The mandible is one of the strongest bones in the craniofacial skeleton. Aesthetically, it defines the lower facial contour in three anatomic planes and structurally it is integral to the masticatory function. In treating patients with mandibular fracture, the overall goal is to restore this lower facial form and return the patient to full masticatory function. In other words, a restored mandible must look and function as a mandible. The patients should be able to open and close their mouth with good occlusion of the dentition and enough strength to chew and swallow food without pain or oral incontinence. The goal of the chapter is to provide a concise and complete overview of the current understanding and practice of mandibular fracture management; it is hoped that after reading this chapter, one would be able to properly diagnose and treat common mandibular fractures effectively and efficiently, and explain the rationales that underpin their management.

● BIOMECHANICS OF THE MANDIBLE AND MECHANOBIOLOGY

The mature mandible is like a long bone bent back on itself, forming a blunted V with identical 160-degree, out-of-plane, oblique extensions on both ends. These ends articulate with the skull base at the glenoid fossa forming the complex ginglymo-diarthroidial temporo-mandibular joints. Like other bones of the body, the mandible is rigid, which means for a large amount of force, it deforms only very slightly. Force is that which makes mass alter its velocity, or $F = ma$, where F is force and m is mass and a is acceleration. The unit of force is therefore product of mass unit and acceleration unit, for example, kg m/sec². $F = ma$ is Newton's Second Law of Motion and 1 kg m/sec² is known as a Newton or N. During normal chewing, the force generated from the contraction of temporalis and

masseter is in the range of 500 N. This magnitude of force causes deformation of the mandible, or ΔL, in the range of 0.6 mm. When ΔL is normalized to the original dimension, L_0, this ratio is known as strain. That is strain, usually represented by ε, $=\Delta L/L_0$. Strain, therefore has no units. When the force causing deformation is normalized to the cross-sectional area on which it is acting, the result is known as stress, S, which has N/m² or pascal (Pa) as its unit. The typical stress experienced by the mandible is in the range of millions of Pa, or mega pascals (MPa). Fundamentally, all stresses can be broken down into three basic types: tensile, compressive, and shear. Tensile and compressive are the principle stresses; they will change the volume of the object they are acting on, although by a very minuscule amount, that is, they cause nonisovolumetric strains. Shear, on the other hand, causes isovolumetric strain which is much less well tolerated. When the mandible is subjected to high enough stress, the deformation will be permanent. In engineering terms, it has exceeded its elastic limit and has undergone plastic deformation. The stress at which the plastic deformation occurs is called yield stress and the corresponding strain is the yield strain. A very important parameter for any material, bone included, is this ratio of stress to strain, S/ε which is known as the elastic modulus, or Young's modulus. The longitudinal elastic modulus for human mandible is 16 to 18 billion Pa, or GPa for giga pascals. If the applied stress continues to increase above the yield stress, the strain will reach a maximum point and the mandible will break apart. The strain at which this fracture occurs is known as the ultimate strain and the responsible stress is the ultimate stress. The ultimate stress, also known as the strength, for human cortical bone is 67 MPa in shear, 135 MPa in tension, and 205 MPa in compression. Bone as a material, can only elongate or compress 1% to 2 % before it will break. That is the ultimate tensile and compressive strain is no more than 1% to 2%; it is therefore understandable why reducing interfragmentary strain by fixation is so important.

There is a key difference between living tissues such as bone and other nonliving rigid materials, and that is bone is continuously remodeled. Because all living tissues undergo cyclic strains, the repeated loading and unloading produce microcracks. These microcracks are initiated from the inevitable imperfections at the nanometer level and create sites for tremendous stress concentration and given enough loading cycles will eventually propagate to macroscopic level failure. This deterioration of material property as a result of cyclic loading is known as fatigue. The higher the stress, the fewer cycles a material can withstand; at lower the stress, more cycles can be tolerated. When the stress is sufficiently low, the number of cycles tolerated approaches infinity. This "tolerable" level is called the endurance limit. For almost all the plates and screws used in fixation of mandibular fractures, the loading is higher than the endurance limit. That is why unless bone heals and resumes the load-bearing function, the plates will fail given enough loading cycles. How does bone overcome this problem of fatigue damage? The answer is Haversian systems. Living bone is not a static entity. It is a "smart material" in that sensors are embedded throughout and they monitor the complete strain state of the bone. There is a constant conversion of liquid to solid (osteogenesis) as well as the reverse (osteolysis). At a particular point in time, within a particular location in the bone, the end outcome of this balance depends on the strain, the age of the individual, and the systemic conditions. Bone will reinforce itself in areas of high strain and remove bone in areas where the strain is too low. There is thus an anabolic window defined by the strain which is critically important in bone homeostasis. Excessive strain, like insufficient strain, will suppress osteogenesis and favor osteolysis. The putative sensors in bone are the osteocytes. There are 20,000 osteocytes in every mm^3 of lamellar bone, and each osteocyte occupies a lacuna and has a life span of 25 years. These osteocytes have several hundred cytoplasmic processes, each housed within a canaliculus measuring only 350 nm in diameter. Through these cytoplasmic processes, gap junctions are formed to allow direct cell-to-cell communication. It has recently been determined that this lacuno-canalicular system will amplify the macroscopic bone strain by 10 to 15 fold. The loading and unloading of bone also forces fluids within the canaliculus to flow, generating fluid shear stress at about 1.6 Pa level. Subjected to this appropriate quantity and duration of fluid shear stress, osteocytes change their transcriptome to stimulate surface osteoblast to produce more bone. Without sufficient cellular strain, the osteocytes will not elicit osteoblasts to form more osteoid; it is therefore undesirable to have excessive amount of rigidity in fracture fixation for the salutary effects of physiologic loading cannot occur, creating a condition called stress-shielding. The ideal fixation system should allow for about 1200 microstrains or 0.12% of strain at the bone level.

PATTERNS OF MANDIBULAR FRACTURES

Fracture is macroscopic material failure; it occurs whenever the stress exceeds the ultimate stress and the resulting strain is greater than the ultimate strain of the material. Due to the particular geometry and the materials property, the human mandible contains areas of stress risers—location where the forces are supported by less cross-sectional areas. The space occupied by muscles, nerves, blood vessels, major salivary glands, and developing tooth buds are necessarily not occupied by bone and this inevitably weakens the mandible at these particular areas. Looking at this from the other perspective, where the ridges and cortical thickenings are, the mandible is relatively stronger. In the midface, these cortical thickenings are called the buttresses. The mandible, all things considered, is a very sturdy bone. The typical areas where the mandible breaks up during sudden impact are subcondylar, angle, body, parasymphyseal, and the alveoar regions. The condylar neck is very narrow and if there is latero-cursive movement at the time of impact, the entire force will be concentrated on one side; this small 0.0003 m^2 area can tolerate a maximum of 18,000 N, given an ultimate shear stress for cortical bone of 67 MPa.

Several classification systems exist for mandibular fractures, some use location, others use dentition, still others use muscular actions. Of all these classification schemes, the most commonly used, and the most helpful, remains to be the classification by location. In an edentulous mandible, the fractures are considered class 3. For mandibles with teeth, if the fracture occurs outside of the tooth-bearing segment, it is a class 1 fracture; and class 2 if it is within the tooth-bearing segment. Due to the muscular actions, the gap of mandibular fractures can either be increased or decreased. If muscular action tends to reduce the fracture gap width, it is considered a favorable fracture. If the gap width increases with the muscular contraction, then it is unfavorable. These can be further divided based on the anatomic plane: horizontal (axial or transverse) and vertical (parasagittal). A fracture at the angle of the mandible, anterior to the masseter-medial pterygoid sling, that extends from superior-anterior to inferior-posterior will have a tendency to be distracted into a wider gap upon contraction of these muscles; it is therefore vertically unfavorable. On the other hand, an angle fracture that is oriented from posterior-superior to anterior-inferior will have the fracture reduce automatically when masseter and medial pterigoid contract. Thus, it is called a vertically favorable fracture. Whether a fracture is favorable or not assists in the management of mandibular fracture; it does not, however, determine if surgical treatment is indicated or not. More importantly, the consideration of muscular actions will give a better understanding, or even relatively accurate prediction, of how the fragments tend to displace once the mandibular integrity is lost. It is particularly important to recognize that in bilateral body or angle fractures, the suprahypoid musculatures such as geniohyoid and genioglossus tend to pull the tongue posteriorly and produce serious upper airway compromise. These patients should be intubated early or transported in either upright or prone position to avoid the soft tissue collapse in the oropharyngeal region due to supine positioning. In bilateral subcondylar and condylar fractures, the posterior vertical support is lost, this reduction in posterior occlusal vertical dimension will result in tilting of the mandibular occlusal plane in a clockwise fashion and produce anterior open bite, or traumatic anterior apertognathia. Should there be unilateral subcondylar fracture or condylar fracture occurring inferior to the attachment of the inferior belly of the lateral pterigoid muscle, the contralateral lateral pterigoid pull upon mandibular opening will cause the lower jaw to deviate toward the side of the fracture. The pull of the ipsilateral inferior belly of the lateral pterigoid muscles tends to displace the proximal fragment medially and anteriorly. Isolated fracture of the coronoid is very rare, and there is usually very little displacement. In the absence of other associated fracture, this frequently requires no surgical treatment and can be managed by placing the patient on a soft diet.

The mandibular fracture pattern in the pediatric population differs from that of the adults due to several reasons. Children do not experience with nearly the same frequency the type of high impact trauma due to motor vehicle collisions or personal violence from altercations. Pediatric mandibles are structurally and geometrically different from adult mandibles. The elastic modulus of younger bones is less than that of the adult bones. They are also more ductile; they have more capacity to undergo plastic deformation before reaching breaking. Stated more precisely, their stress-strain curve has a lower slope and reaches yield point earlier, but the failure point is moved further to the right. As a result, green-stick fractures can occur and may complicate the treatment. In children younger than 6 years, their mandible is packed with developing permanent tooth buds and these liquid-filled sacs alter the biomechanical behavior of the bone. The gonial angle is more obtuse than the 160- to 165-degree range seen in adults, and the length of the ramus is shorter. Condylar fracture and alveolar fracture are more common, usually from blunt trauma due to falls. After the eruption of the maxillary central incisors, around ages 6 to 8 years, they are particularly prone to apical-posterior impaction type of alveolar fractures, especially if the occlusion is Angle's class II division 1, where there is increased overject. Mandibular dentoalveolar fractures are not as common. More inferior frontal impact with the mouth open, such as what happens during tripping and falling, directs the load posteriorly to the condyles and may result in fractures in that region. It is thus important whenever one is treating a child with chin laceration to evaluate the status of the condyle and subcondylar region by observing the occlusion and mandibular opening. Tenderness to palpation in the pre-tragal area is a very sensitive sign of condylar and subcondylar fractures.

SURGICAL AND TOPOLOGICAL ANATOMY

The functional restoration of the mandible requires a sound knowledge of the osteology of the mandible, dental anatomy, occlusion, and muscles of mastication. The mandible articulates with the temporal bone at the skull base. It is unique among all bones in that two symmetrical synovial joints exist and that both must perform in concert; there is never an instance when movement in one joint can occur without some corresponding movement of the other.

The mandibular condyles are irregular ellipsoid with a major axis of 18 to 20 mm and about half of that length for the minor axis. The two major axes point posterior-medially, forming an angle of 165 degrees. The glenoid fossa is just anterior to the osseous external auditory canal; superiorly, it is bordered by the root of the zygomatic process of the temporal bone and anteriorly by the articular eminence. Three named bony openings aligned almost linearly in a sagittal plane about 10 mm medial to the glenoid fossa: foramen spinosum, carotid canal, and jugular foramen. The joint itself has two compartments separated by the meniscus which is attached anteriorly to the superior belly of the lateral pterygoid muscle. Posteriorly, the disc is held by the retrodiscal tissue. The insertion of the inferior belly of lateral pterygoid is the pterygoid fovea. During mandibular opening, the inferior belly of the lateral pterygoid contracts first while the superior belly relaxes, thus allowing the condyle to slide anteriorly and inferiorly down the articular eminence with the meniscus trailing posteriorly. Upon closing, the opposite occurs: the inferior belly of the lateral pterygoid relaxes while the superior belly of the lateral pterygoid contracts, resulting in condyle returning to the original posterior location and the meniscus being pulled anteriorly back onto the top of the condyle.

Below the insertion of the inferior belly of the lateral pterygoid and above the insertion of the masseter, is the "surgical neck" where fractures often occur obliquely from superior-anterior to inferior-posterior. In this subcondylar region, the ramus is robust in the sagittal plane measuring 12 to 14 mm at the narrowest point but only about half of that in the coronal plane. The length of the ramus is about 60 mm from the very top of the condyle (condylion) to the inferior-posterior most aspect of the gonial angle (gonion). At its narrowest, near the level of occlusal plane, the ramus is about 30 mm in the anterior-posterior dimension. Bisecting the ramus, on its medial surface, is the lingula to which the sphenomandibular ligament is attached.

The lingula marks the opening to the mandibular canal, which houses the inferior alveolar neurovascular bundle. Immediately posterior and inferior to this is the mylohyoid groove housing the mylohyoid nerve and artery. There are two thickened bony ridges extending from the coronoid process which is a triangular-shaped traction process formed partly as a result of the action of the temporalis muscle. These ridges extend inferiorly and anteriorly, creating the external and internal oblique ridges with the former being more anterior than the latter which becomes the mylohyoid line to which mylohyoid is attached.

The buccinator and superior constrictor originate from the pterygomandibular ligament which is anchored at the medial aspect of the ramus–body junction, where the internal oblique ridge turns into the mylohyoid line. Three fossae border the mylohyoid line: one above, the sublingual fossa, and two below, the digastric and submandibular. The space between the internal and external oblique ridges begins the dentition, 16 in number, arranged in a more U-shaped rather than the V-shaped configuration of the inferior mandibular border.

On the external surface, the intersection of a horizontal line midway between the superior and inferior borders of the mandible and a vertical line through the interdental space between the first and the second premolars marks the location of the mental foramen through which the terminal branches of the third division of trigeminal nerve exit the mandibular canal while the rest of the inferior alveolar nerve continues anteriorly to supply the incisors and canine. Due to the differential growth, both in quantity (allometry) and timing (heterochrony), between the corpus and the ramus, mental foramen typically points more posteriorly and the mandibular canal may have a more inferior course than the mental foramen.

The nomenclature of the various surfaces of a tooth warrants mentioning. As with any cuboidal/rectangular solid, a tooth has six surfaces, the very top of the crown is the occlusal surface for the molars and premolars (incisal for anterior teeth). The opposite of occlusal/incisal is apical. The external side is the labial surface (facing the lip for the anterior teeth) or the buccal surface (facing the buccal mucosa for the premolars and molars). The internal surface is designated lingual while the side facing midline is called mesial and the side facing away from the midline is distal. Combination of these can denote the specific line angles, ridges, or the cusps such as the mesio-buccal cusp of the mandibular first molar and the disto-occlusal line angle of the second premolar. The soft tissue immediately surrounding the tooth root is the periodontium. There is a cuff of pink keratinized tissue with dense attachment to the alveolar process called attached gingiva, measuring about 2 to 4 mm in healthy adults. At its apical edge is the mucogingival junction, where the attached gingiva meets the mobile, redder, and more reflective oral mucosa. Most intraoral incisions should be made at least 5 to 6 mm apical to the mucogingival junction, so that it can be sutured close at the end of the case.

By convention, the side that the mandible is moving toward is the working side and the side it is moving away from is the balancing side. The condyle on the working side is the rotating condyle and the opposite condyle is the orbiting condyle. When the maxillary and mandibular teeth are in their tightest opposition, the occlusion is known as position of maximum intercuspation, or centric occlusion. This differs from centric relation which is when the mandible is gently guided posteriorly so that the condyles assume the "hinge axis" position. For most individuals, there will be a discrepancy between the centric occlusion and centric relation with the posterior dentition making premature contacts in centric relation and then the mandible slides anteriorly into centric occlusion.

Normal topological anatomy of the lower face must be restored if one wishes to achieve an aesthetically acceptable result in mandibular fracture treatment. The lower facial height, measured from soft tissue subnasale to soft tissue menton should be one third of the total facial height as measured from trichion to menton. The distance from subnasale to stomion should be 50% of the stomion to menton distance. An aesthetically pleasing lateral facial profile should have the following four points in near a straight line: the most anterior points of the upper lip and the lower lip, midpoint of the columella, and the pogonion. The H angle is the angle formed between the Holdaway line and the aesthetic plane and ranges from 4 to 6 degrees. The Z angle is the angle formed by Frankfort horizontal and the line pogonion to the most anterior point of the lip, upper or lower, usually the upper. There should not be mentalis strain at rest while trying to keep the upper lip in contact with the lower lip; and a gentle, graceful, curved crease (the mental crease) should be present just about the depth of the lower buccal sulcus. The cervicomental angle should not be effaced and the inferior mandibular border from gonial angle to chin should be well defined. The maximum mandibular opening should be greater than 40 mm in adults with the head held in neutral position. In the frontal view, the occlusal plane should be level and the bi-gonial width is almost equal to bi-temporal width (90–95 mm), both being less than the bi-zygomatic width of about 110 mm.

If one can look directly at the mandible, the fracture treatment will not be that difficult. To expose the various parts described above is complicated by the investing soft tissues, in particular the nerves. The condyle, the subcondylar region, ramus, and posterior body are covered, from superficial to deep, by skin, subcutaneous tissue, superficial fascia, muscles of facial expression, and a deep fascia known as the parotidomasseteric fascia, facial nerve branches, auriculo-temporal nerve, superficial temporal artery and vein, and finally, at the deepest level, the muscles of mastication (mainly the masseter muscle). The term SMAS, superficial musculoaponeurotic system, is frequently used to denote the superficial fascia and the muscle of facial expression which it envelops. The condyle is surrounded by the joint capsule which is thickened laterally (sometimes referred to as the temporomandibular ligament), it is situated between the two terminal branches of the external carotid artery with the internal maxillary artery medial to the condyle and the superficial temporal artery lateral to it. Excessively vigorous blind dissection medial to the mandibular condyle/subcondylar region is occasionally met with significant arterial hemorrhage from this internal maxillary system and can be quite difficult to directly ligate, thus requiring packing and patient waiting to allow hemostasis. The course of the internal maxillary artery is typically about 3 mm below the lowest point of the sigmoid notch. The temporal and zygomatic branches of the facial nerve cross over the external surface of the zygomatic arch in a region 2 cm posterior to the posterior edge of the lateral orbital rim and 0.8 cm anterior to the root of the auricular helix. The auriculo-temporal nerve, a branch of the third division of trigeminal nerve, travels lateral to the temporomandibular joint (TMJ) capsule, supplying sensation to the joint, the external auditory meatus, and outer surface of the tympanic membrane. It also carries the postganglionic parasympathetic secreto-motor fibers to the parotid gland and plays part in the development of gustatory sweat or Frey syndrome.

The marginal mandibular branch of the facial nerve should be preserved during the exposure of the mandible. The above mentioned relationship holds for the upper cervical region as well: immediately deep to the subcutaneous tissue is the platysma, a member of the mimetic muscles, invested by the superficial fascia. Deep to this is the deep fascia which envelops the major neck muscles such as the sternocleidomastoid and the trapezius. The same deep fascia that invests the parotid gland and the masseter muscle (parotidomasseteric fascia) in the lower facial region extends down in the neck, and is anchored to the inferior mandibular border and the body of the hyoid bone. Similar to the relationship in the midface, the marginal mandibular branch of the facial nerve is immediately deep to this deep fascia. In nearly 100% of the cases, the marginal mandibular branch will cross the inferior mandibular border within 2 cm of the border superficial to the facial vessels, thus it would be safe to carry one's dissection toward the mandible in a plane deep to the facial vessels beginning 2 cm below the mandible.

PATIENT EVALUATION

Patients with mandibular fractures always present with a history of trauma, usually with pain near the fracture site, and sometimes with malocclusion. Trauma of sufficient force to cause fracture of the mandible usually results from either a motor vehicle accident or an altercation. Certainly falls can cause fractures to the symphyseal and subcondylar regions as well. Physical examination can reveal local edema or ecchymosis (which may be hidden below the tongue), a step-off of the teeth adjacent to the fracture, and/or malocclusion. Care must be taken to rule out cervical spine trauma, as this may accompany concomitant facial injury.

Following an accurate clinical diagnosis, radiographic studies are important to clearly localize and characterize the fracture pattern and identify occult fractures not previously suspected. In the absence of numerous superimposed osseous cortices, plain films are excellent for the diagnosis of mandible fractures. Oblique views are used to separate the two bodies from one another to better visualize the region near the angle. An orthopantomogram places an x-ray film behind the patient and creates the image as the

beam rotates around the head. A complete study should include both condyles and the inferior-most portion of the chin. The modality is excellent for the more lateral regions of the mandible, while the central portions often remain hazy. It can accurately demonstrate the molar regions where teeth may lie in the line of the fracture. CT scanning is similarly an excellent modality for mandible fractures and frequently used in conjunction with an orthopantomogram, since axial slices can demonstrate differences in fracture displacement across both cortices.

PATIENT PREPARATION

Because it is always easier to reduce and repair the acute fracture rather than osteotomize and fixate the healed fracture, time to repair plays an important role. Fractures of the mandible should generally be performed within a week or so of injury. Immediate repair can be justified, as can waiting 3 to 5 days to allow for swelling to abate. Prior to surgical intervention, the patient should be instructed to frequently rinse with an antimicrobial solution such as Listerine or Peridex several times a day.

Surgery is best performed under general anesthesia with a reinforced angled endotracheal tube placed through the nose and directed into the trachea with either direct vision using Magill forceps or a thin endoscope over which the tube is placed. It should be sutured to the caudal nasal septum and securely fixated to the midline forehead over several gauze pads with either suture or tape. A throat pack should be placed to avoid aspiration of liquids or dislodged bone or teeth. A toothbrush should be available in the operating room to clean the visible portions of the teeth with a dilute solution of Betadine, saline, and peroxide.

TECHNIQUE

The overall aim in mandible fracture management is to restore the patient's lower facial form and masticatory function. The crucial aspects of this goal involve achieving anatomic reduction and stabilization of the fracture fragments that will reestablish the patient's pretraumatic dental occlusion. If the patient's normal skeletal and dental relationships are reestablished, then the facial height and projection as well as facial contour and symmetry will be restored. This universal concept is applicable to mandible fracture in the various anatomic locations. In general, the options include both nonsurgical and surgical approaches. The nonsurgical approach involve nonoperative interventions while the surgical options include closed reduction with mandibulomaxillary fixation (MMF), open reduction, and internal fixation with or without maintaining MMF or the application of external fixation.

The nonsurgical approach may adequately manage nondisplaced stable fractures that are associated with normal dental occlusion. These favorable fractures are usually beveled and have a fracture line that resists displacement, and the attached muscles tend to impact rather than displace

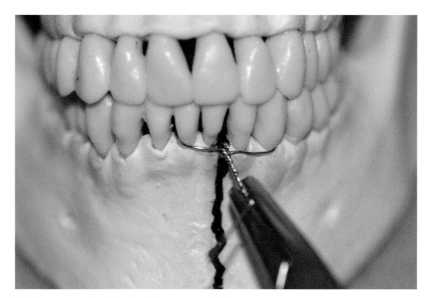

● FIGURE 26-1. Bridle wire placement. (1) The two mandibular segments are manually reduced by applying a compressive force across the fracture site. (2) A piece of 24- or 26-gauge wire is passed around the necks of adjacent stable teeth. (3) The fracture is reduced and stabilized by twisting the wire using a needle driver in a clockwise direction.

the fragment ends. The patient is typically kept on a soft diet for about 4 weeks while maintaining good oral hygiene. The patient is counseled to avoid further trauma to the fracture site and encouraged to restrict excessive or extreme mouth opening.[1] The caveat to this nonsurgical approach is that patients require close follow-up. Serial examination should ensure that the fracture fragments remain anatomically aligned as indicated by preservation of the patient's pretraumatic occlusion. Stability at a nontender fracture site indicates appropriate healing.

Often, there is malocclusion requiring proper reduction by first establishing the preinjured occlusion using MMF. MMF stabilizes and maintains the position of the fracture. When the fracture displacement is minimum, the upper and lower jaws can be kept immobilized in normal occlusion with either arch bars or Ivy loops until fracture healing is demonstrated at around for 4 to 6 weeks.[2] Training elastics allowing restricted mouth opening may be used during the final weeks of MMF. Weight loss may be minimized on the obligatory liquid diet by appropriate dietary counseling, including nutritional and vitamin supplements. The most commonly used methods to achieve MMF include the use of a bridle wire and placement of arch bars or Ivy loops. Stable dentition in both the maxilla and mandible is a necessary prerequisite. The instruments include a stout needle driver, 24- and 26-gauge wires, a wire cutter, and arch bars. An alternative fixation method needs to be considered in children with primary dentition and edentulous patients, which is outlined later in this chapter. A bridle wire can easily be placed around the teeth adjacent to a mandible fracture to achieve temporarily stabilize of a flailing segment. If the adjacent tooth is loose, decayed, or avulsed, one can use the nearest available stable tooth. This technique may be preformed at the bedside under local

anesthesia or certainly under general anesthesia when concomitant injuries are being treated in the operating room. The three essential steps to correctly place a bridle wire are outlined in Figure 26-1.

The bridle wire technique is ideally suited to achieve temporary stabilization of mandible fractures, especially in patients where the definitive fixation needs to be delayed because of concomitant injuries. Additionally, it prevents further soft tissue trauma, assists in airway protection, and helps alleviate pain and muscle cramps from moving unstable mandible segments.

MMF by arch bars is another very common method. Exposure of the teeth is obtained by using a self-retaining cheek retractor supplemented by a tongue retractor. Placement of a mandibular arch bar is outlined in Figure 26-2.

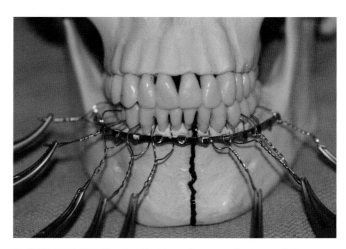

● FIGURE 26-2. Application of a mandibular arch bar.

The first step is to measure and cut a suitable length of arch bar. It should fit from a point distal to the molar teeth on one side to the opposite side. The third and possibly the second molars can be excluded if it is too challenging to pass wire around these teeth. Next, a 24-gauge wire is pre-stressed by stretching and cut into suitable lengths for the circumdental wires, and a 26-gauge wire which will be used to hold the maxillary and mandibular arch bars together. The circumdental loops of wire are placed loosely around the teeth on both sides of one jaw excluding the central incisors, which grip wires poorly and have a tendency to extrude. One passes the gently curved piece of a 24-gauge wire through the interdental space, first distal and then mesial around the lingual aspect of each tooth. The measured arch bar is then placed in these loops of wire and loosely secured. The hooks need to be correctly oriented to allow the box wires or elastics to hold the arch bars together. They are tightened in a clockwise fashion from midline to posterior to avoid excess arch bar anteriorly. The wire ends are cut, forming rosettes which are turned in to the gingiva. After gross reduction of the fracture segments to achieve normal occlusion, the box wires of a 24-gauge wire are placed around four hooks and fully tightened to maintain the teeth in a position of maximal intercuspation. Occasionally, the arch bars have to be cut at the site of the fracture to allow for proper reduction. After pretraumatic occlusion is achieved, these arch bar segments can be held together with 26-gauge wires.

Ivy loops are quicker and easier but incur some limitations (Figure 26-3). They do not provide an addition level of stability offered by arch bars, although both can function as tension bands. Additionally they cannot be used to stabilize an avulsed tooth or alveolar bone segment. Ivy loop placement is outlined in Figure 26-4.

The majority of the fracture will require open reduction and internal fixation. Adequate exposure for open reduction of most mandible fractures can be achieved via a lower buccal sulcus incision. Typically, the patient has

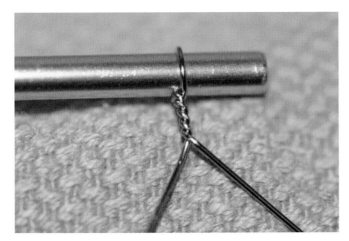

● **FIGURE 26-3.** The Ivy loop is made of 24-gauge wire by first forming a 2-mm eyelet, or loop. This is done by wrapping the central portion of the wire around a small suction cannula.

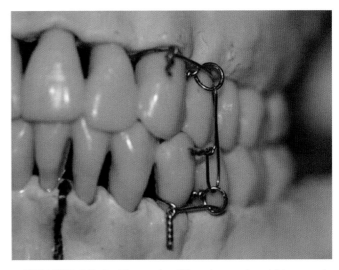

● **FIGURE 26-4.** The ends of the wire are brought around the mesial and distal sides of these two teeth. The posterior end of the wire is passed through the eyelet and tightened to the anterior wire to hold the eyelet securely between these teeth. The jaws are manipulated into the position of normal occlusion. A small segment of 26-gauge wire is passed through the eyelets of opposing maxillary and mandibular teeth and tightened in a clockwise direction.

been intubated with a nasotracheal tube that is secured to the nasal septum with a 2-0 silk suture. A tracheotomy set should always be available for potential airway emergencies. The eyes are lubricated and taped closed for protection during the entire procedure. The oral cavity is irrigated with an antimicrobial solution and the teeth scrubbed with a toothbrush. After arch bars are applied, the patient's face and neck are prepped and draped, carefully avoiding getting prep solution into the eyes. The patient should not remain paralyzed for an extended period of time and the angle of the mouth should be in full view in order to monitor facial nerve activity. The intraoral approach provides rapid access to fractures without significant external scars. The symphyseal, parasymphyseal and mid-body regions can be easily exposed through intraoral approaches, but the angle and ramus require additional buccal cheek retractors for adequate visualization. Internal rigid fixation and stabilization of the fracture fragments is achieved by applying plates and screws. Alternative techniques for stabilization include lag screws that are only applicable to noncomminuted fractures with sufficient overlapping of the fracture surfaces. However, in the presence of other multiple traumatic intraoral lacerations, the bony segments could potentially be devascularized and it is difficult to achieve a watertight closure of the inferior buccal sulcus incision especially with associated tooth avulsions. This may predispose to an increased postoperative infection rate. The intraoral approach exposes only the labial cortex of the fracture and, as such, it is possible to have a significant undetected gap on the lingual surface. Comminuted fractures may require an external approach. Nearly all regions of the mandible can be exposed via external incisions.

Multiple fracture fragments can be better visualized via extraoral approach provided by either a submandibular or a preauricular incision. Open reduction of these comminuted fractures can be best achieved with optimal exposure of the multiple fragments. Once the fracture is adequately exposed, anatomic reduction can be confirmed by direct visualization of both the labial and lingual surfaces. Large fixation plates can be more easily applied than with more limited access available via an intraoral approach. However, both the condyle and subcondylar regions are technically difficult to expose and provide a higher potential for bleeding complications and nerve injuries. The main trunk of the facial nerve is at risk with the preauricular approach, while the marginal mandibular branch which innervates the depressors of the lower lip may be injured with a submandibular incision.

Symphyseal and Parasymphyseal Fractures

True symphysis fractures are rare and may not be appreciated on panorex evaluation due to the central opacification from overlapping midline structures.[3] Nondisplaced symphysis and parasymphysis fractures can be stabilized with MMF alone. However, the pretraumatic occlusion must be maintained overcoming the significant torque due to muscle pull on the anterior mandible. Intraoral exposure via a lower buccal sulcus incision is required for displaced symphysis and parasymphysis fractures. The lower buccal sulcus can be delineated with the aid of retractors (two double hook or army/navy) holding the buccal mucosa of the lower lip in an outward and lateral direction. A curvilinear incision is marked just on the mandibular side of the deepest recess of the inferior buccal sulcus and should leave a cuff of oral mucosa (5 mm) to allow for secure closure. The incision line, including mucosa and muscle is infiltrated with local anesthetic (1% lidocaine, 1:200,000 epinephrine) to achieve vasoconstriction. A lower buccal sulcus incision is made with a number 15 scalpel blade perpendicular to the mucosal surface down to bone. A needle tip electrocautery is useful for this part of dissection. It is essential to leave a cuff of mucosa and underlying mentalis muscle attached to the superior flap to achieve a secure watertight closure. The dissection is carried subperiosteally, sweeping downward and laterally on the labial surface of the mandible with a periosteal elevator to carefully expose the mental neurovascular bundles bilaterally.

The mental foramina are usually located below the first or second bicuspid, midway between the alveolar ridge and the inferior mandible border on each side. The mental nerves must be protected during this entire procedure. The fracture site is identified and its labial surface is fully exposed, enabling all clot and fibrinous material to be cleaned off. One must use the occlusion status in addition to the exposed fracture site to achieve anatomic reduction and avoid any gaping on the unexposed lingual surface. The fracture site can be temporally stabilized with bone clamps applying compression via outwardly angled drill holes. Alternatively, unicortical interosseus wire can be used until internal fixation is achieved. An important step after the fractures are rigidly fixed is test for maintenance of occlusion after releasing MMF. The mandible should open and close easily while both condyles are properly seated in their respective glenoid fossa. Once this maneuver is preformed, elastic bands are reapplied to guide the mandible during the immediate postoperative period. The inferior buccal sulcus wound is irrigated and closed in layers. Interrupted 3-0 absorbable sutures can be used for the muscle closure while a running 4-0 chromic catgut suture can be used to achieve a secure mucosal layer closure. Rigid internal fixation using two plates is necessary to overcome the torsional forces in the symphyseal region. Generally one plate (2.4 mm) is placed along the inferior border and either a monocortical tension band plate (1.5 mm) or the arch bar is used at the superior border. Alternatively, central fractures in this region may be amenable to lag screws fixation with two 35 to 45 mm screws.[4]

Fractures of the Mandible Body

Fractures of the mandible body are located from the cuspid through the first molar and thus may involve a tooth in the line of fracture. Involved teeth require appropriate radiological evaluation in order to decide if tooth extraction is indicated. Nonrestorable teeth need to be removed at the time of fixation in order to minimize postoperative infective complications. Nondisplaced or minimally displaced body fracture may be stabilized with MMF for 4 to 6 weeks. Close follow-up to ensure adequate fracture healing and maintenance of pretraumatic occlusion is required. Training elastics allowing restricted mouth opening may be used during the final weeks of MMF. Displaced body fractures generally require open reduction and internal fixation. An intraoral approach is used with placement of a plate (2 mm) along the inferior border of the mandible. The mandible arch bar may serve as a tension band or alternatively a second, upper border, plate can be placed.[5] The use of monocortical screws at the superior border of the mandible avoids injury to the tooth roots. A submandibular incision (Risdon) provides good exposure of bone fragments in comminuted fractures of the mandible body.[6]

The 6-cm skin incision should be positioned in an existing skin crease about 2 cm below but parallel to curve of the mandibular angle to optimize the resulting external scar. The subcutaneous tissue and the superficial cervical fascia are dissected with cautery until the platysma muscle is reached. Dissection then proceeds carefully to avoid injury to the marginal mandibular branch of the facial nerve that lies below the platysma, just deep to the superficial layer of the deep cervical fascia. It has a variable course; usually no lower than 1 cm inferior to the mandibular border. If necessary, ligation of the facial artery and vein, allows the marginal mandibular branch of the facial nerve to be included in the reflected superior flap. Dissection is then carried through the deep cervical fascia directly to the inferior border of the mandible. The submandibular gland and associated lymph nodes are located just inferior to the lower border of the mandible, while the tail of the parotid gland which is usually posterior to the ramus may wrap around the inferior angle of the mandible. Care must be taken to avoid disrupting the capsules of these adjacent salivary glands because violation could result in transient sialoceles or salivary fistulas.

Fractures of Mandibular Angle

The angle of the mandible is prone to fracture, especially with the weakening presence of third molars. These angle fractures carry the highest complication rate and thus warrant an aggressive approach to delineated involvement of the third molar tooth in the line of fracture.[7] Devitalized molar teeth require extraction at the time of reduction. Open reduction of angle fractures can usually be accomplished via a lower buccal sulcus incision which extends posteriorly. This intraoral approach usually provides adequate exposure. The cheek is retracted laterally while marking the previously described lower buccal sulcus incision, which is carried distally along the external oblique ridge. The superior extent of the incision is limited to the mandibular occlusal plane, avoiding entrance into the buccal fat pad, which could potentially prolapse in to the wound. This incision line extends to posterior buccal mucosa and infiltrated with local anesthetic containing epinephrine to minimize bleeding and achieve optimal visualization. The incision is made through the mucosa and muscle, leaving an adequate superior cuff of tissue for closure. Dissection proceeds in the subperiosteal plane, sweeping the tissues posteriorly and laterally to expose the body and angle of the mandible. Rigid internal fixation usually involves placing a large angled plate (2.4 mm) along the inferior border with a monocortical tension band plate (1.5 mm) at the superior border. The transcutaneous trocar system is extremely useful, if not a necessity, in this location.

A solitary lag screw may be used to stabilize angle fractures, but this method can be technically demanding.[8] Alternatively, nonrigid fixation may be used in favorable fractures by placing a Champy plate along the external oblique ridge of the mandible angle. An open approach to mandibular angle fractures using a submandibular or modified Risdon incision may be required for improved access to achieve precise reduction and stable fixation of multiple fracture fragments. Fractures of the coronoid can involve only the tip of the coronoid process or the whole process. These simple fractures seldom produce malocclusion and can usually be treated nonoperatively. Ramus fractures are often nondisplaced because of the splinting effect from the surrounding masseter and temporalis and medial pterygoid muscles. They are usually vertically or horizontally oriented. It is necessary to ensure that the facial height and pretraumatic occlusion are maintained in these patients. MMF may be adequate stabilization for minimally displaced ramus fractures. However, open reduction and internal fixation via an internal approach is necessary to reduce displaced ramus fractures associated with malocclusion and loss of facial height. Stripping off the buccinator muscle and temporal tendon with a periosteal elevator may be necessary to expose the anterior surface of the ramus. The entire ramus and subcondylar region can be fully exposed by elevating and retracting off the masseter muscle.

Fractures of the Mandibular Condyle

Fractures of the mandible condyle are common (18%) and can be classified into those involving the head, neck, and subcondylar regions. Fractures in these three condyle regions require different approaches. Generally, the treatment of mandible condyle fractures is conservative, aiming to reestablish normal occlusion while preserving the vertical height of the ramus and maintaining the range of motion in the TMJ. Fractures of the condylar head are intracapsular injuries prone to TMJ ankylosis due to hemarthrosis and the immobilization period necessary to achieve adequate fracture healing. These fractures can be treated with soft diet alone if occlusion remains normal. However, if malocclusion is present, MMF is required for a short period of stabilization (2 weeks) after closed reduction which manipulates the jaws in to the pretraumatic occlusion position. An aggressive physiotherapy program is essential to regain normal mouth opening and lateral excursion of the mandible after this type of injury. Similarly fractures of the condyle neck and subcondylar region are generally also treated by closed reduction and stabilization with MMF (2 weeks) followed by physiotherapy. Adequate exposure of condylar neck fractures are challenging with potential risk of facial nerve injury. Open reduction should be reserved for specific circumstances, such as unable to obtain adequate dental occlusion by closed technique. Other less common indications include lateral extra capsular displacement of the condyle, displacement of the condyle in to the middle cranial fossa, and the presence of a foreign body such as a gunshot pellet in the TMJ.[9] Patients presenting with dental malocclusion may have displacement or over riding of the proximal condyle segment. Those patients with unilateral displaced condyle fractures occlude prematurely on the side of the fracture because of vertical length shortening. Patients with bilateral displaced condyle fractures have an anterior open bite or apertognathia, because of premature contact of the posterior teeth. This results from a bilateral decrease in the vertical height of the mandible rami. In panfacial trauma bilateral subcondylar fractures may be associated with midface fractures. Open reduction and rigid internal fixation of the condyle neck fractures are required to reestablish the vertical height of the lower face in these complex injuries. A combined preauricular and modified Risdon approach generally provides the best exposure for type of open complex reduction and internal fixation. The preauricular approach provides good exposure to the condyle and subcondylar regions of the mandible as well as the temporomandibular joint area. A preauricular incision, 3 to 4 cm in length is made in the skin crease that is easily identified by pushing the ear and tragus forward. Dissection is carried along the anterior aspect of the tragus, avoiding the external auditory canal as it courses anteromedially. The main trunk of the facial nerve is relatively safe as long as the dissection is kept within 0.5 cm anterior to the tragus. The incision is carried down to the zygomatic process of the temporal bone. The periosteum overlying the posterior part of zygomatic arch is sharply incised to elevate and reflect all soft tissues from a posterior to anterior direction. The superficial temporal vessels, auriculotemporal nerve, facial nerves and its branches, as well as the parotid gland can be protected in this anterior displaced soft tissue flap. The capsule of the TMJ is visualized in this region. It can be opened via a transverse incision, leaving a 3-mm cuff for closure. Care must be taken to avoid tearing the articulating disc, which is usually attached medially. The condyle is just inferior and may be displaced medially by the attached lateral pterygoid muscle. The condyle head can be grasped and pulled laterally into its anatomic position. It may be necessary to release MMF in order to achieve adequate reduction of the condyle neck fractures. An endoscopically assisted approach can provide assistance with direct fracture reduction, allowing better visualization to achieve precise anatomic alignment of the condyle segments.

There are a number of distinctive situations that require special consideration regarding fixation of mandible fractures. These include mandible fractures in children, the edentulous patient, and teeth in the line of fracture.

Fractures in Children

The mandible of a child differs from an adult mandible in a number of regards. The condyle is the major growth center and during the first three years of life it consists of a delicate vascular sponge covered by thin cortical bone underneath the articular cartilage. Injury to the condyle head during this period may lead to growth disturbance. Also, crushing injury to this highly vascular condyle head may result in an intracapsular hemorrhage and hemarthrosis with a high risk of ankylosis of the TMJ. Incomplete or greenstick fractures, especially in the condylar region, are more common in children as the pediatric mandible is more elastic and tends to bend rather than break.[10] In early childhood, there are numerous primary (deciduous) and unerupted teeth that may weaken the mandible because of lack of cortical bone.[11]

Orthopantomogram examination is a useful evaluation of the state of mixed dentition. These unerupted teeth must also be taken into account when using bicortical screws with plate fixation in order to avoid tooth bud injuries. In addition, stabilization by application of arch bars, Ivy loops, or open interosseous wiring is not recommended before 9 years of age.[12] In this period of mixed dentition, it is difficult to hold wires around the bases of deciduous teeth because of their conical shape with the widest area of the crown located at or below the free gingival margin. Also these teeth tend to extrude when the wires are tightened. Intermaxillary fixation is best achieved by using circummandibular wires connected to wires passed though drill holes at the piriform aperture. In addition a custom-made acrylic trough, a splint can be attached to the teeth. Conservative nonoperative management is applicable to most pediatric mandible fractures. Closed reduction is always preferable if reasonable anatomic reduction of the fracture fragments can be achieved, thus avoiding extensive dissection, periosteal elevation, and interference with growth centers in the mandible.

Condyle fractures in children deserve special mention as indicated above. Subcondylar greenstick fractures are more common than intracapsular fractures and tend to be medially displaced with a resultant lateral cross bite. Treatment of these fractures aims is to preserve the height of the ramus and TMJ function. Closed reduction with a short period of immobilization (1–2 weeks), followed by active exercises is usually sufficient.[11] More extensive injury to the condyle region resulting in bilateral fracture dislocations with telescoping of the fracture fragments. This is a serious threat to growth and normal occlusion. Closed reduction and a longer period of immobilization (3–4 weeks) are often required. Open reduction is reserved for significantly displaced fracture fragments resulting in malocclusion that fail closed techniques.[13] Fractures of the body of pediatric mandible are likely to follow the line of structural weakness due to developing teeth. Their management must take into account the child's state of mixed dentition. Closed reduction and fixation by means of circummandibular wires and lingual splints are appropriate.

Fractures in Edentulous Patients

The edentulous mandible often has loss of height with atrophy of the alveolar ridge. The body is more prone to fracture because of the smaller cross-sectional area and significant atrophy. This region has reduced capacity for repair because the remaining bone is primarily cortical bone. Fixation of edentulous mandible fractures is challenging because of lack of teeth to observe occlusion and anchor MMF. Closed reduction of nondisplaced or minimally displaced fractures may be achieved with circummandibular wiring of Gunning splints or fabricated acrylic saddles for stabilization of the fracture fragments. Fixation using the patient's own dentures with skeletal wires is cumbersome and does not permit any oral hygiene to be accomplished on the lingual aspects unless an opening is made by removing the incisors of the denture. Open reduction with rigid internal fixation is the treatment of choice for displaced fractures in the edentulous mandible. This approach ensures direct visualization to provide optimal stability of the fracture fragments with large plates and screws. If the height of the atrophic mandible allows placement of a second tension band plate, it will help avoid any torsional instability especially on the lateral aspect of the edentulous mandible. This method allows early return of masticatory function. Osteogenesis is stimulated when compressive plates are used. Supraperiosteal placement of large locking reconstructive plates (2.4 mm) ensures rigid fixation, while avoiding compromise to the underlying blood supply of the edentulous mandible.[13] When there is severe atrophy, with a mandible height of less than 10 mm, primary bone grafting should be considered because of demonstrated impaired bone healing. Postoperative complications parallel the extent of bone atrophy in this compromised group. If bone healing fails to occur, the plates are at risk of breaking due to metal fatigue.

Teeth in the Line of Fracture

Mandible fractures with teeth in the line of fracture should be considered compound. They consequently have a higher potential for postoperative infective complications such as osteomyelitis. Usually these patients are admitted to hospital to administer parenteral antibiotic therapy and to optimize oral hygiene with antimicrobial mouthwashes. These fractures require a through radiological evaluation to assess tooth root involvement. Panorex and special periapical dental x-rays are helpful in delineating the involvement of the fracture line with the tooth root.[3] Teeth should be retained whenever possible and removed only when they are nonrestorable or severely broken.[14]

Restorative dentistry should be considered if the involved tooth is intact with a stable root. An asymptomatic impacted tooth in the fracture line of uncomplicated mandible fracture should be left in place.[14] Avulsed teeth should be replanted as quickly as possible with stabilization of the alveolar fragment by means of an arch bar or interdental wires.

Nonrestorable teeth that are likely to contribute to infective complications should be removed. Patients with fractures of the tooth root, those with severe loosening of teeth associated with chronic periodontal disease, those with extensive periodontal injury and broken alveolar walls, and those with displacement of teeth from their alveolar sockets should undergo tooth extraction at the time of fracture reduction.

● COMPLICATIONS

Complications related to mandible fractures and their treatments are not rare, occurring in 14% of all patients.[15] They tend to occur in a predictable pattern, more commonly seen in patients with predisposing risk factors. For example, angle fractures have more associated complications because of the presence of the third molar tooth.[16] Complications related to mandible fracture treatment can be divided into early and late types. Early complications include airway compromise, hemorrhage, malocclusion, and nerve injury. The importance of careful documentation in the initial patient assessment cannot be over emphasized. Late complications include infection, such as cellulitis, abscess, and osteomyelitis. Altered healing may be a late complication encompassing delayed union, malunion, and nonunion. In addition, malocclusion, TMJ ankylosis,

and TMJ dysfunction may be long-term issues. Infection of mandible fractures can be problematic and account for nearly half of all postoperative complications. The spectrum of severity ranges from cellulites, to abscess formation, and potentially subsequent osteomyelitis. Predictably, those patients with poor oral hygiene and nutrition compromised by alcohol or drug abuse, those who present late with subsequent delay in treatment, or those who are noncompliant with therapy are more likely to experience infection complications.[17]

Displaced fractures and those patients with teeth in the line of fracture are at higher risk of infection. The severity of infection dictates the aggressiveness of the required therapy. Early superficial cellulitis of the surrounding soft tissue may respond to antibiotic therapy alone. The choice of antibiotic is determined by the sensitivity of the most likely involved organisms. Oral or intravenous Clindamycin (600 mg q6h) is often initially used until culture results dictate differently. Deep infection, in which the fixation is still stable and intact, may be treated by washout. Debridement of necrotic tissue, removal of involved teeth, and IV antibiotic therapy are also necessary. Fixation hardware if stable often can be left in place if the infection can be adequately controlled. Alternative fixation such as an external fixator may be required when the original fixation is loose and requires removal due to infection. The second most common complication of mandible fracture treatment is altered healing, which includes delayed healing, malunion, and nonunion. Infections are frequently an important cause of nonunion. Fractures of the mandible body have the highest incidence of nonunion (3.2%). Other conditions contributing to nonunion include inadequate immobilization of fractures and teeth involved in the line of fracture. The treatment of nonunion generally consists of washout, debridement of necrotic bone, extraction of involved teeth, and reapplication of rigid internal or external fixation with possible bone grafting. Bone grafting should be delayed until all infection has been eradicated and healthy viable soft tissue coverage can predictable be achieved.

Malocclusion is usually related to inadequate reduction of the fracture fragments. This is often precipitated by maladaption of the fixation plates that do not allow anatomic reduction of the fracture. This can be prevented by releasing the MMF after fixation has been applied and reassessing the occlusion. The mandibular condyles need to be appropriately seated in the glenoid fossae with the dentition in a position of maximum intercuspation. Any discrepancy in the occlusion needs to be addressed at this stage by removing the fixation, reestablishing MMF and reapplying new bone fixation plates to achieve anatomic reduction. Arch bars may need to be cut with fixation on either side of the fracture. These two segments can be held together with loops of 26-gauge wire to achieve optimal reduction of the displaced fracture fragments. Prolonged postoperative immobilization in MMF for more than 6 weeks may lead to stiffness and predispose to dysfunction or TMJ ankylosis.

● OUTCOMES

In general, the treatments of mandibular fractures enjoy a high rate of success with uneventful healing in more than 85% of cases. Positive and negative results from the treatment of mandibular fractures will ultimately be judged by the adequacy of healing. Fractures that heal in the prescribed time course without complication or need for additional procedures are the goal. Specific measures to examine in the postoperative period include pain, dentition, and range of motion. Following an adequate period of healing, patients should be free of both pain in the mandible at rest and with mastication. The dentition that was present before the inciting trauma should be present and healthy after healing. And the excursion of the mandible should be equal to that preoperatively both in the vertical and horizontal planes. Meticulous techniques and attention to details regarding both systemic and local factors will increase further the success rate.

REFERENCES

1. Guerrissi JO. Fractures of mandible: Is spontaneous healing possible? Why? When? *J Craniofac Surg.* 2001;12(2):157.

2. Ellis E 3rd, Moos KF, EL-Attar A. Ten yeast of mandibular fractures: An analysis of 2,137 cases. *Oral Surg.* 1985;59:120.

3. Wilson IF, Lokeh A, Benjamin CL, et al. Prospective comparison of panoramic tomography (zonography) and helical computed tomography in the diagnosis and operative management of mandibular fractures. *Plas Reconstr Surg.* 2001;107:1369.

4. Ellis E, Ghali GE. Lag screw fixation of anterior mandibular fractures. *J Oral Maxillofac Surg.* 1991;49:13.

5. Haug RH, Fattahi TT, Goltz M. A biomechanical evaluation of mandibular angle fracture plating techniques. *J Oral Maxillofac Surg.* 2001;59:1199.

6. Fonseca RJ, Walker RV, eds. *Oral and Maxillofacial Trauma.* 2nd ed. Philadelphia: Saunders; 1997.

7. Ellis E 3rd. Treatment methods for fractures of the mandibular angle. *Int J Oral Maxillofac Surg.* 1999;28:243.

8. Shetty V, Caputo A. Biomechanical validation of the solitary lag screw technique for reducing mandibular angle fractures. *J Oral Maxillofac Surg.* 1992;50:603.

9. Zide MF, Kent JN. Indications of open reduction of mandibular condyle fractures. *J Oral Maxillofac Surg.* 1983;41:89.

10. James DR. Maxillofacial injuries in children. In: Rowe NL, Williams JLI, eds. *Maxillofacial Injuries.* New York: Churchill Livingstone; 1985:538–542.

11. Schweinfurth JM, Koltai PJ. Pediatric mandibular fractures. *Facial Plast Surg.* 1998;14(1):31.

12. Posnick JC, Wells M, Pron GE. Pediatric facial fractures: evolving patterns of treatment. *J Oral Maxillofac Surg.* 1993;51:836.

13. Bradley JC. Age changes in the vascular supply to the mandible. *Br Dent J.* 1972;132:142.

14. Shetty V, Freymiller E. Teeth in the line of fracture: A review. *J Oral Maxillofac Surg.* 1989;47:1303.

15. Moulton-Barrett R, Rubinstein AJ, Salzhauer MA, et al. Complications of mandibular fractures. *Ann Plast Surg.* 1998;41:258.

16. Winzenburg SM, Imola MJ. Internal fixation in pediatric maxillofacial fractures. *Facial Plast Surg.* 1998;14(1):45.

17. Haug RH, Schwimmer A. Fibrous union of the mandible: a review of 27 patients. *J Oral Maxillofac Surg.* 1994;52:842.

chapter 27

Panfacial Fractures

Daniel Y. Maman, MD, MBA / Mark L. Smith, MD, FACS

● INTRODUCTION

The treatment of panfacial fractures requires careful patient assessment, prioritization of injuries and consideration of long-term function and cosmesis. The etiology of panfacial fractures, according to a recent retrospective analysis, are assault (36%), motor vehicle accidents (32%), falls (18%), sports (11%), occupational injuries (3%), and gunshot wounds (2%).[1] In young adults, sports like football, hockey, and baseball account for a high percentage of injuries.

Panfacial injury presents a unique challenge on account of the interrelationship between the bones and the vital structures they house. The superficial facial bones include the frontal bone, nasal bones, zygomas, maxillary bones, and mandible. The deeper facial skeleton consists of the sphenoid, lacrimal, vomer, ethmoid, and temporal bones. The temporomandibular joint (TMJ) on each side is the only facial joint and plays important functions in oration and mastication. The meniscus and mandibular condyle form a hinged joint allowing for rotation. A sliding joint is formed between the meniscus and temporal bone allowing for additional forward translation of the mandible at the end of opening. The direct relationship of the facial bones to vision, breathing, smell, mastication and facial form necessitates an understanding of the relevant anatomy in order to successfully treat panfacial injuries.

● FACIAL ANATOMY

The vertical buttresses of the midface are regions of thick bone designed to resist the forces of mastication and distribute them over the cranial base. They also serve as mitigators of energy in vertically oriented facial trauma. There are five vertical buttresses (Figure 27-1):

1. Frontonasomaxillary buttress
2. Frontozygomaticomaxillary buttress
3. Pterygomaxillary buttress

4. Frontoethmoid-vomerine buttress
5. Posterior mandibular ramus/condyle

The frontonasomaxillary buttress (often referred to as the medial buttress) begins superiorly at the maxillary process of the frontal bone and superior orbital rim, extends inferiorly to the frontal process of the maxilla, and then caudally to lateral piriform rim and the maxillary canine area. The frontozygomaticomaxillary buttress (often referred to as the lateral buttress) begins superiorly with the zygomatic process of the frontal bone, and then moves downward through the lateral orbital rim, across the zygomaticofrontal suture, through the main body of the zygoma and the zygomatic process of the maxilla to the zygomatico-alveolar crest junction below. The pterygomaxillary buttress supports the posterior maxilla via the pterygoid plates of the sphenoid bones. As opposed to the nasomaxillary and zygomaticomaxillary buttresses, the pterygomaxillary buttress is usually not reconstructed in panfacial fractures due to inaccessibility. The frontoethmoid-vomerine buttress is an unpaired midline support below the nasal structures on which the quadrangular cartilage rests. The posterior mandibular ramus and condyle make up the most posterior vertical buttress and serve to establish posterior facial height.[2]

The horizontal buttresses are also referred to as the anterior-posterior buttresses. There are four horizontal buttresses (see Figure 27-2):

1. Frontal buttress
2. Zygomatic buttress
3. Maxillary buttress
4. Mandibular buttress

The frontal buttress is composed of the superior orbital rims and the glabellar region. The zygomatic arch, zygomatic body, and infraorbital rim make up the zygomatic

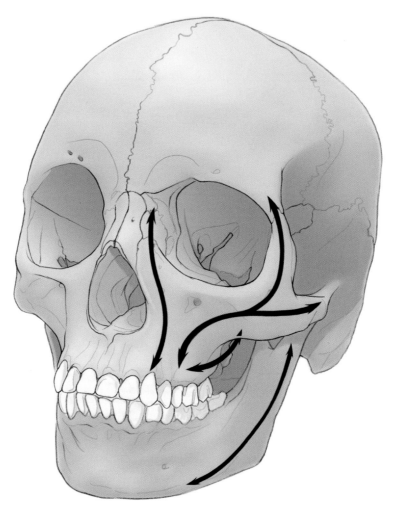

● **FIGURE 27-1.** Vertical buttresses.

buttress. The maxillary and mandibular buttress consists of the arches of the maxillary bone and mandible, respectively. These buttresses offer some protection against horizontal forces, but are significantly weaker and less protective than the vertical buttresses. Therefore, vertically oriented trauma is better absorbed by the facial skeleton, whereas horizontal force often overwhelms the horizontal buttresses and causes fracturing through the vertical pillars. In surgical approaches to the facial skeleton, attempts should be made to restore both the vertical and horizontal buttresses. Reduction at these sites will help ensure appropriate facial height, width, and projection.[2]

The naso-orbitalethmoid (NOE) complex consists of the confluence of the frontal, maxillary, nasal, ethmoid, lacrimal, and sphenoid bones. The frontoethmoid-vomerine and paired nasomaxillary buttresses provide the vertical support structures of the NOE complex. The adjacent more delicate structures are supported and protected by these buttresses. The medial orbit is made up of the lacrimal bone which contains the medial canthal tendon attachment and the lamina papyracea (lateral roof of the ethmoid bone). The ethmoid bone forms part of the floor of the anterior skull base. Injury in this area can result in dural tear and resultant cerebrospinal fluid (CSF) leak. The anterior and posterior

ethmoid vessels exit the skull through foramina located at the frontoethmoid suture, in the posterior-superior portion of the orbit. Shearing of these vessels in NOE fracturing can result in intraorbital hematoma. The optic canal is located more posteriorly and uncommonly involved in NOE fracture patterns. However, bony fragment displacement and nerve edema within the optic canal can lead to optic neuropathy. In this situation, prompt surgical decompression is needed to prevent permanent blindness.

The ethmoid sinuses are a labyrinth of sinuses, separated by the perpendicular plate of the ethmoid bone, forming the *inter*orbital space. This interorbital space is reinforced superiorly by the cribriform plate and posteriorly by the skull base and the sphenoid bone. In severe NOE fractures, collapse of the interorbital space can result in anterior intracranial injury (frontal lobe) and injury or herniation of the intraorbital contents.

The medial canthal tendon (MCT) inserts on the lacrimal bone. The MCT contains three limbs. The superficial heads of the orbicularis oculi muscle create the anterior and superior limbs of the tendon inserting on the anterior lacrimal crest. The deep head forms the posterior limb and inserts on the posterior lacrimal crest. The three limbs of the MCT incase the lacrimal sac within lacrimal fossa and

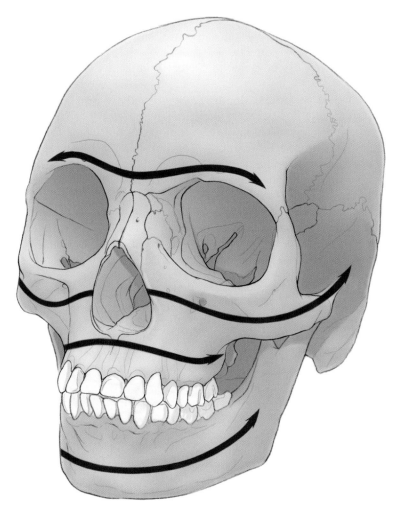

● FIGURE 27-2. Horizontal buttresses.

function to pump and propagate tear transmission through the lacrimal duct system. The MCT also functions (in conjunction with the lateral canthal tendon) to suspend the eyelids against the globe. Other chapters in this textbook dealing with specific types of fractures provide further information on pertinent anatomy.

● PATIENT EVALUATION

Advanced Trauma Life Support (ATLS) protocol takes precedence in the initial evaluation of maxillofacial trauma patients, especially those with panfacial injury. Life-threatening injuries in trauma patients must be diagnosed immediately. Facial fractures are rarely life-threatening when they occur alone, but can present significant challenges when much of the bony support to the airway is fractured and bleeding. During the primary survey, injuries to the face or oropharynx that compromise the airway are assessed. Airway management indications are unchanged in facial trauma. Orotracheal intubation is preferred over blind nasotracheal intubation. Bleeding from severe facial injury, either intraorally or from epistaxis may complicate intubation. Occasionally, severe bleeding is an indication

for intubation to protect the airway. Rarely, large hematomas can extend into the neck or supraclavicular region causing external compression of the pharynx. When a difficult intubation is suspected, a dual setup for intubation and cricothyrotomy is prudent. Cervical spine stabilization should be achieved via standard protocol.

Upon completion of the ATLS primary survey, the secondary survey is initiated and careful assessment of the face is performed. In unintubated alert patients, a history should be elicited that addresses the following areas:

1. Does the patient's dental occlusion and sensation feel normal?
2. Can the patient hear normally?
3. Is the patient's vision normal and extraocular movement intact?
4. Can the patient breathe through both nostrils?
5. Is the patient able to speak normally?
6. Does the patient have any history of previous facial trauma or surgery?

Understanding the mechanism of injury, the magnitude of force, and the vector of impact is helpful in tailoring the clinical examination and ensuring that all injuries are recognized. A history of loss of consciousness or mental status changes can be a clue to intracranial injury. Any functional deficits as elicited by the questions above can be a clue to localizing fracture locations.

A general examination of the face is performed, noting any asymmetries or motor deficits. Subtle findings, such as mild enophthalmos or decreased globe excursion on upward gaze, can have long-term implications if missed. Palpation of the bony skeleton should then occur. Crepitus, severe focal tenderness, abnormal prominences, and bony step-offs are indications of underlying fractures. Focal areas of swelling or hematoma may also be a sign of underlying fracture. Facial nerve motor function is critical to normal facial function and each of the five branches should be assessed on clinical examination. Sensation throughout the face should also be tested to assess for trauma to the three trigeminal nerve branches. Photographs are helpful in preoperative planning and postoperative outcomes assessment.

Each area of the face should then be evaluated systematically. In the forehead, loss of convexity, crepitus, and focal tenderness are suggestive of frontal sinus fractures. Evaluation of the eyes should include visual acuity and movement of the extraocular muscles. Changes in visual acuity may signal injury to the globe or retina, disruption of the optic canal or a neurologic injury. Assessment of upward globe excursion is of particular importance, as entrapment of the inferior rectus muscle in orbital floor fractures is common. Periorbital swelling, ecchymosis, hyphema, proptosis, enopthalmus, and inferior orbital nerve parasthesia are all signs of possible orbital fractures. Eye pain, photophobia, and tearing are signs of possible corneal abrasions. An ophthalmologic examination in the setting of an orbital fractures is prudent. The orbital rims should be palpated for step-offs.

Particular to periorbital and NOE fractures, soft tissue edema may mask findings if only minimal displacement is present. If posterior telescoping of the nasal bones and frontal process of the maxilla are present, clinical diagnosis will be more obvious. Intercanthal and interpalpebral distances should be measured. If the intercanthal distance is more than 50% of the interpupillary distance, suspicion for traumatic telecanthus should be further explored. Telecanthus is a telltale sign of NOE fracture. If the MCT is displaced or cut during impact, telecanthus occurs. Usually, the MCT itself remains intact, and it is the fragment of bone to which it is attached that becomes displaced. Unopposed tension from the orbicularis oculi muscle that remains attached to the lateral orbit by the lateral canthal ligament causes unopposed pull on the tarsal plates and eyelid skin—resulting in the telecanthus. For MCT fracture avulsion to occur, NOE fracturing must occur at four sites: lateral nasal bones, medial orbital wall, nasomaxillary buttress, and frontomaxillary junction.

Integrity of the MCT can be tested manually by placement of lateral traction on the upper and lower eyelids. With instability of the MCT in NOE fracture, lateral displacement will occur with traction. Compression of the

canthal-bearing medial orbital rim with the thumb and index finger may reveal instability and/or crepitus. As with all panfacial fractures, thorough examination of the eye for visual acuity, extraocular muscle function, and pupillary response is essential. Lacrimal function should also be assessed. Lacrimal duct probing and Jones I/II dye tests may be necessary to rule out any injury. The presence of rhinorrhea, not uncommon in NOE fracture, is suggestive of CSF leak. If adequate fluid volume can be collected, testing for beta-2 transferrin is the gold standard for confirmation of CSF rhinorrhea.

Milder NOE injuries result in minimal or no MCT displacement. More severe injuries result in lateral displacement of the MCT segment, resulting in telecanthus. The severity of MCT disruption and bony comminution is the basis for NOE fracture classification (Figure 27-3). All types (I, II, III) may be unilateral or bilateral. Type III is almost always bilateral given the impact force necessary to generate severe comminution.[3]

- **Type I**—Large single segment NOE fracture with no disruption of the MCT attachment
- **Type II**—Comminuted fracturing of the NOE complex with no disruption of the MCT attachment
- **Type III**—Comminuted fracturing of the NOE complex with disruption of the MCT attachment

Preoperatively, distinction is only possible between types I and II. Intraoperatively, the integrity of the MCT and bone to which it is attached is assessed to differentiate between types II and III. For appropriate preoperative planning, the surgeon must only know if the NOE fracture is single segment versus comminuted and unilateral versus bilateral. This knowledge alone dictates the number of incisions and types of surgical approaches described below.

Initially, evaluation of the nose should include notation of any obvious deformity or deviation of the dorsum and nasal tip. Palpation for focal tenderness, crepitus, or instability of the nasal bones should be assessed. Intranasal examination with a speculum may reveal a septal hematoma or deviation suggestive of a fracture. A septal hematoma should be drained immediately, otherwise it may lead to septal cartilage necrosis and eventual saddle nose deformity. Rhinorrhea is a sign of CSF leak, and may indicate a frontal sinus posterior table fracture or cribiform plate fracture. Mobility of the entire nasal pyramid may be caused by a LeFort II or III fracture. (A more detailed nasal examination is discussed in Chapter 24.)

Zygomaticomaxillary complex (ZMC) fractures often result in enophthalmos or malar deformity. A depressed zygomatic arch fracture may cause trismus, while tenderness and crepitus over the midcheek could signify a maxillary sinus fracture. Anesthesia in the distribution of the infraorbital nerve, or its dentoalveolar branches, often accompanies fractures involving the orbital floor, the orbital rim or the anterior maxillary wall.

Overall stability of the midface is assessed via inspection, palpation, and manipulation to rule out LeFort fractures.

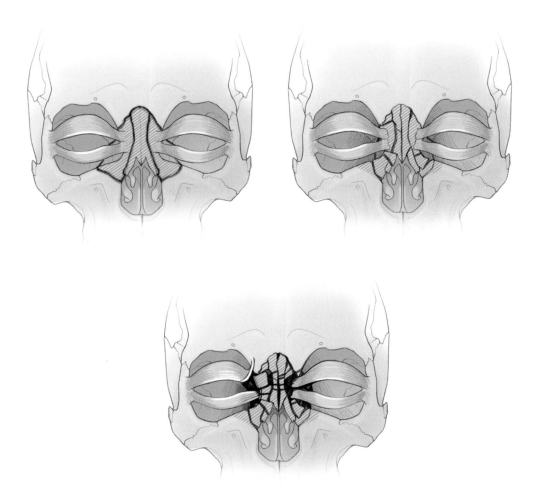

● **FIGURE 27-3.** NOE fracture classification.

This can be done by stabilizing the patient's forehead while grasping the anterior maxillary teeth or alveolar ridge and pulling forward on the maxilla. Mobility of the maxilla is a sign of fracture. Periorbital swelling may be a sign of LeFort II or III fracturing. Retrusion of the midface from a direct inward blow in LeFort fractures creates a "dish face" appearance. The posteriorly displaced maxillary segment may create premature contact between the maxillary and mandibular molars leading to an anterior open bite.

Otoscopic examination should be performed to assess the tympanic membrane and external canal. Hemotypanum and/or otorrhea are a sign of serious injury. The classic "Battle's sign," or posterior auricular ecchymosis, is suggestive of basilar skull fracture. This sign, however, does not develop for 24 to 48 hours after trauma.

Intraoral examination should assess dentition, maxillomandibular occlusion, stability of the alveolar ridge, and integrity of the palate. In the awake and cooperative patient, asking the patient to close their mouth and report if the occlusion feels normal best assesses the dental occlusion. The patient is usually more accurate than the physician given the high variability in preinjury occlusions. The hard palate should be palpated for any step-offs or

sensitivity. The inability to fully open the jaw is suggestive of a mandible fracture, although zygomatic arch fractures may also limit opening. Anterior open bite, posterior open bite, occlusal tilts, and unusual mobility of the mandible are other clues. Impacted molars create a weak point in the mandible and are often involved in the fracture line. Fracture of a tooth may necessitate removal. Intraoral palpation in the gingival buccal groove along the maxilla may reveal contour abnormalities if maxillary fractures are present. Caudal portions of the anterior maxillary sinus, nasomaxillary buttress and zygomaticomaxillary buttress should similarly be palpated.

Diagnostic Imaging

The role of plain radiographic films has diminished in the assessment of panfacial trauma, as almost all patients will undergo a CT scan. Multiple radiographic views are needed to fully assess the complex planes of the facial skeleton. An occipitomental (Water's) view and submental-vertex view are used to visualize zygmaticomaxillary complex fractures. A 15-degree posterior-anterior (Caldwell's) view may reveal injuries to the superior orbit, frontal, and ethmoid sinuses.

Lateral views are helpful to assess the nose, palate, and frontal and maxillary sinuses. More commonly, radiographs may demonstrate air fluid levels within the sinuses, suggestive of nonvisualized wall fractures. A panorex is the single most useful view for assessing the mandible; however, the lateral oblique views provide good imaging of the ramus and body while the frontomastoid (Townes') view shows the condyles. A cervical spine film is helpful to exclude vertebral column injury. Nevertheless, plain radiographs are almost never obtained in modern facial trauma evaluation.

CT imaging provides the most accurate and thorough evaluation of the facial skeleton and is preferable to plain radiographs for evaluating a patient with panfacial fractures.[4] It can also simultaneously evaluate for associated intracranial and cervical spine injuries. CT imaging of the facial skeleton should be done with 1-mm cuts and be weighted for bony evaluation. Axial, coronal, sagittal, and 3D reformatting are helpful in delineating the full extent of facial trauma and for visualizing fracture patterns. CT angiography can give additional information in the setting of expanding facial hematoma or concern for carotid artery injury. Soft tissue structures such as TMJ meniscus, extraocular muscles, and the optic nerve may also be visualized with CT imaging; however, soft tissues are best imaged using MRI. The advent of specialized equipment and software, now allows use of CT and MR imaging to perform sophisticated preoperative planning and intraoperative image-guided reduction of fracture segments.

● PATIENT PREPARATION

Indications for surgical intervention in panfacial trauma are similar to those for individual facial fractures. Importantly, definitive surgery should not proceed until all life-threatening injuries have been addressed. Panfacial fractures often occur in association with other systemic injuries. Delineating the appropriate time for surgical intervention is of key importance. Often times, only one operation is necessary for definitive treatment. However, an initial treatment may be necessary to clinically stabilize the patient prior to undertaking complete surgical repair.

Obviously, general anesthesia should not be induced unless a secure airway is in place. As in all surgery, the risks from general anesthesia must be weighed against any medically confounding variables (eg, heart disease, pulmonary disease). Repair of panfacial fractures is not always necessary, but unaddressed fractures may lead to significant functional and cosmetic disability.

The goal of surgery for facial fractures is to promote healing, restore function, and maximize cosmesis. Soft tissue loss may necessitate delayed treatment of fractures or required the use of distant flaps for coverage. External fixation is another option. Extensive tooth loss may cause difficulty in reestablishing preinjury occlusion. Posterior tooth loss and mandibular condyle fractures lead to loss in the vertical height dimension. Primary bone grafting is indicated to restore buttresses and to replace missing or severely comminuted bone. In non-load bearing regions,

small bone gaps of less than 5 mm may be bridged with a miniplate. Larger gaps or those in load-bearing regions should be filled with bone grafts.

Indications for hospital admission and early repair:

- NOE fractures with CSF leak (need to monitor for continued CSF leak and possible complications such as meningitis)
- Frontal sinus posterior table fractures
- Zygomatic fractures with trismus
- LeFort midface fractures
- Orbital floor fractures with signs of ocular muscle entrapment

Indications for immediate surgical intervention:

- Airway preservation: craniofacial fractures commonly cause airway compromise. Immediate surgical reduction of the fractured facial bones may be necessary to decompress the airway. Commonly, tracheostomy is necessary both for immediate airway restoration and to facilitate future surgical intervention.[5] Submandibular and endotracheal intubations are alternatives.
- Hemorrhage: The facial skeleton is extremely well vascularized, and any associated bony or soft tissue facial trauma can produce massive hemorrhage. Bony reduction or vessel ligation may be necessary in the acute setting. Massive uncontrollable bleeding from facial fractures is rare, but when occurs is best treated by arterial embolization.
- Large open soft tissue wounds with exposure of vital structures (nerves, vessels, ducts)

As long as the indications for immediate surgical intervention discussed above (eg, airway compromise, hemorrhage, exposure of vital structures) are not present, surgery for panfacial fracture repair can be delayed up to 2 weeks. This allows time for adequate and accurate presurgical evaluation, clinical optimization of hemodynamics, decreased facial swelling, and creation of any dental molds that may be necessary during surgery. Surgical repair is not necessary for nondisplaced fractures. Definitive repair in adults is most easily performed in the first 2 weeks after injury, and sooner in children, before callus formation begins.

Dental models can be fabricated to assist in facial skeleton reduction and cases of malocclusion. From these models, acrylic stents for mandibulomaxillary fixation (MMF) and splints for palatal fractures can be made. For edentulous patients, dentures are useful in creating splints and facilitating MMF.

● TECHNIQUE

Preoperatively, patients should be informed of the likelihood of MMF and its planned duration. The risks and benefits of surgery must be discussed and informed consent provided. The risks of surgery for fixation of panfacial fractures include but are not limited to contour deformity,

CSF leak, temporary or permanent parasthesias, anosmia, malocclusion, infection of implants (both alloplastic and autogenous bone), osteomyeltis, malunion, nonunion, meningitis, tooth root injury, plate/screw exposure, ectropion, eye injury, and the need for additional or revision surgery.

CT images should be available in the operating room for referencing. A complete maxillofacial plating system must also be available. Because most panfacial cases require placement of MMF, nasotracheal intubation is preferential (unless tracheostomy exists).

Patients with soft tissue injury may have traumatic lacerations or defects that allow access to the facial skeleton for fracture repair. Otherwise, access must be gained by strategically placed incisions:

Upper face and zygomatic arch: coronal, brow, Gillies temporal incisions
Midface: periorbital (transconjuctival, lower eyelid, upper eyelid, rim incision, brow), intraoral vestibular
Lower face: buccal, preauricular, retromandibular, submandibular

Sequencing of Surgery

Sequencing the repair is the key to treating panfacial fractures. Traditionally, this has been described via two main approaches: bottom-to-top or top-to-bottom. The basic tenet of fracture fixation from stable to unstable while maintaining the occlusal relationship holds true for either technique. There have been no randomized trials comparing outcomes from different technique and, therefore, surgeon preference predominates and is heavily case dependent. Determination of which sequence to use is predicated on the type of injury and where the largest fracture segments and greatest stability are found. The three top priorities are to establish facial width, facial projection, and occlusion.

The bottom-to-top or inside-to-out technique predates the advent of miniplate and screw rigid internal fixation. In this technique, mandibular reduction and preinjury occlusion are achieved via MMF. The bottom-to-top technique establishes the mandible as the foundation for setting the rest of the face. In the case of combined mandibular and palatal fractures, dental impressions and occlusal splints are helpful in trying to properly align maxillary and mandibular fragments in the correct occlusion. Arch bars are applied to the upper and lower jaws. If the mandible is comminuted and the maxillary arch can be easily reduced, it is helpful to fix the palatal fracture first so a stable maxillary arch can aid in the alignment of the mandibular segments. There are fewer muscle forces acting to displace palatal fractures than mandibular fractures.

Mandibular condyle fractures must be repaired prior to placement of MMF in order to ensure proper facial height. If any other mandibular fracture (eg, body, ramus, angle, symphysis) requires rigid fixation, it is done immediately after placement of MMF and before progressing outward

to other facial regions. If there is significant comminution or loss of the mandible bone then the top-to-bottom technique may provide better accuracy in fracture reduction.

Once the mandible is reduced and plated, fixation of the maxillary arch, ZMC, and zygomaticomaxillary buttress is performed. Frontal sinus fractures are reduced, followed by NOE repair. Care must be taken to ensure that the condyles are properly situated in the glenoid fossa. In addition, it is important that the mandible is not over-rotated upward, otherwise the midface height will be shortened and an anterior open-bite deformity may result upon release of MMF. Overall, the bottom-to-top technique is a mandibulo-centric technique that relies on primary reduction of the mandible and maxilla to align and reduce the remainder of the upper face.[6,7]

The opposite approach, or top-to-bottom or outside-in technique, begins with fixation of the frontal sinus and then the bilateral zygomatic regions. Attention to the lateral orbital wall and zygomatic arch helps to properly align the ZMC. This sets the proper width and projection of the facial frame. Once the outer upper facial frame is reduced and fixated, reduction and fixation of NOE fractures should be performed. The maxilla is addressed next and any LeFort fracture patterns would be addressed now. The zygomaticomaxillary and nasomaxillary buttresses should then be repaired. This provides stable support for fixation of maxillary sinus fractures. Palatal fractures are repaired and the reestablished maxillary arch is secured to the zygomaticomaxillary and nasomaxillary buttresses. The mandible is then placed in MMF with the intact maxillary arch and mandibular fractures are plated. In the top-to-bottom approach, mandibular condyle fractures often do not need to be addressed with open technique. The interval of MMF may vary depending on the type of condylar neck facture and the degree of rotation or medially displacement. Edentulous patient creates less concern about restoring precise occlusion since adjustments can be made in their dentures after healing. However, the lack of dentition necessitates the use of splints if MMF is needed for condylar neck fracture treatment. Otherwise, open reduction internal fixation (ORIF) or external fixation is required to repair the condylar neck to maintain posterior facial height.[8]

Manson et al.[6] described a sequencing technique to panfacial fractures that takes a slightly different approach by conceptualizing the face upper and lower facial groups. The upper facial group is divided into the cranial unit and the midfacial unit. The lower facial group is divided into the occlusal unit and mandibular unit. Each unit is fixed according to facial landmarks taking into account facial width, projection and height. After fixating units, the upper and lower facial groups are anatomically linked at the LeFort I level using the medial and lateral vertical buttresses.[9]

In practice, the route of starting with known and working to unknown is usually taken. For example, if a patient has panfacial fractures with severe comminution of the mandible, it would be advisable to start with the upper face and work down to the mandible. This would allow the grossly disrupted and unstable mandible to be fixated to the more rigid and less destabilized midface. Reducing larger fragments that are easy to align, as well as those that can be stabilized to the skull base, helps facilitate the reduction of smaller fracture segments. Key steps in all approaches are wide exposure to identify fractures, restoration of occlusion, reestablishment of facial height, width and projection, and bone grafting for stability.

After internal rigid fixation, soft tissue suspension should be performed, particularly in panfacial fractures where significant soft tissue degloving of the midface is necessary for fracture exposure. Special attention should be paid to the zygomatic arch and infraorbital rim, as failure to resuspend the soft tissues in these areas leads to malar descent with exposure of the bony prominences and associated hardware. Suture through the malar soft tissues may be suspended to the temporal fascia, drill holes in the bone, or the plates themselves.

Zygomaticomaxillary Complex Fractures

The zygomaticomaxillary complex is important in defining facial width and malar prominence. ZMC fractures are the second most common facial fracture in adults, only after nasal fractures. ZMC fractures involve the inferior and lateral orbital rim, the zygoma, and the maxilla. A complete ZMC fracture involves the following four stability points (Figure 27-4):

1. Zygomaticofrontal suture
2. Zygomaticomaxillary buttress
3. Zygomaticotemporal suture
4. Zygomaticosphenoidal suture

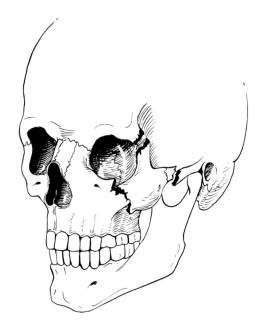

● **FIGURE 27-4.** ZMC complex. *(Reprinted with permission from Stone CK, Humpries RL. Current Diagnosis & Treatment: Emergency Medicine. 6th ed. New York: McGraw-Hill; 2008.)*

The zygomaticomaxillary buttress and zygomaticosphenoid suture where the zygoma attaches to the greater wing of the sphenoid is often considered a single unit, thereby, yielding the name "tripod" fractures. Although, "tetrapod" or "quadripod" may in fact be more accurate nomenclature.[10]

Clinically, these fractures may result in flattening of the zygomatic prominence, infraorbital nerve parasthesias, ocular dystopia, palpable orbital rim step-offs, lateral canthal ptosis, and enopthalmus. Separation at the zygomaticofrontal suture predisposes to downward displacement of the ZMC from unopposed tension exerted by the masseter muscle. If left untreated, unacceptable facial asymmetry may result with permanent enopthalmos and malar flattening.

Displaced ZMC fractures require repair via open reduction and internal fixation. Precise reduction of the zygomaticofrontal suture, zygomaticomaxillary buttress, and zygomatic arch must be performed. Ideally 3 points of fixation, at the zygomaticofrontal suture, the infra-orbital rim and the maxillary buttress, are required to minimize risk of the ZMC rotating during mastication. The inferior orbital rim often requires plating when reconstruction of the orbital floor is necessary.

Numerous surgical approaches to the ZMC exist— coronal, upper or lower eyelid, transconjunctival, brow, and maxillary vestibular incisions are used as needed depending on what other fractures are present. A transverse buccal sulcus incision permits access to the zygomaticomaxillary buttress for plating. L-shaped plates are specifically made for this purpose and should be placed high to prevent injury to the maxillary canine tooth roots. A lower eyelid incision is used for the inferior orbital rim. An upper eyelid or brow incision allows access to the frontozygomatic suture, but is unnecessary if a coronal incision is present.

In the setting of panfacial trauma, segmental fractures through the zygomatic arch are typically exposed through a coronal incision to allow reduction and fixation while avoiding injury to the facial nerve. Isolated arch fractures are uncommon in panfacial trauma; therefore, the Gillies approach using a small temporal incision and a Dingman elevator to reduce the segment is rarely used. A common pitfall in reducing zygomatic arch fractures is aligning the fragments as an arch rather as an anatomically correct flat surface. In the setting of panfacial fractures, this leads to decreased facial projection and increased facial width.

Maxillary (LeFort) Fractures

In 1901, Rene LeFort reported his work on cadaver skulls subjected to blunt forces. He described three predominant predictable midface fracture patterns: transmaxillary (type 1), pyramidal (type 2), and craniofacial (type 3). Importantly, all fracture patterns end posteriorly with separation of the pterygoid plates.

A LeFort I is a transverse fracture pattern beginning medially at the rim of the piriform aperture and then extending laterally through the maxillary sinus, traversing above the maxillary tooth roots. It crosses below the ZMC into the pterygomaxillary junction, with interruption of the pterygoid plates. Intranasally, the base of the nasal septum is fractured. Clinically, mobility of the maxilla upon grasping and rocking of the upper teeth is noted (the forehead must be held stationary). This fracture pattern may result from a traumatic force to the maxillary alveolar rim (Figure 27-5A).

MMF is used to align the fracture segment with the mandible. Almost all LeFort I fractures will require open reduction and fixation. Miniplate fixation is the treatment of choice in acute noncontaminated LeFort I cases. Exposure is achieved through a gingival buccal incision made with a needle-tip electrocautery. This incision is made approximately 0.5 to 1.0 cm labial to the sulcus apex, preserving a mucosal cusp to allow for an easy and well-sealed closure

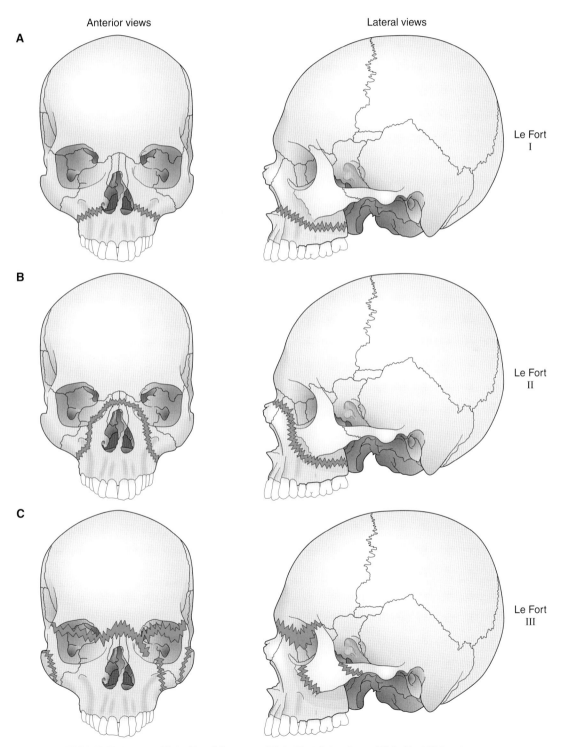

● **FIGURE 27-5.** (A) LeFort I fracture. (B) LeFort II fracture. (C) LeFort III fracture.
(Reprinted with permission from Stone CK, Humpries RL. Current Diagnosis & Treatment: Emergency Medicine. 6th ed. New York: McGraw-Hill; 2008.)

at case completion. The incision is then carried down perpendicular to the alveolar bone. Once the periosteum is opened, a Freer elevator can be used to expose the fracture lines. The length of the incision is surgeon dependent, but may stretch from the first molar all the way to the contralateral side. As the periosteum is elevated, care must be taken not to injure the infraorbital nerve as it exits the infraorbital foramen in the maxilla. The periostial elevator should be used to completely expose the nasomaxillary and zygomaticomaxillary buttresses. The piriform aperture, nasal spine, and premaxilla should also be cleaned so that the entire fracture line can be easily visualized.

Miniplate fixation with low-profile titanium plates secured with monocortical self-tapping screws is the preferred method for ORIF. For adequate stabilization of LeFort I fractures, the medial and lateral buttresses should be plated across the fracture. An L-shaped plate is usually used, with the long limb oriented along the length of the buttress, and the short limb horizontally across the top of the alveolar ridge. When plating, at least two screws should be placed on each side of the fracture. Malleable plating templates can be used to assist in more accurately contouring the titanium plates to lie flush on the bone.

Interosseous wiring is an alternative to miniplates. In this technique, opposing drill holes should be made on each side of the fracture and wire passed through each hole and the twisted tight to bring the fracture edges together. Interosseous wiring is less secure than miniplating and requires longer midface stabilization with MMF.

A LeFort II is a pyramidal shaped fracture pattern that begins superiorly on the nasal bridge, at or below the nasofrontal suture. It then extends laterally through the frontal process of the maxilla and the lacrimal bones. It progresses inferiorly to the inferior orbital rim and/or floor and then across the anterior maxillary sinus. It then extends under the zygoma, across the pterygomaxillary fissure and through the pterygoid plates. With the forehead held steady, the fractured maxilla and nasal complex will move as a unit when grasped and rocked. This fracture pattern may result from a traumatic force to the lower or midmaxilla (Figure 27-5B).

As for all LeFort fractures, fracture disimpaction and MMF is required. Access for ORIF is achieved through ginigival buccal incisions similarly to LeFort I repair as described above. This allows visualization of the LeFort II fracture as it courses across the maxillary sinus, through the zygomaticomaxillary buttress into the pterygomaxillary fissure. Additional incisions are necessary to gain access to the superior portions of the LeFort II. This can be achieved through transconjunctival or subcilliary incisions, allowing access to the orbital rim and floor. If additional access is needed centrally, a transfixation incision to separate the columella from the septum allows further degloving of this region.

Fracture reduction should be performed first prior to any plate fixation. Once adequate reduction has been achieved, the pyramidal shaped LeFort II maxillary segment can be secured laterally to the stable zygomatic portion of the zygomaticomaxillary buttress. Fixation of the inferior orbital rim and/or floor, as well as the frontonasal buttress should then be performed. Monocortical self-tapping screws should be used.

A LeFort III fracture pattern entails a craniofacial dysjunction, with the entire midface separated from the cranial base. The fracture begins medially at the nasofrontal and frontomaxillary suture and extends posteriorlaterally along the medial orbital wall. It traverses the nasolacrimal groove and ethmoid bones until it reaches the lesser wing of the sphenoid in the posterior orbit. The sphenoid bone in the posterior orbit contains thicker bone providing greater protection of the optic nerve as it enters the optic canal. This bony thickness protects the nerve and deflects the fracturing force inferiorly through the inferior orbital fissure and across the orbital floor. It then extends laterally through the lateral orbital wall, through the zygomaticofrontal suture and across the zygomatic arch. Like LeFort II, it then extends under the zygoma, across the pterygomaxillary fissure, and through the pterygoid plates. Intranasally, the fracture extends from the perpendicular plate of the ethmoids, through the vomer and across the base of the sphenoid. A CSF leak can occur. This fracture pattern may result from a traumatic force to the upper maxilla or nasal bridge (Figure 27-5C).

Often times, maxillary fractures occur in more complex patterns than initially described by LeFort. The basis for fracture patterns depends primarily on two factors. First, the anatomy of the midface with its vertical and horizontal buttresses is designed to bolster the midface and orient traumatic forces away from vital intracranial structures. Second, depending on the mechanism of injury and the force generated, maxillary fractures may be unilateral or bilateral. Often, a combination of various LeFort patterns is seen and an associated ZMC fracture is not uncommon.

LeFort III fractures involve a total dissociation of the midface from the cranial skeleton. Stabilization and fixation is necessary to the frontal bone cephalically and mandible caudally. MMF should be achieved after disimpaction of the maxilla. Once satisfactory occlusion is achieved, a bicoronal incision is used to access the upper nasal bones, lateral orbital rim, and zygomatic arch; and lower eyelid or transconjunctival incisions are used to access the orbital floor. Bicoronal flaps are raised via either a linear or zig-zag incision extending from the posterior-superior portion of the auricular helix, over the top of the scalp, to the contralateral side. The flap can be raised centrally either in the subperiosteal or subgaleal plane. The supratrochlear and supraorbital nerves exit the skull just above the superior orbital rim. If dissecting in the subgaleal plane, the pericranium should be incised just above the exit points of these nerves to preserve the blood supply to the flap. However, this eliminates the potential use of the pericranium as a flap in the future. A small osteotomy can be made in the supraorbital foramen to allow the nerve to fall into the orbit, allowing for greater inferior folding of the soft tissue flap.

Laterally, care must be taken not to injure the frontal branch of the facial nerve as it courses superior to the zygomatic arch and lateral brow. The nerve runs on the underside of the superficial temporal fascia (also known as tempoparietal fascia). In order to avoid injury, at approximately 1 to 2 cm above the zygomatic arch, the superficial layer of the deep temporal fascia should be incised, exposing the temporal fat pad. Dissection is then carried down within the fat pad until the superior aspect of the zygomatic arch is reached. Once adequate reduction has been attained, miniplate fixation is performed. In LeFort III fractures, plate fixation is necessary at the bilateral frontozygomatic buttress, nasofrontal buttress, and zygomatic arch. Repair of the orbital floor should then be performed.

Maintenance of fracture immobilization is the most important aspect of postoperative LeFort fracture management. This is primarily achieved in the postoperative period via compliant MMF. The duration of MMF is surgeon and case dependent, but traditionally ranges from 3 to 8 weeks. In general, miniplate fixation allows for earlier MMF removal as compared with interosseous wiring or suspension wiring. During this time, keen oral hygiene with prescribed antiseptic rinses is essential. Chlorohexidiene mouthwash is commonly used. Midface fracture union and callus formation may be tested both clinically and radiographically. Maxillary stability may be tested by grasping the maxillary arch and asking the patient to repeatedly clench and relax their muscles of mastication. Maxillary motion indicates that fracture healing has not yet occurred and arch bar removal at this stage would be detrimental. In the late postoperative period, maxilliary motion is a sign of nonunion or malunion. A CT scan is helpful in confirming the diagnosis.

NOE Fractures

Naso-orbitoethmoid fractures involve concurrent fractures of the nasal, ethmoid, and medial orbital bones. The NOE region is prominent on the facial profile and, therefore, is susceptible to injury. NOE fractures usually occur from a forceful impact at the upper midface, just over the nasal bones and radix. Severe injury to the NOE complex presents one of the greatest challenges in facial fracture management because of the displacing force of the orbicularis oculi muscles and difficulties in restoring proper alignment of the medial canthus. The force required to create NOE fracturing is less than that necessary for frontal or zygomatic fractures. However, as in all panfacial fractures, a thorough history and mental and physical examination is necessary to rule out concomitant injuries. Motor vehicles accidents are the most common mechanism, followed by assault.

NOE fractures can result in significant physical, functional, and cosmetic deformity. Only fractures with no signs of instability on physical examination and no displacement on CT imaging, can avoid repair. Surgical repair in a timely fashion is recommended. Although delay is not life-threatening, scar formation and soft tissue retraction can make later repair more difficult. The primary goal in surgical ORIF is to restore native position of the MCT and the bony segment to which it is attached. Secondary goals

include restoration of preinjury intercanthal distance, symmetric canthal positioning, maintenance of nasal projection, and normal soft tissue contour. Failure to treat can result in long-term severe aesthetic distortion, lower eyelid laxity, and lacrimal gland dysfunction.

ORIF of the NOE complex requires access through multiple incisions. A Lynch incision (direct vertical incision just medial to the MCT) provides direct access to the fracture site; however, the resultant scar is unsightly and easily visible. A bicoronal incision is most often necessary for adequate exposure in conjunction with a periorbital incision (either lower eyelid transconjunctival or lower subciliary incision). The frontonasal suture and superior and medial orbital rims are exposed through the bicoronal incision. In bald or elderly patients, a vertical midline incision in the glabellar region allows direct access via small incision and requires less dissection. The lower eyelid incision allows visualization of the fracture segments along the inferior-medial orbital wall/floor and nasomaxillary junction. Additional exposure may be achieved through medial conjunctival incisions (paracaruncular and transcaruncular approaches). A maxillary gingivobuccal sulcus incision allows access to fractures along the nasomaxillary buttress and piriform aperture. Obviously, any overlying skin lacerations may be used (and extended) for exposure.

Once adequate NOE fracture exposure has been achieved, the medial canthal tendon and its attachment should be delineated. This delineation defines the type of NOE fracture pattern based on the classification discussed above. Usually, the MCT remains fixated to a lacrimal crest bone fragment without being entirely avulsed. However, if avulsed, the tendon leafs should be identified and suture tagged for later canthopexy after bone segment reduction. Overall surgical repair is NOE "type" specific and described below.

A type I fracture is a large single segment NOE fracture. Bone reduction with either digital manipulation or instrumentation should be performed. A penetrating towel clamp or bone reduction clamp can be used to hold the fracture segment in place while fixation is performed. Fracture segments that involve the frontal process of the maxilla or inferior orbital rim, should be miniplated with monocortical screws. Wire fixation with 28-gauge steel wire is an alternative method of fixation.

In rare cases where MCT avulsion from the bony fragment has occurred, refixation to the lacrimal crest is necessary. Two small holes (4 mm apart) should be drilled in the superior-posterior lacrimal crest. A strong permanent suture or 30-gauge steel wire should then be passed through the avulsed canthal tendon and secured to the bone. Of utmost importance is adherence to repair of the MCT to the superior and posterior portion of the lacrimal crest to prevent poor eyelid apposition to the globe and a potential "clothes line" effect.

In type II fractures, there is comminuted fracturing of the NOE complex, but the bony segment to which the MCT is attached remains intact. Surgical exposure is the same as for type I repairs. Meticulous subperiosteal dissection is necessary to delineate the MCT and associated comminuted bony fragments. If entrapment of the medial rectus or superior oblique muscles is encountered, they should be released back into the orbit.

In minimally displaced and minimally comminuted type II fractures, miniplate fixation with monocortical screws can be performed, as done for type I fractures. Fracture segments must be large and rigid enough to support screw placement. In fractures with severe bony displacement or severe comminution with very small bone fragments, transnasal wiring is additionally necessary for fixation. In these cases, an additional exposure of the contralateral medial orbital wall is necessary.

Transnasal wiring is performed using 28- or 30-gauge steel wire. For unilateral fractures, two small holes should be drilled on the ipsilateral canthal-bearing bone segment. Drill holes should be made superior and posterior to the native canthal tendon insertion. Using a large curved needle, the wire is passed through the drill holes, then through the nasal septum, and out through similar drill holes in the contralateral lacrimal crest. The wire or suture may be secured around a monocortical screw inserted on the superior medial orbital rim or to itself. If the NOE fractures are bilateral, central bone fragments are best stabilized to each other with transnasal wiring. The nasal bones may be removed and subsequently replaced, for better visualization during transnasal wiring. During transnasal wiring of bilateral segments, the wire should be placed so that the twist is located intranasally. Once the intercanthal distance of the NOE complex has been reestablished, the NOE complex should be secured to the superior orbital rim and frontonasal suture with either miniplate or wire fixation.

In type III fractures, comminuted fracturing of the NOE complex with disruption of the MCT attachment occurs. The MCT may not be avulsed, but regardless, the bony fragment to which it is attached is too small for fixation. These are the most severe type of NOE fractures and, therefore, have a higher incidence of intraorbital, dural and skull base injury.

Transnasal wiring to reposition the lacrimal crest should be performed as described for type II fractures above. The canthus should be reattached to the bone segment using additional transnasal wires or to the existing wire using suture. As with type II fractures, any additional bone segment fractures can be secured with monocortical screw miniplate fixation. After restoration of the intercanthal distance, the NOE complex should be secured to the superior orbital rim and frontonasal suture with miniplate or wire fixation. In severe comminution with loss of lacrimal bone, monocortical calvarial bone grafts may be used to restore bony contour and provide a site for attachment of the medial canthal tendon. Bone grafting to the nasal dorsum and medial orbital wall and floor may also be needed.

Immobilization of the NOE complex with a nasal splint is recommended. Wired cross-nasal compression splints help the soft tissues to adhere to the underlying bone. Postoperative antibiotics are recommended given the continuity with the sinus cavities. In the immediate postoperative period, the head of the bed should stay elevated greater than 30 degrees. Serial eye examinations should be performed every hour for the first 24 hours, and observation for any increase in intraorbital pressures (ie, from hematoma) is essential.

Postoperative Management

Intraoperative antibiotics, ideally 1 hour prior to skin incision, are almost always used in the operative treatment of panfacial fractures. The question as to whether postoperative antibiotics are necessary is still debated. In general, if the fracture sites were initially exposed to the external environment through open soft tissue wounds or are in continuity with any of the sinuses, nasal cavity, tooth roots, or mouth, broad-spectrum antibiotics are recommended for 7 to 10 days. Postoperatively, patients should be monitored for changes in vision, bleeding, airway problems, CSF leak, fever, and vomiting. If MMF with wires is used, wire cutters should be with the patient at all times, in both the inpatient and outpatient settings. Patients should be instructed on how and when to remove wires if vomiting or airway compromise occurs.

● COMPLICATIONS

Skin and Soft Tissue

Facial incision healing is no different in the treatment of panfacial trauma than in any other type of facial surgery. Skin edges should be handled with great delicacy. A double-layered closure is always preferable to take tension off the skin closure. Soft tissue complications may result from damage during the initial trauma, improper suturing technique, and/or intraoperative trauma from stretching or devascularization.

Dehiscence of intraoral incisions may occur as a result of poor oral hygiene, excessive motion, or poor technical closure. As previously mentioned, correct design of the buccal incision is the key to a good closure. It is important to keep a cuff of mucosa for purposes of suturing on the gingival side of the gingivobuccal incision. Good oral hygiene facilitates wound healing.

Infection

The facial skeleton and soft tissue is relatively well vascularized compared with other areas of the body. However, infections after panfacial fractures still occur. Patients with extensive soft tissue trauma, open fractures, and contaminated wounds are at higher risk. Fractures and fixation hardware continuous with the nasal passage, the sinuses, or the oral cavity can become infected if not empirically treated with antibiotics. If empiric antibiotics are inadequate for preventing or treating infection, incision and drainage may be necessary.

Long-standing or untreated infections may result in osteomyelitis of the facial skeleton. Plates and screws used for bony fixation may be a cause of the infection. Treatment usually involves 4 to 6 weeks of IV antibiotics. If antibiotic treatment is inadequate, bony debridement may be necessary. Internal fixation of involved bone often becomes loose, requiring removal of the infected hardware. Premature removal and/or infection may result in malunion or nonunion. Sinusitis can occur if fracture patterns or surgical hardware block drainage through sinus ostia. In cases unresponsive to decongestants and antibiotics, surgical drainage may be necessary.

Facial Asymmetry and Bony Malposition

Postoperative facial asymmetry may occur in up to 40% of panfacial trauma patients. Any early error in operative reduction may result in a series of compounding errors, often resulting in increased facial width, decreased posterior facial height, or decreased anterior-posterior projection. Telecanthus is common after NOE fracture. For this reason, the surgeon must work carefully, using stable segments and known landmarks to get excellent reduction. Correction of major asymmetry may require surgical intervention with osteotomies and bone grafting.

Neurologic Deficits (Motor and Sensory)

A well-documented preoperative facial neuromotor and neurosensory examination is important, as nerve deficits may be a result of the inciting trauma or operative procedure. In patients with extensive midface and maxillary trauma, neuropraxia or permanent infraorbital nerve damage is common. The infraorbital nerve courses through the inferior orbital fissure and exits the facial skeleton through the infraorbital foramen, just below the orbital rim. As this foramen creates a structural weakness in the maxilla, fractures often occur through this site. The result is ipsilateral anesthesia of the medial cheek, maxillary teeth, and upper lip. Damage to the nerve may occur from the initial trauma or intraoperatively during exposure and fixation of the maxillary sinus or orbital rim. Often, extensive retraction through a gingival buccal incision or periorbital incision can result in a prolonged postoperative neuropraxia.

The supraorbital nerve may be injured in trauma to the forehead region, supraorbital rim, frontal sinus, and in NOE fractures. Intraoperatively, the supraorbital nerve may be injured during bicoronal approaches to the superior or medial orbital rim. This can occur from accidental nerve laceration or from excessive retraction of the forehead flap.

The frontal branch of the facial nerve may be injured during the dissection of bicoronal flaps or from retraction through a lateral brow incision. Injury to the facial nerve may also occur from traction during exposure of the mandibular condyle from a Risdon (submandibular) approach.

Bleeding

The internal maxillary artery provides most of the vascular supply of the midface. Extensive anastomosis of the branches of the external carotid systems occur in the facial skeleton. Facial fracturing may result in profuse bleeding requiring embolization or ligation of the internal maxillary artery. This is also a common site of bleeding during LeFort fracture treatment, as the vessel is in proximity to the posterior fracture line at the pterygomaxillary junction.

Ophthalmologic

Panfacial fracturing and fracture repair involving the orbit may result in injury to the lacrimal duct, optic nerve, globe, cornea, and extraocular muscles. Extraocular muscle entrapment may occur between bone segments or between internal plating systems and bone.

Lower eyelid ectropion is a common complication of periorbital incisions for maxillary fracture exposure. It is believed that a transconjunctival incision decreases the risk of ectropion as compared with subcilliary or lower eyelid incisions. Care should be taken not to aggressively stretch the lower eyelid during retraction. The risk of lower eyelid ectropion may be decreased by not elevating the pretarsal portion of the orbicularis oculi muscle and meticulous dissection and hemostasis of the orbital septum to minimize scar formation. Panfacial fracture patients with lower eyelid laxity or negative vector morphology may benefit from canthopexy after fracture fixation. Adequate malar suspension after facial degloving will minimize downward pull on the eyelid. A Frost suture is left until major swelling subsides to mechanically elevate the lower eyelid and help keep the lamellae of the eyelid properly aligned and to prevent them from adhering to the orbital rim.

Traumatic or iatrogenic blindness is one of the most serious complications associated with facial trauma. Swelling, malpositioned bone grafts and bleeding are potential causes of postoperative vision loss. Scheduled postoperative visual acuity checks by nursing and physician staff are essential. Approximately 30% of postoperative patients may experience transient mild visual acuity changes. Any significant postoperative loss of visual acuity is an indication for immediate orbital re-exploration and decompression.

Malunion/Nonunion

Malunion or nonunion may occur secondary to infection, unstable fixation, or patient noncompliance with MMF. Persistent telecanthus is the most common postoperative complication after NOE fracture repair. It can be the result of either delayed or inadequate repair. Separation or detachment of the transnasal wiring can also occur, reversing the results from initial repair. In all cases, surgical re-exploration and revision is recommended. Lower eyelid laxity, ectropion, and scleral show may occur from incorrect positioning of the transnasal wire.

Lacrimal System Injury

Routine exploration of the lacrimal system in NOE fractures is not indicated because the incidence of injury is low and often asymptomatic. Symptomatic obstruction to the lacrimal system is usually treated secondarily with dacrocystorhinostomy. Occasionally, lacrimal system injury may occur during transnasal wire fixation. Wires positioned too low on the lacrimal crest may cause impingement of the lacrimal sac, resulting in obstruction or epiphora. Prophylactic intraoperative lacrimal duct stenting can be performed to diminish the risk of iatrogenic injury. Obstruction of the nasofrontal duct can also occur. Patients will complain of progressive frontal pressure. Treatment involves duct recannulation or obliteration of the frontal sinus in severe cases.

Dental Injury

Iatrogenic injury to tooth roots may occur from improper placement of arch bars or screws. When fixating maxillary or mandible fractures, use monocortical screws if in proximity to tooth roots and avoid plating directly over them.

Malocclusion is not uncommon and may require dental manipulation and occasionally reoperation.

● OUTCOMES

Given the inherent nature of traumatic facial injuries, prospective studies assessing outcome measures are lacking. Repair of simple panfacial fractures usually results in satisfactory restoration of facial appearance, bony contour, and function. Severe panfacial fractures, despite appropriate operative repair, often have persistent sequelae.

Since the 1980s, miniplate fixation has gained popularity over interosseous wiring. Despite its intended permanence, indications for hardware removal do exist. Palpability of the plates and screws remains the most common indication for removal (35%), followed by loosening of the fixation devices (25%), infection and pain. Cold sensitivity is a rare indication for hardware removal.[11]

REFERENCES

1. Erdmann D, Follmar KE, Debruijn M, et al. A retrospective analysis of facial fracture etiologies. *Ann Plast Surg.* 2008;60(4):398–403.

2. Thaller SR, McDonald WS. *Facial Trauma.* New York: Marcel Dekker; 2004.

3. Sargent LA. Nasoethmoid orbital fractures: diagnosis and treatment. *Plast Reconstr Surg.* 2007;120(7 Suppl 2): 16S–31S.

4. DeMarino DP, Steiner E, Poster RB, et al. Three-dimensional computed tomography in maxillofacial trauma. *Arch Otolaryngol Head Neck Surg.* 1986;112(2):146–150.

5. Babu I, Sagtani A, Jain N, Bawa SN. Submental tracheal intubation in a case of panfacial trauma. *Kathmandu Univ Med J (KUMJ).* 2008;6(1):102–104.

6. Kelly KJ, Manson PN, Vander Kolk CA, et al. Sequencing LeFort fracture treatment (organization of treatment for a panfacial fracture). *J Craniofac Surg.* 1990;1(4):168–178.

7. Markowitz B. Rigid fixation of panfacial injuries. In: Yaremchuk M, Gruss J, Manson P, eds. *Rigid Fixation of the Craniomaxillofacial Skeleton.* Stoneham, MA: Butterworth-Heinemann; 1992.

8. Gruss J, Phillips J. Rigid fixation of lefort maxillary fractures. In: Yaremchuk M, Gruss J, Manson P, eds. *Rigid Fixation of the Craniomaxillofacial Skeleton.* Stoneham, MA: Butterworth-Heinemann; 1992.

9. Moe K. Facial trauma, management of panfacial fractures. September 2009. http://emedicine.medscape.com/article/1283471-overview.

10. Evans BG, Evans GR. MOC-PSSM CME article: Zygomatic fractures. *Plast Reconstr Surg.* 2008;121(1 Suppl):1–11.

11. Orringer JS, Barcelona V, Buchman SR. Reasons for removal of rigid internal fixation devices in craniofacial surgery. *J Craniofac Surg.* 1998;9(1):40–44.

chapter **28**

Pediatric Facial Fractures

Sanjay Naran, MD / Ahmed M. Afifi, MD / Joseph E. Losee, MD, FACS, FAAP

● INTRODUCTION

Pediatric facial fractures are recognized as separate entities from those occurring in the adult. They differ significantly in their epidemiology, diagnosis, and treatment. The aim of this chapter is to highlight differences and review the principles of management of pediatric facial fractures. The pediatric population is defined by the American Academy of Pediatrics as those younger than 21 years of age; however, most of the discussion in this chapter will focus on those before puberty, as it is in this age group that the major differences are most apparent. At or after puberty, the frequency, distribution, and treatment strategy approaches those of the adult population.

Anatomic Differences and Special Fracture Patterns

The higher cranial to facial proportion in children reduces the risk that a frontal impact will cause a facial fracture, but increases the risk of skull fractures and intracranial injuries. At birth, the cranial to facial proportion is 8:1, gradually becoming 4:1 at the age of 5 years and 2:1 at adulthood. This unfolding of the face from underneath the skull increases the risk of facial fractures with age. Consequently, younger children whose trauma is of a magnitude to cause a facial fracture will usually have significant concomitant neurological injuries[1] (Table 28-1). With age, the fracture frequency shifts from the upper face (with frontal and orbital fractures more common in the first 5 years of life), to the lower face (with mandible fractures having a higher incidence after 6 years and into adulthood). Facial bones in children have a higher cancellous to cortical bone ratio and higher cartilage content. This imparts more elasticity to the pediatric facial skeleton, decreasing the probability of fractures. When

fractures do occur they are rarely comminuted and more commonly greenstick and minimally displaced. In addition, patent suture lines commonly separate, leading to unusual fractures not seen in adults.

Developing teeth and sinuses affect the way fractures form and are treated. At birth, sinuses have not yet developed and exist only as a bud of mucosa surrounded by cancellous bone. Therefore, the facial skeleton in the child is composed of solid blocks of bone, in contrast to that of the adult skeleton whose sinuses are surrounded by buttresses that dissipate injury leading to more common fracture patterns. This solid architecture makes the pediatric facial skeleton more resistant to trauma and more liable to unusual fracture patterns. In general, bone-bearing mixed dentition is more resistant to fracture. The shape and position of deciduous and mixed dentition has a major impact on several aspects of fracture reduction and fixation in the mandible and the midface. Most importantly, mixed dentition in the mandible can occupy almost the entire vertical length of the mandible, placing the teeth and the inferior alveolar nerve at risk during screw placement.

Physiological

The speed of bone healing and the remodeling capacity of pediatric facial bones can be incredibly fast. The surgeon should appreciate this healing potential and reduce these fractures as early as possible, utilizing shorter immobilization periods after reduction. After 3 to 5 days, fractures begin to heal, making fracture identification, disimpaction, and reduction harder. On the other hand, the surgeon can accept minor misalignment of the often greenstick fractured segments, knowing that the remarkable remodeling capacity of the pediatric skeleton will compensate for such discrepancy.

TABLE 28-1. Pediatric Facial Trauma at Children's Hospital of Pittsburgh of the University of Pittsburgh Medical Center: Demographic of Age, Fracture Type, Cause of Injury and Associated Injuries

Age Group (n)	Fracture Type (%)	Causes of Injury (%)	Associated Injuries (%)	Required Surgery n (%)	Admitted to ICU n (%)
0–5 y (156)	Orbit (57.3) Skull (41.0) Mandible (22.9) Nasal (20.3) Maxillary (14.0) Dentoalveolar (7.6) Zygomatic (1.9) NOE (0.6)	ADL (38.5) Play (23.7) MVC (21.8) Sports (0.63)	Soft Tissue (96.6) Neurologic (61.4) Musculoskeletal (10.1) Ophthalmological (8.2)	43 (27.6)	44 (28.2)
6–11 y (272)	Orbit (51.0) Nasal (29.6) Skull (27.90) Mandible (27.5) Maxillary (16.8) Dentoalveolar (8.2) Zygomatic (3.7) NOE (1.65)	MVC (31.6) Play (20.5) Sports (13.9) ADL (7.4) Assault (1.2)	Soft Tissue (95.2) Neurologic (54.8) Ophthalmological (17.5) Musculoskeletal (15.3)	91 (36.1)	52 (20.6)
12–18 y (373)	Orbit (45.6) Nasal (39.9) Maxillary (22.8) Mandible (21.2) Skull (15.20) Zygomatic (7.6) Dentoalveolar (6.7) NOE (1.9)	Assault (26) MVC (24.7) Sports (22.2) Play (10.3) ADL (4.9)	Soft Tissue (94.4) Neurologic (43.9) Ophthalmological (22.2) Musculoskeletal (10.3)	143 (38.3)	47 (12.6)

ADL, activities of daily life; MVC, motor vehicle collision; NOE, naso-orbitoethmoid.

From Grunwaldt L, Madia JV, DeCesare GE, et al. Pediatric craniofacial fracture demographics: a five year institutional review of 1508 consecutive patients. Plastic Surgery Research Council, 54th Annual Meeting. Pittsburgh, PA: 2009.

Psychological

The child and the parents' fear and anxiety are unique, leading to an uncooperative apprehensive child and parents with clouded judgment. Handling both the child and his family in the emergency room necessitates wise assessment of the situation, and should be considerate. These children are at risk to develop post-traumatic stress disorder, and every effort should be made to help them overcome the possible functional, aesthetic, and psychological consequences of the fracture.

The Fourth Dimension

Perhaps the most important difference that the surgeon should consider when managing these fractures is that a primary aim of surgery is to not only achieve a three-dimensional fracture reduction, but to allow for normal unimpeded growth of the skeleton, the so-called "fourth dimension." Knowledge of the growth periods of regions within the pediatric facial skeleton is therefore essential (Table 28-2). Our understanding of the effect of

fractures and their management on craniofacial growth is limited because of the paucity of data, following through to adulthood, regarding the growth and development of facial fractures treated in childhood. Data that do exist

TABLE 28-2. Table of Facial Growth

	Onset (y)	Maximum Growth (y)	Growth Complete (y)
Cranium	0	1–2	10
Nose	5	10–14	16
Orbit	0	1–2	7
Frontal Sinus	5	8–16	20
Maxillary Sinus	5	10–12	14
Maxilla	5	8–12	16
Mandible	1–4	8–12	20

From Mathes SJ, Hentz VR. Plastic Surgery. Philadelphia: Saunders; 2006.

focus on pediatric mandible fractures and suggest that these do not result in a higher incidence of orthodontic intervention, and that there do not appear to be any growth disturbances associated with indicated conservative or surgical treatment.[2]

Theoretic growth disruption can occur due to the fracture itself, its operative exposure, or the rigid fixation. Furthermore, scarring within the soft tissues may impede bone growth. When a fracture does require open exposure, soft tissue undermining should be kept to a minimum. Fixation of bone can have deleterious effects secondary to mechanical restriction of growth across the plate and by relieving the bone from the usual stresses stimulating its growth.

PATIENT SELECTION

In general, children are less prone to facial fractures (1%–15% of all facial fractures affect children[3]), due to their protected environment, the decreased facial to cranial proportion, the flexibility of their facial bones and the considerable fat pads around their mandible. Motor vehicle accidents, including all-terrain vehicles, account for the vast majority of these fractures, followed by falls form a height and sporting accidents[1,4] (Table 28-1). Child abuse is a less common cause but one that should be bore in mind.

The resiliency of the pediatric facial skeleton implies that those who do sustain fractures will have been subjected to trauma of such a high force that they are likely to have significant associated injuries (Table 28-1). The injured child with multiple or severe trauma poses a significant challenge to the resuscitating physician. In the presence of extensive craniofacial injury, provision of a safe airway should be the first priority. Children have a relatively larger tongue and tonsils, and a smaller trachea and pharynx that are easily obstructed. In addition, infants younger than 6 months are obligate nasal breathers. Pulling the tongue or mandible forward, removing foreign bodies, and suctioning the upper airway should be done promptly. It is rare to have a grossly mobile maxilla, and this should not be initially considered the cause of any airway compromise. A tracheostomy or endotracheal intubation can provide a definitive airway.

Resuscitation is usually started with a warmed crystalloid at a rate of 20 mL/kg, assessing response by hemodynamic parameters, level of consciousness, and urine output. Once the airway and hemodynamic stability are secured, the secondary survey begins to identify and treat different injuries. In the child with facial trauma, three injuries are particularly common and should be vigilantly looked for: intracranial, ophthalmologic, and cervical-spine injuries.

The examination of the craniofacial skeleton should proceed in an orderly fashion assessing pain, tenderness, swelling, asymmetry, step-offs, crepitus, paresthesia, and facial nerve function. Ophthalmologic and neurosurgical consultations should be obtained if necessary. An intraoral examination is part of the facial examination, and should include a search for mucosal wounds and missing or loose dentition. Assessment of the occlusion is of paramount importance in fractures involving tooth-bearing bones. Orthodontic records, dental models, and photographs are useful in determining pretraumatic occlusion.

PATIENT PREPARATION

Conventional x-ray imaging is largely nondiagnostic in the pediatric population, as fracture lines are difficult to localize in an immature skeleton with high cancellous bone content. CT scans are considered the first-line radiographic modality in diagnosing pediatric facial fractures. Coronal and axial thin-cut sections will accurately define the presence and features of most fractures and will aid in treatment planning. A 3D reconstruction is a helpful modality that is handy to have as a quick reference during surgery. The only conventional x-ray image still recommended is an orthopantomogram (panorex), which provides a panoramic view of the mandible that can diagnose mandible fractures with a reasonable accuracy. It is also commonly used postoperatively to assess reduction, the dentition, and for long-term follow-up of mandible growth.

As stated above, assessment of the occlusion is of paramount importance in fractures involving tooth-bearing bones. In the presence of a traumatic malocclusion, dental models are useful in determining pre-traumatic occlusion. These are fabrication from an alginate impression of the patient's maxillary and mandibular dental surfaces. From these negative models, plaster casts of each dental surface can be created. The two individual models can then be manipulated or cut at suspected fracture lines and re-glued together to obtain a preinjury ideal occlusion. From these altered models, acrylic splints can be made to be used either alone or in conjunction with surgical intervention.

Patients with orbital fractures need proper ophthalmologic evaluations, as these fractures are frequently associated with ocular injuries. Injury to the globe must be identified to prevent vision loss.

TECHNIQUE

Principles of Management and Repair

An infant with a minimal fracture does not require operative intervention, while an older child with a grossly displaced comminuted fracture is best served with open reduction internal fixation (ORIF). Unfortunately, most patients fall in the large watershed area in between, where the experience and preference of the surgeon will oftentimes determine the course of management. Until further evidence is available to provide accurate guidelines as to the degree of reduction accepted, it rests upon the surgeon to decide for each case individually whether closed or open reduction is warranted, and in doing so consider the degree of displacement, the feasibility of open reduction, and the age of the patient.[5]

Conservative (Nonsurgical) Management

Closed reduction or simple observation is often employed in children due to the high frequency of minimally displaced and greenstick fractures. Factors favoring this approach are the younger age of the patient, absence of malocclusion or other functional deficits, and good alignment of the fracture segments. In all cases, the patient must be followed on a yearly basis to monitor skeletal and soft tissue growth.

Surgical Management

The trend in adults to treat most facial fractures with ORIF does not translate to children. ORIF provides perfect reduction of the fracture and often avoids the need for mandibulomaxillary fixation (MMF), which can be a difficult procedure in children with developing teeth; however, this is at the risk of potential growth retardation. Clear indications for surgery are failure of closed reduction and a significantly displaced or comminuted fracture. All cases of internal fixation should be performed with minimal but adequate exposure of the fracture, avoiding unnecessary soft tissue undermining and dissection.

Fixation Hardware

A better understanding of the biological and mechanical properties of hardware has facilitated many innovations and refinements in their material and design. The surgeon should be able to choose the proper shape, size, and type of hardware, which may be easily applied with the least soft tissue dissection, while providing sufficient load sharing. Debate regarding the use of permanent hardware versus absorbable plates continues.[6] Absorbable plates subjugate the need for a second surgery; however, they likely do not provide the same degree of rigid fixation that can be provided by metallic plates. Some argue that metallic hardware should be removed after 3 to 6 months in order to avoid growth disturbances or translocation of the plates (cranial plates have been found to translocate from the external surface of bone to its endocranial or internal surface).

Mandibulomaxillary Fixation

MMF provides accurate reduction and stabilization while avoiding the growth insult of open reduction. However, this technique remains challenging in the pediatric population, particularly those in primary and mixed dentition. The surgeon must be facile in the various different methods of MMF. Arch bars, the most common method in adults, may not suit children due to the conical shape of their deciduous dentition, partially erupted secondary dentition, and carious teeth, all of which do not provide a strong foundation for MMF. In addition, injury to permanent teeth or

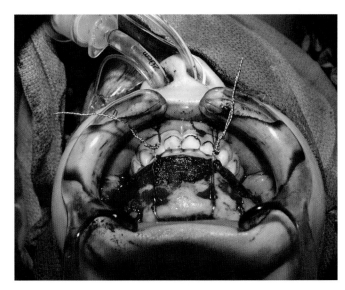

● **FIGURE 28-1.** Alternative forms of MMF: skeletal wires through the piriform aperture and mandible.

their periodontal ligament may result from the circumdental wiring. If used, wires should be placed below the gum line, and should encircle stable or multiple teeth. Similarly, interdental wires provide a minimally invasive method of fracture stabilization; however, one must choose the correct teeth for fixation of the wires.

Challenges associated with circumdental wiring have lead surgeons to use wires that either wrap around the mandible (circum-mandibular) and/or wires that drop down from more stable bones such as the piriform aperture (Figure 28-1). These wires are then connected to each other by another wire to achieve and maintain proper arch relationship. Alternatively, these wire fixation techniques can be used to help maintain the position of arch bars.

As described above, acrylic splints provide another modality to assist in obtaining and maintaining arch relationship, but requires time, special equipment, and expertise to utilize. These splints are fabricated after accurate reduction of the fracture (closed reduction or interdental wiring), should include both lingual and buccal surfaces of the dentition, and should taper posteriorly so as not to create an open bite. They are fixed to the mandible by circum-mandiblar wires. Acrylic splints have significant advantages, namely that they are applicable to all ages (including infants where other forms of MMF are fraught with difficulties or complications), and do not stress the teeth but rather fix them in place. They may also be used in the setting of the edentulous neonate or infant.

Bone Substitutes

While the use of bone grafts in the immature craniofacial skeleton is controversial, due to their unpredictable long-term results and their unknown effect on growth, they remain preferable to alloplastic materials. Common donor sites for bone grafts are the iliac crest, ribs, and the skull. When harvesting an iliac crest bone graft, the surgeon should avoid injury to the superior cartilaginous lip of the iliac crest, which is the growth center. The skull is an excellent source for bone grafts in older ages, and CT scans can be used to detect the presence of a diploic space, which denotes the feasibility of harvesting calvarial bone grafts.

Mandible Fractures

Mandible fractures are one of the more common pediatric facial fractures, representing 20% to 50% of all pediatric facial fractures,[1,3] and are more likely to require some form of surgical reduction or fixation. The goal is to gain adequate reduction with proper occlusal relationship while maintaining the growth potential of the mandible, and avoiding interference with the eruption and development of dentition. The distribution of fractures within the mandible differs from that of the adult (Table 28-3), with the incidence of condylar fractures being higher.[2]

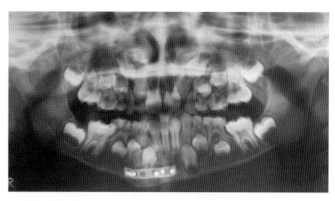

● **FIGURE 28-2.** Pediatric dentition and hardware placement: panorex of a pediatric mandible showing metallic hardware and asymmetry of the mandible.

Many pediatric fractures are either minimally displaced or greenstick fractures, and may be adequately treated conservatively (cervical-spine collar, soft diet, pain control, avoidance of intense physical activity, and observation). The risk of growth retardation imposed by open reduction is justified when occlusion cannot be achieved or maintained by closed reduction or MMF, when the fracture is grossly comminuted or displaced, and in cases of multiple fractures and certain condylar fractures.

As with all pediatric fractures, open reduction with internal fixation of the mandible follows the same principles, including minimal exposure and limited soft tissue dissection and undermining. Awareness of the position of teeth in relation to the age of the patient, especially during drilling and plating the mandible, will further help the surgeon avoid many of the most commonly dreaded complications. To avoid disruption of unerupted dentition, it is recommended to place the plates on the inferior border of the mandible and fix them using monocortical screws[6] (Figure 28-2).

Condylar Fractures

Condylar fractures remain one of the most controversial and difficult to treat types of mandible fractures. There are three main reasons why condylar fractures pose such a challenge; the first is the effect of these fractures on long-term mandibular growth. The condyle is purported to be the primary growth center of the mandible in the postnatal life.[6] Injury to the condyle may lead to growth retardation, and unfortunately no treatment modality has been shown to prevent this. The second reason is the concern for TMJ ankylosis following these fractures. The third reason is the difficult approach used for exposure of the condyle, which puts the facial nerve at risk of injury. MMF has been the most commonly used method for treating these fractures, on the assumption that achieving correct occlusion will reduce the fracture and allow for healing in an acceptable position. However, this remains debatable as MMF only repositions the distal segment and has no effect on the proximal segment.

TABLE 28-3. Mandibular Fractures at Children's Hospital of Pittsburgh of the University of Pittsburgh Medical Center: Demographic of Age and Fracture Location

Age Group (%)	Fracture Location (%)
0–5 y (25.14)	Condylar head (27.27)
	Parasymphysis (20.45)
	Condylar neck (18.18)
	Angle (11.36)
	Body (11.36)
	Ramus (6.82)
	Symphysis (4.55)
	Coronoid (0)
6–11 y (40.57)	Condylar neck (28.17)
	Condylar head (26.76)
	Parasymphysis (16.90)
	Symphysis (8.45)
	Angle (8.45)
	Ramus (5.63)
	Body (5.63)
	Coronoid (0)
12–18 y (34.29)	Condylar neck (31.67)
	Parasymphysis (28.33)
	Angle (16.67)
	Condylar head (6.67)
	Ramus (6.67)
	Body (5.00)
	Symphysis (5.00)
	Coronoid (0)

From Smith DM, Bykowski MR, DeCesare GE, et al. 179 mandible fractures in 96 children: demographics, early outcomes, and a prospective analysis of growth and development. International Society of Craniofacial Surgeons XII Biennial International Congress. Oxford, UK; 2009.

The three main factors influencing the decision to treat conservatively versus surgically are the location of the fracture, the degree of displacement or angulation, and the relation of the condylar head to the glenoid fossa. Condylar fractures are divided according to location into three subsets, fractures of the intra-articular head, fractures of the neck (above the level of the sigmoid notch but outside the capsule), and subcondylar fractures. In general, fractures with normal occlusion, no open bites, and good range of motion are treated with a soft diet and physiotherapy. If the above conditions are not met, high condylar fractures are treated with MMF and low fractures are treated with ORIF. Other indications for ORIF are foreign bodies in the joint, bilateral condylar fractures (in which case at least one should be fixed), and associated midface fractures. In the patient with primary or mixed dentition, almost always, a conservative approach is taken when treating condylar fractures.

Nasal Fractures

Nasal fractures are extremely common, and as a result of its role in growth of the midface, can have dire long-term consequences. Nasal fractures in children present differently than in adults due to their different anatomy.[7] The nasal bones are not united, explaining the possibility of a unilateral nasal bone fracture (a rare occurrence in adults) and the frequency of the open book fracture, a peculiar fracture in children where the nasal bones are splayed open and override the frontal process of the maxilla. The pediatric nasal skeleton also has a higher proportion of cartilage that is highly vascular and grows rapidly. A careful clinical examination, including intranasal examination and palpation for tenderness and mobility, is therefore required. Many surgeons will rely solely on the clinical picture for diagnosis of nasal fractures, with some being more obvious than others (Figure 28-3). Plain x-rays are of limited value in the cartilaginous skeleton of a child. If a naso-orbitoethmoid (NOE) fracture

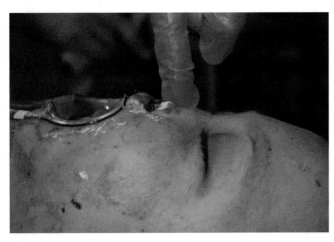

● **FIGURE 28-3.** Nasal Fracture: collapse of the nasal septum.

is suspected, a CT scan should be obtained. Septal hematomas should be suspected and appropriately managed in all nasal injuries, as they may have dire consequences, namely abscess formation, septal perforation, pressure-induced avascular necrosis of the nasal cartilage, saddle nose deformity, infection, fibrous thickening, and nasal obstruction. Septal hematomas usually appear as a bluish red bulge in the anterior part of the septum, can be of variable size and location, and may obstruct nasal breathing. Although usually associated with a fracture of the septum, this is not necessarily true in all cases. Septal hematomas should be drained promptly through an appropriately placed incision in the nasal septum. The incision should provide access to the whole hematoma and should ensure dependent drainage.

While the closed reduction of nasal fractures in adults result in a high percentage of persistent nasal deformities, nasal fractures causing a visible deformity in the pediatric population should be reduced once diagnosed. Although local anesthesia supplemented with IV sedation may be used, children are usually better served by a general anesthetic if feasible. Reduction of the fracture is achieved with the aid of a long straight flat instrument inside the nose (Ash forceps or the back of a scalpel) and digital pressure on the outside. An external and occasionally an internal nasal splint is used for 5 to 7 days.

Naso-Orbitoethmoid Fractures

These involve the nasal bones, the medial orbital wall and the ethmoid bones. They may be associated with fractures of the frontal bone, skull base, infraorbital rim, or blowout orbital fractures. If a NOE fracture is suspected, a CT scan should be obtained (Figure 28-4). Classically, the nasal bones are posteriorly and laterally displaced, and the medial orbital rim bearing the medial canthal ligament is laterally displaced. This results in the classical clinical picture of a depressed nasal dorsum and telecanthus. To judge the presence of telecanthus, one should compare the intercanthal distance with the width of the palpebral fissure (they are normally similar), or use age-specific values of interorbital distance.

The most important determinant for the need to intervene (and for adequacy of treatment) is the position and mobility of the central (canthal bearing) bone fragment.[8] A simple way to test this is by external traction on the medial canthal ligament laterally. This is especially important as telecanthus may not be apparent initially but may develop in the weeks to follow.

NOE fracture reduction can be technically demanding and the degree of displacement and mobility will determine the operative approach, with the most important goal being the restoration of intercanthal distance. In minimally displaced fractures, conservative management is advocated. If operative reduction is planned because of significant displacement, the anatomy of the fracture and the proposed points of fixation will dictate the choice of incisions and follow the same principles as

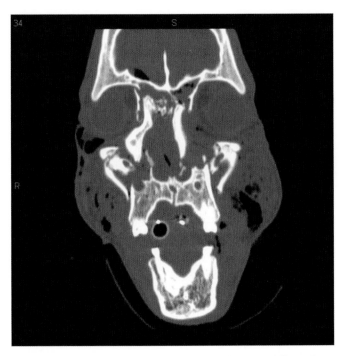

● **FIGURE 28-4.** Naso-orbitoethmoid fracture: bilateral NOE fractures on CT scan.

in the adult. Usually coronal, lower eyelid and gingival buccal sulcus incisions are needed. If the medial canthal ligament is still attached to a bone fragment, that fragment is reduced and fixed. If the ligament has been separated from the bone, transnasal wiring is required. NOE fractures may require bone grafts to fill the gaps in the inferior and the medial orbital walls, as well as to recreate the nasal dorsum and provide stabilization.

Zygomaticomaxillary Complex Fractures

Zygomaticomaxillary complex (ZMC) fractures are not common in children, and when they do occur they are often minimally displaced. They may not follow the standard fracture patterns, and may be associated with other injuries, most notably neurological and ophthalmologic injuries. ZMC fractures lead to a constellation of signs and symptoms, including epistaxis, upper buccal sulcus hematomas, loss of malar eminence, enophthalmos, and an inferiorly displaced lateral canthus.

Minimally displaced ZMC fractures not causing functional (eg, malocclusion or muscle entrapment) or aesthetic (eg, vertical orbital dystopia or cheek retrusion) problems do not require surgical correction. As in the adult, most displaced ZMC fractures will require exposure through a lower eyelid and upper buccal incisions. Despite the age of the patient, standard three-point fixation is commonly used,[7,9] with fixation at the zygomaticofrontal suture, inferior orbital rim, and the zygomaticomaxillary buttress, once the fracture is reduced at the lateral orbital wall (zygomaticsphenoid bone). The orbital floor is explored as part of

the surgery and any fractures or defects are dealt with appropriately.

Orbital Fractures

Patients with orbital fractures need proper ophthalmologic evaluations, as these fractures are frequently associated with ocular injuries. Trapdoor fractures, an entity more commonly seen in children, are fractures that entrap the extraocular muscles as the bone rebounds faster than the soft tissues. Muscle entrapment is diagnosed by limitation of extraocular motion or by a forced duction test. This is a true emergency necessitating immediate surgery to release the trapped muscle and hopefully prevent irreversible muscle necrosis and fibrosis.

Unlike adults, where the size of the orbital wall defect dictates treatment, in children other factors dictate treatment recommendations.[10] Pediatric orbital fractures may be classified into one of three groups (Table 28-4). Pure orbital fractures are the most common pediatric orbital fracture and should be followed conservatively regardless of defect size, unless there is acute evidence of entrapment, enophthalmos, or vertical orbital dystopia (Figure 28-5). Craniofacial fractures involving the orbital roof are common, occurring as oblique fractures in children, and should be treated conservatively with vigilant follow-up, including serial CT scans and detailed physical examinations, with particular attention paid to the potential development of a growing skull fracture. Orbital fractures associated with common fracture patterns (eg, NOE, ZMC) should be treated surgically as part of the concomitant fracture, employing resorbable plating systems when feasible. Operative approach is

TABLE 28-4. Pediatric Orbital Fracture Classification

Type 1	*Pure orbital fractures*
1a	Floor fractures
1b	Medial wall fractures
1c	Roof fractures
1d	Lateral wall fractures
1e	Combined floor and medial wall fractures
Type 2	*Craniofacial fractures*
2a	Growing skull fractures
Type 3	*Orbital fractures associated with common fracture patterns*
3a	Fractures of the floor and inferior orbital rim
3b	Zygomaticomaxillary fractures
3c	Naso-orbitoethmoid fractures
3d	Other fracture patterns

From Losee JE, Afifi A, Jiang S, et al. Pediatric orbital fractures: classification, management, and early follow-up. Plast Reconstr Surg. 2008;122(3):886–897.

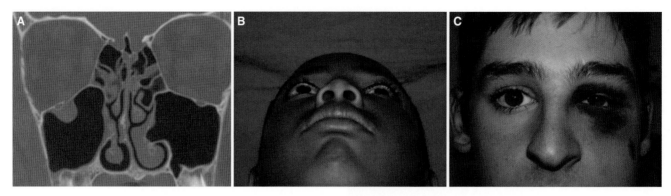

● **FIGURE 28-5.** Orbital fractures: (A) herniation of orbital globe contents on CT through a fracture of the orbital floor. (B) Enophthalmos may be assessed by observing the patient from a worm's eye view. (C) Vertical orbital dystopia may be subtle; a tongue blade may be employed to determine orbital height.

dictated by fracture location and follows the same technique as in the adult.

Frontal Bone Fractures

The frontal sinus begins to pneumatize around the age of 5 years, and is not fully developed until after puberty. Therefore, frontal bone fractures in infants and children are skull base fractures. The large cranium-to-face ratio in young children results in a relatively higher incidence of frontal bone fractures in these patients. In children, fractures are usually linear and extend from the temporal or frontal skull in an atypical oblique fashion to the orbits.

Indications for surgery in frontal bone fractures are significant displacement, intra- or extracranial hematomas, pneumocephalus, brain injury, or persistent CSF leak. The goal of surgery is to "separate the brain from the nose and external environment," manage the brain and dural injury, avoid CSF leak, and correct facial contour. This goal usually necessitates a procedure with neurosurgical colleagues for a combined extra- and intracranial approach. Several factors will affect the decision on how to deal with the fracture, including the exact location and extent of the fracture, integrity of the nasofrontal duct, and associated intracranial and facial bone injuries.[5] A "safe sinus" can be achieved by repairing the fracture if the duct is intact. If the surgeon doubts the integrity of the duct or the possibility of achieving a "safe sinus," one should opt for cranialization or obliteration of the sinus. In all cases, these patients should be carefully followed as they may develop a mucocele years later with drastic sequelae.

● COMPLICATIONS

Complications may occur early in the postinjury period or later whether or not surgical intervention has been preformed. Most complications in the immediate postoperative period relate to imperfect reduction or fixation of the fracture. These may manifest as malocclusion, decreased mouth opening, orbital dystopia, or facial asymmetry.

While infection is a rare complication in the highly vascular craniofacial skeleton, it is one that can have serious consequences and will usually result in removal of implanted hardware and grafts. Antibiotics are therefore usually administered empirically. Further studies are needed in order to better assess the need and benefit of empiric antibiotic treatment.

Careful surgical technique will reduce the occurrence of damage to the mental nerve and permanent dentition while repairing mandibular fractures. Temporomandibular dysfunction, TMJ ankylosis, and growth disruption are the most common long-term complications of condylar fractures. In the case of unilateral injuries, stress imposed on the injured side by the intact TMJ is thought to be the cause of temporomandibular dysfunction. TMJ ankylosis is often the result of articular disc damage and is seen in the setting of severe comminuted fractures of the condyle. Prolonged MMF may also be a contributing factor, again advocating for a short immobilization period.

With orbital fractures, common complications include ocular injury, enophthalmos, diplopia, and residual telecanthus. Injury to the nasolacrimal apparatus and anosmia may also occur. Complications related to nasal fractures again apply here. Growth disruption and midface retrusion may also develop and will require secondary surgery once growth is complete. Blindness, while rare, is a dreaded complication. Persistent enophthalmos or vertical orbital dystopia may also result from inadequate reduction and treatment, or unpredictable postoperative growth and development. Routine postoperative and follow-up ophthalmologic evaluation of visual acuity and ocular function is essential.

Facial asymmetry secondary to resultant midface hypoplasia may develop from midfacial fractures due to disruption of growth centers. Parents should be counseled in regard to growth disruption and deformity, with management tailored at a time when growth is complete.

Of special importance in frontal, skull, and orbital roof fractures in children is the possibility of developing growing skull fractures.[10] This occurs when an associated dural

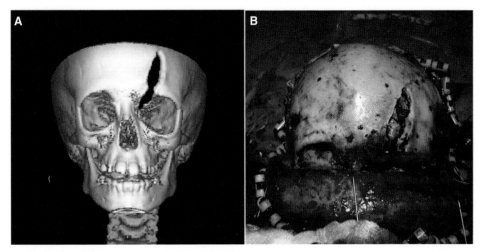

● **FIGURE 28-6.** Growing skull fracture. (A) Three-dimensional CT scan of a growing skull fracture. (B) Intraoperative exposure of the fracture.

injury allows brain pulsations to slowly and persistently separate the fracture, resulting in nonunion and growth of the fracture (Figure 28-6). For this concern, it is suggested that pediatric craniofacial fractures be followed clinically and radiographically. If a growing skull fracture is found, it will often necessitate surgical repair of the dura and reconstruction of the bone.

● OUTCOME

It is the late consequences of pediatric facial fractures that make them unique compared to those of the adult, with disruption of facial growth being the primary concern. Routine follow-up, on a yearly basis, is suggested for pediatric patients, and may include the cooperation of multiple specialties, including a neurosurgeon, ophthalmologist, orthodontist, and a psychiatrist in addition to the plastic surgeon. Serial radiographic studies are useful and cephalometric analysis may be employed to objectively evaluate facial growth.

Follow-up for mandible fractures should be in conjunction with the orthodontist. Occlusion should be checked routinely to ensure that the reduction is stable. Nutrition and oral hygiene should not be overlooked. The maximal incisor opening should also be measured routinely. Growth and development may be followed using panorex radiographs and cephalometric analysis.

Nasal fractures require long-term follow-up in order to assess for late complications such as airway obstruction, saddle nose deformity, maxillary hypoplasia, and other growth disruption. These late complications should preferably be approached in the late teens, when nasal growth is complete and the patient is mature enough to comprehend and elect to undergo surgery.

REFERENCES

1. Grunwaldt L, Madia JV, DeCesare GE, et al. Pediatric craniofacial fracture demographics: a five year institutional review of 1508 consecutive patients. Plastic Surgery Research Council, 54th Annual Meeting. Pittsburgh, PA; 2009.

2. Smith DM, Bykowski MR, DeCesare GE, et al. *179 Mandible fractures in 96 children: demographics, early outcomes, and a prospective analysis of growth and development.* International Society of Craniofacial Surgeons XII Biennial International Congress. Oxford, UK; 2009.

3. Vyas RM, Dickinson BP, Wasson KL, Roostaeian J, Bradley JP. Pediatric facial fractures: current national incidence, distribution, and health care resource use. *J Craniofac Surg.* 2008; 19(2):339–349.

4. Ferreira PC, Amarante JM, Silva PN, et al. Retrospective study of 1251 maxillofacial fractures in children and adolescents. *Plast Reconstr Surg.* 2005;115(6):1500–1508.

5. Hatef DA, Cole PD, Hollier LH Jr. Contemporary management of pediatric facial trauma. *Curr Opin Otolaryngol Head Neck Surg.* 2009;17(4):308–314.

6. Smartt JM Jr, Low DW, Bartlett SP. The pediatric mandible: II. Management of traumatic injury or fracture. *Plast Reconstr Surg.* 2005;116(2):28e–41e.

7. Dufresne CR, Manson PM. *Pediatric Facial Injuries.* Vol 3. 2nd ed. Philadelphia: Saunders Elsevier; 2006.

8. Sargent LA. Nasoethmoid orbital fractures: diagnosis and treatment. *Plast Reconstr Surg.* 2007;120(7 suppl 2):16S–31S.

9. Kelley P, Hopper R, Gruss J. Evaluation and treatment of zygomatic fractures. *Plast Reconstr Surg.* 2007;120(7 suppl 2): 5S–15S.

10. Losee JE, Afifi A, Jiang S, et al. Pediatric orbital fractures: classification, management, and early follow-up. *Plast Reconstr Surg.* 2008;122(3):886–897.

chapter 29

Reconstruction of the Ear

Christopher J. M. Brooks, MD

● PATIENT EVALUATION

The goal of ear reconstruction is to provide a realistic appearing and functional (eyeglass-supporting) auricle in patients who are missing all or part of an ear due either to a congenital malformation or to a secondary insult. The majority of patients who seek *total* ear reconstruction are those with microtia. Microtia affects 0.76 to 2.35 in 10,000 live births and can be unilateral or bilateral. Hispanics and Asians have a significantly higher incidence of microtia than do Caucasians and blacks. Males and the right ear are also disproportionately affected. There is a wide spectrum of severity ranging from complete anotia to minor deformities. Microtia is typically classified into three types: lobule, concha, and small concha. Microtia may also be a part of a larger syndrome with associated anomalies affecting other organ systems, most commonly facial clefts and cardiac defects. Microtia is frequently associated with craniofacial microsomia and many feel that isolated microtia is actually the most mildly affected variant of this malformation. In children with microtia, one of the bigger determinants in patient selection is the age of the patient. The appropriate age will be determined by which reconstructive technique is selected.

The second subset of patients is those who have suffered trauma, burns, cancer, or infection affecting the auricle. Clearly, reconstruction of an ear should be addressed only when the cancer or infection has been cleared and the major threats to life and limb have been addressed. In traumatic, sharp, complete amputation of the ear, replantation should be attempted when possible. In subtotal amputations and avulsions, this is rarely possible due to lack of suitable vessels. Except in the very young, composite grafting is most often unsuccessful. Reconstruction of partial ear defects is also possible using the techniques outlined below.

When examining the auricular deformity, it is important to note what structures are present, what structures are absent, and what structures are present but deformed. The microtic ear is also usually abnormally positioned over the temporal scalp. It is often more inferior and anterior to the normal side. Microtia is classified into different grades depending upon severity (Figure 29-1). Anotia represent the most severe form in which no external ear tissue is present. In grade 1 microtia, the ear is smaller than normal but retains most of the features of a normal ear, including a well-defined lobule, helix, and antihelix. An external auditory canal may or may not be present. In grade 2 microtia, the normal features of the ear are missing. A lobule and remnants of the helix and antihelix remain. In grade 3 microtia, the ear consists of disorganized cartilage beneath a skin envelope attached to a displaced lobule. Usually there is no external auditory canal.

● PATIENT PREPARATION

Given the spectrum of anomalies and the multiple needs of a patient with microtia, referral to a craniofacial team is recommended. This will allow for a thorough physical examination, a genetic evaluation, audiologic evaluation as well as the host of important ancillary services provided by this team approach. A temporal bone CT scan is crucial to determine the status of the middle ear as the severity of the external deformity does not necessarily correlate well with the development of these structures. This may be deferred until the time of reconstruction to minimize early radiation exposure.

This information, together with audiologic evaluation, can determine the need for any otologic surgery to improve hearing. Given that most children with microtia

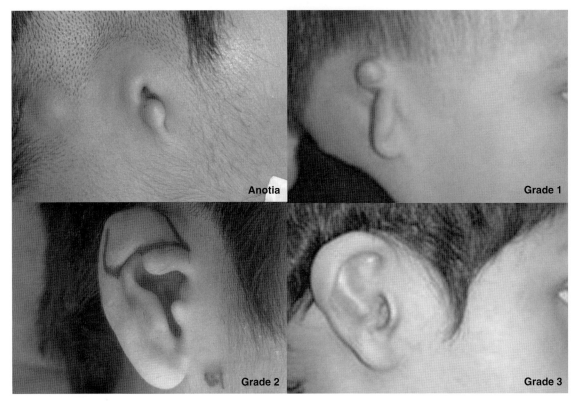

● **FIGURE 29-1.** Classification of microtia severity.

will have some degree of decreased hearing, augmentation of hearing on the affected side coupled with preservation and protection of hearing on the unaffected side is critical. Hyper vigilance against infection is important. The affected side hearing can be augmented by headband-based bone conduction hearing aids, bone anchored hearing aids, atresia surgery, or middle ear surgery.

Once a technique has been selected, and the appropriate age has been reached, surgery can be scheduled. One consideration in the pediatric population can be the school schedule. Scheduling the stages of ear reconstructions to coincide with summer and winter breaks can help minimize absence from school. Typically, after the rib harvest stage of any of the reconstructions, children will require 2 to 3 weeks for recovery before returning to school. Smaller revisions and stages may require less time.

● **TECHNIQUE**

In general, there are three broad categories of total auricular reconstruction: (1) autologous reconstruction, (2) alloplastic reconstruction, and (3) prosthetic reconstruction. Autologous reconstruction is typically a multistaged procedure based around a costal cartilage construct, which is harvested, carved to the desired shape, and buried beneath the skin. The subsequent stage elevates the reconstructed ear and to provide projection. Between two and four stages of surgery are required to complete the reconstruction, with the remaining stages devoted to

positioning of the lobule, creating the tragus, and deepening the conchal bowl. There are several approaches to this type of reconstruction, some of which will be discussed below.

Alloplastic reconstruction provides a realistic appearing ear in as little as one operation, without the associated morbidity and possible donor defect involved with harvesting rib. The material used is high-density porous polyethylene, which has multiple applications in cosmetic surgery and craniofacial reconstruction. The reported advantage of this material is that the porous nature of the product allows tissue ingrowth into the synthetic material, which may render it more resistant to infection or exposure. Its critics argue that the infection and exposure rates resulting in explantation are higher than that seen in autologous reconstruction. Many of the early alloplast ear reconstruction failures occurred prior to the standard use of temporoparietal fascial coverage. Despite its critics, reconstruction with porous polyethylene has evolved since its inception and is widely a viable option in auricular reconstruction.

For prosthetic reconstruction, a silicone framework is created and is affixed in the proper location by adhesives or systems using osseointegrated magnets or clips. This can be performed in one to two steps. Aside from patient preference, there are often valid reasons to select this type of reconstruction. Patients with poor skin secondary to burns, trauma, radiation, or prior attempts at reconstruction may require prosthetic based reconstruction due to the poor quality of the surrounding skin. Also, patients who cannot tolerate a more involved reconstruction due to comorbidities may benefit from a prosthesis. There is some controversy regarding the use of osseointegrated prostheses as a first line therapy in the pediatric microtia patient. While a prosthesis can appear quite realistic, it does require replacement every 2 to 5 years, and more frequently with higher sun exposure and smokers. Many surgeons have been concerned that a prosthetic ear does not become incorporated into the body image. Multiple studies, however, have shown a generally satisfied patient population.

General anesthesia is required for most types of ear reconstruction. Smaller revisions may be done under local anesthesia with or without sedation. Patients are generally positioned supine with both ears prepped into the field to allow reference to the unaffected ear as necessary to maximize symmetry. Access to the chest is necessary for harvesting rib grafts if needed. Sterile technique is mandatory especially when using rib grafts or prosthetic materials such as porous polyethylene. If required, some of the hair may be clipped after induction. Preoperative antibiotics are given, with *Pseudomonas* and possibly methicillin-resistant *Staphylococcus aureus* coverage required for those with a patent ear canal.

For the most part, no special equipment is required. When performing autologous reconstruction with rib, some surgeons like to use special carving tools, but this is not mandatory. If split-thickness skin grafting is being used, a dermatome may be used.

Brent Technique for Autologous Reconstruction

This involves three to four stages typically beginning anytime after 5 years of age.

Stage One. A template for the ear to be reconstructed is created by tracing the contralateral ear on a piece of x-ray film (Figure 29-2). (In those patients with bilateral

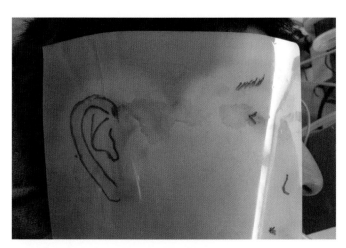

● **FIGURE 29-2.** Planning the position of the ear reconstruction using x-ray film.

microtia, a sibling's or parent's ear may be traced.) This template is then reduced in size by a few millimeters on all borders to account for the thickness of the skin. The template is then reversed and positioned on the affected side using measurements taken from the contralateral side and anatomic landmarks for reference. Again, x-ray film can be used to mark the desired location of the ear using various anatomic landmarks (eyebrow, eyelid commissure, oral commissure) on the normal side and transposing them to the contralateral side. Generally, the angle of the nasal dorsum, the distance to the lateral canthus and the lobular position are utilized. In patients with hemifacial microsomia, this is more difficult due to the diminished size of the face. In these patients, better symmetry can be obtained by referencing the height of the contralateral helical apex.

A chest incision is then created to harvest the *contralateral* ribs 6 through 8 (Figure 29-3A). This allows the use of the synchondrosis of ribs 6 and 7 to be utilized to construct the wide helical base. This base is carved that exaggerates the peaks and troughs so as to maximize surface when placed beneath the thick skin of the scalp. The rib 8 is then used to create the helix. It is attached to the base using clear nylon sutures (Figures 29-3B, 29-3C, and 29-3D). An incision is then created at the posterior aspect of the auricular remnant and a subcutaneous pocket is created. The abnormal vestigial cartilage is carefully excised so as not to damage the overlying skin. The cartilage ear framework is then placed in the pocket which needs to be large enough to accommodate the high-profile construct without undue tension. Suction drains are then placed and the skin is closed.

Stage Two. This stage is performed several months after the first. In this stage, the lobule is simply transposed on an inferior-based pedicle, rotating posteriorly and inferiorly into position. Sometimes it is necessary to create a pocket in the lobule to accept the inferiormost aspect of the cartilage construct.

Stage Three. In this stage, the construct is elevated to achieve projection of the ear. To do this, an incision is created along the posterior margin of the helical construct and dissection continues anteriorly beneath the construct. It is crucial to leave the capsule (think neoperichondrium) along the deep margin of the construct. Once an adequate amount of dissection has been completed, a piece of banked cartilage left over from the first stage in a subcutaneous pocket is trimmed to the appropriate size using the contralateral ear as a reference. It is then placed beneath the main construct, against the capsule, and held in place with nylon suture. Some surgeons opt to place extra cartilage beneath the graft at the initial inset. The postauricular scalp is then elevated and advanced anteriorly as much as possible. The remaining open area is covered with a split-thickness skin graft (Figure 29-4).

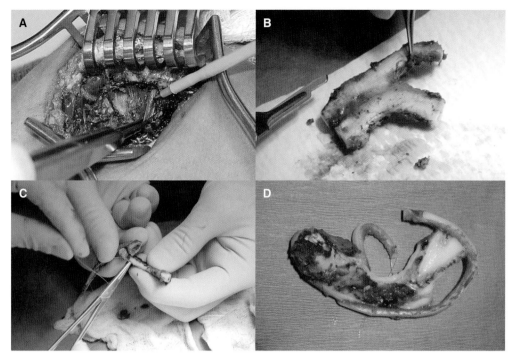

● **FIGURE 29-3.** Fabrication of the autogenous ear framework.

Stage Four. The fourth stage involves creation of the tragus, excavation of the concha and procedures to both the reconstructed ear and the contralateral normal ear to maximize symmetry. The tragus is created by harvesting a composite graft from the contralateral ear. A J-shaped incision is then created on the posterior margin of the tragus. Via this incision, the region of the conchal bowl is deepened by removing the subcutaneous tissue. The composite graft is then placed so as to provide projection to the tragus and a shadow in the area of the bowl. More recently, Brent began adding a segment of tragal cartilage to the original auricular construct. Finally, at this stage, fine-tuning of the contour, projection and position of both the reconstructed ear and the native ear can occur.

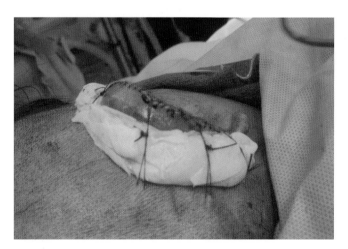

● **FIGURE 29-4.** Skin graft used to cover the posterior aspect of the elevated ear.

Nagata Technique

This technique requires only two stages. Creation of the framework, transposition of the lobule, and creation of the tragus are all accomplished in the first stage. The second stage, done several months later, elevates the construct for projection.

Stage One. Creation of the template and markings for the positioning of the construct are similar to those described for Brent technique. Next, a W-shaped incision is created along the proposed border of the helix and the inferior margin of the posterior lobular remnant. It is critical that a subcutaneous pedicle be left intact immediately posterior to the lobular remnant to provide blood supply to the posterior skin flap. In addition, a small circular incision is made at the anteriormost aspect of the W. This will be closed in a cone to create a depression at the incisura intertragica. Via this incision, the abnormal auricular remnants are excised carefully, and the subcutaneous pocket developed.

The construct in the Nagata technique is a layered construct. It requires more rib cartilage which is why reconstruction must be delayed until around nine years old. Nagata utilizes the *ipsilateral* ribs 6 to 9. The posterior perichondrium is left intact and the harvested segments are turned upside-down. Ribs 6 and 7 become the base. Using the template, depressions are carved into this base to represent the cymba and cavum conchae. The helix is formed from rib 8. The rib 9 is used for the antihelix. Once created, these pieces are stacked on the base to provide an extremely high level of relief. The segments are attached to the base using wire sutures.

Once the construct is created, it is placed in the pocket without disrupting the subcutaneous skin pedicle. The lobule is then transposed similar to a z-plasty and the skin is closed. Bolsters are then placed with mattress sutures for 2 weeks to accentuate the relief.

Stage Two. The elevation of the reconstructed ear takes place 6 months after stage one. An incision is created about 5 mm posterior to the helix. Dissection then continues anteriorly and the construct is elevated with a piece of banked cartilage placed in the subcutaneous tissues in stage one. This cartilage wedge is carved into a semilunar shape, fastened behind the contours of the antihelix to recreate the posterior wall of the concha. This is then covered with a temporoparietal fascia (TPF) flap which is then covered with a delicate, hand-harvested, split-thickness skin graft from the scalp. A tie-over bolster is used to hold this in place.

Firmin Modifications

While Firmin technique, which is the author's preferred method, shares many similarities with Nagata, there are significant modifications. Firmin has classified three types of skin incisions and three types of constructs. A similar z-plasty (type I) incision is used for the lobular microtias and a "transfixion" (type II) incision is used for the conchal types. A type III skin incision is used in cases of anotia or when the ear has a normal size but deformed cartilage. A similar multilayer construct is used though the body of the antihelix together with the superior and inferior crus tend to be a single piece. A type I construct is a complete framework, type II lacks a tragus, and type III lacks a tragus and an antitragus. Lately, an additional piece has been added to the construct behind the root of the helix and the tragus to increase their projection and improve their contour. A subcutaneous pedicle to the skin is not used and fewer wires (and much less time) is required in creation of the construct. Closed suction drains instead of tie-over bolsters are used to help the skin adhere to the framework. The rib used in the second stage for elevation is wired to the *bare* cartilage of the posterior aspect of the base and the TPF flap is frequently, but not always, used to cover this graft. Firmin feels that direct cartilage-to-cartilage contact provides for better adherence and stability.

Alloplast Reconstruction

Reconstruction with porous polyethylene has been presented as the ideal solution to auricular reconstruction. It offers the advantage of a one-stage operation without the donor site defect found with autologous reconstruction. Early results, however, were frequently unsuccessful and many abandoned the approach. There are still many proponents of this technique. Using this approach, the procedure can be performed on as young as 3 years of age, though at this time the implant needs to be made

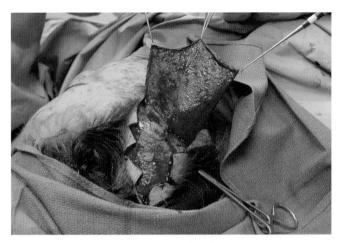

● **FIGURE 29-5.** Elevation of a temporoparietal flap for coverage of an alloplastic ear framework.

15% larger than the contralateral side and patient compliance may be an issue. Markings for the position of the reconstruction are similar to those described in the autologous reconstruction. An anteriorly based conchal flap is elevated by incising the skin immediately posterior to the proposed location of the construct. This incision is then connected to a modified Y-shaped incision in the scalp for harvest of a TPF flap (Figure 29-5). (This flap is now frequently harvested endoscopically.) The abnormal auricular remnants are removed and the anteriorly based conchal flap elevated leaving a subcutaneous pedicle to augment blood supply. The porous polyethylene implant is constructed from its component parts and placed in the appropriate location (Figure 29-6). The entire implant is then draped with the TPF flap. This is crucial and is most likely responsible for the improved success of this technique. The lobule is transposed and the TPF flap is then covered with the conchal flap. The lateral portion of the ear reconstruction is covered with a contralateral, postauricular, full-thickness skin graft for color match. The posterior aspect of the reconstruction is covered with a full-thickness skin graft from the groin. It is felt that the combination of the TPF and the full-thickness skin grafts make the reconstruction more resistant to contracture and the resultant obliteration of the sulcus.

Prosthetic Reconstruction

A variety of methods can be utilized to fix a prosthesis in the appropriate place. Traditionally, adhesives were used, but these have been replaced by methods offering better stability and retention. While subcutaneous magnets offer an attractive option, the majority of prostheses are now secured with osseointegrated posts. For an osseointegrated auricular prosthesis, the mastoid must be of adequate thickness to accept the implants. This is felt to occur by the age of 5 years. Most often, this is a two-staged procedure with the first stage consisting of the placement of the osseointegrated implants. Once

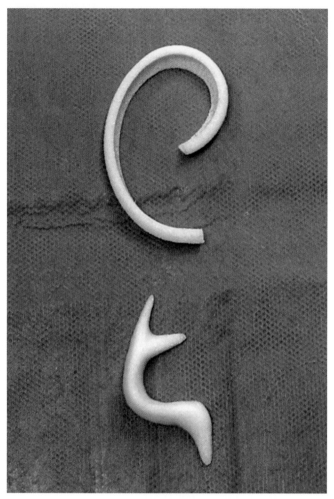

FIGURE 29-6. Components of the alloplastic ear framework. Each may be modified to suit the deformity.

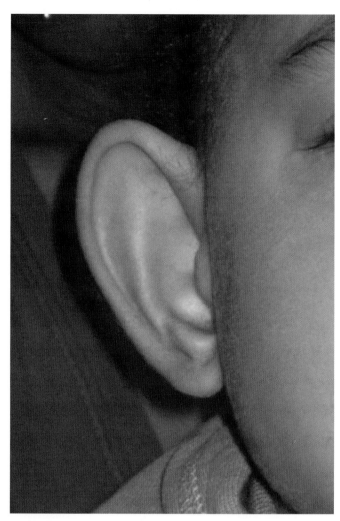

FIGURE 29-7. Effacement of the antihelical fold in prominent ear deformity.

healing occurs, generally 3 to 6 months later, the implants are uncovered and the prosthetic affixed. Patients with extensive trauma or temporal bone resection undergo preopertaive CT scans and Simplant planning studies. Those who have a history of radiotherapy are sometimes treated with a course of hyperbaric oxygen therapy before the first stage.

PROMINENT EAR DEFORMITY

Prominent ear deformity is the result of one or more characteristic findings. Most often there is effacement of the superior crus of the antihelix (Figure 29-7). The severity of the prominence varies according the degree to which the antihelix is flattened. Next, there may be excess height or widening of the conchal bowl. Finally, there may be a combination of the two, which serves to worsen the prominence.

Correction of the prominent ear is directed at the specific deformity of the auricle. If the antihelix is effaced producing prominence at the middle and upper thirds, then the antihelical fold must be created, often exaggerated. The anterior surface of the antihelix is weakened via a small anterior incision high along the antihelix with an "otobrader," mattress sutures are placed from medial to lateral across the posterior aspect of the antihelix to cause it to fold, and additional sutures may be placed from the conchal bowl to the mastoid fascia to hold the reconstructed ear closed to the head. If there is conchal excess, then either conchal excision or conchal setback with suture techniques must be used. Likewise, if there is prominence of the lobule, posterior lobule skin needs to be resected. Often, it is a combination of these techniques which are used to tailor the operation to the individual patient. It should be noted that if prominent ears or other relatively mild deformities are recognized early enough (in the first few weeks of life), custom splints can be used to correct many minor auricular deformities. This is thought to be secondary to the high levels of circulating maternal estrogens during this time period.

● PARTIAL AURICULAR RECONSTRUCTION

Much more common than microtia, partial auricular defects are common after trauma or cancer resection. Each defect is unique and therefore reconstruction is individualized to the specific need. Conceptually, there are two requirements which must be met: ears need structural support and skin coverage. If possible, these needs should be met with local tissues. However, cartilage and skin grafts from distant sites are sometimes required.

Small skin defects with good cartilage support and intact perichondrium can be treated with simple skin grafts. Full-thickness skin from the retroauricular area is often used as it resists contraction and provides a good color match from the same operative field. Two layer defects which have one layer of skin and a small cartilage defect can also be treated with skin grafting, provided that there is adequate support from the surrounding cartilage. Larger defects lacking adequate support or coverage require local flaps, local grafts, distant grafts, or a combination thereof.

Cartilage grafts can be obtained from either ipsilateral or contralateral ear or from the rib. Use of auricular cartilage is preferable, as it provides support but is thinner and more pliable than costal cartilage. Conchal grafts can be obtained from either ear using either a posterior or an anterior approach. The anterior approach allows for direct visualization and the scar is usually quite acceptable. For small (<1.5 cm), full-thickness defects, composite grafts can be used from the contralateral ear. These can be wedge shaped from the scapha and helix, or an ellipse from the conchal bowl. The resultant defect can be closed primarily, closed with a local flap, or covered with a skin graft.

Helical rim defects are most often treated by a procedure known as the Antia-Buch flap. This is a technique which allows advancement of the remaining helical rim both superiorly and inferiorly into the defect. Incisions are created in the remaining helical sulcus through the anterior skin and cartilage but leaving the posterior skin intact. After completely freeing the remaining helical rim from the scapha, the posterior auricular skin is undermined to allow the advancement of the helical rim segments into the defect. This is then closed, usually with the excision of a posterior dogear.

Partial auricular defects are often classified based on their location in the upper third, middle third, lower third, and lobular defects. While countless techniques have been described for reconstruction of these defects, the principles of cartilaginous support and skin coverage remain true. This is most often achieved using a retroauricular flap and a cartilage graft (auricular or costal) in a two-stage procedure. The resultant retroauricular defect can be closed primarily or grafted. Both the Dieffenbach technique and the Converse tunnel technique are variations on this theme.

Earlobe deformities can be the result of trauma or frequently the resection of large keloids which formed secondary to ear piercing. Two-staged operations with formation of a tubed pedicle from the adjacent skin is quite common. In addition, there are some ingenious single-stage, two-flap techniques described by Alanis, by Converse, and by Brent.

● COMPLICATIONS

Complications of this complex, often multistaged operation range from mild annoyances to major disasters. While the carving of the rib cartilage construct can seem daunting to the inexperienced, it is more often complications of the skin envelope which can lead to problems. Areas of skin necrosis can occur and must be dealt with expeditiously to prevent deformation or resorption of the cartilage framework. The necrotic areas must be debrided and covered with healthy vascularized tissue such as fascial or skin flaps The TPF flap is a good bailout, but will obviously make it unavailable for the second stage in the Nagata technique.

Cartilage which has become exposed will quickly be resorbed. Restoration of these contour defects can be difficult. Alloplast that becomes exposed will persist since the underlying framework is avascular (Figures 29-8 and 29-9). The temptation to treat exposure conservatively with dressing changes and antibiotic creams should be resisted. Other problems which can severely compromise the reconstruction are seromas, hematomas, and infection. These issues are uncommon but are mentioned to emphasize the importance of aseptic technique, antibiotic coverage, hemostasis, and drain placement. The closure of the incisions need to be airtight and the drains brought through separate distant incisions. Pressure dressings are typically avoided as they can cause ischemia of the tight overlying skin flaps. As mentioned, Nagata prefers sutured bolsters for the initial 2 weeks—most surgeons

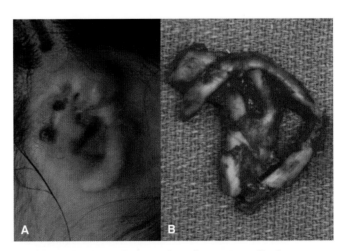

● **FIGURE 29-8.** Deformation of a costocartilaginous framework.

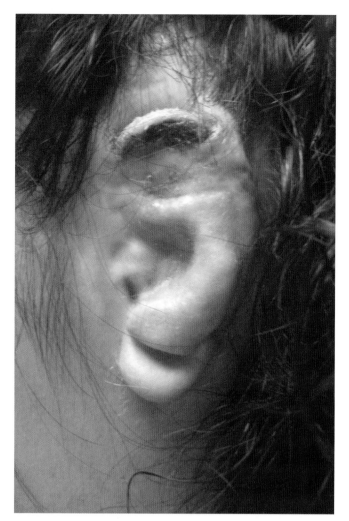

● **FIGURE 29-9.** Skin necrosis over a reconstructed ear.

changes. Hair on the reconstruction can be addressed with laser hair removal as needed. (It should be noted that some tend to use laser hair removal prior to reconstruction to address this potential problem, as they feel the presence of hair overlying the cartilage reconstruction can lead to increased incidence of infection.)

In addition to the complications at the site of reconstruction, donor site morbidity can be a problem. Incidents of pneumothorax, atelectasis, and chest wall deformity are noted. Usually, a pneumothorax is quickly identified and easily treated with a small catheter. It is unusual to require a chest tube and pleurevac. Atelectasis secondary to pain was quite common. The use of local anesthetic (bupivacaine) pumps for the first few days after surgery has dramatically decreased this problem leading to decreased postoperative pain and narcotic use. Anterior chest wall deformities are nearly universal, especially with the larger rib resections required of the Nagata and Firmin techniques. This donor site morbidity is felt to be outweighed by the improvement in the more readily apparent facial morphology. Some groups have reported a decrease in chest wall contour abnormalities when more perichondrium is left behind. In fact, some are now advocating leaving all of the perichondrium behind or creating a Vicryl tube and filling it with diced remnants of cartilage left over from the creation of the construct. Early results of these techniques to diminish donor site contour problems are promising and long-term studies of rib regeneration are ongoing.

● **OUTCOMES ASSESSMENT**

Clearly the measure of outcome in any type ear reconstruction should be symmetry with a pleasing contour and adequate projection. A reconstruction which is incorporated into the overall body image is certainly the goal. Overcoming the psychosocial barriers resulting from the congenital malformation, deformation, or acquired auricular defect can often require a multidisciplinary team approach, a skilled and experienced surgeon, and a patient patient. At the completion of the reconstruction, there is no better indicator of success than when a patient enters the office with hair short or pinned back and a smile on her face.

now substitute closed suction drains, as they are felt to be an ischemic risk. And even with perfect technique, the cartilage framework can warp, deform, or migrate.

Finally, there are smaller complications which are easier to handle. These include wire extrusion, small open wounds, or skin graft loss without cartilage exposure and hair on the reconstruction. Once the cartilage has incorporated, wires can be easily removed. Open wounds without cartilage exposure typically respond well to dressing

SUGGESTED READING _____

Braun T, Gratza S, Becker S, et al. Auricular reconstruction with porous polyethylene frameworks: outcome and patient benefit in 65 children and adults. *Plast Reconstr Surg.* 2010; 126(4):1201–1212.

Brent B. Microtia repair with rib cartilage grafts: a review of personal experience with 1000 cases. *Clin Plast Surg.* 2002; 29(2):257–271.

Brent B. Technical advances in ear reconstruction with autogenous rib cartilage grafts: personal experience with 1200 cases. *Plast Reconstr Surg.* 1999;104:319–334, discussion 335–338.

Byrd HS, Langevin CJ, Ghidoni LA. Ear Molding in newborn infants with auricular deformities. *Plast Reconstr Surg.* 2010; 126(4):1191–1200.

Chen ZC, Goh RC, Chen PK, Lo LJ, Wang SY, Nagata S. A new method for the second-stage auricular projection of the Nagata method: ultra-delicate split-thickness skin graft in continuity with full-thickness skin. *Plast Reconstr Surg.* 2009;124(5):1477–1485.

Federspil PA. Auricular prostheses. *Adv Otorhinolaryngol.* 2010; 68:65–80.

Firmin F. State-of-the-art autogenous ear reconstruction in cases of microtia. *Adv Otorhinolaryngol*. 2010;68:25–52.

Horlock N, Vogelin E, Bradbury ET, Grobbelaar AO, Gault DT. Psychosocial outcome of patients after ear reconstruction: a retrospective study of 62 patients. *Ann Plast Surg*. 2005;54(5):517–524.

Jinguang Z, Leren H, Hongxing Z. Experience of correction of prominent ears. *J Craniofac Surg*. 2010;21(5):1578–1580.

Korus LJ, Wong JN, Wilkes GH. Long-term follow-up of osseointegrated auricular reconstruction. *Plast Reconstr Surg*. 2011;127(2):630–636.

Nagata S. Modification of the stages in total reconstruction of the auricle. Part I. Grafting the three-dimensional costal cartilage framework for lobule-type microtia. *Plast Reconstr Surg*. 1994;93:221–230, discussion 267–268.

Nagata S. Modification of the stages in total reconstruction of the auricle. Part III. Grafting the three-dimensional costal cartilage framework for small concha-type microtia. *Plast Reconstr Surg*. 1994;93:243–253, discussion 267–268.

Nagata S. Modification of the stages in total reconstruction of the auricle. Part IV. Ear elevation for the constructed auricle. *Plast Reconstr Surg*. 1994;93:254–266, discussion 267–268.

Pearl RA, Sabbage W. Reconstruction following traumatic partial amputation of the ear. *Plast Reconstr Surg*. 2011; 127(2):621–629.

Reinisch JF, Lewin S. Ear reconstruction using a porous polyethylene framework and temporoparietal fascia flap. *Facial Plast Surg*. 2009;25:181–189.

Shonka DC Jr, Park SS. Ear defects. *Facial Plast Surg Clin North Am*. 2009;17(3):429–443.

Siegert R, Weerda H, Magritz R. Basic techniques in autogenous microtia repair. *Facial Plastic Surg*. 2009;25(3): 149–157.

Steffen A, Wollenberg B, Konig IR, Frenzel H. A prospective evaluation of psychosocial outcomes following ear reconstruction with rib cartilage in microtia. *J Plast Reconstr Aesthet Surg*. 2010;63(9):1466–1473.

Walton RL, Beahm EK. Auricular reconstruction for microtia. In: Siemionow MZ, Eisenmann-Klein M, eds. *Plastic and Reconstructive Surgery*. Springer Specialist Surgery Series. Part IV. London: Springer; 2010:357–378.

chapter 30

Reconstruction of the Nose

Peter J. Taub, MD, FACS, FAAP

● PATIENT EVALUATION AND SELECTION

The nose is arguably one of the most obvious features of the human body. Its structure is complex and its function is one of the most intricate. As such, reconstruction of the nose following trauma, cancer ablation, infection, or congenital malformation may present difficult challenges for the plastic surgeon. There are essentially three components of the nose: a thin, vascularized lining of mucosa lined with squamous epithelium, a supporting framework of bone and cartilage, and an outer skin envelope with variable colors and textures. When analyzing a defect and planning a reconstruction, tissue loss to each of these layers must be identified, including any losses to surrounding cheek or upper lip. Simple closure of the wound often accomplishes only the functional goal while sacrificing the aesthetic result.

The skin of the nose may be thought of as several adjacent convex and concave subunits.[1] Each subunit has its own characteristic geometry and neighboring subunits are separated by natural lines that reflect light and cast shadows onto the surrounding skin. The various subunits include the midline nasal dorsum, tip, and columella and the paired sidewalls, alar rims, and soft triangles. For example, the dorsum is half of a cylinder and the tip half of a sphere. Each convex subunit has a central highlight and each concave subunit has a central shadow. The combination of highlights and shadows gives the nose its characteristic aesthetic appearance.

Flaps of skin and subcutaneous tissue form a sheet of scar on the recipient bed and undergo centripetal contraction by myofibroblasts during wound healing, resulting in a bulging or "trapdoor" effect. This phenomenon is used to the surgeon's advantage in recreating the contour of a convex subunit, but detracts from the final result if a flap is placed on a concave area. Skin grafts form a similar layer of scar tissue that undergoes contraction, but does not bulge

due to the lack of subcutaneous tissue. This makes full-thickness grafts a better choice for reconstructing concave subunits.

The subunit principle can also be applied secondarily in the case of a large defect spanning several nasal subunits, or a composite defect involving surrounding tissue of the cheek or upper lip. In these circumstances, it is often necessary to perform a staged reconstruction and initially transfer a bulky flap with enough skin area to resurface the missing nasal subunits, surrounding skin, and restore deep tissue loss.

Once the flap is inset, a secondary refining procedure may be performed at a later date. Incisions are made in the desired location along the borders of the subunit based on the contralateral intact side. Through these incisions, the underlying soft tissue may be sculpted, and the surface lines of contour created using quilting sutures. These additional scars may be hidden in the deep contour lines establishing the aesthetic appearance of light and shadow regions.

Similarly, skin quality across the nose is not identical. Several distinct areas exist. The skin over the glabella, upper dorsum, and paired nasal sidewalls is usually thin, smooth, nonsebaceous, and pliable. It moves easily over the underlying bony and cartilage support. The skin covering the majority of the tip and alar regions is thicker, more adherent, and pitted with sebaceous glands. A layer of dense subcutaneous fat is present that provides definition and contour. This area also overlies the lateral crura of the lower lateral cartilages. A third skin type covers the alar margins, the soft triangles, and columella. It is similar in quality and color to the skin of the dorsum, but is firmly fixed to the underlying cartilage.

Local skin damage from radiation injury should be questioned and sought. Often, skin and soft tissues around a defect are unsuitable for reconstruction. It is better to avoid the problem of flap necrosis beforehand than manage it afterwards. In certain instances, pre- and postoperative hyperbaric oxygen therapy may ameliorate the deleterious effects of radiation damage.[2]

Visual inspection and manual palpation of the nose externally, as well as speculum examination with an adequate lightsource intranasally, should evaluate the existing bony and cartilaginous support to the nose. Superiorly, the nasal pyramid is composed of two small bones anchored to the frontal bone superiorly, to the maxilla laterally, and to each other medially. The cartilaginous septum provides most of the support caudally with contributions from the upper and lower lateral cartilages to prevent collapse of the internal nasal valves and nostrils with inspiration. The symmetry of the nose is best appreciated on frontal view, while the height and straightness of the dorsum is best appreciated from the side. The respective contributions of bone loss as well as cartilaginous septal loss should be noted.

Prior to speculum examination, a topical vasoconstrictive spray may be used to better visualize the intranasal anatomy. The caudal edge of the bony pyramid may be noted as well as the support provided by the upper and lower lateral cartilages. The internal nasal valve angle should be noted. The septum should be visualized and palpated and any deformations or communications should be appreciated. Gentle pressure on the septum with a cotton-tipped applicator will identify areas deficient in cartilage and whether sufficient stock remains as a source of graft material.

Much of the lining of the nose is not easily visible on cursory examination. The mucosa extends over the turbinates, which should be inspected for hypertrophy and airway compromise. Preoperatively, the intranasal examination will highlight areas of deficient mucosa that may need to be addressed. In addition, areas of scarring that may contribute to postoperative airway compromise should be noted.

Respiratory function needs to be addressed preoperatively. A thorough history should identify any evidence of difficulty breathing through the nose. Specific questions to ask the patient include when the problem began, whether or not there is a seasonal component to the symptoms, and whether or not the patient uses medications such as antihistamines to address the problem.

Casual observation of the external nasal valves on inspiration may identify weakness of the lower lateral cartilages. Intranasal inspection should be performed on all patients with and without a topical vasoconstrictive agent to shrink the nasal mucosa. This should identify lesions or bands of scar tissue that may need to be addressed in order to improve postoperative nasal function.

The Cottle test attempts to identify collapse at the internal nasal valve. The patient is asked to breathe in and the ease or difficulty of simple air exchange is noted. The maneuver is then repeated while gently pulling on the cheek just lateral to the nostril. Improvement in breathing may be interpreted as a sign of internal valve compromise. It should be noted, however, that some surgeons

question the validity of the test because most symptomatic and nonsymptomatic patients will report benefit with the maneuver.

● PATIENT PREPARATION

There is a well-intended adage that the best procedures should be reserved for the best patients. Often, the ideal reconstructive procedure for any given patient requires multiple stages with close follow-up between each stage and good communication between the patient and the surgeon. In a retrospective analysis of more than 1000 cases, over 70% required at least two procedures and a large percentage even more.[3] Patients in whom follow-up is anticipated to be difficult or comprehension regarding the chronicity of the reconstruction to be lacking may be better served with a lesser procedure.

A variety of conditions may produce defects of the nose. In the case of a malignant neoplasm, confirmation that the malignant process has been completely excised is imperative prior to beginning a lengthy and complicated reconstruction. This is best achieved with lateral and deep biopsies of the wound margin for local involvement and any number of radiographic studies for distant spread.

The initial surgical intervention should achieve negative margins in the case of malignant disease (Figure 30-1). Scars and contractures may be released so that the full size of the defect may be appreciated and the tissues returned to their normal anatomic position. This may be done at a separate procedure following temporary coverage of any raw surfaces with split-thickness skin grafts and/or direct approximation of the wound margins or it may be done as the initial part of the actual reconstruction. Many surgeons prefer the use of Mohs micrographic surgery for the excision of skin malignancies versus wide local excision. The Mohs technique attempts to maximize the amount of normal tissue left in place after surgical resection.

A guiding principle of reconstruction is that destruction of at least half of a subunit warrants reconstruction of the entire subunit. Incisions should ideally be designed

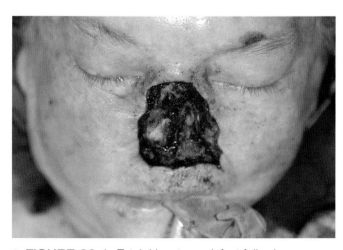

● **FIGURE 30-1.** Total rhinectomy defect following resection of a squamous cell carcinoma.

along the lines separating any two subunits. Recent articles have challenged the need to reconstruct entire subunits with larger defects citing the benefits of retaining as much native, healthy tissue as possible. Newer techniques of laser and dermabrasion make softening the edges between the flap and the surrounding native skin much more effective.[3]

● TECHNIQUES

The reconstruction of nasal deformities is both an artistic and scientific endeavor. The nose is the visual centerpiece of the face and is essential to an aesthetically pleasing appearance. In addition, the nose offers protection to surrounding structures and is vital to maintaining a patent airway. Therefore, reconstruction of the nose must address both functional and aesthetic concerns.

The principles of the reconstructive ladder should be applied to the reconstruction of the nose. Small defects certainly may be left to heal by secondary intention and often this is the ideal course of treatment. Outside of the social stigmata of a nasal dressing, local wound care is usually not difficult. For larger defects, each component of the nose must be considered when the reconstruction is planned.

Mucosal Lining

The replacement of adequate nasal lining is perhaps the most challenging component of complex nasal defects. The ideal donor site for nasal lining replaces the defect with like tissue of equal vascularity and pliability. Any flap used must be thin enough to avoid airway obstruction, pliable enough to conform to an underlying cartilage or bone graft, and vascular enough to provide nourishment to the grafts.[1] Poor perfusion may result in overlying flap ischemia, necrosis, infection, and/or extrusion of the underlying cartilage or bone grafts. Failure of the lining is the most common cause of functional and aesthetic compromise.

Several options exist for nasal lining, including skin grafts, local mucoperichondrial flaps, and foldover flaps. Many techniques date back to the work of Harold Gillies during World War I who popularized the use of the turnover hinge flap, which involves using small, adjacent flaps folded over on themselves with the epithelium facing intranasally. Based on scar tissue, they create a lining of limited length due to the inherently poor blood supply. As a result, all cartilage grafts should be placed secondarily to maximize their viability. Delaying transfer of the flaps may also gain additional length. Skin grafts, on the other hand, require a well-vascularized bed, which is often deficient in the presence of exposed bone or cartilage.

First described by Millard, the ipsilateral septal mucosal flap based on the septal branch of the superior labial artery is a commonly used option.[4] A pedicle slightly larger than 1 cm allows for the elevation and transfer of septal mucosa. The flap can be modified to allow for the simultaneous reconstruction of lining and cartilage support. A composite flap of septal cartilage and mucosa can be rotated out

of the piriform aperture at the posterior septal angle to cover defects of the lower half of the nasal vestibule. In the case of bilateral lining defects, right and left mucosal flaps are elevated and rotated downward and laterally, and the septal cartilage is sculpted to replace the medial crura and columella.

For defects of the nasal margin, remaining intact nasal lining skin above the defect can be brought down as a bipedicle flap to provide vascular squamous epithelium to the desired alar rim level in a bucket-handle fashion. The secondary defect may be closed with a full-thickness skin graft, or by ipsi- or contralateral septal mucosal flaps. The contralateral septal mucoperichondrial flap involves the removal of the central septal cartilage, raising a long dorsally based contralateral mucosal flap, and delivering it through an incision high in the ipsilateral mucosa. The septal cartilage can then be used to fabricate any variety of onlay, cantilever, or strut grafts for support. Other options exist for situations where mucosal lining flaps are unavailable. These include the inferior turbinate flap,[5] and a three-layer sandwich graft of cartilage and skin taken from the root of the ear helix for alar rim defects less than 1 cm.

Skin grafts applied to the surface of a forehead flap, braced by cartilage grafts within the flap is another accepted technique. This composite version of the forehead flap can be prefabricated and banked prior to transfer for several weeks to ensure viability of the flap elements. The nasolabial flap can also be folded on itself to supply both cover and lining and close defects along the alar rim. These techniques are limited by bulk and often require aggressive secondary thinning procedures to prevent airway obstruction. Defects involving the entire nasal unit require large lining flaps such as microvascular free flaps or a depilated scalp flap.

It is not generally necessary to replace the lining of the narrow middle and upper portions of the nasal vault. These areas are often not present in Asians, and are not touched by normal horizontal airflow patterns in the nose. Reconstruction of the nasal septum should be avoided due to the likely possibility of airway obstruction. There is no functional deficit in creating a nose with a single, large vestibule.[6]

Nasal Support

Solid tissue support is essential for maintaining long-term aesthetic results. Bone and cartilage grafts prevent the skin and lining from collapsing under the forces of scar contracture. In addition, they help to ensure airway patency during inspiration by preventing sidewall collapse, and prevent cephalic retraction of the alar rim.[1] Early attempts at reconstruction without using support grafts resulted in disfiguring scar contracture or soft tissue collapse.

Reconstruction of the bony nasal pyramid or dorsum often requires autogenous bone grafts. Sources include the skull, iliac crest (Figure 30-2), and rib cage (Figure 30-3). Bone provides a rigid framework to address collapse of the osseocartilaginous vault as a result of tumor resection

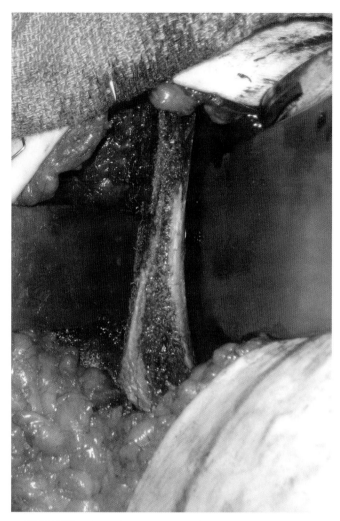

● FIGURE 30-2. Bone harvested from the iliac crest.

or trauma (Figure 30-4). Due to the limited quantities required, most bone graft may be harvested with minimal donor site morbidity.[7] The grafts may be anchored to the maxilla and/or frontal bone using titanium microplates. Alloplastic alternatives include thin sheets of porous hydroxyapatite.[8]

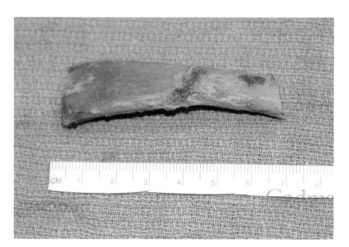

● FIGURE 30-3. Bone harvested from the rib cage.

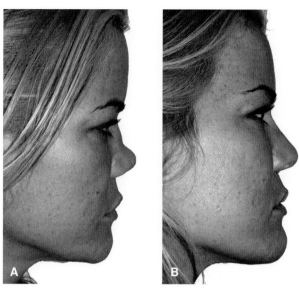

● FIGURE 30-4. Saddle-nose deformity secondary to trauma reconstructed with a costal rib graft.

Cartilage grafts rely on the vascularity of the wound bed and/or the overlying flap. Whenever possible, these grafts should be placed primarily at the time of flap transfer to prevent the need for re-expansion after scarring has occurred which will compromise the final aesthetic result. The nonanatomic placement of bone and cartilage grafts from the existing nasal bone to the alar margin and columella will help maintain the desired dimensions, projection, and contour of the reconstruction.

Common donor sites for cartilage grafts include septal, conchal, and costal cartilage. Each donor site has distinct advantages and disadvantages. Septal cartilage is strong and easily carved (Figure 30-5). It is easily harvested during the fabrication of intranasal lining flaps; however, its supply is limited and may be affected by the initial defect itself. Conchal cartilage has a natural curve that lends itself well to reconstruction of the alar rim, and has minimal donor site morbidity. It is significantly weaker than other donor options and may collapse if the skin envelope is excessively

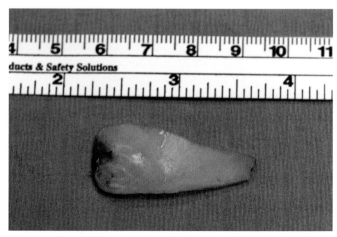

● FIGURE 30-5. Cartilage harvested from the septum.

thick or scarred. Costal cartilage is abundant, strong, and easy to carve, but has the tendency to warp during healing and is moderately prone to reabsorption over time.

Cartilage grafts are perhaps most important when reconstruction of the alar rim is required. Nonanatomic placement of cartilage grafts is a key concept for recreating the support and projection of the alar rim and nasal tip. Arches of donor cartilage are fabricated with a thickness of 1 to 2 mm and bend at one end to recreate the genu of the medial crura. These arches can be anchored to remnants of the existing medial and lateral crura, or fastened to a central columellar strut of stiff cartilage. If necessary, the points of greatest projection are weakened by repeated puncturing with a fine-gauge needle. Batten grafts placed in a subcutaneous pocket along the alar rim are fastened in place with sutures spanning the graft and nasal lining that eliminate any dead space between tissue layers. Other techniques such as tip grafts, spreader grafts, and contouring sutures can be utilized to fine-tune the ultimate aesthetic result.

Current research has focused on the use of technology, specifically in the areas of structural grafting. The use of alloplastic implants with or without acellular human cadaveric dermal grafts (Alloderm) has been reported with successful outcomes.[9] In addition, the applications of tissue-engineered cartilage from the patient's own chondrocytes are being investigated.[10–12] Tissue engineering has the potential to create "autogenous" cartilage grafts in an exact three-dimensional shape with minimal donor site morbidity.

Skin Coverage

The final component of nasal reconstruction, and perhaps the most important to the aesthetic outcome, is the skin coverage.

The type of flap or graft used for reconstruction is dependent on the size, anatomic location, and skin zone of the defect, as well as the quality of surrounding skin. The literature reports a wealth of different flap types and potential graft donor sites for use in all possible defect locations. These techniques can be used alone for superficial defects, or in combination with any of the previously mentioned techniques of nasal lining and structural support in full-thickness defects.

For areas where the skin is thin, smooth, and mobile, such as the nasal dorsum, primary closure is often possible. For larger defects, a skin graft is another option. The choice of donor site depends on the location and size of the defect. Superficial defects of the upper two-thirds of the nose with a vascularized recipient bed can be resurfaced with a full-thickness skin graft. The preauricular skin is an ideal donor site on account of its color, texture, and quality. Grafts up to 2 cm or more can be harvested with primary closure and minimal donor site morbidity. Secondary donor sites include the postauricular and supraclavicular skin. The former may easily conceal an incision but tends to have a less satisfactory color match. The latter has the advantage of being plentiful and blends well in older patients with actinic damage. It is important to remember that skin grafts will appear thin and shiny after transfer due to relative ischemia, and frequently become hyperpigmented or hypopigmented.[6]

Composite grafts of skin and cartilage may be used as a one-stage reconstructive option for defects of the alar rim. The most common donor site for a full-thickness defect is a sandwich graft of cartilage between two layers of skin from the root of the auricular helix (Figure 30-6). Perfusion limits the size of the graft to between 1 and 2 cm. Other composite donor sites include the helical rim, helical crus, antihelix, or tragus. All grafts have the potential for central

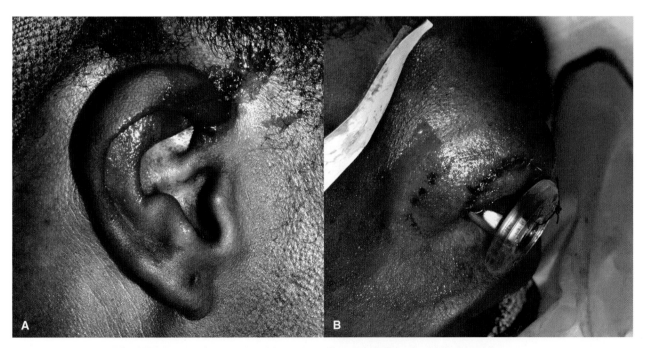

● **FIGURE 30-6.** Composite skin and cartilage graft from the helical root for nasal alar reconstruction.

necrosis. This should be allowed to separate naturally over time and heal by secondary intention. If possible, skin grafts should be secured on the recipient bed with a bolster to limit shear and prevent hematoma or seroma formation. Split-thickness grafts tend to contract over time with a poor aesthetic result. As such, they have little role in nasal reconstruction other than for temporary closure.

Smaller defects of the lower twothirds of the nose may also be reconstructed using full-thickness skin grafts. The forehead is considered to be the gold standard in terms of skin match. Grafts can be harvested from near the hairline with considerably less donor site morbidity than a large flap. Some advocate grafts from the nasolabial fold to match the color, texture, and contour of the alae or nasal tip.[13] These grafts revascularize well with only peripheral perfusion due to the thick dermis of the donor site, and the donor scar is easily camouflaged in the nasolabial fold.

Single-stage local flaps should be the method of choice if the aesthetic and functional goals can be achieved. These flaps range in complexity from a simple rotational flap, V-Y advancement flap, and cheek advancement flap, to the bilobed flap. They should be designed using the contralateral, unaffected side as a model and not the actual defect. A model of the flap may be sterilized for use in the operative field.[14]

The bilobed flap is most useful for small to medium defects of the lower third of the nose. It has the advantage of allowing easier transposition of thick, sebaceous skin under less tension with no dog-ear formation versus rotational flaps. It relies on a random cutaneous vascular pattern. The flap consists of two lobes: one to fill the primary defect, and a second to fill the secondary defect created by the primary lobe (Figure 30-7). This ultimately creates a remote, tertiary defect that may be closed primarily.

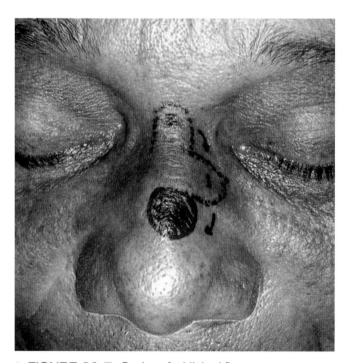

● **FIGURE 30-7.** Design of a bilobed flap.

There are several important keys to success when designing and transferring a bilobed flap. In general, the diameter of the primary lobe should be smaller than the defect, while the secondary lobe should be smaller than the first. Since each flap suffers from loss of effective length during rotation, each lobe must be slightly longer to overcome the difference. Undermining in a supraperiosteal plane promotes adequate perfusion of the flap. Closure should begin with primary closure of the tertiary defect at the glabella.

Skin over the tip and alar margins is thick, sebaceous, and more difficult to manipulate. Smaller defects less than 1.5 cm may be amenable to adjacent tissue transfer with a random cheek advancement flap, lateral nasal flap, or dorsal nasal flap. The dorsal nasal flap is particularly useful in defects of the dorsum and/or tip. The flap is incised along the lateral ridge superiorly, and a backcut is made across the glabellar region. The skin of the upper twothirds of the nose and glabella is then be rotated inferiorly onto the nasal tip (Figure 30-8).

A nasolabial flap from the cheek may be used for superficial coverage of certain nasal defects. The flap is based on the angular branch of the facial artery and is desirable since the donor scar falls within the natural nasolabial crease (Figure 30-9). It may be left longer than required for skin coverage but folded onto itself to provide additional lining. A secondary procedure may then be required to remove the bulkiness of the flap, which may compromise the airflow through the nares.

Paramedian Forehead Flap

The paramedian forehead flap has arguably been considered the workhorse flap for coverage of large nasal defects. It is the preferred method for resurfacing larger defects of the nasal tip, lobule, dorsum, or columella greater than 2 cm in diameter. The flap is versatile and can be designed to cover defects crossing multiple subunits.

Its blood supply is derived from one or both supratrochlear systems and may be considered an axial flap proximally and a random flap distally. The flap may be prefabricated with thin grafts of cartilage and/or split-thickness skin to provide support and/or lining to areas of reconstruction that require more than simple skin coverage. At the time of prefabrication, a gauze dressing spread with petrolatum jelly may be left beneath each "heminostril" to provide a desired curvature to the new alar rim.

Burget described the forehead flap as a three-staged procedure with each stage having individual goals toward the shaping of the final product.[6] Stage one involved elevation and transposition of a viable flap with adequate length. Stage two focused on refining, sculpting, and detailing the flap. Accessory cartilage grafts were added in this stage if necessary. Stage three involved division of the pedicle and final inset of the flap.

The paramedian forehead flap is based proximally with the pedicle centered most commonly over the ipsilateral

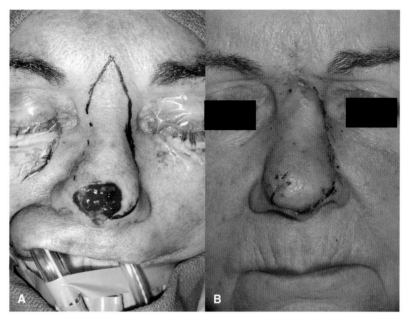

● FIGURE 30-8. Design and inset of a dorsal nasal flap.

supratrochlear artery (Figure 30-10). The vessel consistently lies between 1.7 and 2.2 cm lateral of midline at the medial border of the eyebrow. At this level, the vessel pierces the orbicularis oculi and frontalis muscles and runs vertically in a subcutaneous plane. The course of the vessel can be assessed using Doppler ultrasound. The pedicle should be designed between 1 and 1.5 cm in diameter at the proximal attachment. This allows for more length and prevents tension and strangulation when the flap is rotated inferiorly into position.

Prior to incision, a template of the defect is fabricated from suture foil or glove paper. The flap should be designed with a vertical axis, which may be extended distally into the hairline and proximally over the supraorbital rim if more length is needed. The design should be centered on the previously identified vascular pedicle. Some authors advocate angling the skin flap obliquely near the hairline to prevent the inclusion of hair-bearing skin. Due to the extensive arborization of the musculocutaneous arterial supply of the forehead skin, a randomly based oblique flap

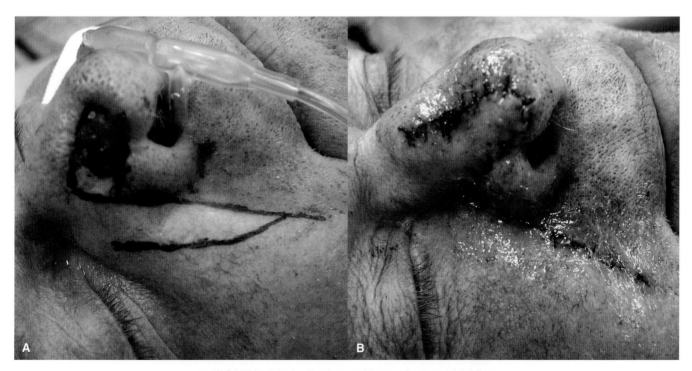

● FIGURE 30-9. Design and inset of a nasolabial flap.

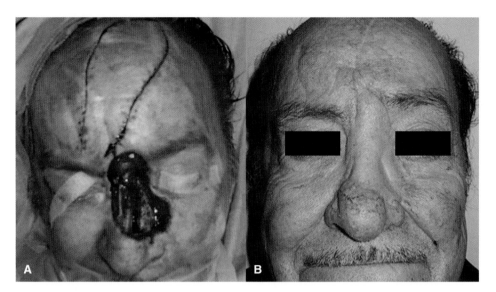

● **FIGURE 30-10.** Use of a paramedian forehead flap for reconstruction of a nasal tip defect.

would easily survive. This, however, creates a more difficult donor site to close primarily and increases the incidence of unilateral brow elevation with scar contracture.

At its distal extent, the forehead flap is elevated in a subcutaneous plane to minimize tissue bulk in the hopes of producing maximal definition at the nasal tip. More proximally, the flap is left bulkier to provide the greatest vascularity. This is rarely a problem since the more inferior portions of the flap are returned to their origin once the flap has had an adequate chance to develop a collateral circulation.

Distal to the origin of the pedicle, the dissection is carried out in the submuscular plane just superficial to the periosteum. Blunt dissection is used to separate the corrugator muscles from the flap to protect the pedicle. Adequate mobilization often requires release of the corrugators near the origin of the supratrochlear artery. Once the flap is elevated along its length, it is rotated into position over the nasal defect taking care not to strangulate the vascular pedicle. Only the very distal 3 to 4 mm of the flap are thinned to facilitate matching of contour with the normal skin of the defect margins. Another technique to gaining flap length involves dividing the frontalis muscle on the under side of the flap horizontally in 1-cm intervals to release the overlying skin and dermis.[15] The superficial course of the blood vessels protects them from injury with this maneuver. If the patient has a history of cigarette smoking, flap transfer should be delayed at least 3 weeks by incising the perimeter of the flap without elevating it, and closing the delayed incisions in layers in an effort to improve blood supply by neovascularization.

The forehead donor site is undermined in a subfascial plane as wide as the temporalis muscle on either side and closed primarily. Any remaining defect is allowed to close by secondary intention with appropriate wound care. This creates a very fairly well hidden forehead scar that may be easily revised at a later date, if needed.

The second stage involves sculpting and refinement of the flap with the placement of secondary cartilage grafts or revision as needed. The flap is elevated by narrowly excising the lateral scars and raising the flap on its attachment at the nostril margin. This gives easy access for thinning and sculpting of subcutaneous tissue to achieve the desired contour. Quilting stitches are placed and removed 1 to 2 days postoperatively to decrease hematoma formation and promote adherence of the flap. The final stage of flap transfer involves division of the pedicle and insetting the tail.

In all cases, most authors recommend waiting at least three, and preferably 12 to 16 weeks between surgical stages to allow for scar maturation between procedures. Epinephrine with local anesthesia is avoided because blanching of the flap intraoperatively is a vital clue to flap ischemia and viability that should not be masked.

Isolated defects involving the alar rim and vestibule may be difficult to reach with the paramedian forehead flap. Frequently, these defects also involve portions of the cheek and apical triangle of the upper lip. In these cases, a viable option for reconstruction is the nasolabial flap, which may be transferred as a peninsula or as an island. Similar to the forehead flap, the template for the skin paddle is designed from the contralateral unaffected side. The medial border of the nasolabial island flap should lie in the nasolabial crease for optimal camouflaging of the donor site scar. The flap is raised deepening the dissection proximally. A wide superolateral pedicle of fat should be maintained between the skin island and the zygomaticus major muscle to preserve the perforators. As in all cases of alar rim reconstruction, a cartilage support graft must be used to prevent airway collapse and contracture of the flap. Occasionally, nonanatomic cartilage grafts are needed over the entire vestibule to maintain shape and projection. A second refining procedure may be required in which the subunit borders are carved into the flap and the wound bed sculpted through these new incisions. Contour is created with buried and quilting sutures.

Maintaining the shape of the skin covering the soft triangles and columella is crucial to repairing defects in this area. Superficial defects can be reconstructed using a composite graft from the antihelix of the ear. A secondary deformity of the ear is sacrificed for quality aesthetic results in the nasal reconstruction. The donor site closure often requires a full-thickness skin graft. Deeper, more complex defects of the columellar region may require unilateral or paired nasolabial fold flaps over an anchored cartilage strut graft.

Free Tissue Transfer

Microvascular free flaps play a role in nasal reconstruction in cases of large defects where tissue loss prevents the use of all other local flaps for nasal lining. Free flaps are transferred with multiple skin islands based on musculocutaneous perforators and used to recreate the nasal lining and columella, as well as any adjacent defects of the nasal floor. Commonly used free flaps are the radial forearm flap, groin flap, and anterolateral thigh flap. These flaps are often bulky and require multiple thinning procedures to maintain a patent airway. The free flaps are frequently anastamosed to the facial vessels. Ideally, cartilage grafts are used for support over the free flap, and a paramedian forehead flap is used for skin covering. In cases of burns and significant facial trauma, a free flap may be used to supply the skin covering, but the aesthetic results are suboptimal. On account of the fine definition and relatively thin soft tissue covering the nose, free tissue transfer is less commonly used to reconstruct the nose. In addition, the forehead flap is usually available and provides a more aesthetic reconstructive option.

● COMPLICATIONS

Because certain areas of the nose require full-thickness skin, there is the potential for a higher rate of graft loss. Should graft loss occur, a search for possible offending causes should be made. In the case of a forehead flap, the distal skin in the region of the hairline is often tenuous due to the random nature of the distal blood supply. This may be minimized by a primary delay procedure. At the time of the delay, the distal skin pattern—either a heminasal outline or full nasal outline—may be incised and partially elevated. A thin skin graft, with or without a cartilage graft for alar rim support, may be fixed to the underside of the flap as a means of prefabrication.

● OUTCOMES ASSESSMENT

Any reconstructive endeavor will ultimately be judged on how closely it recreates the natural appearance of the nose. Minimal incisions, placed along the aesthetic lines of the nose, with minimal subcutaneous tissue is the goal. For large defects, the nasolabial flap usually fulfills these needs well. The reconstruction, however, must not compromise the ultimate survival of the patient. As such, the survival rate among cancer cases must be examined.

REFERENCES

1. Chang JS, Becker SS, Park SS. Nasal reconstruction: the state of the art. *Curr Opin Otolaryngol Head Neck Surg.* 2004;12(4):336–343.

2. Kindwall EP, Gottlieb LJ, Larson DL. Hyperbaric oxygen therapy in plastic surgery: a review article. *Plast Reconstr Surg.* 1991;88(5):898–908.

3. Rohrich RJ, Griffin JR, Ansari M, Beran SJ, Potter JK. Nasal reconstruction–beyond aesthetic subunits: a 15-year review of 1334 cases. *Plast Reconstr Surg.* 2004;114(6):1405–1416; discussion 1417–1419.

4. Millard DR Jr. Various uses of the septum in rhinoplasty. *Plast Reconstr Surg.* 1988;81(1):112–128.

5. Friedman M, Ibrahim H, Ramakrishnan V. Inferior turbinate flap for repair of nasal septal perforation. *Laryngoscope.* 2003;113(8):1425–1428.

6. Burget GC. Aesthetic reconstruction of the nose. In: Mathes SJ, Hentz VR, eds. *Plastic Surgery.* Philadelphia: W.B. Saunders; 2005.

7. Tessier P, Kawamoto H, Posnick J, Roulo Y, Tulasne JF, Wolfe SA. Complications of harvesting autogenous bone grafts: a group experience of 20,000 cases. *Plast Reconstr Surg.* 2005;116(5 suppl):72S.

8. Byrd HS, Hobar PC. Alloplastic nasal and perialar augmentation. *Clin Plast Surg.* 1996;23(2):315–326.

9. Gryskiewicz JM, Rohrich RJ, Reagan BJ. The use of alloderm for the correction of nasal contour deformities. *PlastReconstr Surg.* 2001;107(2):561–570; discussion 571.

10. Anderer U, Libera J. In vitro engineering of human autogenous cartilage. *J Bone Miner Res.* 2002;17(8): 1420–1429.

11. Kita M, Hanasono MM, Mikulec AA, Pollard JD, Kadleck JM, Koch RJ. Growth and growth factor production by human nasal septal chondrocytes in serum-free media. *Am J Rhinol.* 2006;20(5):489–495.

12. Chang CH, Kuo TF, Lin CC, et al. Tissue engineering-based cartilage repair with allogenous chondrocytes and gelatin-chondroitin-hyaluronan tri-copolymer scaffold: a porcine model assessed at 18, 24, and 36 weeks. *Biomaterials.* 2006; 27(9):1876–1888.

13. Hubbard TJ. Leave the fat, skip the bolster: thinking outside the box in lower third nasal reconstruction. *Plast Reconstr Surg.* 2004;114(6):1427–1435.

14. Cook JL. A review of the bilobed flap's design with particular emphasis on the minimization of alar displacement. *Dermatol Surg.* 2000;26(4):354–362.

15. Menick, Frederick J. Nasal Reconstruction: Forehead Flap. *Plast Reconstr Surg.* 113(6):100e–111e, May 2004.

chapter 31

Lip Reconstruction

Naveen K. Ahuja, MD / *Robert J. Morin, MD* / *Mark S. Granick, MD*

● INTRODUCTION

The importance of functional and aesthetically pleasing lips transcends their ability to maintain oral competence. In addition to providing a role in mastication, the lips are an essential part of communication, facial expression, and beauty. Phonation of many sounds requires the advanced function of the lips and their surrounding musculature. The same is true for the ability to create a vast number of human expressions, including smiling and pouting. Finally, the role of lips in facial beauty and human sensuality cannot be underestimated. The ability to restore both the form and function required to perform these advance tasks is an integral skill required of all reconstructive surgeons.

Defects of the lips are most often acquired secondarily. Traumatic injuries do occur; however, defects secondary to oncologic excision are much more common. Squamous cell carcinoma is the most common malignancy and the lower lip is involved approximately 90% of the time. Regardless of the etiology, form must be restored carefully and meticulously. Many techniques have been described and modified over time, but the ultimate goal has remained the same: sensate, functional, and aesthetically pleasing lips. This chapter highlights the essential features and techniques involved in the reconstruction of this complex anatomic structure.

● PATIENT SELECTION

It is important to identify the structures of the lip that are deficient and will require either direct repair or reconstruction. Some defects may be simply superficial and not require reconstruction of the deeper structures. An accurate understanding of the anatomy of the lips is the foundation necessary for a successful reconstruction. The lips exist between the subnasal superiorly, the mental crease inferiorly, and the modioli laterally. They are covered by skin, mucosa, and a unique, keratinized, stratified squamous epithelium known as the vermilion. There is a well-defined border between the skin and the vermilion. If not carefully repaired, the vermilion border is unforgiving when violated. Just above the vermilion border is the white roll, which is prominent because of the underlying orbicularis muscle. The red line is located a few millimeters posterior to where the lips meet during normal closure. This line separates the dry portion of the vermilion from the intraoral mucosa. The central portion of the upper lip forms two philtral peaks that encompass a soft depression known as the philtral groove. The shape of the superior border of the upper lip (which begins laterally at the commissure, rises to a peak at the base of the philtral column, descends to a point in the midline, rises again to the base of the contralateral philtral column, and then descends to the contralateral commissure) is often referred to as the Cupid's bow.

The musculature of the lip is as complex as the function it provides. The orbicularis oris is the dominant muscle that encircles the mouth. It originates at the modiolus: a fibrous structure adherent to the skin just lateral to the commissures bilaterally. The primary function of the orbicularis is to provide the sphincter tone necessary for oral competency. It is also responsible for the ability to pout and to evert the lips. The mentalis muscle originates from the mandibular periosteum and inserts into the chin pad. Contraction of this muscle results in the elevation of the lower lip. The depressor anguli oris, the depressor labii inferioris, and the platysma all contribute to lip depression. The levator anguli oris, the zygomaticus and the levator labii superioris contribute to lip elevation.

The lips have a robust blood supply as demonstrated by both their unique coloration and their impressive ability to avoid infection when injured. The dominant supply comes from the superior and inferior labial arteries that run below the vermilion in a plane between the orbicularis oris and the oral mucosa. These small arteries branch off the facial artery just lateral to the commissures. Most flaps are designed based on the location of these arteries. Due to the extensive collateral network, however, certain flaps can also survive on a random blood supply.

Lip sensation is provided by both the mental and the infraorbital nerves. The mental nerve is a branch of the mandibular division of the trigeminal nerve. The infraorbital nerve is a branch of the maxillary division of the trigeminal nerve. Motor innervation of the lips is provided by the buccal and marginal mandibular branches of the facial nerve. Most of the motor innervation occurs on the posterior surface of the muscles; however, the mentalis muscle is innervated on its anterior surface.

Any patient with a lip defect is in theory a candidate for reconstruction. However, patient comorbidities may often delay or prevent surgery. The ideal patient is either a young, healthy trauma patient or a patient who recently had a resection of a lip cancer with negative margins and no metastatic disease. Unfortunately, the situation is usually more complex. Trauma patients may have other potentially life-threatening injuries, and oncology patients may have inadequately resected disease or adverse effects secondary to other treatment modalities. Major reconstructive lip surgery, especially procedures that irreversibly alter the surrounding normal tissue, should be delayed until the patient can safely tolerate what usually amounts to an elective operation. In addition, the surgeon should be reasonably sure a proper cancer resection has been performed based on a tissue diagnosis and the current recommendations for surgical margins.

● PATIENT PREPARATION

Prior to performing any reconstructive procedure, it is essential to discuss the risks, benefits, common complications, alternative options, and postoperative care with the patient in as much detail as possible. Discussions about postoperative feeding should take place prior to any procedure that may temporarily interfere with mouth opening (eg, Abbe flap) due to pedicled blood supply.

From a technical perspective, patients undergoing lip surgery should be prepped with some form of antiseptic, although the utility of this is questionable due to the nonsterile nature of the mouth. Perioperative antibiotics are usually recommended. Nasotracheal intubation is the preferred method of maintaining an airway, as it allows the lips to be completely accessible and it prevents distortion of the perioral anatomy. If this is not possible, oral intubation is usually tolerated fairly well by placing the tube on the contralateral side. Performing some procedures under local anesthesia with sedation is another option. Finally, the endotracheal tube must be secured in a manner that does not interfere with the operation. Wiring the tube to a maxillary tooth avoids the excessive use of tape and can decrease the incidence of accidental intraoperative extubation.

● TECHNIQUE

Superficial Defects

Small superficial defects of the vermilion or the surrounding lip often heal well by secondary intention. Minimal distortion should be expected, however, as a degree of contraction will occur in all healing wounds. This contraction can be reduced by closing the defect primarily; alternatively, some surgeons advocate using a full-thickness skin graft. In our experience, however, full-thickness skin grafts result in an aesthetically unacceptable result. These techniques should only be used with defects superficial to the orbicularis oris muscle. Deeper defects require a more complicated repair.

Vermilion Defects

Lip vermilion is specialized tissue that is unlike any other soft tissue in the body. It has unique properties of color and texture that result in a suboptimal aesthetic result if reconstructed with any other type of tissue. Additionally, lip vermilion overlies muscle that is essential to maintaining proper sphincteric function of the lip. If at all possible, vermilion should be reconstructed with vermilion.

Small, lateral, superficial defects of the vermilion will usually heal by secondary intention with acceptable results. Similar defects located more medially can often be closed primarily. The skin edges should be approximated carefully and everted in order to prevent lip notching. Anatomic landmarks, particularly the white roll and the vermilion border, should be marked prior to injecting local anesthetic solution, as injection will distort the normal lip anatomy. Alignment sutures can be used in place of marking to assure accurate approximation; even small discrepancies are noticeable at conversational distance. Three-layer closure of the buccal mucosa, orbicularis oris, and skin can then be performed. Mucosal closure should be accomplished with a fast absorbable suture, while the muscle layer is closed with a slowly absorbable suture. Accurate re-approximation of the orbicularis oris muscle will help prevent stomal incompetency. A secure deep closure also minimizes tension on the cutaneous closure, which should be performed using small, permanent suture that is usually removed after 5 days.

Larger defects of the vermilion require more advanced reconstructive procedures, including vermilion advancement flaps or vermilion switch flaps. Vermilion advancement flaps are most useful when repairing midline vermilion defects.[1] After extraoral and intraoral incisions are made, tissue flaps are then created. These flaps include vermilion and are based on the labial artery. The flaps are advanced into the defect and sutured in place. The extraoral incision is extremely important cosmetically; it should be made precisely at the vermilion border and it should be meticulously repaired.

A bipedicled contralateral labial mucosal flap is often used to repair vermilion defects when additional soft tissue bulk is required. Labial mucosa flaps from the opposite lip are raised on a pedicles and rotated 180 degrees to fill the defect. The flap can be divided 10 to 14 days later, at which time the donor defects can be repaired with a vermilion advancement flap. Patient compliance is important for this procedure as lip motion prior to flap division, and inset can compromise the reconstructive result.

When the remaining vermilion is inadequate for a complete reconstruction, tongue flaps can be used in an attempt to reconstruct vermilion. The ventral portion of the tongue is used because it provides a closer tissue match than the dorsal portion. The leading edge of the flap is sutured to the most anterior aspect of the defect, and the pedicle is divided after 2 weeks. Again, patient compliance and a previously discussed nutrition plan are essential. Although these flaps close the defect and provide adequate bulk, reconstruction with tongue tissue provides an aesthetically suboptimal result. In addition, tongue flaps often require moisturizing regimens, as constant exposure to an unnatural environment leads to desiccation and flaking.

Lower Lip Defects Less Than One Third the Width

Reconstruction of defects that involve less than one third of the total width of the lower lip can usually be closed primarily. The three layers involved in the closure are fairly compliant and can usually be brought together without causing microstomia or creating an obvious

size discrepancy between lips. When dealing with these defects one of the most important anatomic landmarks is the mental crease. The mental crease marks the inferior border of the gingivo-buccal sulcus, and incisions through this crease result in suboptimal aesthetic result.

Wedge excision of the lower lip is a relatively straightforward way to remove either cancerous or damaged soft tissue in a manner that facilitates primary closure. Two essential rules should be followed: incisions should not cross the mental crease and the vertex of the wedge should not exceed 30 degrees. If an excision requires either a vertex angle greater than 30 degrees, or an incision through the mental crease, a w-plasty may be performed. The w-plasty is a modified wedge excision which employs a W-shaped excision. The apices of the W are directed inferiorly, and again the vertex angles should not exceed 30 degrees or cross the mental crease. This modification permits the excision of wider defects without compromising aesthetic outcome.

Another option is a rectangular or barrel excision. This procedure can be used when a wedge excision would result in an incision that crosses the mental crease. A rectangular segment of tissue is excised, and a crescent-shaped incision is created around the mental prominence. The incision creates bilateral flaps that are then advanced medially (Figures 31-1A–C and 31-2A, B) to close the defect. Excision of crescent-shaped areas of normal skin

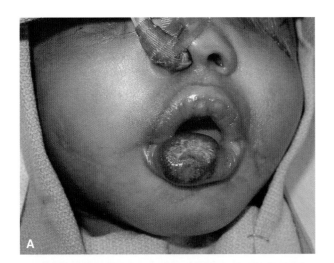
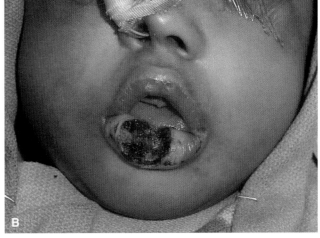
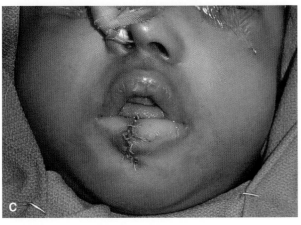

● FIGURE 31-1. (A) A pediatric patient with a large lower lip lesion. (B) The patient following excision of the lesion with markings for bilateral advancement flaps. (C) The patient following closure of the reconstructed lower lip.

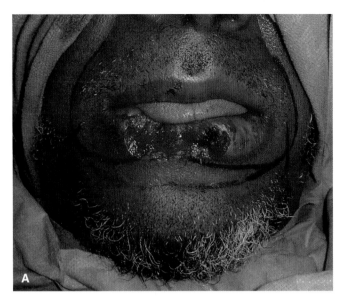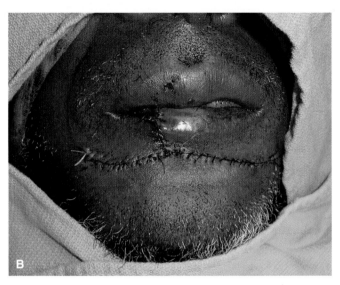

● **FIGURE 31-2.** (A) A patient with a lower lip defect after oncologic resection with markings for bilateral rotation-advancement flaps. (B) The patient following flap inset.

around the mental prominence may be necessary in order to advance the lateral tissue without distorting the normal lower face architecture.

The most important principle to consider when closing these lip defects is the need for a meticulous three-layer closure, including a careful approximation of the muscular layer. Additionally, if these techniques are used to repair traumatic lip defects where the damaged margins are excised, the principles of contaminated wound closure must be applied. These principles include copious irrigation, debridement of nonviable tissue, removal of foreign bodies, and meticulous hemostasis.

Lower Lip Defects Between One Third and Two Thirds the Width

Larger defects, involving one third to two thirds the total width of the lower lip, demand a more complex reconstruction. Previously mentioned techniques inevitably lead to microstomia and occasionally sphincter incompetence when applied to more moderately sized defects. As a result, procedures that recruit tissue from uninvolved parts of the lip can be employed. Lip-switch procedures are the most commonly used methods for the reconstruction of medium-sized defects.

The Abbe flap is one of the most consistent and reliable methods of lip reconstruction (Figure 31-3A–D). The Abbe flap provides healthy lip tissue, including vermilion, from the opposite lip and successfully replaces "like with like." This flap also allows for the transposition of hair-bearing skin, which is an important consideration when operating on men. From a technical perspective, a full-thickness lip flap based on the labial artery is raised from the donor lip. Extreme care is taken to protect the arterial pedicle, as damage to the sole blood supply will likely

result in flap loss. The flap is then rotated 180 degrees and sutured into the original defect. While this flap has been described as a free composite graft, its use as a rotational flap gives predictable results. The pedicle is divided after 14 to 21 days and the flap is inset. It is important to note that ideally, only tissue lateral to the philtrum should be used; violating the anatomic boundaries of the philtrum results in an undesirable cosmetic deformity. Additionally, Abbe flaps should be designed so that the width of the flap is approximately half the width of the defect. This important principle ensures that each lip is shortened by the same amount and prevents aesthetically unpleasing asymmetry. Finally, bilateral Abbe flaps can be used in patients with large, centrally located, lower lip defects. The flaps are raised laterally to the philtral column and rotated medially into place. Surgical scars can usually be hidden in the borders of the aesthetic subunits.

The staircase or stepladder advancement flap is another reconstruction option. Both unilateral and bilateral versions have been described and their use depends on whether the defect is medial or lateral. "Stairs" are created on either one or both sides of the defect; the width of the each stair is approximately half the width of the defect. The height of each stair is approximately 8 mm. Usually two to four stairs are required for closure. This method unfortunately leads to more noticeable scarring than most other procedures.

The Estlander flap is another form of cross lip reconstruction. It differs from the Abbe flap; in that it can be used to reconstruct defects that involve the lateral commissure. An ipsilateral, triangular-shaped flap with curvilinear borders is raised from the upper lip. This flap is then rotated 180 degrees into the defect. Closure is completed in one stage, however, and the modiolus is displaced and the commissure is obliterated. Frequently, the result is a

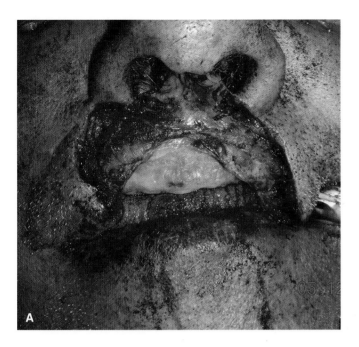

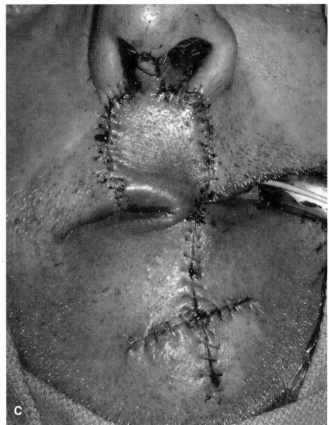

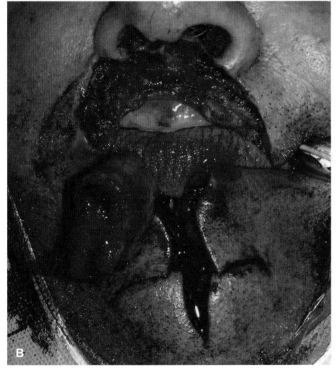

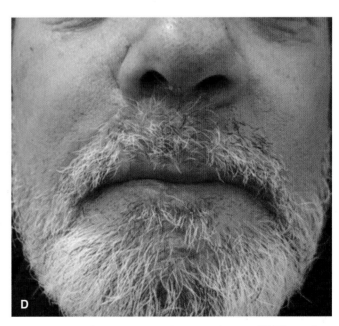

● **FIGURE 31-3.** (A) A patient with a large upper lip defect following resection of recurrent basal cell carcinoma. (B) The patient undergoing harvest of an Abbe flap from the lower lip based on the inferior labial artery. (C) The patient following inset of the Abbe flap into upper lip and primary closure of the lower lip donor site. (D) The final result of the patient several months after the division and inset of the Abbe flap.

new, unnaturally round commissure. Depending on the clinical situation and the patient's preference, this can often be corrected with a secondary procedure.

The Gillies fan flap is a rotation advancement flap that reconstructs lateral defects by recruiting tissue from the mesolabial fold in addition to advancing ipsilateral lip and rotating the opposing lip.[2] When using a Gillies flap, a fan-shaped area of tissue is raised from the ipsilateral upper lip, which is then rotated around a point adjacent to the oral commissure to close a lateral lower lip defect.

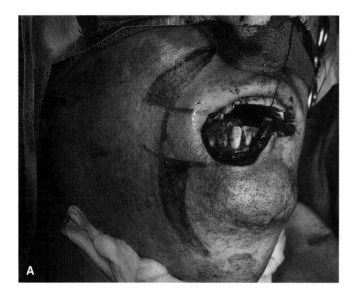

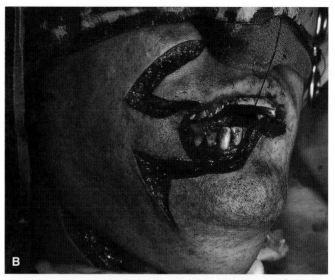

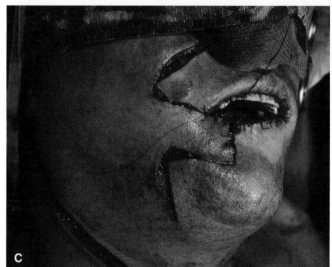

● **FIGURE 31-4.** (A) A patient with a large lower lip soft tissue defect secondary to oncologic resection. (B) The patient demonstrating modification of a unilateral Bernard-Burrow-Webster flap to close the defect. Soft tissue triangles are excised to allow medial advancement without distortion of the cheek. (C) The patient demonstrating inset of the Bernard-Burrow-Webster flap.

The Gillies modification allows for the mobilization of greater amounts of tissue, but suffers from the same rounded commissure seen in the Estlander flap.

Karapandzic further modified the Gillies flap by designing a flap that preserves both neurovascular supply and motor function. Large circumoral incisions are made in the melolabial crease that extend inferiorly to the lower lip (Figure 31-4A–C). Flaps are rotated inferomedially in order to close the defect (Figure 31-5A, B). This procedure, similar to the previous designs from which it was modified, often results in a rounded commissure and microsomia.

Lower Lip Defects Greater Than Two Thirds the Width

Subtotal or total defects of the lower lip often require the most advanced reconstructive techniques. Attempts to use local tissue for near-complete defects have been described. However, there is usually insufficient local tissue to recreate a lower lip without compromising function and creating unacceptable aesthetic results. With that caveat in mind, several local techniques are available. A modification of the Gillies fan flap that entails rotating the flap about the oral commissure can be used to reconstruct extensive defects of the lower lip. Based on the labial vessels, this flap may be raised bilaterally to reconstruct the lower lip. The orbicularis fibers are also rotated with the flap, however, and altered sphincteric function or sphincter incompetence may result.

The Bernard-Burrow-Webster flap is a horizontal, cheek advancement musculocutaneous flap that, if raised bilaterally, can be used to reconstruct the entire lower lip. The creation of a Bernard-Burrow-Webster flap involves creating a horizontal incision lateral to the oral commissure, followed by excising a cutaneous triangle (Burrow's triangle) lateral to the philtral column to allow medial advancement of the flap without otherwise distorting the cheek.[3] Neovermilion creation is then undertaken to complete the reconstruction.

Another well-described method of total lower lip reconstruction with local tissues is the gate flap, originally described by Fujimori et al. in 1968. This flap utilizes

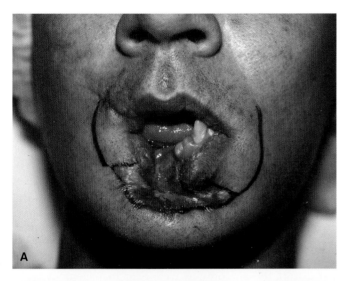

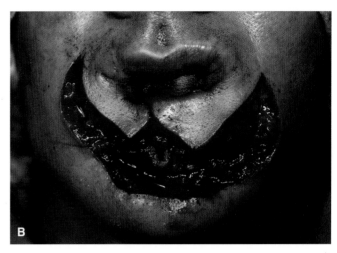

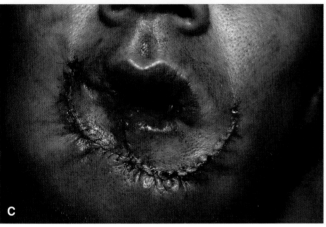

● **FIGURE 31-5.** (A) A patient with a lower lip defect secondary to post-traumatic deformity. (B) The patient demonstrating use of a Karapandzic flap to rotate and advance lateral tissue to fill medial lower lip defect. (C) The patient following closure of the defect demonstrating a moderate amount of microstomia.

bilateral wedges of tissue extending along the nasolabial folds to the inferior border of the mandible that are rotated medially. These two flaps are then sutured together and come together somewhat like a gate, giving this flap its descriptive name. A secondary z-plasty after an appropriate interval improves the cosmesis and overall function of the reconstruction.

Many methods of distant tissue transfer have also been described. All options unfortunately share the need to create a new vermilion with either tongue or mucosal advancement flaps. As stated previously, use of distant tissues in an attempt to accomplish this task is suboptimal.[4] In the event that distant tissue is the only option, several pedicled and free flaps have been described. The deltopectoral and pectoralis major flaps are particularly useful for reconstructing the entire lower lip but primarily provide adynamic bulk. The radial forearm, gracilis, and anterolateral thigh flaps are among the most popular options for free tissue transfer.

The radial forearm free flap is the most commonly performed free tissue reconstruction of the lip.[5] It can be combined with palmaris longus tendon in order to improve sphincter function. Anastomosing the lateral antebrachial cutaneous nerve to the mental nerve can provide sensation. The flap is usually folded over the palmaris tendon, which is sutured to periosteum, to provide support for the lower lip. The tendon may also be sutured to remaining orbicularis fibers to provide a more dynamic appearance. Vermilion reconstruction is performed and hair transplantation can be used to improve skin texture and to help camouflage the scars.

The free gracilis flap, often harvested with a branch of the obturator nerve, has also been successfully used to reconstruct subtotal or total lip defects.[6] The facial artery and vein are used as recipient vessels. The marginal branch of the facial nerve can be anastomosed to the obturator branch of the gracilis flap, allowing for flap innervation. If any orbicularis muscle remains, the remnant fibers can be sutured to the gracilis, which helps provide some sphincter function. Skin grafting and vermilion reconstruction complete the procedure.

Upper Lip Defects

Upper lip reconstruction can usually be accomplished by following the same principles and techniques described for lower lip reconstruction with a few additional considerations. While the upper lip is not as important from a functional perspective, it contains most of the anatomic landmarks and aesthetic subunits responsible for the appearance of the lips. The philtral columns, philtrum, upper vermilion border, and nasolabial folds are all very important in terms of aesthetics. In the event that a large percentage of an anatomic subunit must be violated, it is often better to resect the subunit en bloc and to replace it in its entirety. Additionally, the proximity of the upper lip to the nose makes any scar contracture more noticeable. Distortion of the nasal anatomy can be quite obvious, even to the casual observer.

Upper lip reconstruction is often required as a secondary procedure in patients who previously underwent the repair of a bilateral cleft lip. These patients are often missing bulk in the upper lip and the soft tissue that is present is often scarred and contracted. Use of an Abbe flap in this situation to create a new philtrum usually yields excellent results.

The patient's gender must be taken into consideration during upper lip reconstruction. While the use of hair-bearing skin in men will allow for postreconstruction scar camouflage, transposing hair-bearing skin to the lip in women is less than ideal. For example, the delayed temporal frontal scalp flap is a good option for upper lip reconstruction in men. This flap recruits hair-bearing skin and subsequently produces a better result.

● COMPLICATIONS

Due to the important aesthetic and functional characteristics of the lips, successful reconstruction is both essential and technically difficult. In addition to standard complications including bleeding, infection, and abnormal scarring, there are several well-described complications specific to lip reconstruction. Often, secondary procedures are needed to correct these problems.

Microstomia results when too large a percentage of lip tissue is excised and the defect is closed without introducing new tissue (Figure 31-5C). This may occur following the reconstruction of large defects with local advancement flaps. Microsomia is functionally compromising as it limits the patient's ability to eat, wear dentures, or be orally intubated. It can also be emotionally disturbing to the patient, especially in social situations. Surgical correction of this complication is usually necessary. A procedure that either rearranges or recruits tissue in the deficient area is often employed.

Loss of sphincteric function or oral competency is most commonly seen when dealing with defects that involve large portions of the muscular lower lip. This can result in drooling, impaired phonation, and difficulty eating. Loss of sensation secondary to nerve transection is a well-described complication of any procedure that uses incisions designed to divide tissue in the vicinity of sensory nerves.

A rounded commissure may result if rotational procedures near the commissure are used. Displacement of the modiolus results in the distortion of the normal lateral lip features and can be aesthetically unpleasing. A secondary commissure-plasty is often required to restore the normal appearance. Scar contractures and hypertrophic scarring can distort the anatomy as well. Scar management techniques as well as early scar release are employed to correct this distortion.

Careful planning, extensive knowledge of the anatomy, and meticulous technique are essential when attempting to prevent these complications.

● OUTCOME

Lip reconstruction is a difficult task due to the complex anatomy as well as the high functional and aesthetic demands. Postoperatively, patients should be followed to assess their overall function, especially their ability to maintain oral competence, as well as their natural appearance. An acceptable aesthetic and functional outcome will be achieved if several fundamental principles apply regardless of whether a defect is the result of trauma or oncologic resection. By respecting the concepts of aesthetic subunits, recruiting additional tissue when necessary, and meticulously re-approximating vital structures, both form and function can be restored. When defects cannot be closed primarily, transposition, rotation advancement, and occasionally free flaps may be employed. The anatomic reconstruction of a carefully evaluated lip defect in a properly prepared patient can produce excellent results with a low risk of functionally and aesthetically devastating complications.

REFERENCES

1. Boutros S. Reconstruction of the lips. In: Thorne CH, Bartlett SB, Beasley RW, et al., eds. *Grabb and Smith's Plastic Surgery.* 6th ed. Philadelphia: Lippincott, Williams & Wilkins; 2006.

2. Lesavoy M, Smith A. Lower third face and lip reconstruction. In Mathes SJ, ed. *Plastic Surgery.* Vol. 2. 2nd ed. Philadelphia: Saunders; 2005.

3. McCarn K, Park S. Lip reconstruction. *Otolaryngol Clin North Am.* 2007;(40):361–380.

4. Sarukawa S, Kashiwaya G, Sakuraba M. A new flap design for reconstruction full-thickness defects of the lower lip: The extended upper lip island (EULI) flap. *J Plast Reconstr Aesthet Surg.* 2006(59):1436–1441.

5. Lee J, Fernandes R. Microvascular reconstruction of extended total lip defects. *Oral Surg Oral Med Oral Pathol Oral Radiol Endod.* 2007;104(2):170–176.

6. Ninkovic M, Spanio di Spilimbergo S, Nincovic M. Lower lip reconstruction: introduction of a new procedure using a functioning gracilis muscle free flap. *Plast Reconstr Surg.* 2007;119(5):1472–1480.

chapter 32

Cheek Reconstruction

Richard A. Hopper, MD, MS / *Scott D. Imahara, MD* /
Jon P. Ver Halen, MD / *Joseph S. Gruss, MD, FRCS[C]*

● INTRODUCTION

The functional facial areas of the eyelid, nose, mouth, and ear border the cheek region. Although it does not have the same intrinsic functional properties as these adjacent structures, inappropriate cheek reconstruction will reliably disrupt facial function, resulting in debilitating patient morbidity. Reconstruction of cheek defects requires meticulous preoperative planning, consideration of the effect of scar contracture on the adjacent soft tissue, and precise surgical technique. Successful cheek reconstruction relies on an intimate understanding of the skin quality of the different areas of the face by age, the vascular supply of the tissues, and the optimum orientation and location of scar placement. Despite these challenges, unlike other areas of the face, the cheek has a laxity and compliance that permits a variety of reconstructive options ranging from primary closure to extensive local and regional flaps. The focus of this chapter is reconstruction of the skin and subcutaneous tissues of the cheek. Facial nerve, parotid duct, and bone injuries are covered elsewhere in this text.

● PATIENT EVALUATION

Key to the assessment of patients with cheek defects is their precise location because different areas of the cheek require different reconstructive options. Gonzalez-Ulloa and colleagues[1] provided an original description of the regional esthetic units of the cheek which was later subdivided into three overlapping regions by Zide[2] (Figure 32-1). A modified demarcation of these subunits into three, interdigitated triangular zones has been adopted that aligns with our approach to regional flap selection and rotation (Figure 32-2).

The medial infraorbital triangle (triangle I) is the area bounded superiorly by the lower eyelid, medially by the nasolabial groove and lateral nasal unit, and laterally by a line from the lateral canthus to the lateral oral commissure. In triangle I, the close relationship of the cheek to the inferior eyelid and external nasal valve pose challenges to reconstruction due to the risk of distorting these two important areas to function and symmetry. Although the lower eyelid is not formally part of the cheek, it is often involved in cheek defects. Since this is a vital component in flap design in this region, we designate cheek defects involving the lower lid as triangle Ia.

The lateral preauricular triangle (triangle II) comprises the region encompassed medially by a line drawn from the lateral canthus to the angle of the mandible, laterally by following the pretragal fold, and superiorly by a line joining the lateral canthus to the hairline. The middle buccomandibular triangle (triangle III) is inverted compared to the other two triangles, with its base inferior. It is bounded by the margin of the mandible inferiorly and triangles I and II medially and laterally, respectively.

Each triangular zone has its own particular characteristics which must be taken into consideration in the reconstruction of cheek defects, including superficial differences in skin color and texture, adjacent functional structures, and underlying vascular, nerve, and muscular anatomy. The landmark boundaries of each zone are not rigid, but rather should serve as an anatomic outline of the principles and techniques of cheek reconstruction. The rest of this chapter uses the interdigitated triangular subunit classification of defects to describe a useful approach to skin and soft tissue reconstruction.

The cheek is composed of the overlying skin envelope, subcutaneous fat, the superficial musculoaponeurotic system (SMAS), muscles of mastication and facial expression, and underlying bone support. There is considerable interindividual variability in the quality and characteristics of the

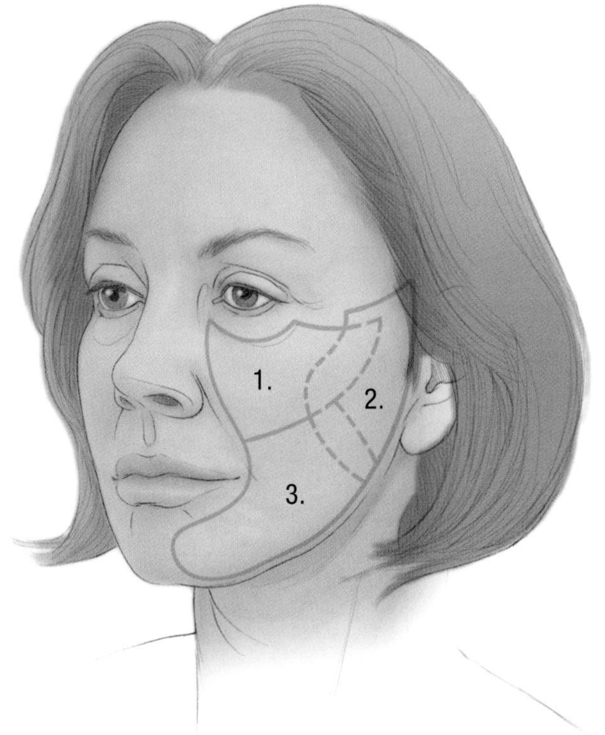

● **FIGURE 32-1.** The aesthetic subunits of the cheek.

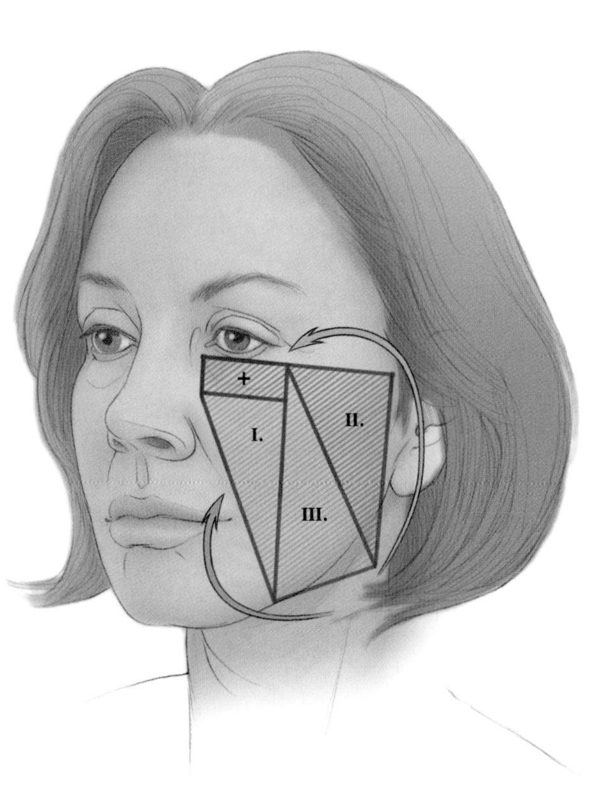

● **FIGURE 32-2.** Reconstructive triangle classification of the cheek.

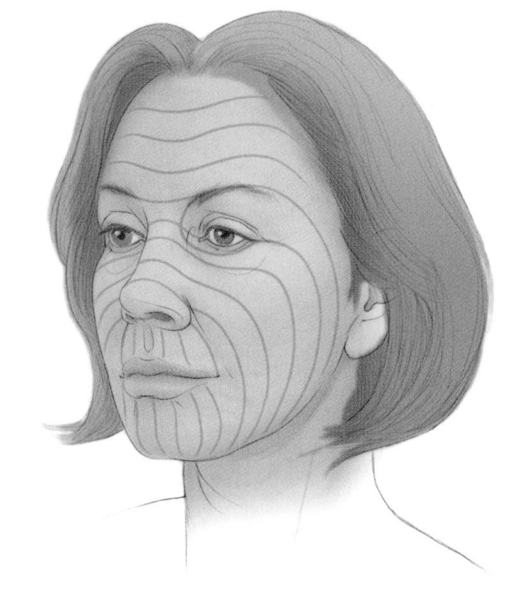

● **FIGURE 32-3.** Facial relaxed skin tension lines. *(From Leach J. Proper handling of soft tissue in the acute phase. Facial Plast Surg. 2001;17(4):227–238.)*

cheek skin. In older patients, the skin envelope is lax, has a paucity of subcutaneous fat, possesses multiple rhytids, and is compliant to stretch. Younger patients in contrast will have more subcutaneous fat and smooth elastic skin.[3] The cheek has a complex pattern of relaxed skin tension lines.[4] Orienting incisions along these lines will optimize the final scar, regardless of age, by minimizing perpendicular stretch (Figure 32-3).

In addition to interindividual variability of the skin, there are also differences in skin quality between different regions of the same patient. Skin within the infraorbital triangle (triangle I; Figure 32-2), including the malar eminence, tends to be relatively thicker, more pigmented, and shiny. Preauricular skin (triangle II) is paler and thinner, with a matte surface texture. Finally, lower cheek skin in triangle III is of intermediate texture, color, and thickness in relation to the other two zones. The terminal hair-bearing skin of the cheek within all three triangles must be carefully observed, including future hair growth in prepubescent males. Patient dissatisfaction will result from reconstruction of a hairless region with skin containing terminal follicles. The transition zone between the lower eyelid and triangle I of the cheek is marked by a change in skin quality (thinner skin in the eyelid), the delicate animation and support provided by the underlying orbicularis oculi muscle, and the attachment of the orbital septum to the arcus marginalis at the inferior orbital rim. Skin and subcutaneous cheek injuries that violate this transition increase the complexity of the reconstruction.

Beneath the skin lies the SMAS, the investing fascial layer of the head and neck.[5,6] This layer is continuous with the platysma in the neck, the temporoparietal fascia in the lateral temporal region, the fascia of the frontalis muscle in the forehead, and galea aponeurotica of the scalp. In the face, the SMAS is located between the subcutaneous fat and deeper structures, including the facial nerve branches, the muscles of the face, the parotid gland, Stensen duct, and the buccal fat pad. Terminal branches of the facial nerve (CN VII) supply all the superficial muscles of facial expression. Freilinger et al. grouped the muscles of facial expression into four layers, with muscles in the three most superficial layers being innervated on their deep surfaces.[7] The muscles in the fourth, or deepest, layer (ie, mentalis, levator anguli oris, and buccinator muscles) are innervated through their lateral or superficial surfaces. The masseter muscle, as well as sensation to the upper lip, infraorbital region, and malar eminence, is innervated by the second division of the trigeminal nerve, the maxillary nerve (CN V2). The infraorbital foramen is located approximately 1 cm below the infraorbital rim, in a line perpendicular to the pupil. The third division of the mandibular nerve (CN V3) provides sensation to the lower lip, mandibular region, and preauricular skin.

The branches of the external carotid artery, and associated minor contributions from the internal carotid artery tree, provide the dominant arterial blood supply to the skin and muscles of the cheek. The facial artery is a branch of the external carotid artery, and enters the cheek by crossing mandible border at 2 to 3 cm anterior to the angle. It then traverses the face obliquely, and provides superior and inferior labial branches below the ala, and the lateral nasal artery above the alar crease before terminating as the angular artery along the side of the nose. The transverse facial artery arises from the superficial temporal artery and crosses the face parallel to the zygoma below the orbit, meeting the angular artery. The dorsal nasal artery emerges along the superior medial surface of the orbit, is a terminal branch of the ophthalmic artery from the internal carotid artery system, and anastomoses with the superior end of the angular artery. These interconnected external and internal carotid artery-supplied systems provide a rich, redundant blood supply to the cheek. Respect for these reliable arterial systems permits the safe elevation and transfer of large local and regional flaps for cheek reconstruction.

The venous drainage from the cheek is predominantly into the external jugular system via the anterior facial vein. A secondary system is via the ophthalmic, infraorbital, and deep facial veins which eventually drain into the intracranial cavernous sinus. Uncontrolled cheek infections therefore have the potential for intracranial extension via the latter route.

PATIENT PREPARATION

Initial interaction with the patient with a cheek defect does not always require immediate, definitive closure. An adequate margin of clean tissue either following trauma or cancer ablation should be confirmed. The planned and potential reconstructive options should be thoroughly discussed with the patient beforehand. Necrotic skin edges can be excised to healthy tissue. A staged or combination approach may be preferable with questionable resection margins or large defects that cross multiple zones. Closure in the emergent setting can usually be accomplished with at least a sterile dressing or skin graft for temporary wound coverage until definitive reconstruction is appropriate. Staged options include the use of tissue expanders to pre-expand local flaps prior to elevation at a second operation.

● TECHNIQUES OF CHEEK RECONSTRUCTION BY TRIANGULAR SUBUNIT

Infraorbital Triangle (Triangle I)

Due to the thicker underlying subcutaneous fat and lack of strong retaining ligaments, the medial aspect of triangle I is relatively mobile, and subunit defects can usually be closed primarily at the nasojugal and nasolabial folds with minimal lateral undermining. Care must be taken, however, to avoid tenting of the nasojugal junction as described in the design of local flaps below. Even small defects, such as benign skin lesion excisions, have the potential to distort the lower eyelid upon primary closure. To avoid this, lesions should be excised as a circular defect and then closed primarily in an orientation that does not distort the eyelid margin. Any residual dog-ear deformities may be excised as needed.

As with most cheek defects, if primary closure is not possible, skin grafting is appropriate in select cases. Examples include defects when tumor surveillance is required after primary ablation, if there are contraindications to a large regional flap such as heavy smoking or poor health, and if a temporizing measure is required prior to planning staged definitive reconstruction. Split-thickness skin grafts in triangle I defects must be used with care, since there is a considerable risk of causing lower eyelid retraction and ectropion, even if the defect does not involve the eyelid itself. Full-thickness skin grafts, which are less prone to contraction, are better suited for skin replacement of superficial defects in this region, but even these grafts can distort the lower eyelid if the defect crosses the cheek–lower lid junction. Appropriate harvest sites for color match include preauricular, postauricular, and supraclavicular skin. Multiple full-thickness skin grafts patching should be avoided, but if necessary, the grafts edges should align with the esthetic subunit borders and be oriented along relaxed skin tension lines (Figure 32-3).

The use of small transposition local flaps within triangle I is restricted by the limited laxity of the adjacent nose and lower eyelid. For medium-sized defects inappropriate for primary closure, wide lateral undermining of the cheek skin in a subcutaneous plane can often close defects in this zone by taking advantage of lateral laxity to advance the skin. These local advancement flaps can easily "tent" in the region of the line of closure at the nasojugal groove. To avoid this potentially difficult secondary deformity, it is extremely important to secure the dermis at the edge of the flap to the periosteum of the nasal bone or piriform

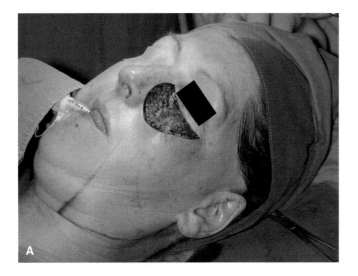
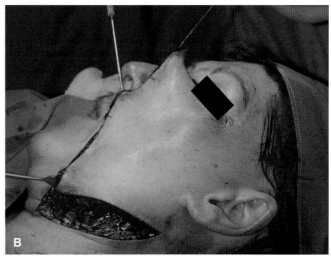
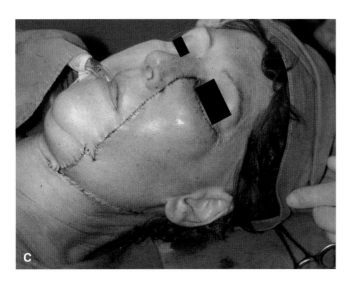

● **FIGURE 32-4.** Reconstruction of complete triangle I defects. (A) A large residual defect within triangle I is shown after lesion excision. (B) A posteriorly based cervicofacial flap was elevated in the subcutaneous plane and perfused by branches of the facial artery. (C) Final flap inset is shown with flap edges created along margins of the aesthetic triangles, including along the nasolabial fold and lateral nasal unit. The flap must be secured to underlying periosteum near the piriform rim and malar eminence to avoid inferior traction on the eyelid. (D) Final result is shown more than 1 year after reconstruction.

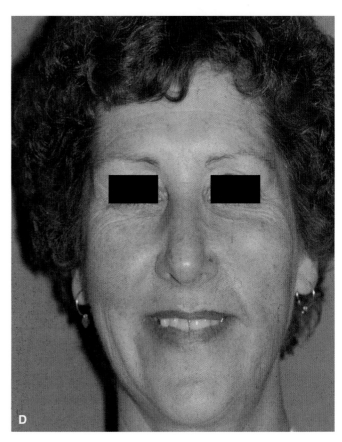

aperture with long-lasting or permanent sutures. All tension on the flap should be on these retaining sutures, such that the nasojugal groove is reformed, and there is no tension on the skin closure line just medial to the groove.

For complete triangle I defects (Figure 32-4), a posteriorly based cervicofacial flap can be employed. When performed correctly, these large flaps are perfused by the facial artery and can provide enough tissue for coverage of the entire triangle I, transferring primary closure of the donor site to the supraclavicular region. The posterior cervicofacial flap can be raised in a plane deep to the SMAS in

the face with subplatysmal extension into the neck for improved flap viability, but with increased risk of damage to the branches of the facial nerve.[8] More commonly, the flap is raised in a subcutaneous plane.

When planning the cervicofacial flap, the desired arc of rotation needs to be determined. For defects not involving the lower eyelid, the flap should be based posteriorly, and can be rotated upward along the nasolabial and mentojugal grooves, limiting the scars to this line as it extends into the supraclavicular region. For triangle Ia defects involving the lower eyelid, the cervicofacial flap is instead based anteriorly, and is rotated in an opposite arc of rotation, superiorly and then medially along the lower eyelid. In these cases, the superior margin of the flap should extend laterally and superiorly above the lateral canthus and into the non–hair-bearing temple region before it heads inferiorly toward the neck via the preauricular crease. The donor site tension is therefore placed either behind the ear or in the lateral neck. This is the Juri[9] modification of Beare's[10] initial description of the flap. By suspending the cervicofacial flap from the temporal region, and again from the infraorbital periosteum, the surgeon can avoid inferior traction on the flap and subsequent eyelid ectropion.

In all cervicofacial flaps for triangle I defects (whether anteriorly or posteriorly based), the distal edge of the flap must be anchored to the periosteum of the malar prominence of the zygoma, the infraorbital rim, the nasal bone, and the piriform aperture. We prefer a series of delayed ties of 3-0 PDS (monofilament polydioxanone) but a Vicryl (polyglactin) suture is also appropriate. Without this detail, the flap will "tent" in this region and distort the shadow of the nasojugal groove and pull inferiorly on the lower eyelid. It must be emphasized that these deep anchoring sutures are not a substitute for full flap dissection and elevation. The tension of closure must be transferred to the donor site in the neck, not placed on the distal flap. The deep anchoring sutures should not provide radial traction on the distal flap which would compromise perfusion; instead, they are used to contour the deep surface of the flap and counter the inferior pull of gravity after the flap has been rotated into the defect.

Preauricular Triangle (Triangle II)

Reconstruction and closure of defects in the preauricular triangle follow principles that are similar to those described for the infraorbital triangle. Skin overlying the preauricular triangle is inherently lax, resulting in an excess of skin and enabling its use as a donor site more often than as a recipient. Moderate-sized defects in zone 2 can often be closed with advancement of anteriorly or inferiorly based undermined subcutaneous flaps, similar to a subcutaneous facelift dissection. Anteriorly based cheek flaps are limited by secondary distortion of the nasofacial groove and oral commissure. The inferiorly based advancement flaps in this zone can be extended well into the neck, as a truncated version of a cervicofacial flap (Figure 32-5).

Defects in the inferior portion of triangle II can be closed with a local transposition flap or a V-Y advancement flap. In both these flaps, the donor site scar should be planned inferior to the defect. This will avoid scarring of the anterior central face, which is visible on frontal view, as well as to minimize edema of the flap and a secondary trap-door deformity. An inferiorly based transposition flap from the postauricular skin can be a reasonable option for inferior preauricular defects, but the patient needs to be aware that the flap will be non-hair bearing.

Two remaining options for reconstruction of triangle II defects are serial excision and tissue expansion, particularly if there are no time constraints such as benign lesions, old defects, or scars.

Buccomandibular Triangle (Triangle III)

Deep defects in triangle III can involve the facial artery, preventing the design of inferiorly based axial cervicofacial flaps, such as those described above. An additional consideration is that reconstruction of full-thickness defects in this zone requires not only skin and soft tissue coverage, but also intraoral buccal lining. Reconstruction of defects involving the orbicularis oris muscle or the lateral commissure of the mouth should first recreate a functional sphincter with labial based dissected muscle slips similar to a macrostomia repair.

Small, partial-thickness triangle III defects may be repaired using local transposition flaps or posteriorly based cervicofacial flap if the facial artery is preserved. Care must be taken to orient incisions along relaxed skin tension lines, in particularly the mentolabial fold whenever possible. Prophylactic w-plasty or z-plasty should be considered for incisions, which cross the mandibular border to minimize linear contracture. Local flap options for intraoral closure that have been described include tongue flaps, turnover or hinge flaps, buccal fat pad flaps, galeal flaps with periosteum, or masseter crossover flaps.[11-17] All of these flaps are then covered by a separate, cutaneous flap. For large full-thickness defects, a variety of regional myocutaneous and composite flaps have been described that enable folding, splitting or paddling, including the deltopectoral fasciocutaneous flap, and the pectoralis major, or trapezius myocutaneous flaps.[18,19]

Combination Zone Defects

Large defects involving both triangles I and II with or without zone 3 pose a particular challenge. A traditional cervicofacial flap in these cases often does not reach the superomedial aspect of the defect adjacent to the lateral nasal unit. In order to advance sufficient tissue from the lower cheek, a well-vascularized robust flap is required. The platysma should be incorporated into the superior portion of the flap, and the pectoral fascia below. This allows elevation of a large inferomedial cervicopectoral flap to be raised based on the anterior thoracic perforators of the internal mammary artery. To avoid vertical banding across the neck, the posterior incision should follow a course under the ear lobule, behind the border of the trapezius, across the acromioclavicular joint and along the lateral pectoralis border. The chest donor defect in these cases typically requires skin grafting. Other options include the medially based deltopectoral flap, the cervicohumoral flap, the trapezius flap, the pectoralis major myocutaneous flap, and the latissimus dorsi myocutaneous flaps.

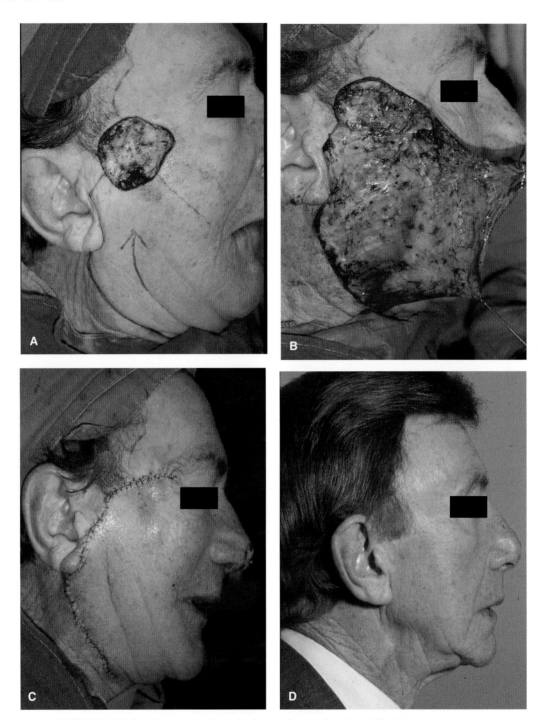

● **FIGURE 32-5.** Reconstruction of a large triangle II defect. (A) Defect appearance after lesion excision. (B) The elevation of an inferiorly based cervicofacial flap in the subcutaneous plane with extension into the neck. (C) Final flap inset with flap margins along the borders the aesthetic triangles. (D) Final result more than 1 year after reconstruction.

Microvascular transfer flaps have largely replaced these large pedicled regional flaps for large defects due to decreased donor site morbidity. For malignant lesions that have undergone or will undergo irradiation, microvascular free flaps have become the mainstay of treatment of complex full-thickness defects. Well-vascularized tissue distant from an irradiated field, with unlimited three-dimensional movement, conformability, and the ability to transfer composite tissue such as bone, have made free flaps particularly attractive in this application. The radial forearm free flap (RFFF) is often utilized as a reconstructive option. The RFFF can be harvested with palmaris longus tendon to enable resuspension of the lateral lip if it is involved, and it can be folded to enable combined inner lining and

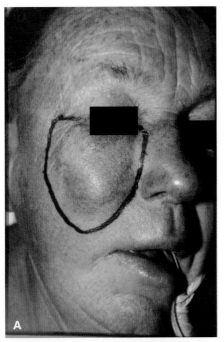

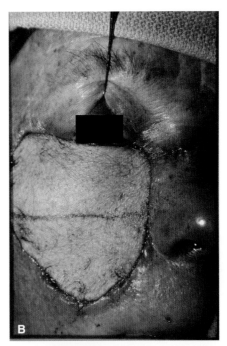

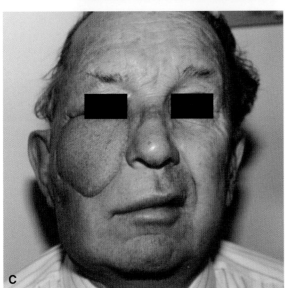

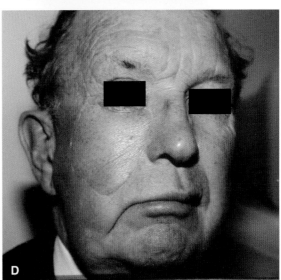

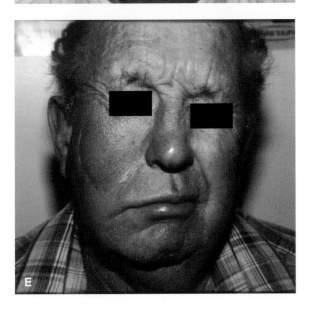

● FIGURE 32-6. Microvascular reconstruction of a large combination zone defect. (A) Preoperative view of a 62-year-old man with a large angiosarcoma involving triangle I and Ia (ie, the lower eyelid) and triangle III. (B) Intraoperative result after lesion extirpation and reconstruction with a parascapular free flap. (C) Early result several weeks after cheek reconstruction. (D, E) Final result more than 1 year after final lower eyelid reconstruction using a Hughes tarsoconjunctival flap.

skin coverage. In addition, thinning of the RFFF can allow cheek reconstruction with satisfactory facial contour. Other microvascular flaps available for application in full-thickness buccal defects include the tensor fascia lata free flap[20] and the parascapular free flap[21] (Figure 32-6).

As stated earlier, staged reconstructive options include the use of tissue expanders to pre-expand local flaps prior to elevation at a second operation. The tissue expanders are placed subcutaneously under the cheek via scalp or facelift approaches, with a remote reservoir placed over the mastoid or under the scalp to allow gradual expansion (Figure 32-7). A combination of flaps or approaches is also possible. A cervicofacial flap can be used to reconstruct the zone 2 and 3 components of the defect, while a delayed two-stage forehead flap could be used to reconstruct the zone 1 component (Figure 32-8).

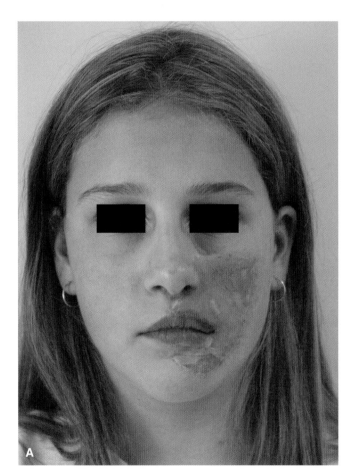

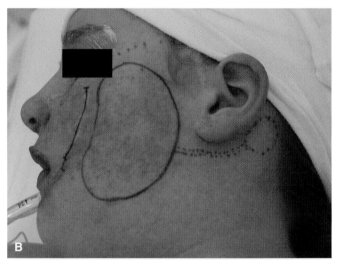

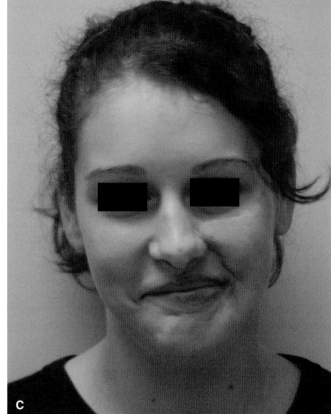

● FIGURE 32-7. Staged cheek reconstruction using tissue expansion. (A) An adolescent girl who underwent excision of a congenital nevus involving triangle I, triangle III, and upper lip as an infant. The cheek had been resurfaced with gluteal full-thickness skin and the upper lip with supraclavicular full-thickness skin. These distant donor sites demonstrate the limitations of poorly matched skin graft in cheek reconstruction. (B) Prior to placement of a cheek tissue expander to pre-expand a posteriorly based cervicofacial flap. The tissue expander fill port is placed distant to the device over the mastoid. (C) Final result after elevation and reconstruction using a pre-expanded cerviofacial flap.

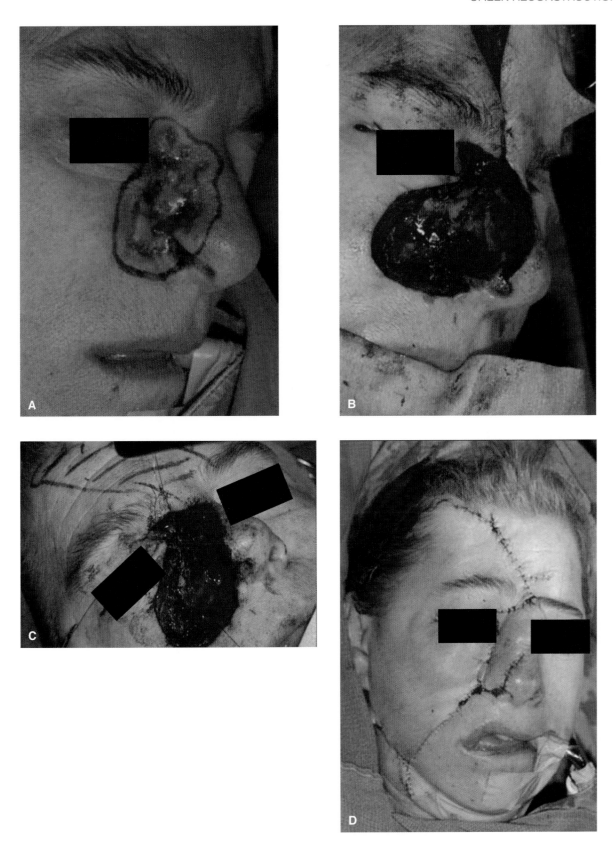

● FIGURE 32-8. Combination flap reconstruction. (A) Operative view of a
squamous cell cancer involving triangle I, the medial canthus, and the lateral nose.
(B, C) Intraoperative view after cancer extirpation demonstrating a large defect including
triangle I, Ia (the lower eyelid), triangle III, full-thickness lateral nose and alar rim.
(D) Final flap reconstruction using a posteriorly based cervicofacial flap for reconstruction
of the cheek elements and a first-stage forehead flap. Note the junction of the two flaps
is placed along the margin of the nasal and cheek aesthetic subunits.

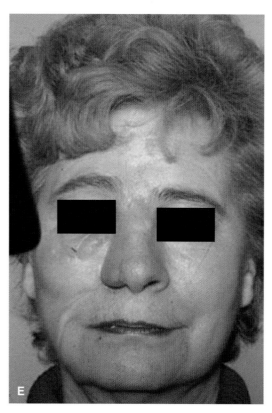

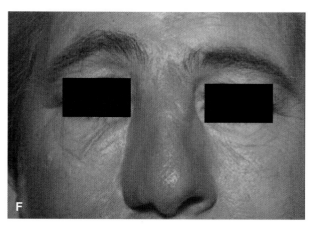

● FIGURE 32-8. (*continued*) (E, F) Final result after second stage division of the forehead flap.

● COMPLICATIONS

Because of the intricate anatomy of the face, numerous complications can occur following reconstruction. Certainly, scars should be placed in the least conspicuous locations. For defects of triangle I, closure of even small defects by primary approximation has the potential to displace the lower eyelid inferiorly, resulting in either eyelid retraction or ectropion. To avoid this, lesions should be excised as a circular defect and then closed primarily in an orientation that does not distort the margin of the lower eyelid. Any residual dog-ear deformities may be excised as needed. Widening of the nasal base can occur with reconstruction of zone 2 defects. Care should be taken to not release the soft tissue attachment of the base of the flap to the piriform rim to avoid this complication. For defects in triangle III, appropriate intraoral, water-tight closure needs to be achieved prior to addressing skin closure. If the oral closure is inadequate, orofacial fistula, flap breakdown, severe contraction, or infection will result.

● OUTCOMES ASSESSMENT

Conceptualizing cheek defects as three interconnected triangular zones facilitates creation of a reconstruction plan that will preserve both form and function. Basic plastic surgery principles must be followed, such as orienting scars along the relaxed skin tension lines or natural esthetic subunit junctions, reconstructing like tissue with like, and transferring the tension of closure to the laxity of the donor site. Variations of the cervicofacial flap with different arcs of rotation based on the location of the defect are the work horses of cheek reconstruction. More complex defects require multiple regional flaps, a staged approach, or microvascular transfer of tissue. Care must be taken in flap planning to avoid distortion of the adjacent lower eyelid, the nasojugal groove, and the oral commissure by tension-free insetting of the flap into the defect with adequate suspension and anchoring the flap to the deep tissues.

REFERENCES

1. Gonzalez-Ulloa M, Castillo A, Stevens E, et al. Preliminary study of the total restoration of the facial skin. *Plast Reconstr Surg.* 1954;13(3):151–161.

2. Zide B. Deformities of the lips and cheeks. In: McCarthy J, ed. *Plastic Surgery*. Philadelphia: Saunders, WB; 1990.

3. Friedman O. Changes associated with the aging face. *Facial Plast Surg Clin North Am.* 2005;13:371–380.

4. Borges A. Relaxed skin tension lines (RSTL) versus other skin lines. *Plast Reconstr Surg.* 1984;73:144–150.

5. Mitz V, Peyronie M. The superficial musculo-aponeurotic system (SMAS) in the parotid & cheek areas. *Plast Reconstr Surg.* 1976;58:80–88.

6. Friedman O. Facelift surgery. *Facial Plast Surg.* 2006;22(2):120–128.

7. Freilinger G, Gruber H, Happak W, Pechmann U. Surgical anatomy of the mimic muscle system and the facial nerve: importance for reconstructive and aesthetic surgery. *Plast Reconstr Surg.* 1987;80(5):686–690.

8. Kroll SS, Reece GP, Robb G, Black J. Deep-plane cervicofacial rotation-advancement flap for reconstruction of large cheek defects. *Plast Reconstr Surg.* 1994;94(1):88–93.

9. Juri J, Juri C. Advancement and rotation of a large cervicofacial flap for cheek repairs. *Plast Reconstr Surg.* 1979;64(5): 692–696.

10. Beare R. Flap repair following exenteration of the orbit. *Proc R Soc Med.* 1969;62(11 Part 1):1087–1090.

11. Chambers RG, Jaques LD, Mahoney WD. Tongue flaps for intraoral reconstruction. *Am J Surg.* 1969;118(5):783–786.

12. Chicarilli ZN. Sliding posterior tongue flap. *Plast Reconstr Surg.* 1987;79(5):697–700.

13. Kim YK, Yeo HH, Kim SG. Use of the tongue flap for intraoral reconstruction: a report of 16 cases. *J Oral Maxillofac Surg.* 1998;56(6):716–719; discussion 720–721.

14. Samman N, Cheung LK, Tideman H. The buccal fat pad in oral reconstruction. *Int J Oral Maxillofac Surg.* 1993;22(1): 2–6.

15. Dean A, Alamillos F, García-López A, Sánchez J, Peñalba M. The buccal fat pad flap in oral reconstruction. *Head Neck.* 2001;23(5):383–388.

16. Stefanovic P, Nikolic Z, Stajcic Z. Reconstruction of full-thickness cheek defect affecting the oral commissure by galeal skin island flap: a case report. *J Craniomaxillofac Surg.* 1992;20(7):317–319.

17. Langdon JD, Ord RA. The surgical management of lip cancer. *J Craniomaxillofac Surg.* 1987;15(5):281–287.

18. Sharzer LA, Kalisman M, Silver CE, Strauch B. The parasternal paddle: a modification of the pectoralis major myocutaneous flap. *Plast Reconstr Surg.* 1981;67(6):753–762.

19. Nakatsuka T, Harii K, Asato H, et al. Analytic review of 2372 free flap transfers for head and neck reconstruction following cancer resection. *J Reconstr Microsurg.* 2003;19(6): 363–368; discussion 369.

20. Endo T, Nakayama Y, Soeda S. Reconstruction of the cheek and palate using a three-paddle tensor fasciae latae free flap. *Br J Plast Surg.* 1991;44(3):234–235.

21. Upton J, Albin RE, Mulliken JB, Murray JE. The use of scapular and parascapular flaps for cheek reconstruction. *Plast Reconstr Surg.* 1992;90(6):959–971.

chapter 33

Eyelid Reconstruction and Ptosis Repair

Lisa R. David, MD, FACS / Claire Sanger, DO

● INTRODUCTION

The primary importance of the eyelid is functional, specifically protection of the cornea. Reconstruction of the upper and lower eyelids is challenging because of the complex anatomy and specialized function of the structures. The goal of any type of eyelid defect reconstruction, regardless of the size and layers involved, is globe protection without visual disruption and restoration of the area to an appearance as close to normal as possible. Surgical technique must include repair of all the missing layers of the defect. The etiology of the defect may often impact the choice of reconstructive techniques. Eyelid defects are usually secondary to trauma, congenital abnormalities, or after cancer treatment. There are a significant number of techniques described for eyelid reconstruction that increases the complexity of the surgical decision making process. Many of these techniques are simply variations of the same principle. General principles include replacing like with like, therefore eyelid skin should be the first choice if it is available. If it is not an option then use skin grafts or regional flaps. If nothing else is available, the final option should be a free flap. Reconstruction of the eyelid can be addressed in a straightforward algorithmic approach based on the depth, location, and size of the defect.[1]

● PATIENT EVALUATION

The etiology of the defect needs to be determined and a history of previous treatment to the region must be obtained. In addition, it is important to identify other factors that will affect the repair including previous surgery, radiation, and skin damage in the area of the planned donor site. A detailed history and physical exam of the eyelids is crucial for treatment planning. On physical examination, the horizontal and vertical extent of the defect should be measured and photographed. The condition of the eye itself must be assessed for symptoms of dry eye, chronic irritation, tear production, visual acuity, and muscle function. Timing of the repair depends on the risk that delay will have on the structures the eyelids protect, specifically the cornea. If this is a secondary reconstruction, obtaining pictures and medical records of the previous defect is essential. The depth of the original injury can often be underestimated when evaluating the secondary defect. As a result, secondary defects once recreated intraoperatively may require more extensive surgical intervention.

Additional Studies

Ancillary testing for eyelid reconstruction depends upon the etiology of the defect. Traumatic and congenital defects require radiographic analysis of the orbital bones. Any bony defect will need to be addressed in addition to the soft tissue defect. If the etiology is postoncologic resection then final pathologic diagnosis with confirmed clear margins is necessary. This is sometimes problematic for patients where there is no access to Mohs microscopic surgery. Choices for management of cancer in this region include Mohs surgery versus frozen section versus permanent histology with delayed reconstruction. However, it is in the patient's best interest to be sure there is no residual cancer prior to starting the reconstruction; otherwise some of the reconstructive options may be lost.

● PATIENT PREPARATION

Reconstruction of the eyelid is a complex process often requiring a staged approach. It is important to discuss with the patient the possible need for multiple procedures. The patient's ability to tolerate more than one procedure may impact your choice of reconstructive options. Even with a planned one-stage procedure, secondary work is often indicated. In addition, a discussion of the type of anesthesia is warranted. The patient's ability to have a local rather than a general anesthesia must be considered in surgical planning. Some patients will have significant medical comorbidities and are unable to undergo general anesthesia. Local anesthesia is often a viable option but it may impact the selection of surgical technique. The postoperative course must be discussed, including a possible period of eye irritation and redness requiring eye drops or patching. Once the patient and his or her family are aware of what the surgery will involve, it is appropriate to proceed with the surgical repair.

● TECHNIQUE

An algorithmic approach incorporating defect size, thickness, and location is the easiest approach (Figure 33-1). Many techniques have been described for all types of eyelid defects. Rather than explain each procedure in detail, this chapter will focus on technique choice. To understand the choice of surgical techniques that follow, it is imperative to understand the complex eyelid anatomy (Figure 33-2). The skin of the eyelid is the thinnest in the body. Deep to the skin is a very thin layer of subcutaneous tissue and deep to that the orbicularis oculi muscle. The tarsal plate is deep to the orbicularis oculi muscle. In the upper eyelid, the levator palpebrae superioris is attached to the superior margin of the tarsus. The ends of the tarsal plates are attached to the medial and lateral orbital margins by the medial and lateral palpebral ligaments. The conjunctiva, the inner lining of the eyelid, runs over the sclera to the cornea and joins it at the limbus. The orbicularis oculi muscle is responsible for opening and closing the eyelids. The levator palpebrae superioris muscle, in conjunction with Muller muscle, elevates the upper lid. The eyelid sensory innervation is from the trigeminal nerve, both the ophthalmic and maxillary division. The motor innervation to the orbicularis oculi muscle is from the facial nerve. The motor innervation to the levator palpebrae superioris is from the oculomotor nerve. The blood supply to the eyelid comes from the medial palpebral branches of the ophthalmic artery and the lateral palpebral branches of the lacrimal artery. The medial canthus is a complex structure attached to the nasal bones and contains the caruncle and the puncta for the upper and lower canaliculi. The lacrimal duct and sac lie medial and caudal to the canaliculus. The lateral canthus is a two-layered ligament attached to the lateral orbital rim that holds the eyelid in place. Technique selection for reconstruction is based on this anatomy and assessment for treatment planning and includes the depth, location, and size of the defect. Procedure selection will be discussed based on these characteristics.

Partial-thickness Loss of the Upper or Lower Eyelid

Partial-thickness defects include loss of a portion of the anterior or posterior lamellae. The anterior lamella consists of the skin and the underlying orbicularis oculi muscle. Reconstruction options include full-thickness skin grafts harvested from the contralateral upper eyelid, postauricular, or neck donor sites. This option is a valuable one especially in an older patient who may only be able to tolerate a procedure that can be done with a local anesthetic (Figure 33-3A, B). Skin grafts are not ideal for all patients because of associated pigmentation, scarring, and cosmesis. For those patients, local skin flaps and myocutaneous flaps are a better option. The horizontal V-Y advancement flap recently described by Marchac is a good example of a local flap for the reconstruction of partial-thickness defects of the anterior lamellae.[2] The Tripier flap is especially useful for congenital deficiencies (Figure 33-4A–C).

The posterior lamella consists of the conjunctiva and tarsus. Defects in this region often result in loss of support to the eyelid and can be very problematic. If the defect is an isolated lining problem, which is rare, then the options for mucosal reconstruction include hard palate mucosa, buccal mucosa, acellular dermis, and skin grafts. If the tarsus is involved, reconstruction with skin, mucosa, cartilage or composite grafts is needed. If enough lower lid support is lost, then a fascial sling is indicated. Key points for the reconstruction of partial-thickness defects are to resurface the cutaneous defect, to put the incisions within natural skin tension lines, and to minimize tension on the eyelid margin.

Full-thickness Loss of the Upper or Lower Eyelid

In cases with full-thickness loss of either of the eyelids, the size and location of the defect dictates what surgical reconstructive options are available as long as there is no history of radiation or previous flaps in the area. If there is a full-thickness defect with less than one third of the eyelid involved and the canthus is spared, then the options include primary closure with or without the release of a portion of the lateral canthal ligament, a local myocutaneous transposition flap, composite grafts, and a sliding flap.[3] If the resection was not performed in a pentagonal pattern, then revision of the defect should be undertaken to create two sides perpendicular to the eyelid margin that turn obliquely to meet at the inferior aspect of the defect. Primary closure is often an option in the elderly patient because of skin laxity in the area. In the patient with less skin laxity, the release of a portion of the lateral canthal ligament can allow the skin to move together with less

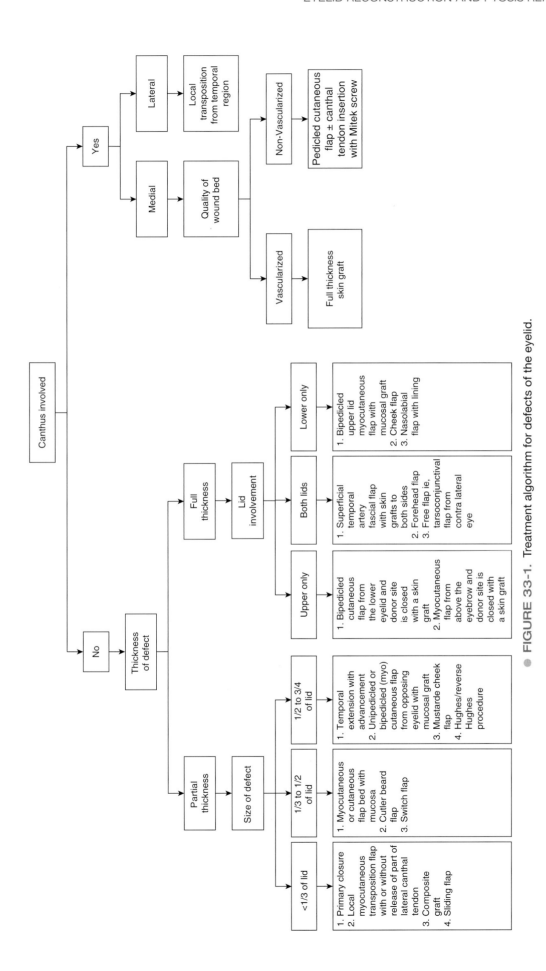

● FIGURE 33-1. Treatment algorithm for defects of the eyelid.

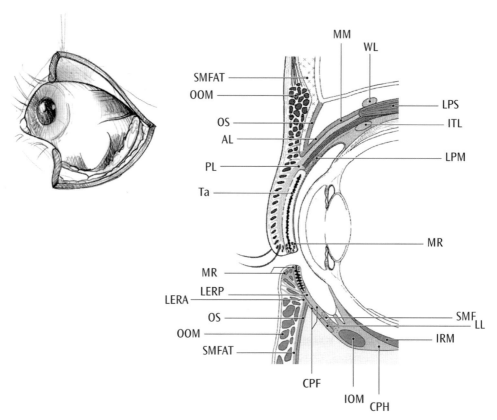

UPPER LID
Mueller's muscle (**MM**); Whitnall's ligament (**WL**); Levator palpebrae superioris (**LPS**); intermuscular transverse ligament (**ITL**); lamina propria mucosae (**LPM**); muscle of Riolan (**MR**); anterior aspect of the tarsus (**Ta**); levator aponeurosis - posterior layer (**PL**); levator aponeurosis - anterior layer (**AL**); orbital septum (**OS**); orbicularis oculi muscle (**OOM**); submuscular fibroadipose tissue (**SMFAT**).

LOWER LID
Smooth muscle fiber (**SMF**); Lockwood ligament (**LL**); inferior rectus muscle (**IRM**); capsulopalpebral head (**CPH**); inferior oblique muscle (**IOM**); capsulopalpebral fascia (**CPF**); submuscular fibroadipose tissue (**SMFAT**); obricularis oculi muscle (**OOM**); orbital septum (**OS**); lower eyelid retractor - anterior layer (**LERA**); lower eyelid retractor - posterior layer (**LERP**); muscle of Riolan (**MR**).

● **FIGURE 33-2.** Cross-section anatomy of the upper eyelid. (*Redrawn from a figure WFUSM Plastic Surgery Collection.*)

tension and is safe as long as only a portion of the ligament is released.[4] A full-thickness defect necessitates repair of the lining as well as the overlying structures. Local V-Y or rhomboid myocutaneous transposition flaps therefore must be lined either with buccal or hard palate mucosa. Composite grafts are an option only if the defect is small enough to ensure its viability.

If there is a full-thickness defect with one third to one half of the eyelid involved and the canthus is spared, the reconstruction usually can be done with eyelid skin, avoiding the use of a remote donor site. Local transposition or advancement flaps within the eyelid are useful here. Lateral defects can be closed using temporal rotation flaps. Local flaps that have been successful with this size defect include a myocutaneous flap lined with mucosa, the Cutler-Beard technique, and the eyelid switch flap (Figure 33-5A–D). The Cutler-Beard flap uses a full-thickness rectangular segment from the lower eyelid and is done in two stages. The eyelid switch flap rotates a small full-thickness flap from the opposite eyelid based on the marginal artery (Figure 33-6A–D). It is also a two-stage procedure.

A full-thickness defect with one half to three quarters of the eyelid involved and the canthus spared usually necessitates utilizing tissue from donor sites outside the eyelid. The options include temporal extension of the defect and advancement, a uni- or bipedicled myocutaneous flap from the opposing eyelid with a mucosal graft for lining, a Mustarde rotational cheek flap, and a reverse Hughes or a Hughes procedure, depending on the eyelid

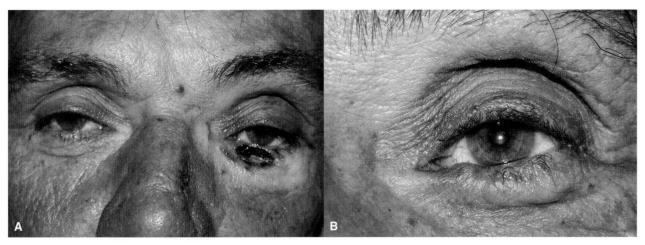

● FIGURE 33-3. (A) Partial-thickness lower eyelid reconstruction utilizing a full-thickness skin graft; and (B) 3-month follow up result. (*WFUSM Plastic Surgery Collection.*)

involved.[5] A Mustarde flap can be useful for both upper and lower eyelid defects (Figure 33-7A–C). For upper eyelid defects, the first stage uses a full-thickness flap from the lower eyelid to reconstruct the upper eyelid based on a pedicle. In the second stage, the pedicle is divided and a rotational cheek flap is used to close the lower eyelid defect. Lower eyelid defects can be reconstructed with a single-stage Mustarde cheek flap (Figure 33-8A–E). The

Hughes procedure originally described for lower eyelid defects is a tarsoconjunctival lining flap from the upper lid to the lower lid covered with a skin graft that is staged with pedicle division a few weeks later.

Complete upper or lower eyelid loss is a difficult problem, which is fortunately uncommon. For complete loss of the lower eyelid, surgical options include a bipedicled upper lid myocutaneous flap with mucosal graft for lining.

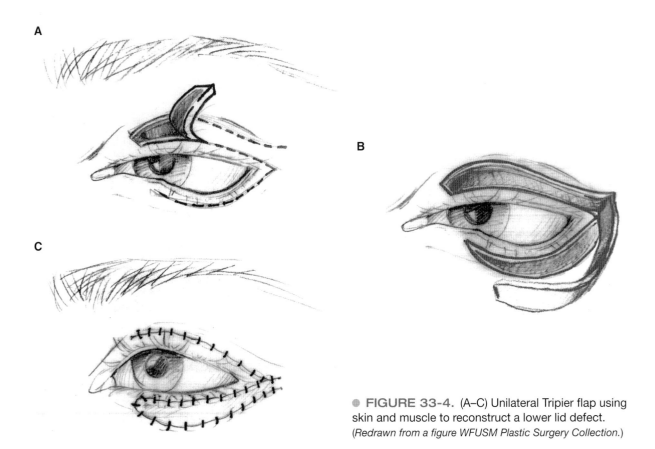

● FIGURE 33-4. (A–C) Unilateral Tripier flap using skin and muscle to reconstruct a lower lid defect. (*Redrawn from a figure WFUSM Plastic Surgery Collection.*)

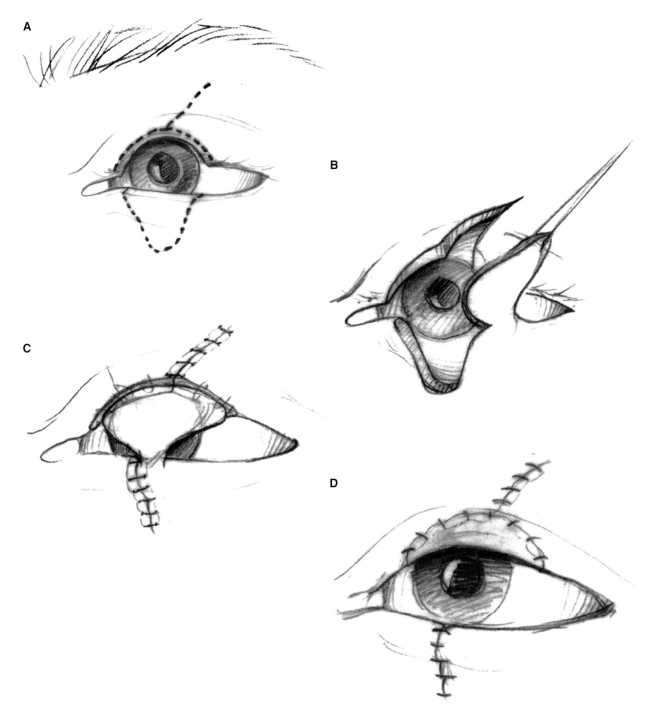

● **FIGURE 33-5.** Eyelid switch flap: a two-stage procedure. (*Redrawn from a figure WFUSM Plastic Surgery Collection.*)

This must be situated above the canthus to prevent ectropion. Other options include a cheek flap with a medial and lateral z-plasty and a graft for lining or a nasolabial flap with lining.[6] Treatment options for complete loss of the upper eyelid include a bipedicled cutaneous flap from the lower eyelid and a mucosal graft for lining. Closure of the donor site can be accomplished with a Mustarde cheek flap for the best results. Other donor site treatment options include a skin graft, composite graft, or a myocutaneous flap from above the eyebrow and skin graft to the donor site. The repairs described below for loss of both eyelids can be used for one eyelid as well.

Complete upper and lower eyelid loss requires a combination of reconstruction techniques, and choice is usually dependent on donor site availability. Treatment options usually include more remote donor sites such as a superficial temporal artery fascial flap with skin grafts on both sides, and a forehead flap. In cases when nothing

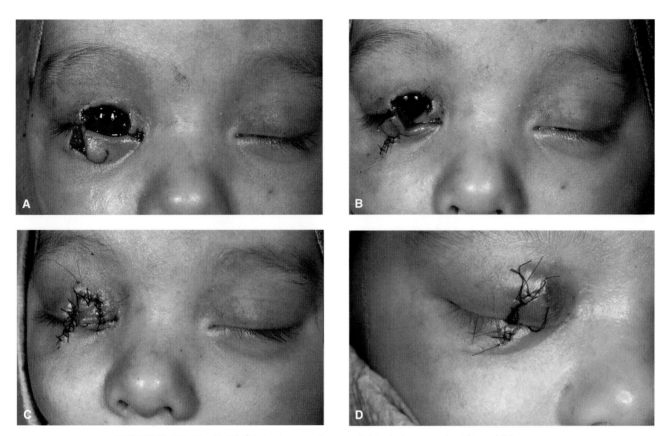

● **FIGURE 33-6.** (A–D) Clinical case of an eyelid switch procedure in a child. (*WFUSM Plastic Surgery Collection.*)

is available regionally, then a free flap such as a tarsoconjunctival flap from the contralateral eye is an option.

The medial and lateral canthi are critical structures to the support and integrity of the eyelid. Medial canthal reconstruction options are dependent on the extent of the defect. If there is a good bed, then a full-thickness skin graft from the upper eyelid is adequate. If there is no vascularized bed, then a unipedicled cutaneous flap from the upper eyelid will be needed. Onishi recently described the use of glabellar combined Rintala flaps with good success in this region.[6,7] If the medial canthal tendon needs to be reinserted, then a screw should be used. The lateral canthus is easier to reconstruct, and a local transposition flap from the temporal area is usually sufficient.

Eyebrow and Eyelash Reconstruction

Cosmesis and a reconstruction that recreates the normal appearance of the eyelid necessitate the reconstruction of the eyebrow and eyelashes if involved.[8] Conservative treatment includes tattooing, but most would agree this is suboptimal. Current techniques include the transplantation of hair follicles, strip grafts, or pedicled flaps that are hair bearing. Follicular grafting can be done for the eyelashes as well, but this is a little more labor intensive. Often repeat grafting is necessitated to get an adequate density of hair follicles.

● COMPLICATIONS

For reconstruction of the eyelid, as with any surgical procedure, complications are better avoided than managed. The key to preventing complications is to remember the anatomy of the eyelid and to replace all of the missing structures. In addition, a tension-free repair is an absolute requirement in this region both because the eyelid skin is thin and because the protection of the globe itself is so critical. Unlike other areas of the face, waiting until the scar has settled 9 to 12 months later before reoperation is often a luxury we do not have in this area because of the associated risk. The globe itself must be protected either with a temporary Frost suture or lateral tarsorrhaphy.

Major complications in this area include ectropion with scleral show and entropion. Ectropion, an eversion of the eyelid margin, most often involves the lower eyelid. It can be best prevented by avoiding tension on the lower eyelid and by adequately supporting the lower lid. Once it occurs, treatment is surgical and may include a z-plasty, a skin graft, or a fascial sling. Entropion is an inversion of the eyelid margin causing corneal irritation by the lashes. In eyelid reconstruction entropion is best prevented with adequate lining as a component of the reconstruction. Once it occurs, treatment is surgical and, in the case of a postreconstruction complication, recreation of the lining defect along with a mucosal graft is usually successful in correcting this secondary deformity.

A

B

C

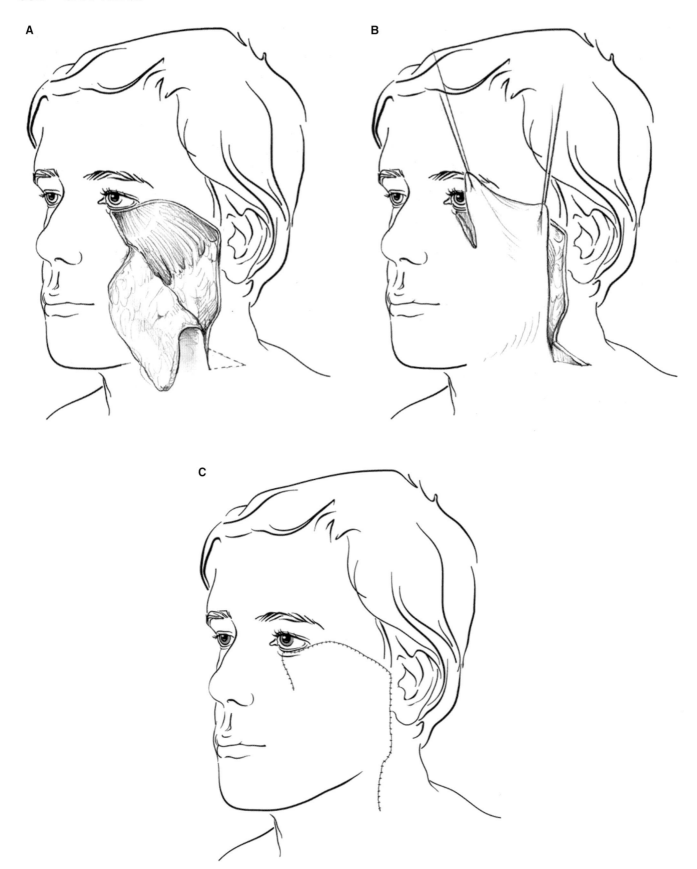

● **FIGURE 33-7.** (A–C) Mustarde rotational cheek flap for reconstruction of a lower eyelid defect. (*Redrawn from a figure WFUSM Plastic Surgery Collection.*)

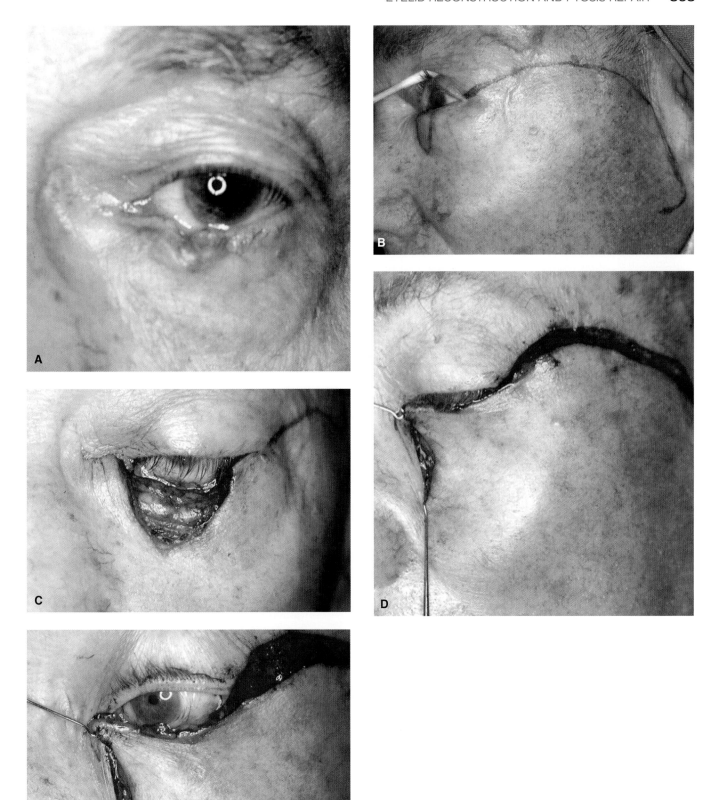

● **FIGURE 33-8.** (A–E) Clinical example of the Mustarde rotational cheek flap closure of an eyelid defect. (*WFUSM Plastic Surgery Collection.*)

Ptosis

The healthy eyelid in primary gaze should be located half way between the pupillary aperture and the corneoscleral junction. The major muscle involved in eyelid elevation is the levator palpebrae superioris and, to a lesser extent, Mueller's muscle. If the eyelid is caudal or inferior to the half way point, it is likely a case of eyelid ptosis (blepharoptosis).[8] In true ptosis one or more of these muscles is affected. A diagnosis of pseudoptosis is made when the eyelid is inferiorly displaced, but the cause is not attributed to the levator complex. It is often a result of enophthalmos due to the displacement of the globe posteriorly into the orbital space.

The etiology of ptosis may be congenital or acquired. In congenital cases, the levator muscle is either fibrosed, not functioning properly, or absent. This can be determined clinically by having the patient look down (downward gaze). If lagophthalmos is present, then congenital ptosis is likely the etiology. Improved long-term results have been achieved when the repair is accomplished within the first year of life, as documented with improved aesthetic outcomes and decreased physiological and developmental side effects.

The most common etiological factor that leads to acquired ptosis is a stretching of the aponeurosis superior to the tarsus but it can result from any injury to the levator aponeurosis. This can be due to traumatic injury, surgical injury, tumor, syndromes such as Horner, myasthenia gravis, third nerve palsy, and mechanical changes with anophthalmos. It is estimated that 40% to 50% of causes are involutional, while approximately 40% are a result of trauma. Depending on the severity of ptosis, severe visual obstruction and even gait disturbances can result and thus necessitate surgical intervention.

● PATIENT SELECTION

Identifying the underlying cause of a patient's ptosis is essential to selecting the most appropriate surgical procedure to correct the condition, to prevent recurrence, and to minimize the risk of postoperative complications. A detailed history should include onset of symptoms, history of trauma, contact lens use, coexisting systemic conditions, previous surgery, and any recent use of botulinum toxin. It is important to determine if there is any fluctuation in the degree or severity of ptosis during the day that may require further work up to rule out the presence of myasthenia gravis. Any use of anticoagulation medications should be documented as well.

Extraocular movement and visual acuity should always be examined and documented prior to any periorbital surgical intervention. A thorough clinical examination can help identify the etiology of the ptosis and guide the surgeon to the most effective surgical treatment. Irregularities in the pupil size or in response to light may indicate a neurological condition. A motility examination may reveal a coexisting Horner syndrome (Mueller

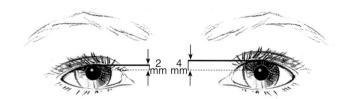

● FIGURE 33-9. Technique for measurement of marginal reflex distance which measures the distance between the upper lid margin and the corneal reflex. (*Redrawn from a figure WFUSM Plastic Surgery Collection.*)

muscle) or Bell phenomenon (third cranial nerve palsy), which can be either a congenital or an acquired condition. Symmetry should be examined and reviewed with the patient. The severity of the ptosis should be quantified by measuring the interpalpebral fissure height, upper lid margin to corneal reflex distance, levator function, and upper lid crease position.

- The *interpalpebral fissure height* is obtained by measuring the height from the lower eyelid to the upper eyelid centrally. This determines the vertical aperture, which is between 8 and 12 mm (average 10 mm) in adults.

- The *upper lid margin to corneal reflex distance* is referred to as the marginal reflex distance (MRD-1) (Figure 33-9). It is measured from the corneal light reflex to the upper central lid margin with the patient in the primary gaze position. The normal upper eyelid in the primary position will rest at or just below the superior corneal limbus with a MRD-1 between 4.0 and 4.5 mm. If the corneal light reflex is obstructed by the upper lid, then the degree of ptosis is severe, and the measurement is obtained by lifting the eyelid until the corneal light reflex is visualized. The MRD-1 is then recorded as a negative value. The MRD-1 is a very important value as it is independent of the position of the lower lid.

- The *levator function* is assessed by measuring the upper eyelid excursion from maximal downward gaze to maximal upward gaze while eliminating any interference from the frontalis muscle by placing pressure on the forehead during the examination. Normal levator function is considered greater than 12 mm excursion. It is classified as good at 10 to 15 mm, fair between 6 and 9 mm, and poor if it is less than 5 mm.

- The *upper lid crease position* is described as the margin crease distance (MCD). The eyebrow is lifted and the patient asked to look down. The measurement is made from the lid crease centrally to the lash line while in downward gaze. A normal MCD should be between 9 and 11 mm. A separation of the levator aponeurosis from the orbicularis muscle is suspected if the MCD is greater than 9 mm. Separation of the levator aponeurosis from the tarsus is suspected if the fold is excessively deep. An absent fold may indicate congenital ptosis.

● PATIENT PREPARATION

Clear and detailed documentation will assist in communication with the patients and their families concerning their condition and the treatment options. It is very helpful to take preoperative photographs of the patient (primary gaze, upward gaze, downward gaze, and eyes closed) to compliment the discussion and for documentation. Photographs help patients to express their concerns, likes, and dislikes concerning the form and function they anticipate postoperatively.

There are several different ways to classify ptosis. To meet the objective of choosing the best surgical intervention, we will classify according to true ptosis and pseudoptosis.

1. *True ptosis* is characterized by an upper eyelid margin in primary gaze below the normal anatomic position as described above. It can result from dysfunction in one or more of the components of the levator complex (levator palpebrae superioris muscle, levator aponeurosis, and the Mueller muscle). Patients may compensate by using the frontalis muscle to lift the upper lid. The etiologic factors can be isolated or be part of a syndrome, and within these two categories it can be congenital or acquired.

2. *Pseudoptosis* is used to describe a condition that appears to give an inferiorly displaced eyelid but in which the etiology is unrelated to the levator complex. Intervention focuses on treating the underlying disorder, which can improve the effect on the eyes. It is often related to conditions that effect orbital volume such as enophthalmos, anophthalmos, phthisis bulbi, microphthalmos, and fat atrophy. In these conditions, the eyelid is usually normal. It is the globe that is incorrectly positioned. Treatment is therefore best focused on addressing the orbital volume and not the levator muscle. Dermatochalasis, redundant upper eyelid skin, can be corrected by blepharoplasty.

● SURGICAL TECHNIQUE

In order to select the correct operation, it is imperative that the anatomical structures directly contributing to the ptosis are identified. The two most important factors for selecting an appropriate surgical technique are the degree of ptosis that is present and the quality of levator muscle function remaining. When a patient has a mild ptosis (2–3 mm) and good levator excursion (10–15 mm) correction can be achieved by plicating, shortening or advancing the levator muscle. For a patient with moderate ptosis (3–5 mm) and good levator excursion the levator muscle can still be plicated or advanced. For a patient with severe

ptosis (>5 mm) and normal levator excursion, levator advancement remains the technique of choice. If the levator excursion is moderate (6–9 mm) in combination with any amount of ptosis, advancing the levator muscle will give the strength and durability needed to correct the ptosis. In the case of a poorly functioning levator muscle, a frontalis sling is required. In summary, if levator function is present, then the levator can be used to correct the ptosis. These procedures can be combined with an upper lid blepharoplasty; however, for purposes of this chapter we will focus on the procedure done for ptosis correction.

Levator Aponeurosis Repair and Advancement

This procedure can be used in varied severity of levator dysfunction and thus is a very important technique to master. The patient should be positioned supine in a comfortable position, tetracaine drops applied, and a sclera shield placed for corneal protection. The intended site for the incision should be marked and then the skin infiltrated with a local anesthetic. The incision should be located approximately 9 to 12 mm above the lid margin centrally as in blepharoplasty cases. The incision is made through the skin and orbicularis muscle to identify the levator aponeurosis. A fine-tipped electrocautery device or tenotomy scissors can be used to dissect the aponeurosis from the orbital septum superiorly and then inferiorly to expose the edge of the tarsal plate where the aponeurosis may still have attachments.

1. **In cases when a levator advancement is planned (levator excursion >6 mm):** The levator aponeurosis is released from the superior edge of the tarsus carefully to limit disruption of the vascular arcade which will increase the risk of bleeding. Just deep to the levator is the Mueller muscle, which should be preserved in the deep layer overlying the conjunctiva. Once lifted off the deep layer and freed medially and laterally, the levator is advanced inferiorly toward and over the tarsal plate. Generally, one can expect a 1:1 result of correction (1 mm of advancement = 1 mm of elevation). For more severe cases, additional advancement will be needed; this should be tested with a cooperative patient after the first stitch is centrally placed securing the levator to the tarsal plate. Many surgeons have a strong preference regarding the type of suture material selected. Absorbable sutures can be used either in a running or interrupted fashion. Care should be exercised in order to maintain inclusion of the tarsus and levator while avoiding full-thickness bites which include the conjunctiva. Excess aponeurosis should be excised after the placement and elevation has been confirmed to be correct. It is acceptable to overcorrect by 1 to 1.5 mm.[9] Excision of the skin should be done very cautiously, as aggressive resection can lead to eyelid entropion and distortion. If recreation

of the lid crease is needed, the skin closure should include intermittent portions of the levator aponeurosis within the stitch.

2. **In cases when a levator plication is planned (ptosis <5 mm and good levator function):** This approach is very similar to that of the levator advancement. The medial and lateral fibers are released, but the attachment to the superior tarsal plate is left intact. Instead of separating the levator from the tarsus, it is plicated on itself at the superior margin of the tarsus. If the bulk of the levator creates a distortion of the overlying skin, it should be trimmed. The degree of plication should be evaluated with a cooperative patient as described previously.

Tarsal Conjunctival Mullerectomy

This technique, also referred to as the Fasanella-Servat procedure, is a reconstructive option when a patient has a mild amount of ptosis (≤2 mm) with good levator function and a positive response to phenylephrine eye drops. The MRD-1 should be measured both before and during the phenylephrine test to determine the severity of ptosis (normal MRD-1 = 4.5 mm). Phenylephrine 2.5% is recommended as it has less propensity for cardiac side effects and has been shown to be equally effective as 10% phenylephrine.[10,11] Systemic absorption can be decreased by occluding the canaliculi during insertion of the drops by pressing on the opening with the index finger. Tetracaine drops and local anesthetic are recommended and should be injected carefully so as not to distort the upper lid margins. A frontal nerve block is another good option.

Once the anesthetic has taken effect, the eyelid is everted to expose the conjunctiva overlying the tarsal plate. Either a resection-ptosis clamp or two identical size mosquitoes are used to clamp the posterior lamella at the level of the superior margin of the tarsal plate (Figure 33-10). Special care is used to be sure the clamps are in line with the curve of the upper lid to prevent distortion. A monofilament suture is placed through the skin under the clamp. The tissue is then excised between the suture and the

clamp. After waiting several minutes to assure hemostasis the clamps are removed and the eyelid reverted to its normal position.[12] The suture is removed 1 to 2 weeks later according to the clinical signs of correction.

Frontalis Sling

For patients who have a poorly functioning levator (<5 mm), upper lid function will need to come from periorbital muscles linked to the upper lid, regardless of the amount of ptosis (Figure 33-11). This is a common situation for congenital cases of ptosis (Figure 33-12). The procedure is performed by connecting the tarsus to the frontalis muscle.[13] Several materials, each with benefits and potential risks, have been used. Autologous material can be harvested from the fascia lata and has a low risk of infection, but it requires a second operative site and scar. Donated fascia lata eliminates a donor site scar in the patient but carries a small risk of transmission of disease. Silicone rods have been used successfully, but they have a slightly higher rate of infection, exposure and material failure. The material is generally connected to the frontalis muscle at the level just superior to the eyebrow and then to the tarsus just above the lash line. The intraoperative level of the corrected eyelid should be 1 mm or so above the desired level as the material will relax in the postoperative period. Regardless of the material chosen, the tension must be adequate to correct the ptosis and not to create compensatory entropion of the upper lid.

● COMPLICATIONS

Complications from upper lid ptosis surgery can be categorized as follows: contour irregularities, under correction, overcorrection, and keratitis. Levator aponeurosis under correction is seen with inadequate advancement, under resection, or dehiscence or loosening of the sutures. This can be salvaged with re-advancement, resection, or replacement of the sutures. A frontalis sling may be needed if the levator is injured or not functioning properly. In the case of overcorrection, conservative treatment with massage and lubricants should be instituted upon detection of

A

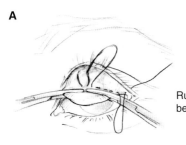

Running suture (full thickness) behind clamps, lateral to medial

B

Trim excess clamped tissue

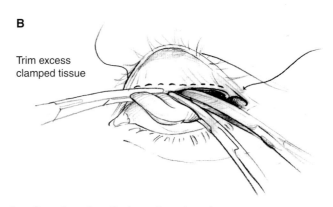

● **FIGURE 33-10.** Fasanella-Servat procedure (tarsal conjunctival muellerectomy).
(Redrawn from a figure WFUSM Plastic Surgery Collection.)

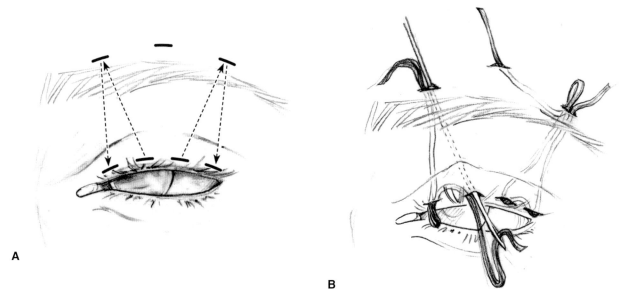

A

B

● **FIGURE 33-11.** (A, B) Frontalis sling procedure used for ptosis repair with history of poor levator function. (*Redrawn from a figure WFUSM Plastic Surgery Collection.*)

the problem to decrease the likelihood of having to do a resection of the levator for correction. Complications with the *tarsal conjunctival Mullerectomy* often involve eyelid contour abnormalities that can be created if the clamp or mosquitoes are not placed complimentary to the contour of the lid. If this is noted in the postoperative period, the stitch should be loosened and the eyelid smoothed to improve the contour. If that does not solve the problem, then the excess tarsus, usually located centrally, can be excised to achieve the correct contour. Under correction will result if there is not enough tissue removed from the posterior lamella or if there is dehiscence of the incision site. Correction can be achieved by repeating the procedure or by addressing the levator. Over or under correction with the *frontalis sling* correction can be done by opening the brow incision and tightening or loosening the sling as needed. Keratitis can occur with any of these procedures from exacerbating a dry eye state, lagophthalmos, suture keratopathy, or granuloma formation. Artificial tears and lubricating ointments will provide relief of the symptoms

and stimulate repair. If the irritation is from the suture, it should be removed but can be avoided if the suture is buried during the initial operation.

● **OUTCOMES ASSESSMENT**

A good aesthetic and functional result is the goal of any reconstructive procedure of the eyelid. The best results come from adhering to the following principles:

1. Avoid tension and reconstruct the defect whenever distortion occurs with primary closure.
2. Full-thickness defects require adequate reconstruction of all the involved layers.
3. Reconstruct with like tissues if available. Use the upper eyelid to replace the lower if needed but avoid the reverse as much as possible.
4. Avoid staged procedures if possible. Flaps with a large base should be utilized in preference to a narrow pedicle.

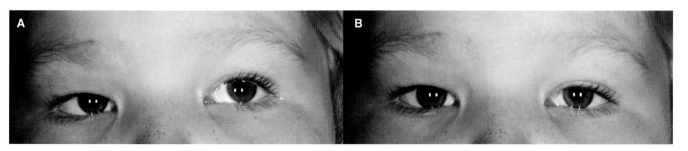

A

B

● **FIGURE 33-12.** Clinical example of congenital ptosis before (A) and after (B) the repair. (*WFUSM Plastic Surgery Collection.*)

5. Attention to the contour intraoperatively will improve the postoperative results.

6. Perform a thorough preoperative examination so as to address the underlying cause of ptosis in order to select the proper technique for repair.

7. Protection of the globe is your primary responsibility.

It should be remembered that the more obvious the residual deformity or reconstruction, the less likely the patient will be happy with the result. The most complex techniques do not always give the best results and a forehead flap or free flap are good examples of such. The more remote the donor site (eg, forehead) the less it will be like the original tissue, and the more obvious it becomes to the patient.

REFERENCES

1. Mathijssen I, van der Meulen JC. Guidelines for reconstruction of the eyelids and canthal regions. *J Plast Reconstr Aesthet Surg.* 2010;63(9):1420–1433.

2. Marchac D, de Lange A, Bine-bine H. A horizontal V-Y advancement lower eyelid flap. *Plast Reconstr Surg.* 2009; 124:1133–1141.

3. Demir Z, Yüce S, Karamürsel S, Çelebioğlu S. Orbicularis oculi myocutaneous advancement flap for upper eyelid reconstruction. *Plast Reconstr Surg.* 2008;121(2):443–450.

4. Lewis CD, Perry JD. Transconjunctival lateral cantholysis for closure of full-thickness eyelid defects. *Ophthal Plast Reconstr Surg.* 2009;25(6):469–471.

5. Morley A, deSousa J, Selva D, Malhotra R. Techniques of upper eyelid reconstruction. *Surg Ophthalmol.* 2010;55(3): 256–271.

6. Onishi K, Maruyama Y, Okada E, Ogino A. Medial canthal reconstruction with glabellar combined rintala flaps. *Plast Reconstr Surg.* 2007;119:537–541.

7. Stein J, Antonyshyn O. Aesthetic eyelid reconstruction. *Clin Plastic Surg.* 2009;36(3):379–397.

8. Ahmad SM, Della Rocca RC. Blepharoptosis: evaluation, techniques, and complications. *Facial Plast Surg.* 2007; 23(3):203–215.

9. Newman M, Spinelli H. Reconstruction of the eyelid, correction of ptosis, and canthoplasty. In: *Grabb and Smith's Plastic Surgery.* 6th ed. Philadelphia: Lippincott Williams & Wilkins; 2006;39:397–416.

10. Fraunfelder FT, Scafidi A. Possible adverse effect from topical ocular 10% phenylephrine. *Am J Ophthalmol.* 1978;85:447–453.

11. Glatt HJ, Fett DR, Putterman AM. Comparison of 2.5% and 10% phenylephrine in the elevation of upper eyelids with ptosis. *Ophthalmic Surg.* 1990;21:173–176.

12. McLeish WM, Anderson RL. *Cosmetic Oculoplastic Surgery: Eyelid, Forehead, and Facial techniques.* 3rd ed. Philadelphia: W.B. Saunders; 1999.

13. Saunders RA, Grice CM. Early correction of severe congenital ptosis. *J Pediatr Ophthalmol Strabismus.* 1991;28: 271–273.

chapter 34

Scalp, Calvarial, and Forehead Reconstruction

Matthew R. Swelstad, MD / *Michael L. Bentz, MD, FACS, FAAP*

● INTRODUCTION

Scalp, forehead, and cranial defects occur from a variety of congenital and acquired processes. Lacerations, burns, and tissue avulsions may require emergent treatment. Tissue defects are also the result of the medical and surgical management of neoplastic conditions of the scalp, including basal cell carcinoma, squamous cell carcinoma, melanoma, dermatofibrosarcoma protuberans, soft tissue sarcomas, and vascular malformations. Excision of premalignant lesions such as giant congenital melanocytic nevi and nevi sebaceous may also require complex closure. Infectious complications from leprosy, herpes, fungi, lupus vulgaris, and lichen planus may also lead to scalp and calvarial defects. External beam radiation used in the medical management of neoplastic and other scalp disorders may lead to scalp ulceration or osteoradionecrosis. A variety of congenital anomalies, such as cutis aplasia, may be associated with defects in the scalp and cranium exposing the underlying bone or dura. The role of the plastic surgeon is to safely and reliably reconstruct these defects while preserving function, maximizing aesthetics, and minimizing risk and morbidity.

Vascular Supply

The vascular supply of the scalp is excellent. It consists of several axial arterial vessels connected by an intricate vascular plexus. Scalp vessels originate from the internal and external carotid arteries. In the forehead, the supraorbital and supratrochlear arteries (branches of the internal carotid) exit their respective foramina in the supraorbital ridge and travel superiorly toward the vertex of the cranium. The external carotid artery branches into four main scalp vessels. The first of these branches is the occipital

artery, which is the predominant blood supply to the posterior scalp. The posterior auricular artery provides blood supply to the scalp over the mastoid and temporal areas behind the ear. The internal maxillary artery courses anteriorly toward the midface and sends off the anterior and posterior deep temporal arteries which supply the temporalis muscle. The superficial temporal artery, which is the terminal branch of the external carotid artery, divides into the frontal branch and the parietal branch. The frontal branch supplies the anterior temporal region and lateral forehead. The parietal branch supplies the posterior temporal and parietal regions.[1] Figure 34-1 illustrates the vascular supply to the forehead and scalp.

Innervation

The forehead is innervated by the supraorbital nerve and the supratrochlear nerve, both branches of the ophthalmic division of the trigeminal nerve (CN V1). The supraorbital nerve exits its foramen in the supraorbital ridge, and divides into a superficial branch and a deep branch. The superficial branch penetrates the frontalis muscle and courses toward the scalp vertex in the subcutaneous plane. It supplies sensation to the overlying forehead skin. The deep branch of the supraorbital nerve travels between the periosteum and deep margin of the frontalis muscle. It provides sensation to the temporoparietal scalp. Innervation to the skin over the lateral orbit and temporal area of the forehead is supplied by the zygomaticofacial and zygomaticotemporal nerves, branches of the maxillary division of the trigeminal nerve (CN V2). The temporal scalp, innervated by the auriculotemporal nerve, is a branch of the mandibular division of the trigeminal nerve (CN V3). The great auricular and

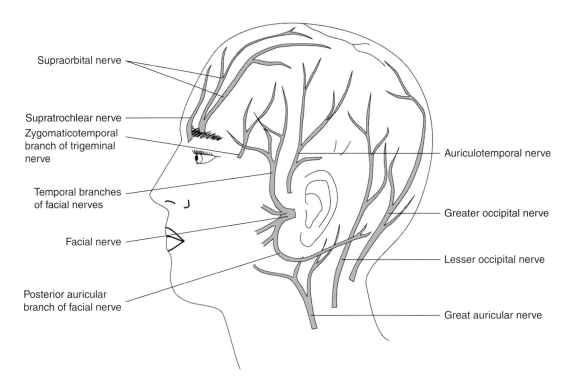

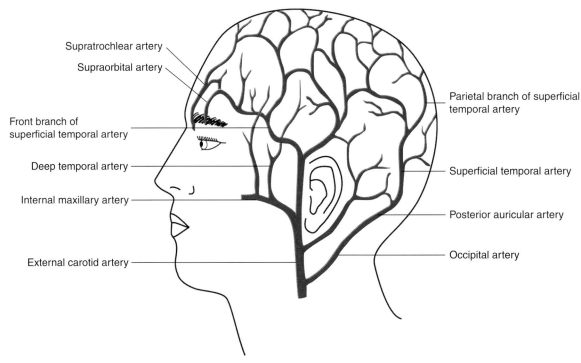

● **FIGURE 34-1.** Schematic drawing of the neurovascular anatomy of the scalp. A thorough understanding of this anatomy allows the surgeon to design flaps with optimal vascularity while minimizing the morbidity of damaging important nerves.

the lesser occipital nerves, both branches of the cervical plexus, exit immediately posterior to the sternocloidmastoid muscle providing sensation to the soft tissue of the ear and post auricular region of the scalp. The greater

occipital nerve, which is a branch of the cervical spinal nerve, provides posterior scalp sensation.[1]

Motor innervation of scalp muscles is supplied by branches of cranial nerve VII (facial nerve). The most

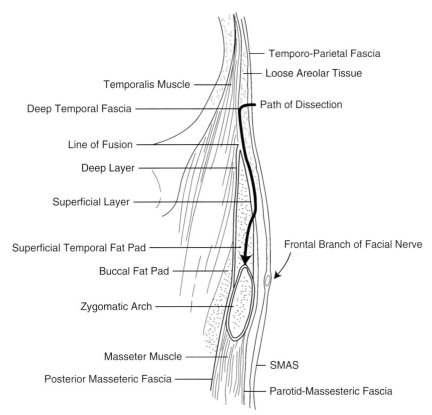

● **FIGURE 34-2.** Schematic drawing of the course of the temporal branch of the facial nerve (CN VII). The temporal branch is vulnerable to injury on account of it superficial location. To prevent damaging the nerve, it is recommended to dissect in a plane immediately superficial to the deep temporal fascia until two centimeters above the zygomatic arch. At this point, one should drop below the superficial leaf of the deep temporal fascia into the temporal fat pad. (*From: Stuzin, JM, Wagstrom L, Kawamoto HK, Wolfe SA. Anatomy of the frontal branch of the facial nerve. Plast Reconstr Surg. 1989;83:265–271.*)

important of these branches in scalp reconstruction is the frontal branch of the facial nerve. The facial nerve exits the cranial base through the stylomastoid foramen. The frontal branch then courses through the parotid gland and eventually into the temporal parietal fascia. Once in the temporoparietal fascia, the frontal branch crosses the middle third of the zygomatic arch in a plane superficial to the deep leaf of the temporal fascia and innervates the frontalis muscle (Figure 34-2).[2] The path of the nerve lies along a straight line between the lobule of the ear and a point 1.5 cm lateral to the upper lateral eyebrow. Damage to the frontal branch of the facial nerve will result in paresis of the ipsilateral frontalis muscle and the inability to elevate the eyebrow. Dissection in the lateral orbital region places this nerve at risk of either transection or traction injury.[3] Command of the anatomy and careful dissection allows the surgeon to navigate this complex anatomical region with success. Figure 34-1 illustrates the nervous supply to the forehead and scalp.

Lymphatic System

The lymphatic system of the scalp is composed of the highly variable nodal basins of the parotid, preauricular, postauricular, mastoid, and occipital regions. More predictable nodal regions exist in the neck as well. Because of the variable lymphatic drainage of the scalp, nodal mapping is performed simultaneously with surgical management of some scalp neoplasms (melanoma) to identify sentinel lymph nodes.

Muscles of the Scalp and Forehead

The scalp and forehead consist of 10 paired muscles, the frontalis, occipitalis, temporalis, procerus, corrugator, depressor supercilii, and the three auricular muscles, the auricularis anterior, posterior, and superior. Each of these muscles is innervated by branches of the facial nerve with the exception of the temporalis. The temporalis muscle is a muscle of mastication, and is innervated by the mandibular division of the trigeminal nerve (CN V3). All of these muscles except for the temporalis muscle lie within the galea aponeurosis layer.[3]

Cranium

The major bones of the cranium include the frontal, occipital, temporal, and parietal bones. Each bone is separated by a suture line, which normally fuses at predetermined ages. The bone itself is composed of an outer cortex and an inner cortex separated by the diploic space. This space is not clinically developed in young children, so reconstructive strategies which utilize the diploic space, such as split calvarial bone grafts, cannot be as easily performed until the space is adequately developed. Several venous channels course within the diploic space. Emissary veins connect the venous system of the scalp to the intracranial venous systems by traversing all three layers of the cranium.[1,2]

PATIENT EVALUATION

When evaluating the patient with trauma to the scalp, it is important to identify the depth of the injury and the tissues involved. The scalp consists of the hair-bearing and non–hair-bearing tissue between the supraorbital rims and the posterior nuchal line of the occiput. The forehead is the non–hair-bearing area of the scalp extending from the temporal hairline laterally, to the anterior hairline superiorly, and to the supraorbital rims inferiorly. The forehead can be divided into five subunits: one central area, two lateral areas, and two eyebrow areas.

The scalp is composed of five basic layers that can be remembered by using the mnemonic **SCALP**. SCALP stands for *S*kin, sub*C*utaneous tissue, galea *A*poneurosis, *L*oose areolar tissue, and *P*eriosteum.[4,5] The skin of the scalp is one of the thickest on the body. It is firmly adhered to the underlying subcutaneous layer and galea aponeurosis. Because no natural surgical plane exists between these layers, flaps such as the temporal parietal fascia flap (which is contiguous with the galea aponeurosis), require sharp dissection during elevation. If the dissection is too superficial, damage to hair follicles in the subcutaneous tissue will result in alopecia. If the dissection is too deep, the temporoparietal fascia vascular supply may be compromised. Excellent surgical planes exist between the galea, the subgaleal fascia and the periosteum. The loose attachments between these layers allows for scalp mobility. With careful technique it is possible to elevate the subgaleal areolar tissue in the interval between the periosteum and galea, creating a thin, translucent, well-vascularized fascia layer that is easily rotated into small local defects to cover exposed bone. The periosteal layer, also known as the pericranium, may also be elevated as a flap. The periosteum is firmly fixed to the underlying cranium. It is very strong and firm and it too may be rotated into adjacent tissue defects.

PATIENT PREPARATION

The patient should be positioned supine on the operating table with the head propped up on a circle of foam small enough to allow maximal exposure of the head but large enough to provide adequate support. Reconstruction may be performed under different types of anesthesia depending upon the patient and the size and location of the defect. Reconstruction of the scalp frequently requires constant turning of the head to visualize more lateral areas of the scalp to facilitate flap elevation and ultimate closure. If an endotracheal tube or laryngeal mask airway is used, special care must be taken to ensure that it is well-secured. The hair does not necessarily need to be shaved and is usually left intact. It should however be thoroughly prepped with an aqueous solution to ensure coverage.

The excellent vascular supply of the scalp may lead to brisk bleeding at the time of the surgery. Electrocautery can be effective in controlling this bleeding, but places hair follicles at risk for thermal injury and subsequent alopecia. To limit bleeding, lidocaine with epinephrine can be injected preoperatively, where epinephrine acts to vasoconstrict the blood vessels. With various concentrations of lidocaine with epinephrine available, one needs to be careful not to exceed the maximum recommended dose particularly in children. Some surgeons also use metal clips applied along the edge of the scalp flaps to temporarily compress the tissue to limit bleeding, while others use sutures placed several millimeters from the wound edge to compress vessels.

TECHNIQUE

Several factors influence scar visibility. First, proper placement and design of incisions may help to conceal alopecia associated with scars. Scars located at the hairline, adjacent to the ear, or within rhytids are usually inconspicuous. In addition, avoidance of hair follicles and minimization of tension at the suture line will help to reduce scar width, alopecia, and visibility. Incisions made within the hair-bearing regions of the scalp should be parallel to the angle of the hair follicles. This will help minimize hair follicle damage. Finally, flap design needs to consider final hair orientation after rotation or transposition. Flaps that surgically alter the natural orientation of the hair follicles will make the reconstruction less aesthetic and may require altering the patient's hairstyle.

Reconstructive Strategies

Plastic surgeons have several reconstructive strategies available to repair defects of scalp soft tissue. Ideally, the soft tissue defect is closed with similar tissue from the adjacent scalp in such a way that the aesthetics and function of the region are preserved. When the defect is not able to be primarily closed using local tissues, the wound may be closed by secondary intention (with/without skin grafts), tissue expansion, pedicled flaps, and microsurgical free flaps.[4,5]

Simple wound closure is the technique of choice for small defects. It involves re-approximating the wound edges with minimal adjacent subgaleal undermining. Advancement flaps may be used to close moderate-sized defects. This may involve significant undermining of adjacent tissue (as well as galeal scoring) with care not to disturb the overlying blood supply. When advancement flaps do not suffice, or if advancement flaps create a significant amount of aesthetic or functional distortion, then rotation flaps or transposition flaps are the next consideration. These local flaps come in a variety of sizes and shapes. For example, hair-bearing transposition flaps work well to reconstruct defects involving the sideburns. The resulting scars are well hidden along the hairlines and the orientation of the hair follicles is similar to normal. Another example is the more technically challenging use of the Orticochea three-flap reconstruction for moderate-sized scalp defects. The Orticochea scalp flaps are large flaps based on axial blood flow from large axial vessels (ie, superficial temporal, occipital, posterior auricular, supraorbital, and supratrochlear vessels).[3]

The galea is an inelastic layer of the scalp that resists stretching. Therefore, scoring of the galea at approximately one centimeter intervals, starting at the edge of the flap and parallel to the defect, may dramatically improve tissue mobility.[4,5] When scoring the galea, care needs to be exercised to release only the galea, and not injure the subcutaneous tissue. Too deep of an incision may damage the vascular supply to the flap or hair follicles leading to scalp necrosis or alopecia. Some surgeons prefer to also score the galea perpendicular to the direction of desired advancement. This can be effective in achieving additional expansion and advancement, but may lead to an increase in flap tip necrosis. All techniques are facilitated by use of a needle tip bovie to minimize secondary scalp bleeding.

When closing defects of the forehead, the surgeon should attempt to reconstruct the anterior hairline. Rotation (and occasionally transposition) flaps are usually the best means to do this. If the defect is large, then back grafting may be necessary in the donor area of the occiput. Other flap options to reconstruct the anterior hairline include the bipedicled Juri flap or pedicled hair bearing island flaps.

Final position of the eyebrow needs to be monitored during forehead reconstruction.[5] Often, some displacement of the eyebrow is necessary to achieve an adequate closure. In the case of glabellar defects, medial displacement of the eyebrows is infrequently permanent. Vertical elevation of the eyebrow commonly improves with time. With experience, the surgeon will be able to determine which changes are temporary and therefore acceptable, and which changes are likely permanent but possibly unavoidable.

Finally, when designing scalp flaps it is important to consider both motor and sensory innervation.[1,5] Cutting across motor nerves, such as the frontal branch of the facial nerve, will result in brow paralysis and potential significant facial asymmetry. Damaging a sensory nerve such as the greater auricular nerve or the deep branch of the supraorbital nerve will result in paresthesia and potentially a painful neuroma. It is not always possible to spare these nerves as part of the primary or reconstructive efforts. When sacrifice of one of these nerves is planned or possible, a discussion with the patient regarding postoperative changes is useful.

Healing by Secondary Intention. Not all scalp soft tissue defects are able to be closed using full-thickness local tissue rearrangement. In these situations, alternative management strategies are employed. One option is to perform local wound care, allowing it to close by secondary intention. Healing by secondary intention is often the treatment of choice in patients where either the risk of surgical reconstruction is too high, or the morbidity of the reconstruction unacceptable. With proper care and time, these wounds will ultimately contract and re-epithelialize. In the hair-bearing scalp, this results in alopecia. In the forehead, healing by secondary intention may produce an excellent result. For this reason, secondary intention healing of small- to moderate-sized forehead wounds is often the treatment of choice.

Skin Grafts. Skin grafting is the process of removing skin from one area of the body and applying it to another. Skin grafts may be harvested remotely as either full-thickness skin grafts or as split-thickness skin grafts. Full-thickness skin grafts are composed of all the layers of the skin, while split-thickness grafts are only composed of the epidermis and a portion of the dermis. Split-thickness skin grafts contract more during the long-term healing phase than full-thickness skin grafts. Split-thickness grafts may also be meshed (multiple small holes are placed in the graft), which allows a given graft to expand over a greater surface area. Meshed grafts also contract more during the healing phase compared to non-meshed grafts. The ability of meshed split-thickness skin grafts to shrink a wound during the healing process can be exploited by the reconstructive surgeon to decrease the final size of the wound.

Skin grafts do not have their own blood supply. They receive nutrition from the underlying wound bed. Therefore, before a skin graft may be used, a healthy vascularized wound base must exist. An example of a good wound base would be the presence of viable periosteum, subgaleal fascia, muscle, or granulation tissue. Denuded bone in the absence of periosteum is not a healthy wound base. To improve the chances of optimal skin graft "take" on exposed bone, the outer cortex of the bone can be removed to facilitate granulation tissue formation. Burring of the outer cortex of the bone followed by several weeks of wound care will accelerate creation of a graftable granular wound base.[6] Figure 34-3 illustrates a case where a scalp rotation flap was used to decrease the size of a large forehead defect. However, exposed bone was still present at the wound base. A subgaleal fascia flap was mobilized and rotated over the exposed bone and immediately skin grafted with good long-term results. Figure 34-4 demonstrates bilateral scalp rotation flaps with galeal scoring for closure of a vertex defect.

Since skin grafts do not usually have viable growth of hair follicles, areas of hair-bearing scalp reconstructed with skin grafts will have noticeable alopecia. The areas of alopecia can occasionally be camouflaged with hair transplantation, serially excised, or closed by local tissue flaps.

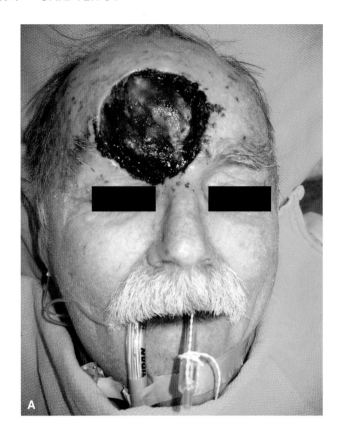

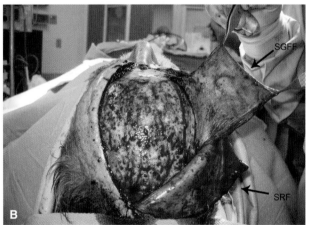

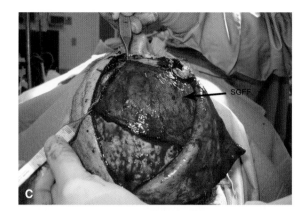

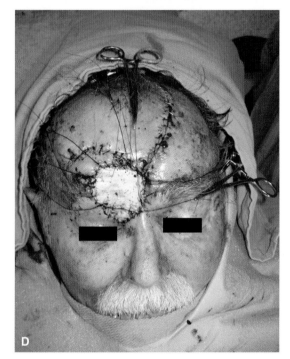

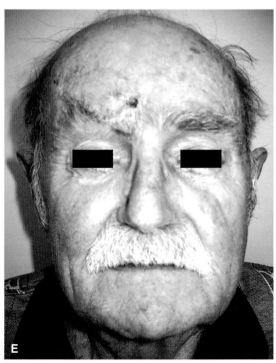

● **FIGURE 34-3.** (A) Intraoperative photographs of a patient with a large forehead defect and exposed bone following Mohs micrographic surgery for a basal cell carcinoma. (B) Elevation of subgaleal fascia flaps and a large posterior scalp rotation flap. (C) Subgaleal fascia flap anteriorly rotated to cover exposed forehead bone. (D) The scalp rotation flap decreased the size of the forehead defect; a skin graft was applied immediately over the subgaleal fascia flap. (E) Six months after surgery.

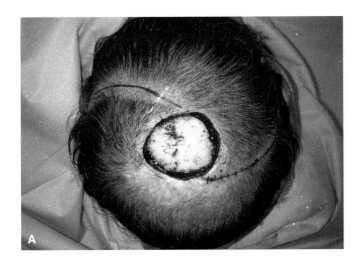

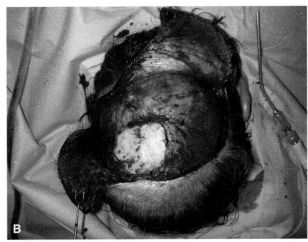

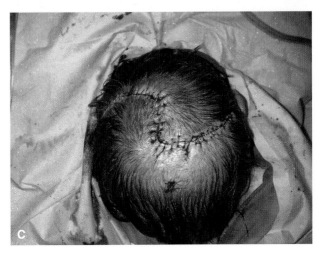

● **FIGURE 34-4.** (A) Intraoperative photographs of a patient with a scalp defect located at the vertex of the cranium following basal carcinoma excision. (B) Two scalp rotation flaps were elevated and the galea scored. (C) Immediate postoperative result.

If these options are insufficient, tissue expansion of adjacent areas is often quite effective.

Tissue Expansion. Tissue expansion allows the reconstructive surgeon to increase the surface area of donor "normal" tissue to be used in the primary or secondary reconstruction process. Inflatable silicone expanders are placed under the adjacent normal galea and scalp. Each expander is injected weekly or biweekly with saline until the amount of expanded tissue is greater than perceived necessary to close the scalp defect. Expanders are then removed, and flaps of appropriate geometry are created with the expanded scalp to close the defect. Expansion is most commonly used in this area to increase available forehead skin for contralateral defects, or to increase hair-bearing scalp, which is then mobilized over areas of scarring and alopecia.[7] Dog ears are often created in the process of expanded tissue rearrangement. These will usually resolve over weeks to months. Aggressive trimming of dog ears is discouraged, however, as this may narrow the flap base and decrease flap perfusion.[4] The most

common complications associated with tissue expansion include infection, extrusion or rupture of the expanders. In addition, patients need to understand and accept their progressively abnormal appearance during the expansion process. Figure 34-5 demonstrates the efficacy of tissue expansion in complex scalp reconstructions.

Cranial Vault Reconstruction. It is important to establish, prior to cranial reconstruction, that overlying soft tissue of the scalp is healthy and is present in adequate supply. Proceeding with cranial reconstruction before a stable soft tissue envelop is created will lead to wound breakdown, infection, and failure of the cranial reconstruction. In addition, patients with a history of prior infections in the surgical field need to be warned of the increased risk of subsequent infections during reconstruction.

The cranium may be reconstructed in a variety of ways. Alloy, titanium, or resorbable plates and screws are used when the cranial bones are present but maligned or fractured. When deficiencies of the cranial

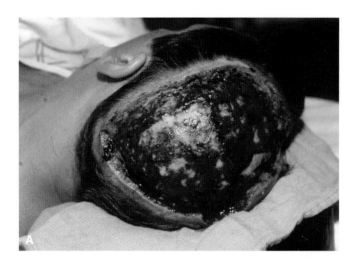
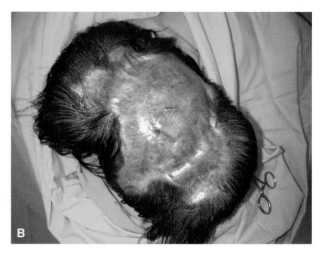
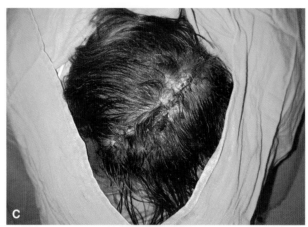

● FIGURE 34-5. (A) Intraoperative photographs of a patient with a large scalp and cranial defect following Mohs micrographic surgery for dermatofibrosarcoma protuberans. A skin graft was applied acutely to cover the defect. (B) After maturation of the skin graft, two tissue expanders were used to increase the amount of adjacent scalp tissue. (C) Postoperative result following removal of the tissue expanders and advancement of scalp flaps.

bone are present, many authors utilize the adjacent cranial bone as a graft source, exploiting that the cranium is composed of an outer and inner cortex separated by a diploic space. Defects up to one half the size of the cranium can be reconstructed by separating the contralateral inner and outer cortex. The outer cortex is then returned to its anatomic position and fixated, while the inner cortex is used to reconstruct the skeletal defect. Transposed bone is then secured in place using resorbable plates in children, and titanium plates in adults. If the defect is larger than one half the size of the cranium, or if the patient does not have a well-developed diploic space, then demineralized cadaveric donor bone may be used. Demineralized bone promotes both osteoconduction and osteoinduction. Sources for additional bone in large reconstructions include autologous split-rib grafts (Figure 34-6) and ilium.

Synthetic materials such as methylmethacrylate, porous polyethylene, and hard tissue replacement are also used. Methylmethacrylate is a nonporous acrylic

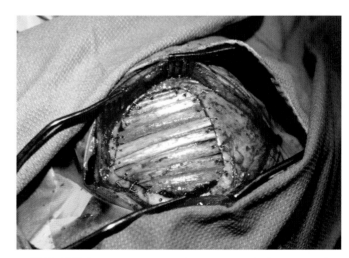

● FIGURE 34-6. Intraoperative photograph demonstrating the use of split-rib grafts for the reconstruction of a large cranial defect.

monomer that is easily molded in the operating room but has a high rate of infection and extrusion. Porous polyethylene (Medpor) and hard tissue replacement polymers (hard tissue replacement) are both synthetic implants with lower rates of extrusion because each allows for vascular ingrowth into the material. These synthetic constructs are computer generated to fit the exact size of the calvarial defect according to preoperative computed axial tomographic imaging. Because they are synthetic, extrusion and infection are still possible. Long-term data assessing these outcomes is still somewhat limited.

Hydroxyapatite cement is also extensively used in cranial reconstructions. Hydroxyapatite cement is composed of calcium phosphate and is easily molded in the operating room. Early studies suggested that hydroxyapatite cement was converted to bone. However, more recent studies suggest that only the outer layers of the hydroxyapatite cement become revascularized while the inner portions remain avascular. The most common form of hydroxyapatite cement used in cranioplasties comes in a paste form. The paste is mixed in the operating room and applied to the defect. When applied to a full-thickness calvarial defect, hydroxyapatite cement may develop microfractures. The significance of these microfractures remains unclear. Some surgeons use hydroxyapatite cement as an onlay for bone augmentation and recontouring.

Flap Reconstruction. Traditionally, large scalp defects have been managed with pedicled flaps or microvascular free flaps. These large flaps are based on axial blood vessels. Flaps are often composed of fascia, muscle, skin, or a combination of all three. In addition to the combined use of local flaps (pericranial flap, subgaleal fascia flap, temporoparietal fascia flap) other useful regional flaps include the temporalis muscle flap, as well as rotational flaps based on the splenius capitus, frontalis, and occipitalis muscles. Examples of distant pedicled flaps used for scalp reconstruction include the extended deltopectoral flap, trapezius flap, latissimus dorsi flap, lateral arm flap, and pectoralis major flap. With the advent of microsurgical techniques, new and more acceptable tissue donor sites evolved. Common free flaps used in scalp reconstruction include the latissimus dorsi, anterior lateral thigh, omentum, radial forearm, rectus abdominus, and the dorsal thoracic fascia flaps. Microsurgical free flaps offer not only reliable soft tissue coverage, but also greater flexibility with flap insetting, positioning, and in selecting donor sites with an optimal match for the given defect.[4,5]

Microsurgical techniques also provide the potential for large pieces of avulsed scalp to be revascularized. This can help avoid the need for more complex secondary scalp reconstructions, with hair growth in the avulsed tissue providing an acceptable reconstruction.[8,9] It may ultimately be possible to perform large scalp and facial reconstructions with transplant allografts, following improvements in the safety of long-term immunosuppression.[5,10]

Cutis Aplasia Congenita. Cutis aplasia manifests as a tissue defect of the scalp (and possibly underlying cranium) ranging from a minor anomaly to a massive deficiency of scalp and cranium that leads to exposed dura. Several management strategies have been employed. In defects with exposed dura, it is important to keep the dura moist at all times to prevent desiccation and cracking. If the dura is not damaged, then spontaneous re-ossification of the cranium may occur over several months based on the osteogenic potential of the dura. Cranioplasty may otherwise be performed after a stable soft tissue envelope has been reconstructed. Healing by secondary intention and re-epithelialization of the wound from the margin is safe. Critical to the success of treatment plans is the need for consistent and meticulous care to protect the integrity of dura during the healing process. In addition, the newly formed skin is often friable and of poor quality. Local flaps may be a good option in some cases, but are more challenging in the neonatal age group. Scalp tissue expansion is usually avoided in neonates since the pressure of the expanders will significantly deform the underlying cranial bone. More recently, dermal substitutes have been used for exposed scalp coverage. Dermal substitutes are easy to apply at bedside, and keep the dura moist. In addition, newly formed skin is more supple and durable when compared with secondary intention healing. Finally, assessment of the underlying intracranial structures should be organized in conjunction with the neonatologist caring for these pediatric patients.

● COMPLICATIONS

The more common complications seen with any surgical procedure, namely bleeding and infection, are certainly seen with scalp reconstruction but may take on more significant weight. Superficial infections are less common in the scalp on account of its robust blood supply. With the need for calvarial bone reconstruction, however, infection that may involve the meninges can be potentially life-threatening. Similarly, bleeding inside the cranial vault has little room for expansion and can produce either a closed-space epidural or subdural hematoma. Thus, careful inspection and hemostasis is critical during reconstruction. If a large area of dura is exposed, it is probably beneficial to place circumferential tie-up sutures from the dura to the surrounding edge of bone to minimize tracking of blood laterally.

Injury to the dura is a potential complication with skull reconstruction. Care should be taken to dissect cautiously when bone is absent. Should a dural injury be discovered, adequate exposure of the entire defect should be achieved. This may require removal of more bone around the area of injury so that sutures can be placed with safety. If the edges can be approximated without undue tension, the wound should be closed with interrupted braided nylon. If the edges remain apart, a patch of either autogenous pericranium or alloplast can be used as an inlay material and sutured to the edges of the defect. Similarly, a patch of pericranium may be used as an overlay even if the edges can be approximated. Sterile sealant can also be used on top of the repair to further minimize cerebrospinal fluid leak.

The use of hydroxyapatite cement in the pediatric population remains controversial, with a concern that hydroxyapatite cement may alter cranial growth, thus creating cranial asymmetries. In cases when hydroxyapatite cement is used as an onlay for augmentation, it may become internalized within the cranial vault as the surrounding cranium grows. To understand why hydroxyapatite onlays become internalized within the cranium, one has to reexamine the mechanisms of calvarial growth. In a child, the cranium grows by deposition of new bone at the outer cortex with simultaneous resorption of the inner cortex. Hydroxyapatite used as an onlay graft prevents new bone formation on the outer cortex but does not prevent resorption of the inner cotex. Over time, the underlying bone is completely resorbed, and a full-thickness cranial defect is created. Therefore, the use of hydroxyapatite as an onlay for cranial augmentation and recontouring

should be delayed until cranial skeletal maturity. This process of internalization is also one of the reasons temporary resorbable plates and screws are used in children, while permanent titanium plates and screws are used in adults.

● OUTCOMES

Success or failure of scalp reconstruction is usually known within the first several days following the reconstruction. A successful outcome results if the flaps remain viable and the wound remains closed and stable. Scars that area able to be hidden further contribute to an aesthetic appearance and an excellent result. Occasionally, the reconstruction is adequate yet the underlying problem recurs, either due to regrowth of tumor or inadequate eradication of infection. A well-designed flap that accurately restructures the soft tissue is of little benefit if the patient continues to have leakage of cerebrospinal fluid from the edges of the wound. Carefully cataloguing the injured tissues within the defect and adequately reconstructing each will go a long way toward a successful outcome.

REFERENCES

1. Knize DM. *Forehead and Temporal Fossa: Anatomy and Technique.* Philadelphia: Lippincott Williams & Wilkins; 2001.

2. Stuzin JM, Wagstrom L, Kawamoto HK, Wolfe SA. Anatomy of the frontal branch of the facial nerve. *Plast. Reconstr. Surg.* 1989;83:265–271.

3. Orticochea M. New three-flap scalp reconstruction technique. *Br J Plast Surg.* 1971;24:184–188.

4. Leedy JE, Janis JE, Rohrich RJ. Reconstruction of acquired scalp defects: an algorithmic approach. *Plast Reconstr Surg.* 2005;116:54e–72e.

5. Temple CLF, Ross DC. Scalp and forehead reconstruction. *Clin Plastic Surg.* 2005;32:377–390.

6. Seline PC, Siegle RJ. Scalp reconstruction. *Dermatol Clin.* 2005;23:13–21.

7. Zuker RM. The use of tissue expansion in pediatric scalp burn reconstruction. *J Burn Care Rehabil.* 1987;8:103–106.

8. Thomas A, Obed V, Murarka A, Malhotra G. Total face and scalp replantation. *Plast Reconstr Surg.* 1998;102:285–287.

9. Sabapathy SR, Venkatramani H, Bharathi RR, D'Silva J. Technical considerations in replantation of total scalp avulsions. *J Plast Reconstr Aesthet Surg.* 2006;59:2–10.

10. Siemionow M, Agaoglu G. Allotransplantation of the face: how close are we? *Clin Plast Surg.* 2005;32:401–409.

chapter 35

Head and Neck Cancer

Stephan Ariyan, MD, MBA

● INTRODUCTION

In the early part of the twentieth century, George Crile[1] noted that most patients with cancer of the upper aerodigestive tract would die as a result of regional metastases to the cervical lymph nodes rather than metastases to distant organs. He therefore recommended the radical resection of the cervical lymph nodes in an attempt to cure these patients. The advances of anesthesia, and the establishment of blood transfusions paved the way for major improvements in the survival of these patients. Further developments in medicine continued into the late 1930s and 1940s that permitted safer extensions of the operations to achieve better cure rates from cancer treatment. The advent of intravenous thiopental (Pentothal) facilitated the induction of anesthesia and permitted the routine use of endotracheal tubes, as originally reported by Crile, for inhalation anesthetics. Once blood could be controlled from entering the tracheobronchial airway, these operations became safer. The further developments of blood-typing techniques and the establishment of blood banks permitted the replacement of blood loss and controlled the incidence of postoperative shock. Finally, early development of antibacterial drugs such as sulfa (and later the antibiotics) allowed control of the wound infections that followed these operations.

These landmark advances in medicine led to the improvement and the safety of major surgical procedures and permitted even more aggressive resections to treat more extensive cancers. Hayes Martin[2] advocated the radical resection of oral cancer together with the underlying mandible, popularizing the "commando procedure," to improve the chances of cure or local control. Subsequently, major advances by plastic surgery permitted early reconstruction, and eventually one-stage operations for the resection of the cancer and the repair of the regional anatomy.

Soon after the discovery of x-ray by Roentgen,[3] there were parallel improvements in the treatment of cancers with radiation therapy. In the early 1920s, orthovoltage machines with 200 kV radiation were developed and used in the treatment of these cancers, but there were many local complications from the radiation damage. Coutard[4] replaced single-dose radiation treatment with that of divided doses over 3 weeks, and the time-dose relationships that were elaborated by Strandqvist[5] led to the widespread acceptance of divided daily doses of radiation over 4 to 6 weeks. Towards the latter half of that century, there were advances in the development of various radioisotopes which led to the use of interstitial implantation to deliver additional radiation when the patient had already had previous external beam treatments. In a further evolution of these techniques, it was possible to add radioactive seeds in the periphery of the surgical resection site to further decrease local recurrence.

Similar advances occurred in chemotherapy subsequent to the discovery of methotrexate in the 1940s. The addition of new drugs and chemical agents have been shown to improve the results of surgery alone or radiation alone. Several successful trials have led to the advocacy of chemotherapeutic agents in the adjuvant setting, thereby permitting the preservation of vital organs, such as the larynx.

The development of these various therapeutic modalities mandates a close communication among the various specialists managing these cancer patients. Most medical centers have developed multidisciplinary tumor boards to evaluate these patients and to recommend appropriate treatment plans. It is the author's belief that these tumor boards should not recommend any one "decision" on management, because cancer is different in each patient and the possible combinations of primary site, lymph node involvement, and ancillary medical problems lead to innumerable possibilities of outcome. Furthermore, most studies of head and neck cancers have been retrospective because no single institution can generate significant numbers of comparable patients in a short period of time to make valid comparisons between different modalities for any given tumor site and stage. Tumor boards should therefore be advisory, providing a consensus of opinion and permitting minority opinions as well. The ultimate decision should still rest with the physician who has the primary responsibility for the individual care of that specific patient.

It is expected that there will be more than 40,000 new cases of cancer of the oral cavity, pharynx, and larynx in 2006.[6] Although we will be able to cure many of these patients, we must also remember that there will be many patients who come to see us when their cancers are too advanced for any hope of cure. In spite of this, some of these patients may be candidates for resections, for adjuvant radiotherapy, or chemotherapy, if only to achieve local control. On occasion, aggressive treatments, such as with intraoperative adjuvant radiation with radioactive seeds implanted following surgical resection of recurrence, have permitted long-term, disease-free survivals. These successes have opened up new avenues in treating patients with advanced cancer. As physicians, our goal is to "cure" patients; whenever we cannot accomplish this, our goal should be to "care" for them. We have a responsibility to provide our patients with comfort from their disability and their pain, and to provide them the opportunity to die with dignity in the company of their families and loved ones. Even though such palliation does not lead to increased survival in these patients with advanced cancer, these treatment modalities may allow the patients to return to their homes and spend the rest of their time in their chosen environment, rather than to spend it in a hospital or nursing home.

● GENERAL PRINCIPLES OF INTRAORAL CANCERS

Leukoplakia is a hyperkeratosis which appears as a white patch on the oral mucosa as a result of chronic irritation. For a number of years, leukoplakia was believed to be a precancerous lesion of the oral cavity. However, Pindborg[7] reported that in one third of the patients who harbor this lesion are cleared of the disorder within 15 years of follow-up. On the other hand, erythroplakia or erythroleukoplakia (white patches of leukoplakia within an area of erythroplakia) has been reported to show a higher risk of malignant transformation. Shafer and Waldron[8] reported that biopsies of erythroplakia were found to represent invasive carcinoma, carcinoma in situ, or severe dysplasia. Therefore, while leukoplakia can be treated conservatively, all lesions of erythroplakia should be biopsied and treated according to the histologic diagnosis.

Epidermoid carcinoma of the oropharynx grows with local invasion, and as it progresses, the cancer cells may spread along the lymphatics to the regional cervical lymph nodes. The various sites of the primary cancer have a

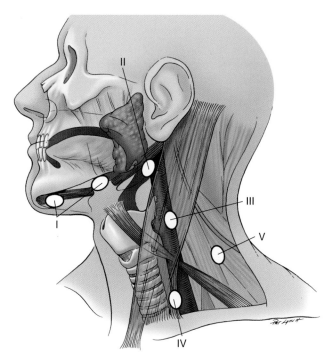

● **FIGURE 35-1.** Sites of cervical metastases to the various nodal groups: I—submandibular, II—jugulodigasrtic, III—midjugular, IV—supraclavicular, V—posterior cervical.

propensity to spread through these lymphatic channels to different chains of cervical lymph nodes (Figure 35-1). An understanding of this course of events is important because the treatment of these cancers is predicated on decisions based on the location and extent of the primary tumor, regional nodal involvement, and distant organ involvement, all of which result in the staging classification, which will be illustrated later.

Lymphatic Spread

Tumor cells may travel along lymphatic channels to reach the cervical nodes. These nodes may become enlarged either because of a reactive response to the bacteria in the oral cavity, which invade the tumor mass to cause a local infection, or because of tumor replacement of the node. Generally, lymph nodes need to enlarge to at least 1 cm in diameter before they can become clinically detectable.

On examination of the neck, the clinical impression of a "fixed" lymph node (ie, a lymph node that cannot be moved around by the examining fingers) is believed to represent the growth of tumor through the capsule of the lymph node and into the adjacent structures. However, this fixation may, in fact, also result from inflammation of the node as a response either to the tumor cells, or to bacterial invasion of the primary tumor. Although preoperative radiation may convert a "fixed" lymph node to a "freely movable" one, this change can also be observed in a number of patients treated with systemic antibiotics alone, and is not diagnostic.

Unknown Primary

Sometimes a metastatic lymph node may be diagnosed in the neck, but the site of the primary tumor cannot be identified. A complete and thorough examination with direct endoscopy and random biopsies will reveal the primary tumor in 60% of the initial cases; among the remaining patients, one third (15%) are identified later, while two thirds (25%) will remain undiagnosed even at autopsy.

These unknown primary tumors are often the result of a very small primary lesion that metastasized early from a region of the pharynx that is rich with lymphatics. The most common sites of these are along the Waldeyer ring: nasopharynx, base of tongue, tonsils, and pyriform sinus. In a smaller number of patients, it may actually represent a regression of the primary tumor after some cells have already metastasized to the lymph nodes. Regardless of the true etiology, the consensus is to treat these patients with cervical lymphadenectomy, or with radiation therapy to the neck, since such treatments result in 25% to 30% of the patients remaining disease-free at 5 years.

Hematogenous Spread

Metastases in lymph nodes do not *cause* distant organ spread, but are *indicators* of the potential for distant metastases having already occurred. Although tumor cells may be spread into the bloodstream as a result of biopsies or surgical removal, there is no correlation between positive blood samples or wound washings and subsequent recurrences or distant metastases.[9,10] It is more likely that the primary tumor is shedding malignant cells in the bloodstream continuously throughout its growth for some time before the diagnosis of malignancy is even made. When lymph nodes are found to be harboring cancer cells, it implies that this cancer is aggressive enough to overcome the immunologic defense of the lymph nodes. Therefore, this would represent a greater likelihood that any other cancer cells that may have entered the bloodstream, and traveled to distant organs, are more likely to be as aggressive and have the same potential to survive in these distant sites as well—presenting at a later date as distant metastases. The most frequent sites of distant organ spread by epidermoid carcinoma of the head and neck are the lungs, bones, and liver. Although distant metastases are detected clinically in 5% to 25% of the patients with oropharyngeal cancers,[11] 10% to 50% of the autopsy specimens have demonstrated such distant metastases.[12–14] Thus, the initial workup should include CT scans of the neck (for evaluation of the lymph nodes) or any painful boney areas (for metastases to bones), chest x-ray, and liver function tests in order to stage the patient according to the TNM (tumor, node, metastasis) system.

● DIAGNOSTIC WORKUP

The proper workup of the patient with a tumor of the head and neck must include a thorough clinical examination together with proper biopsies to determine the extent of the cancer, in order to classify and stage the disease. The occurrence of benign lesions, such as necrotizing sialometaplasia,[15] that resemble malignancies, and the presentation of some early malignancies that look like benign lesions, both serve to preclude accurate assessment of oral and pharyngeal lesions by clinical examination alone. Regardless of the clinical experience and expertise of the treating physician, the use of tissue biopsy remains the essential definitive diagnostic tool.

Biopsy

The biopsy of the tumor may be either *incisional or excisional*. Incisional biopsy of a representative portion of the lesion should include a small segment of adjacent normal tissue in order to differentiate a malignancy from tissue damage due to chronic irritation, previous interventions, or previous radiation therapy. Excisional biopsy should be reserved for solitary lesions that are small, easily accessible, and superficial. In all excisional biopsies, attention must be paid to both the peripheral and the deep margins to ensure adequate and complete removal for microscopic examination of extent of invasion.

Fine-Needle Aspiration. It is absolutely essential to defer any open biopsy of a suspicious neck node or of any mass in the head and neck region until a full and comprehensive diagnostic workup has been completed in an effort to find the primary lesion. Since the primary cancer can be discovered in most of the patients who are initially seen with such masses, this policy of a thorough workup avoids treatment delays, inappropriate incisions, and local recurrences as a result of seeding of tumor cells.

While open biopsy as a first step in diagnosis are to be condemned, the technique of thin- or fine-needle aspiration (FNA) biopsy has been firmly established in the diagnostic workup. FNA defines the disorder as a malignancy or inflammation, can identify the cell type or tissue of origin, has been found to be a reliable technique for diagnosis, and is virtually free of needle tract recurrences in malignant tumors in the neck. This is a simple technique that can be performed readily in the office with a 22-gauge needle (Figure 35-2), and can provide the pathologist with glass slide smears for cytologic examination, and samples for a paraffin block.[16]

Sentinel Node Biopsies. The principle of this technique is based on three tenets: (1) that each anatomic site has specific lymph nodes that filter the efferent lymphatic vessels leading from the tumor; (2) that these lymph nodes can be identified; and (3) that the absence of tumor cells in those lymph nodes is a reliable indicator that there are no other lymph nodes in that group harboring cancer. This technique of localization of the lymph nodes has been employed successfully for the detection of metastatic nodes in the workup of melanomas.[17–20] This has been particularly helpful in tumors located near the anatomic midline, to locate the draining lymph nodes, and

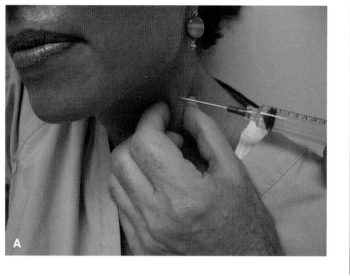
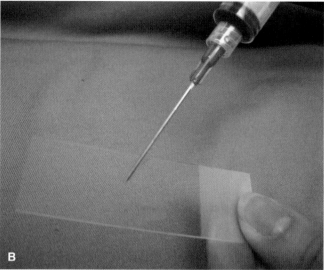
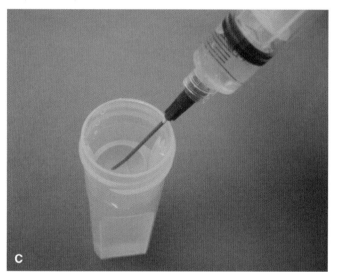
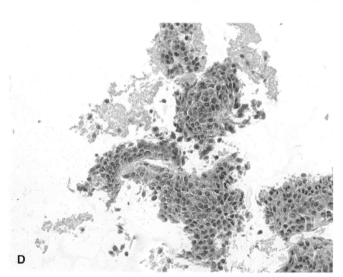

● FIGURE 35-2. FNA can be performed in the office with a three-ring controlled syringe using a 22-gauge needle (A), to prepare smears on a slide (B), as well as needle bore flushes in absolute alcohol (C), to provide histologic diagnosis (D)—in this case of melanoma.

to determine if the drainage involves the lymph nodes of the parotid region (Figure 35-3). Since head and neck cancers are epithelial malignancies in origin, this method of radiolocalization has also been evaluated in oral cavity cancers.[21-22] These authors found that the injected technetium sulfur colloid in the mucosa surrounding the oral carcinomas was readily taken up by the regional nodes. However, they noted that after the tumors had been resected, the changes in the anatomy has the potential to render the uptake of the colloid unreliable for any meaningful localization.[21]

Diagnostic Imaging Tests

With the exception of primary glandular neoplasms (salivary gland, thyroid gland, lymph glands), the vast majority of head and neck cancers are epithelial surface tumors. Therefore, useful radiographic studies are limited to

evaluations of the surface mucosa, sometimes with the use of contrast material such as barium swallow to examine the hypopharynx or the esophagus. Otherwise, diagnostic imaging studies for the tumors of this region are most successful when employing computerized technology.

Computed Tomography and Related Studies. CT scanning is most helpful in the evaluation of the primary tumors, by allowing a non-invasive evaluation of the tumor size, providing information regarding extent of invasion, and evaluating evidence of invasion of bony structures of the maxillofacial area (Figure 35-4). CT scans are also helpful in the evaluation of cervical lymph node metastases, and criteria have been developed that provide for differentiation of normal or "reactive" nodes from those involved with metastatic tumor.[23,24] The criteria for lymph nodes positive for harboring tumor include discrete masses measuring 15 mm or more in diameter, ill-

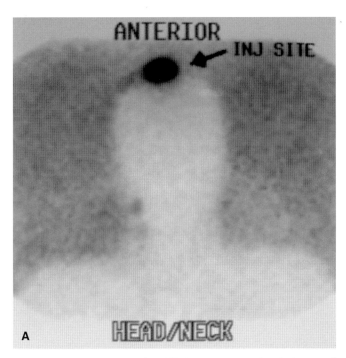
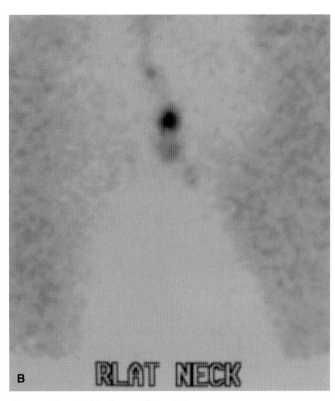

● FIGURE 35-3. A lymphocintigram of a melanoma located in the midline of the vertex of the scalp (A), shows drainage toright neck only, while a lateral view (B) shows drainage to a small node of the parotid gland, a hotter node at the angle of the mandible, and two additional nodes in the middle and lower neck.

defined or irregular borders to nodal masses, and groups of three or more nodes, each in the range of 6 to 15 mm in diameter.

Nuclear Magnetic Resonance Imaging. Magnetic resonance imaging appears to be superior to CT in several respects. Techniques for MRI allow for a better definition of soft tissue and the extent of tumor invasion into the various tissue planes. As such, MRI is superior to CT scanning for soft tissue delineation. The use of MRI of the posterior fossa was first reported by Young et al.[25] to illustrate these advantages. In a subsequent study, Randell et al.[26] compared MRI with CT in a series of 26 patients with tumors in the posterior fossa. While CT was better for demonstrating calcification or bony invasion by tumor, MRI was shown overall to be more much more sensitive for the demonstration of mass effects (Figure 35-5); even identifying some tumors that were not visualized at all by CT. MRI is also excellent for evaluating the neck for large metastatic nodes and determining the extent of tumor invasion of adjacent muscles, vessels and nerves.[27]

MRI has also been helpful in the diagnostic workup of salivary gland tumors. Because the intensity of the signal of the parotid gland is slightly less than that of the surrounding subcutaneous fat, and greater relative to muscle, it can enhance the difference between these adjacent

structures. Additionally, the submandibular gland has a slightly lower signal intensity than the sublingual gland, which may permit the delineation of the deep segment of the submandibular gland from the adjacent sublingual gland. Any tumor within the salivary glands would then be differentiated from the glandular structures.

Technetium Scan. The ability of salivary glands to concentrate technetium-99m pertechnetate (Tc 99m) forms the basis of the use of this nuclear medicine technique in imaging salivary glands. The increased metabolic activity of the cells comprising Warthin tumor produces the characteristic image of increased uptake. Oncocytomas are other lesions that may take up this tracer in excess of surrounding gland. Rarely, oncocytic rests in pleomorphic adenomas, and oncocytic tumor metastases might also mimic this picture. However, aside from Warthin tumor, Tc 99m scans are not very useful in other salivary gland imaging, or in oropharyngeal carcinomas.

● **INTRAORAL CANCERS**

Although the oral cavity and oropharynx are anatomically distinct regions for classification, their management is discussed together because of the many similarities in their diagnostic workup and treatment options. Whereas the oral cavity is defined as the area extending from the

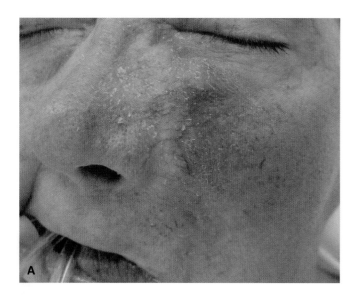

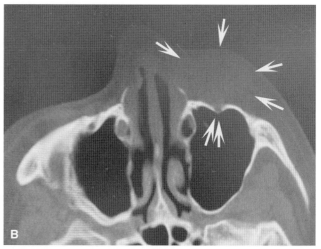

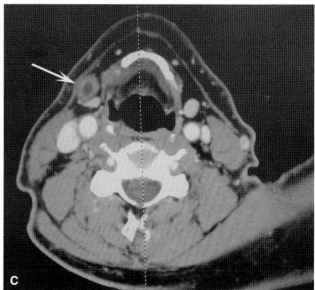

● FIGURE 35-4. A recurrent tumor of the maxillofacial area (A) can be evaluated by CT scan (B) to determine if the tumor (*single arrows*) invades bone (*double arrow* is at infraorbital foramen). A CT scan of the neck (C) of another patient shows an enlarged node with central necrosis (*arrow*).

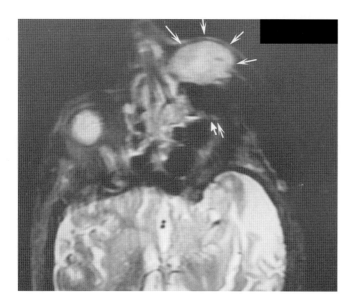

● FIGURE 35-5. MRI scan of same patient as in Figure 35-4A,B shows the extent of the tumor (*single arrows*) much better, and can evaluate the bony wall of the maxillary sinus, and the posterior wall of the sinus (*double arrows*).

vermilion border of the lips to an imaginary plane between the junction of the hard and soft palates above, and the circumvallate papillae of the tongue below, the oropharynx extends from this plane posteriorly and includes the soft palate, tonsils, tonsillar pillars, base of tongue, and pharynx (Figure 35-6).

The most common sites of cancers of the oral cavity are the tongue (36%), floor of mouth (35%), gingiva (16%), buccal mucosa (10%), and hard palate (3%) (Figure 35-7). The overall 5-year survival rates at these sites range from 31% to 66%, but two thirds of these cancers are already in stage III or IV by the time they are first seen by a physician. This delay in treatment has many causes, including minimal symptoms, inadequate routine oral examinations, and reluctance by the patient to acknowledge its presence because of fear of a diagnosis of cancer.[28]

The order of frequency for sites of oropharyngeal cancers are the tonsillar fossa (43%), soft palate (26%), base of tongue (20%), and the pharyngeal walls (11%) (Figure 35-8). The overall 5-year survival rates at these sites range from 17% to 57%. In the past, the differences

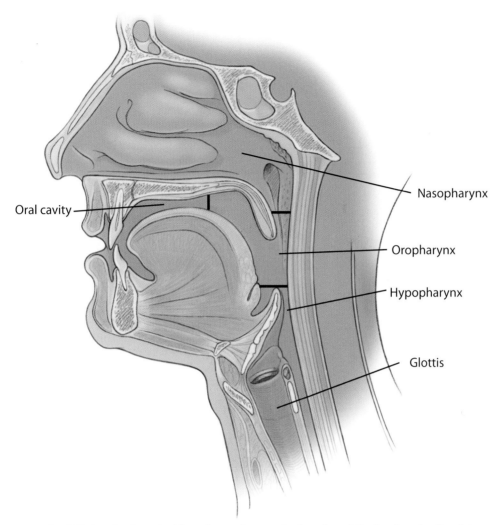

FIGURE 35-6. A vertical imaginary plane at the junction of the hard and soft palates separates the oropharynx from the oral cavity.

in survival statistics between oral cavity and oropharyngeal lesions was believed to be due to the biologically more aggressive nature of cancers of the oropharyngeal area. This is not quite correct. The difference is the delay in the detection of the cancer which leads to the more advanced stage of the oropharyngeal tumors at the time of diagnosis. This delay can account for as much as 20% to 30% of the advanced lesions of the pharynx not being diagnosed until metastases have been detected in the cervical nodes.

The classification of these tumors (T) is based on the measured size of the primary lesion (Table 35-1). Regardless of the size of the primary tumor, any invasion of the tumor into adjacent and deeper structures represents more aggressive behavior and therefore upstages the tumor. The classification of the nodal involvement has been unchanged with the latest (6th edition) American Joint Committee on Cancer system revision of 2002 (Table 35-2). The one major change with the 6th edition is in the separation of the stage IV tumors (Table 35-3) into those that are locally advanced, surgically resectable

(stage IVa), and may be salvaged, from those that are not resectable (stage IVb) but potentially treatable by chemotherapy, and those that have evidence of distant metastases (stage IVc).

Treatment

Stage I Disease. Stage I disease is best treated by local excision. Although radioactive seed implants have also been used successfully for early lesions of the floor of the mouth,[29] it has some distinct limitations because of the expertise necessary to properly plan and execute this treatment. Excision and primary closure of the wound may be successful in very small lesions. However, in larger resections, this type of closure will surely lead to a tethered tongue and deficient articulation.

Tongue Flap. A resection of the ipsilateral anterior tongue can be covered by the lateral rotation of the remaining tongue. The tongue flap can be used quite effectively from the lateral aspects of the tongue to resurface lateral or anterior floor of mouth defects (Figure 35-9).

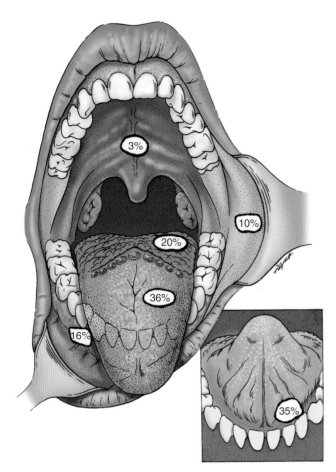

● **FIGURE 35-7.** Common sites of cancer of the oral cavity by order of incidence: anterior tongue, floor of mouth, posterior tongue, gingival, buccal mucosa, hard palate. (*From Chicarilli ZN, Ariyan S. Cancer of the Oral Cavity Basic Principles. In: Ariyan S, ed. Cancer of the Head and Neck. St. Louis, MO: CV Mosby; 1987.*)

TECHNIQUE. A traction suture is placed through the tip of the tongue to stabilize the extended tongue. The flap is taken from the lateral aspect of the tongue, with equal amounts from the dorsal and ventral surfaces. The incisions are angled in to excise a wedge of tongue muscle in the flap, to dissect a flap of adequate thickness (and vascularity), and to permit easy closure of the donor site. As the dissection proceeds posteriorly, the flap should become wider to ensure a more vascular and more reliable flap. Then the flap is transferred to the wound, and the muscle of the tongue flap is anchored securely to the wound margins.

ADVANTAGES. This is a very reliable vascular flap that does not leave a scar on the face or neck. The donor site is closed by direct suturing, and it does not leave a sensory or motor deficit.

DISADVANTAGES. Although we have had very good successes with this flap, there is always the potential that the use of this flap could have some adverse effects on the speech of some patients.

Stage II Disease. Stage II disease can be resected locally, but these larger lesions often encroach upon the mandible and may require rim resections of the mandible[30,31] to get adequate margins (Figure 35-10), while still providing local control rates equal to segmental resection of the mandible.[30] While marginal resections take a vertical segment of the inner table of the mandible, a rim mandibulectomy, on the other hand, takes a horizontal segment of the full thickness of the mandible and has been shown to not weaken the structural integrity of the mandible.[32]

The reconstruction of these surgical defects may be via an apron flap,[33,34] the platysma flap,[35] the sternocleidomastoid musculocutaneous flap,[36,37] or a free flap (for a reconstruction without tethering the tongue). Larger defects may require reconstruction with the pectoralis major myocutaneous flap, latissimus dorsi myocutaneous flap, or free flaps of muscle or bone, with or without overlying skin.

Platysma Flap. The apron flap is actually a musculocutaneous flap incorporating the platysma muscle. It was originally used as a vertical flap overlying the anterior neck (Figure 35-11). This muscle may be used to transport a transversely outlined paddle of skin on the posterolateral aspect of the neck, incorporating the posterior blood supply to the platysma muscle.[38,39]

CLINICAL APPLICATION. The vertical platysma flap is suitable for coverage of small defects in the floor of mouth, undersurface of the tongue, and lower lip. The transverse platysma flap can be used to cover defects on the outer surface of the lips, cheek, and preauricular skin.

TECHNIQUE. A paddle of skin is outlined in the middle portion of the neck (Figure 35-11). The flap is then elevated with skin and underlying platysma muscle, incorporating branches of the facial vessels for blood supply. The base of the flap is de-epithelialized and turned under the mandible to reach the floor of mouth and resurface the defect. The skin remains at the distal end of the flap. The de-epithelialized base of the flap is covered with the raw surface of the root of the tongue. The donor site on the anterior neck is covered with a skin graft.

The transverse platysma flap can be outlined as parallel incisions cutting through the skin, subcutaneous fat, and the platysma muscle fibers (Figure 35-12). Once the submuscular plane is reached, the flap is dissected up to its base, taking care to not cut into the undersurface of the muscle, and to avoid damage to its intramuscular blood supply. The donor site can then be closed with neck advancement flaps.

ADVANTAGES. This flap provides thin, pliable tissue for the small defects of the anterior portion of the oral cavity, and the incorporation of the platysma muscle improves the vascularity of the flap. The transverse platysma flap donor site can be closed with a cervical advancement flap resulting in a very acceptable linear scar of the neck.

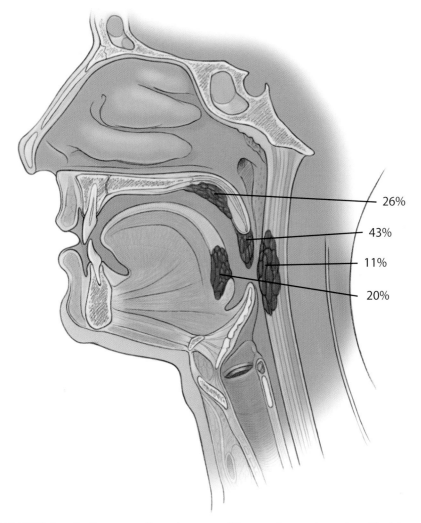

26%

43%

11%

20%

● **FIGURE 35-8.** Common sites of cancer of the oropharynx by order of incidence: tosillar fossa, soft palate, base of tongue, posterior pharyngeal wall. (*From Chicarilli ZN and Ariyan S: In Ariyan S, ed., Cancer of the Head and Neck, CV Mosby, St. Louis, 1987.*)

DISADVANTAGES. The flap is unreliable in patients with previous radiation therapy to the face and neck, as it has probably caused fibrosis to the delicate blood supply. In addition, patients with previous neck dissections most likely have significant scarring of the platysma muscle, precluding its use in the flap. The donor site of the full apron flap requires coverage with a skin graft.

Sternocleidomastoid Flap. The sternocleidomastoid (SCM) muscle has three blood supplies: (1) a branch of the occipital artery superiorly, (2) the superior thyroid artery in the midportion, or (3) the thyrocervical trunk inferiorly (Figure 35-13). This flap can be used for reconstruction, incorporating a superiorly based flap with a skin paddle inferiorly (Figure 35-14), which can then be transported under the mandible to reconstruct a surgical defect in the floor of the mouth. Alternatively, an inferiorly based flap with the skin over the mastoid portion of the flap (Figure 35-15) can be transported to reach the floor of the mouth, or twisted 180 degrees on its vertical axis to reach the lateral pharynx or tonsillar fossa.

TECHNIQUE. Once the skin incisions are made along the outline of the skin paddle, another skin incision is made along the midaxis of the SCM muscle along its entire length (Figure 35-16) to expose the anterior and posterior borders of the attachments of the cervical fascia. The skin paddle should be sutured securely to the underlying SCM muscle fascia to protect the delicate musculocutaneous vessels from shearing while being transferred during the reconstruction. This is even more important over the supraclavicular area, where there is abundant loose areolar tissue and very thin delicate blood vessels to the skin. Traction sutures placed at the distal end of the muscle pedicle, can help to elevate the flap from the deeper layer of the investing fascia once the fascia is cut along the anterior and posterior borders of the muscle. The muscle pedicle should be dissected out only as is needed to reach the recipient wound; in this fashion, the middle blood supply may often be preserved. The flap may then be transferred under the mandible into the floor of mouth, to securely anchor the muscle pedicle to durable structures along the periphery of the wound (periosteum or adjacent muscular fascia).

TABLE 35-1. Primary Tumor (T) Classification of the Oral Cavity and Oropharynx

Tis: Carcinoma in situ
T1: Tumor ≤2 cm in greatest dimension
T2: Tumor >2 cm but <4 cm in greatest dimension
T3: Tumor >4 cm in greatest dimension
T4: Tumor invading adjacent structures
(Lip) Tumor invades through cortical bone, inferior alveolar nerve, floor of mouth, or skin of face (ie, chin or nose)
4a: (Oral cavity) Tumor invades through cortical bone into deep muscles of tongue maxillary sinus, or skin of face
4b: Tumor invades masticatory space, pterygoid plates, or skull base, and/or encases carotid artery

From Greene FL, Page DL, Fleming ID, et al. AJCC Cancer Staging Manual. 6th ed. New York: Springer; 2002.

TABLE 35-2. Nodal (N) Classification of Cancers of the Oral Cavity and Oropharynx

N0: No regional nodal metastases
N1: Metastases in a single ipsilateral lymph node, ≤3 cm in greatest dimension
N2: Metastases in a single ipsilateral lymph node, >3 cm, but <6 cm in greatest dimension; or multiple ipsilateral lymph nodes, none >6 cm; or contralateral or bilateral lymph nodes, none >6 cm in greatest dimension
N3: Metastases in any lymph node >6 cm in greatest dimension

From Greene FL, Page DL, Fleming ID, et al. AJCC Cancer Staging Manual. 6th ed. New York: Springer; 2002.

TABLE 35-3. Stage Grouping of Cancers of the Oral Cavity and Oropharynx

Stage	N0	N1	N2	N3	Any M
T1	I	III	IVa	IVb	IVc
T2	II	III	IVa	IVb	IVc
T3	III	III	IVa	IVb	IVc
T4a	IVa	IVa	IVa	IVb	IVc
T4b	IVb	IVb	IVb	IVb	IVc

is no significant fibrosis from the previous radiation. However, this flap should not be used in any patient who has clinical evidence of radiation thickening of the skin, as this represents fibrosis of the fine vessels to the skin, as well as scarring of the muscle.

ADVANTAGES. This flap permits the transfer of local tissue in one stage without delay. The donor site of the skin can be closed with advancement flaps, and skin grafts can be avoided.

DISADVANTAGES. Even with careful selection of the patients, a third of the flaps exhibit epidermal loss. In such cases, the remainder of the flap remains intact (including the dermal portion of the skin) and will re-epithelialize without additional surgical intervention. Another disadvantage is the cosmetic deficiency in patients with a thin neck as a result of the transfer of the muscle.

Pectoralis Major Flap. The pectoralis major muscle is a flat muscle on the chest that has a large and easily identifiable dominant blood supply from the thoracoacromial artery, a branch of the sublavian artery. The reliability of a large portion of skin elevated on only a narrow portion of this muscle was first reported by Ariyan and Krizek[41] in 1977. The vascular anatomy of this muscle was defined as having its dominant blood supply from the thoracoacromial artery, its minor blood supply from the lateral thoracic artery, and additional segmental blood flow from the perforator vessels from the internal mammary arteries.[41,42]

The pectoralis major flap can be used for large defects of the oral cavity, pharynx, orbital exenterations, temporal bone resections, and large craniofacial resections.[43-45] In thin patients, it has also been used successfully for pharynoesophageal reconstructions. The safety, reliability, and versatility of this flap for various reconstructions has been validated by a number of other authors.[46-48]

TECHNIQUE. The vascular pedicle is first outlined on the chest by an axis drawn from the shoulder tip to the xyphoid—the thoracoacromial vessels exit the midportion of the clavical at a perpendicular to this axis, and then follow distally along this line (Figure 35-17). The skin paddle is drawn to the size necessary for the planned reconstruction, centered on this vascular axis.

This is essential in order to prevent shearing the small vessels to the skin paddle by traction on the muscle pedicle when the patient moves the neck in the early postoperative period. Since the skin paddle of this flap is usually small (often only 3 × 6 cm), the donor site can usually be closed by advancement of local tissue.

CLINICAL APPLICATION. This flap is suitable for reconstruction of small defects in the oral cavity, lateral tongue, retromolar trigone, and tonsillar fossa. I have often used this flap successfully on either end of the muscle pedicle, even in patients with previous radiation therapy to the neck,[37,40] with the following proviso: that the skin and muscle are still soft and pliable, and radiation is not suspected until the patient's history determines it to be so. This is because a soft neck probably signifies that there

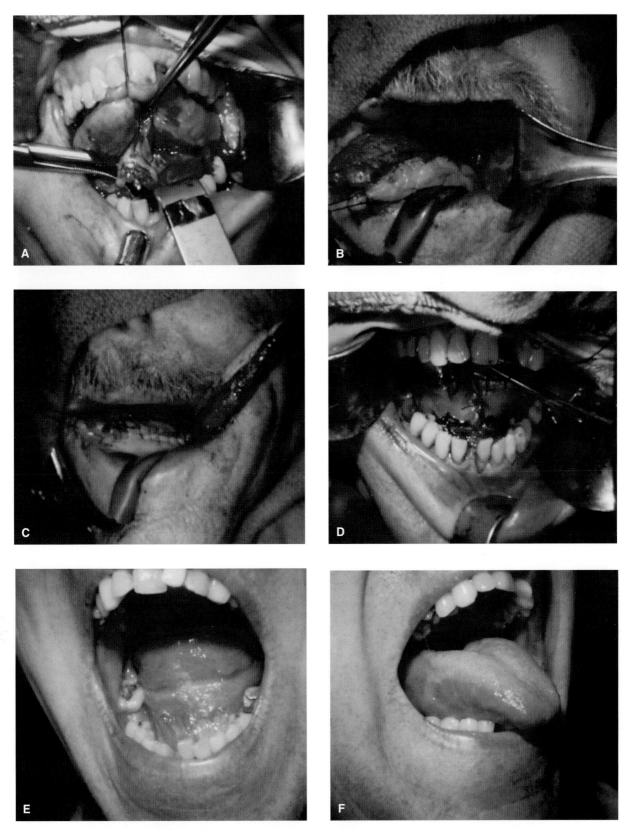

● **FIGURE 35-9.** Resection of a tumor of the floor of mouth (A) can be reconstructed with one or two local flaps from the lateral portions of the tongue. The lateral flap (B) is raised with a wedge of the underlying tongue musculature, based on its posterior blood supply (C). The flaps can then be sutured together and to the wound margins (D). When the flaps mature, they are soft, pliable, and allow for good protrusion of the tongue tip, without loss of length (E, F).

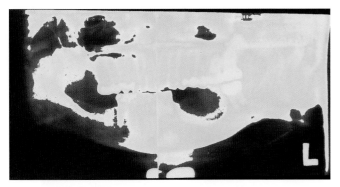

FIGURE 35-10. A cancer of the floor of mouth can be resected with a full thickness of the body of the mandible, while preserving the cortical base and the integrity of the mandibular arch. (See also Figure 35-16).

To be sure that the flap is elevated without injury to the blood supply, it is best to visualize the vessels directly. This is most readily done by making an incision along the lateral aspect of the skin paddle, down to the underlying pectoralis major muscle, and splitting the muscle along its fibers until the subpectoral fascia is penetrated. A large retractor is then placed in this subpectoral plane and the muscle is separated and elevated from the chest wall by finger dissection in this loose areolar plane—this is a bloodless finger dissection. The vascular pedicle is then easily visualized directly in this subpectoral plane, and protected during the remainder of the dissection of the flap.

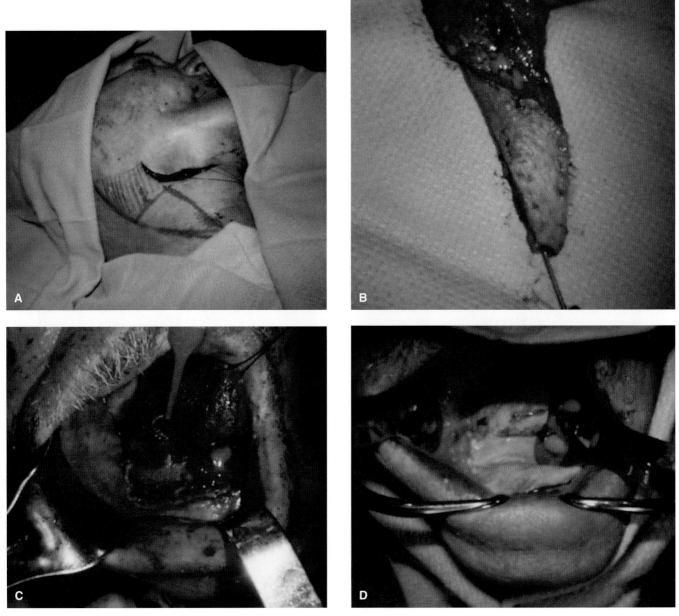

FIGURE 35-11. A small paddle of skin (A) can be transferred on a vertically oriented pedicle of platysma muscle (B), to reconstruct a resection of the floor of mouth (C), and can be seen at 4 years following the surgery (D).

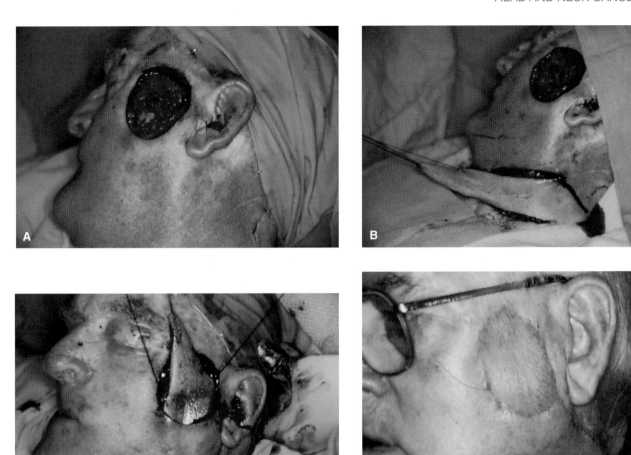

● **FIGURE 35-12.** A radical resection of a tumor overlying the parotid gland
(A), is reconstructed with a segment of skin across the neck incorporating the underlying
transverse portion of platysma muscle (B). The flap is tunneled under the facial skin
(C), the skin of the buried portion of the flap is removed leaving only platysma muscle, the
complete the repair in one stage (D). The flap donor site in the neck is closed primarily.

As the dissection is carried along the periphery of the flap, sutures are placed to anchor the skin paddle to the underlying muscle fascia to prevent inadvertent shearing of the small vertical musculocutaneous blood vessels. The muscle pedicale that is dissected along with the skin paddle needs only to be as wide as is necessary to incorporate the thoracoacromial vessels, generally about 4 to 6 cm (Figure 35-18). Once the muscle pedicle is dissected up to the clavicular border, the muscle is then dissected off the clavicle, freeing its attachment to this bone, and separating it by a few centimeters. However, the vessels should not be skeletonized during this dissection, but should be left attached to the subpectoral fascia under the clavicle, to allow the tethering which would protect the vessels from shearing injury. This fascial attachment allows the detached muscle pedicle to turn above and

over the clavicle, with only the vessels and accompanying fascia to lie over the bone. In this fashion, the clavicular bulge from the muscle pedicle may be avoided.

The entire skin paddle is drawn to lie over the pectoralis major. If a larger skin paddle is required, a portion of it may be extended beyond the inferior margin of the pectoralis major. However, it should incorporate the underlying fascia of the external oblique muscle, and half or more of the skin paddle should still remain over the pectoralis major.

Finally, unless an extraordinarily large skin paddle is required, the donor site can be readily closed by dissection along the chest wall laterally, and advancement of this large chest flap.

CLINICAL APPLICATION. The pectoralis major is very useful for the reconstruction of large defects at a number of

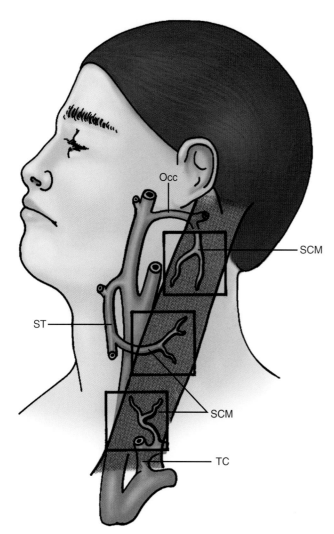

● **FIGURE 35-13.** The three blood supplies to the sternocleidomastoid (SCM) muscle include the branches of the occipital artery (Occ) above, the branch of the superior thyroid artery (ST) in the midportion, and the branch from the thyrocervical trunk (TC) in the lower portion. (*From Ariyan S. One-stage reconstruction for defects of the mouth using a sternomastoid myocutaneous flap. Plast Reconstr Surg. 1979;66:618.*)

surgical resection sites. Within the oral cavity it provides sufficient bulk following total glossectomy. Since it has been demonstrated that this muscle flap can provide nutrient flow to the rib through the periosteal blood supply,[49] this musculocutaneous flap can be harvested with a segment of underlying rib for replacement of bone and soft tissue of the mandible and malar region.

Most patients who have cancers of the oropharyngeal area are underweight because of difficulty with swallowing. As a result, the flap can be used to facilitate reconstruction of the pharyngoesophagus in thin patients (Figure 35-19). Two musculocutaneous pedicles can be harvested, either in tandem (with the intervening skin removed) or side-by-side (one on the thoracodorsal blood supply and one on the lateral thoracic blood supply) for through-and-through resections of the cheek.[50]

Furthermore, this flap has had significant applications in the reconstructions of very large defects of the skull base in temporal bone resections (Figure 35-20), radical orbital resections (Figure 35-21), and fronto-orbitomaxillary resections[45] (Figure 35-22).

ADVANTAGES. The pectoralis major flap is very reliable, and surgeons do not need additional instruments or surgical skills, as would be necessary for microsurgical free flaps. These reconstructions can be performed virtually in any operating room around the world. The muscle in the flap provides additional blood supply if the site of reconstruction has been previously treated with high dose radiation, and the flap can tolerate additional postoperative radiation. In older female patients, the skin paddle can be harvested from the medial and parasternal aspect of the chest so as not to distort the breast form. In younger women, the skin can be designed in the inframammary area to maintain the shape of the breast mound.[51]

DISADVANTAGES. While hair-bearing tissue may be transferred to the intraoral area in hairy males, this is not quite as problematic in the oropharyngeal reconstructions as it may seem. The hair on the chest is very short, and the individual hair follicles are very fragile, break off, and fall out before they get long.

Reconstructions of the frontal, orbital, or maxillary areas may require the muscle pedicle to be left exposed on the surface of the face, requiring a secondary procedure to divide and inset the flap, at which point the pedicle may be discarded.

Trapezius Flap. The trapezius is a flat triangular muscle overlying the neck, shoulder and upper back. The muscle is supplied with three blood vessels: the upper cervical portion of the muscle is supplied by a branch of the occipital artery; the distal portion of the shoulder segment overlying the acromion is supplied by a branch of the suprascapular artery; and the remainder of the muscle over the back is nourished by the dominant blood supply from transverse cervical artery. This blood supply travels along the undersurface of the muscle, descending the back along the paraspinous region.

The trapezius myocutaneous flap, described by Demegasso and Piazza,[52,53] was designed entirely on the transverse cervical blood supply, to transport a skin paddle to various sites of the oropharyngeal area. McGraw and associates[54,55] reported the use of this flap designed transversely along the shoulder, as in epaulettes of a uniform (Figure 35-23A), on its occipital blood supply. Ariyan[56] reported the application of this design entirely on the transverse portion of the muscle to the shoulder tip, preserving the transverse cervical artery, but transecting the suprascapular artery at the tip of the shoulder. Since the transverse cervical artery descends along the undersurface of the muscle along the back, Mathes and Nahai[57] described the design of the flap along the paraspinous back (Figure 35-23B), providing a long flap nourished by

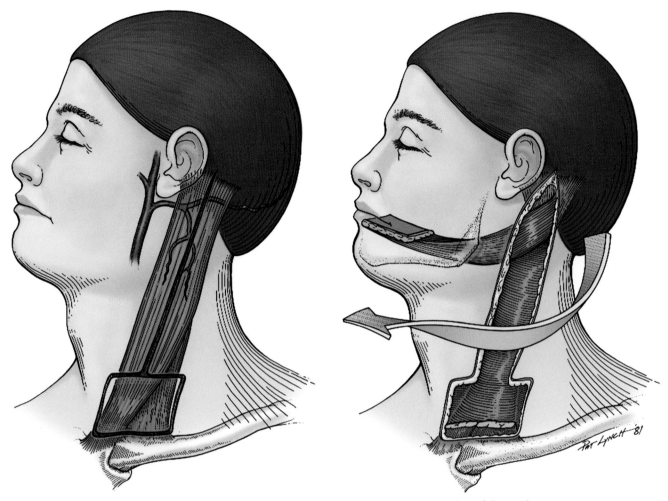

● **FIGURE 35-14.** A segment of skin outlined on the inferior portion of the neck overlying the SCM can be elevated with the muscle as its pedicle based superiorly with the branch of the occipital artery.

this axial blood supply. Proposing that the blood to the flap would flow retrograde from the back if the transverse cervical artery has been transected in the neck during a radical neck dissection, Gardiener et al.[58] subsequently reported the successful use of a trapezius myocutaneous flap designed transversely on the shoulder, after dissecting and freeing and preserving the descending portion of the blood vessels as a "mesentery." Finally, as with many myocutaneous flaps, the trapezius was demonstrated by Panje and Cutting[59] to be capable of incorporating the attached acromion to reconstruct a segment of resected mandible.

Technique. The outline of the anterior border of the muscle is marked on the skin of the neck and shoulder. The anterior border of the skin paddle is along this border of the muscle, and the posterior border of the skin is marked according to the width of the flap that is desired (Figure 35-24). The distal end of the flap is marked according to the length to which the flap must reach to the recipient defect.

The incisions along the skin markings are deepened to include the muscle as the pedicle. If the distal end of the

flap is beyond the crest of the acromion, then the fascia of the deltoid and part of the periostium covering the acromion should be incorporated with the muscle. As the muscle is dissected up to its base in the neck, the transverse cervical artery and vein are identified deep to the trapezius and above the levator scapulae muscles, and preserved. The dissection then continues medially up to the base of the neck and the muscle may be left attached to include the branch of the occipital artery, or the muscle may be detached here to be transported as an island vascular flap.

If the acromion or the transverse spine of the scapula is needed, then the muscle is not detached from the bone at the distal end of the flap. A segment of the needed bone is marked with a surgical pen and the segment of bone is cut with a power tool and left attached to the muscle pedicle.

If a large segment of skin or a long pedicle is required, then the skin paddle is marked on the back of the chest, descending in a vertical direction along the paraspinous portion of the muscle. To do so, the operation begins with prepping the head and neck area, the entire arm, as well as the axilla, anterior chest, and posterior chest within the field of surgery. The sterile drapes are stapled

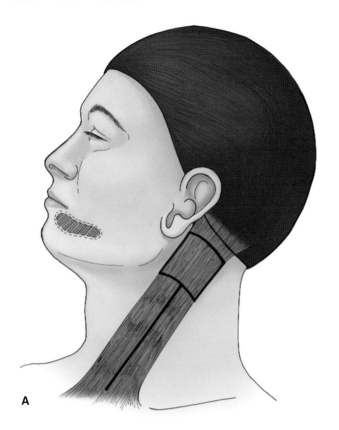

A

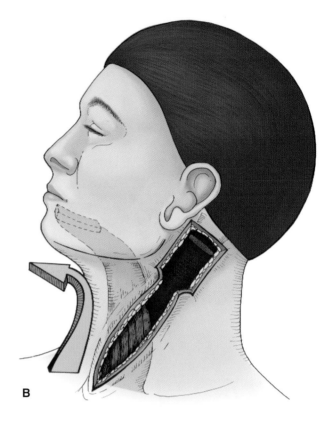

B

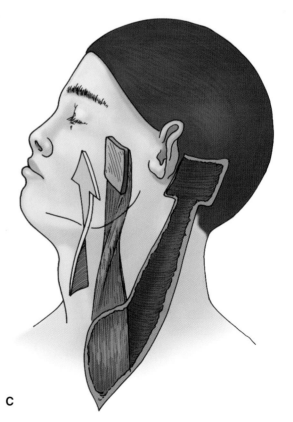

C

● **FIGURE 35-15.** A segment of skin outlined on the mastoid attachment of the muscle (A) can be elevated with the blood supply provided by the thyrocervical trunk inferiorly to reach the floor of mouth (B) or the lateral pharynx (C).

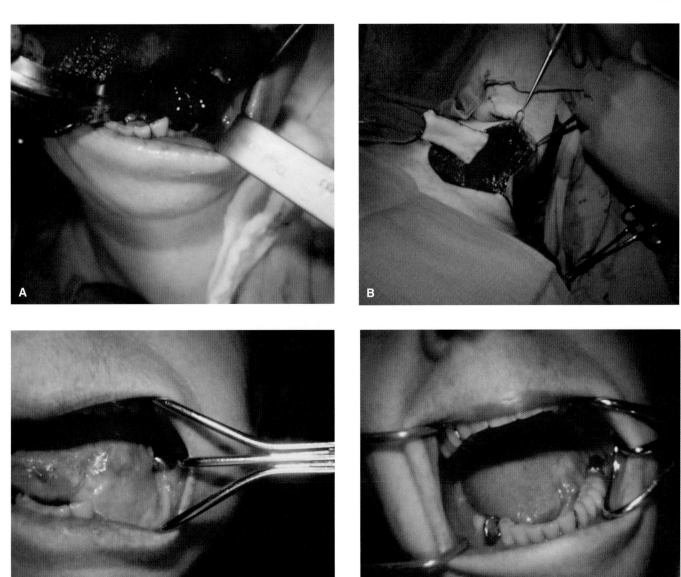

● **FIGURE 35-16.** A cancer of the floor of mouth was resected (A) together with a full thickness of the alveolar portion of the mandible while preserving the cortical base and the integrity of the mandibular arch (as in Figure 35-10). A skin paddle overlying the lower portion of the sternocleidomastoid muscle was elevated on its superior blood supply (B), transferred under the mandible to reconstruct the floor of mouth and undersurface of tongue seen at 10 months (C). The dental occlusion can be restored with a dental bridge (D) to the posterior molar that was preserved.

to the back, and the patient is returned to the supine position in order to continue with the surgical draping. After the resection is completed, the patient is turned onto the opposite side and the flap margins are outlined on the back with a marking pen. The incisions are made through the skin, deepened through the muscle, the submuscular plane is entered, and the flap is dissected up to the neck, identifying and protecting the vascular pedicle along the undersurface of the muscle.

CLINICAL APPLICATION. This flap can be harvested as a transverse flap along the shoulder for reconstructions of the cheek and neck. The posterior vertical variant of the flap can be used for reconstructions of the base of skull, or occipital portion of the cranium. The flap can incorporate the transverse spine for repair of the body of the mandible, or the acromion for reconstruction of the symphyseal portion of the jaw.

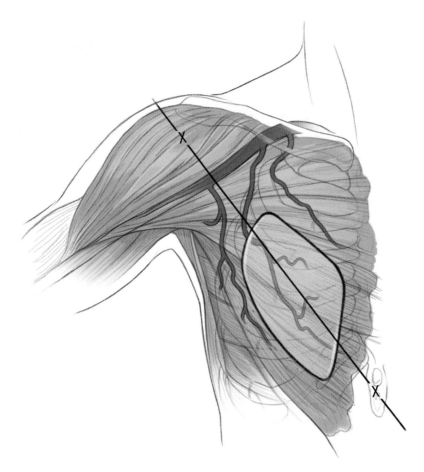

● **FIGURE 35-17.** The skin paddle of the pectoralis major flap is outlined on the underlying blood supply, centered on an axis from the shoulder tip to the xyphoid. Only that narrow portion of the muscle that is needed is taken as a vascular pedicle, and the muscle is separated from the clavicular attachments, leaving the flap as a true vascular island flap.

ADVATAGES. The flap can be used for one-stage reconstructions without necessitating delaying incisions. The donor site of the descending vertical flap can be closed primarily without difficulty. Unless a large portion of skin is necessary, the donor site of the transverse variant of the flap on the shoulder can also be closed primarily.

DISADVANTAGES. The transposition of the flap to reach the area of reconstruction often results in bulk at the base of the neck, which may limit the extent of reach of the flap. If the muscle at the base of the flap is cut to convert it into a vascular island flap, it results in a more mobile and versatile flap, but it requires a more tedious dissection. If the descending vertical flap is required, the patient must be turned midway during the operation to the lateral decubitus position to harvest the flap.

Latissimus Dorsi Flap. The latissimus dorsi is a large flat muscle along the lateral and posterior chest wall (Figure 35-23B). The primary blood supply is from the thoracodorsal vessels which attach to the muscle approximately 10 cm from the insertion of the muscle to

the humerus. The vessels travel axially along the undersurface of the muscle in the direction of the muscle fibers. The muscle also has a secondary segmental blood supply from perforating vessels along the paraspinous origins of the muscle. Following the development and popular use of this myocutaneous flap for breast reconstruction, Quillen[60,61] reported the use of this flap for reconstructions in the head and neck area. In a fashion similar to the pectoralis major muscle, the axial dominant blood supply of the latissimus dorsi bifurcates at the muscle attachment to permit the use of two separate segments of the split muscle to transfer two skin paddles if such is necessary.[62]

TECHNIQUE. The preparation of the patient for the use of this flap requires prepping the entire arm, axilla, and chest, both anteriorly and posteriorly. The drapes are then stapled to the back and the patient is returned to the supine position. Once the resection is performed, the head and neck wound is evaluated to determine the size of the skin paddle and the volume of muscle bulk that is required. The skin paddle is marked along the lateral border of the

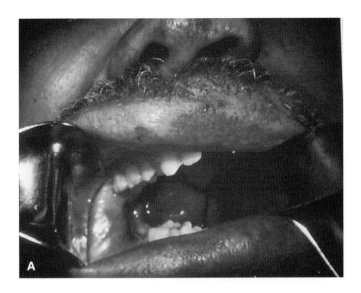

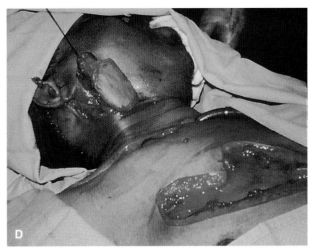

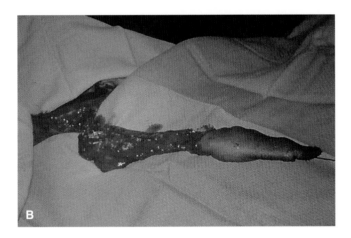

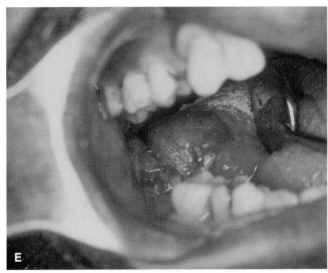

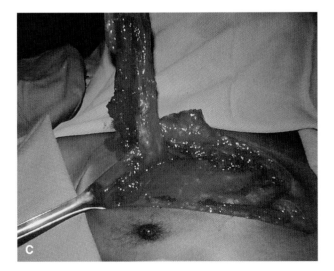

● FIGURE 35-18. A cancer of the right lateral floor of mouth and tongue (A) was resected leaving a large defect. This was reconstructed with a paddle of skin outlined on the vascular axis of the pectoralis major muscle (B), a narrow portion of which was elevated as the pedicle of the flap. The clavicular portion of the muscle was removed, leaving only the vessels and fascia attached (C) to cross over the clavicle, and under the neck skin (D). The healed flap provides sufficient tissue (E) to replace the missing portion of the lateral tongue.

muscle at the necessary distance from the axilla to provide enough length to the muscle pedicle to reach the site of the reconstruction.

The skin incision is begun along the lateral border of the muscle, and the dissection is carried into the axilla. The

thoracodorsal vessels are readily identified along the undersurface of the muscle, and the dissection is continued up toward the apex of the axilla to the level of the subscapular artery. The vascular branches to the serratus anterior and terres major muscles are identified, and may be transected to provide further mobility of the muscle pedicle. If the thoracodorsal vessels had been divided by a previous surgical procedure in the axilla, then the branch to the serratus anterior is preserved, which should be sufficient to provide retrograde arterial flow into the latissimus dorsi. The vascular pedicle to the flap must not be skeletonized, but dissected free while preserving a portion of the surrounding fascial tissue to prevent traction damage to the blood vessels.

Once the vascular blood supply is identified and dissected free, the remainder of the skin incision is completed around the skin paddle to the latissimus dorsi muscle fascia, a longitudinal segment of a portion of the muscle is split along its fibers, and the tendinous portion of the insertion is transected to free up the flap. At this point, a tunnel is prepared from the axilla, along the plane under the pectoralis muscle toward the midportion of the clavicle.

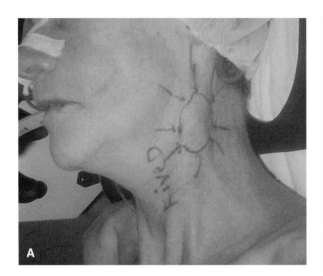

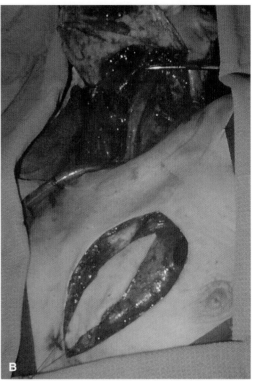

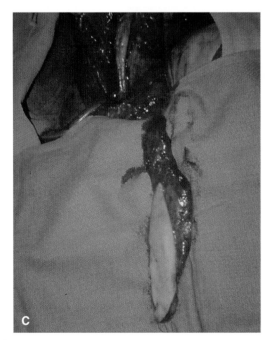

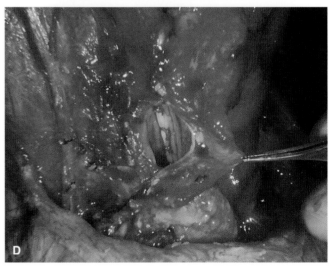

● FIGURE 35-19. A patient with a pharyngeal fixed tumor (A) had a laryngopharyngectomy needed a reconstruction of the cervical esophagus (B) which was performed with a pectoralis major flap with a thin skin paddle located over the parasternal medial chest. This skin paddle was elevated with only a narrow portion of the muscle (C) incorporating the thoracoacromial vessels, and the clavicular attachments of the muscle were excised, brought over the clavicle and the cervical skin tube constructed over the narrow posterior pharyngeal mucosa (D).

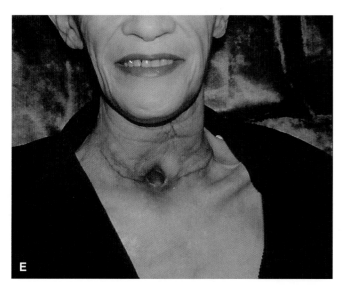

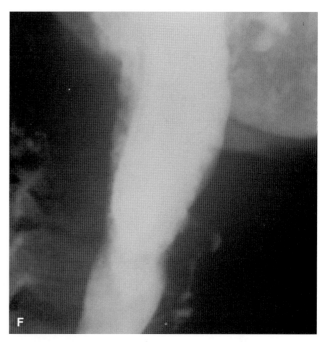

● **FIGURE 35-19.** (*continued*) The reconstructed flap healed without any bulk over the clavicle or neck (E), and the barium swallow (F) demonstrated a very patent pharynx.

This tunnel must separate the attachment of the pectoralis major from the clavicle to allow passage of the flap into the region of the neck for the reconstruction. The donor site can often be closed readily by direct advancement of the chest flap.

CLINICAL APPLICATIONS. The latissimus dorsi may be used for most of the applications that have been described for the pectoralis major flap. It can provide a large amount of skin and soft tissue for large surgical defects (Figure 35-25). In fact, when the advantages and disadvantages are evaluated, it is best applied to those cases in which the patient chooses not to have an incision along the anterior chest, or those cases in which the pectoralis major is not available due to previous surgery or congenital absence.

ADVANTAGES. The latissimus dorsi can provide very large amounts of tissue for reconstruction and has a large arc of rotation. It is as reliable as the pectoralis major flap. Some women patients may prefer to have a surgical scar along the posterior chest.

DISADVANTAGES. The major disadvantage of this flap is the positional change of the patient from the supine to the lateral decubitus position required during the reconstructive portion of the procedure in order to get access to the skin and muscle along the back. The flap must also be tunneled under the subpectoral space and over the clavicle to gain access to the neck. This process mandates a pedicle of muscle to lie over the clavicle, which then leads to bulky tissue at this juncture after the transfer.

● **MICROVASCULAR FREE FLAP RECONSTRUCTION**

Microvascular surgery is a technique of transfer of tissue from one part of the body to another part, when the vascular pedicle of the flap cannot reach the distance. In those cases, the vessels can be transected and reattached at the more distant site. The advent of microsurgical techniques led to the development of various donor sites for the harvesting of this tissue. While it is true that myocutaneous flaps can be transferred by microsurgery to more distant sites, most of the reconstructions of the head and neck with the myocutaneous flaps employs the regional donor sites described above. However, the need for thinner, more pliable, and less bulky donor sites led to the trials and acceptance of several other donor sites which can provide sufficient tissue for reliable reconstructions in the oropharyngeal area.

While microsurgery has traditionally employed the use of fine 8-0 to 10-0 sutures for the circumferential repair of the vessels under the operative microscope, many surgeons have learned to modify this technology to facilitate this delicate and time-consuming procedure. One of the things learned from digital replantation was that the operative microscope often required repositioning several times during the procedure, which usually takes time. On the other hand, the use of operating loupes allows for repositioning of the operator's head to change the field of vision instantly. A comprehensive review of the free flaps performed at one institution demonstrated equal success and survival of free flaps within the head and neck performed with either the microscope or the

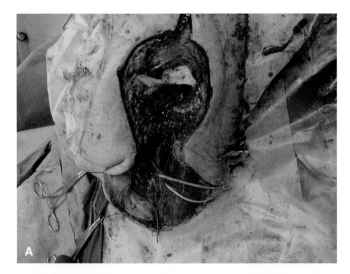

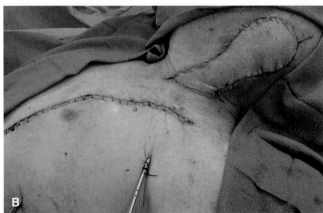

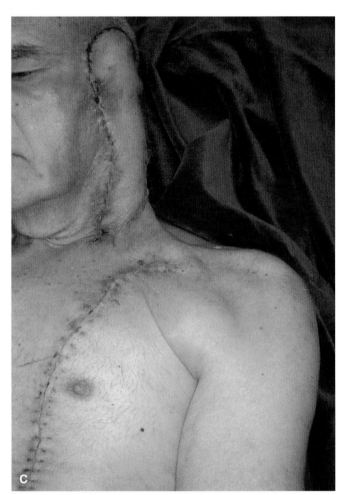

● **FIGURE 35-20.** A recurrent squamous cell carcinoma with invasion of the mastoid bone required a radical temporal bone resection (A). This was covered with a large pectoralis major myocutaneous flap tunneled under the neck (B) skin for a one-stage reconstruction (C).

operating loupes.[63] Use of operating loupes made the procedure far less tedious, and shortened the operating time.

Another modification that has simplified the surgical procedure has been the development of the microvascular anastomotic coupling device (microcoupler). The microcoupler is a pair of rings composed of high-density polyethylene with a central opening, and multiple interlocking stainless steel pins along the perimeter of both rings. This allows the surgeon to pass each of two ends of vessels through the center of each ring, splay them open, impale the end of each vessel on one of the two opposite rings, and approximate and lock the two rings for the completion of the anastomosis in one maneuver. The success and reliability of this coupler has been reported in a large series of clinical cases,[64] as well as in some head and neck cases.[65] Although the coupler has been used mostly for the anastomosis of veins, we have found the device to be equally as successful for the arterial anastomosis,[66] and therefore use it for the entire microvascular anastomisis on as many of the free flaps as we can (Figure 35-26).

Jejunal Free Flap. Longmire[67] was the first surgeon to report in 1946 the reconstruction of the esophagus with an antethoracic transposition of a pedicled loop of jejunum for the repair of a strictured esophagus. Subsequentlty, Seidenberg[68] and his colleagues reported the first repair of an esophagus with the microvascular transfer of an isolated segment of jejunum in 1959, followed by a report of Jurkiewicz[69] in 1965. There have been subsequent reports of larger series demonstrating the reliability and success rates of free tissue transfers of a loop of jejunum for pharyngoesophageal reconstruction, as well as a flat patch of jejunum developed by the longitudinal opening of a segment of jejunum along its antimesenteric side.[70]

TECHNIQUE. Once the tumor has been resected, the appropriate vessels in the neck are prepared for the vascular anastomosis of the free flap. While any artery and vein can be used for these anastomoses, I believe it is more prudent to use larger vessels, particularly in patients who have been previously treated with radiation therapy, which can result in thickening of the walls of these vessels. Therefore, my

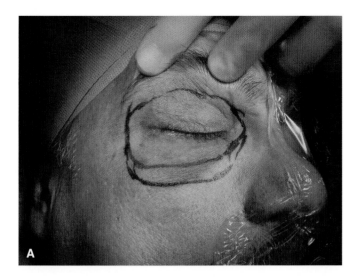
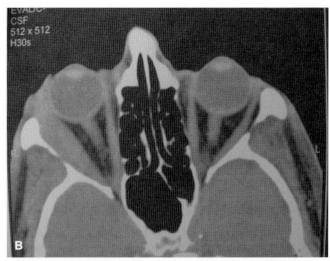
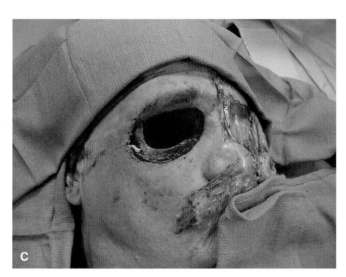
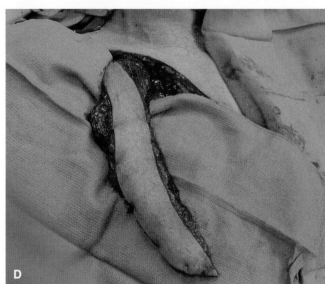

● **FIGURE 35-21.** A recurrent epidermoid carcinoma of the periorbital tissue (A) demonstrated invasion of the intraorbital contents (B), requiring a radical orbital exenteration (C). This was reconstructed with a narrow pectoralis major myocutaneous flap (D),

preference is to use the internal jugular vein (or one of its large branches, eg, facial vein) and the external carotid artery (or one of its tributaries, eg, superior thyroid, ascending pharyngeal). Finally, the length of the esophageal segment that needs repair is measured.

The segment of bowel is then harvested from the abdomen. A suitable segment of the jejunum is selected, with a good vascular arcade, generally just distal to the ligament of Treitz (Figure 35-27). First, the vessels are skeletonized meticulously, cutting and tying the branches with fine ligatures. Once this has been completed, the two ends of the segment of bowel are clamped and transected. The unclamped segment of bowel is examined for proper color, circulation, and bleeding from the mucosal edges. This isolated segment is left attached by its main blood supply to provide circulation, while the reanastomosis is performed of the two ends of the main loop of bowel.

The isolated segment of the jejunum can then be monitored for those few minutes to verify the proper circulation. The proper artery and vein of this isolated segment are then transected and tied, and the segment of bowel is transferred to the recipient site in the head and neck area. In this fashion, there will be minimal warm ischemia time to the bowel.

The jejunal segment is then secured to the superior portion of the wound with a suture to prevent motion during the vascular repair. A nasogastric tube is passed into the pharynx, through the segment of jejunum, then out the distal esophagus into the stomach before the repair. If this is a tube repair of an esophagus, it is easier to perform the proximal suture line first, as this is the more difficult part of the procedure. The distal repair may be performed next, before the vascular anastomosis. Alternatively, some surgeons prefer to repair the vessels next in order to

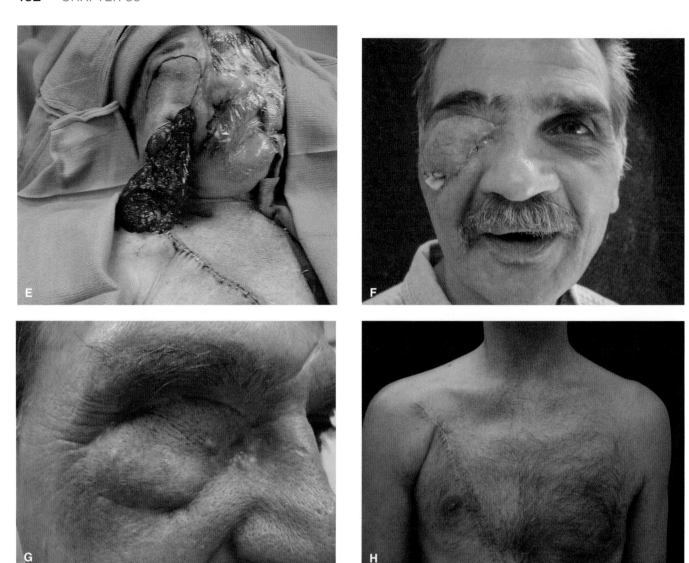

● **FIGURE 35-21.** (*continued*) routed above the clavicle and filling the orbital contents
(E). At 12 days, the pedicle was transected at the infrorbital rim and inset over a penrose
drain (F), and the remainder of the pedicle was discarded. The reconstructed flap is
durable (G), and the chest donor site (H) is healed by direct closure.

visualize the mucosal bleeding of the revascularized segment of bowel, after which they repair the distal end of the bowel.

The vessels are then repaired. The vein may be repaired first and examined for patency of the retrograde flow through the suture line, followed by the arterial repair. Alternatively, the artery may be repaired first, flow allowed through the segment of bowel, and the venous outflow visualized to verify proper flow. In this case, the arterial flow must be stopped with a vascular clamp while the vein is subsequently repaired. Once the flow is established, the segment of bowel is observed for color and peristalsis to verify viability. If the distal end of the bowel lumen has not been repaired completely, the mucosa can be inspected for mucosal color and bleeding of the edges.

Another option is to have a second, but smaller, segment of bowel left attached to the vascular pedicle—this

segment serving only as a monitor of flow and mucosal bleeding. At the end of the surgical reconstruction, this segment can then be discarded, or the segment can be left exiting the skin flap coverage, to serve as a monitor of the bowel viability over the next 7 to 10 days. At that time, the vascular pedicle at the exit site is clamped, transected, tied, and this segment of bowel is discarded.

CLINICAL APPLICATION. The jejunum is best suited for reconstruction of a circumferential resection of the cervical esophagus. It is also applicable for the repair of a patch of pharynx, resection of the buccal mucosa, and even floor of mouth.

ADVANTAGES. This flap allows for the repair of a mucosa-lined tube of the esophagus to be repaired with like-tissue. There is no longitudinal suture line that can potentially

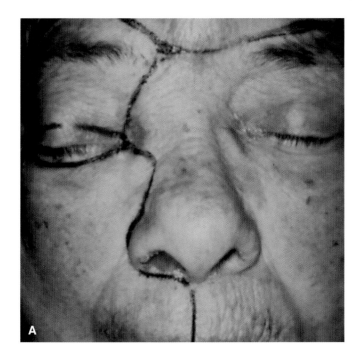

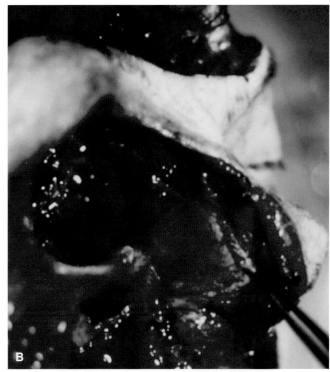

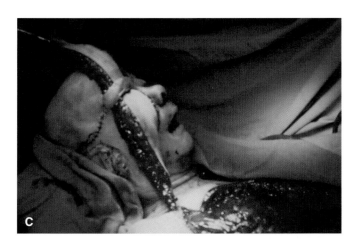

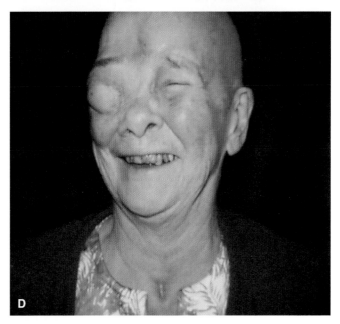

⬤ **FIGURE 35-22.** A recurrent epidermoid carcinoma (A) involved the ethmoid, frontal, and maxillary sinuses, with invasion of the orbital contents. The tumor was removed with a radical craniofascial resection (B). The resulting large facial deficit was filled in with and extended pectoralis major myocutaneous flap (C) in one stage. The flap pedical was left attached outside the neck for 2 weeks, at which time it was divided and inset as a second stage, and the pedicle was discarded (D).

leak saliva and oral bacteria into the closed contents of the neck. The segment of bowel can tolerate a full course of postoperative radiation therapy.

DISADVANTAGES. The harvesting and repair of the donor bowel is time-consuming, although this can be circumvented by using two surgical teams—one to perform the resection of the recipient site and microvascular repair in the head and neck, the second to harvest and repair the donor bowel in the abdomen. There is always the risk of subsequent intra-abdominal adhesions in the postoperative period, with risk of bowel obstruction.

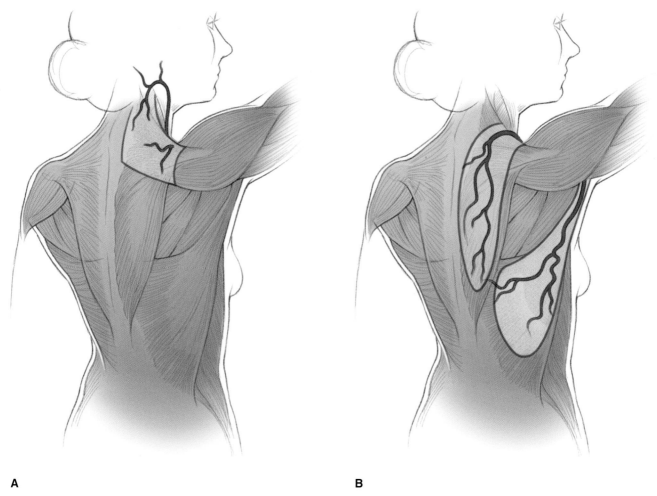

A   **B**

● **FIGURE 35-23.** (A) The trapezius muscle with the occipital artery at the base
of the skull, the suprascapular artery at the shoulder tip, and the transverse cervical
artery in the middle, descending the back along the undersurface of the muscle.
(B) The distal trapezius outlined posteriorly over the descending portion of the transverse
cervical artery. The latissimus dorsi flap along the posterolateral chest is supplied by the
thoracodorsal vessels.

Radial Forearm Free Flap. The fasciocutaneous flap
from the anterior surface of the radial forearm can be
particularly useful for head and neck reconstruction. The
flap has been shown to be easy to harvest, reliable for
repair, and possess robust durability for the reconstruction of various sites of the body.[71,72] It has been used for
the repair of the cervical esophagus with an excellent
outcome.[73]

TECHNIQUE. The surgical defect of the resection site is measured and the necessary flap is outlined overlying the radial
artery on the distal volar forearm (Figure 35-28). It is preferable to outline the required flap with its central axis
directly over the radial artery as much as possible, even
though this is not essential, as the flap is harvested with the
fascia and accompanying vascular connections.

It is better to begin the dissection from the ulnar side of
the flap, and dissect toward the radial artery, as the fascia
is more readily identified here. The muscle fascia does not

need to be harvested, because the risk of a hematoma is
otherwise greater, risking a greater loss of the skin graft
that is applied. The correct plane is just above the flexor
retinaculum until the radial artery is approached, at which
time the dissection goes through this plane, down and
around the radial artery and its accompanying veins. The
artery at the distal limit of the flap is clamped, transected,
and ligated.

The dissection is then carried more radial to the artery,
and becomes more superficial again, coming up to the
flexor retinaculum. As the dissection of the flap is completed in this direction, every attempt is made to not damage the sensory branch of the radial nerve (small branches
are cut).

The flap dissection is carried more proximally where one
to two subcutaneous veins may be preserved with the flap.
This is not essential because the two radial artery venae
commitantes are sufficient for the anastomoses in most
cases. However, it is recommended these subcutaneous

veins be included with the flap as a precaution in the event the other veins are damaged in the neck, or are deemed to be insufficient.

The skin is incised proximal to the skin flap markings to access the vessels deep to the flexor muscles in order to provide sufficient length to the pedicle. Once the vessels in the neck are judged to be properly prepared, the radial artery and the veins of the flap are cut, and the proximal ends ligated.

The flap is brought to the recipient site, and the perimeter of the flap is sutured securely to the margins of the wound with 3-0 silk, or polyglycolic acid absorbable suture. It is essential that the suture line is secure and somewhat watertight so that salivary fluid and oral bacteria do not continue to contaminate the neck in the postoperative period. Once the flap is secure, the vascular pedicle is repaired. This can be performed either with microsutures or with the microcoupler as discussed above.

Finally, the donor site on the forearm needs to be repaired. If the harvested flap is small, the donor site can be closed in some cases with transposition and advancement flaps of the forearm. Otherwise, the surgical donor wound is covered with a split thickness skin graft (Figure 35-29). If the flexor retinaculum was preserved, then the healed skin graft can glide over the flexor tendons without adherence.

CLINICAL APPLICATION. The radial forearm free flap is best suited for the reconstruction of any defect that requires thin, pliable tissue. This flap is ideal for the floor of mouth (Figure 35-30), some repairs of partial resection of the tongue, alveolus, retromolar trigone, and buccal surface. This flap can also be used for the repair of fistulae of the pharynx, partial resections of the cervical esophagus, and even for circumferential resections (Figure 35-31).

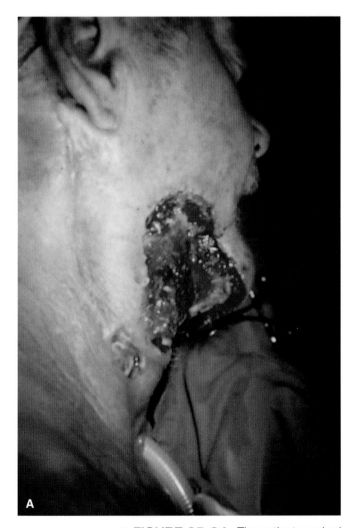
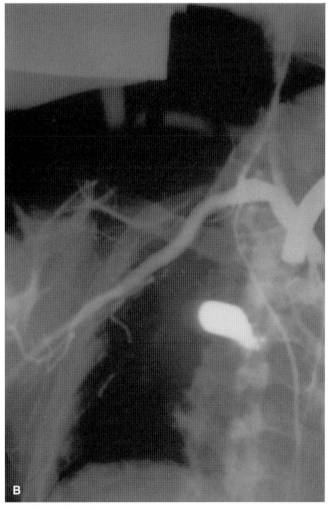

● FIGURE 35-24. The patient required a resection of recurrent carcinoma of the soft tissues of the submandibular area (A). If the transverse cervical artery is known to have been previously transected in the neck (B), then the vessel can be identified along the anterior margin of the undersurface of the muscle. Since this blood flow is now retrograde from the back of the chest, the vessels are protected by direct vision, while the posterior skin incision is made.

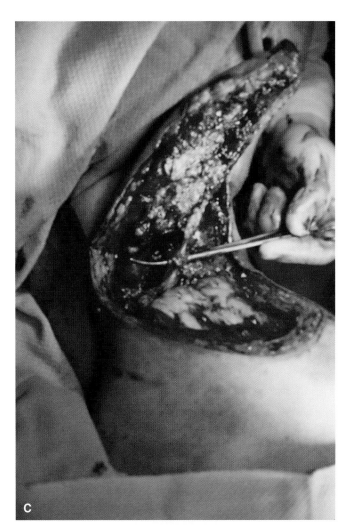

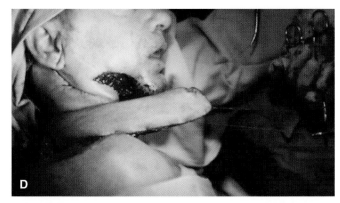

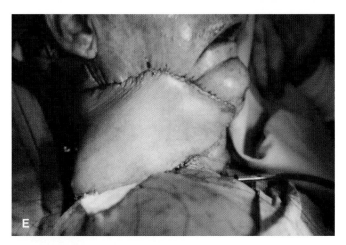

● **FIGURE 35-24.** (*continued*) The incision is deepened through the muscle fibers until these vessels are approached (while still visualizing them directly), and the distal portion of the vessels (C) are freed more posteriorly under the trapezius. This is continued until enough of the vessel length is freed from the muscle to allow for transposition of the flap (D, E).

ADVANTAGES. Provides thin pliable skin and soft tissue of varying sizes to reconstruct small- and moderate-sized defects of the oral cavity. The donor site is easily managed by direct closure or with a skin graft, in which case a small splint will allow the patient to use the hand for meals. I have also used a single large flap to resurface an extensive resection of the entire forehead from one temporal hairline to the other.

DISADVANTAGES. The donor site on the forearm is visible, and a failed skin graft can develop hypertrophic scars. There can be symptomatic neuromas if there is damage to the radial sensory nerve.

Scapular Free Flap. This flap of soft tissue is based over the axial blood supply of the circumflex scapular artery, a branch from the subscapular artery that penetrates the triangular space formed by the teres major, the teres minor, and the triceps muscles to reach the skin over

the posterior shoulder.[74] The circumflex scapular artery then bifurcates into a transverse scapular branch and a descending parascapular branch. This split of the main axial vessel allows the surgeon to develop two separate skin paddles. In fact, there is a third vascular branch that enters the scapula along its descending lateral border to provide endosteal blood supply, which allows the harvesting of a third flap incorporating a segment of bone.[75] This flap was very helpful for the reconstruction of major soft tissue resections removed with a portion of the mandible in advanced oral cancers.

TECHNIQUE. The shoulder ipsilateral to the side of the proposed mandibular rersection is prepped and draped while the patient is turned to the opposite lateral decubitus position. The patient is then placed supine for the resection of the tumor and mandible. Subsequently, the patient is returned to the lateral decubitus position for harvest of the flap. To locate the triangular soft tissue

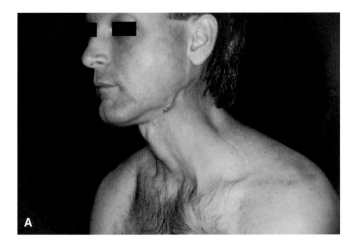

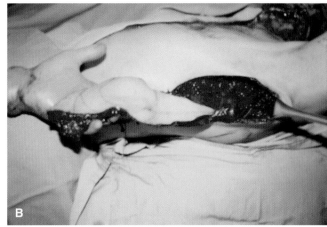

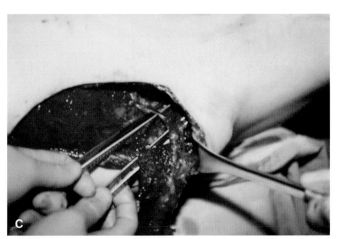

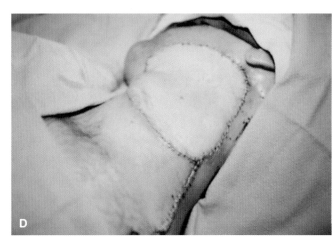

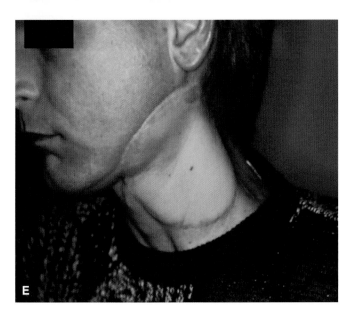

● **FIGURE 35-25.** A recurrent epidermoid carcinoma involving the skin and soft tissues of the mandibular and cervical regions (A) in a patient in whom the pectoralis major had been previously used. The defect was resurfaced with a latissimus dorsi myocutaneous flap (B), with careful dissection and preservation of the thoracodorsal vessels (C), for one-stage repair (D). The flap is not bulky (E), and because it has fresh muscular blood supply, can tolerate postoperative radiation therapy.

through which the vascular pedical traverses, the index finger of the surgeon is placed in the posterior axillary fold, and the thumb is placed on the posterior of the shoulder until it falls in the depression between the teres major and teres minor. This locates the site of penetration of the circumflex scapular artery, and is marked. The

two branches are then drawn horizontally and vertically overlapping their ends over this point (Figure 35-32), and the lateral border of the scapula is marked, if a segment of bone is needed. Either one or two skin paddles are then drawn overlying the vessels, depending on the needs of that particular reconstruction.

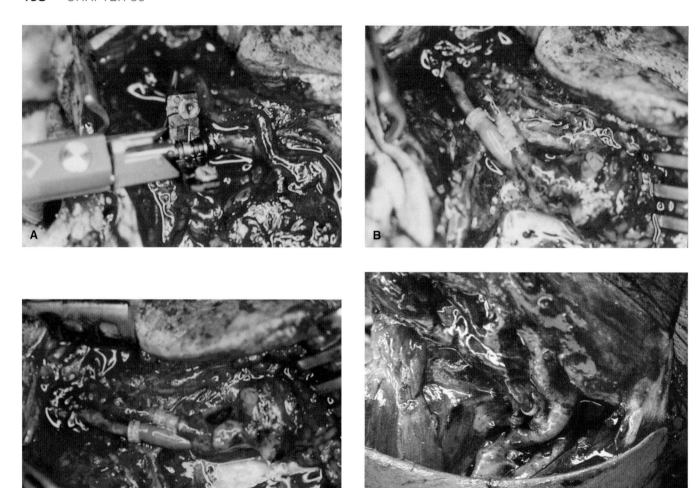

● **FIGURE 35-26.** (A) Microcoupler applicator device holding two arterial ends on the pins of the microcouplers prior to closing. (B, C) Pairs of artery and vein anastomosed with microcouplers. (D) A free flap in the floor of mouth has been repaired using the microcoupler to anastomose the radial artery (*center*) to the superior thyroid artery, and the two venae comitantes to branches of the facial vein.

The dissection of the skin paddle begins from distal to proximal at the level of the deep fascia. The vessels are easily identified in this fascial plane, as the vascular pedicle needs to be dissected into the soft tissue triangle. If a segment of the bone is required, care must be taken to not damage the short arterial branch that enters the bone. The segment of bone is cut with a power saw to the size and shape required for the reconstruction. The circumflex scapular artery is then dissected far enough in the space between the teres major and minor muscles to provide a pedicle of 4 to 8 cm, including the two accompanying veins.

CLINICAL APPLICATION. This is the ideal flap when an abundant supply of tissue is required with a repair of the mandible. A composite resection of a segment of mandible, together with the a through-and-through resection of the cheek can be reconstructed with a segment of bone and two skin paddles, one for external coverage and one for buccal lining.

ADVANTAGES. The vascular pedicle is quite reliable, and a significant amount of skin can be harvested for large areas of resection. The donor sites can be closed with local advancement flaps without the need for skin grafts.

DISADVANTAGES. The position of the patient needs to be changed during the procedure, between the resection of the operative site and the harvesting of the flap. Furthermore, the ablative and reconstructive teams are not able to work simultaneously. If a segment of scapula is incorporated, the bone in most patients is usually not thick enough to permit osseointegrated dental implants.

Fibula Free Flap. The fibula free flap has evolved into the bone of choice for the reconstruction of the mandible

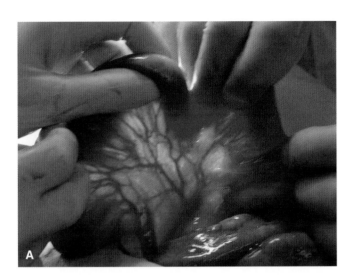

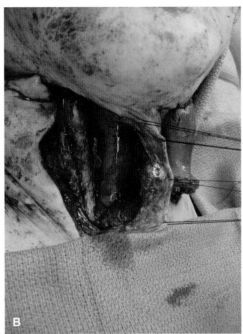

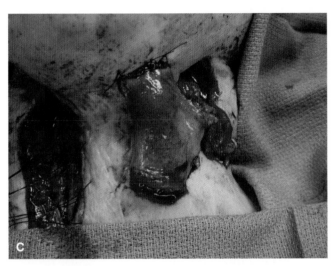

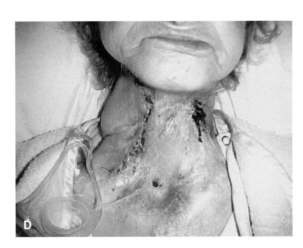

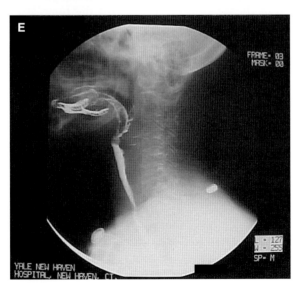

⬤ **FIGURE 35-27.** (A) A donor segment of jejunum is identified based on a proper vascular arcade. (B) The proximal portion of the segment is repaired to the base of tongue and oropharynx, the distal end to the esophagus, and the mesenteric artery and vein are anastomosed to the ascending pharyngeal artery and internal jugular vein. (C) A secondary loop of bowel is left attached to the exterior of the neck for monitoring of the viability of the primary segment of bowel. (D) The final healed wound after the secondary segment has been removed. (E) A barium swallow showing the continuity of the pharyngoesophagus.

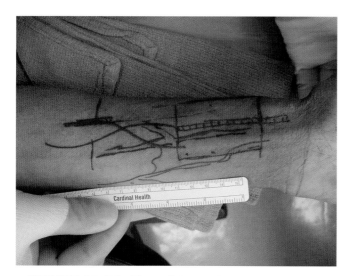

● **FIGURE 35-28.** The radial artery is outlined on the distal volar forearm, as well as any veins that can be seen or palpated. The size and shape of the required flap is outlined over this artery, and the proximal skin incision for the dissection of the vascular pedicle is marked in a lazy-S pattern.

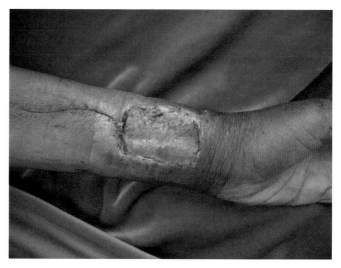

● **FIGURE 35-29.** If the skin paddle is small, the donor site may be closed with advancement flaps. If the flexor retinaculum is preserved, the skin graft will heal to this tissue and allow the flexor tendons to glide underneath it without attachment to the overlying skin.

since its introduction in 1989.[76] What makes this flap ideal is the abundant length that can be harvested, up to 25 cm, and the thickness of the cross-section of the bone. This choice of reconstruction of the mandible is ideal for osseointegrated dental implants. In addition, skin overlying the midportion of the fibula has cutaneous perforating vessels that can provide a small segment of thin skin for intraoral lining.

TECHNIQUE. The leg is prepped circumferentially up to the groin, and a sterile thigh touriquet is applied. The cutaneous perforating vessels are identified with a doppler probe and marked on the skin overlying the midportion of the bone, and the skin paddle is outlined (Figure 35-33). The leg is elevated to exanguinate it by gravity, and the tourniquet is inflated. In this fashion, there is still some blood in the vessels to help to visualize the structures at the time of the dissections. First, the anterior skin incision is made down to and including the underlying muscle fascia. The skin paddle is dissected with the fascia to protect the perforating vessels, until the septum is reached. Here the dissection is carried into the muscles of the lateral compartment with a needle-tip electrocautery to harvest the bone with a thin 5-mm layer of muscle left attached to the bone to protect the periosteal blood supply. The dissection is carried through the septum of the lateral and anterior compartments, and the dissection is continued with a muscular cuff. When the interosseous septum is reached, this structure is incised carefully to avoid damage to the vessels lying deeper to it.

Next, the posterior skin incision is made through the fascia. The soleus is separated from the bone with electrocautery, and the flexor hallucis longus muscle is incised. The proximal osteotomy is performed at the level of the neck of the fibula, while the distal osteotomy is performed at the length of bone necessary, leaving at least 4 to 6 cm of fibula above the lateral malleolus to retain ankle stability. The bone is then pulled laterally to expose the tibialis posterior muscle, which is dissected with the electrocautery. As this dissection is carried proximally, the bone will be released further, exposing the vascular pedicle. Proximally, the vessels are carefully visualized during the dissection as it traverses toward the bone. If a longer vascular pedicle is needed, and there is sufficient bone, the proximal periosteum is dissected with the vascular pedicle off the bone, and this segment of stripped bone can be transected with a sagittal saw. The segment of bone can be shaped to the pattern of the resected mandible by performing osteotomies. The vascular pedicle is dissected at the subperiosteal plane off the bone at the site of each planned osteotomy. The segments of bone can then be plated to complete the shape.

CLINICAL APPLICATION. This flap can be used for the reconstruction of segmental, hemi-, or subtotal resections of the mandible. It is particularly useful for one-stage reconstructions of mandible requiring a limited amount of intraoral lining.

ADVANTAGES. The bone can be resected with minimal disability to the patient. It can provide large lengths of thick bone that can be shaped with variable osteotomies. There is sufficient cross-sectional area to permit the placement of osseointegrated dental implants. Thin pliable skin can be harvested with the bone to provide intraoral lining. The flap can be harvested by a second team of surgeons, while the first team is completing the resection of the tumor, and preparing the neck vessels for the microvascular anastomosis.

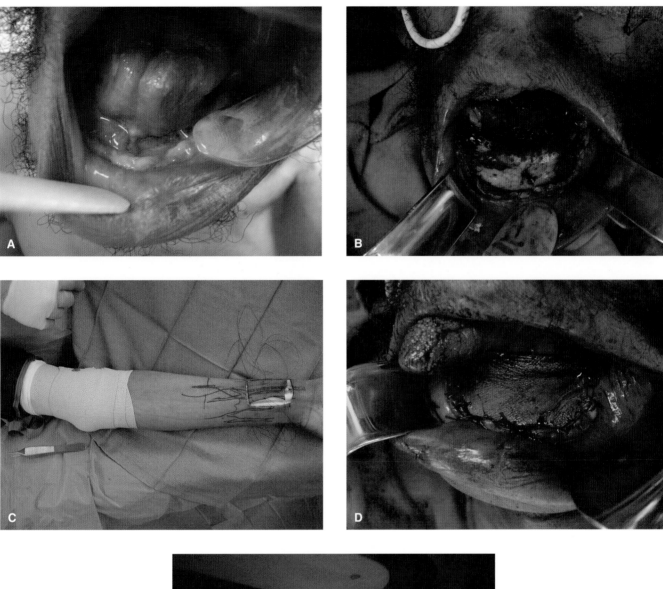

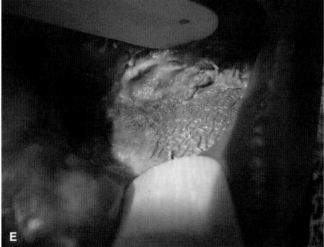

● FIGURE 35-30. The resection of an ulcerated carcinoma of the floor of mouth (A) results in a moderate-sized defect requiring coverage of the mandible (B). The flap is marked on the forearm and elevated, preserving the flexor retinaculum (C), and transferred to the floor of mouth (D). One week later, the flap and margins (E) show appropriate healing.

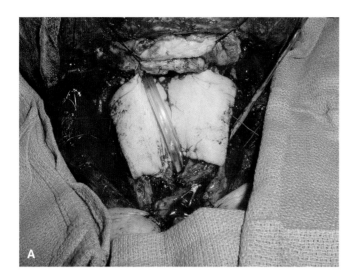
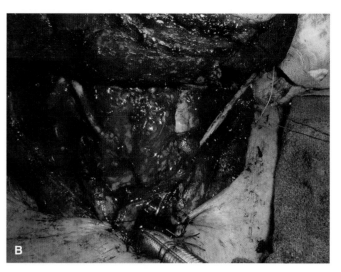
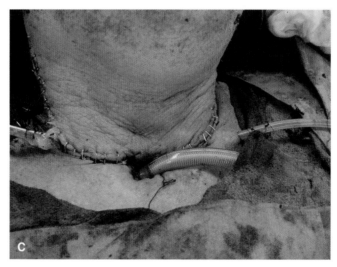

● FIGURE 35-31. A laryngopharyngectomy that required a circumferential resection of the cervical esophagus (A) is repaired over a nasogastric tube, with the suture line anteriorly (B). The cervical apron flap is then brought down to cover the repair (C).

DISADVANTAGES. While most patients are able to ambulate within a week of the operation, some patients may need an extended period of time to regain sufficient ambulation to become independent again. Ankle instability is otherwise uncommon.

● COMMENTS

While there has been a trend in publishing the successful series of a number of microvascular free flap reconstructions, there is no single flap that is the "universal flap of choice." Surgeons who participate in reconstructions of the head and neck area must be sufficiently experienced with all of the techniques mentioned in this chapter in order to select the proper flap for each individual case, based on the particular needs—whether that is based on size of tissue, structures needed, previous flaps that have been already harvested, previous surgical scars, previous radiation to the donor or recipient sites, or patient concerns about the location or extent of scars necessary for the donor flap.

A previous review of this author's first 360 cases of reconstruction reveals that the myocutaneous flaps were used in about half of the patients, and microvascular free flaps in the remainder, particularly when thin introral lining was required, or when bone was necessary for mandibular resections (Table 35-4). On a worldwide basis, myocutaneous flaps are utilized more readily by surgeons, particularly because they do not require special instruments or microscopes. However, the reliability of performing the free flaps with operating loupes has extended the use of these flaps for specialized needs. Nevertheless, there are numerous reports attesting to the far more extensive use of the pectoralis major flap in South America,[77] Asia,[78] and Eastern Europe.[79] The myocutaneous flaps have robust blood supplies that allow the use of intraoperative brachytherapy with radioactive seeds,[29] and the addition of postoperative radiation far

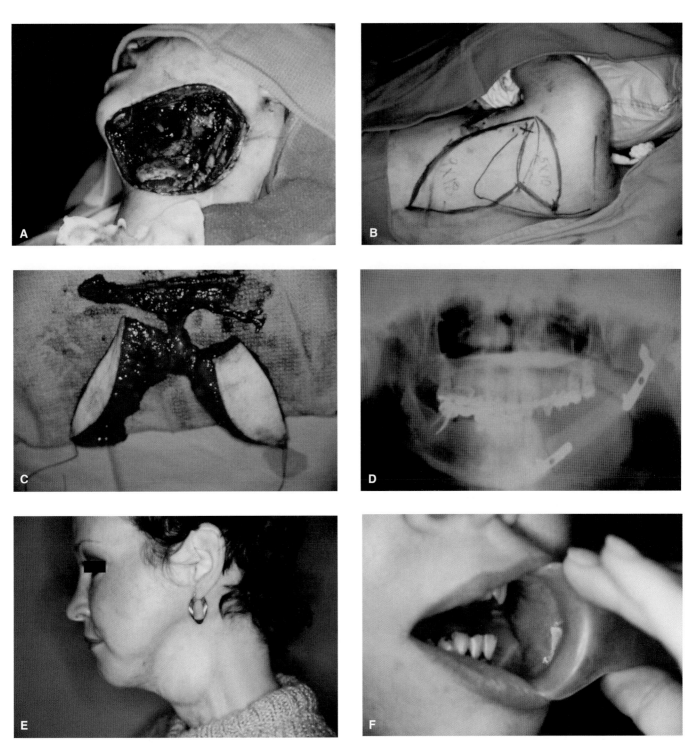

● FIGURE 35-32. A patient with a recurrent epidermoid carcinoma of the floor of mouth with invasion of the mandible and tumor involvement of the soft tissues of the face required through and through resection (A). Two skin paddles incorporating the scapular and parascapular vascular axes (B) were outlined, and these two separate flaps were harvested with a segment of scapular bone (C) on a third vascular pedicle. The segment of bone was plated to the mandible (D). At 1 year, there is good contouring to the one skin paddle on the neck (E), as well as the second skin paddle in the lateral floor of mouth (F) covering the bone flap.

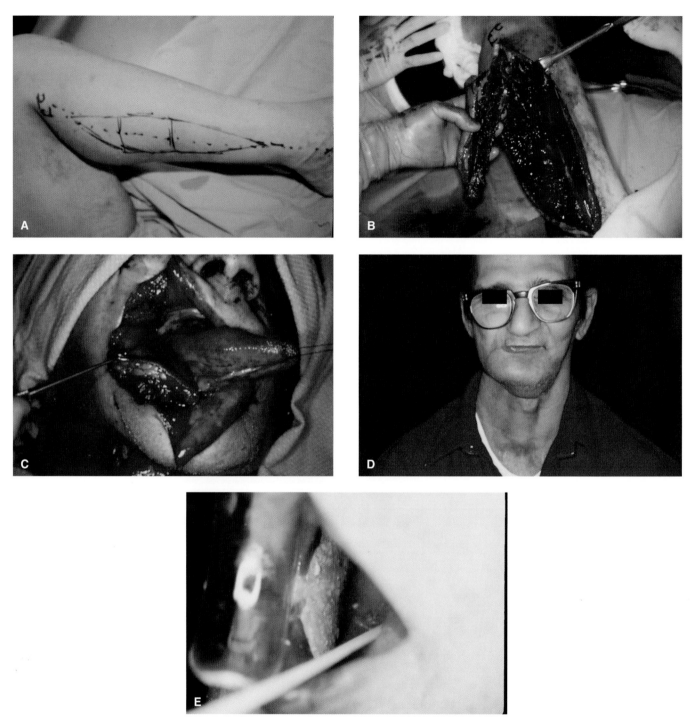

● FIGURE 35-33. A paddle of skin from the leg (A) is harvested with a segment of fibula (B), to reconstruct a defect of the lateral floor of mouth (C) and body of the mandible. At 1 month, there is good reconstitution of the mandible (D), and the floor of mouth (E).

better than cutaneous flaps.[80] We have also demonstrated that a reconstruction with these myocutaneous flaps permits future resection of recurrent tumors, reelevation of the residual myocutaneous flap, and reconstruction with this same flap, thereby avoiding the dissection of a new flap.[81]

Patients with head and neck cancer should be seen and evaluated by a multidsiciplinary team of physicians. All treatment options should be considered and reviewed, and the recommendations should take into account the special needs of each individual patient. If an extensive resection is performed, the head and neck surgeons should remain facile with all the various techniques of flap reconstructions, and should continue to select those reconstructive methods that best fit the surgical requirements of each case.

TABLE 35-4. Distribution of Flaps Used for 364 Reconstructions of the Head and Neck

| | | | COMPLICATIONS | | |
| | | | Skin Paddle | | Flap |
	Number	Percent	Pt	TH	TH
PLATYSMA	9	11%	1		
transverse					
SCM	33	42%			
superior	−23		9		
inferior	−10		5		
PECT. MAJOR	125	9%			
oropharynx	−53		6	1	
neck	−15		1		
esophagus	−8				
orbitofacial	−25		1		
temp. bone	−19				
jaw/rib	−5		1	1	
TRAPEZIUS	18				
LAT. DORSI	12	8%	1		
FREE FLAP	133	7%			
lat. Dorsi	−12				3
jejunum	−1				
omentum	−2				
radial forearm	−70		1		1
rib	−3				
scapula	−15		2		
cut.	−7				
osteocut	−8				
fibula	−32				
osteo	−16				1
osteocut	−16		1		
TOTAL	364	10%	29	2	5

REFERENCES

1. Crile GW. Excision of cancer of the head and neck: with special reference to plan of dissection based on one hundred and thirty-two operations. *JAMA.* 1906;47:1780.

2. Martin HE, Del Valle B, Ehrlich H. Neck dissection. *Cancer.* 1951;4:441.

3. Roentgen WC. On a new kind of rays. (Read before the Wurzberg Physical and Medical Society. Translated by Arthur Staton). *Nature.* 1895;53:274.

4. Coutard H. Results and methods of treatment of cancer radiation. *Ann Surg.* 1937;106:584.

5. Strandqvist M. Studien uber die cumulative wirkung der roentgenstrahlen bei fraktionierung. *Acta Radiol.* 1944;(Suppl 55):1.

6. Jemal A, Siegel R, Ward E, et al. 2006 statistics: cancer for the year. *CA Cancer J Clin.* 2006;56:106.

7. Pindborg JJ, Jolst O, Renstrup G, et al. Studies in oral leukoplakia: a preliminary report on the period prevalence of malignant transformation in leukoplakia based on a follow-up study of 248 patients. *J Am Dent Assoc.* 1968;76:767.

8. Shafer WG, Waldron CA. A clinical and histopathologic study of oral leukoplakia. *Surg Gynecol Obstet.* 1961; 112:411.

9. Arons MS, Smith RR, Myers MH. Significance of cancer cells in operative wounds. *Cancer.* 1961;14:1041.

10. Griffiths JD, McKinna JA, Rowbotham HD, et al. Carcinoma of the colon and rectum: circulating malignant cells and five-year survival. *Cancer.* 1973;31:226.

11. Merino OR, Lindberg RD, Fletcher GH. An analysis of distant metastases from squamous cell carcinoma of the upper respiratory and digestive tracts. *Cancer.* 1977;40:145.

12. Dennington ML, Carter DR, Meyers AD. Distant metastases in head and neck epidermoid carcinoma. *Laryngoscope.* 1980;90:196.

13. Papac RJ. Distant metastases from head and neck cancer. *Cancer.* 1984;53:342.

14. Probert JC, Thompson RW, Bagshaw MA. Patterns of spread of distant metastases in head and neck cancer. *Cancer.* 1974;33:127.

15. Gahhos F, Enriquez RE, Bahn SL, Ariyan S. Necrotizing sialometaplasia: report of five cases. *Plast Reconstr Surg.* 1983;71:650.

16. Goldberg NH, Cuono CB, Ariyan S, et al. Improved reliability in tumor diagnosis by fine needle aspiration. *Plast Reconstr Surg.* 1981;67:492.

17. Morton DL, Wen DR, Wong JH, et al. Technical details of intraoperative lymphatic mapping for early stage melanoma. *Arch Surg.* 1992;127:392.

18. Reintgen D, Cruse CW, Wells K, et al. The orderly progression of melanoma nodal metastases. *Ann Surg.* 1994;220:759.

19. Albertini JJ, Cruse CC, Rappaport D, et al. Intraoperative radiolymphoscintigraphy improves sentinel lymph node identification for patients with melanoma. *Ann Surg.* 1996;223:217.

20. Cascinelli N, Belli F, Santinami M, et al. Sentinel lymph node biopsy in cutaneous melanoma: the WHO melanoma program experience. *Ann Surg Oncol.* 2000;7:469.

21. Chiesa F, Mauri S, Grana C, et al. Is there a role for sentinel node biopsy in early N0 tongue tumors? *Surgery.* 2000;128:16.

22. Alex JC, Sasaki CT, Krag DN, et al. Sentinel lymph node radiolocalization in head and neck squamous cell carcinoma. *Laryngoscope.* 2000;110:198.

23. Mancuso AA, Harnsberger HR, Muraki AS, et al. Computed tomography of cervical and retropharyngeal lymph nodes: normal anatomy, variants of normal: application in staging head and neck cancer. 1. Normal anatomy. *Radiology.* 1983;148:709.

24. Mancuso AA, Maceri D, Pice D, et al. CT of cervical lymph node cancer. *Am J Roentgenol.* 1981;136:381.

25. Young JEM, Archibald SD, Shier KJ. Needle aspiration cytologic biopsy in head and neck masses. *Am J Surg.* 1981;142:484.

26. Randell CP, Collins AG, Young IR, et al. Nuclear magnetic resonance imaging of posterior fossa tumors. *Am J Neuroradiol.* 1983;4:1027.

27. Runge VM, Nelson KL. Contrast agents. In: DD Stark, Bradley WG, eds. *Magnetic Resonance Imaging.* 3rd ed. St. Louis, MO: Mosby; 1999:264.

28. Shah JP, Cendon RA, Farr HW, et al. Carcinoma of the oral cavity: factors affecting treatment failure at the primary site and neck. *Am J Surg.* 1976;132:504.

29. Son YH, Ariyan S. Intraoperative adjuvant radiotherapy for advanced cancers of the head and neck: preliminary report. *Am J Surg.* 1985;150:480.

30. Barttlebort SW, Bahn S, Ariyan S. Rim mandibulectomy for cancer of the oral cavity. *Am J Surg.* 1987;154:423.

31. Flynn MB, Moore C. Marginal resection of the mandible in the management of squamous cell carcinoma of the floor of the mouth. *Am J Surg.* 1974;128:490.

32. Barttelbort SW, Ariyan S. Mandible preservation with oral carcinoma: rim mandibulectomy versus sagittal mandibulectomy. *Am J Surg.* 1993;166:411.

33. Edgerton MT, DesPrez JD. Reconstruction of the oral cavity in the treatment of cancer. *Plast Reconstr Surg.* 1957;19:89.

34. DesPrez JD, Kiehn CL. Method of reconstruction following resection of anterior oral cavity and mandible for malignancy. *Plast Reconstr Surg.* 1959;24:238.

35. Futrell JW, Johns ME, Edgerton MD, et al. Platysma myocutaneous flap for intraoral reconstructions. *Am J Surg.* 1978;136:504.

36. Ariyan S. One-stage reconstruction for defects of the mouth using the sternocleidomastoid myocutaneous flap. *Plast Reconstr Surg.* 1979;63:618.

37. Ariyan S. Further experiences with the sternocleidomastoid myocutaneous flap. A clinical appraisal of 31 cases. *Plast Reconstr Surg.* 1997;99:61.

38. Ariyan S. The transverse platysma myocutaneous flap for head and neck reconstruction. *Plast Reconstr Surg.* 1997;99:340.

39. Ariyan S. The transverse platysma myocutaneous flap for head and neck reconstruction. An update. *Plast Reconstr Surg.* 2003;111:378.

40. Ariyan S. Further experiences with the sternocleidomastoid myocutaneous flap. *Plast Reconstr Surg.* 2003;111:381.

41. Ariyan S, Krizek TJ. Reconstruction after resection of head and neck cancer. CINE CLINICS session presented at the annual meeting of the American College of Surgeons; Dallas, TX; October 1977.

42. Ariyan S. The pectoralis major myocutaneous flap. *Plast Reconstr Surg.* 1979;63:73.

43. Ariyan S. Further experiences with the pectoralis major myocutaneous flap for immediate repair of defects from excision of head and neck cancers. *Plast Reconstr Surg.* 1979;64:605.

44. Ariyan S. Pectoralis major, sternocleidomastoid, and other musculocutaneous flaps for head and neck reconstruction. *Clin Plast Surg.* 1980;7:89.

45. Ariyan S. The pectoralis major for single-stage reconstruction of difficult wounds of the orbit and pharyngoesophagus. *Plast Reconstr Surg.* 1983;72:468.

46. Theogaraj SD, Merritt WH, Acharya G, et al. The pectoralis major myocutaneous flap in single stage reconstruction of the cervical esophagus. *Plast Reconstr Surg.* 1980;65:267.

47. Baek S, Lawson W, Biller HF. An analysis of 133 pectoralis major myocutaneous flaps. *Plast Reconstr Surg.* 1982;69:460.

48. Ahmad QG, Navadgi S, Agarwal R, et al. Bipadle pectoralis major myocutaneous flap in reconstructing full thickness defects of cheek: a review of 47 cases. *J Plast Reconstr Aesthet Surg.* 2006;59:166.

49. Cuono CB, Ariyan S. Immediate reconstruction of a composite mandibular defect with a regional osteomusculocutaneous flap. *Plast Reconstr Surg.* 1980;65:477.

50. Ariyan S. Reconstruction of the oropharyngeal area. In: Ariyan S. *Cancer of the Head and Neck.* St. Louis, MO: CV Mosby Company; 1987:251.

51. Ariyan S, Cuono CB. Myocutaneous flaps for head and neck reconstruction. *Head Neck Surg.* 1980;2:321.

52. Demergasso F, Piazza MV. Colajo cutaneo aislado a pediculo muscular en cirugia recunstructiva por cancer de cabeza y cuello. Technica original. XLVII Congresso Argentino de Cerugia Forum de Investigaciones. *Rev Argent Cirug.* 1977;32:27.

53. Demegasso F, Piazza MV. Trapezius myocutaneous flap in reconstructive surgery for head and neck cancer: an original technique. *Am J Surg.* 1979;138:533.

54. McGraw JB, Dibbell DG, Carraway JH. Clinical definition of independent myocutaneous vascular territories. *Plast Reconstr Surg.* 1977;60:341.

55. Sharzer LA, Horton CE, Adamson JE, et al. Intraoral reconstruction in head and neck cancer surgery. *Clin Plast Surg.* 1976;3:495.

56. Ariyan S. One stage repair of the cervical esophagostome with two myocutaneous flaps from the neck and shoulder. *Plast Reconstr Surg.* 1979;63:426.

57. Mathes S, Nahai F. Muscle flap transposition with functional preservation: technical and clinical considerations. *Plast Reconstr Surg.* 1981;67:177.

58. Gardiner LJ, Ariyan S, Pillsbury HC. Myocutaneous flaps for challenging problems in head and neck reconstruction. *Arch Otolaryngol.* 1983;109:396.

59. Panje WR, Cutting C. Trapezius osteomyocutaneous island flap for reconstruction of the anterior floor of the mouth and mandible. *Head Neck Surg.* 1980;3:66.

60. Quillen CG, Shearin JC, Georgiade NG. Use of the latissimus dorsi myocutaneous island flap in the head and neck area: case report. *Plast Reconstr Surg.* 1978;62:113.

61. Quillen CG. Latissimus dorsi myocutaneous flaps in head and neck reconstruction. *Plast Reconstr Surg.* 1979;63:664.

62. Tobin GR, Spratt JS, Bland KI, et al. One stage phayngoesophageal and oral musculocutaneous reconstruction with two segments of one musculocutaneous flap. *Am J Surg.* 1982;144:489.

63. Ross DA, Ariyan S, Restifo R, et al. Use of the operating microscope and loupes for head and neck free microvascular transfer. A retrospective comparison. *Arch Otolaryngol Head Neck Surg.* 2003;129:189.

64. Ahn CY, Shaw WW, Berns S, et al. Clinical experience with the 3M microvascular coupling anastomotic device in 100 free tissue transfers. *Plast Reconstr Surg.* 1994;93:1481.

65. DeLacure MD, Wong RS, Markowitz BL, et al. Clinical experience with a microvascular anastomotic device in head and neck reconstruction. *Am J Surg.* 1995;170:521.

66. Ross DA, Chow JY, Shin J, et al. Arterial coupling for microvascular free tissue transfer in head and neck reconstruction. *Arch Otolaryngol Head Neck Surg.* 2005;131:891.

67. Longmire WP Jr. A modification of the Roux technique for antethoracic esophageal reconstruction-anastomosis of the mesenteric and internal mammary blood vessels. *Surgery.* 1947;22:44.

68. Seidenberg B, Rosenak SS, Hurwitt ES, et al. Immediate reconstruction of the cervical esophagus by a revascularized isolated jejunal segment. *Ann Surg.* 1959;149:162.

69. Jurkiewicz MJ. Vascularized intestinal graft for reconstruction of the cervical esophagus and pharynx. *Plast Reconstr Surg.* 1965;36:509.

70. Coleman JJ. Reconstruction of the pharynx after resection for cancer. A comparison of methods. *Ann Surg.* 1989;209:554.

71. Song R, Gao Y, Song Y, et al. The forearm flap. *Clin Plast Surg.* 1982;9:21.

72. Soutar D, Sheker LR, Tanner NS, et al. The radial forearm flap. A versatile method of intra-oral reconstruction. *Br J Plast Surg.* 1983;36:1.

73. Cicarilli ZN, Ariyan S, Cuono CB. Free radial forearm free flap versatility for the head and neck and lower extremity. *J Reconstr Microsurg.* 1986;2: 221.

74. dos Santos L. The vascular anatomy and dissection of free scapular flap. *Plast Reconstr Surg.* 1984;73:599.

75. Swartz WM, Banis JC, Newton ED, et al. The osteocutaneous scapular flap for mandibular and maxillary reconstruction. *Plast Reconstr Surg.* 1986;77:530.

76. Hidalgo DA. Fibula free flap: A new method of mandible reconstruction. *Plast Reconstr Surg.* 1989;84:71.

77. Vartanian JG, Carvalho AL, Carvalho SM, et al. Pectoralis major and other myofascial/myocutaneous flaps in head and neck cancer reconstruction: Experience with 437 cases at a single institution. *Head and Neck.* 2004;26:1018.

78. Mehta S, Sarkar S, Kavarana N, et al. Complications of the pectoralis major myocutaneous flap in the oral cavity: a prospective evaluation of 220 cases. *Plast Reconstr Surg.* 1996;98:31.

79. Milenovic A, Virag M, Uglesic V, et al. The pectoralis major flap in head and neck reconstruction: First 500 patients. *J Craniomaxillofac Surg.* 2006;34:340.

80. Ross DA, Hundal JS, Son YH, et al. Microsurgical free flap reconstruction outcomes in head and neck cancer patients after extirpation and intraoperative brachytherapy. *Laryngoscope.* 2004;114:1170.

81. Havlik R, Ariyan S. Repeated use of the same pectoralis major myocutaneous flap in difficult second operations. *Plast Reconstr Surg.* 1994;93:481.

chapter 36

Oral Cancer

Suhail K. Mithani, MD / Anthony P. Tufaro, DDS, MD, FACS

● INTRODUCTION

The oral cavity is the most prevalent site for primary cancers within the head and neck and represents the sixth most common malignancy in the United States. The American Cancer Society and the National Cancer Institute's Surveillance, Epidemiology, and End Results (SEER) report indicates that approximately 5% of all newly diagnosed cancers in the United States are cancers of the oral cavity and adjacent structures. The most common primary malignancy of the oral cavity is oral squamous cell carcinoma (OSCC), accounting for 90% of lesions, with the majority of patients presenting with advanced stage disease. Due to the advanced stage at the time of presentation, only half of all patients with newly diagnosed oral cancer remain alive 5 years from the time of their diagnosis.

There is no single etiologic agent that is solely responsible for cancer of the oral cavity. Carcinogenesis is likely due to a combination of intrinsic and extrinsic factors which function synergistically over a long period of time. The strongest correlation for development of oral cancer is exposure to extrinsic carcinogens, such as tobacco and alcohol. While the use of tobacco exposure remains the leading risk factor for the development of oral cancer, with alcohol second, the two in combination have a synergistic effect. Recently, it has been discovered that Epstein-Barr virus, HIV, and human papilloma virus infections are also associated with oral cancers.

Oral cancer is predominantly a disease of middle to later age, with a median age at presentation of 68 years in the United States. Oral cancer demonstrates a male predominance, but the incidence in women has progressively increased in recent years. In 1934, 15% of newly diagnosed cases were women. This has increased to 47% in 1998. This change may be due to inherent genetic susceptibilities in women, but its exact etiology remains the topic of active investigation. Changes in social behaviors such as smoking and alcohol use may also be the cause of these changes in demographics.

● PATIENT EVALUATION AND SELECTION

The oral cavity is bordered by the mucosal surface of the lip anteriorly, the hard palate superiorly, and the floor of the mouth inferiorly. The posterior extent of the oral cavity is the junction of the hard and soft palates superiorly, and the circumvallate papillae inferiorly. The anterior tonsillar pillar created by the mucosal reflection of the palatoglossus muscle is the most posterior aspect of the oral cavity. Tumors arising from the tonsillar fossa and posteriorly are managed differently than OSCC.

The oral cavity is divided into various subsites (Figure 36-1), which are useful in identification and classification of OSCC. They vary in their incidence of development of OSCC and in approaches of surgical management. They include the mucosal lip anteriorly, the buccal mucosa laterally, the lower gingiva inferolaterally, the retromolar trigone posterolaterally, the upper gingival laterally, the hard palate superiorly, the floor of the mouth inferiorly, and the oral anterior two thirds of the tongue.

The lymphatic drainage of the oral cavity progresses initially to the ipsilateral facial, submental, submandibular, and jugulodigastric nodes (ie, levels I, II, and III of the neck), and progresses to levels IV and V (infraomohyoid and posterior triangle nodes) (Figure 36-2). The midline is drained by bilateral lymphatics.

Most patients with oral cancer present with advanced stage disease, with regional, or less commonly distant, metastases at the time of diagnosis. These patients typically present with signs or symptoms of their metastatic

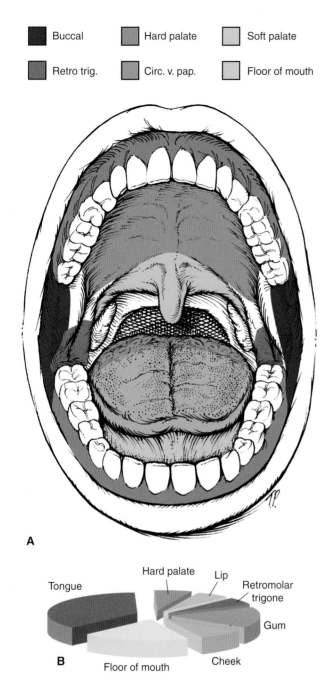

Buccal   Hard palate   Soft palate

Retro trig.   Circ. v. pap.   Floor of mouth

A

Tongue   Hard palate   Lip   Retromolar trigone   Gum   Cheek   Floor of mouth

B

● **FIGURE 36-1.** Oral cavity subsites.

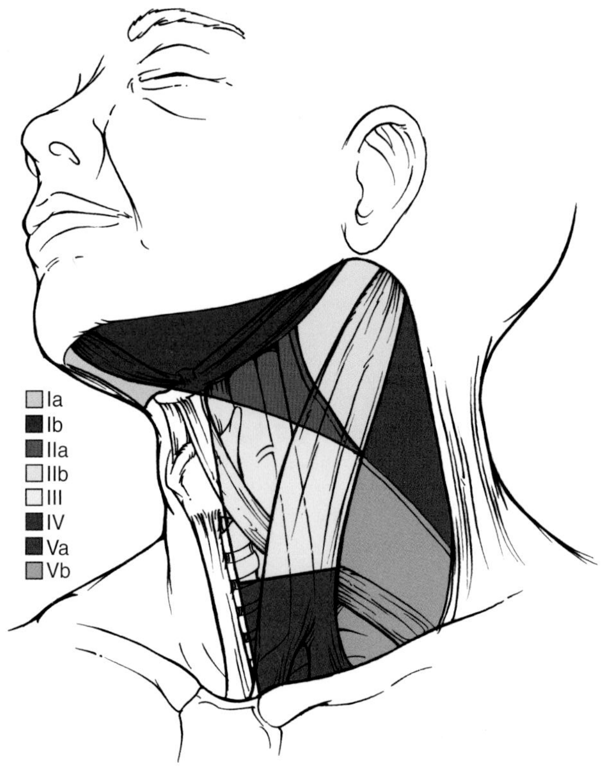

☐ Ia
■ Ib
■ IIa
☐ IIb
☐ III
■ IV
■ Va
☐ Vb

● **FIGURE 36-2.** Lymph node drainage of the head and neck. Node levels. I: Submental and submandibular nodes. Level II: Upper internal jugular nodes, posterior to the back of the submandibular salivary gland, anterior to the back of the sternocleidomastoid muscle and above the level of the bottom of the body of the hyoid bone. Level III: Middle jugular nodes, between the level of the bottom of the body of the hyoid bone and the level of the bottom of the cricoid arch, anterior to the back of the sternocleidomastoid muscle. Level IV: Low jugular nodes, between the level of the bottom of the cricoid arch and the level of the clavicle, anterior to a line connecting the back of the sternocleidomastoid muscle and the posterolateral margin of the anterior scalene muscles; they are lateral to the carotid arteries. Level V: Posterior triangle nodes, posterior to the back of the sternocleidomastoid muscle, and posterior to the line described in level IV. Level VI: Posterior triangle nodes, posterior to the back of the sternocleidomastoid muscle, and posterior to the line described in level IV.

disease (palpable lymph nodes, pulmonary nodule). Occasionally these patients present with symptoms that are associated with local invasion of the primary tumor (bleeding, mass effect, dysphagia, and odynophagia).

Key to reduction of morbidity and mortality in oral cancer is early diagnosis and appropriate management (Figure 36-3). Physical examination of the oral cavity in high-risk patients is the most important aspect of early recognition of oral cancer and precancerous lesions. Most early stage oral cancers are less than 2 cm in diameter. The most common locations of OSCC are the floor of the mouth, the ventrolateral tongue, the lingual aspect of

the retromolar trigone, the hard palate, and the anterior tonsillar pillar.

The anterior oral cavity and ventral aspect of the tongue can be evaluated by asking a patient to open the oral vestibule and direct the tip of the tongue dorsally until it contacts the hard palate. By grasping the anterior third of the tongue and directing it anteriorly, the posterior floor of mouth, the retromolar trigone, and the posterior ventrolateral tongue can be visualized. As an adjunct, a mirror can be used to visualize the lingual aspect of the retromolar trigone. Complete examination includes manual palpation of all mucosal surfaces for

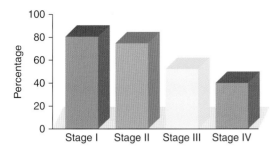

● **FIGURE 36-3.** Oral squamous cell cancer survival by stage.

irregularity, firm areas that may represent submucosal disease, and the cervical region for adenopathy.

● PREOPERATIVE EVALUATION

For small lesions felt to have a high risk of malignant potential by patient history or clinical appearance, surgical excision with 1-cm margins is the preferred method to achieve definitive diagnosis. For larger lesions, transoral biopsy using local anesthetic is warranted and can provide sufficient pathologic evidence to make a diagnosis. Fine-needle aspiration of suspicious nodal disease can provide adequate tissue for pathological analysis. Pan endoscopy is advocated for patients with larger tumors. This technique allows the accurate evaluation of the extent of the primary lesion and thus more accurate staging and at the same time identification of possible synchronous lesions

In addition to tissue diagnosis, radiographic imaging can help delineate the extent of the disease, identify metastases, and identify synchronous lesions (up to 15% occurrence). CT scan of the head and neck for tumor extent and metastatic disease is indicated for all but the most limited tumors and is absolutely warranted in the setting of advanced stage disease (ie, palpable nodes). MRI with gadolinium contrast is beneficial when bony or perineural invasion is clinically evident or suspected. MRI may provide better soft tissue imaging than CT, making it more desirable for head and neck imaging of malignancies of the tongue. Chest x-ray is the imaging modality of choice for initial evaluation for metastatic pulmonary disease. Suspicious lesions may be further evaluated by CT scan of the chest. PET-CT may also be of benefit if a suspicious lesion is identified by chest x-ray, but its cost coupled with the equivocality of its benefit over CT scan for oral malignancy limits its value.

Staging and Survival

Oral cavity cancer is staged using the TNM (tumor, node, metastasis) system following guidelines of the American Joint Committee on Cancer (Figure 36-4). Initial staging of malignancy is based on clinical evaluation and radiographic imaging. Final staging is based on pathological evaluation and histology if surgical excision is performed. The single-most important factor impacting long-term

outcome is the stage of disease at the time of diagnosis. Additionally, the presence of lymph node metastasis is an important prognostic sign. The presence of cervical node metastasis decreases survival by 50% when compared with patients without cervical nodal metastasis and identical tumor characteristics. Prognosis varies also by site of tumor within the oral cavity. Stages I and II cancers account for nearly 75% of newly diagnosed OSCC of the lip. This group of tumors tend to present at an earlier stage, and therefore are amenable to successful treatment with cure rates of 90% to 100%. Early cancers of the retromolar trigone, hard palate, and upper gingiva are also amenable to successful treatment at rates approaching that of cancer of the lip; however, these lesions are often identified at a later stage. Survival is diminished in early cancers of the anterior tongue, the floor of the mouth, and buccal mucosa; however, local control rates of up to 90% can be achieved with appropriate multimodality therapy.

Stage III disease accounts for approximately 20% of newly diagnosed OSCC. Invasive lesions of the retromolar trigone without spread to cervical lymph nodes are curable, and demonstrate local control rates of up to 90%. Locally advanced lesions of the hard palate, upper gingiva, and buccal mucosa have a local control rate of up to 80%. In the absence of clinical evidence of spread to cervical lymph nodes, moderately advanced lesions of the floor of the mouth, and anterior tongue are generally curable, with survival rates of up to 70% and 65%, respectively.

● TREATMENT MODALITY SELECTION

Stages I and II tumors of the oral cavity are can be cured by surgery or radiotherapy alone. Tumor depth of invasion greater than or equal to 3 mm in T1 and T2 disease significantly increases the risk of regional lymph node metastasis. Advanced cancers (stages III and IV) of the lip and oral cavity require multiple modality therapy with limited exceptions. Furthermore, because locoregional recurrence and development or progression of metastatic disease is likely, advanced stage patients with oral cancer should be considered for clinical trials of radiation modifiers or combination chemotherapy in addition to surgery and/or radiation therapy.

● SURGICAL MANAGEMENT

Surgical management of cancers of the oral cavity is dictated by the site of tumor, its location and relationship to adjacent structures. Extent of surgical resection is dictated by the goal of the operative procedure (ie, curative or palliative). There are several surgical approaches to the oral cavity: peroral, mandibulotomy, lower cheek flap, visor flaps, and upper cheek flap.

Peroral Resection

Most small and moderate-sized tumors, T1 and T2, of the oral cavity can be resected using a peroral technique

Primary Tumor (T)

TX Primary tumor cannot be assessed

T0 No evidence of primary tumor

Tis Carcinoma in situ

T1 Tumor ≤ 2 cm in greatest dimension

T2 Tumor > 2 cm, but ≤ 4 cm in greatest dimension

T3 Tumor > 4 cm in greatest dimension

T4 (*lip*) Tumor invades through cortical bone, inferior alveolar nerve, floor of mouth, or skin of face, i.e. chin or nose

> **T4a** (*oral cavity*)
> Tumor invades adjacent structures (e.g. through cortical bone, into deep [extrinsic] muscle of tongue [genioglossus, hyoglossus, palatoglossus, and styloglossus], maxillary sinus, and skin of face)
>
> **T4b**
> Tumor invades masticator space, pterygoid plates, or skull base and/ or encases internal carotid artery

Note: Superficial erosion alone of bone/ tooth socket by gingival primary is not sufficient to classify a tumor as T4.)

Distant Metastasis (M)

MX Distant metastasis cannot be assessed

M0 No distant metastasis

M1 Distant metastasis

Regional Lymph Nodes (N)

NX Regional lymph nodes cannot be assessed

N0 No regional lymph node metastasis

N1 Metastasis in a single ipsilateral lymph node, ≤ 3 cm in greatest dimension

N2 Metastasis in a single ipsilateral lymph node, > 3 cm, but ≤ 6 cm in greatest dimension; or in multiple ipsilateral lymph nodes, ≤ 6 cm in greatest dimension; or in bilateral or contralateral lymph nodes, ≤ 6 cm in greatest dimension

> **N2a**
> Metastasis in a single ipsilateral lymph node > 3 cm but ≤ 6 cm in dimension
>
> **N2b**
> Metastasis in a multiple ipsilateral lymph nodes, ≤ 6 cm in greatest dimension
>
> **N2c**
> Metastasis in bilateral or contralateral lymph nodes, ≤ 6 cm in greatest dimension

N3 Metastasis in a lymph nodes > 6 cm in greatest dimension

In clinical evaluation, the actual size of the nodal mass should be measured and allowance should be made for intervening soft tissues. Most masses > 3 cm in diameter are not single nodes but are confluent nodes or tumors in soft tissues of the neck. The 3 stages of clinically positive nodes are: N1, N2, and N3. The use of subgroups a, b, and c are not required but are recommended. Midline nodes are considered homolateral nodes.

Stage	Groupings			Stage	Groupings		
0	Tis,	N0,	M0	**IVA**	T4a,	N0,	M0
					T4a,	N1,	Mo
I	T1,	N0,	M0		T1,	N2,	M0
					T2,	N2,	M0
II	T2,	N0,	M0		T3,	N2,	M0
					T4a,	N2,	M0
III	T3,	N0,	M0	**IVB**	Any T, N3, M0		
	T1,	N1,	M0		T4b, any N, M0		
	T2,	N1,	M0	**IVC**	Any T, any N, M1		
	T3,	N1,	M0				

● FIGURE 36-4. AJCC staging of oral cavity and lip lesions.

(Figure 36-5). Lesions of the anterior two thirds of the tongue can be safely resected through the open mouth. The surgery is best done under general anesthesia. A nasal endotracheal tube facilitates complete visualization. For tumors of the lateral border of the tongue, a wedge resection of the tongue is achieved with a transversely oriented incision. This will shorten the tongue somewhat but will give the patient a better overall functional outcome. A longitudinally oriented excision will result in an elongated, "serpentine" tongue that can interfere with function.

One-centimeter margins are marked out and the resection carried out with cautery. Care should be taken to avoid injury to the lingual and hypoglossal nerves. Functional deficits in either or both of these nerves lead to significant disability. Frozen sections are sent from the deep muscular and mucosal margins. The defect is closed in layers after careful hemostasis is established.

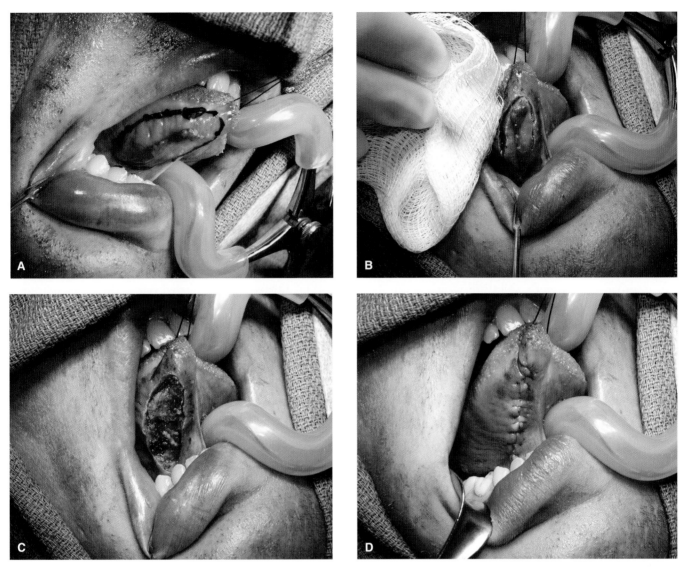

● **FIGURE 36-5.** Peroral resection of tongue lesion. (A) The extent of resection is outlined with marking pen; 1-cm margins are desired. (B) Initial incision. (C) Defect after removal of lesion. (D) Result after primary closure. Note transverse closure to optimize postoperative function.

Absorbable sutures are used in the muscular layer and the mucosa. Burying the knots on the mucosal closure will decrease abrasion of adjacent tissues. Clear liquids and oral rinses can begin in 24 hours.

Most thin T1 and T2 lesions of the anterior floor of mouth and the buccal mucosa are amendable to resection and either direct primary closure or healing via secondary intention. Resections that extend into the deeper structures, musculature, if left to heal by secondary intention will cause significant scarring and possible limitation of function. These resections may be reconstructed with a full-thickness skin graft from the supraclavicular fossa, or other sites in the head and neck. It should be sutured in place and reinforced with a bolster dressing. This technique should help avoid significant scar contracture.

Resections of the hard and soft palate present with unique problems for reconstruction. Often, the size of the resection will preclude the use of local tissue flaps for closure. The options are healing by secondary intention, skin graft, or primary closure. The process of secondary intention healing is quite efficient and made much less painful for the patient when a stent is used. The patient is referred to their dentist prior to resection for the stent fabrication. At the time of surgery, the stent is placed. This technique is also very effective when a skin graft is placed. The stent can protect the skin graft and decrease patient discomfort. Primary closures in the area of the hard palate will often leave an area of denuded periosteum at the donor site. Here, again, the use of a preoperatively fabricated stent will facilitate wound healing and decrease patient discomfort.

Malignant lesions of the alveolus and floor of mouth are often adherent to the adjacent bone. There must be a complete evaluation of the bone preoperatively. When tumor develops adjacent to dentition, often the malignant lesion will extend down the periodontal ligament and into the soft cancellous bone rather than direct invasion through the cortical bone.

In patients where there is significant tumor burden adjacent to bone, a marginal resection may be done. The bone will represent the "deep margin." A marginal mandibular resection will leave the inferior border intact and reduce the functional deficit.

Marginal resections are very difficult in the edentulous mandible where residual bone stock is often atrophic. Patterns of bone resorption with time may leave the patient with a pencil thin mandible that is prone to fracture, particularly if any bone is attempted to be resected.

It is important to round all bony surfaces after the marginal resection. This will reduce the possibility of erosion and exposure. The rounded bone edges will decrease stress and potential for fracture. This small step will improve the patient's ability to wear prosthesis in the postoperative period. The defect created by the marginal resection can often be closed with the local tissue. The resection decreases the height of bone and mobilization of buccal soft tissue and the floor of mouth will often allow for primary closure. A radial forearm free tissue transfer is an excellent option for more complicated reconstruction. A marginal resection is contraindicated in cases of gross tumor invasion into bone as identified on radiographs or clinical examination, tumor metastasis (ie, renal cell, prostate) to bone, or evidence of invasion of the inferior alveolar canal and its contents, which may present as paresthesia.

Mandibulotomy

Tumors arising in the middle and extending into the posterior third of the tongue and floor of mouth, or lesions arising or extending into the oropharynx will need wider access for oncologic resection. The use of mandibulotomy will allow wide and safe access to the posterior oral cavity back to the prevertebral space (Figure 36-6). A panoramic radiograph of the mandible is obtained preoperatively to plan proper placement of the osteotomy to avoid tooth roots and other anatomic and dental obstacles (eg, bridgework, infected teeth, impacted teeth).

The osteotomy is planned just anterior to the mental nerve. This will allow for an easier osteotomy between the premolar roots and the canine, which have a natural divergence. This approach will preserve the inferior alveolar nerve and sensation to the lip and gingiva. If the mandibulotomy is placed in a more posterior position, the osteotomy will be in the direct portal of any radiation that may be needed in the postoperative period and, as stated earlier, the inferior alveolar nerve will be transected. Placement of the mandibulotomy in a more anterior position will usually require extraction of a tooth to facilitate the bone cut. If the tooth is not extracted, the roots of the anterior teeth are at high risk of injury and it opens the possibility of infection.

The mandibulotomy is carried out by dividing the lower lip and elevating a cheek flap. The mental nerve is identified and a site selected for the osteotomy. The site is marked on the bone. A bone plate is fixed to the inferior border of the mandible with 2-mm screws placed in a bicortical fashion. The planned osteotomy should fall directly under the central hole of a 7-hole plate. This will allow for three screws on either side of the osteotomy. The holes are drilled and the screws placed. A smaller plate is now place in the tension band position again with the central hole of a 5-hole plate over the osteotomy. These screws are placed in a monocortical fashion to avoid injury to the dental roots. The holes are drilled and the screws placed.

The plates are now removed and held on the back table. The osteotomy is carried out with a sagittal saw. As the alveolar ridge is approached, the bone is scored and the final osteotomy is carried out with fine osteotomes. The mandible is now able to be opened and excellent access is given to the floor of mouth, posterior tongue, and pharynx. Using cautery, the mucosa is carefully opened. As the mylohyoid muscle is divided, close attention must be paid to the hypoglossal and lingual nerves. They are found very superficially crossing from lateral to medial across the floor of the mouth. At the termination of the resection the soft tissue is re-approximated with absorbable sutures. The muscles can be re-approximated with interrupted sutures in an effort to reconstruct the diaphragm of the floor of the mouth and ensure return to normal function. The bone plates are reapplied to the mandible in the predrilled holes. There should be a small bone gap to account for the thickness of the saw blade. Using this technique, the patient's occlusion will be unchanged from presurgical occlusion.

Resection of the Maxilla for Oral Cavity Tumors

Resection of the maxilla is indicated for the management of tumors arising on the gingiva, hard or soft palate, or buccal sulcus (Figure 36-7). The maxillary ostectomy is indicated for tumors adherent to or invasive to the bony maxilla. Depending on the extent of invasion, the maxillary resection may be as simple as an alveolectomy for small lesions progressing up through palatal fenestration, partial or medial maxillectomy to complete maxillectomy. For this discussion, we will limit the extent of resection to more localized tumors.

The surgical plan begins with axial and coronal CT as well as a panoramic dental radiograph. Dental impressions preoperatively for the fabrication of stents are often important.

Small lesions are addressed with mucosal incisions down to bone with adequate margins. The bone is scored or sectioned with a cutting burr or saw. The final cuts are finished with fine osteotomies. The small defect can be dressed with petrolatum gauze and allowed to granulate in. The dressing is removed at 1 week and the area will

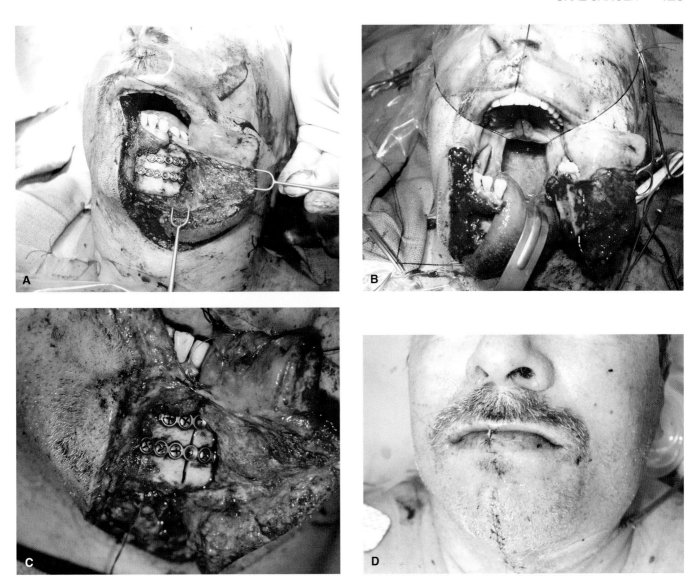

● **FIGURE 36-6.** Mandibulotomy for access to lesion in the posterior oral cavity. (A) Mandible preplated with osteotomy site marked. Adaptation of plate prior to osteotomy is critical in successful reconstruction. (B) Access to posterior oral cavity after Mandibulotomy. (C) Fixation of Osteotomy. (D) End of Surgery.

re-mucosalize. A dental stent or obturator will reduce discomfort and speed healing.

Large tumors will need to be addressed with an upper cheek flap, Weber-Ferguson incision, for access. Attention to detail for placement of the skin incision is of great importance. The incision will be in the central gaze of all people the patient comes in contact with, and the incision should be placed along the lines of esthetic units. The cheek flap is elevated with adequate soft tissue margins. The infraorbital nerve is preserved if possible. The denuded portions of the cheek flap can be skin grafted. The maxillary sinus can be covered with a skin graft if the mucosa is removed. The skin graft is held in place with petrolatum gauze and a prefabricated stent is used to cover the defect and stabilize the packing. The stent and packing are removed at 1 week. The patient is instructed in daily irrigation and can obtain a final prosthesis in 2 to 4 months, depending on healing.

Neck Dissection

The presence of nodal metastasis has a profound negative effect on patient survival, decreasing 5-year, disease-specific survival by 50%. The American Cancer Society states that more than 40% of patients with oral cavity and pharyngeal squamous cell carcinomas present with regional metastasis at their initial examination. The risk of occult metastasis is relatively high for most primary oral cavity cancers. The risk of oral cavity occult metastasis is directly related to the thickness of the primary tumor. Tumors of 3 to 5 mm in thickness have an occult metastatic rate of about 30%.

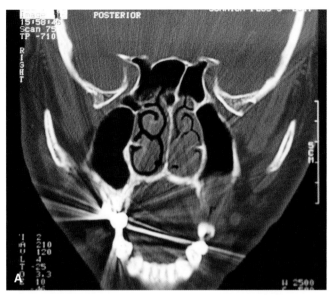
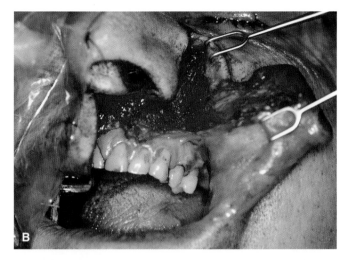
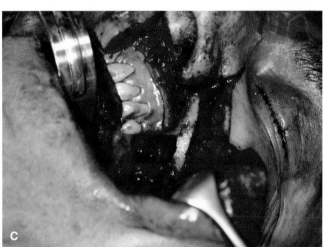
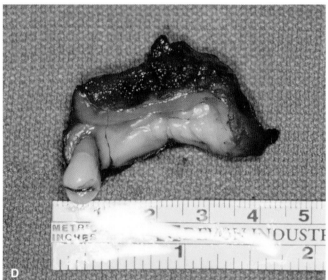

● **FIGURE 36-7.** Partial alveolectomy for oral cavity lesion. (A) Lesion arising from left hard palate abutting maxillary alveolus. (B) Access to the maxilla utilizing a modified Weber-Ferguson incision and gingivabuccal sulcus incision. (C) Defect after removal of portion of maxillary alveolus and palate. (D) Pathologic specimen.

Levels I, II, and III are at the highest risk for occult metastasis from oral cavity primary tumors. The supraomohyoid neck dissection has been shown to be effective for the management of the clinically N0 neck in patients at risk for occult metastasis. Approximately 30% of these patients will have positive nodal disease at pathologic evaluation. In patients with clinical evidence of cervical nodal metastasis, a therapeutic neck dissection, including levels I to V, is indicated (Figure 36-8). Most often a therapeutic neck dissection for an oral cavity primary is a modified neck dissection sparing the sternocleidomastoid muscle, the internal jugular vein, and the spinal accessory nerve.

Technique: Supraomohyoid Neck Dissection

The incision is placed in a natural skin crease and extends from the mastoid area to the midline approaching the hyoid bone. The incision is two finger breaths below the angle of the mandible. The incision is carried through the platysma muscle, and superior and inferior subplatysmal flaps are raised. The greater auricular nerve and the marginal mandibular branch are identified and preserved. The marginal mandibular branch is found directly on the capsule of the submandibular gland and is elevated with either bipolar cautery or scissors. The nerve is retracted in a cephalad direction. Next, the fascia overlying the anterior border of the sternocleidomastoid muscle is incised and the muscle freed of the investing fascia. The spinal accessory nerve is identified as it passes deep to the posterior belly of the digastric muscle. The nerve is traced to the point it enters the SCM. The nerve is freed using scissors. The fibrofatty node–bearing tissue from level IIB is passed deep to the nerve and the dissection proceeds down the internal jugular vein to the omohyoid muscle. The omohyoid is followed to the hyoid bone. The fibrofatty

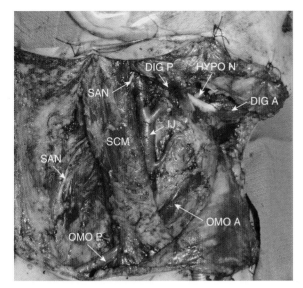

FIGURE 36-8. Neck dissection. Structures identified: SAN, spinal accessory nerve; SCM, Sternocleidomastoid muscle; DIG P, digastric muscle posterior belly; DIG A, digastric muscle anterior belly; HYPO N, hypoglossal nerve; IJ, internal jugular vein; OMO A, omohyoid muscle anterior belly; OMO P, omohyoid muscle posterior belly.

tissue from the submental area is elevated using electrocautery. Care is taken to maintain good hemostasis in this area to avoid injury to the lingual and hypoglossal nerves. Cautery is used to dissect from anterior to posterior along the anterior belly of the digastric muscle. The dissection proceeds until the posterior edge of the mylohyoid muscle is identified. The mylohyoid is retracted to expose the submandibular gland. The gland is retracted posteriorly and the lingual nerve is identified in the cephalic portion of the submandibular triangle. Care is taken to identify the secretomotor fibers going into the gland. They are clamped, divided, and ligated. The hypoglossal nerve is identified as it crosses deep to the digastric tendon. The facial vein and artery are identified and divided. Wharton duct will pass between the two nerves. The specimen is elevated posteriorly and the contents of levels I, II, and III are delivered in continuity.

Technique: Modified Radical Neck Dissection

The upper transverse incision is the same as for the supraomohyoid dissection. A vertical incision is carried down to the midpoint of the clavicle in a lazy-S. This should be planned to lie over the sternocleidomastoid muscle. This will protect the deeper vascular structures if there is a dehiscence of the incision line, particularly if radiation may be used in the postoperative period. The operation begins in level V. The posterior flap is elevated and care is taken to avoid injury to the spinal accessory nerve. It can be found by identifying the trapezius muscle and finding the nerve on the deep surface of the muscle, where the nerve enters at the junction of the middle and distal

thirds of the muscle. Once the nerve is found and freed from investing tissue, the dissection starts in the apex of the posterior triangle taking the fibrofatty node–bearing tissue off of the deep muscles, the splenius capitis, and levator scapulae. The dissection proceeds inferiorly and is passed under the spinal accessory nerve down to clavicle. The specimen is elevated anteriorly and the posterior belly of the omohyoid is identified. This muscle will be freed and elevated so that the entire aspect of level IV can be removed. The dissection should slow in this area to avoid injury to the brachial plexus, phrenic nerves, and internal jugular vein. As the internal jugular vein is approached, in the left neck, all tissue must be divided between clamps and ligated in an effort to avoid lymphatic leak from injury to the thoracic duct. The entire specimen is passed deep to the SCM and combined with the tissue from levels I, II, and III. The dissection then proceeds as the supraomohyoid dissection. The flaps are closed over closed suction drains. The platysma muscle is closed with interrupted sutures.

Adjuvant Therapy

Complete discussion of this topic is beyond the scope of this chapter. However, in general, terms external beam radiation is indicated for patients with multiple positive nodes, nodes completely replaced by tumor, extra nodal extension of disease, and perineural and perivascular tumor invasion. Recent reports have indicated that patients at high risk for local regional failure may benefit from chemotherapeutic agents in conjunction with surgery and radiation. The use of chemotherapy may improve local regional control but shows little or no improvement in survival.

COMPLICATIONS

There is a broad range of complications of surgery of the oral cavity. They range from failure to affect an oncologic cure, to local wound breakdown and subsequent infection, and sequelae of radiation therapy resulting in injury to bone in the irradiated field. Due to the often times difficult nature of achieving ideal and appropriate resection in the face of advanced or invasive disease, these complications are at times unavoidable; however, they may be minimized by careful planning, attention to detail, and adherence to the oncologic principles set forth in the previous sections.

Wound Infection

Wound dehiscence can result in infections which are difficult to be treated with only antibiotics and may be complicated by development of a salivary fistula. The most critical aspect in prevention of wound breakdown is meticulous attention to the suture line, which must be approximated completely, with apposition of tissue in a watertight fashion along the entire length of the incision.

Oral incision lines are constantly bathed in the salivary microbiologic milieu which is conducive to infection of the underlying soft tissue and bone if the suture line is compromised in any way. Meticulous attention to the suture line is especially critical in patients after oncologic resection due to the impaired wound healing associated with subsequent radiation therapy after surgery. Additionally, appropriate preoperative antibiotics have been shown to diminish the likelihood of infection, but are not a substitute for appropriate closure. Broad-spectrum antibiotics and debridement of infected tissue with packing and healing with secondary intention is the initial management of wound infection. Bony hardware in the region of wound infection must be removed with attempts at reconstruction deferred until infection is managed. In the setting of intractable wounds, flap reconstruction is often required to facilitate infection resolution.

Osteoradionecrosis

Radiation therapy is an important adjuvant to surgical resection for management of oral cancer, especially for local control of advanced disease, but it is not without its sequelae. Tissues surrounding the irradiated field are subject to devitalization, hypovascularity, and hypoxia. In the oral cavity this can retard wound healing of the soft tissue and lead to devitalization and necrosis of the bone, also known as osteoradionecrosis (ORN). ORN and inevitable wound breakdown is highly associated with development of infection. The incidence of ORN increases with increased radiation exposure (>6000 cGy) and occurrence can either be spontaneous or associated with local trauma such as tooth extraction, biopsy, or surgery that stresses the regenerative capacity of the bone. The mandible is the most commonly affected bone by ORN after oral cancer resection. The incidence of ORN can be greatly diminished by thorough dental evaluation and extraction of infected or nonrestorable dentition in all patients with oral cancer who may conceivably receive radiation therapy. Extraction of diseased teeth should be carried out at least 3 weeks prior to radiation. All patients who receive radiation therapy should undergo prophylactic fluoride therapy daily for life to prevent radiation caries.

The management of ORN involves hyperbaric oxygen and limited sequestrectomy for early stage disease and radical debridement of nonviable or infected tissues for more advanced disease, which may involve bone, subcutaneous tissue, and/or skin. Reconstruction can employ bone graft, but the hypoxic nature of the wound bed especially in the setting of further irradiation, makes this an inadequate option for reconstruction. Free vascularized bone flaps are the optimal choice for reconstruction of ORN of the mandible requiring extensive debridement.

● OUTCOMES ASSESSMENT

Aside from the development of immediate or delayed complications described above, the assessment of surgical outcomes is directly related to the recurrence of tumor. This may be local recurrence in the vicinity of the oral cavity, regional recurrence in the draining lymph node basins, or metastatic recurrence in sites distant to the original tumor.

Local Recurrence

Return of tumor to the site of original resection is termed *local recurrence*. Diagnosis is made by clinical evaluation of the site of primary disease or patient complaints similar to the initial presentation of disease. Its incidence is highest in the first 2 years after initial resection and is highly unlikely to occur after 5 disease-free years. Local recurrence is likely due to incomplete initial resection with residual micro- or macroscopic disease present at the time of initial extirpation. Adherence to the principle of achieving 1-cm margins in all planes is the most likely method to prevent local recurrence. Often, oral cancer is associated with a desmoplastic reaction in the surrounding tissues, making the margin of tumor spread indistinct and difficult to define clinically. When it is unclear whether appropriate margins have been achieved with wide excision, intraoperative frozen section with pathologic analysis should be undertaken in the plane which is in question. A 1-cm additional margin should be taken beyond the extent of pathologically positive frozen section. Management of local recurrence follows the same principles as primary resection with a goal of achievement of at least 1-cm margins. Oftentimes, resection of local recurrence is complicated by intervening radiation therapy which creates concerns about wound healing and underscores the importance of adequate resection at the time of initial procedure. The management of local recurrence is a significant problem and should be addressed as soon as possible. The surveillance schedule for the first 2 years after initial management is directed at early diagnosis, with clinical examinations every 3 months, and imaging studies (CT, MRI, ultrasound) on a 6- or 12-month basis.

Regional Recurrence

Regional recurrence is defined as development of malignant spread of disease to the lymph nodes of the regional nodal basin after resection of the initial disease. This can be associated with local recurrence, but oftentimes it is not. A diagnosis of regional recurrence is made by clinical examination and imaging studies which are routinely performed in the postoperative period after resection. Avoidance of regional recurrence is best made by appropriate selection of patients for neck dissection at the time of initial operation. Patients with cervical lymph nodes larger than 1 cm in size or that are fixed often have nodal metastases. Suspicious lymph nodes should be biopsied preoperatively by fine-needle aspiration. Patients with biopsy-proven nodal disease should undergo uni- or bilateral neck dissection at the time of initial operation, depending on the distribution of nodal disease.

Additionally, patients with primary tumors that invade more than 3 mm into the basement membrane should undergo a staging supraomohyoid neck dissection, due to their propensity to have occult metastases.

SUGGESTED READING

Bessell A, Glenny AM, Furness S, et al. Interventions for the treatment of oral and oropharyngeal cancers: surgical treatment. *Cochrane Database Syst Rev.* 2011;9:CD006205.

Edge SB, Byrd DR, Compton CC, Fritz AG, Greene FL, Trotti A, eds. *AJCC Cancer Staging Manual.* 7th ed. New York: Springer-Verlag; 2009.

Noonan VL, Kabani S. Diagnosis and management of suspicious lesions of the oral cavity. *Otolaryngol Clin North Am.* 2005;38(1):21–35, vii.

Ow TJ, Myers JN. Current management of advanced resectable oral cavity squamous cell carcinoma. *Clin Exp Otorhinolaryngol.* 2011;4(1):1–10.

Pentenero M, Gandolfo S, Carrozzo M. Importance of tumor thickness and depth of invasion in nodal involvement and prognosis of oral squamous cell carcinoma: a review of the literature. *Head Neck.* 2005;27(12):1080–1091.

chapter 37

Intraoral Reconstruction

Frederic W.-B. Deleyiannis, MD, MPhil, MPH, FACS

● INTRODUCTION

Oral cavity cancer and its treatment affect some of the most fundamental functions of life, including eating, communicating, and interacting socially. The treatment, which may consist of surgery, radiation, or chemotherapy, often is functionally and cosmetically devastating. Facial disfigurement, decreased understandability or absence of speech, and difficulty with swallowing and chewing are common side effects of treatment. These disabilities can alter patients' self-esteem, limit their activity and employment, and decrease social interactions with family and friends.[1]

● PATIENT SELECTION

The goals of reconstruction are to restore an individual to his premorbid function and quality of life. Successful reconstruction requires careful consideration of both the surgical defect and patient-specific variables, such as general medical health, radiation status, and dental rehabilitation needs. Cardiac, vascular, and pulmonary disease, as well as alcoholism, are common in head and neck cancer patients, and may independently impact survival and limit reconstructive options.[2] For example, an individual with severe, lower extremity, peripheral vascular disease would likely not be a good candidate for a fibular free flap. Radiation induces soft tissue fibrosis, in particular, perivascular fibrosis. Therefore, a history of prior radiation and the anticipated decreased vascularity may guide reconstructive options toward using a pedicled or free flap instead of a skin graft.[3]

The anticipated defect should be classified on the extent of the bony, soft tissue, and neurologic component. When possible, respected tissue should be reconstructed with tissue that duplicates both the appearance and the function of the resected tissue. Epithelium can be used to resurface

muscle or mucosal defects. Muscle can be used to restore bulk and motion, and palatal and mandibular skeletal defects can be reconstructed with bone. Skin grafts, local or regional flaps, prosthetic devices, and free tissue transfer are among the range of options that the reconstructive surgeon must possess to customize the reconstruction to an individual patient.

● PATIENT PREPARATION

Oral cavity reconstruction should occur at the same time as tumor resection. Patients undergoing a glossectomy, mandibulectomy, and/or resection of their palate often will require a tracheotomy to manage the airway. Another important factor to consider is the status of the neck and whether a lymph node dissection is needed or has been previously done. Neck dissection can influence the reconstructive decision in many ways, including the need to cover the vessels of the neck (ie, if neck skin has been resected) and the choice and side of inflow and outflow vessels for a free flap. If the reconstructive team is not performing the tumor resection, the preoperative surgical plan should be discussed with the head and neck surgical team to clarify the expected extent of the defect, to plan the surgical incisions, and to position the patient so that two teams can work simultaneously. Positioning the patient 180 degrees from the anesthesia team will allow sufficient room for the extirpative team to work in the head and neck and the reconstructive team to simultaneously harvest a free flap from the upper extremity, abdomen, or lower extremity.

● TECHNIQUE

Primary Repair

Small defects of the oral cavity following extirpation of smaller lesions may require little or no reconstruction,

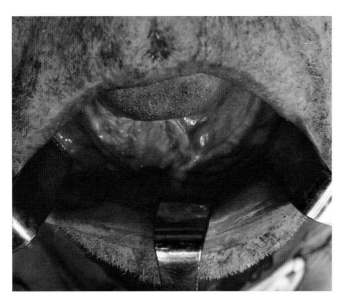

● **FIGURE 37-1.** Healed split-thickness skin graft used to reconstruct a marginal mandibulectomy and floor of mouth defect.

depending on the anatomic location. For instance, the hard palate will heal by secondary intention when surgical resection preserves the palatal bone. Similarly, small defects involving the infrastructure of the oral cavity may be left to heal by secondary intention. This includes small defects of tongue or floor of mouth, and certainly includes defects that involve the anterior tonsillar pillar and tonsil. Some degree of scar contracture is to be expected. When contracture would limit function, the use of a skin graft or other reconstructive technique is preferred. Excision of limited lesions involving the free edge of the soft palate may be closed without sacrificing function. Rhinolalia and nasal regurgitation of fluid is unusual since spontaneous compensation for the defect usually occurs.

Limited defects in the buccal mucosa may be closed primarily with satisfactory results, or alternatively, left to heal by secondary intention. The size of the lesion is the limiting factor. When more than 3 cm of buccal mucosa is removed, some tethering is to be expected with resultant trismus. Use of a local flap is an acceptable alternative. Application of a split-thickness skin graft serves to replace the mucosal defect. Care must be taken to ensure that it is of adequate size, fairly thick (0.018 inch), and properly immobilized to achieve good healing (Figure 37-1). Although some shrinkage may occur, this technique should not result in limitation in opening the mouth.

Tongue Flaps

The tongue provides a ready source of well-vascularized soft tissue for reconstruction of the oral cavity. The use of tongue flaps to reconstruct large defects results in some sacrifice of tongue mobility with subsequent articulation and swallowing difficulties. In these cases, a fasciocutaneous free flap is often a better choice for reconstruction.

The anterior mobile tongue may be useful for reconstruction of the buccal mucosa, floor of mouth, mandibular alveolus, or retromolar trigone. The lingual artery and the hypoglossal nerve are usually intact. A midline or lateral glossotomy is undertaken. The tongue to be used as a flap is sculptured as flat as possible and rotated 60 to 90 degrees into the defect. The mucosal pedicle is 4 to 6 mm in thickness. A bolus or stent is not recommended. The remaining portion of the tongue is closed primarily, which results in a narrow tongue.

An anteriorly based dorsal tongue flap can be used to reconstruct anterior defects of the hard palate (Figure 37-2). The base of the flap should be between 2.5 and 3 cm, and the length (usually 5–6 cm) should be sufficient to avoid tension on the pedicle and on the motion of the tongue. Five to 7 mm of mucosa and muscle should be included in the flap, and the tongue tip should be preserved as much as possible. Division and inset of pedicle is done at second stage approximately 3 weeks after the inset.

Split-Thickness Skin Grafts

The use of split-thickness skin grafts to resurface defects in the oral cavity offers a number of important advantages. Large quantities of skin are readily available. Extremely limited short-term morbidity is experienced at the donor site. Reconstruction is accomplished without employing bulky, adynamic flaps, and rapid healing may be expected if proper technique is used in applying the split-thickness skin graft.

Under most circumstances, the graft is obtained from the lateral aspect of the thigh. A thickness of 0.018 inch is ideal because thick grafts are much easier to handle and sew than thin grafts and have less of a tendency to contract. Complete hemostasis is mandatory before the grafting procedures commence. Complete immobilization of the graft against the recipient bed is critical to successful skin grafting. The graft is sewn circumferentially. The sutures are left long enough so that they can be tied over a bolster (Figure 37-3).

Pectoralis Major Myocutaneous Flaps

The pectoralis major myocutaneous (PMMC) flap is the most frequently used myocutaneous flap in head and neck reconstruction.[4] The blood supply of the PMMC flap is provided by the lateral thoracic artery and the pectoral branch from the thoracoacromial artery. The thoracoacromial artery is a branch of the subclavian artery. The pectoral branch passes beneath the clavicle through the clavipectoral fascia at approximately the junction of the medial two thirds with the lateral one third. It then takes an oblique course under the pectoralis muscle and gives off muscular branches that supply the muscle and pierce the muscle to supply the overlying skin.

The PMMC flap should be designed on the anterior chest wall to conform to the size and shape of the defect

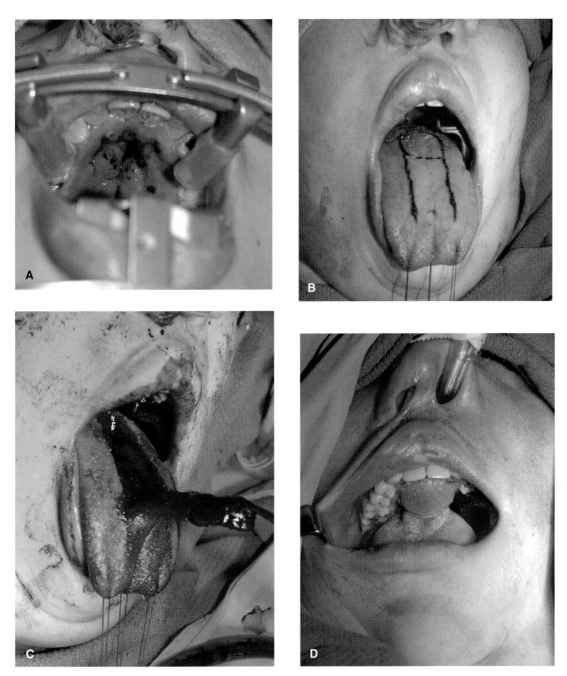

● **FIGURE 37-2.** (A) A patient with an anterior palatal fistula with markings for turnover flaps of oral mucosa to be used for nasal closure. (B) The design for an anteriorly based dorsal tongue flap. (C) The tongue flap being raised. (D) The flap after inset. Note that the flap still maintains a connection to the tongue.

(Figure 37-4). To ensure that the length of the musculovascular bundle will be adequate to reach into the oral cavity, one should fabricate a template of the flap with a surgical towel cut to the anticipated size and length. The point of rotation of the flap can be designed as superior as the point of exit under the inferior edge of the clavicle of the pectoral branch of the thoracoacromial artery. If the PMMC flap is to be mobilized this far superiorly, the lateral thoracic artery must be divided. This may compromise the blood supply of the flap in some patients. Under most circumstances, the PMMC flap begins at the level of

the nipple and is carried inferiorly to the lower borders of the rib. The skin paddle may be extended over the rectus sheath, but these portions of skin are supplied by a random vascular pattern and are less reliable. After the skin incisions around the skin paddle are carried through the subcutaneous tissue, the muscle is incised medially from its sternal attachments and elevated from the chest wall. The neurovascular bundle is identified by direct visualization and palpation. For further mobilization, the humeral attachments of the muscle are divided. An oblique incision from the superior lateral edge of the skin paddle to

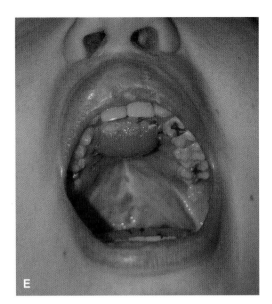
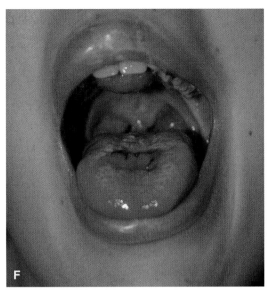

● **FIGURE 37-2.** (*continued*) (E) The tongue flap after division with closure of the palatal fistula. (F) The tongue donor site after flap division and inset.

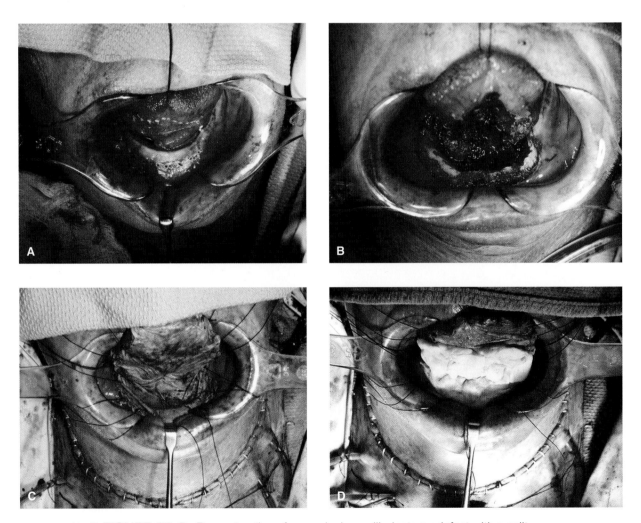

● **FIGURE 37-3.** Reconstruction of a marginal mandibulectomy defect with a split-thickness skin graft. (A) A patient with a T2 carcinoma of the floor of mouth. (B) The marginal mandibulectomy defect, including resection of the floor of mouth and ventral tongue. (C) Split-thickness skin graft (0.018 inch) used to resurface the defect. (D) The Xeroform bolster and tie-over sutures used to secure the skin graft.

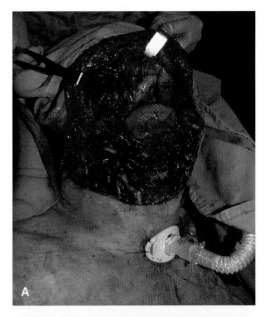

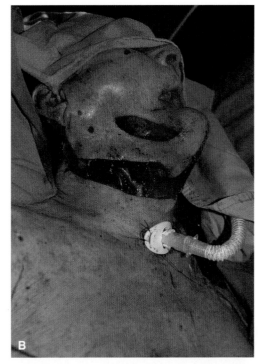

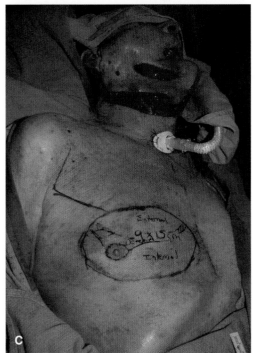

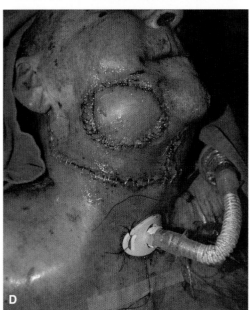

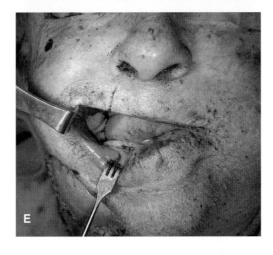

● FIGURE 37-4. (A) Photograph demonstrating resection of the lateral mandible and floor of mouth. (B) The resection of the skin overlying the mandibular body. (C) The design of a pectoralis flap utilizing two skin paddles (one for the floor of mouth, and one for the skin). The area to be de-epitheliazed (including the nipple) is marked. The superior incision is designed to preserve the blood supply and the possibility of raising a deltopectoral flap. (D) The inset of the cutaneous paddle of the flap. (E) The inset of the intraoral paddle of the flap. The lateral bony mandible has not been reconstructed.

the axillae can be used to improve exposure. This incision should be located approximately at the sight of a lower transverse incision that would be used if a deltopectoral flap were designed. By not dividing the second and third intercostals perforators when raising the PPMC flaps and by not incising the skin supplied by the second and third intercostals perforators, one still has the future option of designing an ipsilateral deltopectoral flap. The donor area from the PMMC flap can be closed primarily, leaving little chest deformity.

Multiple modifications of the PMMC flap have been described. The skin paddle can be modified to resurface two epithelial defects (ie, skin and mucosa, when a through-and-through defect has been created) (Figure 37-4). The pectoralis muscle can be employed without the cutaneous portion of the paddle. In this way the flap is far less bulky. If an epithelial surface is required, a split-thickness skin graft can be applied directly to the muscle. When the muscle is used intraorally, it will re-epithelialize with mucosa if allowed to heal by secondary intention.

Several other pedicled flaps have been used for oral cavity reconstruction, most notably the latissimus dorsi flap. The latissimus dorsi shares many of the advantages of a pectoralis myocutaneous flap, including a large arc of rotation, reliable vascularity and possibility of inclusion of muscle with or without a skin island. However, it necessitates turning the patient to harvest the flap, and is generally second to the pectoralis myocutaneous flap for oral cavity reconstruction.

Soft Tissue Reconstruction With Free Flaps

Free flaps are often the ideal reconstructive modality for defects involving large resections of the soft tissues of the oral cavity. The most common free flaps for soft tissue reconstruction are the anterolateral thigh flap, the radial forearm free flap, and the rectus abdominis flap.

The *anterolateral thigh flap* is a perforator flap, derived from the descending branch of the lateral circumflex femoral artery. Its advantages include a long pedicle (Figure 37-5) with a suitable vessel diameter and the possibility of harvesting the flap with thigh musculature (the vastus lateralis muscle, rectus femoris muscle, and/or the tensor fasciae lata) or as a sensate flap (by incorporating the anterior branch of the lateral cutaneous nerve of the thigh). Because of its distance to the head and neck, its harvest can be performed simultaneously with tumor extirpation. Flap elevation begins by mapping the cutaneous perforators with a pencil Doppler probe. These perforators are located by first marking the midpoint between the anterior superior iliac spine and superolateral corner of the patella (Figure 37-5). A circle centered at this midpoint is then drawn with a radius of 3 cm. The majority of the cutaneous perforators are located in the inferolateral quadrant of this circle. The flap is then harvested with its center over these perforators and its long axis parallel to that of the thigh. The flap can be elevated with or without

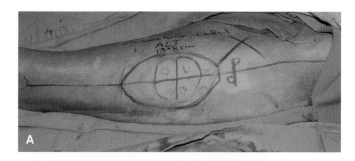

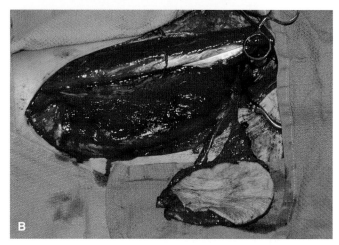

● **FIGURE 37-5.** (A) Photograph demonstrating the design of an anterior lateral thigh flap for coverage of a near-total glossectomy defect. (B) The anterior lateral thigh flap harvested with isolation of its pedicle.

the fascia lata (suprafascial dissection). The flap's skin and subcutaneous tissue are raised until the perforator(s) to the skin is defined. Once the skin vessel(s) is seen, it is dissected until the main pedicle is reached. If the skin vessel(s) is a musculocutaneous perforator(s) (the majority of patients), then the harvest includes an intramuscular dissection through the vastus lateralis muscle. If the skin vessel is a septocutaneous perforator, then the dissection is simpler and proceeds between the vastus lateralis and rectus femoris muscles. The length of the pedicle is 8 to 16 cm, with a vessel diameter of larger than 2 mm. A skin defect of less than 9 cm in width can be closed primarily without any reported evidence of compartment syndrome. Larger defects require skin grafting. A distinct disadvantage is the thickness of the flap in overweight individuals. However, the flap can be trimmed to the subdermal fat level for use as a thinner flap (4 mm).

The radial forearm free flap is a fasciocutaneous free flap deriving its blood supply from branches of the radial artery that run in the intermuscular septum between the brachioradialis and flexor carpi radialis muscle. The major advantage of the radial forearm free flap is the large amount of thin forearm skin that can be harvested for reconstruction. The main disadvantage of the radial forearm free flap is the potential poor cosmesis at the donor forearm site.

For through-and-through cheek defects, the radial forearm free flap can be folded to create separate skin paddles for cutaneous and oral mucosa reconstruction. A segment of radius vascularized by vessels passing from the radial artery through the lateral intermuscular septum and perforating vessels through the muscle belly of the flexor pollicus longus may be transferred with the radial forearm flap and be used for mandible bony reconstruction. The antebrachial cutaneous nerves of the forearm can be incorporated into the flap to make the radial forearm free flap a sensate flap. However, spontaneous return of flap sensation has been documented in patients who underwent reconstruction of the oral cavity with noninnervated flaps. Compared with an anterolateral thigh flap, a radial forearm free flap is often thinner, but has similar indications for reconstruction.[5] By harvesting additional subcutaneous tissue extensions and folding these extensions under the cutaneous portions of the radial forearm free flap, additional bulk can be added to the reconstruction of the mobile tongue or base of tongue. The bulk of vascularized fat does not diminish with time, as is the case with vascularized muscle that undergoes denervation atrophy.

The *rectus abdominis musculocutaneous free flap* is based on periumbilical perforators from the deep inferior epigastric arteries. Incorporation of the periumbilical perforators permits an orientation of the skin paddle virtually in any direction from the midline. After the perforators are identified, the anterior rectus sheath is incised medial to the linea semilunaris and lateral to the linea alba. To preserve the strength of the abdominal wall, the anterior rectus sheath should not be harvested below the arcuate line. Inferiorly, the anterior rectus sheath is incised vertically to completely expose the rectus muscle. The deep inferior epigastric pedicle is identified after the rectus muscle is bluntly dissected free from the posterior rectus sheath. The vascular pedicle, up to 15 cm in length, is exposed all the way to the origin of the vessels from the external iliac artery and vein. The intercostals nerves that supply the rectus muscle and overlying skin are mixed sensory and motor nerves, but microanastomosis to a sensory nerve in the head and neck has not yet resulted in a report of restoration of sensation. Closure of the abdominal wall can be accomplished with direct approximation of the residual anterior fascial margins. Most surgeons would agree that unless patients are engaged in vigorous physical activities, harvest of a unilateral rectus muscle has little functional impact. Probably the biggest disadvantage of using the rectus abdominis flap is its bulky nature. However, for near-total and total glossectomy defects, the rectus abdominis can be a useful option (Figures 37-6 and 37-7).

● COMPLICATIONS

Complications are defect-specific and vary according to the type of reconstruction. In some circumstances, there are clear advantages to be realized through the use of regional flaps to replace extirpated tissue. Conversely, however, the use of a bulky, adynamic flap may severely compromise the function of the residual innervated and mobile tissue. A small finger of residual tongue may perform its duties of mastication and speech quite well unless it is tethered to the alveolus by primary closure or immobilized through attachment to an adynamic myocutaneous flap.

The most common source of skin graft failure in the oral cavity is inadequate immobilization. This results in shearing, which prevents successful revascularization by the capillary buds. A collection of fluid, either hematoma or seroma, under the graft also will lead to skin necrosis because the distance through which the capillary buds must grow prevents reestablishment of a vascular supply within the critical time period. Placement of the graft over an avascular recipient bed will also result in graft failure. Infection and residual cancer are other causes of graft failure. When circumstances require that the graft replace gingiva or extend onto the defect created by a marginal mandibulectomy, immobilization may be facilitated by the preoperative construction of a surgical stent. Split-thickness skin graft reconstruction is contraindicated in patients who have received prior radiation therapy if the graft is to be placed over exposed bone to prevent osteoradionecrosis.[3]

An Allen test should be preformed prior to harvesting a radial forearm free flap to ensure the postoperative viability of the hand. During a radial forearm free flap harvest the paratenon of the flexor tendons should be preserved to minimize the risk of tendon exposure and of skin graft failure. After a rectus free flap, the greater the amount of fascia and muscle removed, the higher the risk of developing a hernia or bulge. Both complications can be avoided by proper repair of the abdominal wall. To repair the fascia after flap removal and to prevent the formation of a hernia or bulge, some surgeons use nonabsorbable mesh to replace the anterior rectus sheath that has been harvested. Success rates for free tissue transfer should exceed 95% in experienced hands.

● OUTCOMES

Repair of Glossectomy Defects

Restoration of tongue function after ablative surgery remains a major challenge for the reconstructive surgeon. The ultimate goal is to restore form and function, but the complex set of intrinsic and extrinsic muscle that provide coordinated motor activity cannot be duplicated by reinnervated muscle flaps. It is unrealistic to expect a unidirectional, reinnervated muscle, such as the rectus abdominis, to mimic the complex, pattern of muscle contraction in the native tongue. The attainable goals of tongue reconstruction are to preserve the mobility of the remaining tongue, to restore bulk so that the neotongue can contact with the palate to assist in articulation and swallowing, and to restore sensation.

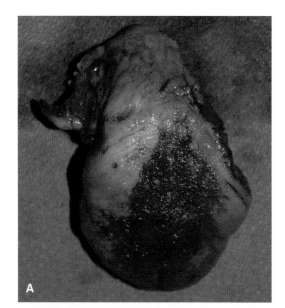

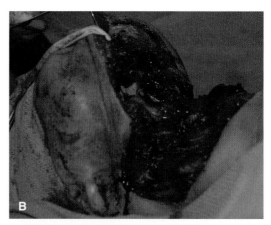

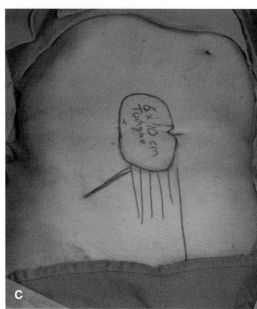

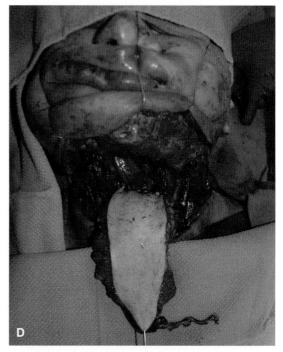

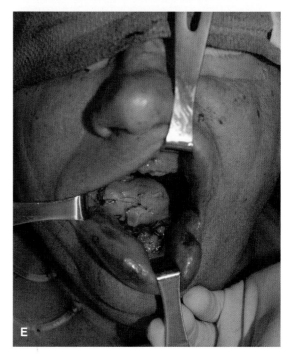

● FIGURE 37-6. (A) A near-total glossectomy specimen. (B) A glossectomy defect. (C) The design of a myocutaneous rectus abdominis free flap. (D) The rectus flap inset into the vallecula for reconstruction of the base of tongue. (E) The rectus inset into the floor of mouth for reconstruction of the anterior tongue.

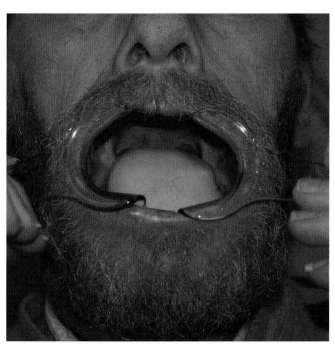

● **FIGURE 37-7.** A total tongue reconstruction with a myocutaneous rectus abdominis free flap.

The extent of the glossectomy and the presence or absence of an associated mandibulectomy defect determine the surgeon's approach to reconstruction. Because of the different functions of the two regions, the tongue is divided into the mobile anterior part and the tongue base. The mobility of the anterior tongue is critical for articulation, mastication, and the oral phase of swallowing. The tongue base is critical in completing the pharyngeal phase of swallowing. The approach to reconstructing the mobile tongue should involve the use of thin, sensate, pliable tissues that maintain maximum mobility and potentially restore sensation. Defects of the tongue base present a separate problem. Volume of the tongue base must be restored so that the tongue base can contact the pharyngeal walls and generate a driving force to drive the food bolus through the pharynx.

To help prevent aspiration and improve swallowing, a number of additional surgical measures should be considered at the time of reconstruction. According to the two pump theory of swallowing, the tongue base acts first as a piston driving the food bolus into the oropharynx. The second pump is the negative pressure in the hypopharynx generated by the anterior elevation of the larynx caused by contraction of the hyomandibular musculature. A glossectomy often involves disruption of the hyomandibular muscle complex. Therefore, to help restore laryngeal elevation, the hyoid should be anteriorly suspended from mandible. This can be accomplished by passing two large prolene sutures around the body of the hyoid and through drill holes created in the anterior, inferior border of the mandible. In patients who are at the greatest risk for aspiration because of the amount of tongue resected,

a tubed epiglottic laryngoplasty may be employed. This involves incising the interarytenoid mucosa and the lower portion of the aryepiglottic folds bilaterally and sewing the sides together to create a tube. This procedure will preserve speech but will also require the use of a tracheotomy. In patients who have undergone an extensive tongue resection, in particular a total glossectomy, management must be individualized on the basis of the patient's pulmonary reserve and general health. Because of the concerns of aspiration some patients may require a total laryngectomy.

Partial Glossectomy Defects

Defects following excision of small lesions of the oral tongue and tongue base may be satisfactorily closed primarily. In 1998, in a prospective study McConnel et al. compared three methods of reconstruction with respect to speech and swallowing function: primary closure, distal myocutaneous flap, and microvascular free flap.[6] The results demonstrated that patients with relatively small resections of the oral tongue (<30%) and tongue base (<60%) who underwent primary closure had better swallowing outcomes and speech intelligibility than patients who underwent distal or free flap closure. Flap reconstruction usually is needed if greater than 50% of the tongue is resected. Hemiglossectomy defects can be closed primarily, but flap reconstruction for hemiglossectomy defects may improve swallowing function. In 2002, Hsiao et al. compared the swallowing and speech of six patients who underwent hemiglossectomy and were closed primarily to six patients who were reconstructed with a radial forearm free flap.[7] Patients who had flap reconstruction had better swallowing but poorer speech. The authors speculated that a flap adds bulk, thus improving pharyngeal clearance by maintaining the tongue-to-mouth roof contact that is necessary for swallowing, but that a nonfunctional flap hinders articulation by restricting the mobility of the remaining portion of the tongue.

When small mobile tongue defects are combined with segmental mandible defects, primary consideration is given to maintaining the mobility of the tongue. Composite skin-bone free flaps, such as the osteocutaneous radial forearm or fibula free flap, can be contoured to replace the soft tissue defect and restore mandibular continuity; but if the position of the skin paddle leads to tethering of the tongue, one should consider reconstructing the floor of mouth and tongue separately from the mandible.

The combination of a segmental mandibulectomy defect with hemiglossectomy defect involving the mobile tongue or both the mobile tongue and base of tongue is a more challenging reconstruction. The reconstructive options begin with first choosing the optimal flap for tongue reconstruction and then considering the options for the mandible. Two free flaps, in particular a forearm flap or an anterolateral thigh with a fibular flap, may be necessary for complex composite defects.

Tongue base defects may be difficult to close primarily if a large portion of the oropharynx has also been resected. The anterior mobile tongue can be advanced posteriorly to assist in closure of posterior defects, but additional tissue must be introduced if closure causes significant distortion of the mobile tongue. A sensate forearm flap is the most useful flap to reconstruct such defects. If the patient is not a good candidate for a free flap, a pedicled pectoralis myocutaneous flap is a good alternative.

Total Glossectomy Defects

Total tongue reconstruction involves creating bulk for the neotongue and positioning the neotongue so that the vertical height is sufficient to achieve contact with the palate. Free musculocutaneous flaps, in particular the rectus abdominis free flap (Figure 37-7), have the advantage that the muscle of the flap can be used as a platform for positioning the overlying fat and skin component. Drill holes placed in the mandible can be used to secure the muscle. The tendinous inscriptions in the rectus abdominis flap offer a better purchase for sutures than those directly placed in muscle. Fasciocutaneous free flaps, such as radial forearm, ALT, scapular, or parascapular flaps, can also be de-epitheliazed and folded on themselves to create additional bulk and to help maintain the position of the neotongue.

Prosthetics After Tongue Reconstruction

In some circumstances the reconstructed tongue may have insufficient bulk. Speech and swallowing can be improved in some patients through the use of a fabricated prosthetic tongue to be attached to a dental prosthesis. Residual dentition facilitates retention of the prosthesis. The prosthetic tongue is modified with a central groove for swallowing, while a fuller model is employed for speech.

An alternative way to address the abnormally large oral cavity resulting from a glossectomy is to employ a palatal-drop prosthesis. This prosthesis is constructed for the maxillary arch. The palatal aspect of the prosthesis is built up gradually until the patient achieves the best possible speech and swallowing ability. Dropping the level of the palate compensates for the lack of tongue volume.

Hard Palate Defects

Mucosal defects of the hard palate do not require any form of reconstruction; they will heal by secondary intention. Patient comfort may be increased by the use of a surgical obturator constructed preoperatively and inserted at the time of surgery. Use of a surgical obturator allows return to oral feeding in the immediate postoperative period. The surgical obturator is removed 5 days postoperatively and is converted into an interim obturate, which may be removed periodically for oral hygiene.

Defects that extend through the palatal bone into the overlying antrum or nasal cavity require either a prosthesis or reconstructive surgery. A number of surgical techniques have been described. Small defects frequently can be closed using a turnover flap for nasal lining and a palatal flap based on the greater palatine artery for oral closure. These techniques are similar to those described for closure of a palatal fistula after repair of a cleft palate. Recent reports suggest that the placement of acellular dermis (alloderm) between the nasal and oral closure may help the closure of palatal fistulas by acting as a scaffold for soft tissue ingrowth. Basic reconstructive principles would suggest that palatal closure requires a two-layer closure of the oral and nasal mucosa. Palatal defects may also be closed with tongue flaps (Figure 37-2). Palatal defects combined with alveolar defects may be closed with the temporalis muscle. However, when the alveolar ridge is intact, one must pass the muscle through a fenestration in the maxillary sinus or advance or remove the maxillary tuberosity.

When local flaps or regional flaps are insufficient, reconstruction of hard palate defects may require free tissue transfer. Large palatal defects often involve resection of the alveolus, maxilla, and the soft tissues of the face and orbit. Radial forearm, rectus abdominis, fibula, scapular, and iliac crest free flaps have been used for successful reconstruction. When the hard palate has been resected without the loss of tooth-bearing segments, a soft tissue flap, such as a radial forearm fasciocutaneous flap, is a good option of reconstruction. When the hard palate has been resected with significant portions of the alveolus, adequate teeth and/or retentive surfaces may not be available to provide stability to a conventional denture. Soft tissue reconstruction alone leaves a blunted buccal sulcus and palatal arch which may not be able to retain a prosthesis or denture. Functional dental rehabilitation in some patients can best be achieved by reconstructing the defect with vascularized bone. The bone from an osteocutaneous radial forearm free flap or from an osteocutaneous fibular free flap can be used to reconstruct the alveolus with the skin paddle used for palatal reconstruction. Futran et al. reported their experience with 27 patients who underwent midface reconstruction with the fibula free flap.[8] Osteotomies were made in the fibula to create the missing tooth-bearing segments. Eighteen patients received secondary osseointegrated implants, and 14 patients were using implant-borne prostheses. The authors noted that in more extensive resections where there was also a need for reconstruction of the zygomatic complex, infraorbital rim, and floor, the utility of fibula free flap was limited.

Recently, Cordeiro and Santamaria proposed a classification system and algorithm for reconstruction of maxillectomy and midfacial structures.[9] The temporalis muscle, soft tissue free flaps (rectus abdominis and radial forearm), nonvascularized bone (rib or calvarium), and vascularized bone flaps (osteocutaneous radial forearm free flap) was used to construct a variety of maxillectomy defects. Palatal defects were closed only with soft tissue (Figure 37-8). The nonvascularized and vascularized bone was used for the osseous reconstruction of the zygoma and orbit.

Defects in the bony hard palate or maxillary alveolus are suited to prosthetic rehabilitation. The prosthodontist

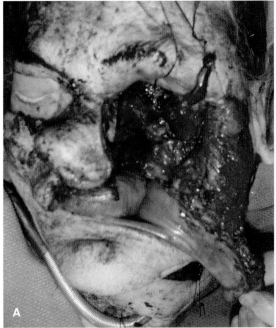

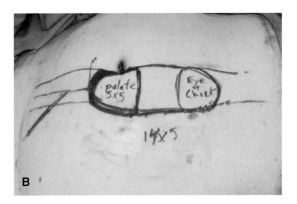

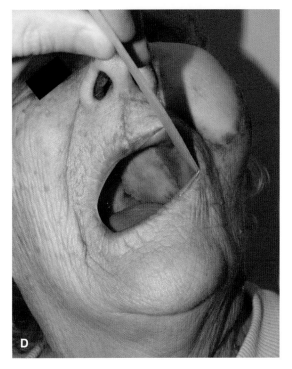

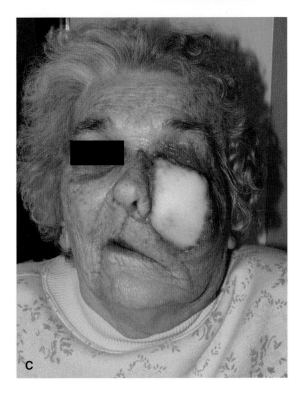

● FIGURE 37-8. (A) Photograph demonstrating a total orbitomaxillectomy defect. (B) The flap design utilizing two cutaneous skin paddles—one for orbit and cheek skin reconstruction and one for the palate reconstruction. (C) Postoperative the patient in (A). (D) Postoperative the palatal reconstruction.

should be consulted prior to surgical treatment. Dental records including casts, roentgenograms, and jaw relationship records are obtained. The surgeon can indicate to the prosthodontist preoperatively the tissue to be resected. In this way, it is possible to construct a surgical obturator prior to the operation. Restoration of residual dentition should be done preoperatively whenever possible. When resection of the alveolus is necessary, bone cuts should be planned to allow a margin of good alveolus adjacent to the teeth that are retained. When intact dentition remains, the bone cuts should be placed through the socket of an adjacent tooth

and not in the interdental space. Failure to observe this precaution frequently results in the subsequent loss of the residual tooth.

Soft Palate Defects

Reconstruction of soft palate defects has traditionally relied on prosthetic rehabilitation. However, a number of surgical options may be entertained. Palatal island flaps alone or in combination with a pharyngeal flap, buccal mucosal flaps, and free flaps have been used to reconstruct soft palate

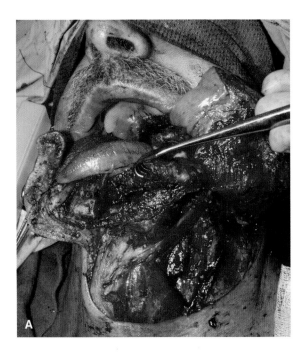

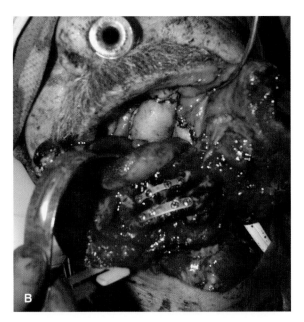

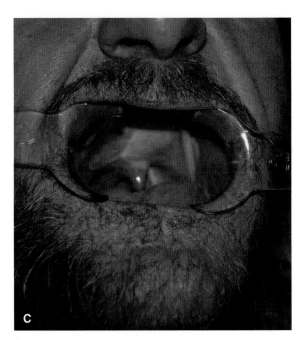

● FIGURE 37-9. (A) The exposure and resection of the hemi-soft palate through a lip splitting approach and midline mandibulotomy. (B) A radial artery free forearm flap inset into the soft palate defect. A superiorly based pharyngeal flap has also been inset for nasal lining and to help suspend the radial artery flap. (C) Postoperative the patient in (A) at 1 year.

defects. Both inferiorly and superiorly based pharyngeal flaps have been described. These flaps have in common the ability to afford the patient acceptable velopharyngeal competence without creating complete nasal obstruction. Brown et al. utilized speech and swallowing domains of the University of Washington Quality of Life questionnaire to assess outcomes of two different forms of palatal reconstruction after resection for cancer.[10] They were able to document better outcomes when a pharyngeal flap was used to supplement radial forearm flap reconstruction (Figure 37-9). The authors proposed that the pharyngeal flap decreases the level of velopharyngeal incompetence by maintaining the radial forearm flap in a posterior position.

Resection of the lateral soft palate is the most commonly encountered defect of the soft palate. They are usually the result of a composite resection of a primary cancer of the retromolar trigone or tonsillar fossa that extends to the soft palate (Figure 37-9). In addition to or instead of soft tissue reconstruction, rehabilitation of the lateral palatal defect can be achieved with a speech prosthesis. The prosthesis is connected to a maxillary plate so that it extends through the palatal defect and is superior to the residual palate. Upon function, the remaining palatal tissue makes contact with the prosthesis, achieving oral-nasal separation.

Most patients, following soft palate resection, have long-standing middle ear abnormalities secondary to Eustachian tube dysfunction. The condition of the tympanic membrane and middle ear should be examined regularly. Myringotomy tubes may be indicated.

REFERENCES

1. Weymuller EA, Yueh B, Deleyiannis FW-B. Quality of life in patients with head and neck cancer. In: Myers EN, Suen JY, Myers JN, Hanna EYN, eds. *Cancer of the Head and Neck.* 4th ed. Philadelphia: Saunders; 2003:809–825.

2. Deleyiannis FWB, Carolyn C, Lee E, et al. Reconstruction of the lateral mandibulectomy defect: Management based on prognosis and the location and volume of the soft tissue resection. *Laryngoscope.* 2006;116(11):2071–2080.

3. Deleyiannis FWB, Dunklebarger J, Russavage J, et al. Reconstruction of the marginal mandibulectomy defect: an update. *Am J Otolaryngol.* 2007;28(6):363–366.

4. Koh KS, Eom JS, Kirk I, et al. Pectoralis major musculocutaneous flap in oropharyngeal reconstruction: revisited. *Plast Reconstr Surg.* 2006;118(5):1145–1149; discussion 1150.

5. Huang CH, Chen HC, Huang YL, Mardini S, Feng GM. Comparison of the radial forearm flap and the thinned anterolateral thigh cutaneous flap for reconstruction of tongue defects: an evaluation of donor-site morbidity. *Plast Reconstr Surg.* 2004;114(7):1704–1710.

6. McConnel FMS, Pauloski BR, Logemann JA, et al. Functional results of primary closure vs flaps in oropharyngeal reconstruction A prospective study of speech and swallowing. *Arch Otolaryngol Head Neck Surg.* 1998;124: 625–630.

7. Hsiao HT, Leu YS, Lin CCL. Primary closure versus radial forearm flap reconstruction after hemiglossectomy: functional assessment of swallowing and speech. *Ann Plast Surg.* 2002;49:612–616.

8. Futran ND, Wadsworth JT, Villaret D, Farwell G. Midface reconstruction with the fibula free flap. *Arch Otolaryngol Head Neck Surg.* 2002;128:161–166.

9. Cordeiro PG, Santamaria E. A classification system and algorithm for reconstruction of maxillectomy and midfacial defects. *Plast Reconstr Surg.* 2000;105:2331–2346.

10. Brown JS, Zuydam AC, Jones DC, Rogers SN, Vaughan ED. Functional outcome in soft palate reconstruction using a radial forearm free flap in conjunction with a superiorly based pharyngeal flap. *Head Neck.* 1997;19:524–534.

chapter 38

Mandibular Reconstruction

Joseph J. Disa, MD, FACS

INTRODUCTION

The mandible defines the profile and appearance of the lower third of the face. It is essential for proper occlusion, mastication, deglutition, and speech. The ultimate outcome of segmental mandibular resection depends on the location and amount of mandible removed. Segmental defects of the mandible can result from the extirpation of benign and malignant tumors and from trauma.

Segmental defects that are traumatic in nature generally result from penetrating trauma. High-velocity gunshot or shotguns wounds or injuries occurring in a combat environment typically are associated with contamination and a large zone of injury. Immediate reconstruction with vascularized or nonvascularized bone grafts in this setting is not likely to be successful; therefore, wound stabilization with serial debridement is necessary to optimize the chances for a successful outcome. In this setting of a surgically created mandibular defect (after tumor removal), immediate reconstruction is ideal. This will eliminate the problems with soft tissue contracture that inevitably occur in the setting of delayed reconstruction.

They can be broadly classified into central, lateral, or hemimandibular. Central defects involve the anterior arch of the mandible, lateral defects involve the mandibular body and ramus to varying degrees, and hemimandibular defects involve the body, ramus, and condyle. Removing the central segment of the mandible without reconstruction will result in loss of lip support, chin projection, and potentially oral competence (the so-called Andy Gump deformity). Lateral mandible resection does not result in a defect of the same severity, there will be a loss of lower lateral facial projection and potential malocclusion due to the unopposed action of the contralateral muscles of mastication. In general, segmental defects of the mandible should be reconstructed if the patient's medical condition permits.

PATIENT EVALUATION

Preoperative evaluation of the patient undergoing mandible reconstruction is based on a multidisciplinary team approach. This includes head and neck surgeons, reconstructive surgeons, pathologists, medical and radiation oncologists, maxillofacial prosthodontists, speech and occupational therapists, internists, psychologists, and social workers. A careful preoperative medical evaluation is necessary because of the frequent associated comorbidities seen in this patient population. Close communication with the extirpative surgeon will help to anticipate the extent of resection and allow for proper flap selection. Potential donor and recipient sites need to be assessed for suitability. The fibula donor site is evaluated for the skin quality and the presence of arterial or venous insufficiency. In the absence of normal pedal pulses on clinical examination, a conventional or magnetic resonance arteriogram or other suitable study should be obtained to determine the patency of the vascular system. The radial forearm donor site is evaluated with an Allen test to determine the patency of the palmar arches. Preoperative dental evaluation is done to establish premorbid occlusion, manage diseased dentition, and begin the planning of dental rehabilitation[1]

PATIENT PREPARATION

In addition to standard preoperative radiography used by the surgical oncologist, a lateral cephalogram and 1:1 CT scan of the mandible are obtained. These studies are used to create templates used intraoperatively. Direct measurements from the surgical specimen determine mandibular segment length while the templates will determine the angles of the osteotomies necessary for accurate graft shaping (Figure 38-1).

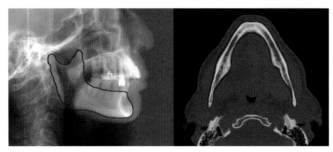

A

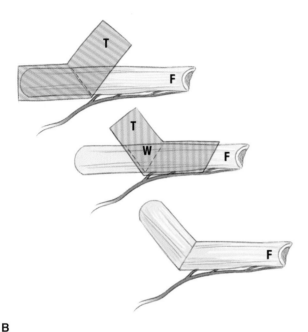

B

● **FIGURE 38-1.** (A) The preoperative lateral cephalogram and 1:1 CT scan of the mandible are used to create templates which will aid in graft shaping. (B) Diagram demonstrating how the template (T) is used to design a wedge (W) osteotomy in the fibula free flap (F). The result is an osteotomy which will allow the fibula to have the same basic shape as the patient's native mandible.

● HISTORICAL PERSPECTIVE

Mandible reconstruction techniques were developed in the early twentieth century. Over the past century significant developments have occurred. Initial attempts at mandible reconstruction utilized nonvascularized bone grafts. Cortical bone from the rib and tibia were initially used with limited success. Later, cancellous bone from the iliac crest proved more useful as this graft material is more cellular and more easily revascularized. External fixation of bone grafts was described during World War I; and internal wire fixation of the grafts and the use of antibiotics were major developments during World War II. With the passage of time, more aggressive surgical resections and the use of postoperative radiation therapy led to problems with bone graft absorption and infection.

Following the initial use of bone grafts, the era of prosthetic and allograft mandible reconstruction followed. This 40-year period utilized various prosthetic materials, including metallic trays, Silastic, Dacron, and Teflon. Although these materials offered good restoration of mandibular contour and continuity, long-term outcome was largely unsuccessful with a high incidence of exposure, fracture, and infection of the materials. In the 1980s, stainless steel and titanium mandibular reconstruction plates were developed and used with some success, particularly in lateral mandibular defects. Plate fracture and exposure remained a problem, and long-term success approximated 50% for anterior arch reconstruction and up to 85% for lateral reconstruction.

The use of regional, pedicled osseocutaneous flaps was the next major advancement. The ability to transfer living bone attached to its muscular pedicle into the defect was felt to be a major advancement. Various flap–bone combinations included pectoralis major with rib, sternocleidomastoid with clavicle, trapezius with scapula, and temporalis with parietal bone from the skull. These techniques suffered from the poor quality of the transferred bone, unreliable blood supply to the bone segments, and less than ideal bone–soft tissue orientation, resulting in suboptimal function and aesthetics.

The greatest development and current gold standard for mandible reconstruction involves the use of microvascular free tissue transfer. Microvascular technique has allowed for the transfer of vascularized bone grafts with or without associated soft tissue to the mandibular defect. These techniques allow for the selection of the ideal bone and soft tissue replacement depending on the needs of the defect. The initial development of the vascularized iliac crest graft, and later vascularized fibula, radial forearm, and scapula grafts have improved both the functional and aesthetic outcome in mandible reconstruction. Refinements in these techniques over the past three decades have led these techniques to be the standard of care in most major centers.

With the exception of traumatic mandible defects, the best time to reconstruct the mandible is at the time of segmental resection. Delaying reconstruction will result in scarring and fibrosis in the remaining bone and soft tissue envelope. This may severely impact the functional outcome of the reconstruction particularly if reconstruction occurs after radiotherapy. Trismus of the remaining mandible is possible further complicating the reconstruction. Immediate reconstruction with well vascularized hard and soft tissue will augment primary wound healing, and optimize functional outcome.

Reconstructive Goals

Segmental resection of the mandible can lead to a bony defect (as in benign disease) or a composite defect consisting of bone, oral cavity mucosa, tongue and supporting structures, and even external skin. The use of osteocutaneous free flaps is a source of composite tissue for these complex reconstructions. Usually one well-planned flap can provide adequate composite tissue for the reconstruction. Vascularized bone will replace the missing mandibular segment; proper alignment of the bone will optimize occlusion and minimize trismus. Reconstruction of intraoral soft tissues needs to maximize mobility of the tongue and buccal mucosa in order to optimize speech and swallowing. An adequate buccal sulcus will allow for dental rehabilitation, and in the instance where a large amount of intraoral soft tissue and/or external skin replacement is required, a second flap either pedicled or free may be required. External skin replacement results in a color mismatch with the native facial skin and will detract from the aesthetic result.

TECHNIQUE

Non–Free Flap Mandible Reconstruction

The vast majority of segmental mandibular defects are reconstructed with free tissue transfer. The non–free flap options, which are occasionally employed, include nonvascularized bone grafts, prosthetic plates and soft tissue flaps, and regional osteomusculocutaneous flaps.

Nonvascularized Bone Grafts. A requirement for considering nonvascularized bone grafts for mandible reconstruction is the presence of adequate blood supply in the surrounding soft tissues. Therefore, pathologic conditions, including prior irradiation, extensive scar tissue from prior surgery, trauma or infection, or inadequate soft tissues will not likely support healing of a nonvascularized bone graft. The main indication for nonvascularized grafts include, small bone-only defects of the ramus and body resulting from the treatment of benign tumors or mandibular fracture nonunion.

Corticocancellous iliac crest or rib grafts are typically used and these are rigidly fixed with mandibular reconstruction plates. The use of particulate cancellous grafts packed into alloplastic or allograft trays with or without the use of concomitant hyperbaric oxygen has also been described.[2] Although nonvascularized techniques have been successful, in an era when vascularized grafts are readily available and reliable, the role of nonvascularized reconstruction is limited.

Prosthetic Plates and Soft Tissue Flaps. Typically, titanium reconstruction plates (>2 mm) are used. They are shaped against the native mandible whenever possible. Placing drill holes through the plate into the native mandible prior to resection will allow for accurate fixation and retention of the position of the remaining mandible. The plate should be placed along the inferior border of the mandible to maintain facial height, avoid tooth roots, and keep it away from the oral mucosa.

If there is not adequate soft tissue to cover the reconstruction plate, the use of a regional or distant soft tissue flap is indicated. Regional soft tissue flaps include the pectoralis major, latissimus dorsi, trapezius, sternocleidomastoid, or platysma. In general, these flaps are hampered by their excess or bulk, limited arc of rotation, donor site morbidity, and lack of reliability of the skin island. Perhaps the best soft tissue flap for covering a reconstruction plate in the lateral or posterior position is the radial forearm free flap. Boyd et al. have reported a 96% success rate.[3] The advantages of this technique include excellent aesthetic and functional outcomes in debilitated elderly patients and poor prognosis patients with lateral and posterior low volume defects. The major downside is the tendency toward plate exposure, fracture, and loosening.

Regional Osteomusculocutaneous Flaps. Several regional osteomusculocutaneous flaps have been described for mandible reconstruction, including flaps based on the pectoralis major, sternocleidomastoid, and trapezius. Realistically, the best flaps are the pectoralis major with an associated portion of the fifth or sixth rib used for anterior mandible reconstruction, or the trapezius with a portion of the scapula spine used for short lateral mandibular defects. The limited amount of bone with its inherent poor blood supply due to it being attached to the distal portion of the flap, limited insetting flexibility, and excessive soft tissue bulk make these flaps a poor second choice when compared with free tissue transfer.

Free Flap Mandible Reconstruction

The advantages of free flap mandible reconstruction compared with other methods are numerous. Vascularized bone allows for the replacement of living bone with living bone. Bone healing resulting in a stable union between the flap and the native mandible can be expected within 2 to 3 months for the majority of patients, regardless of preoperative or postoperative radiation therapy. Various free flap donor sites allow for flap selection based on the requirements of the defect. As a result, a single flap is adequate in the majority of situations. Depending on the flap used, vascularized bone will provided adequate stock for the placement of osteointegrated dental implants.

There are four donor sites used most commonly for free flap mandible reconstruction: fibula, iliac crest, radial forearm, and scapula (Figure 38-2). Each donor site differs with respect to quality and quantity of the bone and skin island, length of the vascular pedicle, and the ability to support osteointegrated dental implants. Additionally, the location of the donor site may or may not facilitate a two-team approach. The anatomic requirements of the defect coupled with donor site factors determine flap selection (Table 38-1).

Fibula Flap. The fibula is the flap of choice for most segmental mandible defects due to its versatility. The flap is based upon the peroneal artery and associated veins (Figure 38-3). The flexor hallucis longus muscle can be harvested with the flap to provide extra bulk. The skin island is supplied by perforating vessels traveling

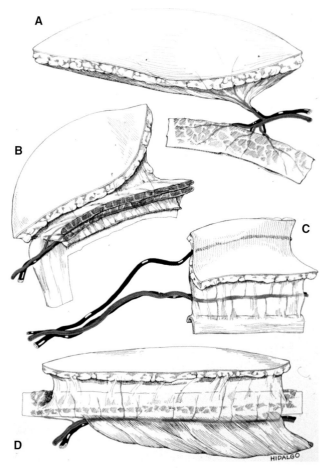

● **FIGURE 38-2.** Diagrammatic representation of the four basic free flaps used in mandible reconstruction; (A) scapula, (B) iliac crest, (C) radius, and (D) fibula.

within the posterior crural septum. The skin island can be positioned either in the oral cavity or externally. The fibula has two distinct qualities that allow it to be used for lateral, anterior, or hemimandibular defects. First, it has the greatest amount of bone available of any osseous free flap. Depending on the length of the donor leg, the flap can provide more than 20 cm of useable bone. Secondly, the fibula has both an intraosseus and segmental blood supply. Therefore, multiple osteotomies can be accomplished to facilitate shaping without fear

of devascularizing the bone.[4] Another advantage of the fibula flap is the quality of the bone is general adequate to allow for the placement of osteointegrated dental implants.

The position on the leg is remote from the recipient site; therefore, a two-team approach with simultaneous flap harvest and tumor ablation can be accomplished. Depending on surgeon preference, the fibula osteotomies and graft shaping can be accomplished in situ while the flap is being perfused, or after the flap has been detached. Donor site morbidity is minimized by preserving 5 to 7 cm of distal fibula at the ankle and 4 to 6 cm of proximal fibula at the knee (Figure 38-4).

The main disadvantage of the fibula is the skin island. With careful preservation of the posterior crural septum and the perforating vessels to the skin island, it is reliable in more than 90% of patients. Incorporation of the flexor hallucis longus with the flap may enhance the reliability of the skin island as well as providing extra bulk for the reconstruction. The anatomy of the posterior crural septum limits the amount of flexibility for positioning of the skin island relative to the bone. Therefore, careful design of the skin island is necessary not only to ensure it has adequate blood supply, but also that it can be positioned properly to meet the needs of the defect.

Iliac Crest. The shape of the iliac crest makes it useful for reconstruction of hemimandibular defects. The thickness makes it acceptable for osteointegrated dental implants. The blood supply to the iliac crest free flap is via the deep circumflex iliac artery and vein. The vascular pedicle is short, thus limiting placement options without vein grafting, and the bone lacks a segmental blood supply, thus limiting the opportunity for graft shaping with osteotomies. The skin island is relatively thick and immobile limiting its utility for intraoral reconstruction. Donor site morbidity is significant with the potential for numbness in the hip region, bulging, and hernia formation. Modifications of this flap include using only the inner table of the iliac crest. This reduces donor site morbidity, but also reduces the quality of the bone available for osteointegration.[5] The versatility of the fibula flap has led the diminished use of the iliac crest in most situations (Figure 38-5).

TABLE 38-1. Comparison of Donor Sites[a]

	Bone	Skin	Pedicle	Location[b]	Osteointegration
Fibula	+++	++	++	+++	+++
Iliac Crest	+++	+	+	++	+++
Radius	+	+++	+++	++	−
Scapula	++	++	++	−	+

[a]Comparison of donor sites with respect to quality of bone, skin, and pedicle; location of donor site allowing for a two-team approach; and ability to receive dental implants. Donor site characteristics are rated as excellent (+++), good (++), poor (+), and negative (−).
[b]Location refers to the ability for simultaneous tumor ablation and flap harvest.

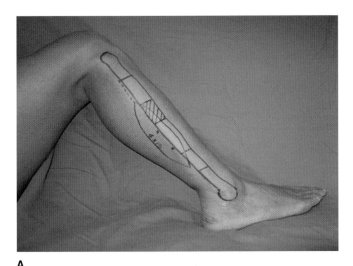

A

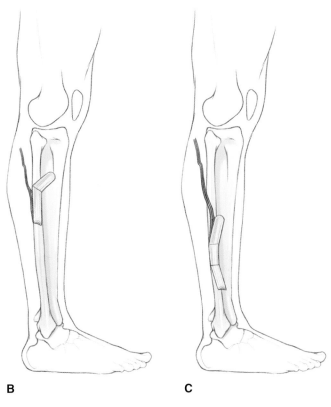

B   C

● **FIGURE 38-3.** (A) Planning the fibula free flap. Care is taken to avoid injuring the superficial peroneal nerve which crosses in the region of the neck of the fibula. The skin island is centered over the posterior border of the fibula so the perforating vessels nourishing the skin island can be captured. (B, C) The bone used for the fibula flap can be harvested either proximally or distally on the leg. This allows for lengthening the vascular pedicle based on the distance from the flap to the recipient vessels which will be used for the microvascular anastomoses. (D) Miniplate rigid fixation of the bone segments after osteotomy.

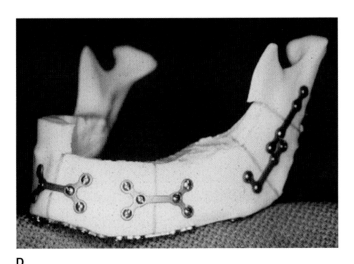

D

Radial Forearm. The radial forearm osteocutaneous flap is based on the radial artery associated venae comitantes and cephalic vein. Harvest of the lateral antebrachial cutaneous nerve allows for this flap to be reinnervated. This

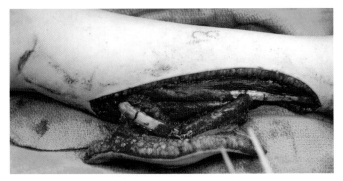

● **FIGURE 38-4.** Shaping the fibula free flap while it is still being perfused in the leg.

flap has the best donor site vessels and skin island quality of all of the free flaps used for mandible reconstruction. The vascular pedicle has excellent length and vessel caliber, the skin island can be large, thin, and pliable (ideal for intraoral resurfacing). The major drawback of the forearm is the poor quality of available bone. Up to approximately 10 cm of unicortical radius can be harvested with the soft tissue component of the flap. Osteotomies cannot be reliably performed in the unicortical segment of radius due to the risk of devascularizing the bone. The amount of bone available is typically not sufficient for the placement of dental implants (Figure 38-6).[6]

The major drawback of the radial forearm donor site is the risk of radius fracture after removing a segment of the radius. Techniques to reduce this risk include adjustments in the size and shape of the radial osteotomies, immediate bone grafting, and the use of rigid fixation. The forearm flap is best suited to lateral or ramus defects where bone requirements are secondary to soft tissue requirements.[6]

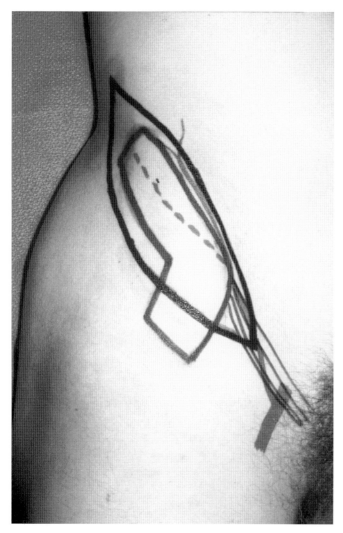

● **FIGURE 38-5.** Design of the iliac crest flap.

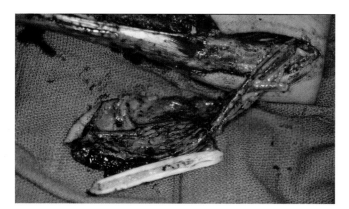

● **FIGURE 38-6.** Radial forearm flap. Note the poor quality bone, but excellent soft tissue and vascular pedicle.

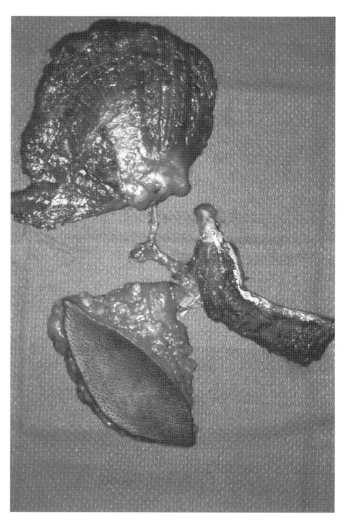

● **FIGURE 38-7.** The scapular vascular axis allows for harvest of bone, muscle, and skin all from the same pedicle.

Scapula. The scapula flap is based on the circumflex scapular vessels. Vessel length and caliber are good and can be extended by proximal dissection. The circumflex scapular vascular axis is versatile because a single blood supply can supply not only bone form the scapula, but also a large quantity of soft tissue. Scapular bone, serratus anterior muscle, latissimus dorsi muscle with or without a skin island, and either a transverse (scapular) or axial (parascapular) skin paddle can all be harvested off the same vessels. This allows for the correction of large and complex defects (particularly those requiring massive soft tissue corrections) with a single flap (Figure 38-7).

The major disadvantages of the scapular flap are the limited amount and poor quality of available bone. The bone does not tolerate osteotomies well and typically is insufficient for the placement of dental implants. Also the location of the donor site precludes a two-team approach toward flap harvest and tumor ablation. The major indication for the scapula flap is a posterior defect with a minimal bone requirement (not requiring an osteotomy) and massive soft tissue requirement (both intraoral and external skin).[7]

Condyle Reconstruction

Due to the unreliability of prosthetic condyles, condyle reconstruction is generally accomplished in one of two ways. Either the native condyle is autotransplanted into the glenoid fossa, or the end of the vascularized bone flap is fashioned into a condyle. Tumors involving the mandibular ramus or angle may necessitate condyle removal with the surgical specimen. If the condyle is not involved with the disease process as judged by the clinical impression of the oncologic surgeon and frozen section pathologic evaluation of the marrow space, then the condyle and condylar neck can be resected from the specimen and transplanted back to the end of the reconstructed mandible using rigid fixation. Surgical oncologists find disarticulation of the condyle and removal with the specimen less likely to injure the facial nerve in resection of tumors high on the ascending ramus of the mandible. The possible exception to this is the pediatric patient where the mandibular condyle is a growth center of the mandible that does not close until late in the teenage years (Figure 38-8).

If transplantation of the condyle is considered to be unwise from an oncologic perspective, the proximal end of the reconstructed mandible can be rounded to mimic the condyle. It can then be covered with fascia, left alone, and anchored into the glenoid fossa. Leaving a small gap (~1 cm) between the ends of the reconstructed mandible and the roof of the glenoid fossa will reduce the risk of ankylosis. Patients generally function well with only one intact temporomandibular joint. There is a slightly higher risk of trismus and malocclusion in this setting compared with condyle preservation or transplantation. As mentioned, prosthetic condyles are typically avoided due to the risk of infection, extrusion, or erosion into the temporal fossa.[8]

Flap Selection

Each of the flaps described have characteristics that make them useful for mandible reconstruction. Depending on the location and type of defect, one flap may be more or less useful than another. In general, the characteristics of the fibula make it the first choice for the majority of defects. The selection of the appropriate donor site is based on the bone and soft tissue requirement of the defect. Short lateral segment, long segment, or anterior bone defects, with or without a soft tissue requirement, are best treated with a fibula free flap (Figure 38-9). In the setting of a massive soft tissue requirement, the fibula free flap in conjunction with a soft tissue flap such as the radial forearm flap may be the best choice. Short segment defects involving the ramus with or without the condyle, associated with large soft tissue and external skin defects, benefit from reconstruction

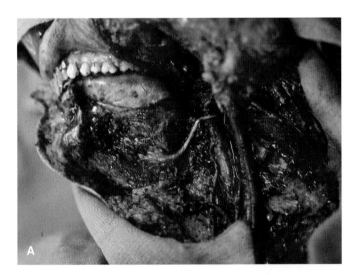
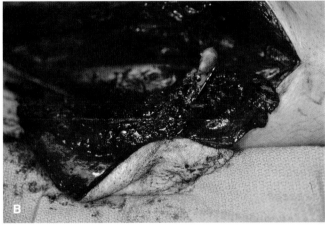
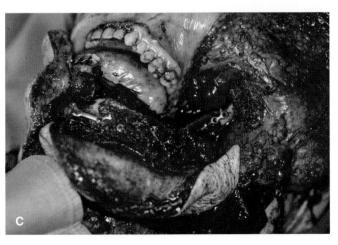

● **FIGURE 38-8.** (A) Hemimandibular defect after segmental resection. (B) Hemimandible reconstruction with fibula free flap. Note skin island and condyle autotransplantation onto the flap. The flap is still connected to the donor site in the leg. (C) The fibula free flap is rigidly fixed to the native mandible and the condyle transplant is seated into the glenoid fossa. Microvascular anastomoses are accomplished prior to inset of the flap skin island.

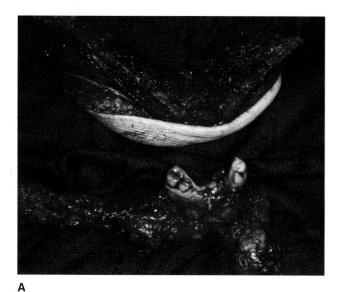 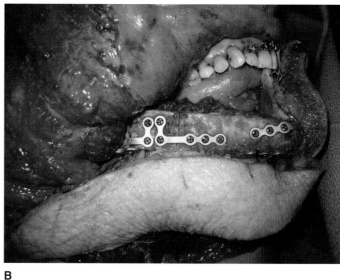

A **B**

● **FIGURE 38-9.** (A) Anterior arch resection and fibula free flap after osteotomies and rigid fixation. Note preservation of mandible shape. (B) Lateral mandible reconstruction with fibula free flap. Individual segments are rigidly fixed to each other and the native mandible.

with a scapular flap. Short segment ramus defects with or without the condyle with a large intraoral lining requirement are best treated with the radial forearm osteocutaneous flap. The ilium has no advantages that make it useful for anterior defects. It is also a second choice for lateral defects due to the poor quality skin and donor site morbidity. Its best use is for lateral or hemimandibular defects when the fibula is not available (Figure 38-10).[7]

Dental Rehabilitation

Mandible reconstruction with vascularized bone is the best method of achieving a stable reconstruction that can tolerate the load created by mastication. The two main

methods of dental rehabilitation include simple dental prosthesis and osteointegrated dental implants. After segmental mandibulectomy, the vascularized free flap can restore incisal opening and occlusion. Soft tissue from the flap can replace the intraoral soft tissues thus creating a stable base for the prosthesis. A simple dental prosthesis is useful to provide lip support and replace dentition. Dental prostheses are typically anchored to remaining dentition. They provide aesthetic correction, but in general are not stable enough to support the load generated by mastication. The best functional and aesthetic results are seen with the use of osteointegrated dental implants. The fibula and iliac crest provide the best bone stock for the use of dental implants (Figure 38-11).[9] Although the placement

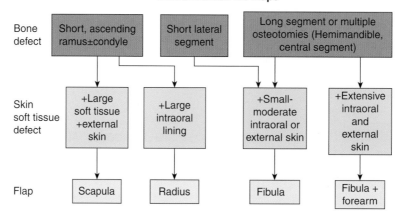

● **FIGURE 38-10.** Algorithm for flap selection based on the requirements of the defect.

COMPLICATIONS

General complications following mandible reconstruction include wound healing problems, leakage of saliva, and hardware exposure, and partial or complete flap necrosis if used in the reconstruction. Use of a prosthetic plate and a soft tissue flap either regional or free has been shown to have a higher overall failure rate of 20%. When used to replace the central segment of the mandible, the failure rate approaches 40%, as compared with approximately 5% for a lateral defect.[3] However, given the overall success with free tissue transfer, prosthetic plate reconstruction of the mandible should be limited to lateral or ramus defects in patients who are not candidates for a vascularized bone flap.

A significantly higher rate of complications has been reported in patients receiving postoperative radiation.[10] These include orocutaneous fistula, osteoradionecrosis, hardware exposure, and/or cervical contracture. The use of a vascularized flap in the form of free tissue transfer has been shown to reduce the rate and/or severity of some of these complications following reconstruction of the mandible.[11,12]

OUTCOMES

The outcome of mandible reconstruction is evaluated by bone retention, speech and swallowing, and aesthetic appearance. Bone retention has been evaluated in mandible reconstruction. Preservation of bone height over time is an indicator of bone mass retention. It has been shown that fibula free flaps maintain bone height in more than 90% of patients with follow up ranging from 2.5 to 10 years.[13] This seems to be independent of irradiation, dental implantation, and the location of the reconstruction. In a series of more than 150 patients during a 10-year period, speech, swallowing, and aesthetics were evaluated.[7] Speech was found to be normal (36%), near normal (27%), intelligible (28%), and unintelligible (9%). The best speech results were seen in lateral and hemimandibular reconstructions and the worse in anterior reconstructions.

In general, the more intraoral soft tissue required, the worse the speech, particularly if the tongue is involved. The skin island from the fibula flap is much less mobile than normal intraoral soft tissues. The findings with diet were similar, 45% of patients returned to an unrestricted diet, 45% soft diet, and 5% each required a liquid diet or tube feeding. Like speech outcome, the best results were seen in the later and hemimandibular reconstructions and the worst with anterior reconstruction particularly if there is tongue involvement. Aesthetic assessment in this same group of patients revealed an excellent aesthetic result in 32% of patients, 27% good, 27% fair, and 14% poor results. The best results were lateral and hemimandibular reconstructions, and the worse anterior and those requiring an external skin island either from the native flap or a second flap. The color and texture mismatch from an external skin paddle greatly detracts from the overall aesthetic result (Figure 38-12).

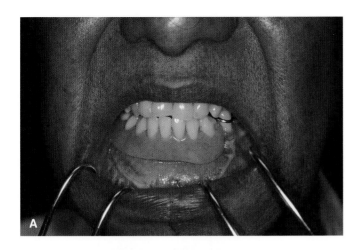
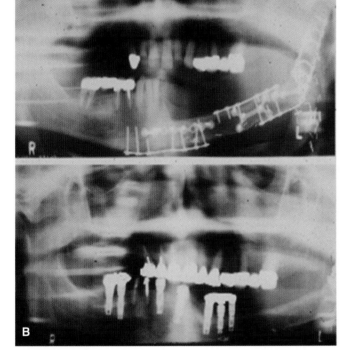

● **FIGURE 38-11.** (A) Anterior mandible reconstruction with removable dental prosthesis sitting on flap skin island and anchored to remaining dentition. (B) Hemimandibular reconstruction with fibula free flap (*above*) and 10 years later after removal of hardware and placement of osseointegrated dental implants.

of dental implants at the time of the mandible reconstruction has been described, most surgeons favor delaying placement until adequate bone healing. Implants placed at the time of reconstruction will lengthen the procedure, potentially compromise bone viability, and may result in implant malposition. Placing dental implants in patients who have been irradiated is controversial due to the high risk of failure of osteointegration and the potential to fracture the reconstructed mandible. In the nonirradiated patient, any hardware in the way of the implant will need to be removed prior to implantation.

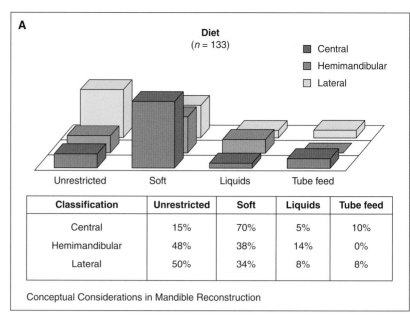

A

Diet
(*n* = 133)

Legend: ■ Central ■ Hemimandibular ☐ Lateral

Classification	Unrestricted	Soft	Liquids	Tube feed
Central	15%	70%	5%	10%
Hemimandibular	48%	38%	14%	0%
Lateral	50%	34%	8%	8%

Conceptual Considerations in Mandible Reconstruction

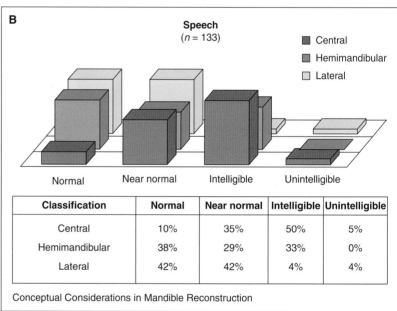

B

Speech
(*n* = 133)

Legend: ■ Central ■ Hemimandibular ☐ Lateral

Classification	Normal	Near normal	Intelligible	Unintelligible
Central	10%	35%	50%	5%
Hemimandibular	38%	29%	33%	0%
Lateral	42%	42%	4%	4%

Conceptual Considerations in Mandible Reconstruction

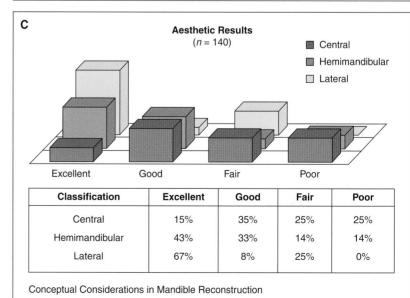

C

Aesthetic Results
(*n* = 140)

Legend: ■ Central ■ Hemimandibular ☐ Lateral

Classification	Excellent	Good	Fair	Poor
Central	15%	35%	25%	25%
Hemimandibular	43%	33%	14%	14%
Lateral	67%	8%	25%	0%

Conceptual Considerations in Mandible Reconstruction

● **FIGURE 38-12.** (A–C) Functional and aesthetic outcome in 150 consecutive mandible reconstructions with vascularized free flaps.

REFERENCES

1. Hidalgo DA. Aesthetic improvements in free-flap mandible reconstruction. *Plast Reconstr Surg.* 1991;97:707.

2. Marx RE, Ames JR. The use of hyperbaric oxygen therapy in bony reconstruction of the irradiated and tissue-deficient patient. *J Oral Surg.* 1982;40:412.

3. Boyd JB, Mulholland RS, Davidson J, et al. The free flap and plate in oromandibular reconstruction: long term review and indications. *Plast Reconstr Surg.* 1995;95:1018.

4. Hidalgo DA. Fibula free flap: a new method of mandible reconstruction. *Plast Reconstr Surg.* 1989;84:71.

5. Shenaq SM, Klebuc MJ. The iliac crest microsurgical free flap in mandibular reconstruction. *Clin Plast Surg.* 1994;21:37.

6. Zenn MR, Hidalgo DA, Cordeiro PG, et al. Current role of the radial forearm flap in mandibular reconstruction. *Plast Reconstr Surg.* 1997;99:1012.

7. Cordeiro PG, Disa JJ, Hidalgo DA, et al. Reconstruction of the mandible with osseous free flaps: a 10-year experience with 150 consecutive patients. *Plast Reconstr Surg.* 1999;104:1314.

8. Hidalgo DA. Condyle transplantation in free flap mandible reconstruction. *Plast Reconstr Surg.* 1994;93:770.

9. Frodel JL Jr, Funk GF, Caper DT, et al. Osseointigrated implants: a comparative study of bone thickness in four vascularized bone flaps. *Plast Reconstr Surg.* 1993;92:449.

10. Deutsch M, Kroll SS, Ainsle N, et al. Influence of radiation on late complications in patients with free fibular flaps for mandibular reconstruction. *Ann Plast Surg.* 1999;42:662.

11. Celik N, Wei FC, Chen HC, et al. Osteoradionecrosis of the mandible after oromandibular cancer surgery. *Plast Reconstr Surg.* 2002;109:1875.

12. Cannady SB, Dean N, Kroeker A, et al. Free flap reconstruction for osteoradionecrosis of the jaws–outcomes and predictive factors for success. *Head Neck.* 2011;33(3):424.

13. Disa JJ, Hidalgo DA, Cordeiro PG, et al. Evaluation of bone height in osseous free flap mandible reconstruction: an indirect measure of bone mass. *Plast Reconstr Surg.* 1999;103:1371.

chapter 39

Reconstruction of the Paralyzed Face

Christopher A. Derderian, MD / Oksana Jackson, MD

● PATIENT EVALUATION AND SELECTION

There are 17 paired and one unpaired facial muscles that serve two critical roles (Figure 39-1). From a functional standpoint they protect the eye, maintain patency of the nasal airway and preserve oral continence. Their integral role in the complex nuances of communication through articulation of speech and facial expression are underscored by the frustration patients with facial paralysis convey when seen in consultation. To best serve these patients, the surgeon must possess an advanced appreciation of the anatomy of the facial nerve (Figure 39-2) and the facial musculature and its function (Table 39-1). Likewise, knowledge of the common etiologies and presentations of facial paralysis (Table 39-2) and an arsenal of surgical techniques to effectively address the patient's concerns are needed.

Obtaining a detailed history of the paralysis is critical. The time and rapidity of onset, related injury or illness, treatments attempted and diagnostic tests performed prior to presentation should be determined. A standard facial nerve examination noting symmetry, muscle tone, twitching/spasms, and the absence or presence of synkinesis can usually pinpoint the location of nerve injury. Several facial nerve grading scales are commonly used today, including the House-Brackmann and Sunnybrook scales, and can be particularly useful in documenting recovery after acquired facial nerve injury and Bell palsy.

The etiology of facial nerve paralysis can be broadly divided into congenital and acquired forms. The vast majority is acquired; however, many of the patients seen by plastic surgeons have a congenital cause. Hemifacial microsomia is the most common cause of unilateral congenital facial paralysis, and Möbius syndrome is the most common bilateral cause. First described by the German neurologist Paul Julius Möbius in 1888, Möbius syndrome consists of congenital bilateral CN VI and VII paralysis, and is associated with trunk and limb anomalies in one-third of patients. Its etiology is unknown, and it is rare, occurring in 1:200,000 births. Bell palsy is the most common acquired cause, and it is believed to have some association with viral illness, specifically herpes simplex virus infection. The distinguishing characteristics of Bell palsy are: acute onset of paralysis (24–72 hours), ipsilateral periauricular numbness and pain, altered taste, decreased tear production, and hyperacusis.

The management of the patient with facial paralysis depends on whether or not the integrity of the nerve can be reestablished, if spontaneous recovery may occur, and the duration of the paralysis. For example, in the setting of Bell palsy, it may take up to a year for the patient to recover function and no surgical intervention would be recommended during this time, whereas with tumor ablation or trauma patients, no waiting period is entertained if the nerve has knowingly been injured or sacrificed and repair or grafting would be employed acutely. The limiting temporal factor to be considered is the time to loss of motor endplates and fibrosis of the facial musculature that generally occurs 1 to 2 years after denervation. However, the time for nerve growth through reestablished branches or grafts must be taken into account; therefore, the general treatment algorithm is divided into two groups: those with paralysis for less than 1 year (early) and more than 1 year (late) (Table 39-3).

In addition to these objective data, a critical component of the evaluation is a detailed discussion with the patient regarding the most troublesome aspects of their paralysis. Practical considerations are the patient's occupation, duration of the treatment, number of stages, and commitment

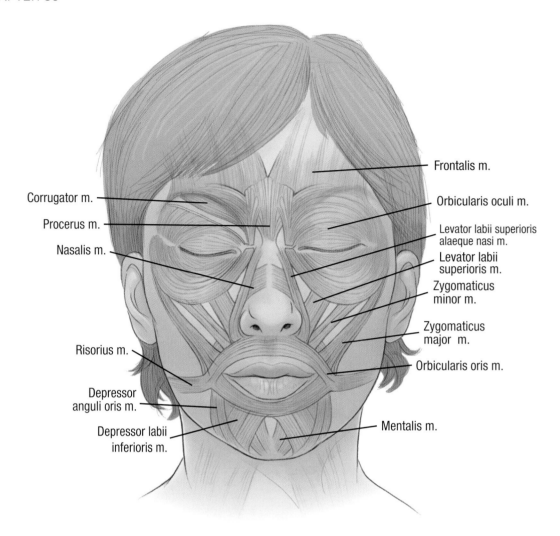

● **FIGURE 39-1.** Anatomy of the facial musculature. (*Adapted from McCarthy JG, Galiano RD, Boutros SG, eds. Current Therapy in Plastic Surgery. Philadelphia: Elsevier/Mosby; 2005:195.*)

to any rehabilitation or learning programs required to maximize results. In selecting the procedures the surgeon must also consider the patient's age, comorbidities, length of operation, soft tissue quality, and nerve and muscle donor site availability. Each region of the face should be treated separately and the most concerning areas addressed first.

● **PATIENT PREPARATION**

In the time leading up to definitive surgical treatment, conservative measures must be instituted to minimize permanent functional losses. These are largely related to eye protection. Maintenance of eye moisture using drops, ointments, lid taping, contact lenses, moisture chambers, eye patches, or temporary tarsorrhaphy sutures may be used to protect the eye and improve patient comfort.

The procedures described below typically require general anesthesia. When performing facial nerve mapping or functional muscle transfer, clear communication with the anesthesia team regarding the need to hold paralysis is critical. For cross-facial nerve graft harvest or gracilis harvest

for functional muscle transfer, a two-team approach is ideal with separate setups to minimize the operative time and the risk of infection in the donor sites. Microvascular anastomosis can be performed under loupe magnification or using an operating microscope. Microvascular instruments and suture and experienced surgical and nursing teams are required.

● **TREATMENTS**

Conservative Treatment

For many patients, despite a thorough workup, there is no known etiology of their facial palsy, and a period of observation is warranted to see if spontaneous resolution occurs. These patients may fall under the diagnosis of exclusion: idiopathic facial paralysis or Bell palsy. There is strong data indicating efficacy in the early use of steroids in the treatment of Bell palsy. The recovery is significantly more rapid and complete when the patient is treated with steroids within 72 hours of onset of symptoms. The use

Type I, 13% Type II, 20% Type III, 28%

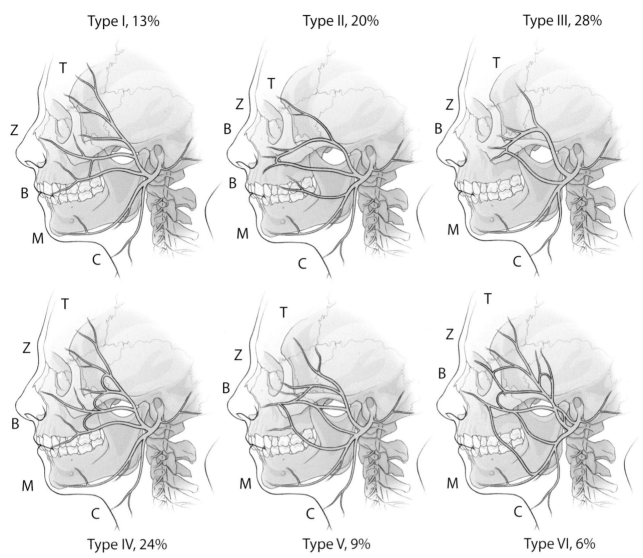

Type IV, 24% Type V, 9% Type VI, 6%

● **FIGURE 39-2.** The considerable variability seen in facial nerve branching patterns is depicted above. (*Adapted from Davis RA, Anson BJ, Budinger JM, Kurth LR. Surgical anatomy of the facial nerve and parotid gland based upon a study of 350 cervicofacial halves. Surg Gynecol Obstet. 1956;102(4):385–412.*)

of antivirals is not indicated unless a concurrent viral syndrome is noted at onset.[1] The remainder of the treatment is conservative: protection of the eye as listed above and physical therapy. Bell palsy is typically self-limiting with spontaneous resolution within 6 months; however, 5% to 10% of patients are left with some degree of severe paralysis that may require intervention.

Physical therapy may be beneficial in many patients recovering from acute facial nerve injuries or postreconstruction, and techniques such as electrostimulation, surface electromyograph biofeedback, and various exercise regimens may augment recovery. Neuromuscular retraining can improve the outcome after Bell palsy, by speeding and strengthening muscle recovery and overcoming synkinesis. Patients with partial paralysis can learn to strengthen alternative muscles on the weakened side and damped

forceful normal motions, thus improving facial balance and symmetry. Botox injections are a useful adjunctive treatment to physical therapy for patients who develop synkinesis during facial nerve recovery. They can also be used in unilateral forehead or lower lip palsies to achieve better symmetry. They need to be repeated approximately every 3 to 6 months; but if the result is favorable, neurectomy or myectomy can be performed surgically for a permanent result.

Surgical Treatment

The goals of reconstruction are divided into regions—brow, eyes, cheek, and lips. The ultimate goals are to restore static and dynamic symmetry and function. The patient's concerns should be addressed and her expectations should be

TABLE 39-1. Action of the Facial Musculature

Scalp
Frontalis: raises brows and wrinkles forehead as in surprise

Eye
Orbicularis oculi: sphincter of eyes, closes lids, compresses lacrimal sac
Corrugator: draws eyebrows downward and medially as in frowning or suffering

Nose
Procerus: draws medial angel of eyebrow downward
Anterior and posterior dilator naris: enlarge nares in hard breathing and anger
Depressor septi: constricts nares
Nasalis: draws alar wings toward septum and depresses cartilage

Mouth
Levator labii superioris: raises upper lip
Levator labii superioris alaeque nasi: raises lip and dilates nares
Zygomaticus minor: with the 2 levator labii muscles, forms nasolabial furrow; deepened when in sorrow
Levator anguli oris: with the 2 levator labii muscles and the zygomaticus minor, expresses contempt or disdain
Zygomaticus major: draws angle of mouth up and back as in laughing
Risorius: retracts angel of mouth
Depressor labii inferioris: draws lip down and back as in irony
Depressor anguli oris: depresses angle of mouth
Mentalis: elevates and protrudes lower lip
Orbicularis oris: a complex muscle with layers, some parts intrinsic to the lips, the others derived from the following facial muscles: buccinator, levator anguli oris, depressor anguli oris, and zygomaticus major and minor: closes lips, protrudes lips, and pressure lips to teeth
Buccinator: compresses cheek, hold food under teeth in mastication, important in blowing when the cheeks are distended with air

Adapted from Pansky B, House EL. Review of Gross Anatomy. New York: Macmillan; 1964:2246.

tempered so that well-defined, achievable outcomes will result in patient satisfaction.

The Brow

Paralysis in the distribution of the temporal branch of the facial nerve results in inability to elevate the eyebrows and wrinkle the forehead, and eventual brow ptosis. The options for treatment include direct, coronal, or endoscopic brow lift to the affected side, and frontal branch neurectomy, frontalis myectomy, and Botox injection to the unaffected side.

TABLE 39-2. Etiology of Facial Palsy and Respective Incidences

Etiology	Percent of Cases
Bell palsy	51%
Trauma	23%
Herpes zoster	7%
Tumor	5%
Birth (congenital and acquired)	4%
Infection	3.5%
Other	6%

Adapted from May M, Schaitkin BM. The Facial Nerve. 2nd ed. New York: Thieme; 2000:181.

Unilateral frontalis muscle paralysis can cause over a 10 mm difference in brow height. Larger discrepancies in brow height tend to occur in older patients who also tend to have deep creases within the brow. Excision of a segment of skin and frontalis above and parallel to the affected brow with placement of the scar in a preexisting skin crease is the most powerful method of brow elevation. Important aspects of this technique are to overcorrect slightly, repair the frontalis muscle and suspend the soft tissue from the underlying periosteum, and minimize the visible scar with appropriate positioning in a preexisting crease.

Coronal endoscopic brow lift has the advantage of an inconspicuous scar but provides limited lift, rarely greater than 5 mm change.[2] It is best used in younger patients with minor asymmetry and in whom the scar from a direct brow lift may be more conspicuous. The use of selective frontal branch neurectomy, frontalis or corrugator myectomy, or Botox injections to the unaffected side are adjuncts to supplement coronal or endoscopic lifts that have some application in select patients.[3]

The Eye

Eyelid closure is controlled by the orbicularis occuli muscle which has palpebral (involuntary blink), preseptal (voluntary blink), and orbital (forceful closure) portions. Paralysis of this muscle results in incomplete eyelid

TABLE 39-3. Treatment Algorithm for Treatment of Facial Palsy by Duration of Paralysis

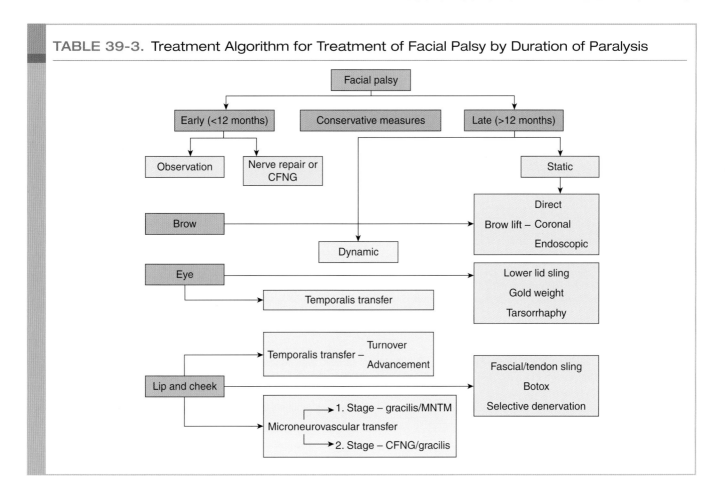

closure, referred to as lagophthalmos. This is caused by inability to close the upper eyelid due to the unopposed action of the levator palpebrae superioris and from paralytic ectropion of the lower eyelid, and it results in discomfort from dry eye, corneal irritation, exposure keratitis, and epiphora. Initial conservative treatments address symptom relief and protection of the cornea, but chronic impairment requires surgical intervention to restore anatomic relationships, protect the globe, and restore function. Lagophthalmos may be surgically treated by a variety of procedures including lid loading, palpebral springs, temporalis muscle transfer, fascial or tendon slings, or tarsorrhaphy, and multiple techniques used in combination are often required.

Eyelid loading consists of the placement of a gold or platinum weight between the orbicularis and tarsus in the upper lid to facilitate upper eyelid closure while preserving the normal levator palpebrae superioris function in eye opening (Figure 39-3). Gold weights significantly decrease ocular care needs long term, although replacement of the weight is occasionally required. Commonly, a lower eyelid procedure is required to augment eyelid loading and achieve complete closure. The mass of the gold weight is determined preoperatively by taping sample weights to the upper lid and testing opening and closure in the upright position. In the patient with an intact Bell's reflex, the goal is to use the lightest possible weight that will bring the upper eyelid within 2 to 4 mm of the lower eyelid. If too large a weight is selected, ptosis can occur and there is an increased likelihood of detachment or erosion of the weight.[4] Palpebral springs are an alternative technique to assist in upper eyelid closure, but are fraught with technical complications, including ptosis, spring breakage, malposition, and extrusion. While several groups have reported success with this technique, it should only be attempted by those with experience in its use.

Lower eyelid support procedures to treat paralytic ectropion and aid in eye closure include static sling suspension, temporalis transfer, tarsal strip, and tarsorrhaphy. During normal eyelid closure, the lower lid moves very little in the vertical dimension, and forced closure of the lower lid raises it only 2 to 3 mm. Thus, a static support procedure such as a fascial or tendon sling can provide a good aesthetic and functional result. The sling is tunneled through the lower lid near the lash margin and secured medially to the medial canthal ligament and laterally to the orbital rim near Whitnall tubercle (Figure 39-4). When selecting the lateral position for anchoring, the vector should adhere to the same principles for negative and positive vector selection adhered to in lateral canthopexy, and slight over correction is preferred.[5]

Temporalis muscle transfer uses autologous tissue to create a dynamic support system. A 1.5- to 2.0-cm strip of

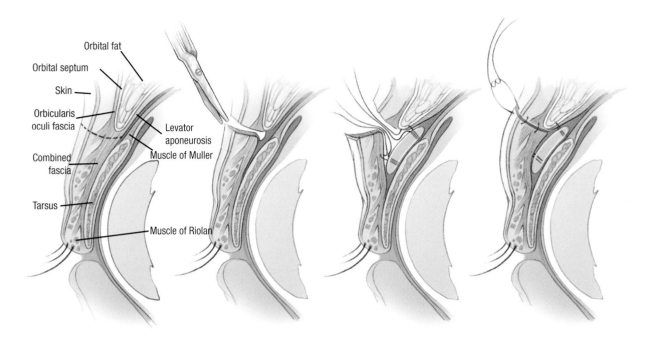

● FIGURE 39-3. Sequence for placement of gold weight loading of the upper lid to aid in eye closure. (*Adapted from May M, Schaitkin BM. The Facial Nerve. 2nd ed. New York: Thieme; 2000:709.*)

temporalis fascia and muscle is elevated and split into two limbs that are tunneled into the upper and lower lids. This procedure has the advantage of providing an architectural and functional mechanism with restoration of lid position, lid support, and spread of tear film. The disadvantages are a lateral temporal bulge, lid movement with mastication, and distortion of the palpebral aperture with contraction. Lateral tarsorrhaphy uses excision of skin, conjunctiva, and muscle from the lateral canthal region to create raw surfaces that are sutured to one another. The result is a tighter lid with a shorter palpebral aperture. This is typically held in reserve for patients with significant corneal exposure after more conservative procedures have failed.

The Cheek and Lips

Inability to smile and lack of oral competence are typically the most problematic and socially stigmatizing symptoms for the facial paralysis patient. There are many techniques to improve appearance and function of the midface, and they range in complexity from static slings to functional muscle transfer. Again, the patient's anatomy, tissue quality, comorbidities, and functional and aesthetic goals are weighted in considering reconstructive options. An understanding of the anatomy of the smile as described by Rubin is critical to achieving a symmetric, dynamic, and natural appearing smile reconstruction (Figure 39-5A).[6] In muscle transfer procedures, critical evaluation of each patient's unique smile features is essential in planning muscle insertion points and muscle orientation, in order to achieve a successful outcome with motion that best mirrors the unaffected side (Figure 39-5B).

Static Reconstructions

The traditional and least complex reconstructions are those utilizing a static sling with the goal of improving symmetry at rest and oral competence. Many tissues have been used for slings, including tensor fascia lata, tendon grafts, and more recently, acellular dermal allograft. Establishing solid anchor points on both the proximal and distal ends of the graft to prevent recurrence, appropriate vector selection, and over correction are the key technical elements. Typically, the sling is sutured at the oral commissure at the site of insertion of the zygomaticus major and minor, and levator labii superioris muscles. Bone-anchored sutures to the body of the zygoma or permanent sutures to the temporal fascia may be used to anchor the superior end of the sling. The critical maneuver is overcorrection to account for future lengthening of the graft and descent of the commissure over time.

Dynamic Procedures

Temporalis Transfer. Temporalis muscle transfer, as either a turnover flap or an advancement flap, is the most popular local flap option in use today (Figure 39-6). When used as a turnover flap, the central portion of the temporalis muscle is dissected away from the midtemporal fossa, rotated over the zygomatic arch, and tunneled to the commissure, typically using the deep temporal fascia as an extension of the muscle. The fascia is dissected away from the muscle and permanent sutures are placed at the fascial fusion point to bolster the strength of its attachment to the muscle. The fascia is then sutured around the oral commissure. As

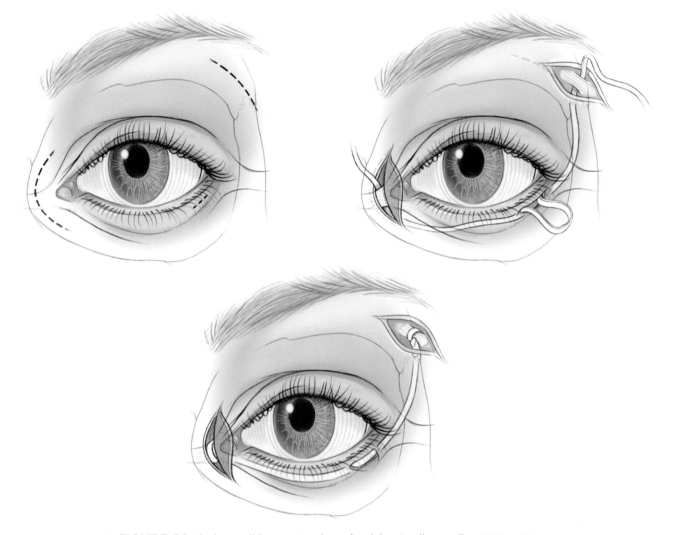

● FIGURE 39-4. Lower lid support using a fascial or tendinous sling. (*Adapted from Zuker R, Manktelow R, Hussain G. Facial paralysis. In: Mathes SJ, ed. Plastic Surgery. Vol 3. 2nd ed. Philadelphia: Saunders-Elsevier; 2006.*)

in static slings, the key aspects of this reconstruction are correct vector and insertion points and overcorrection of the commissure at rest because descent of the commissure is expected. The temporalis advancement flap consists of an intraoral approach to the coronoid process which is removed with insertion of the temporalis muscle. Once the muscle is completely mobilized, it is advanced toward the commissure, and a back cut along the posterior part of the origin of the temporalis is often needed to accommodate the advancement. The inferior end of the muscle is then sutured to the commissure directly or using a bridging piece of tendon or tensor fascia lata. A variation of this technique, the lengthening temporalis myoplasty described by Labbé, removes a section of the zygomatic arch to access the coronoid process and preserves the temporalis tendon for insertion into the oral commissure (Figure 39-6).[7] The advantages of temporalis muscle flaps are a single-stage procedure, shorter operative time, and a less technically demanding procedure. The disadvantages include the need for masticatory effort to animate the

reconstruction and involuntary facial movement with mastication, and in the case of the muscle turnover flap, a conspicuous soft tissue bulge at the arch that increases facial width, and temporal hollowing from loss of temporalis muscle bulk.

Microneurovascular Muscle Transfer. The current gold standard for dynamic reconstruction is microneurovascular muscle transfer in which a segment of muscle from elsewhere in the body brought to the face with its vascular and neural supply. The muscle is attached medially at the corner of the mouth and upper lip and laterally to the parotid fascia just below the malar prominence; thus its orientation and subsequent vector of motion can be more precisely controlled than a local muscle transfer. The advantages, therefore, are a greater ability to simulate the motion on the unaffected side of the face and create a symmetric smile.

This modality may be used for patients who have either unilateral or bilateral facial paralysis. When cases

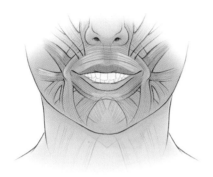
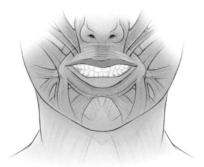
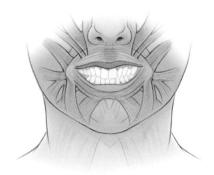

Mona Lisa:

67%
Corners of mouth pulled up and outward
Dominant zygomaticus major

Canine:

31%
Exposure of the canines
Dominant levator labii superioris

Full Denture:

2%
Strong action of all upper lip
elevators and lower lip depressors

A

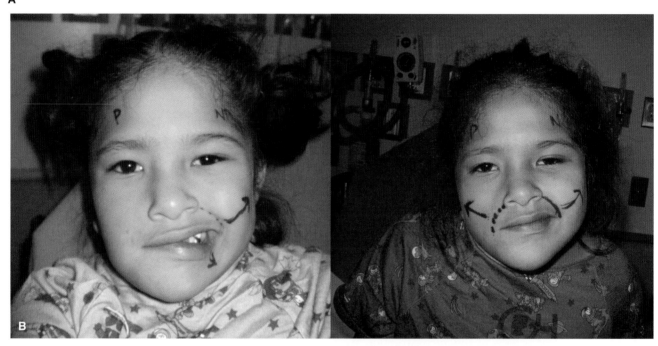

● **FIGURE 39-5.** (A) Anatomy of the smile (B) Preoperative markings to establish the vector of smile on the unparalyzed side prestage 1 cross-facial nerve graft (*left*), and to project the nasolabial fold and smile vector onto the paralyzed side prestage 2 free muscle transfer (*right*). (*Part A: Adapted from Rubin LR. The anatomy of a smile: its importance in the treatment of facial paralysis. Plast Reconstr Surg. 1974;53(4):384–387.*)

are unilateral, the cross-facial nerve graft technique of innervation of the free muscle transfer is preferred. The advantages of utilizing the cross-facial nerve graft are primarily that contraction of the transplanted muscle is spontaneous and emotionally driven, and although physical therapy can greatly improve the outcome by strengthening muscle activity, a lengthy period of relearning is not necessary to initiate motion or coordinate this motion with smiling on the unaffected side of the face. When the neural input is supplied by the cross-facial nerve graft,

the procedure is usually done is two stages, spaced 6 to 12 months apart.

When paralysis is bilateral, the motor nerve to the masseter muscle may be used bilaterally to innervate the muscle transfer in separate single-stage procedures to power muscle contraction and animation of each oral commissure. When compared with the cross-facial nerve graft, the use of the motor nerve to the masseter to power a gracilis free flap results in much greater excursion of the oral commissure and a more symmetric smile, but

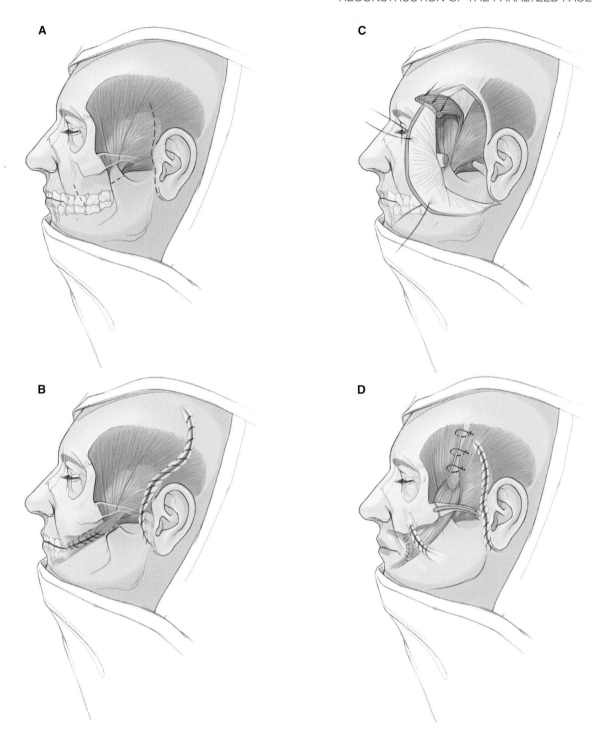

● **FIGURE 39-6.** Temporalis muscle transfer. (A) The incision design for access to the temporalis muscle. Access for the Labbé procedure is gained by reflecting the zygomatic arch inferiorly to expose the coronoid process of the mandible. (B) Advancement of the temporalis insertion to the oral commissure. (C) Muscle flap alternative to the Labbé advancement technique. (D) Position of the turned over and not advanced temporalis muscle, repositioned zygomatic arch, and closed access incisions at the end of the procedure. (*Adapted from Byrne PJ, Kim M, Boahene K, Millar J, Moe K. Temporalis tendon transfer as part of a comprehensive approach to facial reanimation. Arch Facial Plast Surg. 2007;9(4):234–241.*)

spontaneity is compromised. There are some instances where a patient with a unilateral paralysis may be better served by use of the motor nerve to the masseter and these include patients who frequently smile (eg, salesperson), those with heavy faces that require greater force to animate, advanced age, and those who prefer a single-stage procedure. Otherwise, the utility of a spontaneous smile achieved through a cross-facial nerve graft is thought to outweigh the benefit of greater excursion with motor nerve to the masseter.[7–8]

Two-Stage Free Muscle Transfer. In the first stage of a two-stage free muscle transfer, a midfacial branch of the facial nerve on the unaffected side of the face that creates the desired smiling motion upon stimulation is selected and anastomosed to a nerve graft harvested from elsewhere in the body. The patient is marked preoperatively, noting the vector of the normal smile and position of the nasolabial fold. The facial nerve is approached through a preauricular incision with a submandibular extension in a neck crease. Subcutaneous dissection is performed to the anterior border of the parotid gland, and then the midfacial branches of the facial nerve are dissected and mapped with the assistance of electrostimulation. A zygomaticobuccal branch is chosen that optimally elevates the oral commissure and upper lip along the pre-marked vector, creating a pleasing smile without any other facial muscle contraction. It is important to identify a second nerve branch to be preserved that produces a similar motion.

Typically the sural nerve in the lower extremity is chosen as the donor nerve due to its predictable course, available length, and ease of harvest. The nerve can be rapidly and easily harvested with a tendon stripper through two to three small transverse incisions. Alternatively, an open approach can be used, first identifying the nerve just above the lateral malleolus, and then tracing its course up the posterior leg and between the gastrocnemius muscles either via a single longitudinal incision or multiple stair step incisions up the leg. The nerve graft is tunneled from the midcheek across the upper lip and banked in the contralateral upper buccal sulcus in the supraperiosteal plane (Figure 39-7). The end is marked with a colored suture or staple to assist with identification during the second stage. The nerve can also be brought below the chin and banked in the contralateral preauricular region, although this requires a longer nerve graft and subsequently, a longer time for reinnervation. A meticulous epineural repair is then performed with the assistance of an operating microscope to the chosen facial nerve branch.

A Tinel sign is followed clinically in the office to monitor fascicular advancement through the graft, and the second stage is planned when the Tinel sign has reached the distal end of the nerve graft, usually 6 to 9 months after the first procedure. A critical part of planning the second stage is again assessing the characteristics of the smile on the unaffected side of the face, specifically the vector of

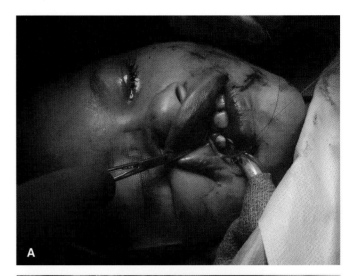

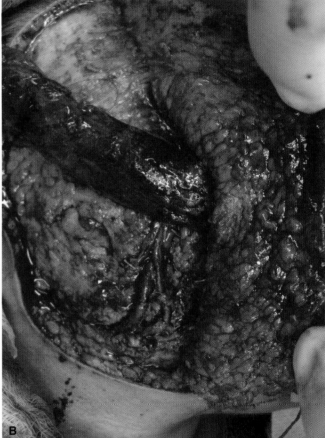

● **FIGURE 39-7.** (A) Position of cross-facial nerve graft in the gingivobuccal sulcus of the upper lip. (B) Inset position of the gracilis microneurovascular free muscle transfer.

motion, strength of motion, relative movement of the upper lip and oral commissure, and the position and depth of the nasolabial fold. Preoperatively, these features are marked on the unaffected side of the face and transposed to the affected side to guide muscle positioning (Figure 39-5).

The gracilis muscle is the preferred donor muscle for reanimation. It can be harvested in the supine position and is distant from the facial site such that two teams can work simultaneously. In addition, its pedicle is a good size match for the facial vessels, it has a reliable pattern of innervation, and its harvest causes no functional deficit. Many other donor muscles, however, have been used successfully for reanimation, including the pectoralis minor, latissimus, serratus anterior, rectus abdominus, and extensor carpi radialis brevis. The gracilis muscle is approached through a longitudinal incision on the inner thigh, and a segment of the muscle is harvested based on the location of the pedicle. The length of this segment is determined by measuring the distance from the oral commissure to the root of the helix. The muscle is also split longitudinally and only 50% to 75% harvested to diminish bulkiness in the cheek. The edge of the muscle to be sewn to the mouth is reinforced with mattress sutures as described by Zuker et al. to minimize tearing of the delicate muscle fibers, dehiscence, or malposition of the muscle at the insertion site.[5,8]

Exposure in the face is again achieved through a preauricular incision with a submandibular extension, and the cheek flap is elevated above the parotid fascia. The facial vessels are identified and isolated at the anterior border of the masseter muscle, and the dissection is continued to the oral commissure and into the upper lip. Three to four inset sutures are then placed in the lower lip, oral commissure, and upper lip sequentially to recreate a pleasing smiling motion that matches the vector and creases of the contralateral smile when traction is placed on these sutures. The inset sutures are brought through the muscle and tied and then the arterial and venous anastomoses are completed, followed by coaptation of the cross facial nerve graft to the gracilis motor nerve in the upper buccal sulcus. Lastly, the muscle inset is completed by sutures in the preauricular region to the parotid fascia; the muscle origin is spread out to avoid bulkiness in the lateral cheek and some tension, enough only to slightly elevate the commissure, is placed on the muscle (Figure 39-7).

Postoperative management includes close monitoring of flap perfusion in an ICU setting for 2 days and a soft diet for several weeks. Muscle activity is seen approximately 6 to 8 months postoperatively, although electrical activity can be detected earlier with a surface electromyograph device. Therapy is begun at this time and helps to strengthen and tailor the muscle activity over the following year. When successful, this procedure can produce a pleasing, spontaneous, and emotionally driven smile, and can have a profound impact on the psychological well-being of patients (Figure 39-8). The disadvantages include a lengthy time period and two procedures to complete the reconstruction, and there is often great variability in outcomes between patients.

The asymmetry of the lower lip seen in unilateral facial paralysis is primarily caused by the depressor labii inferioris on the unaffected side. This is typically not noticeable at rest, but can be quite striking with smile and speech. Even patients with successful reanimation procedures for smile can look quite asymmetric due to the unopposed depressor function. It is usually easier to ablate the function of the unaffected side than to restore the affected depressor function. Resection of the depressor labii inferioris on the normal side or selective denervation of this muscle are effective treatment methods. Use of local anesthetic in the depressor prior to ablation is an easy and useful tool to evaluate if a desirable smile will be produced from selective ablation of depressor function.[9] Botox can similarly provide a temporary cessation in depressor function to determine if the desired affect will be achieved by a permanent ablative procedure.

COMPLICATIONS

Complications after reconstruction for facial paralysis range from acute postoperative problems such as facial hematoma, infections, and arterial or venous thrombosis after free muscle transfer, to a variety of delayed complications relating to muscle or tendon malposition or malfunction that result in less than optimal aesthetic or functional results. Gold weights and palpebral springs of the upper eyelid are subject to exposure and may require replacement. Static slings of the eyelid or cheek may stretch and lengthen with time requiring secondary tightening procedures. Late complications of free muscle transfer are challenging to correct and include excess muscle bulk in the cheek, disruption of the muscle insertion from its perioral attachment, scarring of the muscle to the overlying skin causing irregular dimpling with motion, and the most concerning, inadequate motion after reconstruction. The first three complications can be improved by revisional procedures. The last complication of inadequate motion may be related to muscle viability or neural input and requires either a second muscle transfer, repeat cross-facial nerve graft, or transfer of the gracilis nerve from the cross-facial nerve graft to the motor nerve to masseter to achieve greater power for the reconstruction.

OUTCOMES ASSESSMENT

Successful outcomes and high patient satisfaction after facial paralysis reconstruction are dependent on a realistic reconstructive plan, careful preoperative planning, and good surgical technique. A multispecialty approach is often beneficial and coordinated care by plastic surgeons, ophthalmologists, oculoplastic surgeons, neurologists, physical therapists, and psychologists can improve patient outcomes in complex cases. In dynamic reconstructions, patient motivation and compliance with therapy regimens are critical in maximizing and optimizing motion. Reconstruction of the paralyzed face can successfully improve function, and also can have significant effects on the psychological, emotional, and social well-being of patients affected with this disorder.

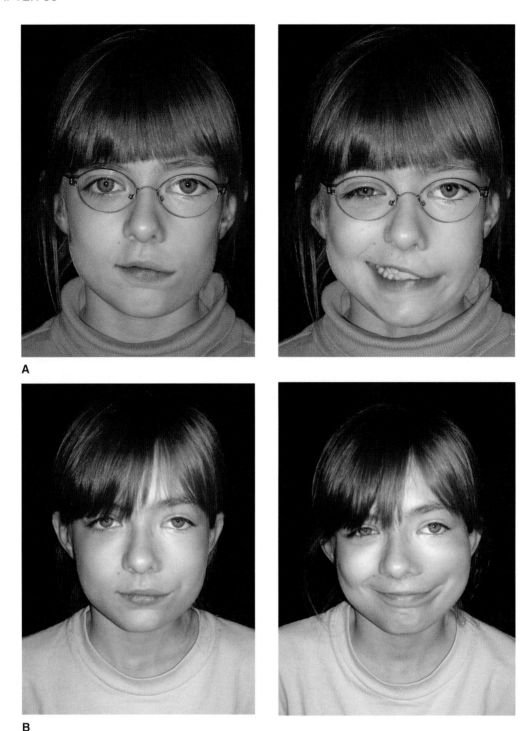

● FIGURE 39-8. Before (A) and after (B) photos of a representative patient with unilateral facial paralysis. This patient was treated with a two-staged cross-facial nerve graft and gracilis microneurovascular free muscle transfer. Note the symmetry in excursion of the oral commissure and vector of smile.

REFERENCES

1. Sullivan FM, Swan IR, Donnan PT, et al. Early treatment with prednisolone or acyclovir in Bell's palsy. *N Engl J Med.* 2007;357(16):1598–1607.

2. Takushima A, Harii K, Sugawara Y, Asato H. Anthropometric measurements of the endoscopic eyebrow lift in the treatment of facial paralysis. *Plast Reconstr Surg.* 2003;111(7):2157–2165.

3. Moody FP, Losken A, Bostwick J 3rd, Trinei FA, Eaves FF 3rd. Endoscopic frontal branch neurectomy, corrugator myectomy, and brow lift for forehead asymmetry after facial nerve palsy. *Plast Reconstr Surg.* 2001;108(1):218–223.

4. Rofagha S, Seiff SR. Long-term results for the use of gold eyelid load weights in the management of facial paralysis. *Plast Reconstr Surg.* 2010;125(1):142–149.

5. Zuker R, Manktelow R, Hussain G. Facial paralysis. In: Mathes SJ, ed. *Plastic Surgery.* Vol 3. 2nd ed. Philadelphia: Saunders-Elsevier; 2006:883–916.

6. Rubin LR. The anatomy of a smile: its importance in the treatment of facial paralysis. *Plast Reconstr Surg.* 1974;53(4):384–387.

7. Labbé D, Huault M. Lengthening temporalis myoplasty and lip reanimation. *Plast Reconstr Surg.* 2000;105(4): 1289–1297; discussion 1298.

8. Marcus J, Borschel G, Zuker R. Facial paralysis and facial reanimation. In: Bentz M, Bauer B, Zuker R, eds. *Principles and Practice of Pediatric Plastic Surgery.* Vol 2. St. Louis, MO: QMP, Inc; 2008:1001–1028.

9. Godwin Y, Tomat L, Manktelow R. The use of local anesthetic motor block to demonstrate the potential outcome of depressor labii inferioris resection in patients with facial paralysis. *Plast Reconstr Surg.* Sep 15 2005;116(4):957–961.

chapter 40

Alopecia

Edward H. Davidson, MA (Cantab), MBBS / Keith Jeffords, MD, DDS / Ernest K. Manders, MD

● INTRODUCTION

Hair, especially that of the scalp, is an important component of body image. Perception of age, well-being, and psyche are in part conveyed by the presence and style of the hair. Furthermore, the hair of the eyebrows and eyelashes provides a role in maintenance of ocular health that goes beyond solely appearance. As such, hair loss can represent a distressing cosmetic and functional problem. Alopecia, or hair loss, may be partial or complete, affecting any part or all of the nonglabrous skin, and has a multitude of causes.

The history of alopecia addressed as a medical problem dates to classical times. Grafting of hair has since evolved in technique and grown in popularity for correction of hair loss along with the emergence of tissue expansion and the use of local soft tissue flaps across the spectrum of alopecia etiologies. Male pattern baldness as well as the deformities of burns, trauma, and congenital hair absence may often be treated effectively with modern surgical techniques.

● PATIENT EVALUATION AND SELECTION

The role of the plastic or reconstructive surgeon embarking on hair restoration surgery must first be to evaluate the hair loss. It is crucially important for the surgeon to know why hair is being lost. If a medical treatment is indicated, then it will surely be more efficacious than any attempt at a surgical solution. Moreover, attempts at restoration surgery may very well fail if an underlying continuing medical condition is not, at least first, adequately treated. This tenet is particularly pertinent to scarring, or cicatricial, forms of alopecia in which there is a potentially permanent and irreversible destruction of hair follicles and their replacement with scar tissue. A classification of alopecia etiopathogenesis and recommended treatments is presented in Table 40-1.

As well as the cause, the extent of the hair loss is a fundamental consideration. Presently, all hair restoration surgery techniques rely on autotransplantation or transposition of the patients' preexisting hair. Tissue-engineered hair and cadaveric allografts are yet to become a surgical reality. Identification of adequate donor hair is therefore a prerequisite to restoration both by grafting and tissue expansion. In the case of male pattern baldness, for example, in which hair is most commonly first lost at the temporal sides of the hairline and at the vertex, correction requires sufficient area of donor hair. Fortunately for both patient and surgeon, an area of scalp may be doubled without any observable diminution of hair density. Since treatment of this patient group is complicated by the progressive nature of balding, it is important for the surgeon to counsel any patient that their relationship will be ongoing, possibly for the lifetime of the patient. Today the timing of surgical intervention should depend on the needs of the patient, and the techniques employed should be chosen with consideration of possible progression of hair loss in male patients. For example, hair restoration early can, for example, create a "donut" deformity as the native hair continues to be lost around an island of transplanted hair. Similarly, the "plugged" look is the result of thinning of native hair surrounding foci of grafted follicles. Hence, age and patient expectations along with the natural history of male pattern hair loss are also important factors in the patient evaluation and selection process.

If medical treatment is not indicated, or there is medical resolution of any ongoing pathologic process, and the extent of hair loss is amenable to improvement without unacceptable compromise of the existing healthy tissue, then the patient may be considered a worthy surgical candidate.

TABLE 40-1. Etiopathogenesis and Treatment

Diagnosis	Medical Treatment	Surgical Treatment
Scarring (cicatricial)		
Hereditary or developmental	—	Yes
Trauma (including traction)	—	Yes
Burns	—	Yes (upon resolution of neoplastic process)
Neoplastic		Yes (upon resolution of inflammatory process)
Inflammation of dermis (eg, syphilis, tuberculosis, herpes zoster, sarcoidosis, pyoderma, gangrenosum, pemphigoid cicatrical pemphigoid, and morphea)	Appropriate treatment of underlying neoplasia	Yes (if medical treatment fails)
Nonscarring		
Autoimmune alopecia areata (may be areata, in patches; totalis, affecting all of the scalp; or universalis, affecting the entire body)	Appropriate treatment of underlying inflammatory process	Yes
Androgenic (male pattern baldness)	Triamcenalone or hydrocortisone	Yes (if conservative therapy fails)
Stress-induced (emotional stress, starvation, crash diets, malaria, tuberculosis, typhoid etc, after surgery, hepatic, or renal failure)	Adjuvant minoxidil, and/or finasteride; consider addition	Not usually indicated
Iron and zinc deficiency	Remove stressor; hair addition	Yes (if conservative therapy fails)
Postpartum	Treat deficiency	Not usually indicated
Thyroid or pituitary disorder	Watchful waiting	Not usually indicated
Collagen vascular disease	Treat underlying cause	Only if resolution does not occur following cessation of treatment
Drug-induced (anticancer chemotherapy, antithyroid drugs, cholesterol-lowering agents, warfarin)	Steroids, disease modifying agents, immunosuppressant monoclonal antibodies Await spontaneous resolution at termination of therapy; wigs	

● HAIR REPLACEMENT THERAPY WITH ADDITIONS

All patients should be counseled about the use of hairpieces and additions. For many patients, these are a practical and satisfactory alternative to surgical therapy. That said, there are drawbacks to the use of this alternative. Expense is an important consideration. Hair replacement organizations have estimated in the recent past that a customer would be worth $40,000 or more over his lifetime use of their products. Hairpieces cost from several hundred dollars each to more than $2000 each. The user must purchase two at the same time, so that his or her appearance is not altered if one is damaged or being cleaned. Hairpieces are typically styled when in place on the wearer and then must be cared for appropriately. Depending on the use and the ambient temperature and humidity where worn, hairpieces are typically cleaned at least every 5 months for a fee. They last for 3 to 5 years and must then be replaced.

Attachment has been provided by several means. Rings through the scalp are not popular now. Most additions depend on adhesives or on their being woven into the native hair at the edge of the area of alopecia. Both systems of attachment require continuing care. Adhesive methods often employ a skin adhesive applied to the skin and a double-sided sticky tape applied to the underside of the hairpiece. Meticulous cleansing and preparation can consume 3 to 4 hours once a week. The wearer still lives with fear of dislodgement.

The weave attachment is an attractive product because it allows patients to participate in physical activities, such as waterskiing, without concern for dislodgement. However, the weave must be tightened as the hair grows, so every 6 weeks or so, a visit to the provider is required to maintain the proper adherence and appearance. There is typically an appreciable charge for this service.

It should be obvious from this discussion that surgical treatment can be cost-effective and relatively trouble free once accomplished. Even given the limitations and costs enumerated above, wearing a hairpiece is a good alternative for many patients.

Special mention should be made of the condition seen in some older women in whom there is a global thinning of the hair. There is a special prosthesis that is custom created for this problem and which is very effective. The hair addition prosthesis is a net with strands of hair attached. The hair is matched to the wearer. It is laid down over the patient's scalp and the native hair is combed up through the interstices in the net. Together with the hair attached to the net strands, a very nice augmentation is achieved. After fitting the hair net prosthesis, a stylist then cuts the hair appropriately. This can be worn for extended periods and cleaned with a regular shampoo in the shower.

● PATIENT PREPARATION

Preoperative workup might well include a biopsy of the skin at the site of which there is hair loss as well as appropriate laboratory blood tests to rule out medically treatable conditions as detailed in Table 40-1.

The role of topical agents, such as minoxidil, and antiandrogenic therapies, such as finasteride, remain controversial because of concerns for cost, effort in use, and limited effectiveness for many patients. They may be useful adjuncts, especially in the treatment of male pattern baldness where they may delay surgical intervention until the degree of progression and patient concerns dictate an intervention.

A preoperative assessment, including clinical history and physical examination, is vital to assess the patient's fitness for surgery. Adequate counseling is essential to ensure patient expectations are realistic and that consent is appropriately informed. Clinical examination for delineation of the affected areas to be treated and selection of donor sites is important for gaining informed consent as well as for preoperative planning. Demonstrating the operative plan and the anticipated result for the patient in front of a mirror is probably the best way to gain a realistic understanding of the results of surgery in the patient's mind. In terms of reconstructive goals in male pattern baldness hair restoration procedures, framing the face by reinvigoration of the anterior hairline should be prioritized over reconstruction of the vertex density.

Prior to surgery, as well as postoperatively, it is prudent to encourage the patient in lifestyle practices that promote hair health. Namely, the use of a good shampoo appropriate to their hair type; diet rich in proteins, iron, zinc and water; avoidance of psychological stress, anxiety, and trichotillomania; avoidance of vigorous combing, excessive shampooing, drying, bleaching, dying, perming or straightening; and avoiding the use of rubber bands, buns, and braids.

● TECHNIQUE

When surgical intervention is warranted, the options available to the reconstructive surgeon for hair rejuvenation are outlined below. Tissue expansion is the preferred technique for large areas requiring repopulation with hair while follicular unit grafts are better suited for more focused, smaller areas. The combination of these two techniques may be indicated; for example, the use

of tissue expansion of the scalp in male pattern baldness with adjuvant follicular unit grafts to shape the anterior hairline. The use of pedicled hair-bearing tissue flaps is now a less commonly employed strategy.

Hair Transplantation

Hair transplantation began with the demonstration by Orentreich that hair follicles show donor dominance when transferred to a different site in the scalp. Donor dominance means that the dermis and hair follicle within it display the hair growth characteristic of the donor area rather than the recipient area after transfer. This is to be expected in view of more modern knowledge that has mapped higher levels of distribution of the enzyme 5-alpha reductase to the areas of characteristic male pattern hair loss. Simply put, the transferred hair follicles are programmed differently than those of the area of normal androgenic baldness. For all hair transplantation, the patient should be told that only one session of grafting is unlikely to achieve the desired results, especially if treating area of total hair loss. Many hair transplant surgeons have routinely counseled patients that up to four sessions of transplantation would be necessary to get an attractive result. Typically, the procedures can be carried out using a combination of local nerve blocks and infiltration of local anesthesia to donor and recipient tissues. Inpatient admission is usually unnecessary and upon completion of the procedure grafts are dressed with an antibacterial ointment and a dressing. Patients may shower the next day. Manipulation of the scalp should be minimal at this juncture in recovery. Patients should be counseled that after hair transplantation, hair growth will not be obvious to them until 3 to 6 months after transplantation and that the hair may not be long enough for styling in the way they want until 6 to 9 months after transplantation.

For male pattern baldness, the patient is prepared before operation with a marking of the intended hairline, with the patient's input and understanding. It should be stressed to the patient that in the case of a mature man, the hairline is expected to be fairly high on the forehead. Pre-pubertal hairlines are unnatural and are to be avoided. When designing the anterior hairline, grafts should be placed at least 8 to 9 cm above the glabella, no farther forward than the preexisting hairline and rather than being straight, a feathered pattern creating an irregular 1 cm hairline transition zone should be used with preservation of some temporal recession.

Follicular Unit Micrografts and Minigrafts (Strip Method). Hair transplantation potentially allows for hair to be transplanted from and placed in any area of the nonglabrous skin without any visible scar (Figures 40-1A, B and 40-2A, B). Whilst usually necessitating a scar, albeit one that is hidden if the hair of the donor region is sufficiently long and dense (ie, if worn >1 cm long in the scalp),

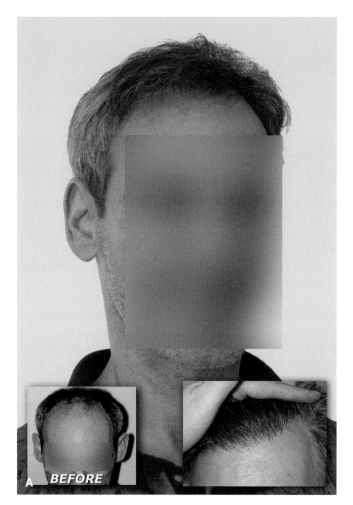

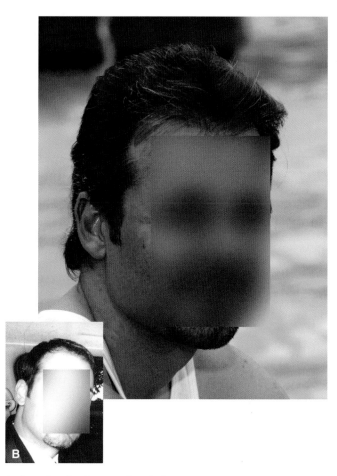

● **FIGURE 40-1.** (A) Photographs before and after of patient requesting hair restoration surgery at the anterior hairline. (B) After patient seeking restoration of the anterior hairline.

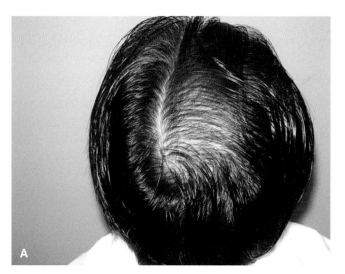

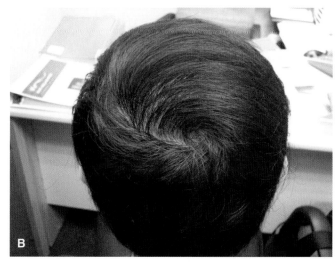

● **FIGURE 40-2.** (A) A patient seeking hair restoration for the vertex scalp. (B) After micrograft transfer to the vertex scalp.

micrografts and minigrafts have become the standard for hair transplantation. This technique, though time consuming and labor intensive, allows for much more efficient harvesting of donor hair with minimal transaction compared with traditional "punch" excision techniques. Typically, a donor ellipse of hair is harvested, hence the resultant scar from which follicles are dissected. An ellipse or longer strip is harvested from the region between the occipital protuberance and 1 cm above the top of the ears (the area above the ear and below the occipital protuberance may thin over time). An alternative to the ellipse method uses a multiblade scalpel that will cut several strips about 2 mm thick from the occipital scalp with one pass of the knife. The multiblade knife must be oriented so that the continuity of the hair shafts and their respective follicles is maintained in each strip of tissue.

Following excision from the posterior scalp micrografts (one or two hairs) or minigrafts (three or four hairs) are then dissected in 1.5- to 3-mm slices from the donor ellipse or strips. Grafts are held by the perifollicular fatty tissue under the hair bulbs or surrounding tissue and must remain moistened with saline as well as ideally being kept at 4°C until insertion. Slits are created 1.5 mm apart using an 18- to 20-gauge needle or thin blade (eg, 22.5 Sharpoint blade or Ziering SP88 and the Ziering SP89) down to the subcutaneous fat (4–6 mm)

at an angle of 30 to 60 degrees facing forward at the anterior hairline and toward the center of the scalp to mimic natural hair growth. As a slit is made, the graft is immediately inserted by sliding the graft along the side of the blade with the help of a jeweler's forceps. The application of pressure can also help with the placement process and prevent "popping," extrusion of the newly placed grafts. The process is time consuming and laborious. It is typical for a committed hair transplant surgeon to have from three to five assistants who prepare and place grafts under his or her direction.[1-3]

Follicular Unit Extraction. Follicular unit extraction has become the method of choice for primary grafting for male pattern baldness. Sometimes called a "scalpel-less hair transplant," grafts are obtained using small, round punches (1–2 mm) harvesting 1 to 2 hair units. The donor sites are shaved close to the scalp. For larger sessions, the posterior hair is trimmed with a military-type haircut. For smaller sessions, the long hair of the occipital scalp is retracted with hair clips and a small portion of the scalp is trimmed. Then the donor area is concealed by covered hair.

The donor area is infiltrated with local anesthesia. Then these small punches are used to harvest follicle directing the punch toward of the visible hair down the hair shaft (Figure 40-3A–C). Hair is harvested every 4 to

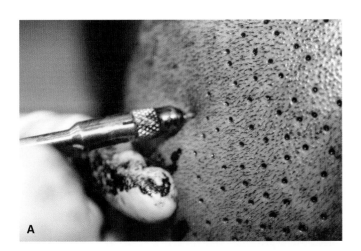

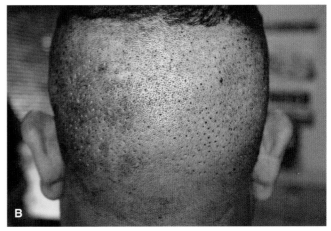

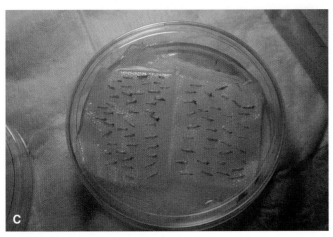

● **FIGURE 40-3.** (A) Recovery of unit follicular grafts with a punch. (B) Appearance of the donor site after harvest. (C) The follicular units awaiting implantation.

5 hair units. No sutures are required. The donor areas are covered with antibiotic ointment. Each donor site contracts and granulates, resulting in a favorable donor field.

The follicular units are then trimmed of excessive fat and readied for transplantation. As with micrografting techniques, the grafts are inserted into the recipient sites using jeweler's forceps. Hair growth takes weeks to months.

This technique can be used for small grafting sessions as in grafting for eyebrows. Larger sessions are used for male pattern baldness. There is no linear scar in the occipital scalp, and patients have minimal postoperative pain. This technique is more expensive than the strip method because of the lengthy time of harvesting individual hair units. However, the patient benefits from no visible scar and reduced recovery time.[4]

Pedicled Hair-bearing Tissue Flaps

The use of pedicled flaps for the reconstruction of areas of alopecia has become increasingly less common, except in clinical situations that require urgent coverage. Flaps used in urgent situations are usually local advancement or transposition flaps. These have been described in detail in multiple sources in the plastic surgery literature. Generally, these flaps do not require delay, but the surgeon should be wary of creating a flap whose tip crosses the midline, especially in an elderly patient. Vascular anastomoses across the midline in aged patients may not support distal tissues.

A variety of pedicled flaps have been described for treatment of male pattern hair loss. Now largely obsolete and out of popular favor due to the stigma of leaving sometimes visible scars, these include local temporal area flaps to more complex flaps like the Juri temporoparietal-occipital flap that benefits from routine delay. Many an unwary surgeon has been confronted with a difficult donor site closure when using scalp flaps for alopecia reconstruction. This is particularly true of the Juri flap when designed by an overly ambitious surgeon.

Today, flaps for aesthetic reconstruction are used less often. They can still achieve excellent results but do present the problem of moving a limited amount of hair-bearing scalp while imposing a donor site defect which may be difficult to close and which may leave an undesirable scar. In addition, the angle of exit of the hair shafts from the skin of the flap may be the complete opposite of the native angle of exit, as in the case of the Juri flap. Today, if flaps are used for aesthetic reconstructions, their use can be significantly enhanced by prior expansion.

Tissue Expansion

Tissue expansion has been extremely valuable in the treatment of soft tissue defects. Physiologically this process is more sophisticated than a simple stretching of the tissue; expansion is the result of formation of new cell growth and increase tissue mass. This requires time and

both patient and surgeon must be ready to commit to the time it takes. Hair follicles are preserved in expansion of the skin and, although new follicles are not thought to be created, this may not be true in the case of scalp expansion in children. An area of scalp may be doubled without producing a visible thinning of hair density.

The fundamental principles of tissue expansion have been described previously; briefly, tissue expansion involves at least three stages: insertion, expansion, and reconstruction. Preoperative planning specifically with reference to expander selection, design of the placement, and timing of surgery is the lynch pin of successful outcome. Among the first questions the surgeon should ask are where he and the patient wish the final scars to lie. The limitations of surgery in this regard should be discussed with the patient. Expanders are almost always placed beneath the galea and above the fascia of underlying muscle. In the area of the anterior scalp and forehead, expanders may be place on top of the frontalis so that innervated motion of the reconstructed forehead is preserved. The dissection between the subcutaneous fat and the underlying frontalis is easier in a child than in an adult. Once the incision has been made and carried to the preferred depth, a pocket is created to allow implant insertion. Inflation of the expander generally begins 7 days after insertion and proceeds at weekly or twice a week intervals. For patient convenience, expansion can usually be performed at home by the patient and his family and friends. Implant expansion should proceed until adequate soft tissue has been generated to accomplish the reconstructive goal. Any type of rotation, advancement, or transposition flap may be designed with the expanded tissue.

After completion of expansion, incision in the line of the previous insertion site will permit removal of the deflated expander. At this time, the bald scalp at the temple areas is surgically removed and the expanded hair-bearing scalp surrounding each of the defect sites is advanced as indicated generally by the arrows to form advanced temple hairlines. The anterior-posterior width of expander assures that with expansion of the hair-bearing scalp surrounding and behind the defect areas sufficient additional hair-bearing scalp is formed to be brought forward and completely cover the defects. The expanded tissue is easily bunched along the new hairline and sutured to the remaining skin at the top of the forehead. In time, the expanded tissue grows flat on the skull with a minimum scar at the hairline. If desired, the expanded forelock may be advanced anteriorly a slight distance.

The precise technique will obviously vary in terms of geometry, expander selection, and expansion course dependent on anatomic location. Three common patterns of expansion for male pattern baldness are detailed here.

Expanded Juri Flap. Use of the Juri flap is made more difficult by the need for several steps for delay and by the difficulty in closing the donor site. It is this latter problem that limits the width of the hair-bearing flap that the surgeon can use. The alternative to these problems lies in the use of a tissue expander prior to fashioning and rotating the Juri flap. Placed under the temporo-parietal-occipital area of the Juri flap (best accomplished with an expander with a slight bend or dogleg), the expansion begins in a week and is continued until the difference of the measurement of the arc over the expander, minus the width of the base of the expander at the level of the skull, equals the width of the desired flap for transfer. With the scalp flap width is achieved by the expansion, this calculation ensures that the surgeon will be able to close the defect without and tension or struggle.

The flap does not require delay for rotation. Its capsule should not be incised at the base, because laboratory studies using radioactive microspheres have demonstrated that the blood flow to an expanded flap is doubled if the capsule is left intact. The rotation is easy and the inset rapid. The result is most gratifying with placement of a broad, hair shaft–dense flap at the anterior hairline.[5]

Temporal Recession. Temporal recession results in a central projecting area of hair bearing scalp with alopecia on each side. In the case of this form of male pattern hair loss, a specialized soft tissue expander having three spaced arms extending from one side of the base with concave recesses between the arms and a single interior cavity may be used (Figures 40-4 and 40-5A–C).[6] The tissue expander is implanted by forming an incision (as indicated) along the patient scalpline at the depths of the recessed hairline, lifting the hair bearing scalp from the skull to form a subgaleal pocket having the shape of the expander and then inserting the expander into the pocket so that the fingers and recesses are positioned to conform closely to the anterior hairline. The hairline incision is then sutured closed to confine the deflated expander within the pocket.

After an appropriate interval, saline solution is injected into the single interior cavity of the expander through the port so that expander and overlying hairy soft tissue are expanded above the base which is supported on the skull. Repeated injection of saline solution into the expander lifts the cover and expands the overlying tissue, thereby increasing the area of the hair-bearing scalp around the two temple bald recess defects.

Expansion is continued until the measured arc length of the expanded scalp indicates sufficient expansion has occurred to cover the temple recesses. Generally, the difference of the measurement of the arc over the expander, minus the width of the base of the expander at the level of the skull, should equal the width of the desired flap for transfer of the width of the advancement needed. Almost any degree of scalp expansion can be easily concealed by wearing a hat, such as a baseball cap, to lessen patient embarrassment during the period of expansion. Only forehead expansion is harder to conceal, but even this altered appearance can be minimized with the use of bouffant caps like those commonly worn in the operating room.

At the time of advancement, the central hairline is reconstructed first and the closure is conducted from central to lateral. There will be dog ears laterally. These may be neglected and will generally go flat. The surgeon should not discard scalp-bearing hair. Allow time for contraction and the dog-ear will shrink. Avoid scars that are perpendicular to the hairline as these will always widen and present a problem in the long term.

Reconstruction of Hippocratic Baldness. Sculpture depicts Hippocrates, the father of medicine, as being bald across the top of his head. The term "Hippocratic baldness" has come to signify complete vertex hair loss. It can now be addressed with micrografts, but the mathematics of follicular transplantation work against obtaining a result that closely approximates a normal expected density of hair across the top of the head. Tissue expansion can accomplish a normal-appearing distribution of hair across the top of most patients' heads. This is because an area of scalp can be expanded to twice its normal area with no visible diminution of hair density. By expanding the remaining privileged areas of the temporal, and lower parietal and occipital scalp, the surgeon can usually create enough scalp with normal-appearing hair density to cover the entire top of the head (Figures 40-6A–C).

The tradeoff for the patient is 2.5 months of visible deformity after the first 6 weeks of expansion, when change is usually not apparent. Not much is visible during the first 6 weeks of expansion while the patient is instructed to simply let his hair grow long. After this he may wish to wear bouffant-type hats or hats of another design to disguise the expansion. This can be accomplished so that the only unusual feature is that of wearing a hat indoors. At about 4 months after expander placement in the typical patient, the expanders can be removed with total reconstruction of the vertex scalp

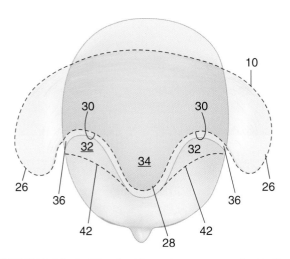

● **FIGURE 40-4.** The double-croissant expander for the anterior hairline.

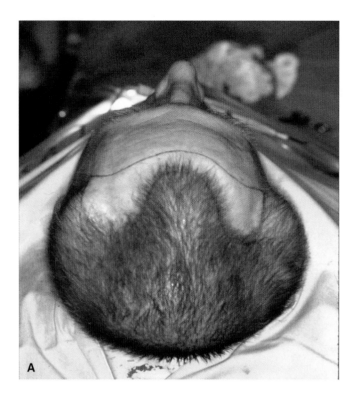
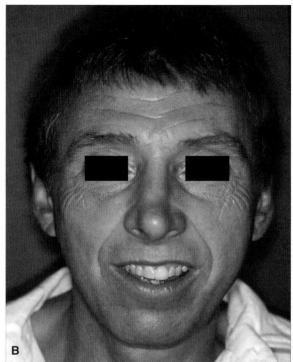
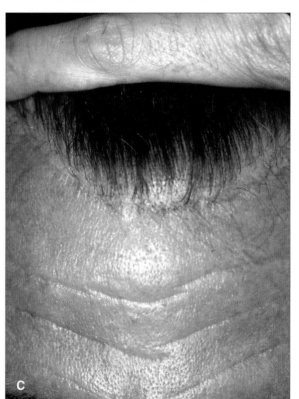

● FIGURE 40-5. (A) A patient with a double-croissant expander, as pictured in Figure 40-3, expanded and ready for advancement. (B) The patient after advancement. (C) A close-up view of the anterior hairline scar.

and fashioning of a new anterior hairline. Because this scalp is privileged and spared complete androgenetic hair loss, the result should be lifelong. Any further hair loss in a patient reconstructed as described here can be treated with a simple midline excision of a thinning area in the outpatient clinic under local anesthesia.

Initially the patient is counseled and the process of expansion explained. The hairline should be set in front of a mirror, recalling the admonition that it should be a mature hairline. Two differentially expanding expanders are placed through a transverse incision centered on the midline at the occipital hairline. Using male Van Buren urethral sounds, the pockets in the subgaleal space are created and the expanders placed with the aid of Scudder bowel clamps with rubber catheter segments placed over their arms. The incision is closed securely and inflation

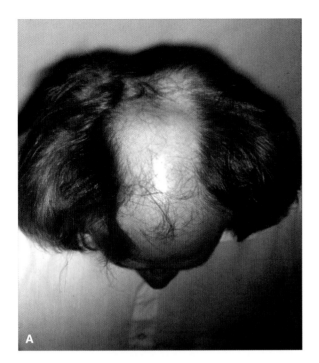

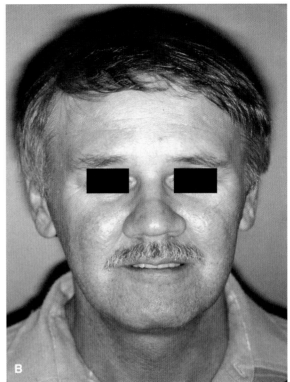

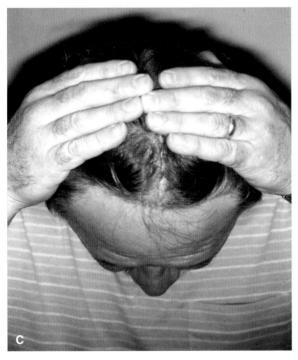

● **FIGURE 40-6.** (A) A differential tissue expander in place with more temporal expansion and the method of treating male temple baldness. (B). After advancement as described in the text and in reference 5. (C) Showing the anterior hairline and the method of closure.

begun in a week. The classic measurements described above are made and when they indicate that enough tissue is generated, then the advancement is made in the operating room.

The advancement incisions begin with an extension of the insertion incision and removal of the expanders. A midline incision across the vertex to the intended anterior hairline is created. The incision posteriorly is extended along the hair-bearing edge of the expanded scalp to a point of incision on the temporal hairline. This point is determined by projecting a 7 cm line perpendicular to

the midline of the scalp to the most anterior point of contact with this line on the temporal hairline. At this point the surgeon directs a straight line incision extending obliquely caudally and slightly posteriorly over the greatest height of the expander in the area of the temporal scalp. The temporal scalp posterior to this incision will then advance upward and to the midline to create a new anterior hairline. The extent of expansion and the placement of this incision allow creation of the desired anterior hairline, even permitting major advancement. Resection of the two "rabbit ears" of bare scalp based at the anterior hairline and closure in the midline over a drain complete the operation. The patient should shower the next day. Patients are typically thrilled at the result, both immediately and in the long term.[7,8]

● COMPLICATIONS

Regardless of the reconstructive technique chosen, postoperative complications in the practice of hair restoration are few. Avoidance of specific complications including the plugged look and so-called donut formation (following transplantation of a vertex in a continuingly balding patient) has been discussed above. Donor site hair sparseness may result from mathematical error. The scalp of the majority of Caucasian patients has 60 to 100 follicular units/cm^2; and if this is reduced by more than 50% (in tissue expansion or by harvest of isolated punch grafts), the hair density of the donor area will be visibly affected. Those with poor donor site density (<40 follicular units/cm^2) are therefore poor candidates. This potential complication is avoided in micrograft and minigraft transplantation as the donor site is, by the very nature of the technique, removed. Overly deep insertion of grafts has been reported to result in the formation of ingrown hairs and cysts hence technical vigilance is a must. Assuming a good sterile operative technique, hair restoration surgery is rarely complicated by infection and, though there are some advocates for their use, prophylactic antibiotics are not generally required. Retraction of expanded tissue has been described but with adequate expansion, this should be negligible and not problematic. Scar widening is a potential complication whenever the skin barrier is breached, and these procedures are no different. As part of preoperative counseling, patients should be consented for possible complications pertaining to scaring, infection hematoma formation where appropriate, as well as for the potential need for revision procedures.

● OUTCOME ASSESSMENT

In practice, assessment of operative outcomes of hair restoration surgery is largely subjective. Patient satisfaction comes first. Independent of that, qualitative comparison of pre-and postoperative photography is currently the mainstay of outcomes documentation. More objective quantitative is truly difficult.

● ACKNOWLEDGMENT

The authors wish to thank Ms. Kathy Smith of the Nu/Hart Hair Clinics, Inc. 200 Fleet Street, Penthouse Suite, Pittsburgh, PA 15220.

REFERENCES

1. Uebel CO. Micrografts and minigrafts: a new approach for baldness surgery. *Ann Plast Surg.* 1991;27(5):476–487.

2. Barrera A. Advances in aesthetic hair restoration. *Aesthet Surg J.* 2003;23(4):259–264.

3. Avram M, Rogers N. Contemporary hair transplantation. *Dermatol Surg.* 2009;35(11):1705–1719.

4. Rassman WR, Bernstein RM, McClellan R, et al. Follicular unit extraction: minimally invasive surgery for hair transplantation. *Dermatol Surg.* 2002;28(8):720–728.

5. Sajjadian A, Manders EK. Surgical and medical treatment for male pattern hair loss. In: Peled I, Manders EK, eds. *Aesthetic Surgery of the Face.* London: Martin Dunitz; 2004.

6. Manders EK. Tissue Expander and Method of Treating Male Temple Baldness. U.S. Patent No. 4,955,395.

7. Manders EK, Graham WP 3rd, Schenden MJ, Davis TS. Skin expansion to eliminate large scalp defects. *Ann Plast Surg.* 1984;12(4):305–312.

8. Manders EK, Mottaleb M, Hetzler PT. Soft tissue expansion. In: Marsh JL, ed. *Current Therapy in Plastic and Reconstructive Surgery: Head and Neck.* Philadelphia: B.C. Decker; 1989:88–98.

chapter 41

Breast Cancer

Gretchen Ahrendt, MD, FACS

● BACKGROUND

Breast cancer remains the most commonly diagnosed cancer in women, with an estimated 212,920 new cases for 2006.[1] The widespread application and improvements in screening mammography have contributed to an increase in the diagnosis of nonpalpable early-stage breast cancer, and ductal carcinoma in situ (DCIS) accounts for 28% of all new breast cancer diagnoses. Although breast cancer mortality has declined in recent years, more than 41,000 women are expected to die annually of their disease. Early diagnosis and multimodality treatment, including appropriate use of surgery, adjuvant systemic therapy, and radiation therapy, have contributed to the recent declines in mortality. Emerging molecular profiling of breast cancer subtypes has demonstrated that breast cancer is a heterogeneous group of diseases with variable clinical outcomes. Although additional research is needed to fully appreciate the complexity of the molecular subtypes of breast cancer, current treatment strategies can be more individually tailored to improve outcomes by identifying patients who maximally benefit from systemic treatment.

● BREAST CANCER RISK FACTORS

Most recognized breast cancer risk factors are related to prolonged estrogen exposure (Table 41-1). Nonmodifiable estrogen exposure risk factors include early onset of menarche, late onset of menopause, nulliparity, and delayed onset of first childbirth. The average age at first childbirth has been increasing, particularly among women in higher socioeconomic classes who are already at increased risk of developing breast cancer.[2] The use of exogenous estrogen, alone or in combination with progesterone, for the management of menopausal symptoms is a modifiable breast cancer risk factor. Results of the Women's Health Initiative demonstrated that the prolonged use of estrogen or combined estrogen plus progesterone hormone replacement therapy (HRT) increased breast cancer risk over never-users.[3] Cessation of HRT resulted in a return of breast cancer risk to baseline levels after 5 years. The use of HRT in postmenopausal women to manage menopausal symptoms needs to be balanced with the increased relative risk of breast cancer. The long-term use of HRT solely for the management of perimenopausal symptoms is no longer advised.

There is mounting evidence that postmenopausal obesity contributes to breast cancer risk.[4] The excess risk appears to be limited to never-users of HRT. Postmenopausal women with a body mass index greater than 30 who have never used hormone therapy have a 1.7- to 2.3-fold increased risk of ductal estrogen receptor positive and progesterone receptor positive (ER+/PR+) tumors compared with lean women. Body mass index was not found to relate to breast cancer risk among current HRT users. Premenopausal women with increased dietary fat intake, particularly animal fat and high-fat dairy foods, have an increased breast cancer risk.[5] Alcohol consumption of more than 10 g per day is also associated with increased risk of ER+ breast cancer.[6] There appears to be an interaction between alcohol consumption and use of HRT on breast cancer risk. Diet, weight gain, hormone use, and alcohol intake are potentially modifiable risk factors that should be discussed with patients as additional breast cancer risk factors.

Women with a first-degree relative with a history of breast cancer are at increased risk for developing the disease. Most women, however, overestimate the magnitude of this risk.[7] A family history of sporadic postmenopausal breast cancer in a first-degree relative modestly increases breast cancer risk, and many women with a family history of breast cancer never develop the disease.

TABLE 41-1. Breast Cancer Risk Factors Stratified by Relative Risk

Factor: Relative Risk

Age >30 y at first pregnancy: 1.1–2.0
Early onset of menarche (<12 y)
Delayed menopause (>age 55 y)
Nulliparity
Recent and long-term use of hormone replacement
Post-menopausal obesity
Excess alcohol use
High socioeconomic status
Single first-degree relative with breast cancer: 2.1–4.0
Atypical ductal or lobular hyperplasia
Age >65 y: >4.0
Inherited susceptibility (*BRCA1* or *BRCA2*)
More than one first-degree relatives with early-onset breast cancer
Personal history of breast cancer

A family history of early onset breast cancer affecting more than one generation should raise the suspicion of a hereditary breast cancer syndrome. Overall, hereditary breast cancer accounts for less than 10% of all breast cancers; however, recognizing a familial pattern should prompt a discussion of genetic counseling and testing. Patients found to carry a deleterious mutation in the *BRCA1* or *BRCA2* gene have a 45% to 85% risk of breast cancer and a 11% to 40% risk of ovarian cancer.[8] The management of breast cancer in women with a documented deleterious mutation in the *BRCA1* or *BRCA2* gene may include surgical risk reduction in addition to treatment of the primary tumor.[9,10]

Breast cancer risk assessment tools are available to assist the clinician and patient in quantifying the short-term and long-term personal risk of developing breast cancer. Tools available for breast cancer risk assessment include the Gail model, Claus family history model, and BRACAPro.[11] It is essential to provide patients with an accurate assessment of breast cancer risk based on objective data to provide reassurance to those who over-estimate their risk and to offer enhanced screening, chemoprevention, or risk-reduction surgery to those at genuinely increased risk.

● IN SITU BREAST CANCER

DCIS and lobular carcinoma in situ (LCIS) are distinct clinical entities with different treatment algorithms. DCIS typically presents in a screening population as mammographically detected microcalcifications without associated breast symptoms or physical findings. Fine, pleomorphic, linear, and branching calcifications are classified as suspicious or highly suspicious for DCIS and biopsy is warranted. The coexistence of a mass lesion with calcifications should increase suspicion for the presence of invasive carcinoma. Most mammographically detected calcifications can be sampled via stereotactic core-needle biopsy, permitting an accurate histologic diagnosis prior to surgical excision.

DCIS is a heterogeneous pre-invasive malignancy with variable potential to develop invasive carcinoma. The pathologic requirement for the diagnosis of DCIS is an intact basement membrane. DCIS is classified by histologic subtype, nuclear grade, and the presence or absence of necrosis. High-nuclear grade DCIS with comedo necrosis is associated with the highest risk of local recurrence or future invasive carcinoma (Figure 41-1A,B).

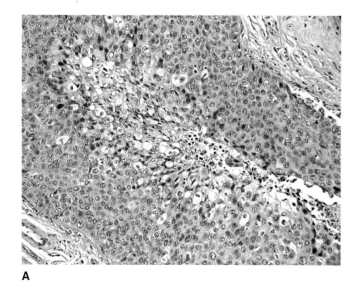

A

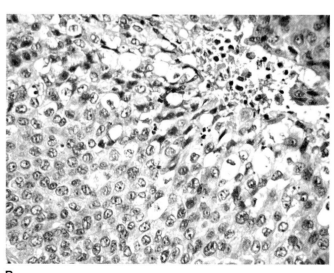

B

● **FIGURE 41-1.** (A,B) High-grade DCIS with central necrosis. Low-power (A) and high-power (B) view. Note intact basement membrane. (*Courtesy of Mamatha Chivikula, MD, Department of Pathology, Magee-Womens Hospital of UPMC.*)

Non–high-grade DCIS retains the risk of subsequent invasive carcinoma; however, the time course for disease progression is variable and for practical purposes nonquantifiable for an individual patient.

The management of DCIS focuses on local surgical excision of the diseased breast segment with attention to obtaining a surrounding margin of histologically normal breast tissue. Regional lymph node staging is not indicated for the majority of patients with DCIS, as the disease is confined to the duct lumen and does not have access to the lymphatic space. Lymph node staging with sentinel node biopsy should be considered in patients undergoing mastectomy for extensive DCIS, patients who present with a palpable mass where there is a suspicion of underlying invasive carcinoma, and large volume partial breast resections of high-grade DCIS. Approximately 20% of these patients will be found to have invasive ductal carcinoma on final pathology and the finding of a negative sentinel node obviates the need for a second operative procedure for axillary staging.

Most patients require mammographically guided wire localization of the microcalcifications immediately prior to surgery to direct excision of this nonpalpable lesion. Patients need to be advised that mammography frequently underestimates the extent of DCIS, particularly when there is extensive noncalcified disease. Meticulous pathology assessment of the specimen with attention to the extent of DCIS found in the specimen and proximity to inked margins will guide the need for additional therapy. There is no standard definition for what constitutes a negative surgical margin; however, DCIS less than 1 mm from the inked specimen edge is generally felt to represent a positive finding. Patients with close or positive surgical margins are advised to have additional surgery to exclude residual disease in the breast. Most patients can be managed with a margin-directed re-excision to achieve clear margins. A postexcision mammogram is recommended to document complete excision of all calcifications prior to initiating radiation therapy.

Adjuvant whole breast radiation is recommended following local excision of DCIS to reduce the risk of local recurrence. Excision alone is associated with 10-year recurrence rates of 25% to 30%,[12,13] and approximately 50% of patients who recur after breast-conserving treatment for DCIS will have invasive carcinoma at the time of recurrence. Whole breast radiation decreases the risk of local recurrence by 40% to 50%.[14] To date, no subset of women with DCIS has been identified for which radiation is not beneficial, although the absolute benefit is highest in patients with the highest risk of local failure. The Van Nuys Prognostic Index incorporates age at diagnosis, extent of DCIS, proximity of DCIS to the closest surgical margin, and DCIS grade and necrosis to classify patients as at low, intermediate, or high risk for local recurrence.[15] The index was developed at a single institution based on retrospective analysis of selected patients and has not been validated prospectively. However, it can be useful in counseling patients about their individual recurrence risk.

Clinical trials are in progress to determine if there is a subset of low-risk DCIS for which radiation therapy can be omitted. A recent prospective study of local excision alone with protocol mandated margins of less than 1 cm met early stopping rules due to ipsilateral recurrence rates of 2.4% per year corresponding to a 12% 5-year recurrence rate.[16] Although DCIS is a nonlethal breast cancer, up to 50% of recurrences are associated with invasive breast cancer with the associated risk of axillary or systemic metastasis. At present, radiation therapy is recommended for the majority of women following local excision for DCIS.

Total mastectomy with immediate reconstruction remains an alternative to breast-conserving therapy for DCIS. Indications for mastectomy include diffuse malignant microcalcifications not amenable to surgical excision with an acceptable cosmetic deformity, failure to achieve negative resection margins after attempts at breast conservation, and patient preference. Scleroderma remains a contraindication to radiation therapy and mastectomy may be the most reasonable option for this special population. Inability to achieve clear margins following multiple attempts at local excision occurs infrequently; however, depending on breast size and patient expectations, mastectomy with reconstruction may result in a superior long-term cosmetic result than continued attempts at re-excision.

Skin-sparing mastectomy via a periareola incision permits dissection of all glandular tissue with preservation of the natural skin envelope and inframammary crease. The boundaries of dissection of the breast glandular tissue are identical to those for standard total or modified radical mastectomy. Rates of local recurrence following skin-sparing mastectomy are comparable with conventional mastectomy procedures.[17] In rare circumstances, a clear plane of dissection cannot be developed due to the presence of DCIS in the most anterior breast tissue, and skin excision overlying the breast parenchyma is necessary. Preservation of the natural skin envelope provides a template for reconstruction, achieving remarkable symmetry to the normal contralateral breast. Sentinel lymph node biopsy can be performed via the periareola incision or, if necessary, via a separate axillary incision. Nipple-sparing and areola-sparing mastectomies are gaining in popularity and selection criteria and long-term outcomes for these procedures are emerging.[18,19]

Oncoplastic breast conserving surgery refers to local tissue rearrangement following the wide segmental excision of breast cancer to improve the cosmetic outcome.[20] In women with large invasive carcinomas, neoadjuvant chemotherapy can be used to locally down-stage the primary tumor to improve the likelihood of successful breast-conserving surgery. At present, there are no systemic treatments to reduce the volume of DCIS to make breast preservation more feasible for patients with extensive disease. As an alternative to mastectomy, large volume full thickness segmental excisions combined with local breast flap advancement can increase the options for

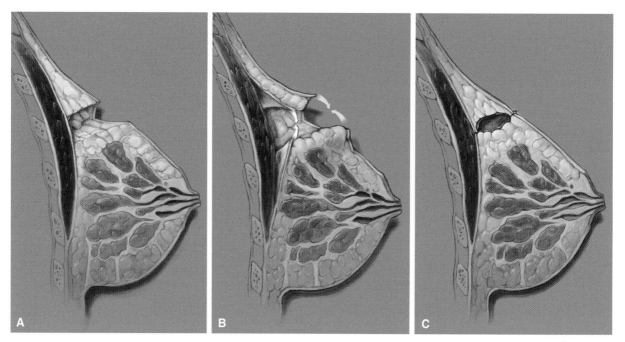

● **FIGURE 41-2.** (A) Full-thickness parenchymal resection from skin to pectoralis fascis. (B) Fibroglandular tissue mobilized off the pectoralis fascia to permit advancement over chest wall. (C) Closue of defect. (*Reproduced with permission of Benjamin O. Anderson, MD.*)

breast conservation in patients with extensive segmental DCIS (Figure 41-2). These procedures include use of a parallelogram skin incision (Figure 41-3), batwing mastopexy (Figure 41-4), donut mastopexy, and reduction mammoplasty.

Preoperative consultation with radiology to plan tumor localization with multiple localizing wires for extensive areas of calcification will increase the chances for negative surgical margins. Patients benefit from consultation with plastic surgery to discuss contralateral symmetry

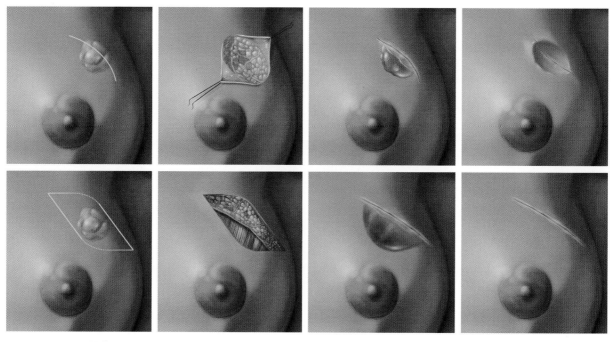

● **FIGURE 41-3.** Standard lumpectomy with resulting deformity (*top row*). Parallelogram mastopexy lumpectomy (*bottom row*). (*Reproduced with permission of Benjamin O. Anderson, MD.*)

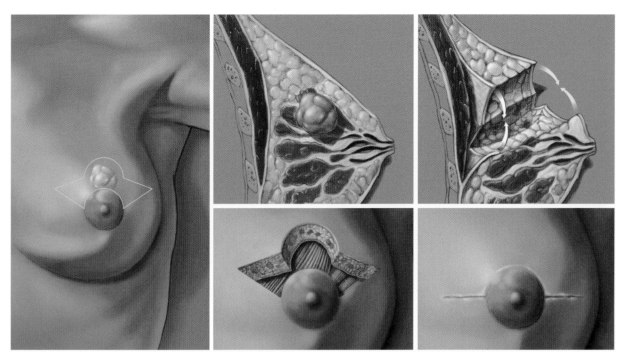

● FIGURE 41-4. Batwing mastopexy lumpectomy. Permits partial- or full-thickness parenchymal resection of centrally located tumors. (*Reproduced with permission of Benjamin O. Anderson, MD.*)

procedures. It is advisable to await final pathology results to determine margin status before proceeding with any contralateral procedures. Positive resection margins following large-volume oncoplastic resection are generally an indication for mastectomy.

The selective estrogen receptor modulator, tamoxifen, has been shown to reduce the risk of ipsilateral DCIS recurrence and contralateral breast cancer events following breast-conserving surgery.[21] Tamoxifen reduces the occurrence of both DCIS and invasive carcinomas, although this benefit is limited to patients with ER+ DCIS. Patients treated with breast-conserving therapy for ER+ DCIS should be counseled about the use of tamoxifen. Trials are in progress evaluating the efficacy of aromatase inhibitors for the management of DCIS in postmenopausal women. Taken together, breast cancer specific survival following local therapy for DCIS approaches 100%.

● **LOBULAR CARCINOMA IN SITU**

LCIS is characterized by a monotonous proliferation of neoplastic cells within the acini of lobules with distention of these structures (Figure 41-5). Loss of cellular cohesion can be observed. There are no clear mammographic, ultrasound, or physical findings associated with LCIS and typically it is discovered on examination of biopsy specimens obtained for other indications. LCIS has traditionally been viewed as a marker of increased risk of breast cancer in both the index and contralateral breast and not as a precursor lesion to invasive breast cancer. LCIS identified following a core-needle biopsy performed for a mammographic abnormality should be further evaluated with surgical excisional biopsy due to the small but measurable risk of associated carcinoma.[22] Attempts to achieve clear surgical margins are not warranted, as it is accepted that LCIS is often multicentric and bilateral. LCIS is almost uniformly ER+, and patients benefit from tamoxifen for breast cancer chemoprevention.

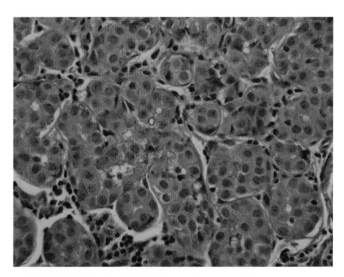

● FIGURE 41-5. LCIS high power view. Monotonous proliferation of neoplastic cells with lobular distention. (*Courtesy of Mammath Chivakula, MD, Department of Pathology, Magee-Womens Hospital of UPMC.*)

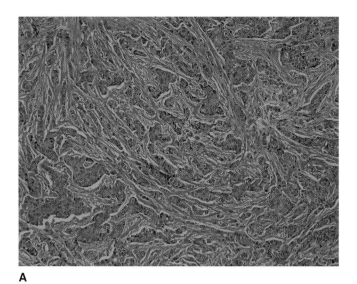
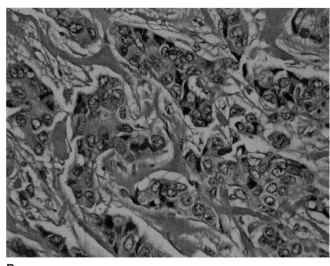

A

B

● **FIGURE 41-6.** (A,B) Invasive ductal carcinoma low-power (A) and high-power (B) views. (*Courtesy of Mammath Chivakula, MD, Department of Pathology, Magee-Womens Hospital of UPMC.*)

There is growing evidence that LCIS represents a spectrum of lobular intraepithelial neoplasia, similar to the heterogeneity observed in DCIS. A more appropriate classification suggested is a three-tiered system with lobular intraepithelial neoplasia 3 associated with the highest level of subsequent breast cancer risk.[23] Pleomorphic LCIS, which may represent a nonobligate precursor of invasive LCIS, may be best managed similarly to DCIS.[24,25] Close communication between the surgical oncologist and pathologist is warranted for cases of LCIS to determine whether additional excision may be warranted.[23]

● INVASIVE CARCINOMA

The identification of mammary stromal invasion differentiates in situ from invasive carcinoma (Figure 41-6). Invasive carcinoma has the potential to metastasize to regional lymph nodes or to distant sites, most commonly bone, lung, liver, and brain. Comprehensive treatment involves multimodality therapy, including surgery and radiation, for local and regional disease and systemic therapy. The majority of invasive carcinomas are ductal in origin and include the special histologic variants: tubular, mucinous, papillary, and medullary. Invasive lobular carcinomas represent approximately 20% of invasive carcinomas. It is recognized that the histologic variants of invasive carcinoma have different metastatic potential; however, local and adjuvant therapy are not primarily influenced by histologic classification.

Patients may present with a screening detected lesion or a palpable mass. The diagnostic evaluation should include a diagnostic mammogram with magnified and spot compression views of the abnormality. The presence of associated calcifications should be noted as this

is often an indication of concomitant in situ carcinoma. Ultrasound is a useful complementary diagnostic study to confirm the size and position of the mass within the breast and is essential in patients with dense breasts and a palpable lesion not visualized on mammography. Ultrasound can be useful for evaluation of the regional axillary lymph nodes prior to surgery. Metastatic axillary nodes will appear abnormally rounded with a thickened cortex and loss of the normal fatty hilum. Ultrasound directed fine-needle aspiration or core-needle biopsy of abnormal nodes is useful to determine whether the patient is a candidate for sentinel node biopsy or if an axillary node dissection is indicated.

Percutaneous image directed core-needle biopsy with stereotactic or ultrasound guidance is the preferred approach to the diagnostic evaluation of a suspicious screening detected or palpable mass. The large, bore core needles currently in use (typically 14-, 11-, or 9-gauge) permit accurate preoperative diagnosis of the lesion to guide patient counseling and surgical planning. Appropriate radiologic-pathologic correlation is indicated following core-needle biopsy. A finding of benign histology with a suspicious lesion mandates further evaluation with surgical excision.

Dynamic contrast-enhanced breast MRI is used with increasing frequency to locally stage primary breast cancer and assist with operative planning. MRI relies on the acquisition of breast images before and after the administration of intravenous gadolinium contrast. Malignant lesions will demonstrate rapid contrast enhancement due to neovascularity and abnormal permeability of the neoplastic vessels (Figure 41-7). Benign breast findings may also show enhancement on MRI and there can be considerable overlap in the pattern of enhancement between benign and malignant lesions. MRI has a high false-positive rate and

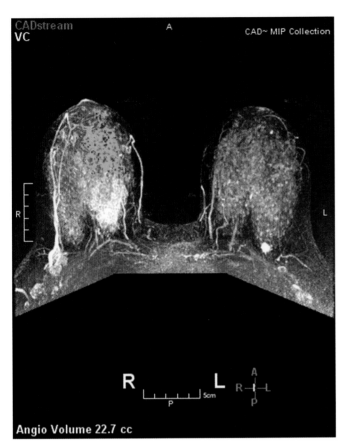

● **FIGURE 41-7.** Contrast-enhanced breast MRI demonstrating diffuse regional enhancement consistent with extensive carcinoma.

biopsy of abnormal MRI detected lesions is essential to avoid unnecessary surgery.[26]

It is accepted that MRI is more sensitive than mammography for detecting cancer in women with heterogeneously and homogeneously dense breasts and may help to delineate the extent of disease in this patient population. MRI may also demonstrate occult foci of multifocal or multicentric disease that could alter the planned operative procedure.[26] MRI is more sensitive than mammography in screening high-risk patients, particularly documented BRCA1/2 mutation carriers.[27] MRI has also proven to be effective for identification of a primary tumor in patients presenting with axillary lymph node metastases, and in monitoring response to neoadjuvant chemotherapy.[28] Breast-conserving therapy consisting of partial mastectomy followed by adjuvant whole breast radiation is the preferred approach for the local management of early-stage breast cancer. Nonpalpable lesions may require imaged-guided, preoperative wire localization to guide local resection. Intraoperative ultrasound can effectively be used to locate a nonpalpable mass and plan the surgical incision and resection and is a patient-friendly alternative to wire localization. Axillary sentinel node dissection is the preferred staging procedure for patients presenting with a clinically negative axilla. The sentinel node(s) represents the first node to receive

lymphatic drainage from the breast and can be identified with the injection of radiolabeled tracer and/or vital blue dye into the breast prior to the planned procedure. The patient receives an injection of technetium-99 labeled sulfur colloid into the breast, usually in the department of nuclear medicine, prior to surgery. Lymphazurin blue dye in injected intraoperatively. The dual technique of radioisotope and blue dye yields the highest sentinel node localization rates with the fewest false-negative sentinel nodes. Through a minimal axillary incision, the sentinel node can be localized with the use of a hand-held gamma probe and the direct visualization of blue-stained lymphatics or node(s). The sentinel node accurately reflects the status of the axilla with a false-negative rate of less than 5% in experienced centers.[29] Patients with a negative sentinel node can be spared complete axillary node dissection with a lower risk of upper extremity lymphedema.[30] The risk of axillary recurrence following a negative sentinel node procedure is less than expected, based on published false-negative rates.[31]

Breast cancer staging is based on the American Joint Committee on Cancer (AJCC) TNM (tumor, node, metastasis) system.[32] The sixth edition of the AJCC breast cancer staging manual introduced substantial modifications to incorporate the detailed lymph node information obtained from sentinel node sectioning. Isolated tumor deposits identified with immunohistochemical stains for cytokeratin can be identified and remain of uncertain clinical significance. The current staging classification standardizes the reporting of these findings to permit prospective evaluation of the impact of isolated tumor cells on relapse-free and overall survival.

Patients found to have axillary sentinel node metastases are recommended to have a complete levels I and II axillary lymph node dissection. Approximately 50% of patients will have no additional metastases identified in the remaining axillary nodes (non-sentinel nodes) on completion dissection. Intense efforts have been applied to identify factors that predict nonsentinel node metastases. In general, the risk of nonsentinel node metastasis increases with the size of the primary tumor, size of the metastasis in the sentinel node, and the number of positive sentinel nodes. A Web-based nomogram is available to provide an estimate of the probability of nonsentinel node metastasis.[33] The predicted probability of additional positive nodes can be used to guide discussions regarding further axillary surgery or alternatives such as axillary radiation. Attempts to identify a subset of patients who can omit axillary dissection with the finding of a positive sentinel node have failed to identify a subset with no risk of additional disease. Adjuvant whole breast radiation is routinely recommended following partial mastectomy to decrease the risk of local recurrence. A total dose of 50 Gy delivered in 25 fractions to the entire breast often with a local boost to the surgical site is standard. Although all patients with invasive breast cancer have lower rates of local recurrence following breast radiation, the magnitude of benefit is proportional to the level of risk. The risk of local recurrence in patients older than 70 years old with small, histologically favorable, node-negative, ER+ tumors may be sufficiently low to omit adjuvant radiation.[34] It is important to evaluate comorbidities and life expectancy in elderly breast cancer patients to compare their risk of breast cancer recurrence with competing causes of mortality.[35]

Accelerated partial breast radiation is an alternative to whole breast radiation, and is increasingly being utilized. Partial breast radiation can be delivered using multiple interstitial catheters, a balloon-based catheter, or with conformal external beam approaches.[36] The advantages of partial breast radiation include the ability to target the radiation dose directly to the primary tumor bed, which represents the area at highest risk for true local recurrence as well as the ability to complete treatment over a 5-day period. Most series of partial breast radiation are single institution phase I/II studies and include highly selected patients with limited follow-up.[37–39] The long-term local recurrence risk for patients managed following partial breast radiation is unknown and patients are encouraged to participate in available clinical trials comparing partial breast radiation to standard external beam radiation. Total mastectomy remains an alternative to breast conservation therapy for surgical management of invasive carcinoma. The liberal use of neoadjuvant or primary chemotherapy in patients with large or locally advanced breast cancer has enabled more women to undergo breast conservation. Patients presenting with large primary tumors, unfavorable tumor to breast size ratio, localized skin involvement, or metastatic axillary adenopathy may potentially undergo breast preserving surgery following response to neoadjuvant chemotherapy. Administration of chemotherapy prior to surgery also provides important information about the response of the tumor to the agents utilized. Anthracycline-based chemotherapy is recommended in tumors that overexpress HER2/neu or simultaneously overexpress topoisomerase II.[40] Tumors with p53 mutations generally have lower response rates.[41] High-grade, ER− tumors with high proliferative rates are more likely to have a complete pathologic response than low-grade ER+ lesions. Although tumor response to chemotherapy is high for ER− tumors, disease-free survival is significantly higher in ER+ disease.

Patients with large tumors that respond poorly to systemic therapy, inflammatory carcinomas, and tumors associated with extensive malignant microcalcifications are best managed with mastectomy and lymph node staging. When a mastectomy is the recommended surgical management, there are often still indications to proceed with chemotherapy initially. Patients with inflammatory breast cancer present with skin thickening, erythema, and edema or peau d'orange skin changes. This clinical presentation is due to the presence of tumor in the dermal lymphatic system and/or the result of significant lymphatic obstruction in the breast from tumor or axillary lymph node involvement. Inflammatory cancer is viewed as inoperable disease due to the extensive skin involvement with tumor and these patients are best managed with primary systemic chemotherapy. The vast majority of cases will have resolution of the underlying skin changes although there may be residual microscopic or macroscopic disease in the breast. Due to the extensive skin involvement at presentation, mastectomy and axillary node staging is the recommended surgical management. These patients are advised to forego immediate breast reconstruction due to the indication for postmastectomy radiation to minimize the risk of local or regional recurrence.

Patients presenting with tumors fixed to the chest wall or with fixed axillary adenopathy are felt to have locally advanced breast cancer (LABC) and also benefit from primary systemic therapy before operative intervention. The success of breast conservation surgery in this population is not established although could be entertained in patients who experience a complete clinical response to chemotherapy. Most patients who present with LABC will ultimately require a mastectomy for definitive surgical management. Like inflammatory carcinoma, the decision for postmastectomy radiation is based on disease stage at presentation. For this reason, patients with LABC who undergo mastectomy are advised to delay breast reconstruction.

The accepted indications for postmastectomy radiation include pathologic tumor size larger than 5 cm, four or more pathologically positive lymph nodes, and positive surgical margins.[42] Relative indications include patients with multicentric disease with total tumor volume approaching 5 cm and close surgical margins. In addition, there is evidence that postmastectomy radiation in women with one to three positive nodes reduces local-regional recurrence and improves overall breast cancer survival.[42] As the indications for postmastectomy radiation expand, it is increasingly difficult to advise patients undergoing mastectomy whether to have an immediate reconstruction. The long-term cosmetic and functional outcome for the reconstructed breast following radiation is generally inferior to the nonradiated reconstruction. Although autologous tissue flaps may tolerate radiation therapy better than implant-based reconstructions, achieving good symmetry and minimizing fibrosis in the reconstruction cannot be guaranteed. Planning targeted radiation therapy to the chest wall is complicated by the presence of a reconstructed breast mound, and higher doses of radiation may be administered to the underlying lungs or heart. Preoperative consultation with radiation oncology and a thorough evaluation of the axillary lymph nodes will help guide the decision for immediate or delayed reconstruction.

There is increasing interest in the use of delayed-immediate reconstruction techniques.[43] This strategy refers to the placement of a tissue expander at the time of mastectomy as a temporizing device in order to offer a skin-sparing procedure. Once the final pathology results are available, a determination can be made as to the indications for postmastectomy radiation. In patients who do not require radiation, reconstruction can proceed with tissue expansion and implant placement or autologous tissue flap based on patient preferences. If radiation is recommended, the tissue expander can be removed, or left in place expanded throughout treatment. Once radiation is complete, a decision regarding the most suitable reconstruction can be made.

ADJUVANT THERAPY

The majority of patients with invasive breast cancer are offered adjuvant systemic treatment to reduce their risk of relapse. Patients with a 10% or greater risk of systemic relapse are recommended to receive adjuvant treatment. Decisions for systemic therapy are based on prognostic and predictive factors including age, lymph node status, tumor size and grade, hormone receptor status and, HER2/neu overexpression. The clinical challenge is to identify the individual patients with the highest risk of relapse who have the most to benefit from cytotoxic treatment. Based on evidence from randomized clinical trials, patients with node-positive breast cancer benefit from receiving adjuvant chemotherapy, even in the setting of ER+ disease. Adjuvant hormonal therapy is recommended for patients with ER+ or PR+ breast cancer.

Patients with small, node-negative, ER+ breast cancer represent a subset of patients with an overall low-risk of systemic failure. However, some ER+ breast cancer patients will experience systemic relapse and ultimately die of their disease. Molecular profiling of the primary tumor can identify low-, intermediate-, and high-risk patients for systemic relapse. A multimarker gene assay has been validated to predict risk of relapse as well as response to therapy.[44] Gene expression profiling has demonstrated that differential expression of certain genes is a more powerful prognostic indicator than traditional factors such as tumor size and lymph node status. Currently, this panel is in use for women with node-negative ER+ breast cancer and can provide meaningful information that may influence treatment decisions.

The Early Breast Cancer Trialists' Collaborative Group reported in their recent overview analysis that anthracycline-based polychemotherapy results in a 38% reduction in the risk of death for patients older than age 50 years and a 20% reduction in the risk of death for 50 to 69 years olds.[45] These benefits of chemotherapy are independent of the use of endocrine therapy (tamoxifen), estrogen

receptor status, nodal status, or other tumor characteristics. For ER+ patients, the use of tamoxifen for 5 years reduced the annual breast cancer death rate by 31%, independent of age, use of chemotherapy, PR status, or other tumor characteristics. Five years of tamoxifen is superior to 2 years and the survival benefit persists after treatment is discontinued. This overview underscores the importance of systemic therapy in the multimodality approach to breast cancer treatment.

For years, tamoxifen was the endocrine therapy of choice for patients with ER+ invasive breast cancer. Recently, the aromatase inhibitors, including anastrazole and letrozole, have been shown to be superior to tamoxifen in disease-free survival and in reducing the number of contralateral breast cancer events.[46] Aromatase inhibitors block the peripheral conversion of estrogen precursors to estrogen but do not block ovarian estrogen production. They are, therefore, only effective and recommended for postmenopausal women. Aromatase inhibitors are associated with fewer adverse events compared with tamoxifen, including fewer endometrial cancers, thromboembolic events, vaginal discharge, and hot flashes, although fracture risk is slightly increased.

The era of targeted therapies for breast cancer is rapidly emerging and the drug trastuzumab (Herceptin) has emerged as major advance in the systemic treatment of breast cancer. Trastuzumab, a humanized mouse monoclonal antibody, targets the HER2/neu protein which is overexpressed in 25% to 30% of breast cancers. Initially used for the treatment of metastatic breast cancer, recent studies have confirmed the efficacy of this drug in the adjuvant setting. With short-term follow-up, 1 year of trastuzumab (combined with conventional chemotherapy) reduces the risk of local, regional, or systemic relapse by 50% in patients with HER2/neu positive breast cancer.[47,48] For high-risk HER2/neu–positive breast cancer patients, the addition of trastuzumab is now a standard option.

CONCLUSION

Care of the breast cancer patient is genuinely multidisciplinary and close communication and integration of the treatment plan across disciplines will maximize outcomes for the patient. Improvements in screening have contributed to earlier detection, allowing many patients to have minimal surgery. There is a growing trend toward targeted therapies, including partial radiation and more selective systemic agents. Further advances in treatment will rely on an improved understanding of the biology of individual tumors and the further development of tailored agents directed at unique targets.

REFERENCES

1. Ries LAG, Harkins D, Krapcho M, et al., eds. *SEER Cancer Statistics Review, 1975–2003*. Bethesda, MD: National Cancer Institute. http://seer.cancer.gov/csr/1975_2003/.

2. Chlebowski RT, Chen Z, Anderson GL, et al. Ethnicity and breast cancer: factors influencing differences in incidence and outcome. *J Natl Cancer Inst*. 2005;97(6):439–448.

3. Chlebowski RT, Hendrix SL, Langer RD, et al. Influence of estrogen plus progestin on breast cancer and mammography in healthy postmenopausal women: the Women's Health Initiative Randomized Trial. *JAMA*. 2003;289(24): 3243–3253.

4. Suzuki R, Rylander-Rudqvist T, Ye W, et al. Body weight and postmenopausal breast cancer risk defined by estrogen and progesterone receptor status among Swedish women: A prospective cohort study. *Int J Cancer*. 2006;119(7): 1683–1689.

5. Cho E, Spiegelman D, Hunter DJ, et al. Premenopausal fat intake and risk of breast cancer. *J Natl Cancer Inst*. 2003;95(14):1079–1085.

6. Suzuki R, Ye W, Rylander-Rudqvist T, et al. Alcohol and postmenopausal breast cancer risk defined by estrogen and progesterone receptor status: a prospective cohort study. *J Natl Cancer Inst*. 2005;97(21):1601–1608.

7. Metcalfe KA, Narod SA. Breast Cancer risk perception among women who have undergone prophylactic bilateral mastectomy. *J Natl Cancer Inst*. 2002;94(20):1564–1569.

8. Kramer JL, Velazquez IA, Chen BE, et al. Prophylactic oophorectomy reduces breast cancer penetrance during prospective, long-term follow-up of BRCA1 mutation carriers. *J Clin Oncol*. 2005;23(34):8629–8635.

9. Rebbeck TR, Friebel T, Lynch HT, et al. Bilateral prophylactic mastectomy reduces breast cancer risk in BRCA1 and BRCA2 mutation carriers: The PROSE Study Group. *J Clin Oncol*. 2004;22(6):1055–1062.

10. Rebbeck TR, Lynch HT, Neuhausen SL, et al. Prophylactic oophorectomy in carriers of BRCA1 or BRCA2 mutations. *N Engl J Med*. 2002;346(21):1616–1622.

11. Domchek SM, Eisen A, Calzone K, et al. Application of breast cancer risk prediction models in clinical practice. *J Clin Oncol*. 2003;21(4):593–601.

12. Silverstein MJ, ed. *Ductal Carcinoma In Situ of the Breast*. 2nd ed. Philadelphia: Lippincott Williams & Wilkins; 2002: 303–321.

13. MacDonald HR, Silverstein MJ, Mabry H, et al. Local control in ductal carcinoma in situ treated by excision alone: incremental benefit of larger margins. *Am J Surg*. 2005; 190(4):521–525.

14. Fisher B, Costantino J, Redmond C, et al. Lumpectomy compared with lumpectomy and radiation therapy for the treatment of intraductal breast cancer. *N Engl J Med*. 1993;328(22):1581–1586.

15. Boland GP, Chan KC, Knox WF, et al. Value of the Van Nuys Prognostic Index in prediction of recurrence of ductal carcinoma in situ after breast-conserving surgery. *Br J Surg*. 2003;90(4):426–432.

16. Wong JS, Kaelin CM, Troyan SL, et al. Prospective study of wide excision alone for ductal carcinoma in situ of the breast. *J Clin Oncol*. 2006;24(7):1031–1036.

17. Singletary SE, Robb GL. Oncologic safety of skin-sparing mastectomy. *Ann Surg Oncol*. 2003;10(2):95–97.

18. Simmons RM, Hollenbeck ST, Latrenta GS. Two-year follow-up of areola-sparing mastectomy with immediate reconstruction. *Am J Surg*. 2004;188(4):403–406.

19. Petit JY, Veronesi U, Orecchia R, et al. Nipple-sparing mastectomy in association with intra operative radiotherapy (ELIOT): a new type of mastectomy for breast cancer treatment. *Breast Cancer Res Treat*. 2006;96(1):47–51.

20. Anderson BO, Masetti R, Silverstein MJ. Oncoplastic approaches to partial mastectomy: an overview of volume-displacement techniques. *Lancet Oncol*. 2005;6(3):145–157.

21. Fisher B, Dignam J, Wolmark N, et al. Tamoxifen in treatment of intraductal breast cancer: National Surgical Adjuvant Breast and Bowel Project B-24 randomised controlled trial. *Lancet*. 1999;353(9169):1993–2000.

22. Arpino G, Allred DC, Mohsin SK, et al. Lobular neoplasia on core-needle biopsy–clinical significance. *Cancer*. 2004;101(2):242–250.

23. Bratthauer GL, Tavassoli FA. Lobular intraepithelial neoplasia: previously unexplored aspects assessed in 775 cases and their clinical implications. *Virchows Arch*. 2002;440(2): 134–138.

24. Hwang ES, Nyante SJ, Chen YY, et al. Clonality of lobular carcinoma in situ and synchronous invasive lobular carcinoma. *Cancer*. 2004;100:2562–2572.

25. Reis-Filho J, Simpson P, Jones C, et al. Pleomorphic lobular carcinoma of the breast: role of comprehensive molecular pathology in characterization of an entity. *J Pathol*. 2005;207(1):1–13.

26. Bedrosian I, Mick R, Orel SG, et al. Changes in the surgical management of patients with breast carcinoma based on preoperative magnetic resonance imaging. *Cancer*. 2003;98(3):468–473.

27. Kuhl CK, Schrading S, Leutner CC, et al. Mammography, breast ultrasound, and magnetic resonance imaging for surveillance of women at high familial risk for breast cancer. *J Clin Oncol*. 2005;23(33):8469–8476.

28. Yeh E, Slanetz P, Kopans DB, et al. Prospective comparison of mammography, sonography, and MRI in patients undergoing neoadjuvant chemotherapy for palpable breast cancer. *AJR Am J Roentgenol*. 2005;184(3):868–877.

29. Lyman GH, Giuliano AE, Somerfield MR, et al. American Society of Clinical Oncology guideline recommendations for sentinel lymph node biopsy in early-stage breast cancer. *J Clin Oncol*. 2005;23(30):7703–7720.

30. Mansel RE, Fallowfield L, Kissin M, et al. Randomized multicenter trial of sentinel node biopsy versus standard axillary treatment in operable breast cancer: the ALMANAC Trial. *J Natl Cancer Inst*. 2006;98(9):599–609.

31. Veronesi U, Galimberti V, Mariani L, et al. Sentinel node biopsy in breast cancer: early results in 953 patients with

negative sentinel node biopsy and no axillary dissection. *Eur J Cancer.* 2005;41(2):231–237.

32. National Cancer Institute. Stage information for breast cancer. *Breast Cancer Treatment (PDQ®).* http://www.cancer.gov/cancertopics/pdq/treatment/breast/HealthProfessional/page3.

33. Van Zee KJ, Manasseh DM, Bevilacqua JL, et al. A nomogram for predicting the likelihood of additional nodal metastases in breast cancer patients with a positive sentinel node biopsy. *Ann Surg Oncol.* 2003;10(10):1140–1151.

34. Hughes KS, Schnaper LA, Berry D, et al. Lumpectomy plus tamoxifen with or without irradiation in women 70 years of age or older with early breast cancer. *N Engl J Med.* 2004;351(10):971–977.

35. Smith BD, Gross CP, Smith GL, et al. Effectiveness of radiation therapy for older women with early breast cancer. *J Natl Cancer Inst.* 2006;98(10):681–690.

36. Vicini F, Winter K, Straube W, Wong J, et al. A phase I/II trial to evaluate three-dimensional conformal radiation therapy confined to the region of the lumpectomy cavity for Stage I/II breast carcinoma: initial report of feasibility and reproducibility of Radiation Therapy Oncology Group (RTOG) Study 0319. *Int J Radiat Oncol Biol Phys.* 2005;63(5):1531–1537.

37. Jeruss JS, Vicini FA, Beitsch PD, et al. Initial outcomes for patients treated on the American Society of Breast Surgeons MammoSite clinical trial for ductal carcinoma-in-situ of the breast. *Ann Surg Oncol.* 2006;13(7):967–976.

38. Zannis V, Beitsch P, Vicini F, et al. Descriptions and outcomes of insertion techniques of a breast brachytherapy balloon catheter in 1403 patients enrolled in the American Society of Breast Surgeons MammoSite breast brachytherapy registry trial. *Am J Surg.* 2005;190(4):530–538.

39. Kuske RR, Winter K, Arthur DW, et al. Phase II trial of brachytherapy alone after lumpectomy for select breast cancer: toxicity analysis of RTOG 95–17. *Int J Radiat Oncol Biol Phys.* 2006;65(1):45–51.

40. Scandinavian Breast Group Trial 9401, Tanner M, Isola J, Wiklund T, et al. Topoisomerase IIalpha gene amplification predicts favorable treatment response to tailored and dose-escalated anthracycline-based adjuvant chemotherapy in HER-2/neu-amplified breast cancer: Scandinavian Breast Group Trial 9401. *J Clin Oncol.* 2006;24(16):2428–2436.

41. Xu Y, Yao L, Ouyang T, et al. p53 Codon 72 polymorphism predicts the pathologic response to neoadjuvant chemotherapy in patients with breast cancer. *Clin Cancer Res.* 2005;11(20):7328–7333.

42. Nielsen HM, Overgaard M, Grau C, et al. Loco-regional recurrence after mastectomy in high-risk breast cancer–risk and prognosis. An analysis of patients from the DBCG 82 b&c randomization trials. *Radiother Oncol.* 2006;79(2):147–155.

43. Kronowitz SJ, Hunt KK, Kuerer HM, et al. Title delayed-immediate breast reconstruction. *Plast Reconstr Surg.* 2004;113(6):1617–1628.

44. Paik S, Tang G, Shak S, et al. Gene expression and benefit of chemotherapy in women with node-negative, estrogen receptor-positive breast cancer. *J Clin Oncol.* 2006;24(23):3726–3734.

45. Early Breast Cancer Trialists' Collaborative Group (EBCTCG). Effects of chemotherapy and hormonal therapy for early breast cancer on recurrence and 15-year survival: an overview of the randomised trials. *Lancet.* 2005;365:1687–1717.

46. Baum M, Buzdar A, Cuzick J, et al. Anastrozole alone or in combination with tamoxifen versus tamoxifen alone for adjuvant treatment of postmenopausal women with early-stage breast cancer: results of the ATAC (Arimidex, Tamoxifen Alone or in Combination) trial efficacy and safety update analyses. *Cancer.* 2003;98(9):1802–1810.

47. Romond EH, Perez EA, Bryant J, et al. Trastuzumab plus adjuvant chemotherapy for operable HER2-positive breast cancer. *N Engl J Med.* 2005;353(16):1673–1684.

48. Piccart-Gebhart MJ, Procter M, Leyland-Jones B, et al. Trastuzumab after adjuvant chemotherapy in HER2-positive breast cancer. *N Engl J Med.* 2005;353(16):1659–1672.

chapter 42

Alloplastic Breast Reconstruction

Louis P. Bucky, MD, FACS / Alexander J. Gougoutas, MD

● INTRODUCTION

With the exception of nonmelanoma skin cancers, breast cancer is the most common cancer seen in women in the United States, with an incidence of 1 in 8 (13%). In this same population, it is succeeded only by lung cancer as the second most common cause of cancer deaths. In 2010, there were more than 200,000 new cases of breast cancer in the United States alone.[1] Breast reconstruction will play an integral role in the increasing number of these patients who will require mastectomy for definitive treatment. This demand, in combination with the well-described psychosocial benefits of reconstruction, has led to the development of numerous reconstructive techniques, all in pursuit of a reproducible and aesthetically pleasing result.

To date, breast reconstruction is accomplished with either rotational or free autologous tissue transfer, prosthetic tissue expanders and implants, or a combination of both. Despite the diversity of available reconstructive techniques, it is evident from a review of the 2010 American Society of Plastic Surgeons statistics that alloplastic expander/implant reconstruction is by far the most common technique employed, accounting for nearly 70% of all reconstructions.[2]

Alloplastic reconstruction accomplishes the recreation of the absent breast mound and can be performed either in the immediate postmastectomy setting or in a delayed fashion. Immediate reconstructions typically are accomplished in one or two stages. In the case of single-stage, immediate reconstruction, a permanent silicone or saline implant is placed following completion of the mastectomy, frequently with the addition on an acellular dermal matrix (ADM). In two-stage, immediate reconstruction, a temporary tissue expander is placed at the time of mastectomy. A second-stage procedure is typically performed at least 3 months after mastectomy, at which time the tissue expander is replaced with a permanent silicone or saline implant. Delayed reconstructions are usually performed at least 6 to 8 months postmastectomy, almost invariably in two stages. Though immediate and delayed reconstructions each have their own advantages and disadvantages, two-stage, immediate reconstruction with tissue expander/implant exchange is by far the most common reconstruction performed and will be the focus of the discussion to follow.

Alloplastic reconstruction confers several unique advantages over autologous reconstruction. These include less scaring; the use of local, texture, and color-matched skin; avoidance of donor site morbidity; as well as a shorter operative time, hospital stay, and overall recovery.[3] Furthermore, advances in expander/implant technology as well as refinements in mastectomy and reconstructive techniques have increased the predictability, reproducibility, and aesthetics of implant reconstruction.

Textured anatomic expanders offer several advantages over their original, smooth, round design. The potential advantages of these devices include a reduction in both capsular contracture and lateral subluxation of the expander. Shaped or anatomic devices can preferentially expand the breast's lower pole, giving it a more natural appearance. Use of the nipple-sparing mastectomy not only may eliminate the need for future nipple-areola reconstruction but also preserves the breast's skin envelope in its entirety, obviating the need for any skin recruitment. The selective addition of an ADM to the reconstruction can create greater definition of the inframammary fold, conceal implant wrinkling or folding, reduce muscle dissection, and potentially decrease the rate of capsular contracture—all of which may provide a better aesthetic appearance. Finally, the selective transfer of autologous fat may serve to blunt contour abnormalities and improve the periprosthetic soft tissue envelope.

All the aforementioned advances have greatly improved the aesthetics of implant-based breast reconstruction. This is particularly true in patients undergoing bilateral reconstructions where achieving symmetry, often the most formidable challenge of unilateral reconstruction, is simplified. This point warrants some discussion as the incidence of contralateral prophylactic mastectomy (CPM) and bilateral prophylactic mastectomy (BPM) has increased dramatically over the past decade.[4,5]

The increased incidence of CPM and BPM likely stems from a multitude of factors. The relatively recent discovery of the *BRCA1* and *BRCA2* genes has allowed physicians to identify a subpopulation of patients at high risk for developing breast cancer. These high-risk patients may derive a significant psychological benefit from elective BPM. Similarly, patients with unilateral disease may elect to undergo CPM to reduce the anxiety associated with the possibility of developing contralateral breast cancer in the future. Finally, there is an abundance of evidence demonstrating improved outcomes, namely a decreased risk of contralateral cancer development, in high-risk patients with unilateral disease who elect to undergo CPM.[6-9] This same decreased risk has also been demonstrated in high-risk, disease-free patients who elect to undergo BPM.[10,11]

The benefits of prophylactic mastectomy have led to a growing population of patients seeking bilateral mastectomies, many of whom are ideally suited for implant-based reconstructions. Furthermore, many of these patients, including, but not limited to, those undergoing prophylactic mastectomy or with small, peripherally located tumors, are candidates for nipple-sparing mastectomy. This technique confers many potential benefits to the ultimate reconstruction, including preservation of the nipple-areola complex and limited skin resection. As a result, many nipple-sparing mastectomies and subsequent reconstructions can be performed in one stage.

PATIENT EVALUATION AND SELECTION

Patient evaluation and selection begins during the initial consultation, a forum in which patients can voice their expectations and be informed of the goals of reconstruction. These goals are: (1) to give the patient an aesthetically pleasing appearance when either fully clothed or when wearing a revealing brassiere or bathing suite; and (2) to allow the patient to get dressed normally every day, free of the potential psychological burden that either the absence of a breast or usage of a cumbersome, unnatural prosthesis may impart. Selection of appropriate candidates for alloplastic reconstruction is based largely on the likelihood of accomplishing these two fundamental goals.

Multiple factors impact the ultimate aesthetic outcome of breast reconstruction, all of which must be taken into consideration. The key to appropriate patient evaluation and selection is understanding those factors that are within the surgeon's control and those that are not. Factors generally beyond the surgeon's control include body habitus, previous radiation therapy, adjuvant chemotherapy, future radiation therapy, previous breast surgeries and scar patterns, unilateral versus bilateral reconstruction, past medical history, general healing capabilities, and a patient's reconstructive preferences. Factors generally within the surgeon's control include selection of mastectomy and reconstructive techniques employed and timing of the reconstruction.

Physical evaluation of potential candidates for alloplastic reconstruction begins and ends with the breasts themselves. In cosmetic breast augmentation, the base width of the breast is the keystone for implant selection. Alloplastic reconstruction, however, must take into consideration not only the base width of the breast but also chest wall dimensions. This stems from the fact that the base of the reconstructed breast parenchyma, namely the expander/implant, will be strictly limited to the muscular confines of the chest wall.

Patients ideally suited for implant-based reconstructions are those with symmetric, small to moderate-sized breasts who seek bilateral reconstruction. A unique group of patients are those seeking reconstructions who have undergone prior breast augmentation. In the case of patients with prior subpectoral breast implants, alloplastic reconstruction is typically far easier as the subpectoral pocket has been previously dissected and expanded. The opposite is true for those patients who have undergone prior subglandular augmentation. In these cases, subpectoral dissection can be more challenging, as the muscle has been compressed against the chest wall by the overlying capsule.

While there are no absolute contraindications to alloplastic breast reconstruction, successful outcomes are predicated on appropriate patient selection. It should be stressed that not all patients are candidates for implant/expander reconstructions. The most fundamental requirement for successful prosthetic reconstruction is adequate soft tissue coverage of the implant/expander. In the case of inflammatory breast cancers, resection of large volumes of skin at the time of mastectomy are often required in addition to frequent adjuvant radiation. This results in a paucity of skin available for prosthesis coverage and thus expander/implant reconstruction alone in these cases is ill advised.

Historically speaking, prior radiation or the need for adjuvant radiation therapy was considered a contraindication to alloplastic breast reconstruction. This stemmed from the higher incidence of both postoperative complications and suboptimal aesthetic outcomes in irradiated patients. Recent data, however, suggests that patient satisfaction and aesthetic results in those undergoing expander/implant reconstruction and adjuvant radiotherapy do not differ significantly from those who do not require radiation.[12-14] While the debate is still ongoing, many believe that adjuvant radiotherapy is at most a relative contraindication to alloplastic reconstruction.

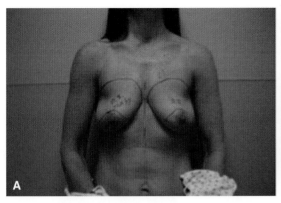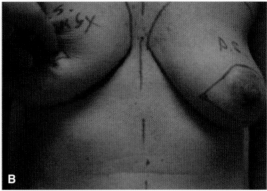

● **FIGURE 42-1.** Preoperative markings. The patient's midline is marked from sternal notch to xiphoid (A) and all anatomic boundaries of the breast are marked with particular attention to the inframammary crease (B).

● PATIENT PREPARATION

Tissue expander breast reconstruction is performed under general anesthesia, and in bilateral cases, will typically require 1 to 3 hours to complete. If performed in the immediate setting, this is in addition to time required by the oncologic surgery team and thus a 4 to 5 hours total operative time should be anticipated. Patient-specific preoperative evaluation should be critically reviewed with both the oncologic surgeon and anesthesiologist prior to the day surgery.

Marking of the patient is performed in the preoperative holding area. In the cases of immediate reconstruction, mastectomy technique and incisions are coordinated with the oncologic surgery team. The patient is marked while standing up with arms at their sides. After marking the midline from sternal notch to xiphoid, all anatomic boundaries of the breast are marked with particular attention to the inframammary crease (Figure 42-1). Preexisting differences in breast morphology and position should be carefully noted.

The availability of all necessary expander/implants should be confirmed prior to surgery. If use of an ADM is anticipated, ordering of the product should be done well in advance, as many institutions do not have stock supplies. In addition to a lighted retractor and light source, a basic plastics instrument tray is typically all that is required.

Patients are positioned supine. In the case of immediate, single-stage reconstruction or second-stage expander/implant exchanges, arms should be positioned at 90 degrees to allow upright positioning of the patient to evaluate symmetry. In the cases of first-stage expander placement, arms may be positioned at 90 degrees in order to facilitate lymph node access during dissection.

● TECHNIQUE

As immediate, two-stage expander/implant reconstructions are by far the most common type of reconstruction performed both at our institution and in the community at large, we will focus on this technique. Though

there are many variations on creation of the submuscular pocket, as a rule, we opt for total muscle coverage using the pectoralis major and serratus anterior muscles. We take exception to this rule in those patients who have a high riding pectoralis, that is, where the inferior most insertion of the pectoralis on the chest wall is superior to the inframammary fold. In these cases, we will frequently employ the use of an ADM sling.

At the completion of the mastectomy, the junction of the pectoralis major and serratus anterior muscles is well exposed. This is the anatomic starting point for creation of the submuscular pocket. Elevation of the pectoralis major begins laterally at its junction with the serratus anterior (Figure 42-2). Using electrocautery, dissection is carried down to the chest wall between these two muscles, creating a window just large enough to facilitate exposure and accommodate the tissue expander (typically the inferior third to half of the pectoralis major is separated from the serratus anterior). Elevation of the pectoralis off of

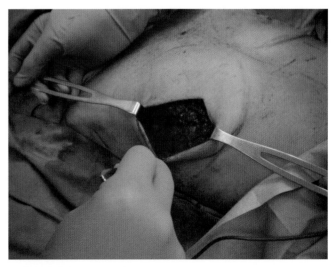

● **FIGURE 42-2.** Elevation of the pectoralis major. Elevation of the pectoralis major begins laterally at the junction with the serratus anterior.

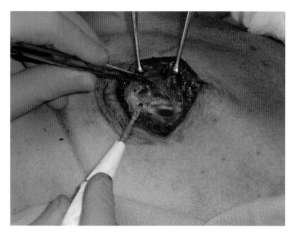

● **FIGURE 42-3.** Continued elevation of the pectoralis major. Elevation of the pectoralis major proceeds from lateral to medial with the aid of a lighted retractor (not pictured).

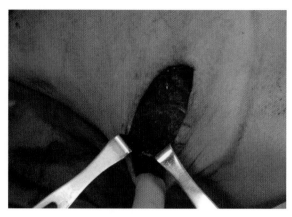

● **FIGURE 42-4.** Elevation of the serratus anterior. Just enough serratus is elevated to provide lateral muscular coverage of the tissue expander.

the chest wall proceeds from lateral to medial with aid of a lighted retractor for visualization (Figure 42-3). All intercostal perforating vessels are carefully identified and coagulated as the dissection proceeds. Medial elevation of the pectoralis is carried to the midline with minimal elevation off the sternum. Inferiorly, elevation of the pectoralis proceeds to the level of the inframammary crease. In those patients with an inframammary crease that sits below the inferior most insertion of the pectoralis, extended subcutaneous dissection over the rectus fascia is required. Once elevation of the pectoralis is complete, attention is turned to elevating the serratus anterior.

Elevation of the serratus begins at the window created between the lateral pectoralis and serratus muscle itself. Dissection is started immediately superficial to an underlying rib to prevent inadvertent penetration of the pleural space. Once again, dissection is carried straight down to chest wall. Elevation of the serratus then proceeds medial to lateral. Care must be taken to follow the curvature of the chest wall as the subserratus plane is often poorly defined and dissection in the wrong plane may lead to penetration of the thorax. Just enough serratus is elevated to provide coverage of the portion of the expander extending beyond the lateral border of the pectoralis (Figure 42-4).

After air is evacuated from the expander, it is placed in the submuscular pocket with the valve facing anteriorly (Figure 42-5). The edges of the pectoralis and serratus anterior muscles are then approximated with absorbable suture to provide complete muscular coverage of the expander (Figure 42-6). It is our practice to select an expander that is smaller than the base width of the breast if it extends beyond the chest wall—a frequently encountered scenario in women with larger breasts. This practice generally errs on the creation of a constricted soft tissue pocket that may require lateral capsulectomy at the time of implant exchange. This situation is, however, aesthetically preferable to an expanded

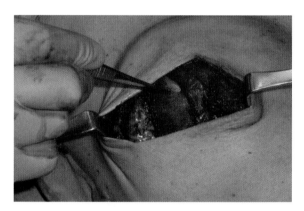

● **FIGURE 42-5.** Placement of the tissue expander. The tissue expander is placed beneath the pectoralis major muscle with the valve facing anteriorly (pictured at the tip of the surgeon's forceps).

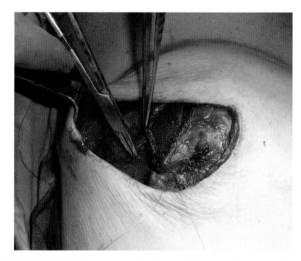

● **FIGURE 42-6.** Approximation of the serratus anterior and pectoralis major. The pectoralis and serratus muscles are approximated with a running, absorbable suture to provide complete muscular coverage of the expander.

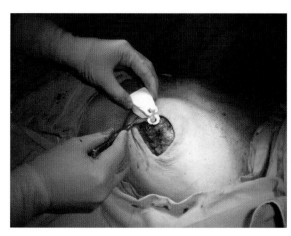

● **FIGURE 42-7.** Locating the fill port. The fill port is localized with a surface magnet.

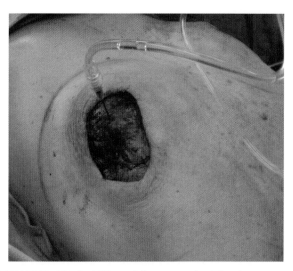

● **FIGURE 42-8.** Filling of the expander. The tissue expander is filled using a 60-cc syringe connected via a two-way valve (not pictured) to a small-bore needle inserted into the expander fill port.

soft tissue pocket requiring capsuloraphy at the time of implant exchange, the ultimate results of which are far less predictable.

In the cases of a high-riding pectoralis muscle, we employ the use of an ADM. In these cases, elevation of the pectoralis and serratus muscles proceeds as previously described; however, the inferior border of the pectoralis is released from the chest wall. The ADM, once reconstituted in sterile saline, is sewn between the inferior border of the window shaded pectoralis and the projection of the inframammary crease along the chest wall. We frequently will also employ the use of an ADM as an overlay to reinforce an attenuated pectoralis muscle or as lateral sling to limit lateral serratus dissection.

Depending on the appearance and redundancy of the mastectomy skin flaps the expander is then inflated with a variable volume of sterile saline. This is accomplished by first locating the fill valve with the locating magnet provided with the expander (Figure 42-7). Once the valve is accessed, 50 to 200 cc of sterile saline are injected with a sterile filling system composed of a 60-cc syringe attached via a T-connector to a reservoir of sterile saline and small-bore needle (Figure 42-8). Partial filling of the expander at the time of its placement serves to expand the overlying musculature while preventing skin contracture. Initial overexpansion, however, may cause undo tension on skin flaps already compromised by the mastectomy and thus initial fill volumes should be tailored to each patient.

Following placement of a 10-Fr round JP, the mastectomy skin flaps are closed with interrupted, absorbable, deep dermal sutures followed by a running subcuticular suture (Figure 42-9). Excessive tension on the mastectomy skin flaps following closure should prompt removal of saline from the expander, as this may increase the likelihood of skin flap necrosis.

Expansion is usually begun 2 to 3 weeks postoperatively when the skin flaps have healed and the patient is comfortable. Roughly 60 cc of sterile saline is injected into

the integrated valve of the expander at biweekly intervals. This interval may be increased depending on patient tolerance. Blanching of the skin or excessive pain at the time of expansion indicates overfilling and should prompt removal of volume to prevent potential skin necrosis. The second stage of the reconstruction should occur approximately 4 to 6 weeks from the time of the final expansion or completion of adjuvant chemotherapy.

At the second stage of reconstruction, the skin and subcutaneous tissue is elevated off the underlying pectoralis muscle. The pectoralis is then incised along the direction of its fibers and the expander is removed. Necessary dissection and capsulotomies are completed to facilitate correct positioning of the permanent implant. Selection of the permanent implant is based on the base width of the expander and the appearance of the chest wall with the expander in place. Typically high profile, permanent gel implants with base widths similar to those of the expander

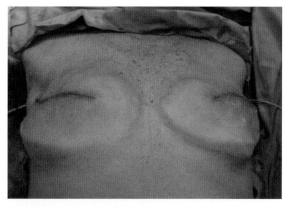

● **FIGURE 42-9.** Skin closure and drain placement.

are utilized. Once the permanent implant is placed, the overlying musculature is approximated with interrupted, absorbable sutures followed once again by a two-layered closure of the skin flaps. The patient is then positioned upright to evaluate symmetry.

Achieving symmetry, particularly in patients undergoing unilateral breast reconstruction, remains a formidable challenge and frequently requires a contralateral balancing procedure. In those patients with large, ptotic breasts this may include a reduction, mastopexy, or mastopexy with an implant. In those patients with smaller breasts, a contralateral augmentation is often required. We typically perform any required balancing procedure at the second stage of reconstruction. This practice avoids any potential contralateral complications at the time of mastectomy and expander placement. Additionally, delay of any necessary balancing procedure until the second stage of reconstruction assures healthy mastectomy skin flaps and, most importantly, allows settling of the reconstructed breast, thus conferring the best chance of achieving acceptable symmetry. Even with this protocol, however, patients who require a contralateral balancing procedure rarely achieve the symmetry of those who undergo bilateral reconstruction, where long-term symmetry is typically far easier to achieve regardless of native breast size and shape.

The use of autologous fat grafting with implant reconstruction has significant potential benefits. These include blunting of any intrinsic irregularities, such as rippling, tapering of the interface between the implant, and the patient's chest wall (the so-called "step-off deformity"), and improved periprosthetic soft tissue coverage. ADMs can similarly be utilized in selective cases to help improve the soft tissue envelope surrounding an implant.

● COMPLICATIONS

As with any surgical procedure, alloplastic breast reconstruction is not without its own set of potential complications, some of which may result in significant patient morbidity. A recent review found a 15.2% postoperative complication rate in all patients undergoing expander/implant reconstruction.[15] These complications include, but are not limited to, mastectomy skin flap necrosis, seroma/hematoma, capsular contracture, implant infection, migration, exposure, and deflation.

Several patient risk factors have been identified which increase the likelihood of developing one or more postoperative complications, and thus appropriate candidate selection for alloplastic reconstruction requires a detailed knowledge of a potential patient's medical and social history. Both smoking and diabetes have repeatedly been demonstrated to be independent risk factors for postoperative complications most notably mastectomy skin flap necrosis and delayed wound healing. Though the data is less clear, other patient factors, including obesity, age older than 65 years, hypertension, laterality of

reconstruction (unilateral versus bilateral), and adjuvant chemotherapy may also independently increase the likelihood of developing postoperative complications.

With reported rates as high as 24%,[16] perhaps no complication has been the source of more study in alloplastic breast reconstruction than infection. Infection may be limited to superficial skin and subcutaneous tissues or may extend deeper to involve the mastectomy pocket musculature and underlying prosthesis. Infection manifests as a spectrum of signs and symptoms ranging from asymptomatic peri-incisional erythema to frank sepsis with hemodynamic compromise. Regardless of how it manifests, an infected prosthesis may, if left untreated, have devastating effects on both the ultimate aesthetic result of the reconstruction and the patient's general health and therefore requires urgent attention.

Limited peri-incisional cellulitis without systemic symptoms may be managed initially with oral antibiotics. Failure to respond should prompt hospital admission for intravenous antibiotics and infectious disease consultation. Radiographic imaging with either ultrasound or CT may help identify periprosthetic collections requiring drainage. Persistent local and or systemic signs/symptoms of infection despite intravenous antibiotics or periprosthetic fluid collections suggest an infected prosthesis.

Traditionally speaking, a presumed expander/implant infection mandated removal of the prosthesis followed by a minimum healing period of 6 months prior to any attempt at implant replacement. The last decade, however, has seen an increasing trend toward attempted implant salvage rather than explantation. Salvage procedures are surgeon specific and entail implant removal, copious irrigation, varying degrees and methods of capsulectomy, and reinsertion of either the original or new implant.

If successful, salvage procedures may spare the patient additional future surgeries as well as the psychological burden of being without a breast during the healing phase. Not all patients are, however, candidates for salvage and such procedures should generally be avoided in those with frank exposure, advanced local infections or signs/symptoms of systemic infection.

Mastectomy skin flap necrosis is another relatively common complication of alloplastic breast reconstruction with reported rates as high as 20%.[17] Flap necrosis, depending on area and thickness, may have profound implications for the ultimate aesthetic outcome of the reconstruction as it results in a loss of soft tissue domain. Furthermore, a breach in the skin's immunoprotective barrier places the underlying prosthesis at risk for exposure and subsequent infection, particularly in cases where the prosthesis has not been placed completely submuscularly. Avoiding both over aggressive thinning of the skin flaps and excessive tension on skin closure can decrease the likelihood of skin flap necrosis. While new technologies are being developed to help determine skin flap viability and guide skin resection, flap necrosis remains a source of significant morbidity in expander/implant reconstructions. In light of this fact, management of skin flap necrosis continues to be the source of much study.

Recent reports suggest that in the absence of infection, skin flap necrosis with eschar formation need not necessarily hinder the expansion process. Eschar excision can be performed 4 weeks post operatively at which time volume is removed from the expander to facilitate a tension-free closure. Once fully healed expansion is resumed, typically 6 to 8 weeks postoperatively.[17]

Capsular contracture is an additional source of potential morbidity in patients undergoing implant-based reconstruction. The etiology and biology of capsular contracture are poorly understood and treatment options are limited. While grade 1 or 2 capsular contracture can often be managed nonoperatively, symptomatic, grade 4 contracture almost universally requires extensive capsulectomies or complete capsulotomy in addition to implant exchange. The incidence of capsular contracture in nonradiated patients who have undergone expander/implant reconstruction is estimated at 15% to 20%.[12] This number increases dramatically in patients who require postoperative radiation therapy.

It is well established that radiation therapy increases the likelihood of postoperative complications in those who undergo expander/implant breast reconstruction. Depending on the study, complications including pain, capsular contracture, implant exposure, infection, migration, and failure are seen in between 17% to 80% of irradiated patients.[3] It is for this reason that radiation therapy has, historically speaking, been considered a contraindication to alloplastic reconstruction. As previously mentioned however, an increased complication rate in irradiated patients does not necessarily translate to less patient satisfaction when compared with nonradiated patients. Therefore, alloplastic reconstruction in patients requiring radiation therapy may, in select cases, be acceptable.

As the use of radiation therapy in breast cancer patients is increasing,[18] so too is the number of irradiated patients seeking alloplastic reconstruction. The decision to offer expander/implant reconstruction to those patients who will require radiation should not be taken lightly, as these cases are among the most challenging a reconstructive surgeon will encounter. Expander selection, timing of and incision utilized for expander exchange, as well as selection of the permanent prosthesis may need to be modified in this unique population. Patients should be made aware during the initial consultation that failure of alloplastic reconstruction may require the pursuit of autologous alternatives.

OUTCOMES

Two-stage expander/implant reconstruction remains the most popular method of postmastectomy breast reconstruction and, in the hands of experienced surgeons, can yield consistently pleasing aesthetic results with high overall patient satisfaction. Successful reconstruction hinges not only on meticulous surgical planning, technique, and proper device selection but also on appropriate candidate selection and patient education. Patients need to understand the realistic alternatives to and potential consequences of alloplastic reconstruction. Additionally, they need to understand that expander/implant reconstruction represents a long-term commitment, often requiring multiple stages and many months to complete. It should also be stressed that implants may fail and require replacement, though typically not before 10 to 15 years following placement.

Understanding a prospective patient's expectations is crucial to a reconstructive success as the definition of such may differ between surgeon and patient. For example, a multiple-stage reconstruction requiring numerous revisions to achieve ideal symmetry, while a success in the eyes of the surgeon, may be less of a success in the eyes of a patient willing to sacrifice a degree of symmetry for less operations and an easier overall convalescence.

A recent review of 410 expander/implant reconstructions over a 12-year period demonstrated that 95% of patients were satisfied with the aesthetics of their reconstruction.[12] This same review demonstrated that an aesthetically pleasing result can be achieved in the vast majority of patients requiring postoperative radiation, despite an overall high complication rate in this subgroup. While alloplastic reconstruction traditionally yields the best aesthetic results in small-breasted patients with minimal ptosis, satisfying outcomes can also be achieved in heavier-set patients with larger, ptotic breasts.[12] And while autologous reconstruction may arguably yield better overall aesthetics when compared with alloplastic reconstruction, studies indicate that overall patient satisfaction may still be greater in the latter group.[19]

As reconstructive techniques continue to be refined and expander/implant technology continues to improve, so too will the aesthetics of expander/implant reconstructions. Improved aesthetic outcomes, while only part of overall reconstructive success, will undoubtedly lead to an increase in overall patient satisfaction and ensure the continued popularity of alloplastic breast reconstruction.

REFERENCES

1. National Cancer Institute. Definition of breast cancer. Breast Cancer. http://www.cancer.gov/cancertopics/types/breast.

2. American Society of Plastic Surgeons. *Report of the 2010 Plastic Surgery Statistics*. ASPS National Clearinghouse of Plastic Surgery Procedural Statistics; 2011.

3. Agha-Mohammadi S, De La Cruz C, Hurwitz DJ. Breast reconstruction with alloplastic implants. *J Surg Oncol.* 2006;94(6):471–478.

4. Tuttle TM, Habermann EB, Grund EH, et al. Increasing use of contralateral prophylactic mastectomy for breast cancer

patients: a trend towards more aggressive surgical treatment. *J Clin Oncol.* 2007;25(33):5203–5209.

5. Jones NB, Wilson J, Kotur L, et al. Contralateral prophylactic mastectomy for unilateral breast cancer: an increasing trend at a single institution. *Ann Surg Oncol.* 2009; 16(10):2691–2696.

6. Herrinton LJ, Barlow WE, Yu O, et al. Efficacy of prophylactic mastectomy in women with unilateral breast cancer: a cancer research network project. *J Clin Oncol.* 2005;23(19):4275–4286.

7. Van Sprundel TC, Schmidt MK, Rookus MA, et al. Risk reduction of contralateral breast cancer and survival after contralateral breast cancer and survival after contralateral prophylactic mastectomy in BRCA1 or BRCA2 mutation carriers. *Br J Cancer.* 2005;93(3):287–292.

8. Guiliano AE, Boolbol S, Degnim A, et al. Society of surgical oncology: position statement on prophylactic mastectomy. *Ann Surg Oncol.* 2007;14(9):2425–2427.

9. Goldflam K, Hunt KK, Gershenwald JE, et al. Contralateral prophylactic mastectomy. Predictors of significant histologic findings. *Cancer.* 2004;101(9):1977–1986.

10. Rebbeck TR, Freibel T, Lynch HT, et al. Bilateral prophylactic mastectomy reduces breast cancer risk in BRCA1 and BRCA2 mutation carriers: the PROSE study group. *J Clin Oncol.* 2004;22(6):1055–1062.

11. Lostumbo L, Carbine N, Wallace J, et al. Prophylactic mastectomy for the prevention of breast cancer. *Cochrane Database Syst Rev.* 2004;4CD002748.

12. Cordeiro PG, McCarthy CM. A single surgeon's 12-year experience with tissue expander/implant breast reconstruction: part II. an analysis of long-term complications, aesthetic outcomes, and patient satisfaction. *Plast Reconstr Surg.* 2006;118(4):832–839.

13. Krueger EA, Wilkins EG, Strawderman M, et al. Complications and patient satisfaction following expander/implant breast reconstruction with and without radiotherapy. *Int J Radiation Oncology Biol Phys.* 2001;49(3):713–721.

14. Percec I, Bucky LP. Successful prosthetic breast reconstruction after radiation therapy. *Ann Plast Surg.* 2008; 60(5):527–531.

15. McCarthy CM, Mehrara BJ, Riedel E, et al. Predicting complications following expander/implant breast reconstruction: an outcomes analysis based on preoperative clinical risk. *Plast Reconstr Surg.* 2008;121(6):1886–1892.

16. Nahabedian MY, Tsangaris T, Momen B, et al. Infectious complications following breast reconstruction with expanders and implants. *Plast Reconstr Surg.* 2003;112(2): 467–476.

17. Antony AK, Mehrara BM, McCarthy CM, et al. Salvage of tissue expander in the setting of mastectomy flap necrosis: a 13-year experience using timed excision with continued expansion. *Plast Reconstr Surg.* 2009;124(2): 356–363.

18. Frassica DA, Zellars R. Radiation oncology: the year in review. *Curr Opin Oncol.* 2002;14(6):594–599.

19. Spear SL, Majidian A. Immediate breast reconstruction in two stages using textured, integrated-valve tissue expanders and breast implants: a retrospective review of 171 consecutive breast reconstructions from 1989 to 1996. *Plast Reconstr Surg.* 1998;101(1):53–63.

chapter 43

Autologous Breast Reconstruction

Joshua Fosnot, MD / Joseph M. Serletti, MD, FACS

● INTRODUCTION

Breast cancer is a devastating disease which will affect one out of every eight women in their lifetime, sometimes at a young age. Although frequent, the disease is often curable; thus, most women live many years following treatment for their breast cancer. To avoid the debilitating psychosocial and aesthetic effects of mastectomy, an increasing number of women elect for reconstruction of a breast mound either at the time of mastectomy or in a delayed fashion. There are many options for breast reconstruction, utilizing either alloplastic materials or autologous tissue. Expander/implant reconstruction by far remains the most common method for reconstruction; however, autologous reconstruction has increased as methods for transferring the tissue evolve to reduce donor site morbidity and improve outcomes. In this chapter, we explore the various methods of autologous tissue reconstruction and discuss the relative risks and benefits of each in an effort to present the breadth of options to restore a woman's sense of self following treatment for breast cancer.

● PATIENT EVALUATION AND SELECTION

A breast cancer patient may seek information regarding reconstruction from a plastic surgeon at different stages in the treatment of her disease with varying levels of understanding of the types of reconstruction available. Breast reconstruction demands an open dialogue with regard to all of the patient's options with associated risks and benefits regardless of what the surgeon is most capable of or what his or her preferred method of reconstruction is. It is important to listen to the patient's wishes and expectations and formulate a plan for moving forward. This is paramount to avoiding untoward outcomes and disappointment with the final result.

Three types of reconstruction are available to the majority of patients: an implant-based reconstruction, autologous tissue reconstruction, or a combination of the two methods. Implant reconstruction has the advantage of being a quicker procedure, shorter recovery, and avoids an additional surgical site. For the right patient, it can offer an excellent result with minimal morbidity. Implant-based reconstructions, however, have risks associated with implant malfunction, such as infection, capsular contracture, and rupture. In addition, it can be risky in patients who have a history of or will require postmastectomy radiation.

Autologous tissue reconstruction, on the other hand, avoids the complications of implants and offers the unique ability to replace "like with like." This may lead to improved overall patient satisfaction in many patients. In addition, autologous reconstruction may be particularly beneficial in unilateral reconstruction in which the reconstructed breast will behave much more like the contralateral native breast over an implant-based reconstruction. The reconstruction has the potential to be lifelong. Despite these benefits, there are risks associated with tissue reconstruction.

Risk Factors for Poor Outcomes

Patient comorbidities play a critical role in the likelihood of complications postoperatively and should be recognized prior to undertaking any operation. Most notably, smoking and obesity have repetitively been implicated as independent risk factors for wound complications, such as wound infection, mastectomy flap necrosis, abdominal flap necrosis, and fat necrosis.[1,2] These risk factors are particularly detrimental in pedicled transverse rectus abdominis myocutaneous (TRAM) flap reconstruction and are generally considered relative contraindications to this procedure.

While not necessarily an absolute contraindication, a hypercoagulable state places a patient at higher risk for thrombosis during free or pedicled flap autologous reconstruction. Patients should be asked specifically about a history of deep venous thrombosis, pulmonary embolism, or genetic diseases such as factor V Leiden. Although no studies definitively support the practice, if patients are willing to accept an increased risk of flap failure and wish to proceed, more aggressive anticoagulation should be considered postoperatively.

Prior surgical history is important to ensure the pedicle of interest or recipient site has not been sacrificed. This is particularly true for abdominal incisions, which may have transected the epigastric artery or vein. A previous subcostal incision almost certainly transected the superior epigastric vessels, making this an absolute contraindication for a pedicled TRAM, whereas an inguinal hernia or paramedian incision may have transected the inferior vessels making a free TRAM based on the pedicle on that side impossible. A prior coronary artery bypass graft (CABG) may make the internal mammary vessels unavailable for recipients of a free flap. In addition, a common CABG conduit is the internal mammary artery, in which case a pedicled TRAM is contraindicated.

As with any major operation, patients should be counseled on the risks of medical complications, including, but not limited to, heart attack, stroke, and pulmonary embolism. Proper patient selection plays a role in minimizing these risks.

Adjuvant Therapy

Although many women with breast cancer undergo chemotherapy, it does not appear to play a significant role in increasing complications in breast reconstruction.[1] It is prudent, however, to avoid operations while on chemotherapy to allow for normal wound healing. Radiation therapy, on the other hand, can have a significant deleterious effect on autologous reconstruction. The use of radiation therapy for the treatment of breast cancer is increasing and while plastic surgeons have no control over its utilization, they do have control over the timing of reconstruction in relation to radiation therapy. Whether administered before or after reconstruction, radiation therapy leads to decreased overall aesthetic outcomes.[3] Fat necrosis, volume loss, and asymmetry are also more likely in flaps that are subsequently irradiated. Although there is some literature to suggest that radiation field design may be compromised by breast reconstruction, to date there are no reports of higher recurrence rates or worse oncologic outcomes in women who receive adjuvant radiation therapy after breast reconstruction.[3] Although aesthetically patients may benefit from delaying reconstruction until after any radiation therapy is complete, this must be balanced with the ability to forgo a second major operation with immediate reconstruction. Ultimately, this is only accomplished between open dialogue between patient and surgeon.

● PATIENT PREPARATION

Imaging

Little in the way of preoperative imaging is necessary prior to proceeding for reconstruction, although this statement is admittedly controversial in perforator flaps. Some authors conclude that preoperative Doppler or CT angiogram is important to identify the perforator vessels when performing a deep inferior epigastric perforator (DIEP) flap.[4] While imaging may make the surgeon more comfortable that a large perforator is available and in the end may shorten operating room time, it is unclear whether the added risk and expense of a contrast enhanced CT has any significant impact on patient outcome or overall expenditure.

Timing

Breast reconstruction may be performed at the same time as mastectomy, or at a later date in delayed fashion. While delayed reconstruction generally should not be performed until several months following mastectomy, there is no temporal limit. In fact, many patients opt for reconstruction 10 or 15 years following cancer treatment. The benefit of immediate reconstruction is multifactorial. First, the native skin envelope can be preserved if the oncologic surgeon is comfortable performing a skin-sparing mastectomy. As a result, the flap skin needed is often only a small, natural-appearing circle used to replace the lost nipple-areola complex. Second, the native skin tends to be more pliable and predictable than that used in delayed reconstruction where new skin flaps are raised from a previously operated, often irradiated field. Due to the resultant discrepancy of skin quality between sides in a unilateral delayed reconstruction, there is a tendency for asymmetry in the long term. Third, symmetry is easier to obtain due to the unaltered native inframammary fold position in immediate reconstruction. In delayed reconstruction, the new inframammary fold must be approximated either by comparison to the contralateral breast, or by the impression left by a well-fitting brassiere. While usually this does not result in any noticeable problems, this does introduce more unpredictability. Lastly, immediate reconstruction allows for completion of two major operations at one time. This efficiency should not be minimized as breast cancer patients often navigate a long journey to complete their treatment. In the end, whether immediate or delayed, long-term outcomes remain excellent.

Operative Planning

Regardless of type of autologous reconstruction performed, several general principles apply. Anatomical landmarks are more easily recognized when a patient is awake and mobile (rather than under drapes). For this reason, marking of the patient for flap design should be done in the preoperative holding area prior to induction of general anesthesia. The width of the flap should be estimated to allow for tension-free donor site closure, yet provide adequate volume.

When asleep, the patient should receive a Foley catheter for monitoring of adequate urine output during these sometimes long procedures. Preoperative antibiotics should be administered within one hour of incision, and may require repeat dosing intraoperatively if the case is prolonged. Antibiotics have been shown to decrease wound infections when used in this manner.

● TECHNIQUE

Latissimus Dorsi Myocutaneous Flap

The latissimus flap was one of the autologous flaps originally described for breast reconstruction. Although it has largely been replaced by lower abdominal island-based flaps for routine reconstruction, it remains an excellent option for breast reconstruction. In particular, in salvage situations where a previous flap was lost, it serves as a reliable and hardy alternative. Due to lack of volume, this flap is often paired with an implant whereby the flap provides a skin envelope and the implant provides the volume. This approach also serves well in delayed reconstruction to an irradiated field in which skin area is needed for coverage.

A skin island can be designed over almost any portion of the muscle; however, skin overlying the most inferior portions of the muscle may be problematic due to compromised blood supply. For breast reconstruction, the skin island is usually placed in a transverse orientation over the superior aspect of the muscle. This allows for the donor scar to be potentially hidden by an overlying back of a brassiere or by the back of a two-piece bathing suit.

In both immediate and delayed reconstruction, surgery may begin with the patient in either the supine or decubitus position. In delayed reconstruction, the chest wall skin is elevated off of the pectoralis muscle to redefine the perimeter of the breast pocket. The flap's skin island is incised, and skin flaps are elevated to expose the needed boundaries of the latissimus muscle. The lateral thoracic skin is elevated so as to create a subcutaneous tunnel between the latissimus dissection and the mastectomy defect (Figure 43-1). In most patients, the thoracodorsal vessels do not need to be dissected, and the insertion of the muscle is left intact. Some surgeons prefer to divide the motor nerve so as to avoid potential motion of the breast reconstruction with shoulder movement. In delayed reconstructions, the thoracodorsal vessels may have been previously injured from the axillary dissection. Despite division of these vessels, the latissimus dorsi is believed to remain reliable through retrograde flow by its serratus branches. In cases of delayed reconstruction, the latissimus muscle should be examined preoperatively. Absence of motor activity within the muscle should raise suspicion about the patency of the thoracodorsal vessels. Flap viability in these patients should be ensured during surgery; questionable viability may require microsurgical intervention to establish a more profound blood supply. When an implant is used, it is placed underneath the pectoralis and latissimus muscles.

Pedicled Transverse Rectus Abdominis Myocutaneous Flap

The transfer of a lower abdominal skin island is the most common method of autologous breast reconstruction, whether as a pedicled TRAM, free TRAM, DIEP, or superficial inferior epigastric artery (SIEA) flap. Considering all alloplastic and autologous methods, most surgeons agree that the abdominal tissue is unmatched in its ability to create a soft, pliable, and natural breast mound with excellent potential for symmetry to an intact opposite breast.

The superior rectus blood supply is provided by the superior epigastric vessels, which are terminal branches of the internal mammary vessels. The inferior muscle is supplied by the inferior epigastric vessels, which originate from the external iliacs. These two systems anastomose with each other through choke vessels within the center of the muscle. The entire muscle can, therefore, be elevated on either blood supply. The overlying skin and adipose tissue within the transverse skin island of the TRAM flap receives its blood supply from perforating vessels through the rectus abdominis muscle. The skin island in the pedicled TRAM flap is based on the superior epigastric vessels as it is transferred to the chest defect.

For a standard lower transverse abdominal based flap, the upper border of the flap is typically 1 to 2 cm above the umbilicus, the lower border close to the pubic hairline, but no lower than what will allow easy closure. Typically, the resultant flap is a standard ellipse (Figure 43-2). The midline should be marked from sternum to pubis to aid in symmetrical closure. The skin island is viewed as four separate zones or quadrants based on its attachment to one vascular pedicle. Zone 1, directly overlying the rectus muscle and vascular pedicle, is the area of greatest perfusion; however, the adjacent zones 2 and 3 are generally reliable for adequate perfusion and subsequent survival. The zone furthest from the muscle (zone 4) is usually unreliable and is discarded before insetting a pedicled TRAM flap.

The pedicled TRAM flap begins with the elevation of the skin superior to the TRAM skin island. A subcutaneous tunnel is created between the abdominal dissection and the mastectomy defect. This tunnel is kept as medial as possible to maintain a significant portion of the inframammary fold, but large enough to allow passage of the TRAM skin island. The skin island can be pedicled on one rectus abdominis muscle or two. A vertical anterior sheath fasciotomy allows for expose of the upper rectus muscle of interest. In preparing the skin island for transfer, all attachments except those of the skin island to the rectus muscle(s) are divided. Whether designed as a unipedicled flap or as a bipedicled flap, some surgeons harvest the entire muscle(s); whereas, others preserve a lateral and medial band of muscle, harvesting only central

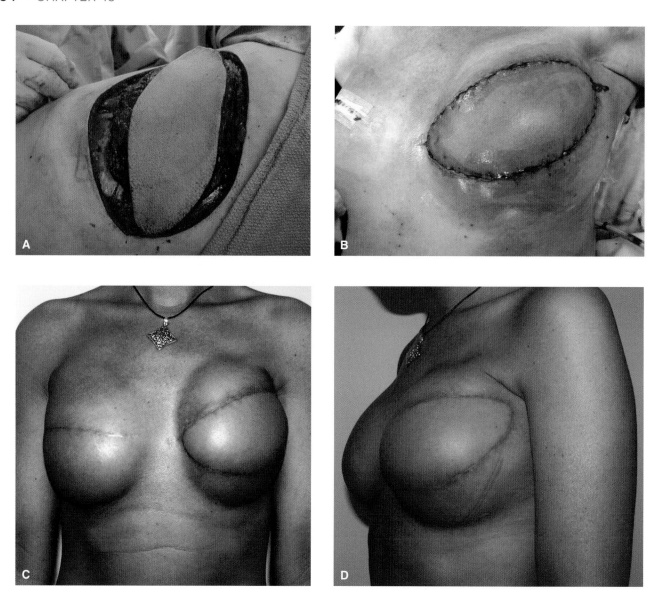

● FIGURE 43-1. This patient underwent bilateral mastectomy with tissue expander/implant reconstruction. On the left, she had been previously irradiated requiring excision of a larger island of skin, thus a latissimus flap was used to cover the prosthesis. (A) The flap is elevated on oblique angle and brought through a lateral subcutaneous tunnel into (B) the mastectomy defect. (C, D) Postoperative result following exchange to implants.

or medial portions of the rectus muscle (Figure 43-3). By definition, a section of the anterior rectus fascia is taken as part of the specimen. In high-risk patients, alterations to technique for the pedicled TRAM flap can be used to augment the blood supply to the skin island. These alterations include a bipedicle blood supply whereby both rectus muscles are harvested. Alternatively, the pedicled TRAM flap can be "supercharged" by dissecting lengths of the inferior epigastric vessels and anastomosing them to the thoracodorsal vessels. To improve abdominal donor site results, muscle-sparing techniques have been used to preserve some muscle and fascia. Once the flap is transferred to the chest, the abdominal wall defect is closed. Onlay and inlay mesh can be used to reinforce

the abdominal wall closure. The lower abdominal skin defect is closed by mobilizing the upper abdominal skin flap inferiorly. The previously separated umbilicus is re-inset into the anterior abdominal skin of the superior skin flap. After closure of the abdominal site is complete, the patient is placed in the sitting position, and the TRAM skin island is trimmed and contoured to match the opposite breast.

Free Transverse Rectus Abdominis Myocutaneous Flap

Although pedicled TRAM reconstruction is still quite common, free flap reconstruction has become

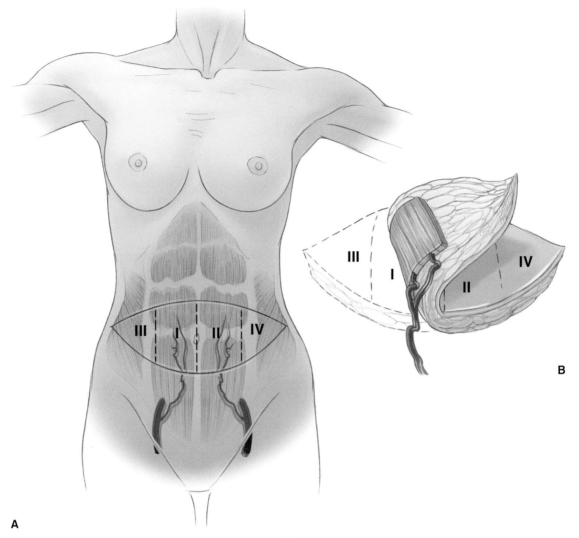

● **FIGURE 43-2.** (A) The typical design of a TRAM flap is elliptical in shape and includes around the umbilicus although the height is dependent on the relative skin and soft tissue laxity of the abdomen. Sometimes a more elliptical design is used (shown by the *dotted line*). (B) The TRAM flap is broken into four vascular zones of perfusion. Zone 1 is the most reliable, lying directly over the vascular pedicle.

increasingly popular. Whereas the pedicled TRAM flap is based on the superior epigastric vessels, the free TRAM flap is based on the deep inferior epigastric vessels. In a pedicled TRAM, the primary portion of the skin island is in the second angiosome, receiving blood via "choke" vessels in the muscle. The TRAM flap island is in the primary angiosome of the inferior epigastric blood supply giving the free TRAM a more robust blood supply. Patients with a history of smoking, hypertension, obesity, chronic obstructive pulmonary disease, previous abdominal surgery, and even diabetes have been considered high-risk patients in regard to the pedicled TRAM flap. The improved blood supply and more limited donor site defect achieved with the free TRAM flap technique has allowed TRAM flap breast reconstruction in these higher-risk patients with acceptable complication rates.[5,6] Insetting of the free TRAM flap is easier and less restrictive as compared to the pedicled flap.

The upper edge of the TRAM skin island is incised, and an upper abdominal flap is raised to the xiphoid and the costal margins in similar fashion to the pedicled TRAM; however, the upper abdominal fascia is not incised. The lower portion of the skin island is then incised. The lateral portion of the skin island closest to the selected muscle is elevated to the first row of lateral perforators, and the fascia is incised. A muscle-splitting dissection is performed, and the inferior epigastric vessels are identified and dissected to the external iliac vessels. There is usually a single inferior epigastric vein at this level or a large vein with a smaller counterpart entering the external iliac vein. A decision as to whether to use an ipsilateral or contralateral free flap has usually been made preoperatively, based on the shape of the contralateral breast and the choice of recipient vessels.

The opposite side of the skin island is elevated to the first row of medial perforators exiting from the selected

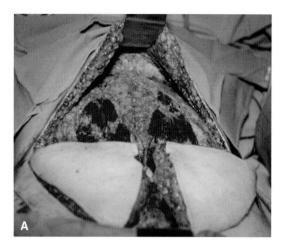

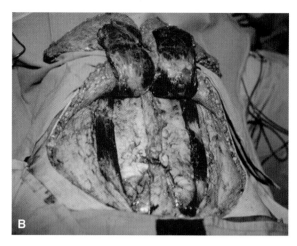

● **FIGURE 43-3.** This patient underwent a bilateral pedicle TRAM breast reconstruction. (A) Dissection of each hemi flap and the corresponding superior pedicle. (B) Note that this is a muscle sparing procedure in which neither rectus muscle is completely sacrificed. (C) The flaps are transferred up to the chest via subcutaneous tunnels medially. (*Photos courtesy of M. Nahabedian, MD.*)

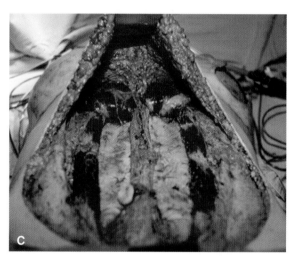

muscle. This maneuver separates the skin island from the vasculature of the opposite rectus. The anterior rectus fascia is incised here, and a medial muscle-splitting dissection is performed. The flap is now ready for division and transfer (Figure 43-4). The vascular anastomosis and inset of the flap is discussed later in this chapter. After the tissue is harvested, a fascial defect remains in the lower abdominal wall. This is typically repaired by primary closure and either onlay or inlay mesh. The abdominal donor site is closed in a manner similar to that of an aesthetic abdominoplasty.

Deep Inferior Epigastric Perforator Flap

The DIEP flap uses the same skin island as described above, but does not sacrifice any of the rectus muscle or anterior rectus fascia. The muscle fibers are temporarily splayed apart to allow for removal of the inferior epigastric vessels and selected perforators. Criticisms of both pedicled and free TRAM flaps have mostly centered on the abdominal wall donor site. The DIEP offers one technical variation that minimizes donor site morbidity.[7] Proponents of this technique suggest that it results in less postoperative pain, a shorter hospitalization, a more

prompt recovery with little or no functional deficit in the abdominal donor site. Because this flap relies on one or two perforators, it may be less suitable for high-risk patients.

Upon selecting the right or left side, the lateral edge of the ipsilateral part of the skin island is elevated off of the fascia. Using loupe magnification and atraumatic technique, the surgeon identifies an acceptably large perforator (or perforators). The anterior rectus fascia is incised above the perforator for a short distance and below it to just above the inguinal region. The fascia is reflected off of the muscle in a lateral direction. The muscle is splayed for a short distance around the perforator, identifying its connection to the inferior epigastric system. The lateral edge of the muscle is elevated off of the posterior rectus sheath for further identification and dissection of the inferior epigastric vessels. Care is taken to maintain all of the intercostal motor nerve supply to the rectus muscle. After completion of the flap dissection, the inferior epigastric vessels are divided proximally and passed through the opening in the muscle at the level of the perforator. The flap is separated from its remaining attachments to the abdominal wall and passed to the chest for anastomosis and inset. The incision in the anterior rectus fascia

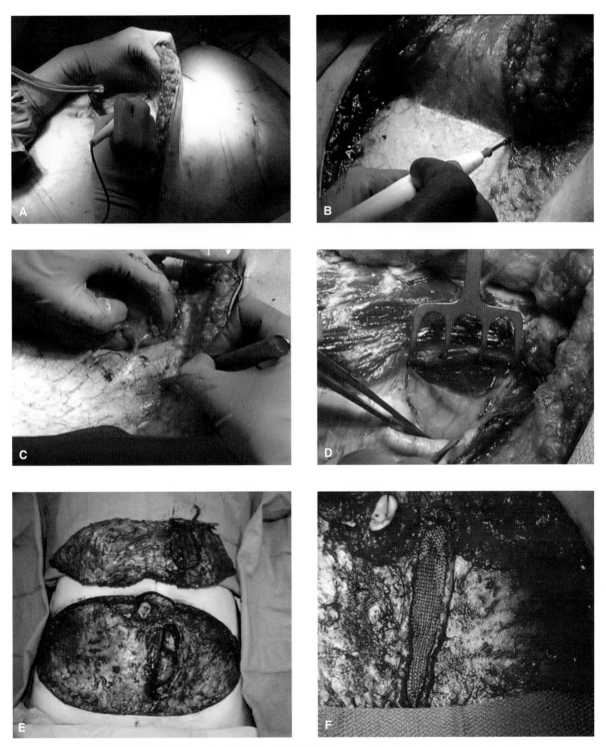

● **FIGURE 43-4.** In a standard free TRAM (A) the superior abdominal flap is raised starting from the superior aspect of the TRAM flap. This will eventually allow for closure of the donor site defect. (B) The lateral aspects of the TRAM flap are raised up until the lateral row of perforators. (C) A fasciotomy is made above and below the perforators. (D) The inferior epigastric pedicle is identified and the rectus muscle is sacrificed in a manner which allows for inclusion of the perforators and vascular pedicle. In most cases, some of the muscle is spared. (E) The resultant flap is shown with muscle and pedicle included. (F) The donor site fascial defect is closed in this case with mesh for added strength. The flap is then ready for anastomosis and inset.

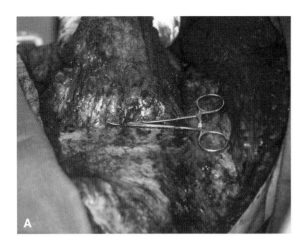

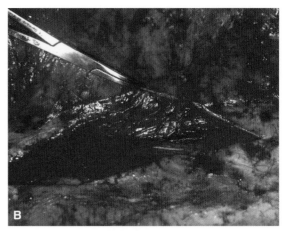

● FIGURE 43-5. (A) In a DIEP flap, the perforators are identified individually to assess the adequacy of their caliber for reliable perfusion. (B) The fasciotomy is made above and below the perforator(s) of interest. The perforators are followed down through the muscle to the deep inferior epigastric vessels without sacrificing any muscle. (C) The resultant flap carries with it no attached muscle and the patient is left with an intact functional rectus muscle.

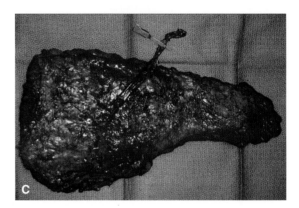

is closed directly, without the need for mesh, and the entire muscle with its nerve supply has been preserved (Figure 43-5).

Superficial Inferior Epigastric Artery Flap

In a small percentage of patients, the superficial inferior epigastric vessels are sufficient in caliber to support half of the transverse lower abdominal flap. The benefit lies in the very nature of the size and location of these extrafascial vessels. The dissection does not violate the fascia or muscle of the abdominal wall, leading to decreased donor site morbidity.[8] The downsides include increased vascular complications such as thrombosis and fat necrosis, as well as limited flap size.[9] Generally, a hemiflap is all that is available for inset given the angiosome distribution of the superficial inferior epigastric vasculature. In addition, the angiosome distribution of the SIEA appears to be highly variable such that simple inspection of the caliber of the vessel may be inadequate to reliably predict a dependable outcome.[10]

The patient is marked and the case started in the same fashion as the free TRAM or DIEP. The superficial vessels, if present, are encountered via the inferior flap incision at the midpoint between the anterior superior iliac spine and pubic tubercle in the subcutaneous tissue (Figure 43-6). If it appears that these vessels will be

large enough, the dissection is carried inferiorly to their origin at the superficial femoral vessels roughly 2 to 3 cm below the inguinal ligament. The flap dissection is then carried out by harvesting the typical lower abdominal ellipse of tissue without violating the fascia. The vessel origins are then taken and the flap is ready for anastomosis and insetting.

Superior Gluteal Flap

Many patients either do not have sufficient abdominal tissue or have had prior abdominal surgery such as an abdominoplasty or previous TRAM, effectively eliminating the option of a subsequent TRAM for reconstruction. In these circumstances, a gluteal flap is an excellent choice. A significant advantage of this technique is the more rapid recovery and decreased postoperative discomfort in comparison with the TRAM flap. Unfortunately, the adipose tissue in the gluteal flap is more septate and less pliable than in both the native breast and the TRAM flap which makes insetting more challenging, and the final result is somewhat firmer than most natural breasts.

The free superior gluteal myocutaneous flap is based on the superior gluteal vasculature to the gluteus maximus muscle and its overlying skin. With the patient in the decubitus or prone position, a line is drawn from the

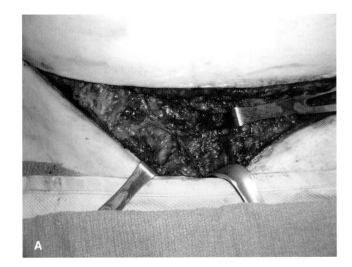

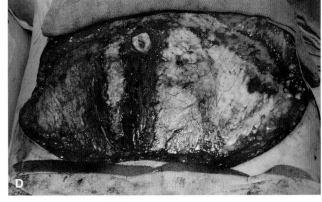

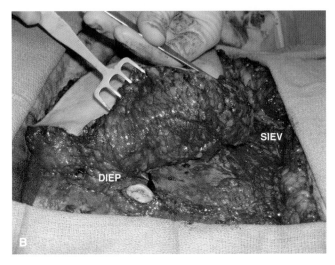

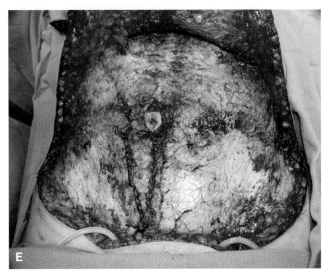

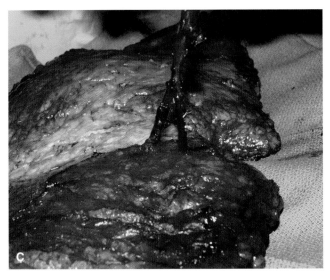

● **FIGURE 43-6.** (A) The superficial inferior epigastric vessels are encountered with minimal dissection in the subcutaneous fat of the inferior flap margin. (B) In this left hemiflap, either the DIEP perforators or the superficial inferior epigastric vessels could be used to support the free flap. Note that the superficial inferior epigastric vessels stay extrafascial, whereas the DIEPs perforate the fascia. The DIEP vessels can be temporarily clamped to ensure the flap is viable via the SIEA. (C) The flap is taken as an SIEA with excellent pedicle length. (D) This patient ultimately underwent bilateral reconstruction with a muscle-sparing free TRAM on the contralateral side. Note the difference between the left and right sides upon completion of flap harvest. (E) The right TRAM requires fascial closure, the left SIEA does not.

posterior superior iliac spine to the top of the greater trochanter. Dividing that line into thirds, the superior gluteal pedicle is located near the junction of the superior and middle thirds. The skin island can be centered along this oblique line or may be rotated to a more horizontal position overlying the upper portion of the gluteus maximus

muscle. As patient positioning generally does not allow access to the contralateral breast during flap harvest, the dimensions of the contralateral breast should be appreciated prior to positioning to help guide the size of the flap needed for symmetry. The superior and inferior edges of the skin island are incised and skin flaps are subsequently raised, leaving an appropriate amount of adipose tissue attached to the muscle for volume. The superior edge of the gluteus maximus is identified and elevated off of the gluteus medius. Dissection then follows to the lateral margin of the muscle as it heads toward the greater trochanter. The lateral muscle here is divided. The superior gluteal vessels are identified on the undersurface of the gluteus maximus and are followed to their origin off of the internal iliacs. This origin is approximately 5 cm lateral to the sacral edge between the gluteus medius and the piriformis muscle. Because the vessels here are fragile, it is imperative that they are dissected carefully. A pedicle length of 2 to 3 cm is typically obtained. The lower edge of the flap with its attached muscle is incised and the gluteus maximus muscle is divided at that level. The vessels are divided, as are the remaining soft tissue attachments to the flap. While the donor site is being closed, the flap is taken to the side table for further dissection to gain pedicle length. The patient is returned to the full supine position for flap anastomosis and inset. Due to the short pedicle length, the internal mammary vessels are preferred, allowing for medial placement of this tissue. Some surgeons regularly use vein grafts with this flap to overcome the difficulties with the short pedicle.

The superior gluteal flap can also be harvested as a perforator flap. Analogous to muscle preservation in the DIEP flap, all of the gluteus maximus muscle is preserved in the superior gluteal artery perforator flap. One or more perforators from this system to the skin can be identified just lateral to the origin of the superior gluteal vessels. The upper and lower edges of the skin paddle are prepared just as in the gluteal flap. Beginning at the lateral edge of the skin island, a subfascial dissection is performed until an acceptable perforator is identified. The muscle fibers are splayed, and the perforator is dissected away from its muscle attachments to where it joins a major muscle branch of the superior gluteal vessels. This major muscle branch is followed proximally to the main gluteal vessels which are then divided as close to the origin as possible. All other attachments of the skin island to the muscle are divided, and the flap is passed to the chest for anastomosis and inset.

The perforator flap leads to a considerably longer pedicle length, upward of 6 cm. This makes performing the anastomosis more straightforward than the standard free gluteal flap procedure. Without the bulk of the muscle, insetting the flap is easier and the intraoperative result more closely mimics the matured postoperative result of a standard gluteal flap procedure. Preserving all of the gluteus maximus muscle has significant functional considerations and leaves a less depressed contour deformity in comparison to the gluteal flap.

Inferior Gluteal Flap

The inferior gluteal flap is a myocutaneous flap based on the inferior gluteal blood supply to the gluteus maximus muscle. The skin island is transversely positioned over the lower half of the gluteus maximus muscle, ending just above the gluteal crease. The skin and muscle are elevated to expose the inferior gluteal vessels, which are the terminal branches of the internal iliacs. This inferiorly designed flap has the advantage of a somewhat longer vascular pedicle but the disadvantage of a more conspicuous donor deformity and scar. Harvesting this flap also usually divides the posterior femoral cutaneous nerve, leaving an area of numbness on the posterior aspect of the thigh. Although there are varying opinions, the majority of surgeons choose the superior gluteal flap over the inferior design as their first choice when a free TRAM flap cannot be used. The inferior gluteal flap can be achieved as a perforator flap as well (Figure 43-7).

Lateral Thigh Flap

The lateral thigh flap is a laterally oriented modification of the free tensor fascia lata myocutaneous flap. This flap is specifically designed to take advantage of excess tissue in the upper lateral thigh for breast reconstruction. A transverse skin island is harvested with the underlying tensor fascia lata. The pedicle to this flap is composed of the lateral femoral circumflex vessels, which can be dissected back to the profundus for a pedicle length of 6 to 8 cm. Patients selected for this technique must have sufficient soft tissue in the upper thigh and generally speaking, this method is considered only if a TRAM or gluteal flap is not available.

Rubens Flap

The Rubens flap, or deep circumflex iliac soft tissue flap, is a variation of the deep circumflex iliac artery or iliac crest flap but without the bone. There can be significant redundant skin and adipose tissue overlying the iliac crest. This soft tissue is supplied by perforating branches of the deep circumflex iliac vessel. A transverse skin island overlying the iliac crest is designed and the circumflex iliac vessels are approached as in the free iliac crest flap. Instead of bone being taken, a subperiosteal dissection is performed, capturing the perforating vessels to the skin. This flap provides a moderate amount of soft tissue with a reliable vascular pedicle. This flap has particular usefulness when the TRAM flap has already been used, since this lateral tissue is often preserved.

Transverse Upper Gracilis Flap

In addition to the lateral thigh and Rubens flaps, the TUG flap is an excellent option for autologous breast reconstruction in patients who are not candidates for transverse lower abdominal based flaps. Here, an upper inner thigh flap based upon the medial femoral circumflex vessels is oriented transversely, with the widest portion directly over the gracilis muscle. The patient is placed in the supine position with legs abducted and knees slightly bent. The anterior portion of the flap is dissected first, superficial to the fascia of the thigh muscles.

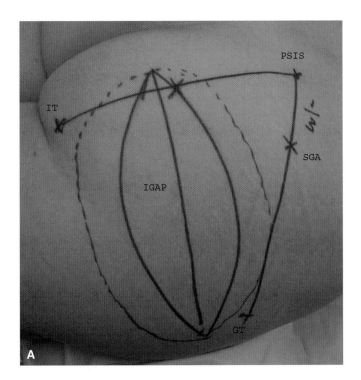

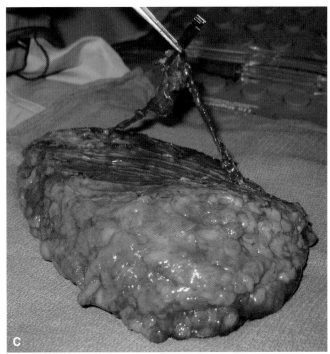

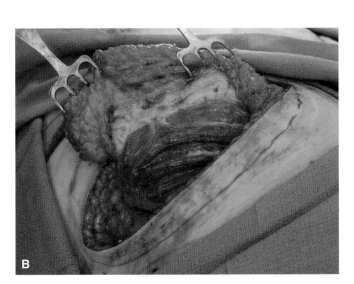

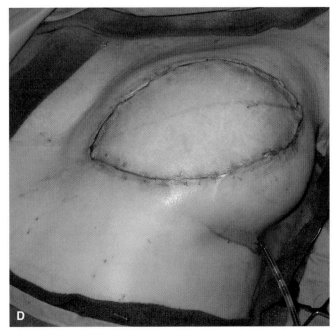

● **FIGURE 43-7.** (A) Depicted are the standard landmarks in a gluteal flap. The superior gluteal artery (SGA) is dopplerable roughly one third the distance between the posterior superior iliac spine (PSIS) and the greater tuberosity (GT). Depicted here is the typical transverse flap design of an inferior gluteal artery perforator flap which is more inferiorly positioned, closer to the ischeal tuberosity (IT). (B) Several perforators are visible entering this inferior gluteal artery perforator flap. (C) The flap is taken with two large perforators, converging to the inferior gluteal artery pedicle. (D) The IGAP flap is shown following anastomosis and inset.

Upon reaching the adductor longus, the fascia is incised allowing for exposure of the gracilis pedicle under the adductor longus muscle. At this point, the posterior end of the flap can be elevated and the gracilis can be divided proximally and distally. The vascular pedicle can be further dissected if needed for length. The pedicle is generally 5 to 6 cm and insetting of the flap provides excellent contour due to the crescent shape of the flap. In addition, this flap offers a simultaneous inner thigh lift as the donor site is closed (Figure 43-8).

Recipient Site and Insetting

The axilla is fairly well exposed during a modified radical mastectomy making the thoracodorsal system useful as a recipient site; however, in most circumstances, the internal mammary vessels have become the primary recipient site for free flap breast reconstruction. Outcomes between the two recipient sites have proven to be similar and the internal mammary site allows for more medial positioning of the flap, leading to improved symmetry and

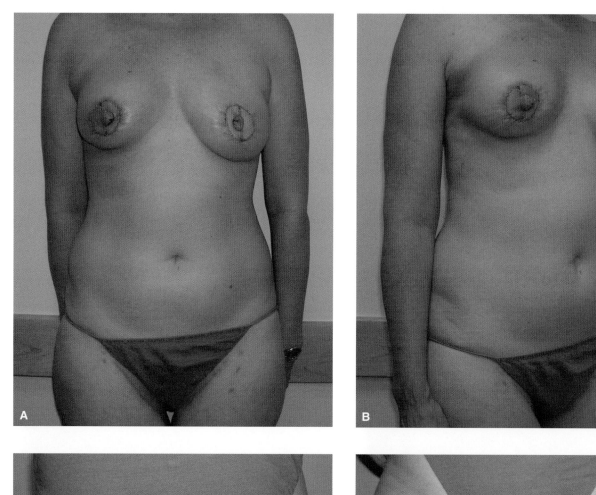

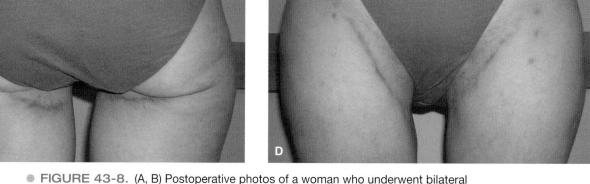

● **FIGURE 43-8.** (A, B) Postoperative photos of a woman who underwent bilateral autologous breast reconstruction using transverse upper gracilis flaps. In this photo, this patient had also undergone recent bilateral nipple-areola reconstruction, but has yet to undergo tattooing. (C, D) The donor site is fairly inconspicuous and offers the benefit of a bilateral medial thigh lift. (*Photos courtesy of Liza C. Wu, MD.*)

aesthetics.[11] In addition, using the internal mammary site avoids having to access the axilla in a simple mastectomy and avoids the risk of injury in cases where reoperating in the axilla for further nodal resection is possible at a later date. The internal mammary system also requires less pedicle length compared to the thoracodorsal, which is particularly helpful in short pedicles such as those found in either the superior or inferior gluteal flaps.

The internal mammary vessels can be approached through a rib-sparing or rib-harvesting procedure. For a rib-sparing procedure, the intercostal space, typically between the third and fourth, is identified. The overlying pectoralis major muscle is split and the intercostal muscle is removed. The internal mammary vessels are found immediately under the intercostal muscles overlying the pleura. In a rib harvesting procedure, the pectoralis muscle overlying the third or fourth costal cartilage is split and the rib is exposed. The perichondrium is incised along the midanterior surface from the junction of the sternum to the costochondral junction. The perichondrium is separated off of the cartilage anteriorly and 2 to 3 cm of costal cartilage is removed with a rongeur. Next, the posterior perichondrium is incised lateral to the internal mammary vessel and reflected lateral to medial. The vessels are found immediately posterior to the perichondrium above the pleura. In both techniques, care must be taken to avoid transection of the small intercostal vessel branches coming off of the internal mammary system. Once the vessels are identified and separated from the internal mammary lymphatics, the length of dissection is increased by harvesting additional rib or intercostal muscles superiorly or inferiorly. Compared with most other recipient vessels throughout the body, the internal mammary artery is more susceptible to injury and thrombosis during its dissection. Minimal use of vascular forceps is recommended. The internal mammary vein tends to be larger on the right side than on the left side. The free flap is temporarily positioned to allow easy performance of the anastomoses. The artery and vein are typically handsewn with 8-0 or 9-0 nylon. The coupler device can be used on the vein as an alternative (Figure 43-9). Following completion of the vascular anastomoses, the flap is inset by closing in multiple layers.

Nipple-Areola Reconstruction

Following re-creation of the breast mound with autologous breast reconstruction, many women opt to undergo re-creation of the nipple-areola complex as a final step in restoring body image. Techniques employed in the past have included grafting from skin, buccal mucosa, labia minora or majora, thigh, buttocks, groin, upper eyelids, or earlobes. Although the technique varies, the principles remain the same: to provide color, texture, size, and projection which are all in line with the patient's aesthetic wishes. The most common method used today consists of local skin flap rearrangement to create texture and projection followed by tattooing for color (Figure 43-10).[12] Nipple-areola reconstruction in most cases is performed more than 3 to 4 months following mound reconstruction or after adjuvant therapy is completed. This allows for complete healing of the flap and ensures stable mound symmetry which is a key prerequisite prior to recreating a nipple-areola complex. Immediate nipple-areola re-creation at the time of flap has been reported but is by far less common. It should also be noted that although mastectomy has classically included excision of the native nipple-areola, there has been an increasing interest and study of the safety and efficacy of nipple-sparing mastectomy.

● COMPLICATIONS

A broad category of wound complications may arise, including seroma, delayed wound healing, hematoma, and mastectomy skin flap necrosis. As a whole, the noninfectious wound complications may be as high as 28% to 43%; however, the vast majority of time, these heal without intervention or long term sequelae.[6] Wound infection occurs 3.5% to 9.5% of the time but is usually limited to simple cellulitis easily treated with antibiotics. Vascular complications such as thrombosis or ischemia may lead to flap loss or fat necrosis; however, complete flap loss is rare. Close observation of these flaps is paramount in the immediate postoperative period as arterial or venous thrombosis can be salvaged with rapid surgical intervention.

Donor site morbidity is an unfortunate downside of autologous reconstruction not seen with expander/ implant reconstruction. Hernias may require reoperation for repair. In addition, following manipulation of the abdominal wall, many patients may experience a permanent decrease in abdominal wall strength.

● OUTCOMES ASSESSMENT

The mastectomy defect can be devastating both physically and psychologically. Numerous studies have documented significant improvement in self-confidence and mental health following breast reconstruction.[13] Although not routinely done, efforts to reestablish innervation to free flaps has been shown to improve patient satisfaction overall.[14] No one procedure outshines another in all circumstances; however, certain patients clearly benefit from careful procedural selection. In the end, the overall plan for reconstruction must be an open dialogue between surgeon and patient, one which ultimately involves listening and education.

Aesthetic complications should be discussed with the patient preoperatively. These include breast mound asymmetry, contour irregularities, contracture and volume loss related to radiation or fat necrosis, poor wound healing, and scaring. With proper planning, these setbacks can be ameliorated with revision surgery, reduction, implant augmentation and newer techniques such as fat grafting for contour irregularities. Proper counseling of patients preoperatively once again is imperative, as accurate expectations will most often yield the greatest patient satisfaction.

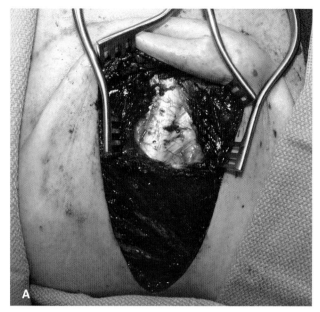

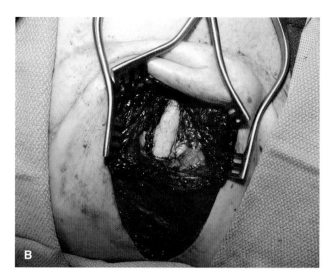

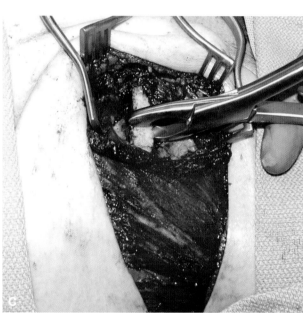

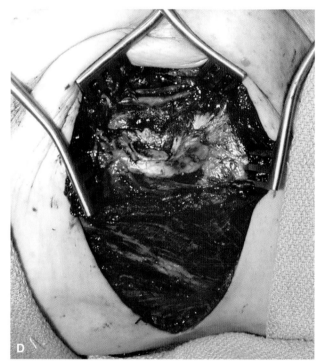

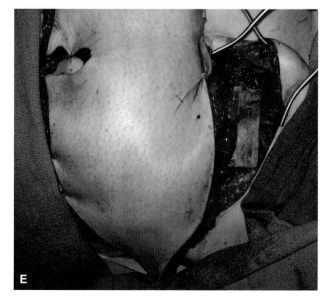

● **FIGURE 43-9.** (A) Shown here is the dissection of the third rib in preparation for exposure of the internal mammary vessels for a recipient site. The overlying pectoralis muscles are splayed apart to allow adequate exposure (B). (C) The perichondrium is incised to allow for removal of the costochondral junction. (D) Following removal, the internal mammary vessels are exposed. Further proximal and distal dissection is generally needed. (E) The flap is anastomosed in standard fashion.

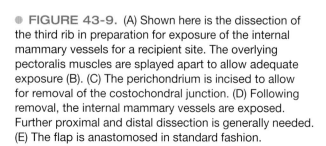

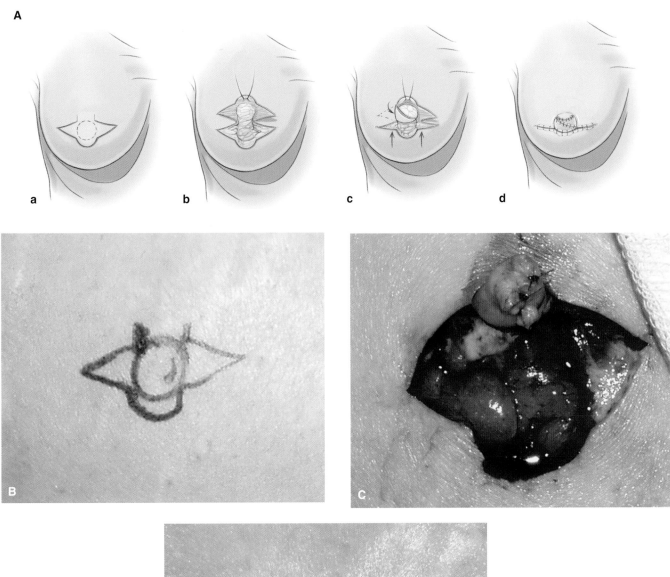

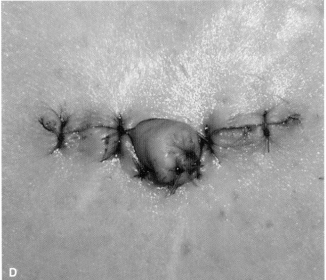

● **FIGURE 43-10.** (A, a–d) Schematic representation of the modified skate flap for nipple-areola reconstruction. The lateral "V" shaped flaps become the walls of the nipple projection, whereas the "C" shaped flap becomes the top. The dissection plane is deeper in the center to add bulk. The blood supply comes from the uncut superior pedicle. (B–D) The same skate flap shown on a typical patient. This is followed by tattooing for color.

● CONCLUSION

Autologous breast reconstruction can be performed using a wide variety of flaps which all offer the ability to reliably recreate a breast mound following mastectomy. This has the unique ability to replace "like with like" and although it is not free of complications, can be performed in a variety of settings with the expectation of excellent patient satisfaction.

REFERENCES

1. Selber JC, Kurichi JE, Vega SJ, Sonnad SS, Serletti JM. Risk factors and complications in free TRAM flap breast reconstruction. *Ann Plast Surg.* 2006;56(5):492–497.

2. Vyas RM, Dickinson BP, Fastekjian JH, Watson JP, Dalio AL, Crisera CA. Risk factors for abdominal donor-site morbidity in free flap breast reconstruction. *Plast Reconstr Surg.* 2008;121(5):1519–1526.

3. Kronowitz SJ, Robb GL. Radiation therapy and breast reconstruction: a critical review of the literature. *Plast Reconstr Surg.* 2009;124(2):395–408.

4. Masia J, Kosutic D, Clavero JA, Larranaga J, Vives L, Pons G. Preoperative computed tomographic angiogram for deep inferior epigastric artery perforator flap breast reconstruction. *J Reconstr Microsurg.* 2010;26(1):21–28.

5. Andrades P, Fix RJ, Danilla S, et al. Ischemic complications in pedicle, free, and muscle sparing transverse rectus abdominis myocutaneous flaps for breast reconstruction. *Ann Plast Surg.* 2008;60(5):562–567.

6. Mehrara BJ, Santoro TD, Arcilla E, Watson JP, Shaw WW, Da Lio AL. Complications after microvascular breast reconstruction: experience with 1195 flaps. *Plast Reconstr Surg.* 2006;118(5):1100–1109; discussion 1110–1111.

7. Man L-X, Selber JC, Serletti JM. Abdominal wall following free TRAM or DIEP flap reconstruction: a meta-analysis and critical review. *Plast Reconstr Surg.* 2009;124(3):752–764.

8. Wu LC, Bajaj A, Chang DW, Chevray PM. Comparison of donor-site morbidity of SIEA, DIEP, and muscle-sparing TRAM flaps for breast reconstruction. *Plast Reconstr Surg.* 2008;122(3):702–709.

9. Selber JC, Samra F, Bristol M, et al. A head-to-head comparison between the muscle-sparing free TRAM and the SIEA flaps: is the rate of flap loss worth the gain in abdominal wall function? *Plast Reconstr Surg.* 2008;122(2):348–355.

10. Holm C, Mayr M, Hofter E, Raab N, Ninkovic M. Interindividual variability of the SIEA angiosome: effects on operative strategies in breast reconstruction. *Plast Reconstr Surg.* 2008;122(16):1612–1620.

11. Saint-Cyr M, Youssef A, Bae HW, Robb GL, Chang DW. Changing trends in recipient vessel selection for microvascular autologous breast reconstruction: an analysis of 1483 consecutive cases. *Plast Reconstr Surg.* 2007;119(7): 1993–2000.

12. Farhadi J, Maksvytyte GK, Schaefer DJ, Pierer G, Scheufler O. Reconstruction of the nipple-areola complex: an update. *J Plast Reconstr Aesthet Surg.* 2006;59(1):40–53.

13. Alderman AK, Kuhn LE, Lowery JC, Wilkins EG. Does patient satisfaction with breast reconstruction change over time? Two-year results of the Michigan Breast Reconstruction Outcomes Study. *J Am Coll Surg.* 2007;204(1):7–12.

14. Temple CL, Ross DC, Kim S, et al. Sensibility following innervated free TRAM flap for breast reconstruction: Part II. Innervation improves patient-rated quality of life. *Plast Reconstr Surg.* 2009;124(5):1419–1425.

chapter 44

Reduction Mammaplasty

Michael N. Mirzabeigi, MD / Liza C. Wu, MD, FACS

● INTRODUCTION

Macromastia, or breast hypertrophy, can prove to be a troublesome condition for many women. Plastic surgeons are frequently called upon to provide the only known definitive treatment of macromastia, which is direct excision of tissue. Reduction mammaplasty (mammoplasty), otherwise known as breast reduction, serves to improve the aesthetics of the breast as well as alleviate functional sequelae that can result from excessive breast enlargement. This is achieved by generally targeting three goals for the patient: (1) reduce breast size, (2) improve breast shape, and (3) improve nipple-areola position. In order to safely achieve these goals, surgeons must carefully select patients who are appropriate candidates for surgery, and in a manner fitting for each patient, surgeons must select a suitable technique for reduction.

● PATIENT EVALUATION AND SELECTION

Symptoms

The etiology of this condition is believed to be secondary to an exaggerated response to circulating estrogen, progesterone, and/or prolactin. The resultant breast hypertrophy can lead to a litany of well documented problems. Patients often complain of musculoskeletal pain of the neck, shoulders, and back. Many patients may also present with intertriginous rash (eg, dermatitis or fungal growth) at the inframammary sulcus, painful shoulder grooving (secondary to pressure from the brassiere overlying the distribution of the trapezius muscle), and kyphosis. Furthermore, psychosocial issues can be prevalent in this patient population with concerns for self-image, confidence, ability to find properly fitting clothes, and sexual dysfunction.

Patient Selection

Reduction mammaplasty is ultimately elective surgery; therefore, patients should not have significant comorbidities which would place them at high risk for anesthetic complications. Otherwise, there are some more specific issues to be considered during the preoperative evaluation. First, patients should be strongly counseled to discontinue smoking for at least 1 month (some would suggest 3 months) prior to undergoing surgery or risk a higher rate of wound complications. Also, patients should be at an age in which the decision can be made autonomously and with full knowledge and understanding of the risks and benefits. Unless there is a compelling or profound disturbance caused by the macromastia, patients should wait until at least 18 years of age to ensure some level of stability in breast size, and moreover, to promote a properly informed decision by the patient.

Once it has been determined that a patient is an appropriate candidate for surgery, a concerted effort should be made in an attempt to assist the patient with the precertification of insurance coverage. This process varies depending on the insurance carrier; however, insurance companies have relatively predictable requests. First, the patient must demonstrate clinical macromastia via some estimation of resection volume or relative breast size as a function of body surface area. Many insurance carriers require documentation of symptoms, which is noted to be persistent over more than one office visit (eg, 6 months of documented symptoms). Oftentimes there is also a request to document a nonsurgical attempt to alleviate symptoms via weight loss programs and/or physical therapy. Among other reasons, these attempts often fail as macromastia can be largely independent of weight loss and pendulous breasts make exercise difficult.

Interestingly, it has recently been established that increased BMI and amount of tissue resection are risk factors for postoperative wound complications. As reduction mammaplasty can be an impetus for weight loss, these patients do not need to be discouraged from surgery; however, a higher rate of wound complications can be expected.

● PATIENT PREPARATION

Patients should undergo a thorough preoperative evaluation, in which it is important to ascertain as well as guide patient expectations. The preoperative evaluation consists of a comprehensive exploration of breast symptomology. Any personal or family history of breast cancer should be investigated. A thorough breast examination should also be performed. Any breast masses, nipple discharge, and skin changes should be noted. The shape, size, and consistency of the breast tissue should be examined. The most relevant measurements, such as the nipple to notch distance, should be recorded at this time.

Although preoperative brassiere size is often used as a measurement, it is unadvisable to make any strong prediction or speak in definitive terms regarding a final brassiere size. Manufacturers do not utilize a universal system, and even still, there is a variation of brassiere size choice amongst women with a similar breast size. Furthermore, the postoperative scarring that is to be expected of the procedure must be thoroughly discussed. For patients older than 40 years old, or those younger with a positive family history of breast cancer, a recent mammogram should be provided prior to surgery. Breast asymmetries are not uncommon, and can also be related to spinal curvature. Preoperative asymmetry, and the potential for a reasonable level of postoperative asymmetry, should be thoroughly explained.

The potential for loss of nipple sensation, one of the more concerning complications following reduction mammoplasty, should be discussed as well. Patients should be counseled that a minority of patients lose nipple sensation. It should also be stated there is a time-dependent component for a return to nipple sensitivity.

● TECHNIQUE

Anatomy

The redundant and multivector nature of the blood supply to the breast parenchyma and nipple-areola complex affords a diverse array of technique designs. Before choosing a technique for reduction, it is essential to have an understanding of the blood supply to the breast.

The dominant blood supply to the breast is supplied by perforating branches of the internal mammary artery (also known as the internal thoracic artery). In addition to the internal mammary perforators, there is a vascular supply from the pectoral branch of the thoracoacromial artery, lateral thoracic artery, and inferior mammary

arteries (branches of the anterior intercostals arteries). There is variation, particularly in the ancillary blood supply, and anatomic studies have demonstrated that the internal mammary system is the most reliable vascular supply.

Sensory innervation to the nipple-areola is provided primarily from the anterior and lateral rami of the 4th intercostal nerve. Additional innervation can be provided by 3rd and 5th intercostal nerves as well. In more recent literature, important fibrous and ligamentous structures of the breast have been described by Wuringer. These suspensions have been increasingly discussed in the literature as they can be used to locate important neurovasculature to the breast. Wuringer horizontal septum, arises from the pectoral fascia at the 4th and 5th rib, traveling perpendicular from the chest wall to the nipple-areola complex. This fibrous septum runs horizontally through the breast parenchyma dividing it into superior and inferior segments. The septum carries the perforators from the anterior intercostal arteries as well as the main sensory supply to the nipple-areola, namely the 4th intercostal nerve which runs with 4th intercostal artery. Also of anatomical importance, Wuringer described a medial vertical ligament which contains the perforators of the internal mammary system, again, typically the dominant supply to the breast.

Pedicle Design

There are multiple pedicle designs which are possible given the aforementioned robust blood supply. These named pedicle types include superior, superomedial, medial, inferior, and central. Traditionally, surveying of the plastic surgery community has demonstrated that the inferior pedicle approach is the most prevalent technique. The inferior dermoglandular pedicle relies primarily on the lower anterior intercostals perforators, consisting of one or more perforators from intercostals spaces 4 through 6. The central pedicle relies on same blood supply as the inferior pedicle; however, it has been described as solely relying on the glandular rather than dermoglandular blood supply. In other words, it relies on the glandular blood supply via the named supply of Wuringer horizontal septum.

The medial pedicle relies on perforators from the internal mammary system as the dominant pedicle source. Oftentimes, the superomedial pedicle can also incorporate perforator vessels from the lateral thoracic artery, lateral intercostals artery, or thoracoacromial artery.

Skin Resection Pattern

Essentially pedicle design and skin resection pattern are independent of one another. Nonetheless, repeated association of a pedicle with a particular skin resection pattern in the literature gives them, in a sense, some degree of association. Skin resection patterns can be largely divided into three categories: (1) Wise or inverted T pattern, (2) vertical reduction pattern, and (3) minimal scarring techniques.

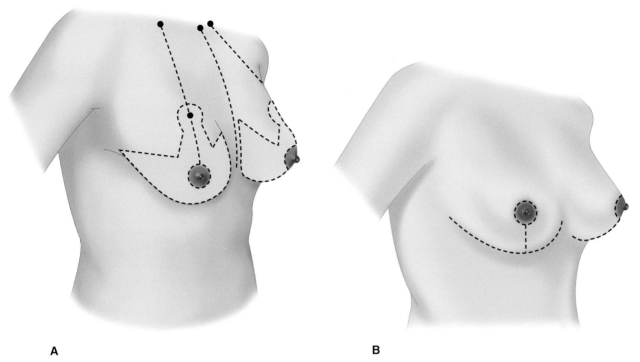

A

B

● **FIGURE 44-1.** Inferior pedicle reduction mammaplasty. (A) Markings for Wise pattern reduction. (B) T-shaped incision on final closure. (*Reprinted with permission from Brunicardi F, Andersen D, Billiar T. Schwartz's Principles of Surgery. 9th ed. New York: McGraw-Hill, 2009.*)

Wise Pattern. The Wise or inverted T pattern remains the most widely utilized skin resection pattern. Typically this is performed via keyhole pattern in which the superior aspect of the keyhole is placed a few centimeters above the nipple-areola complex. The nipple-areola is then transposed cephalad into the keyhole (Figure 44-1).

Vertical Scar Pattern. The vertical reduction method has gained traction and is increasingly more prevalent. These methods eliminate the horizontal inframammary scar that is typical of inverted T or Wise pattern reductions (Figure 44-2).

Miscellaneous Skin Resection Patterns. While vertical reductions have been described to eliminate the inframammary scar, other authors have described efforts to eliminate the vertical scar (see operative technique section below). Additionally, Hammond described a short scar periareola reduction.[1] A Y-scar vertical mammplasty has also been described for grade I ptosis and resections less than 400 g.[2]

Skin Markings

Prior to anesthesia administration, the patient is placed in a standing or upright seated position. The midline of the chest is marked from the sternal notch inferiorly to the umbilicus. Next, the breast meridian is marked by drawing a line from the midclavicle through the nipple-areola complex, extending onto the upper abdomen. Attention should then be turned to marking the new nipple-areola complex, which should be approximately at the midhumeral point. Critical to the placement of the future nipple-areola is the utilization of Pitanguy point, and this landmark can be located by transposing the inframammary fold onto the anterior portion of the breast at the midclavicular line. This can be done by placing one hand in the inframammary fold and palpating with the examiner's opposite hand from the anterior aspect of the breast. The new nipple can be marked at this point ±2 cm above or below this point, depending on the patient and technique (Figure 44-3).

Vertical pattern reductions often result in the inframammary fold traveling cephalad, and therefore, it is reasonable to mark the new nipple 1 to 2 cm lower than one would for a Wise pattern. The superior aspect of the future areola can be marked approximately 2 cm above the future nipple. A cookie-cutter template is used to mark the new nipple-areola diameter. Cookie-cutter templates typically range from 38 to 45 mm in diameter.

The lateral limbs can be marked by rotating the breast medially and laterally, then marking for the limb when the tissue is in line with the meridian. From this point skin markings are dependent on pedicle/skin resection design, and these will be briefly mentioned for each respective technique.

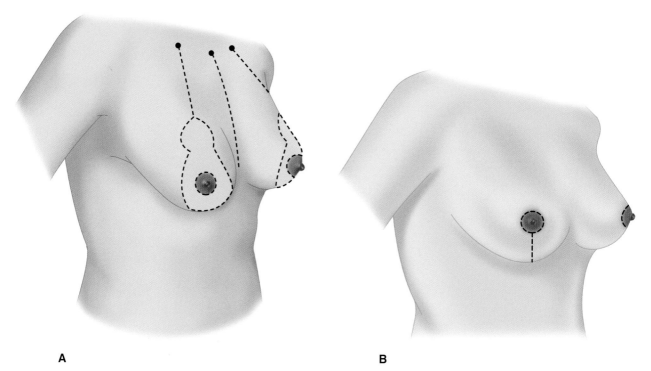

A   **B**

● **FIGURE 44-2.** Vertical reduction mammaplasty, Lejour technique. (A) Markings for vertical reduction. (B) Closure of the vertical mammaplasty. There is bunching up of skin and tissue along the vertical limb that will resolve over time; in addition, the new inframammary fold will declare itself superior to the original one. (*Reprinted with permission from Brunicardi F, Andersen D, Billiar T. Schwartz's Principles of Surgery. 9th ed. New York: McGraw-Hill, 2009.*)

Operative Technique

It is preferred that the patient undergoes general anesthesia; however, this procedure can be performed under conscious sedation. Approximately 60 minutes prior the initial skin incision, intravenous prophylactic antibiotics are administered. Typically a first generation cephalosporin is utilized (eg, cefazolin). Compression devices are placed on the lower extremity for deep vein thrombosis prophylaxis. The patient is then prepped and sterilely

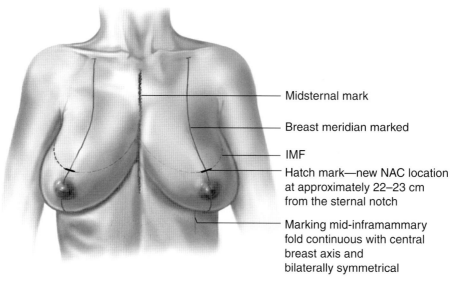

— Midsternal mark

— Breast meridian marked

— IMF

— Hatch mark—new NAC location at approximately 22–23 cm from the sternal notch

— Marking mid-inframammary fold continuous with central breast axis and bilaterally symmetrical

● **FIGURE 44-3.** Commonly utilized landmarks and reference points for skin markings. (*From Shermak MA. Body Contouring. New York: McGraw-Hill; 2010.*)

draped. The skin markings and underlying parenchyma can be infiltrated with 0.25% lidocaine and 1:400,000 epinephrine solution. A Penrose drain can be used as a tourniquet around the base of the breast in order to help control blood loss as well as ease in the de-epithelization and incision of periareola skin markings. The following will describe any skin markings or intraoperative steps unique to each respective technique listed. Following parenchymal resection and glanduloplasty, regardless of technique, the skin edges are closed with buried 3-0 intradermal monofilament suture and running 4-0 subcuticular monofilament suture.

Inferior Pedicle and Wise Pattern. A keyhole pattern is planned using the marking for the new nipple-areola placement. An inferior dermal pedicle is then planned started at the inframmary fold (caudal to the nipple-areola complex) then ascending vertically, stopping approximately 1 cm above the current nipple-areola complex. The dermoglandular pedicle is marked as a vertical strip (8 cm width ±2 cm, widest at the base). This dermoglandular pedicle is then de-epithialized with a 10-blade knife and bleeding is controlled with Bovie electrocautery. The skin and parenchyma are then excised en bloc laterally and superiorly into the keyhole pattern. Vascularized glandular parenchyma under the dermal flap is preserved with tapering of the dermoglandular flap superiorly toward the nipple-areola. The nipple-areola complexis then transposed superior into the "empty keyhole," and the lateral limbs of the keyhole are reapproximated.

The inferior pedicle can be enhanced by augmenting the blood supply with medial vasculature. The medial vertical ligament of Wuringer is incorporated, which preserves the perforators from the internal mammary system. This is done by locating the internal mammary perforators in the medial vertical ligament and creating a 1 cm thick medial flap in conjunction with an inferior pedicle design.

Inferior pedicle-based reductions have been previously criticized as creating a wide, flat, and boxy breast. This phenomenon of "bottoming out," or pseudoptosis, particularly concerning in larger breasts, prompted technical modifications. These modifications have been reported to minimize this aesthetic complication and mitigate these shortcomings. One approach is to plicate the inferior pedicle which decreases inferior pedicle length. This is done by folding the dermis on top of itself at the base of the pedicle. The dermal pedicle is then sutured to the pectoral fascia 2 to 4 cm above the inframammary fold in order to lift the breast. The end goal of these maneuvers is to lift the inframammary fold and narrow the breast, particularly in the inferior aspect. There have also been descriptions of an acellular dermal matrix placed as an inferior hammock to improve outcomes in inferior pedicle mammaplasty. However, acellular dermal matrix is both a foreign body and a costly expenditure that likely does not have a justifiable role in reduction mammaplasty.

Superior Pedicle With Wise Pattern. Superior pedicle techniques are preferred by those who argue that most patients are deficient in the superior pole and that inferior tissue contributing to ptosis should resected. A keyhole wire can be used the mark the new nipple-areola and lateral limbs. The lateral limbs are typically around 5 cm. Horizontal markings then connect the medial limb to the medial inframammary fold, and another horizontal line is drawn to connect the lateral limb to the lateral inframammary fold. The new periareola marking provided by the cookie-cutter template is incised superficially through the epidermis. De-epithelialization begins at the "upper keyhole" and proceeds inferiorly between the lateral limbs, then down to the periareola region, de-epithelializing around to leave about 1 cm around the old nipple-areola complex. Using the horizontal markings, the inferior tissue is excised en bloc down to the pectoral fascia. The dermis of the lateral keyhole limbs is then divided, and the nipple is then transposed directly superiorly on along the hemiaxis of the breast. The nipple is secured with intradermal sutures, and the remainder of the skin edges are approximated.

Medial/Superomedial Pedicle. The medial/superomedial approach has been advocated because is promotes superomedial fullness. Fullness in this region is generally thought to be an aesthetic goal in breast surgery. A keyhole pattern is marked in manner similar to the superior pedicle described above. The pedicle is then designed by dividing the keyhole longitudinally in line just lateral to the new nipple-areola border. The pedicle is then raised with approximately 2 to 3 cm of thickness at the nipple-areola complex and beveled toward the base. The lateral remainder of the keyhole and inferolateral tissue is excised en bloc with skin, fat, and parenchyma. The 9 o'clock of the pedicled nipple-areola is rotated to 12 o'clock of the keyhole excision.

Vertical Scar Reduction. Vertical scar reduction techniques are typically associated with a superior and/or medial dermoglandular pedicle. Lista et al. describe an interesting intraoperative anatomical landmark to dictate pedicle choice. A mosque-shaped dome is marked around the nipple-areola complex with point A (12 o'clock) being marked the transposed inframammary fold.[3] This represents the superior aspect of the new areola (again, the nipple should be marked lower in vertical than in Wise resection patterns). Points C and D are marked inferiorly at the base of the mosque-shaped dome. The skin markings then taper downwards in a narrow semicircle to point B which is marked in the breast meridian, 2 to 4 cm above the inframammary crease. The new nipple-areola complex is marked with a cookie cutter. If any part of the nipple-areola marking lies above the level of points C and D, then a superior pedicle is used, otherwise a medial pedicle is chosen. The resection is then performed in a manner similar to the above descriptions.

The medial and lateral pillars of the breast parenchyma are approximated to shape the breast for greater projection. The skin is then gathered in the vertical wound so as to eliminate a horizontal inframammary scar. The wound is temporarily approximated with skin staples, and the vertical short is shortened with interrupted four-point gathering box stitches. This is done by taking two sequential bites on either side of the wound parallel to the deep dermis.

There are three classically described approaches which have been described in the literature regarding vertical reduction: Lassus technique, Lejour technique, and Hall-Findlay technique. The most recent permutation of this technique was described by Hall-Findlay, which was born from the Lejour description. The Hall-Findlay modification varies from the Lejour technique by utilizing a mosque-dome skin resection pattern and full-thickness medial dermoglandular pedicle. Similar to Lassus, the Hall-Findlay technique also makes a point to avoid liposuction prior to en bloc resection, skin undermining, and pectoral fascia suspension sutures.

Some would argue that vertical scar reduction is more limited with regard to the amount of skin and tissue that can be removed compared with the more traditional inferior pedicle Wise reduction. Proponents of the vertical techniques disagree plus they believe that the vertical technique results in improved long-term projection. This improved projection is theoretically the result of the coning of the breast as the medial and lateral pillars are sutured together. By resecting excess tissue and approximating these pillars, the breast is given a conical shape with improved projection. While there is certainly merit to this argument, a well-approximated, tensionless inframammary scar is more desirable than a forced, bunched, and ultimately, hypertrophic vertical scar. Thus, it is reasonable to avoid an inframammary scar; however, this is dependent on surgeon familiarity with the vertical technique and proper patient selection.

Central/Septum-based Approach.

Recently Hamdi et al. has published a series detailing septum-based mammaplasty, which utilizes Wuringer horizontal septum. This can be done to augment a medial or lateral pedicle. Again this septum relies on the anterior intercostal arteries.[4] In a similar manner, a double pedicle technique in which the central septum-based pedicle augments a superior pedicle can be utilized.

No Vertical Scar.

A new nipple-areola complex is marked as in the techniques described above. A new inframammary fold is then drawn approximately 7 cm below (yet about a centimeter above the current nipple-areola complex). A vertical scar can be avoided by essentially creating a superior skin flap superior to the nipple-areola complex. This is analogous to a thick, robust mastectomy skin flap. A new nipple-areola is excised with a full-thickness circular excision through the skin flap.

The entire region below the skin flap (ie, the old nipple-areola complex periareola region is de-epithelialized). The nipple-areola complex is then transposed superiorly to the full-thickness, circular excision previously placed on the skin flap.[5]

Free Nipple Grafting.

Free nipple grafting has been used in cases of gigantomastia and severe ptosis. Arbitrary cut-off values (ie, >12 or 15 cm of nipple transposition) have traditionally been used to dictate when free nipple grafting may be indicated. The thinking has been that distant nipple transposition risks an insufficient subdermal plexus, kinking, and/or compression of the dermoglandular pedicle. Therefore, a free nipple graft, essentially serving as a full-thickness dermal graft, would result in lower rates of necrosis. While free nipple grafting may have some residual role in the reduction armamentarium, multiple large outcomes studies have been published on pedicled dermoglandular vascular supply for severe cases of gigantomastia and severe ptosis. Therefore, as one becomes more comfortable in performing a preferred technique, most can be applied to these more extreme cases. In doing so, one can minimize the risk of nipple-areola necrosis, discoloration, hyposensitivity, and poor projection which can accompany free nipple grafting.

Suction-assisted Lipectomy.

An alternative to en bloc excision of tissue is to offer patients suction-assisted lipectomy, which is essentially a scar-less solution for breast reduction. While suction-assisted lipectomy does not have a prominent role in reduction mammoplasty, it may be appropriate for a small niche of carefully selected patients. Patients who would be reasonable candidates for suction-assisted lipectomy are generally young, limited to grade I ptosis, have an acceptable skin brassiere/skin envelope, and do not desire a change to their nipple-areola complex. It is also often used as an adjunct to the surgical resection methods.

Incidental Cancer Detection.

Tissue specimens from en bloc excision should be sent to pathology. The rate of incidental breast cancer finding has been traditionally reported to be around 0.5%; however, a large prospective study revealed the rates of carcinoma to be 4% (including rates of 12.4% for carcinoma and atypical hyperplasia combined).[6] For this reason, it is recommended that resected breast specimens should be routinely sent for a formal evaluation. Aside from the less common finding of invasive occult malignancy, formal sectioning of specimens can reveal proliferative or atypical hyperplasia findings which can identify patients at an increased risk for future carcinoma. Interestingly, there has also been data to suggest that the risk of breast cancer is decreased following reduction. This is logically the result of a decrease in the volume of breast tissue.[7]

Drains and Antibiotics.

To date, there has been no evidence to suggest that the usage of either drains or postoperative antibiotics are efficacious following reduction mammoplasty. Studies examining this issue have found that neither drains nor postoperative antibiotics conferred a reduction in complications to patients. While many surgeons use both of these measures, at the current time, these are not evidence-based strategies.[8]

Postoperative Care. Most often, postoperative care can safely be performed on an outpatient basis, thus patients should plan accordingly. Patients are sent home in a soft support bra along with a pain control pump which delivers local anesthetic to the wound. Pain control pumps have been associated with decreased narcotic use and shortened time in the postanesthesia care unit. Upon discharge patients should be instructed to wear a soft bra and avoid strenuous exercise for 3 months. They should be followed on a outpatient basis with a return to the office at approximately 1 week, 6 months, 1 year, and then as needed.

COMPLICATIONS

Local wound complications can be expected in a small percentage of patients postoperatively, and it is important to manage these complications appropriately. Wound dehiscence, particularly at the T junction of Wise pattern incisions, is a more frequent local wound complication. This can often be managed conservatively with observation or wound packing, if necessary. Patients can also present with seroma or hematoma formation. It is advisable to drain these collections in either the office or with a return to the operating room. Prolonged serosanguinous collections place the patient at risk for infection.

Nipple-areola necrosis is the most troublesome and irreversible of the complications. Partial necrosis can be managed more conservatively, whereas total nipple-areola necrosis ultimately results in loss of the nipple. Following debridement and wound healing of the necrosed nipple-areola, nipple reconstruction techniques (as described for breast reconstruction) and areola tattooing can be performed. In some instances, a healthy but hypochromic nipple may result postoperatively. If this is of concern for the patient, this can be addressed with tattooing after healing is complete.

Another complication which can result following reduction is loss of nipple sensitivity. Some monofilament testing has suggested that superior pedicle reductions result in lower nipple sensation as compared with other pedicle designs.[9] In another study, medial and inferior pedicle reductions demonstrated no difference in sensibility, and both pedicle types resulted in an approximately 90% rate of total nipple-areola sensation postoperatively.[10,11] As a whole, clinical outcomes studies have not provided clear evidence to suggest that one pedicle is superior over another in having a higher likelihood of sensation preservation. Theoretically, the 4th intercostal nerve (the main sensory component to the nipple) runs with the anterior intercostals artery, therefore the chance of this complication is affected by reduction size and preservation this neurovascular bundle.

Related to the issue of sensibility, a concerning complication for fertile women is the loss of lactational function. Level III evidence has suggested that superior, medial, and inferior pedicles were all comparable to a control group of women regarding the ability to lactate. All groups in the previously mentioned study all had a lactation success rate of approximately 60% to 65%.[12] The continued ability to lactate is likely a function of the about of remaining lobules rather than pedicle choice, and generally speaking, reduction does not preclude the large majority of women who wish to do so.

OUTCOMES ASSESSMENT

Regardless of the technique used, few other procedures, cosmetic or reconstructive, produce such high rates of patient satisfaction. Large series of postoperative patient surveys have demonstrated a satisfaction rate this has been reliably above 90%.[13,14] In conjunction with satisfactory results, patients have noted improved self-esteem measures. Given that there is also a functional improvement component, the overall patient satisfaction and aesthetic satisfaction outcomes are not entirely equivalent. Nonetheless, in an examination into strictly aesthetics, patients were pleased with the aesthetic outcomes. The most common cause of aesthetic dissatisfaction amongst the patients and independent plastic surgeon reviewers was scarring, and to a lesser extent, high nipple position.[15]

Symptom Improvement

A recent prospective study examined 1 year of consecutive reduction mammaplasty patients. All patients completed an assessment that used five independently validated measures of quality of life. Uniformly, patients scored higher with each of these instruments which demonstrated marked improvements in musculoskeletal pain and psychosocial measures. This same study predicted a gain of 5.32 quality-adjusted life-years as a result of reduction mammaplasty.[16] Even with smaller reductions, these improvements in musculoskeletal pain are accompanied by daily and athletic functional improvements.

In addition to the well-documented amelioration of musculoskeletal pain, Ducic et al. examined the chronic headache/migraine pain in this patient population as well. In a retrospective study of 84 patients, 53% noted a significant reduction in the severity and frequency of migraines/headaches.[17]

REFERENCES

1. Hammond DC. Short scar periareolar inferior pedicle reduction (SPAIR) mammoplasty. *Plast Reconstr Surg.* 1999;103:890–901.

2. Hidalgo DA. Y-scar vertical mammaplasty. *Plast Reconstr Surg.* 2007;120:1749–1754.

3. Lista F, Ahmad J. Vertical scar reduction mammaplasty: A 15-year experience including a review of 250 consecutive cases. *Plast Reconstr Surg.* 2006;117:2152–2165.

4. Hamdi M, Van Landuyt K, Tonnard P, et al. Septum-based mammaplasty: A surgical technique based on Wuringer's septum for breast reduction. *Plast Reconstr Surg.* 2009;123: 443–454.

5. Keskin M, Tosun Z, Savaci N. Seventeen years of experience with reduction mammaplasty avoiding the vertical scar. *Aesthetic Plast Surg.* 2008;32:653–659.

6. Ambaye AB, MacLennan SE, Goodwin AJ, et al. Carcinoma and atypical hyperplasia in reduction mammaplasty: increased sampling leads to increased detection. A prospective study. *Plast Reconstr Surg.* 2009;124:1386–1392.

7. Boice JD, Persson I, Brinton LA, et al. Breast cancer following breast reduction in Sweden. *Plast Reconstr Surg.* 2000;106:755–762.

8. Noone RB. An evidence-based approach to reduction mammaplasty. *Plast Reconstr Surg.* 2010;126:2171–2176.

9. Schlenz I, Rigel S, Schemper M, Kuzbari R. Alteration of nipple and areola sensitivity by reduction mammaplasty: A prospective comparison of five techniques. *Plast Reconstr Surg.* 2005;115:743–751.

10. Nahabedian MY, Mofid MM. Viability and sensation of the nipple-areolar complex after reduction mammaplasty. *Ann Plast Surg.* 2002;49:24–31.

11. Mofid MM, Dellon AL, Elias JJ, Nahabedian MY. Quantitation of breast sensibility following reduction mammaplasty: A comparison of inferior and medial pedicle techniques. *Plast Reconstr Surg.* 2002;109:2283–2288.

12. Cruz NI, Korchin L. Lactational performance after breast reduction with different pedicles. *Plast Reconstr Surg.* 2007;120:35–40.

13. Cardenas-Camarena L. Reduction mammoplasty with superolateral dermoglandular pedicle: details of 15 year of experience. *Ann Plast Surg.* 2009;63:255–261.

14. Davis GM, Ringler SL, Short K, et al. Reduction mammaplasty: long-term efficacy, morbidity, and patient satisfaction. *Plast Reconstr Surg.* 1995;96:1106–1110.

15. Goodwin Y, Wood SH, O'Neill TJ. A comparison of the patient and surgeon opinion on the long-term aesthetic outcome of reduction mammaplasty. *Br J Plast Surg.* 1998;51:444–449.

16. Thoma A, Sprague S, Veltri K, et al. A prospective study of patients undergoing breast reduction surgery: health-related quality of life and clinical outcomes. *Plast Reconstr Surg.* 2007;120:13–26.

17. Ducic I, Iorio ML, Al-Attar A. Chronic headaches/migraines: extending indications for breast reduction. *Plast Reconstr Surg.* 2010;125:44–49.

chapter 45

Advances in Mastopexy

Scott L. Spear, MD / Mark Warren Clemens, MD / Adam D. Schaffner, MD, FACS

● INTRODUCTION

The passage of time may result in the loss of skin elasticity and shape of the female breast. Gravity, weight loss, pregnancy, and breastfeeding all may lead to increasingly pendulous ptotic breasts with further loss of firmness, projection, and downward pointing nipples. Many women may express satisfaction with their bra cup size, but still wish to lift the breast in order to restore a more youthful appearance. The challenge remains restoring a more youthful breast and preserving nipple sensation while minimizing complications, side effects, and scars. The four main variations on mastopexy, in order of ascending complexity are primary mastopexy, augmentation/mastopexy, mastopexy after augmentation, and secondary augmentation mastopexy. This chapter will focus on appropriate patient selection and evaluation followed by some of the most current, safe, and effective surgical techniques for mastopexy.

● PATIENT SELECTION AND EVALUATION

Preoperative evaluation begins with a systematic evaluation of the patient's ptosis. A thorough history and physical examination includes particular attention to oncologic history and previous breast surgeries. All women as appropriate should undergo baseline mammograms prior to surgery as recommended by published guidelines.

There are a number of variables that may increase the risks of performing a mastopexy, including, but not limited to, smoking, collagen vascular diseases, diabetes, or previous breast surgery such as breast augmentation or breast reduction. Smokers are counseled regarding the increased risk of flap necrosis and are encouraged to stop smoking for a minimum of 2 weeks before surgery. Since the blood supply to the nipple-areola complex is impaired to some extent in such patients, the procedure is performed very carefully with minimal undermining. Previously augmented patients have some degree of inferior pole tissue thinning from the implant and, for the same reason, a cautious and conservative approach is necessary in these patients.

The preoperative evaluation includes an assessment of the size and surface area of the breast, the elasticity of the skin, and quality of the breast parenchyma, as well as the relationship between the nipple, the breast gland, and the inframammary fold. The assessment begins with two key elements: nipple position and its distance from the inframammary fold, as classified by Regnault, and the amount of breast tissue that overhangs the inframammary fold. Using the Regnault classification, breast ptosis is rated as grade 1 ptosis, nipple lying at the inframammary fold; grade 2, nipple below the inframammary fold but still on the anterior portion of the breast; and grade 3 ptosis, where the nipple is at the most inferior portion of the breast (Figure 45-1).[1] Glandular ptosis or pseudoptosis is when a significant amount of the breast tissue falls below the inframammary fold, but the nipple is still located at or above the inframammary fold. Breast ptosis can be a complex problem to describe and solve as it involves more elements than just the relationship between the nipple position and the inframammary fold designated by the Regnault classification. There is a broad spectrum of patients who are possible candidates for mastopexy that have the same Regnault classification, but have very different anatomy and present with very different challenges. For example, a young patient with a small tuberous breast deformity and a Regnault grade 2 ptosis with a short nipple to inframammary fold distance and a tight skin envelope represents an entirely different problem

Dr. Spear is a paid consultant to LifeCell and Allergan corporations. Drs Clemens and Schaffner have no disclosures.

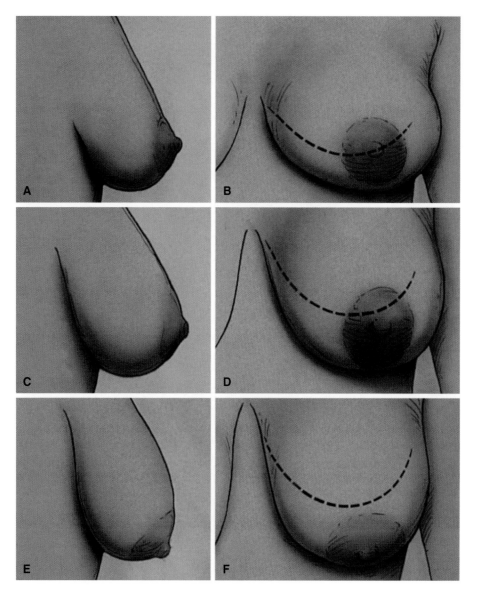

● **FIGURE 45-1.** Regnault classification: (A, B) breast ptosis is rated as grade 1 ptosis, nipple lying at the inframammary fold; (C, D) grade 2 nipple below the inframammary fold but still on the anterior portion of the breast; and (E, F) grade 3 ptosis, nipple is at the most inferior portion of the breast.

compared with a postpartum woman with C-cup grade 2 ptosis, a long nipple to inframammary fold distance, and loose skin envelope with deflated breasts.

There are four basic situations where patients will request a mastopexy. The first is the patient interested in a bilateral mastopexy for an ample breast plus/minus a small reduction. Principal goals within this patient are to lift and reshape. Second is the unilateral mastopexy performed opposite a reconstruction or nonptotic breast. The goals there focus mainly on achieving improved symmetry. Third is the augmentation/mastopexy, which is intended to enlarge the breast while reducing the skin envelope and moving the nipple. And last is the revision mastopexy, which aims to correct the goals that were not adequately addressed in the primary procedure. All of these factors influence the mastopexy plan and pattern.

● **BILATERAL MASTOPEXY FOR THE AMPLE BREAST**

Patient Preparation

The authors' preferred short scar technique includes a superior pedicle and a vertical skin excision pattern from the nipple extending vertically down to just above the inframammary fold.[2,3] If required, a small transverse skin excision can be added in the inframammary fold to eliminate any excess skin and dog-ear(s). Creation of glandular flaps and joining medial and lateral pillars narrows and cones the breast, increases projection, and partially contributes to superior pole fullness. Vertical mastopexy incorporates all of these principles, and therefore represents a type of technique, not just a scar pattern.

Planning begins with the patient standing upright. First, draw the midline, breast meridians, and inframammary folds. A line is drawn tangential to the inframammary folds across the front of the chest to the midline for use as a reference. The midline is marked from the sternal notch to the xiphoid process toward the umbilicus. Careful attention is paid to marking the breast meridians, as there are often lateral asymmetries of the nipple-areola complex that might be improved by adjusting the planned excision (Figure 45-2).

The degree of ptosis is then evaluated noting the relationship of the nipple to the inframammary fold, the distance between the nipple and inframammary fold, and the volume of breast that overhangs the fold. The distance from the nipple to the inframammary fold is measured with the skin placed on tension to simulate the stretch that

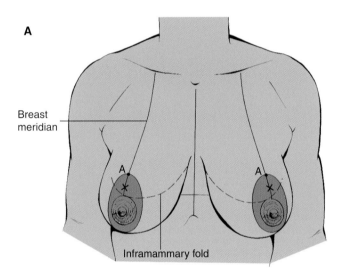

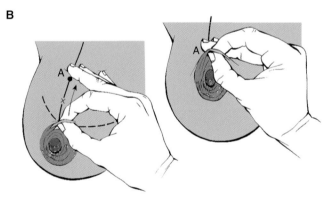

● **FIGURE 45-2.** (A) Marking the patient. The inframammary fold and breast meridian are marked first. Point X represents the new nipple position. It is often marked 2 to 3 cm above the inframammary fold. Point A represents the top of the areola located 2 cm above the nipple site or 4 to 5 cm above the inframammary fold. (B) Tailor-tacking. The desired upper border of the areola can be defined by lifting the edge of the areola between the thumb and index finger and pinning it on the upper breast. (*Modified from Spear SL, Venturi ML. Augmentation with periareola mastopexy. In: Spear SL, ed. Surgery of the Breast: Principles and Art. 2nd ed. Philadelphia: Lippincott Williams & Wilkins; 2006.*)

will be caused after skin excision. Sternal notch to nipple distance differs among patients with different heights, and as such, the absolute numerical measurement is not as helpful as the previously mentioned measurements. However, the nipple to inframammary fold distance is used as a guide to assess symmetry of the nipple-areola complex in each patient. Based on these measurements, an appropriate excision pattern is planned. First, superomedial traction is applied to the breast and vertical marks are drawn on the lateral surface of the breast skin over the projected breast meridian. Next, superolateral traction is applied to the breast and similar vertical marks are drawn on the medial surface of the skin over the projected breast meridian. The key to marking the pillars is estimating how much the medial and lateral portions of the breast can be mobilized to the breast meridian (Figure 45-3). These markings extend from the circumareola marks and join in a V or U shape just above the inframammary fold. These lines are then pinched together to check if skin closure is possible. The length of the vertical limb is directly related to the amount of ptosis, but never extends beyond the inframammary fold. If there is significant asymmetry between the two breasts, it follows that the planned skin excisions may be different. It is made clear to the patient before surgery that while the intent of the procedure is to achieve a more symmetrical result, perfect symmetry is never achieved.

As part of the initial skin marking in the examination room, the nipple-areola complex is manually stretched superiorly and tailor-tacked with the examiners finger tips so that the upper border of the planned new areola position can be marked on the chest with the nipple at or slightly below the center of the projected dimensions of the breast mound (Figure 45-2). Gentle downward traction is placed simultaneously on the superior pole breast skin to simulate the tension that will be created by the mastopexy. It is important to note that the vertical component of the excision will reduce the diameter of the circumareola aperture by a distance measuring approximately one third of the width of the vertical excision (circumference = $\pi \times$ diameter). It is this reduction in width which helps cone and project the breast.

Operative Technique

Circumvertical Technique. The procedure itself begins with the patient in the supine position with arms tucked or abducted less than 90 degrees. Be sure not to over abduct the arms in order to minimize the risk of any nerve injury. Pad both hands, elbows, and any other pressure points. A 38 or 42 mm cookie cutter is centered over each nipple without undue tension on the skin. After de-epithelializing the skin between the reduced areola and the outside border of the new areola window, the outer circumference of the dermis is incised, ensuring the incision is about 5 to 7 mm away from the skin edge in order to leave an adequate dermal cuff in which to place a purse-string suture if desired. Skin edges may be conservatively undermined

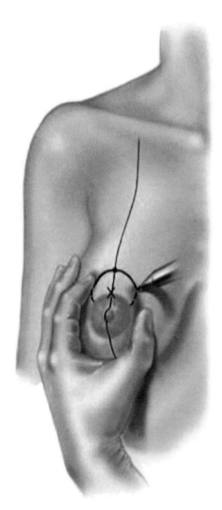
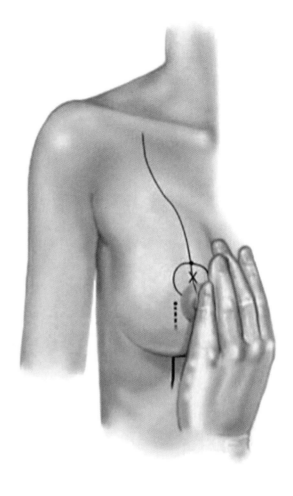

● **FIGURE 45-3.** After the superior edge of the areola is marked, the new areola is drawn while the breast mound is gently pinched. A gentle "push-pull" method should be used to tentatively mark the medial and lateral extent of skin excision. (*Reprinted with permission from Spear SL, Giese SY. Simultaneous breast augmentation and mastopexy. Aesthetic Surg J. 2000;20:155.*)

(approx. 0.5 cm thickness) from the glandular tissue to minimize skin retraction and aid in closure.

Along the vertical component, after the skin incision is made, the skin is de-epithelialized or removed as marked. A decision at this moment must be made whether to imbricate the breast or mobilize flaps based medially and/or laterally. Our preference is to split the lower pole of the breast along or near the medial edge of the window created by the inferior skin excision, thus allowing the mobilization of all the exposed breast tissue on a laterally based flap. The lower pole breast tissue is elevated inferiorly at the level of the pectoralis fascia. This leaves the nipple-areola complex on a superiorly based pedicle. The central portion of the inferior pole may either be resected or included as part of the lateral and/or medial flaps. De Mey et al. noted a critical length of the pillars to be an average of 7 cm from inferior border of the areola to inframammary fold.[4]

In their technique, Graf and Biggs advocate the use of a pectoralis muscle sling to act as support and minimize breast ptosis recurrence.[5] Their technique involves the creation of three flaps: a centrally/inferiorly chest wall-based flap and medial and lateral pillars. The central flap is attached superiorly and held in place by a bipedicled loop of pectoral muscle over which the medial and lateral pillars are closed. Ritz et al.[6] similarly describe using a bipedicled pectoral fascia flap to hold an inferiorly pedicled flap. Unfortunately, these techniques do violate the pectoralis muscle and fascia which may raise oncologic concerns when performing lumpectomy, mastectomy, or even radiographic studies. Additionally, we have found that the central flap is not actually truly inferiorly based and adequately mobilizing the flap off of the chest wall may additionally compromise its blood supply.

We do, however, find the creation of glandular flaps to be a very powerful tool, but we prefer a different approach. We too mobilize and attach glandular tissue to the chest wall in a retroglandular space, which serves to augment projection. We do this by recruiting tissue based on a lateral flap (Figure 45-4). Absorbable sutures

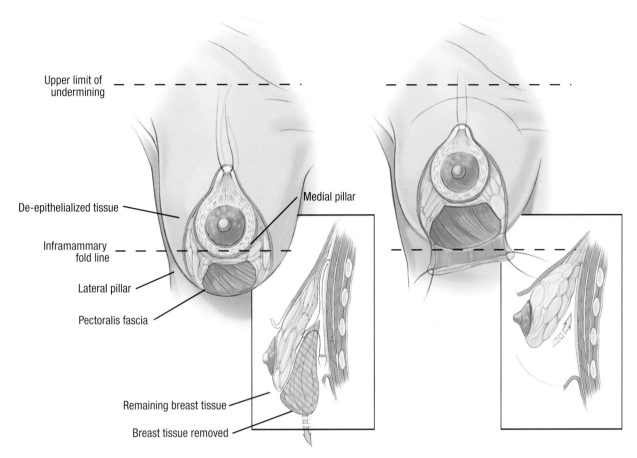

Upper limit of
undermining

De-epithelialized tissue

Inframammary
fold line

Lateral pillar

Pectoralis fascia

Medial pillar

Remaining breast tissue

Breast tissue removed

● **FIGURE 45-4.** Creation of lateral and medial glandular flaps mobilized and attached to the chest wall in a retroglandular space serves to augment projection. Note that the longer lateral flap is mobilized and rotated/advanced superomedially to fill out the central region of the breast behind and above the nipple-areola. The medial glandular pillar is then approximated to the base of the lateral flap. Plication of the pillars from the inframammary fold to just below the areola is then performed in a vertical fashion to cone the breast.

placed high on the chest attach this flap to the pectoralis fascia to overcorrect the lift and compensate for postoperative settling. The lateral flap is mobilized and rotated/advanced superomedially to fill out the central region of the breast behind and above the nipple-areola. The medial glandular pillar is then approximated to the base of the lateral flap. Plication of the pillars from the inframammary fold to just below the areola is then performed in a vertical fashion to cone the breast. The re-approximated pillars may be reinforced with several rows of absorbable sutures, which adds additional projection to the mound and creates a column of breast tissue.[7]

Excess skin may be evenly distributed along the entire vertical incision. If there is too much excess tissue to be absorbed by the vertical incision, the skin generated at the lower pole may be drawn together in a purse string. Alternatively, any residual dog-ear may be excised leaving a small transverse scar in the inframammary fold. No matter what, the final vertical scar should be entirely contained above the inframammary fold. To counteract

unavoidable settling, the superior pole should be overly full in relation to the inferior pole at the end of the procedure.

Final nipple position should be in the vicinity of the apex of the breast. If the circumference of the new areola risks being significantly larger than desired, a "blocking" suture can be used by purse-stringing the dermal cuff with a permanent 3-0 or 4-0 suture.[8] We have adopted the interlocking Gore-Tex suture technique described by Hammond for that purpose (Figure 45-5). Finally, the skin is closed with interrupted and running buried absorbable monofilament suture (Figure 45-6).

Wise Pattern Technique. The inverted T skin pattern remains the most commonly performed type of mastopexy in the United States.[9] We believe that in the vast majority of cases, a circumvertical technique is sufficient, leaving a formal Wise pattern only to be used to treat the most severe grades of ptosis such as in the massive weight loss patient.

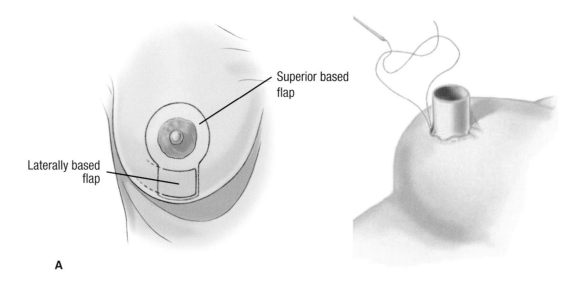

A

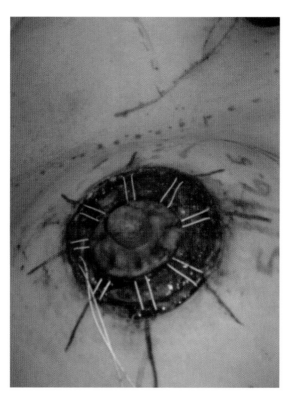

B

● **FIGURE 45-5.** (A) Purse-string suture. A 3-0 or 4-0 Gore-Tex suture on a straight needle is run circumferentially around the areola in the deep dermis and sewn down with the nipple marker in place to set the aperture. (B) Clinical view. *(Part A: Reprinted with permission from Spear, S. L., and Giese SL, Giese SY. Simultaneous breast augmentation and mastopexy. Aesthetic Surg J. 2000;20:155.)*

Preoperative evaluation and markings proceed similar to a short scar mastopexy with the following exceptions: (1) the horizontal component of the skin pattern is placed at the level of the inframammary fold and the final skin closure should remain within this position (Figure 45-7); (2) after skin incisions have been performed, dissection may proceed with either a superior, superomedial, inferior, or central pedicle to supply the nipple-areola complex; and (3) medial and lateral pillars consisting of skin and breast parenchyma are then elevated just above the level of the pectoralis fascia for advancement or transposition, as described in the circumvertical technique. Excess tissue may be trimmed from the cut edge of the lateral flap and/ or from the inferior aspect of both flaps.

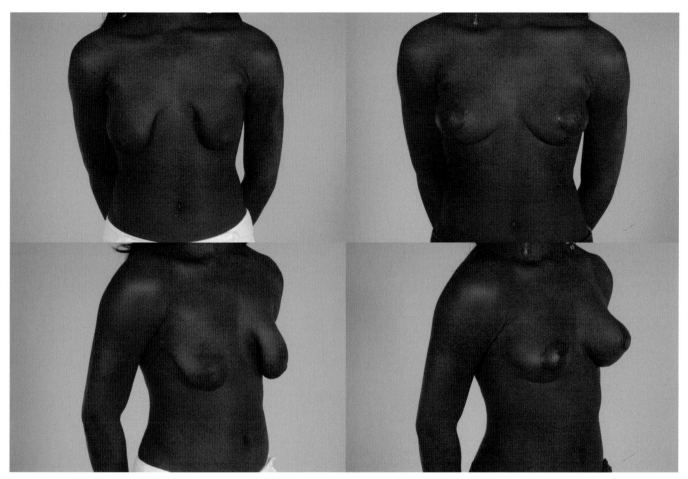

● **FIGURE 45-6.** (Left) Preoperative view of a 19-year-old woman with third-degree ptosis and tuberous breast deformity. (Right) Postoperative view, 6 months after undergoing bilateral vertical mastopexies.

Once the vertical and horizontal limbs are sutured closed, the nipple areolar complex is inset at the apex of the keyhole pattern with the inferior border of the areola set 5 to 7 cm superior to the inframammary fold.

Concentric Technique. When planning the mastopexy pattern, a concentric pattern may at first seem desirable with respect to limiting the amount of scars placed on the breast; however, this is at the cost of placing more tension on the closure and may lead to a flattened breast, poor scarring, and/or a distorted nipple-areola complex, and is not advised for a mastopexy alone.[10] A circumvertical excision pattern increases projection by narrowing and coning the breast and provides the most control in terms of shaping the breast. Even in situations where an acceptable result using a concentric pattern could be achieved, we will often add a conservative vertical excision to improve the overall shape of the breast.

We rarely perform an isolated concentric mastopexy. The most common indications for concentric mastopexy are for attempting to match a reconstructed breast, gynecomastia, and unilateral or bilateral mastopexies done for asymmetry in conjunction with breast augmentation (Figure 45-8). Concentric mastopexy may also be successful when combined with implant explantation.[9] It should not be attempted for substantial grade 2 or 3 ptosis.

● **AUGMENTATION/MASTOPEXY**

The single-stage augmentation/mastopexy has the unenviable distinction as one of the most litigated procedures in plastic surgery.[11] An increased risk of skin and nipple necrosis, distortion of the nipple-areola complex, poor scarring, and even implant extrusion results from an increasingly compromised blood supply and greater stress on the closure.

The inherent risks of this procedure have not affected its popularity among patients. Between 1997 and 2007, there has been a 395% increase in the frequency of breast augmentation and an equal increase in breast lift procedures.[12] The number of combined augmentation/mastopexy procedures has similarly increased in frequency because of the convenience of a single-stage operation. We have previously written extensively on the subject of augmentation/mastopexy.[13,14]

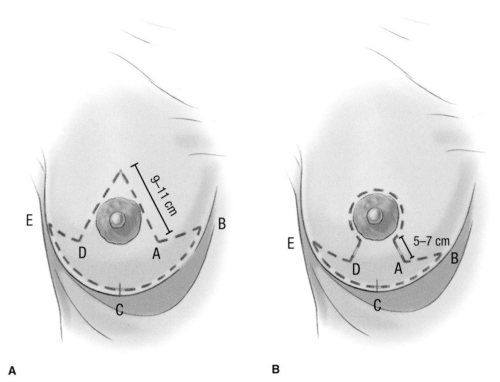

A　　　　　　**B**

● FIGURE 45-7. The standard Wise pattern skin excision pattern may be drawn one of two ways. (A) An inverted V is drawn with vertical limbs measuring between 9 and 11 cm. Later in the procedure, the nipple is externalized at the apex of the design. (B) A keyhole may be incorporated into the initial markings with vertical limbs measuring 5 to 7 cm. Note essential limb measurements: segment *AB* should be ≥*BC*, and segment *DE* should be ≥*CE*.

● FIGURE 45-8. Preoperative markings for the concentric mastopexy include the inframammary fold; (A) the superior extent of the excision, representing the new superior edge of the areola; (B) approximately 6 cm up from the inframammary fold, marked as needed to correct glandular ptosis; (C) the lateral extent of the incision, marked also to leave the desired amount of lateral breast skin; and (D) 8 to 10 cm from the midline, marked as needed to leave adequate medial breast skin. (*Reprinted with permission from Spear SL, Giese SY, Ducic I. Concentric mastopexy revisited. Plast Reconstr Surg. 2001;107(5):1294–1299.*)

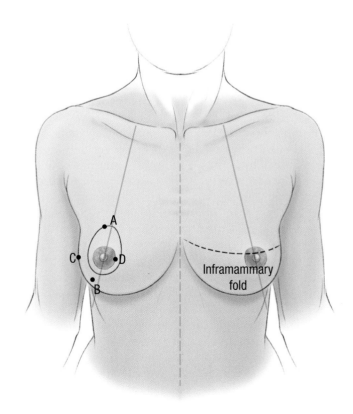

A single-stage procedure may seem attractive to both surgeon and patient, but its successful execution is contingent upon careful preoperative planning and attentive implementation to reduce the severity and frequency of complications. If the primary goal is to correct significant asymmetries, particularly if this involves a significant reduction or a reduction/mastopexy procedure on one side, the safest plan may be to perform the mastopexies first followed by breast augmentation at a second stage. Attempting to account for too many variables in one setting may lead to unpredictable and disappointing results.

Our approach to augmentation mastopexy is focused around several principles: placing the implants first and then tailoring the skin envelope to accommodate the larger breast volume, addressing breast asymmetries by employing different mastopexy patterns when appropriate, tailor-tacking the skin with the patient in the upright position in the operating room prior to committing to the planned mastopexy pattern, and conservative superficial undermining of the skin to preserve perfusion to the nipple-areola complex and to reduce wound healing complications.

Patient Preparation

When evaluating a patient for augmentation/mastopexy, several key factors should be taken into account. An implant alone may be sufficient to address some mild forms of ptosis. However, the more the skin and glandular tissue overhangs the inframammary fold, the less likely an implant will be able to completely fill out the breast in a cosmetically acceptable fashion unless skin is excised.[15] Similarly, the lower the nipple, the less likely a prosthesis will raise the nipple adequately onto the surface of the breast. In these cases, the circumareola or vertical technique are most helpful for addressing a greater degree of ptosis.[16]

After evaluating the degree of breast and nipple ptosis and forming an operative plan, measurements for the implant are made. The base width of the breast is measured as well as the superior pole pinch thickness. The difference between these values is used as a guide to determine the upper limit for the diameter of the implant. Using the implant diameter measurement, the height of anticipated breast is marked from the inframammary fold. Markings are made to visualize the implant position on the chest wall and predict appropriate nipple placement.

Unlike breast reduction procedures, the nipple-areola complex is invariably marked to lie somewhere above the inframammary fold in augmentation/mastopexy. While the most serious error is to place the nipple too high, the most common error is inadequate elevation of the nipple. It is important to note the presence of tan lines. Citing the upper border of the areola needs to take these borders into consideration. It is also useful to have the patient wear a bra and mark the upper boundaries of the breast that the bra covers. These maneuvers can serve as important guides to avoid placing the nipple too high. As a general principle,

the final extent and pattern of the excision should not be committed to until the implants are placed. The skin envelope and nipple position are then tailor-tacked with the patient sitting upright and then adjusted to the dimensions of the newly augmented breast. Only then is the final nipple position determined.

The decision-making process in selecting the appropriately sized implant is more complex in one-stage augmentation mastopexy than staged augmentation after mastopexy alone. Because the skin envelope will be reduced, it is important to measure not only the base width of the breast in its native state, but also the base width while tailor-tacking the skin to simulate the breast dimensions after mastopexy. This will effectively narrow the base width and provides a closer approximation of what the outer limits of the implant diameter should be. For example, if the breast is 14 cm wide with a 2 cm pinch thickness and has a base width of 13 cm when simulating the mastopexy, then an implant diameter of 11 cm might be more appropriate than one with a diameter of 12 cm. In terms of implant projection, for deflated breasts, we prefer the higher profile models to fill out the loose skin envelope. Once these parameters are defined, a discussion with the patient regarding her ideal breast size refines the final choice of implant.

Augmentation/Mastopexy Technique

A concentric mastopexy for augmentation/mastopexy works well for a patient where the nipple lies near or just below the inframammary fold with the inferior border of the areola no lower than the inferior curve of the breast on frontal view, and where there is less than 4 cm of breast overhanging the inframammary fold, leaving an initial nipple to inframammary fold distance of no more than 9 cm (Figures 45-9 and 45-10). In planning a circumareola mastopexy, as a guideline, the ratio of the outer to the inner diameter of the circumareola markings should ideally be no greater than 2:1 and certainly no greater than 3:1. A periareola augmentation/mastopexy must take into account the implant's tendency to dilate the areola while filling out the native breast skin and increasing breast volume. The ideal scenarios for periareola mastopexy and augmentation are (1) the areola being too large preoperatively, (2) the nipple and/or breast being too ptotic for correction with an implant alone, and (3) the breast(s) being tuberous.[17]

The short scar technique is appropriate for the majority of patients with a moderate amount of ptosis (Figure 45-11).[18–21] In patients where it is unclear whether any mastopexy procedure will be necessary, the procedure begins with a periareola incision for placement of the implant without any de-epithelialization.[22] The incision is usually made along the inferior border of the areola and dissection is carried down to the pectoralis major muscle. If the ptosis is severe and the surgeon is confident that a vertical technique is required, then the safest

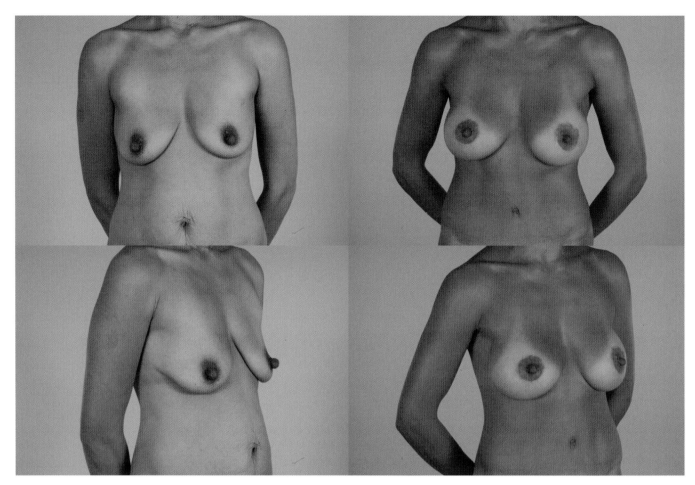

● **FIGURE 45-9.** (Left) Preoperative view of a 37-year-old woman with second-degree ptosis and breast asymmetry. (Right) Postoperative view, 14 months after undergoing bilateral augmentation with 265-cc silicone implants and bilateral concentric mastopexies.

way to enter the breast is in a vertical manner within the planned area of de-epithelialization. Theoretically, this dissection would be parallel to the neurovascular supply to the nipple. However, if there is any question regarding the need for a vertical excision, then a periareola approach is used.

At our institution, we prefer a dual-plane approach when placing the implant partially retropectorally.[23] The inferior third of the pocket is dissected in the subglandular plane while the upper two thirds or so of the pocket lies in the subpectoral plane. Meticulous hemostasis and irrigation with a triple-antibiotic solution are routinely performed to minimize the risk of capsular contracture or infection.[24] After completing the dissection, the implant is soaked in antibiotic solution, the field is re-prepped with a Betadine paint stick, and gloves are changed prior to implant placement. After the insertion of the implant, the incision is stapled closed and the patient is positioned sitting fully upright.

The design is tailor-tacked with the patient sitting upright once the implant is in place. Only then is de-epithelialization performed as necessary. The strategy should be to avoid making unnecessary scars on the breast in borderline cases.[25,26] Minimal undermining in the subcutaneous plane is performed to re-drape the skin. Care is taken not to dissect deep and violate the breast parenchyma in order to preserve blood supply to the nipple. Usually only 1 to 2 cm of undermining is required. The amount of excess skin that can safely be removed is now more accurately determined. These areas are de-epithelialized and then minimal subcutaneous undermining is performed around the areola after incising the dermis leaving a 5 to 7 mm dermal cuff. The vertical closure is usually 6 to 8 cm in length, depending on the implant and final total breast size. Greater vertical lengths are addressed with small transverse triangular excisions based at the inframammary fold. Sometimes, a small amount of excision of breast tissue is required both in the vertical and transverse components of the design. Note that these maneuvers should be conservative as they increase the risk of implant exposure and vascular compromise. All incisions are then closed using buried interrupted

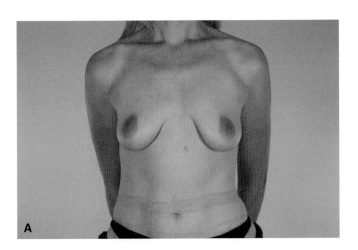
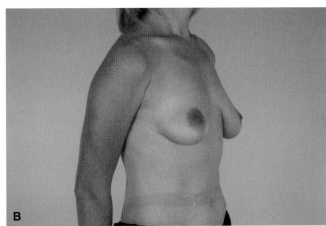
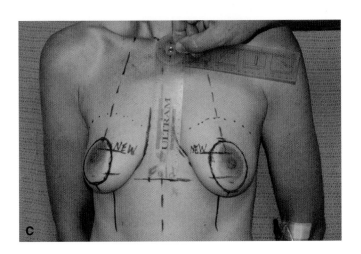
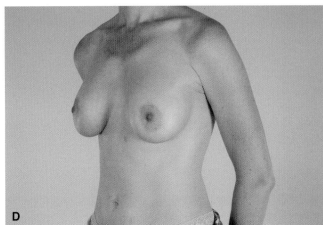
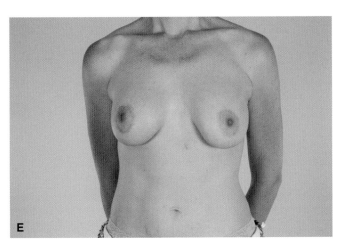
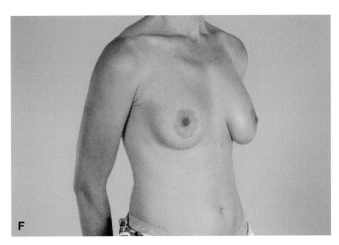

● **FIGURE 45-10.** (A,B) Preoperative view of a 37-year-old woman with second-degree ptosis and breast asymmetry. (C) Preoperative markings. (D–F) Postoperative view, 9 months after undergoing bilateral augmentation with 240-cc silicone implants and bilateral concentric mastopexies.

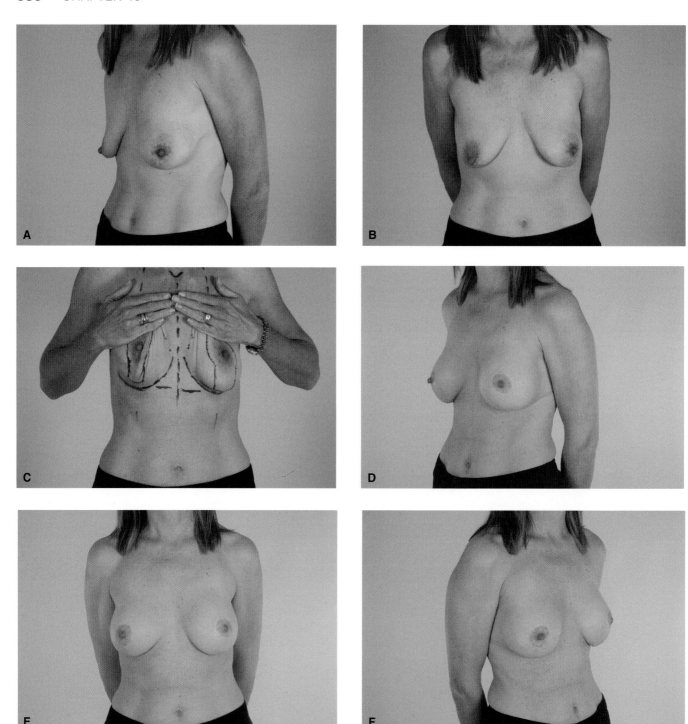

● **FIGURE 45-11.** (A, B) Preoperative view of a 49-year-old woman with third-degree ptosis and breast asymmetry. Patient had previously received a left 180-cc saline implant 25 years earlier from breast asymmetry. (C) Preoperative markings. (D–F) Postoperative view, 3.5 years after undergoing bilateral augmentation with a left 286-cc and right 234-cc silicone implants and bilateral vertical mastopexies.

and running Monocryl suture. The nipple position is then reassessed and remeasured and may be fine-tuned as required. Finally, the skin is closed with interrupted and running buried Monocryl suture. All patients are placed in a soft bra and followed closely in the first few days to monitor the nipple and flaps.

● **COMPLICATIONS**

Regardless of the pattern used, each can be associated with potential complications. Inappropriate use of the concentric excision can lead to poor scarring, areola distortion, and flattening of the breast may occur. Lejour found that

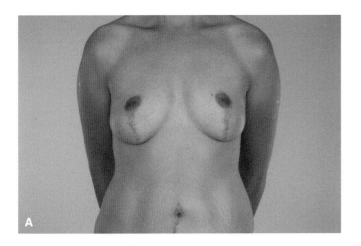

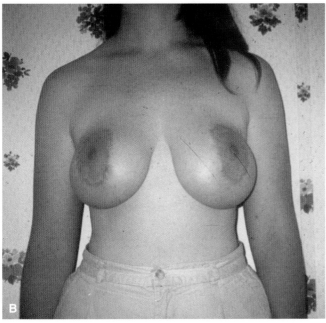

● **FIGURE 45-12.** Examples of poor mastopexy outcomes: (A) over-elevation of the nipple; and (B) unacceptable scarring.

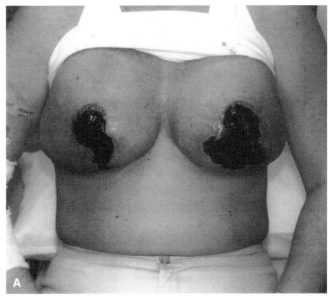

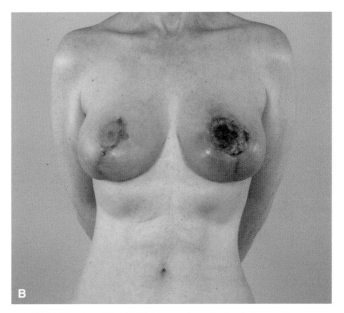

● **FIGURE 45-13.** (A,B) Examples of nipple loss after mastopexy or augmentation/mastopexy.

in her experience of 152 consecutive circumvertical mastopexy patients, complications included four seromas, six hematomas, and one infection.[27]

A malpositioned nipple-areola complex is usually the result of unsuccessful preoperative planning and/or committing to the planned excision without intraoperative tailor-tacking. These maneuvers are critical because it is not always possible to accurately predict the new dimensions of the breast once the implant is placed. Most commonly, the nipple is inadequately raised, which can be addressed with a simple revision. However, a nipple-areola that is too high is a more difficult problem because surgical correction is difficult and may leave the patient with a visible scar in the superior pole of the breast—a scar that may be visible in a swimsuit or low-cut dress (Figure 45-12). More dreaded than the malpositioned

nipple is frank nipple necrosis (Figure 45-13). In patients who have previously undergone breast reduction, the risks may be significant. In secondary cases, when in doubt, the mastopexy may be performed using de-epithelialization only, without undermining the skin. If re-draping is necessary, undermining should always be performed conservatively (1–2 cm) in a superficial subcutaneous plane.

Specifically, with regard to the augmentation/mastopexy patient, these procedures have a higher rate of complication. A review from 1993 to 2001 yielded 34 consecutive revision augmentation/mastopexies with the most common problems being recurrent ptosis (55%),

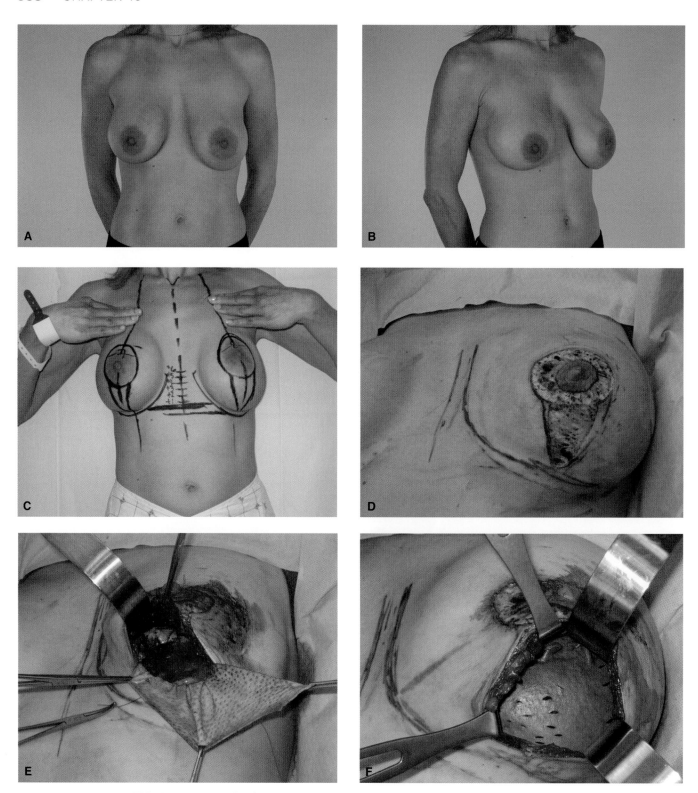

● FIGURE 45-14. (A,B) Preoperative view of a 42-year-old woman who presented 11 years after breast augmentation with subglandular saline implants complaining of droopiness and upper pole emptiness. She has 36C cup breasts and second-degree ptosis with asymmetry. (C) Preoperative markings for a circumvertical mastopexy with augmentation. (D) Intraoperative view of initial de-epithelialization of design. (E) Placement of strattice as an interpositional graft by parachuting. (F) Strattice in place with no ripples.

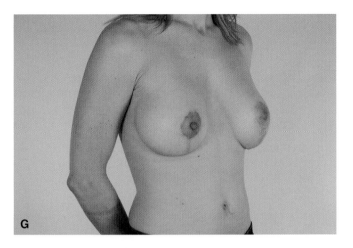

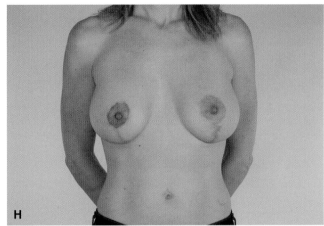

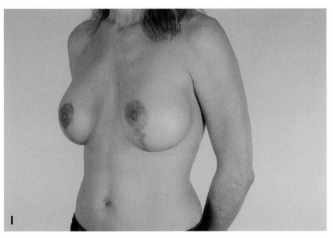

● FIGURE 45-14. (*continued*) (G–I) Postoperative view, 13 months after undergoing bilateral augmentation/mastopexy with 457-cc silicone implants placed subpectorally with bilateral vertical mastopexies.

capsular contracture (55%), implant malposition (35%), size change (30%), poor scars (25%), and nipple malposition (10%), and an average interval to revision of 7 years. If these complications occur, revision surgery can often be very challenging and may require incorporating acellular dermal matrix into revisionary augmentation/mastopexy for capsular contracture, rippling, implant malposition, and reinforcing thinned breast tissues from large breast implants (Figure 45-14). The benefits of acellular dermal matrix include improved control and support of implant position, and better implant coverage. In cases of difficult and recurrent capsular contracture, acellular dermal matrix may be inset as a large interpositional graft.

● CONCLUSION

Mastopexy can be a safe and gratifying procedure for both patient and surgeon when performed with thoughtful planning and careful execution. Patients should be well-informed preoperatively that breast asymmetries may be improved upon but is rarely completely corrected. A symmetric approach is preferred for mild asymmetries while different excision patterns may be required for significant asymmetries. Nipple-areola malposition may be avoided by careful intraoperative tailor tacking. Safe and successful surgeries can be reliably achieved for both mastopexy and augmentation/mastopexy with adherence to these principles.

REFERENCES

1. Regnault P. The hypoplastic and ptotic breast: a combined operation with prosthetic augmentation. *Plast Reconstr Surg.* 1966;37:31–37.
2. Lassus C. Breast reduction: evolution of a technique—a single vertical scar. *Aesthetic Plast Surg.* 1987;11:107.
3. Lejour M. Vertical mammaplasty: update and appraisal of late results. *Plast Reconstr Surg.* 1999;104:771–781.
4. Berthe JV, Massaut J, Greuse M, et al. The vertical mammaplasty: A reappraisal of the technique and its complications. *Plast Reconstr Surg.* 2003;111(7):2192–21929; discussion 2200–21922.
5. Graf R, Biggs TM. In search of better shape in mastopexy and reduction mammoplasty. *Plast Reconstr Surg.* 2002;110(1):309–317; discussion 318–322.
6. Ritz M, Silfen R, Southwick G. Fascial suspension mastopexy. *Plast Reconstr Surg.* 2006;117:86.
7. Hidalgo DA. Vertical mammaplasty. *Plast Reconstr Surg.* 2005;4:1179–1197.

8. Benelli L. A new periareolar mammaplasty: the "round block" technique. *Aesthetic Plast Surg.* 1990;14: 93–100.

9. Rohrich RJ, Beran SJ, Restifo RJ, Copit SE. Aesthetic management of the breast following explantation: Evaluation and mastopexy options. *Plast Reconstr Surg.* 1998;101(3):827–837.

10. Baran CN, Peker F, Ortak T, Sensöz O, Baran NK. Unsatisfactory results of periareolar mastopexy with or without augmentation and reduction mammoplasty: enlarged areola with flattened nipple. *Aesthetic Plast Surg.* 2001;25(4): 286–289.

11. Spear SL, Boehmler JH 4th, Clemens MW. Augmentation/mastopexy: a 3-year review of a single surgeon's practice. *Plast Reconstr Surg.* 2006;118(7 Suppl):136S-147S; discussion 148S-149S, 150S-151S.

12. American Society for Aesthetic Plastic Surgery Website. http://www.surgery.org/media/statistics. Accessed January 10, 2010.

13. Spear SL, Venturi ML. Augmentation with periareolar mastopexy. In: Spear SL, ed. *Surgery of the Breast: Principles and Art.* Vol 2. 2nd ed. Philadelphia: Lippincott Williams & Wilkins; 2006:1393–1402.

14. Spear, SL. Augmentation/mastopexy: "Surgeon, beware". *Plast Reconstr Surg.* 2003;112(3):905–906.

15. Brink RR. Evaluating breast parenchymal maldistribution with regard to mastopexy and augmentation mammaplasty. *Plast Reconstr Surg.* 2000;106:491–496.

16. Cardenas-Camarena L, Ramirez-Macias R. Augmentation/mastopexy: how to select and perform the proper technique. *Aesthetic Plast Surg.* 2006;30:21–33.

17. Spear SL, Giese SY, Ducic I. Concentric mastopexy revisited. *Plast Reconstr Surg.* 2001;107(5):1294–1299.

18. Ceydeli A, Freund RM. "Tear-drop augmentation mastopexy": a technique to augment superior pole hollow. *Aesthetic Plast Surg.* 2003;27:425–432; discussion 433.

19. Gruber R, Denkler K, Hvistendahl Y. Extended crescent mastopexy with augmentation. *Aesthetic Plast Surg.* 2006; 30:269–274; discussion 275–266.

20. Nigro DM. Crescent mastopexy and augmentation. *Plast Reconstr Surg.* 1985;76:802–803.

21. Persoff MM. Vertical mastopexy with expansion augmentation. *Aesthetic Plast Surg.* 2003;27:13–19.

22. de la Fuente A, Martin del Yerro JL. Periareolar mastopexy with mammary implants. *Aesthetic Plast Surg.* 1992;16: 337–341.

23. Tebbets JB. Dual plane breast augmentation: Optimizing implant-soft-tissue relationships in a wide range of breast types. *Plast Reconstr Surg.* 2001;107(5):1255–1272.

24. Adams WP Jr, Rios JL, Smith SJ. Enhancing patient outcomes in aesthetic and reconstructive breast surgery using triple antibiotic breast irrigation: six-year prospective clinical study. *Plast Reconstr Surg.* 2006;118(7 Suppl):46S–52S.

25. Elliott LF. Circumareolar mastopexy with augmentation. *Clin Plast Surg.* 2002;29:337–347, v.

26. Gasperoni C, Salgarello M, Gargani G. Experience and technical refinements in the "donut" mastopexy with augmentation mammaplasty. *Aesthetic Plast Surg.* 1988;12:111–114.

27. Lejour M. Vertical mammaplasty: early complications after 250 consecutive cases. *Plast Reconstr Surg.* 1999;104: 764–770.

chapter 46

Breast Augmentation

Vu T. Nguyen, MD

INTRODUCTION

Augmentation mammaplasty is currently the most popular cosmetic surgical procedure in the United States, and has consistently been so since 2006. Data from the 2010 American Society of Plastic Surgeons' national clearinghouse of plastic surgery statistics show that some 289,000 women underwent augmentation in 2009, a 36% increase since the year 2000.[1] These statistics clearly indicate that augmentation mammaplasty is an integral part of the practice of many plastic surgeons, and will remain so for years to come. However, these statistics should not give surgeons the impression that this procedure is altogether straightforward in regard to its preparation, execution, outcomes, and potential complications. In fact, no plastic surgery procedure has provoked as much controversy and scrutiny, both in the medical literature as well as in the lay public, than that of breast augmentation. The lessons learned from this unique history have taught us how to better approach and inform our patients of the risks and benefits of this popular procedure. Therefore, as we continue in the practice of breast augmentation, it is inherent upon us to minimize complications and unnecessary reoperations, as well as ensure its safe and reliable practice, particularly in light of its known intrinsic issues and somewhat checkered past.

PATIENT EVALUATION AND SELECTION

A wide variety of body and breast types present for augmentation mammaplasty. Furthermore, there exists a dizzying array of options in regard to incision placement, implant location, and implant types, including choice of filler material, surface texture, shape, and size. Given these various options, it should become apparent that no one technique or approach can possibly suffice for all patients and all situations. Instead, practitioners need to become facile with a number of available options; and in conjunction with the patient, make decisions based on a careful evaluation of the patient's specific breast characteristics; noting to the patient the particular benefits and trade-offs of each. It bears repeating that each patient be approached individually, based on not only their physical characteristics but also their desired outcome. Some patient profiles do, however, become apparent. Younger patients in their 20s who present for augmentation are oftentimes single and nulliparous. The body habitus is a relatively thin, athletic, or even muscular physique. Expectations are therefore usually high, and aesthetic concerns are yet unconstrained by more long-term or oncologic issues. This is in contrast to the 30- to 40 year-old age group, who are often seeking augmentation following age-related changes or postpartum-related involution. While expectations are oftentimes more reasonable, concerns regarding cancer surveillance and detection come into play. Additionally, secondary agendas for breast augmentation may play a role, including marital difficulties, issues with social insecurity, and professional career advancement. Beginning the patient evaluation with a frank discussion regarding the motivation behind augmentation can only assist in building rapport between physician and patient, and potentially minimize complications due to unreasonable expectations or other psychosocial issues.

While many patients presenting for consultation regarding breast augmentation appear young and healthy, a complete medical history is a requisite for all patients. Beyond the routine evaluation of a patient's age, past medical/surgical history, list of medications, and allergies, a thorough investigation into potential factors that could contribute to acute postoperative problems should occur (eg, bleeding, infection, delayed wound healing, etc). This includes but is not limited to their history of smoking, diabetes, and possible coagulopathies. A history specific to breast-related illness should also be elucidated; focusing on prior breast-related symptoms, diagnoses, imaging, and procedures. A personal or family history of breast cancer must be noted and if appropriate should prompt a discussion regarding the necessity of genetic testing. In regards to presurgical mammography, screening recommendations are available via the American Cancer Society and the American College of Radiology. Additionally, a discussion regarding the effect of breast implants on breast imaging and cancer surveillance should take place. Patients should be aware that all breast implants interfere with mammography, and that additional views are necessary in order to increase the amount of visualized tissue. Using Eklund views, up to 85% of breast tissue may be imaged with implants in the submuscular position, as compared to up to 64% of breast tissue in the subglandular position.[2] Despite these limitations, current evidence indicates that breast implants do not adversely affect the surveillance of breast cancer, stage at diagnosis, or survival rate.

A discussion regarding the more frequent complications associated with the use of breast implants must include the issues of capsular contracture, implant failure/rupture/deflation, device palpability, rippling, scalloping, deformation, malposition, and asymmetry. The potential for these complications must be addressed on an individual basis and in relation to the type of implant, the patient's anatomy, and their individual breast characteristics. An honest discussion regarding the impact of implants on a particular patient and their breasts is important to mitigate potential problems that arise only after the surgery is performed. Tebbetts, for example, includes a comprehensive list of potential complication unique to implant-based breast augmentation as part of his documentation and informed consent process.[3]

Additional unique complications may include widening and other associated changes of the nipple-areola complex. While sensation is usually not permanently affected, there is some indication that increasing implant size has some effect on diminished sensation. Similarly, lactation is not usually impaired, especially when extensive dissection through breast parenchyma is avoided. However, patients should be advised to refrain from undergoing breast augmentation within 6 months of lactation to prevent the possibility of milk pooling within the breast pocket. Lastly, studies have shown that silicone implants do not increase silicone levels in breast milk above baseline levels, which are in fact lower than those found in infant formula and cow's milk.

While some surgeons may advocate a more cursory or gestalt approach to the physical examination, measuring and documenting these physical findings allows for decision making based on objective parameters. Beginning with height, weight, chest, and bra size; the recording of these values assists in the important practice of reviewing one's own experience, and over time in making adjustments to

technique and approach. Moreover, documenting and conveying these findings to the patient allows the physician the opportunity to point out areas of potential concern. Inherent, yet often unnoticed, asymmetries in regard to breast size, nipple location, breast diameter, and inframammary fold position are the rule and not the exception; and should be highlighted to the patient and trigger a discussion regarding their impact on the final outcome.

Tebbetts, again, has been an advocate for the objective measurement and analysis of breast characteristics. His High Five decision support process uses five measurement and five critical decisions, in order to consolidate the preoperative planning process.[4] Even this method, however, is likely too cumbersome for the vast majority of surgeons to embrace in their everyday practices. Therefore, each individual surgeon must over time develop their own practical system of examination; encompassing at the minimum, assessment of the dimensions of the breast, native breast volume, nipple and inframammary fold position, and the presence of any breast mass. Additional important elements may include the amount of breast skin laxity, overall skin quality, amount of postpartum involution, presence of striae, and other characteristics of the skin envelope. Many advocate measurement of the breast diameter, sternal notch-to-nipple distance, nipple to inframammary fold distance, medial and lateral pinch, and upper pole pinch tests. The chosen implants can then be narrowed in on using a combination of these measurements (ie, breast diameter: one half medial and one half lateral pinch amounts) and the desired outcome of the patient. In regard to the latter parameter, this is of critical importance as it is a major source of patient dissatisfaction. Size, or more accurately inadequate or unwanted size, is viewed as one of the most common reason for early reoperation following breast augmentation. Efforts to estimate a patient's desired amount of augmentation have resulted in a multitude of systems, including custom digital imaging and the use of various spacers (eg, rice bags) and implants placed within a bra to simulate the augmentation. No system is ideal; however, a component of the Bodylogic system uses a four-part visual scale accompanied by descriptive text in order to define the patient's desired outcome.[5]

Type 1—I desire a gentle filling out of my breast in a way that is completely natural with no excess fullness in the upper pole of my breast. I understand that perhaps a bigger implant could potentially be used but my wishes are more for a conservative augmentation.

Type 2—I would like the biggest implant that can be used without creating a breast which has an unnatural look, ie, an excess rounded appearance in the upper pole of the breast. I do not want it to be obvious that I have had a breast augmentation.

Type 3—I desire a large breast augmentation and do not mind if it has a mildly unnatural look, ie, a noticeably rounded contour in the upper pole of the breast.

Type 4—I want to use the biggest implant possible knowing that it will create a distorted unnatural look and it will be obvious that I have had a breast augmentation.

Additional adjuncts for size determination include the use of magazine/internet photographs, the amount of padding if any used by the patient, and their size during pregnancy, including any relevant photographs. Regardless, despite the fact that no guarantees can or should be made regarding the final outcome; all efforts need to be made to ensure that decisions made intraoperatively are consistent with the patient's overall desired outcome.

● PATIENT PREPARATION

Similar to virtually all plastic surgery procedures, the preoperative preparation and patient education prior to embarking on surgery far outweighs what occurs within the operating room. This process is only further obfuscated by the myriad of surgical options available in augmentation; including incision placement, pocket location, implant type, and size. Moreover, each of these variables must be assessed within the context of the patient's own desires, the potential benefits, and the possible trade-offs. Key amongst these is recognizing the particular consequence of choices made, especially regarding their inevitable long-term effect upon the patient's native breast dimensions and tissue characteristics. The general rule being that the choice of implant, incision, and pocket position must be tailored to the individual characteristics and anatomy of the patient and their breasts. Pushing beyond those anatomical limits can risk serious consequences in terms of short-term complications and long-term outcomes. In the end, the goal must be to provide the most optimal long-term soft tissue coverage of the implant, while at the same time fulfilling the objectives and desires of the patient.

Incision Placement

Options for incision placement include inframammary, periareola, axillary, and transumbilical approaches, with the latter two most often requiring endoscopic assistance. Choice depends on the surgeon's training and experience in a given technique coupled with individual patient's desires, anatomical limitations, and surgical demands. In particular, the patient's particular breast habitus may facilitate, or limit, the use of one or more approaches to the breast. Similarly, the need for more direct access and/or additional adjustments to the implant pocket and breast assists in determining what is ideal for a given situation.

Inframammary. The most direct approach, inframammary, takes advantage of the fact that many patients present for augmentation with a demonstrable inframammary fold and some degree of breast ptosis. This incision provides the most direct visual access to both the submammary, as well as the subpectoral, spaces without the excessive dissection of breast parenchyma. Therefore, hemostasis and precise pocket dissection are facilitated; as is the incremental release of the pectoralis muscle needed in dual-plane–type augmentations. The location also allows for a generous incision length. When combined, these factors make the inframammary approach amenable to virtually any type or size of implant, including textured, anatomic, cohesive gel, and even form-stable silicone implants. The scar itself, when placed at the inframammary fold or just above, is usually imperceptible; seen only when the patient is supine or recumbent and one is looking from below. Finally, it can be used in a wide variety of patients, especially those with a well-defined fold and/or small areola size. Caution, however, should be exhibited in patients with severely hypoplastic breast and in constricted or tuberous breast patients, as the new position of the inframammary fold may be difficult to discern (and therefore risking a more visible scar on the breast), and due to the extensive amount of parenchymal adjustment sometimes necessary in these cases.

Periareola. While the inframammary approach is more straightforward, the periareola incision is likely the most versatile. It can be used in a large variety of patients, including those presenting with thin native breast tissue and minimal ptosis, ill-defined or asymmetric inframammary folds, and those requiring more extensive parenchymal alterations (eg, tuberous breasts, revisions, capsulorrhaphies, capsulectomies, etc). The exception to this being those individuals with smaller areola sizes (eg, 3.0 cm diameter areola roughly equates to a 4.5 cm hemi-incision) and with light or indistinct areola margins. Otherwise, it provides for a well-concealed scar when placed exactly at the margin of the areola and breast skin. Incisions placed just within the margin risk hypopigmentation, while those just outside the areola may be complicated by a hyperpigmented and more visible scar. Through this incision, a wide variety of parenchymal adjustments can be made, in addition to alterations to the height of the inframammary fold. Furthermore, the periareola approach can be incorporated into various mastopexy-type incisions and facilitates revisional surgery due to its central location within the breast. Concerns regarding this technique mainly include its proximity to the nipple. This includes the possibility for diminished sensation and the inability for lactation. More pressing may be its implication toward higher capsular contraction rates due to the adjacent nipple and/or the need for parenchymal division, and subsequent bacterial contamination during insertion of the implant. Additionally, advocates of the dual-plane technique warn against the possibility of "upstaging" of the procedure due to the necessary release of parenchymal attachments between the pectoralis muscle and the overlying breast tissue. Depending on the plane of dissection, this may result in a greater than expected cephaled retraction of the pectoralis, and therefore a lesser amount of soft tissue coverage of the implant inferiorly.

Axillary. The axillary approach was developed in the 1970s, and gained more widespread popularity during the 1990s following the introduction of the endoscopic-assisted method. Originally, this technique necessitated a somewhat blind and blunt approach to pocket dissection. Detractors complained of an inability to precisely control the pocket dissection and an increased concern over acute postoperative complications, including bleeding, pain, edema, and ecchymosis. Limitations in surgical control also led to complaints of implants positioned too high secondary to inadequate pectoralis division, or too low due to overdissection of the pocket and inadvertent lowering of the inframammary fold. With the addition of endoscopic assistance, advocates of the approach argue that what was once a blind and blunt type of procedure has been converted to a more direct and precise form of dissection, while still retaining the benefits of the original approach. This includes the absence of any scar on the breast, the lack of violation of any breast parenchyma, and the ability to place the implant in either a subpectoral or subglandular pocket. At the same time, use of the endoscope allows more direct visualization, critical for the accurate dissection of the pocket and division of the pectoralis fibers, control of the fold position, and of course hemostasis. These benefits are balanced by a number of limitations of this approach. While it can be used in a wide variety of breast types, the axillary approach is not recommended when extensive alterations to the breast parenchyma are necessary (eg, tuberous breasts, revisions requiring capsulectomy or capsulorrhaphy). Additionally, this approach is not amenable to performing either a dual-plane type II or III dissection. Due to the remote site and incision size limitations within the boundaries of the axilla, certain implants are not recommend with this approach, including larger silicone (>500 cc), textured, anatomic, and form-stable implants. During the initial portion of the dissection, there is a risk of injury to the intercostobrachial cutaneous nerve, resulting in anesthesia over the upper, inner aspect of the arm. Furthermore, even advocates of this approach recognize that patients should be informed that there is always the possibility that a conversion to a more direct approach may be necessary during the operation and that they will likely require a secondary incision for any subsequent revisional procedure. Finally, logistical issues are present, including the need for specialized surgical training, the fixed-cost investment in equipment, additional staff training in order to troubleshoot potential intraoperative technical problems, and the distinct potential for greater operative and anesthetic times.

Transumbilical. Lastly, the most recent advent in incision type is the transumbilical approach to breast augmentation, introduced in 1993. Since its introduction, refinements in technique and instrumentation have made it an option for surgeons seeking a remote site of access that does not have the same potential for exposure of the incision site during certain social or sporting activities,

as in the axillary approach. However, it shares some of the same limitations as its similarly endoscopic-assisted cousin. This includes restrictions on implant type, limited to essentially saline implants; the overall decrease in pocket control, leading to issues with asymmetry and possibly increased revision rates; and the inability to perform additional adjunctive measures to the breast. Patients should again be informed of the risk of conversion to a more direct approach, and the need for a secondary incision for revisional operations. Finally, while technically possible, there is noted difficulty in creating a subpectoral pocket. This factor, when combined with the need for saline implants, potentially limits the population of patients to those with adequate native soft tissue coverage; in order to limit the issues of implant palpability or visibility.

In the end, the choice of incision type must again be individualized taking to account the surgeon's level of comfort and experience and weighing the benefits and trade-offs of each approach. All are acceptable methods when taking into account a particular patient's breast habitus and desires. In regards to patient choice in the matter, an interesting and revealing practice is to inquire as to which incision would be most desired, not if the incision healed well and resulted in an almost imperceptible scar, but instead if due to differences in patient biology, the incision healed poorly. The answer often comes as a surprise to not only the practitioner, but also the patients themselves.

Implant Position

Choices regarding the position of the implant relative to the surrounding soft tissues are best made in regard to optimizing coverage of the implant. Doing so reduces the potential trade-offs of implant palpability and/or visibility, and respects the character of the tissues in regard to their inevitable evolution over time. Options for implant pocket location include subglandular, subfascial, subpectoral, total submuscular, and dual-plane techniques. Of these, only subglandular, subpectoral, and dual-plane techniques are widely practiced. Subfascial positioning represents a modification of the subglandular technique, adding a thin amount of additional tissue coverage. The total submuscular technique was developed as a method of providing increased lateral coverage of the implant, utilizing a portion of the serratus anterior muscle, in addition to the pectoralis, to provide total muscular coverage. Due to trade-offs of increased technical difficulty, inadequate lower pole projection and inframammary fold definition, and late superior displacement over time, in addition to a lack of significant benefits; this method is less frequently used.

Subglandular. Initial attempts at augmentation placed implants in the subglandular, also known as the retromammary, plane. This technique is still widely practiced, and is ideal in situations of breasts with adequate soft tissue coverage; as evidenced by a 2.0 cm or greater pinch test of the upper pole. This provides adequate coverage for the implant and reduces the risk of implant palpability and visible irregularities often seen in thin-breasted individuals. Potential benefits include less postoperative pain and therefore more rapid recovery, and the avoidance of implant distortion seen sometimes with pectoralis muscle contraction. Trade-offs include the increased risk of implant edge palpability/visibility (particularly with saline-filled and/or textured implants), increased interference with screening mammography, and potentially increased rates of capsular contracture. In addition, caudal migration of the implant over time may place additional pressure on the overlying tissues increasing the amount of ptosis, and in extreme cases result in a "rocks in a sock" type of deformity.

Subpectoral. In order to address these issues, the subpectoral, or retropectoral, technique was developed. Overall, the subpectoral position affords a softer, more natural appearing augmentation. While this technique does provide more soft tissue coverage, particularly in those patients with thin breast tissue and inadequate upper pole pinch tests, it too has its own host of benefits and trade-offs. Studies have reported a lower incidence of capsular contracture; however, it is not known whether this is due to a true reduction in capsule formation or simply a situation of decreased detection. And as previously indicated, the subpectoral position facilitates a greater amount of breast tissue being visible during mammography. Potential trade-offs relate directly to the relationship between the pectoralis muscle and the implant. Primary among these is the sometimes visible distortion of the implant and breast shape with pectoralis muscle contraction. Ironically, this is most often seen in those women with thin breast tissue coverage, for which subglandular placement would risk increased implant palpability/visibility. In contrast, in patients with increased amounts of glandular tissue, particularly those with a moderate amount of breast ptosis or postpartum atrophy, the support added by subpectoral placement may result in increased separation of the implant from the overlying ptotic breast tissue and risk development of a "Snoopy" deformity. Finally, in situations where division of the origins of the pectoralis muscle is not performed; lateral and superior displacement of the implant can occur over time, widening the intermammary space between the breasts and reducing the appearance of cleavage. In order to address this issue, various amounts of pectoralis muscle release have been advocated, except in cases of thin soft tissue coverage at the inframammary fold (inferior pinch test <0.5 cm). This likely represented the impetus for the development of the dual-plane technique.

Dual Plane. This latest method of implant placement reports to offer many of the benefits of the above mentioned techniques, while minimizing the potential trade-offs. Elements of the dual-plane technique include (1) the division of selective origins of the pectoralis muscle, (2) a varying amount of dissection between the pectoralis muscle and the breast parenchyma in order to adjust the amount of muscle retraction and thereby the breast's relationship to the implant, and therefore (3) the placement of the implant partially behind the pectoralis muscle and partially behind the breast parenchyma. The main purpose of the technique is to allow a maximal amount of implant coverage via its partial subpectoral placement, while at the same time allowing varying degrees of interface between the implant and the breast parenchyma; as determined by the amount of native breast ptosis and/or laxity. Type I dual plane refers to a complete division of the pectoralis origins across the inframammary fold, without any dissection within the subglandular plane (Figure 46-1). This technique is applicable to the majority of augmentation patients who present with all of their native breast tissue situated above the inframammary fold and a relatively tight breast skin envelope (eg, areola to inframammary fold distance of 4.0–6.0 cm). Type II dual plane is recommended in conditions where the majority of the breast exists above the inframammary fold and the tissues are more mobile with looser attachments (eg, areola to inframammary fold distance of 5.5–6.5 cm). While the same pectoralis origins are released, dissection is also performed at the subglandular plane up to the inferior level of the areola, allowing for a controlled amount of pectoralis retraction and increased amount of parenchymal-implant interaction. Finally, type III dual-plane techniques are applicable in situations of ptotic breasts where up to a third of the tissue is situated below the inframammary fold and the breast envelope is markedly stretched (eg, areola to inframammary fold distances of 7.0–8.0 cm), or in cases of constricted or tuberous breasts with corresponding short areola to inframammary fold distances of only 2.0 to 5.0 cm. Subglandular dissection is performed to the level of the superior aspect of the areola, allowing for an even greater amount of implant projection and interface with the overlying breast parenchyma. Regardless, shared amongst the different levels of the dual-plane technique is the strict preservation of the pectoralis origins along the sternal edge. Doing so does limit the amount of cleavage attainable, but does so at the benefit of providing maximal medial implant coverage, minimizing the possibility of medial implant show, limiting the window shading of the pectoralis muscle following its release along the inframammary fold, and preventing symmastia.

In summary, the choice of implant placement must be made with the goal of optimizing long-term soft tissue coverage, while appreciating the trade-offs of particular techniques. Paramount is the recognition that areas of overdissection or thinning of the breast parenchyma have long-term consequences as the implant inevitably exerts continued pressure on the overlying tissues, and that the correction of these problems may be difficult to potentially impossible. Therefore, the patient's desired outcome must be tempered by what their tissue characteristics

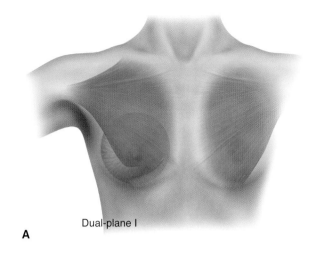

A Dual-plane I

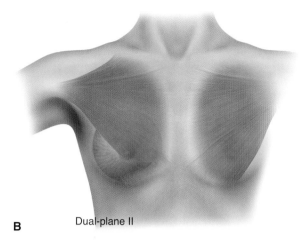

B Dual-plane II

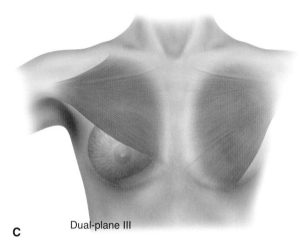

C Dual-plane III

● **FIGURE 46-1.** Dual-plane technique. (*Reprinted with permission from Adams WP Jr. Breast Augmentation. New York: McGraw-Hill; 2011.*)

and dimensions will allow, via the process of adequate preoperative planning and patient education.

Implant Selection

Implant selection from the patient's point of view is driven by several factors, including aesthetics, size, and safety. From the practitioner's viewpoint, much of implant choice and development has been based upon the incidence of capsular contracture. And with the return of silicone implants to the market in 2006, there again is a somewhat perplexing amount of implant choices available. Currently, the majority of implants placed within the United States are round, smooth-walled implants, with an equal distribution between silicone and saline-filled devices. Options due exist, however, in regard to choice of filler material, shell design, implant shape, and of course size.

Silicone vs Saline. While there are obvious differences between the two types of implants, patients tend to fall into one of two categories: those who are comfortable with using silicone and those who are not. Patient education into the history and safety of silicone implants is of vital importance in order to allow patients the option

of an informed choice regarding what they choose to put into their bodies. That being said, neither implant is inherently "safer" or "better" than the other. Benefits and trade-offs exist that must be taken into account, along with the patient's particular breast characteristics.

In some aspects, silicone represents the ideal filler material—inert and similar in consistency and weight to breast tissue. While its early history was plagued with high rates of capsular contracture, the current fourth generation of silicone implant has demonstrated relative low rates, likely due to its low-bleed polymer shell and cohesive gel filler material. Trade-offs include a slightly higher cost, the phenomenon of silent implant rupture, and the need for larger access incisions limiting its use in the majority of axillary and transumbilical cases.

In direct contrast, saline implants enjoy the ability to be placed via smaller incisions and through the full array of access sites. Improved design has corrected early problems associated with valve failure and subsequent deflation. Trade-offs exist, however, due to the inherent nature of a liquid-filled device. Underfilling of the implant, while providing some aspect of softness, is associated with wrinkling and folding of the device, and likely contributes to an increased rate of rupture. In contrast, overfilling can create a scalloping effect along the edge of the device as the shell stretches to accommodate the increased volume. These issues contribute to an overall increased rate of implant palpability and visibility, particularly when using a subglandular pocket. In addition, when appropriately filled, saline devices are again noticeably firmer and slightly heavier than their silicone counterparts.

Smooth vs Textured. Texturing was originally designed in an effort to mimic the decrease capsular contracture rate seen with polyurethane foam-coated implants used during the 1980s. Due to questions of safety regarding their degradation, these devices were removed from the US market in 1991. Regardless, evidence does exist that the textured surface may decrease the rate of capsule formation; however, its benefits appear to be lost when the implant is placed in a submuscular position. Additional attributes include a reduced propensity for migration and/or rotation, explaining its frequent association with anatomic or shaped implants. Downsides include the potential for increased rippling and palpability, particularly in the subglandular position.

Round vs Shaped. While the original Cronin and Gerow implants were both anatomic in shape and textured, issues with high capsular contracture drove manufacturers to create round, smooth-walled implants that could move within their pockets in an effort to reduce capsule formation. With the exception of the previously mentioned polyurethane-coated implants, this type of implant has dominated the US market ever since. Advocates of shaped or anatomic implants purport the benefits of a more "customized" device in certain anatomical situations, such as reduced upper pole fullness in women with thin superior tissues and greater lower pole projection in cases of mammary ptosis. This is, however, at the cost of contour irregularities due to rotation of the implant and therefore the need for exacting pocket dissection. Additionally, arguments exist whether round implants assume an anatomic shape regardless when vertical and in vitro.

Size. It bears mentioning again the critical nature of size in implant selection. In general, the implant most often should fit within the limits of the native breast dimensions. To do otherwise risks issues of contour irregularities, including lowered inframammary folds, lateral arm impingement, high and/or excessively full upper poles, and symmastia. Regardless, the bigger the implant, the more likely that issues of edge palpability and visibility are to occur. Furthermore, over time, the native breast tissue invariably undergoes progressive thinning due to the constant forces of the implant and gravity, which are only exacerbated in situations of larger implants. Therefore, the demands of the patient must always be weighed against the potential short and long-term trade-offs inherent in choosing an implant for augmentation. With careful patient preparation and thorough education on the potential risks and trade-offs, patients most often accept limitations in exchange for minimizing implant palpability/visibility in the short term, and providing the best possible soft tissue coverage in the long term.

● TECHNIQUE

Safe surgical technique begins outside of the operating room. The operative plan, including choices made regarding incision location, pocket position, and implant type, must be documented and reviewed well before embarking on the operation. It is recommended that the choice of implant be "bracketed" by ordering an implant size/type above and below the optimal designated implant. It is also prudent that a third implant be available in the sizes selected, in the rare case of implant rupture or contamination.

Preoperative markings may be done either the day before or the day of surgery. These should be performed in an upright fashion, marking the sternal midline, level of the existing and desired inframammary folds, medial and lateral extents of the implant pocket, any key anatomical landmarks, and the proposed incisions. Any adjustments to the native breast contour should be marked, and may prompt a final discussion regarding the benefits and trade-offs of the proposed operative plan.

Perioperative antibiotic prophylaxis is recommended due to the correlation between bacteria (mainly *Staphylococcus epidermidis*) within the lactiferous ducts of the breast, subclinical infection, and capsular contracture. If utilizing general anesthesia, lower extremity compression devices or pharmacoprophylaxis for deep vein thrombosis is highly recommended. Arms should be securely fastened onto the operative armboards in order to allow sitting up during the operation to assess for symmetry.

Inframammary. When using the inframammary approach, location of the incision relative to the existing inframammary fold is a key factor. In patients with a defined, symmetric, and ideally located inframammary fold, the incision can be placed directly within the fold. However, most situations have some degree of variability. A fact which must be taken into account is that augmentations frequently have a slight lowering effect on the inframammary fold. This situates the final location of the incision usually up onto the dependent portion of the breast, which is much more preferable and less visible than an incision on the chest wall. If planning to adjust the location of the fold, then the incision should be placed in the new, proposed inframammary fold location, taking into account the factors stated above. Incision length is mainly determined by the type of implant, with saline implants requiring a smaller (eg, 3 cm) incision versus larger incisions for silicone and textured implants. Finally, the medial aspect of the incision should not extend beyond the medial border of the areola, in order to prevent its visibility with certain articles of clothing (Figure 46-2).

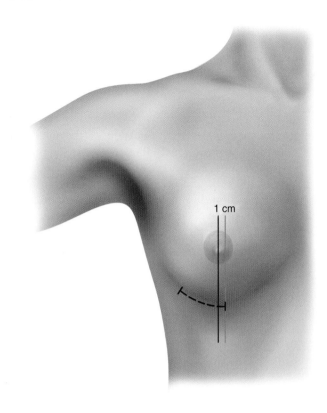

● **FIGURE 46-2.** Inframammary incision. Generally, the most medial extent of the incision is no greater than 1 cm medial to the nipple, with the remaining incision lateral to the nipple. (*Reprinted with permission from Adams WP Jr. Breast Augmentation. New York: McGraw-Hill; 2011.*)

If plans are to maintain the current position of the inframammary fold, dissection must then be directed perpendicularly or cephalad in order to prevent inadvertent undercutting and lowering of the fold (Figure 46-3). With upward retraction using an army-navy–type retractor, access to the subglandular pocket is relatively straightforward. Following division of the fascia, upward retraction also tents up the inferior border of the pectoralis muscle, aiding in its identification. Access to the subpectoral pocket is usually achieved just lateral to the medial costal origins, with further superior pocket dissection greatly facilitated using a lighted retractor. Verification of the pectoralis can be done by lightly touching the muscle in question with the electrocautery, and confirming the proper location and direction of muscular contraction. Additionally, when in question, a small amount of cephalad submuscular dissection can be performed, verifying the subpectoral location via its loose areola tissue, relatively avascular plane of dissection, and the visible rib cartilages and intercostal spaces (Figure 46-4). Further medial and judicious lateral dissection may be performed bluntly at this point, but sharp dissection using the cautery is preferred for hemostasis. Once a precise pocket is created, decisions regarding pectoral division plus/minus dual-plane dissection are performed. Complete division of the inferomedial origins

of the pectoralis is carried out using the cautery and at a location 0.5 to 1.0 cm off of the chest wall (Figure 46-5). This helps to prevent inadvertent lowering of the inframammary fold medially, and assists in identification and ligation of bleeding vessels. More medial division or attenuation of the sternal origins of the muscle is up to the discretion of the surgeon, but does place the patient at risk for increased implant palpability/visibility and symmastia. Once subpectoral dissection is complete, dual-plane techniques may be then performed. It is worth noting that although definitions do exist for the differing levels of this technique, the actual release of the overlying parenchymal attachments to the pectoralis muscle are done in an incremental fashion, with small amounts of dissection resulting in significant retraction of the pectoralis muscle superiorly. In any of the above stated techniques, one can always dissect further; however, reversing the result is technically difficult to impossible. After pocket dissection is complete on both sides, they should be manually palpated for symmetry and any areas of focal constriction. The use of implant sizers is often helpful to define the optimal implant.

Following confirmation of adequate hemostasis, generous irrigation of the pockets should be performed. While previous studies have demonstrated the benefits of povidone-iodine–containing solutions, the FDA in 2000 restricted their use despite the lack of any data linking extraluminal contact with implant shell failure. Regardless, if povidone-iodine solution is utilized, the off-label indication should be documented and discussed with the patient. More commonly, irrigation is performed with approximately 250 cc of a solution consisting of bacitracin, cefazolin, and gentamicin. Insertion of the prosthesis should be performed with a minimal amount of contamination and contact. These methods include the use of talc-free gloves, exchanging of gloves prior to implant handling, wiping the incision site with povidone-iodine or antibiotic solution-soaked sponges, and/or the application of an occlusive dressing around the incision site. Once placed and/or inflated, the implant should be confirmed of its correct anterior-posterior orientation. Symmetry should be assessed with the patient upright. Any final adjustments to the pocket are made, and the incision is closed in layers. Postoperative dressings run the gamut from simple surgical bras to complex dressings and wrapping schemes. While no postoperative dressing regimen is a replacement for accurate, on-table surgical technique; in certain situations, they can assist in maintaining the results achieved within the operating room.

Periareola. Periareola incisions have the benefit of healing almost imperceptively when placed exactly at the inferior areola margin, with likely the lowest rate of hypertrophic scarring. Limitations are based on the size of the areola and the corresponding type and size of the implant. Following skin incision, two approaches exist for parenchymal access—trans- and peri-parenchymal. In the former, dissection is performed directly

A

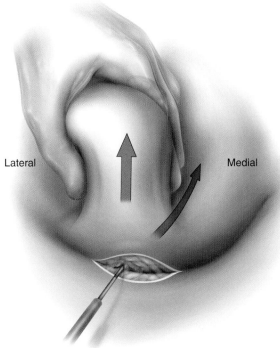

Lateral

Medial

B

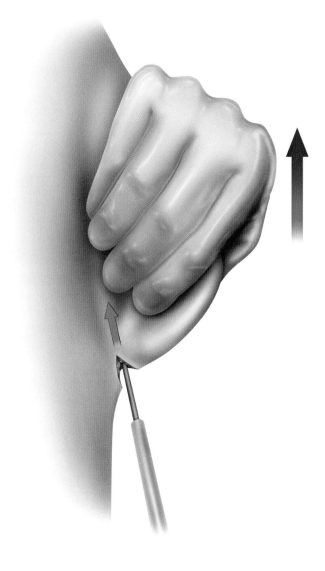

C

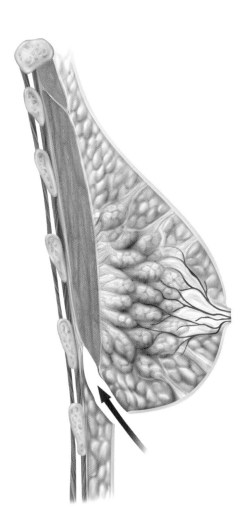

● **FIGURE 46-3.** Inframammary approach. (A, B) After
the initial incision is made, cautery dissection is immediately
performed in a cephalad direction to avoid inadvertent
lowering of the inframammary fold. (C) If performing a
subpectoral pocket dissection, the inferolateral edge of
the pectoralis muscle is identified and dissection proceeds
cephalically beneath the muscle. (*Reprinted with permission from
Adams WP Jr. Breast Augmentation. New York: McGraw-Hill; 2011.*)

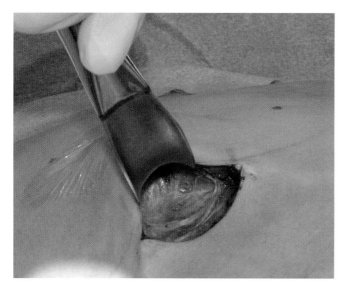

● FIGURE 46-4. Subpectoral pocket dissection. With anterior retraction of the pectoralis muscle, note the relatively avascular plane between the pectoralis major muscle and the underlying chest wall. (*Reprinted with permission from Adams WP Jr. Breast Augmentation. New York: McGraw-Hill; 2011.*)

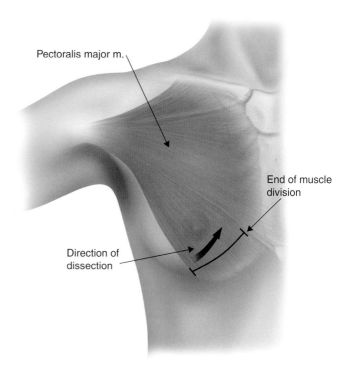

● FIGURE 46-5. Pectoralis major muscle division. Note the preservation of 0.5 to 1.0 cm of pectoralis along the inferomedial origin of the muscle, as well as preserving all of the muscle attachments to the sternal edge. (*Reprinted with permission from Adams WP Jr. Breast Augmentation. New York: McGraw-Hill; 2011.*)

perpendicular toward the pectoralis muscle, with further dissection within the subglandular space. With the latter, dissection is performed inferiorly along a subcutaneous plane in order to reach the inferior aspect of the breast. Both approaches allow varying degrees of access for parenchymal alteration or inframammary fold adjustment. Care must be taken, however, in that both also create potential spaces within the breast that can lead to malposition of the implant. Additionally, transparenchymal dissection automatically creates as type II dual-plane dissection and may be too aggressive in circumstances of thin soft tissue coverage. Finally, this route of access exposes the implant to greater amounts of contamination or seeding, due to the adjacent nipple and parenchymal division; and has been theorized to lead to increasing rates of capsular contracture.

Axillary. Initially, a greater amount of preparation, planning, equipment, and technique are necessary when using the axillary approach. An early decision must be made whether to perform this technique with or without the aid of endoscopy. Traditional techniques necessitated blunt dissection and stretching of the pocket and associated muscular attachments. Complications included higher rates of bleeding, hematoma, asymmetry, and malposition. Advocates of the endocopic technique note its similarity with more conventional approaches to breast augmentation—eg, direct visualization, sharp dissection of tissue, and overall control of hemostasis and pocket dissection. Limitations of this technique may include the choice of implant type and pocket location, with most practitioners utilizing smooth-walled, saline implants (due to the limited incision size and remote

location) and correspondingly a subpectoral placement. Silicone implants may be used, but often must be limited in size (<500 cc).

Initial preparation includes marking of the axillary incision while standing. The incision should be horizontally oriented and high within the axilla, with its anterior limit at the posterior margin of the pectoralis muscle (Figure 46-6). Intraoperative positioning of the patient should be with arms extended 90 degrees, with access to the axilla and adequate space above both arms for positioning of the surgeon. Correspondingly, the endoscopic monitor should be situated at the foot of the bed to facilitate direct line of sight and dissection. Additional key instrumentation includes a short 10 mm diameter/30 degree-angle endoscope, light source, suction, digital camera, and ideally a composite retractor that incorporates all of these elements.

Following incision and cautery dissection of the subcutaneous tissue, scissors can be used to dissect a space toward the posterior aspect of the pectoralis muscle. Of note, maintaining dissection anteriorly limits disruption of the intercostobrachial cutaneous nerve. Division of the perctoralis fascia should occur on a line a parallel to the posterior border of the muscle, and the subpectoral space confirmed with digital palpation of the loose areola tissue and relatively avascular plane. Again, at this point, further dissection may be performed bluntly

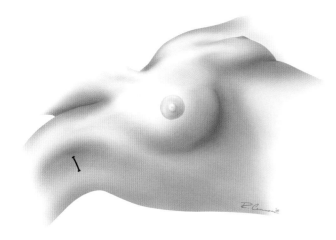

(using a curved Emory or Agris-Dingman dissector) and/or more sharply under direct endoscopic visualization. Division of pectoralis muscular origins proceeds as previously stated, with the axillary technique limited to type I dual-plane dissections, followed by confirmation of adequate hemostasis and pocket irrigation. It is worth noting that exchanging instrumentation is greatly facilitated by the removal and replacement of an instrument prior to withdrawing the retractor or other device from the plane of dissection. This limits the amount of time spent re-manipulating the soft tissues in order to regain access to the pocket. Insertion of a saline prosthesis is also aided by double-rolling the implant around the central valve into a cigar-shape device. Any issues regarding control of the operation (eg, hemostasis) necessitates conversion to a more open approach.

● **COMPLICATIONS**

Any surgical procedure that carries with it an approximate 50% complication rate and/or a 30% reoperation rate would likely be construed by many as ill advised, notwithstanding it being an operation that is both elective and cosmetic. These numbers outline the current statistics associated with breast augmentation; again highlighting the fact that this is anything but a simple and straightforward procedure. A look at the list of adverse events included in the product data sheet associated with breast implants include implant rupture, capsular contracture, reoperation, implant removal, pain, changes in nipple and breast sensation, infection, scarring, asymmetry, wrinkling, implant displacement/migration, implant palpability/visibility, breastfeeding complications, hematoma/seroma, implant extrusion, necrosis, delayed wound healing, breast tissue atrophy/chest wall deformity, calcium deposits, and lymphadenopathy. Review of the Mentor and Allergan 10-year Core Studies reveal

that the risk of any complication following primary augmentation was 36.6% at 3 years (Mentor) and 45% at 7 years (Allergan), with the most frequent being reoperation (15.4% and 30.1%, respectively), followed by grade III/IV capsular contracture (8.1% and 15.5%).[6,7] Within the above stated list exist both unavoidable and avoidable complications. An obvious goal, therefore, must be to reduce and/or eliminate those avoidable occurrences that may lead to later reoperation.

Reoperation for these avoidable complications (eg, change in size) most likely represents a failure of planning and/or education on the part of the surgeon. During the preoperative evaluation, the clinician must recognize what is achievable in regards to the patient's own tissues. The patient must then understand and accept the limitations, risks, and trade-offs of the choices made. Otherwise, pushing beyond those physical limitations increases the risk of complications. This process of discovery and subsequent discussion then assists both the patient and the surgeon in anticipating long-term consequences of those choices.

Broadly speaking, there is nothing done in the process of breast augmentation that improves the tissue quality of the patient's breasts. Additionally, the placement of an implant, particularly a large implant (>350 cc) in conjunction with age-related changes in the breast, will likely diminish the quality of those tissues over the long term.

Implant Rupture

While not the most common complication associated with augmentation mammaplasty, it is often the one that concerns the patient most; in addition to being one that is frequently misunderstood by the patient. Likely due to the history and misinformation surround silicone implants, patients often arrive with preconceived notions regarding both the incidence and consequences of implant rupture. Based on the manufacturers' core study data, including an MRI-evaluated cohort, rupture in silicone implants occurred in 0.5% of patients at 3 years and 8.6% at 7 years, underscoring the fact that rupture is an intrinsic component of implants. Patients should be educated that implants are not lifetime devices, particularly when viewed with the fact that 36% are placed in women age 30 to 39 years, followed by the 20- to 29-year-old cohort (30%) and the 40 to 54 age group (28%). The longer the interval from surgery, the greater the risk of rupture. Consequences of implant rupture are for the most part local (ie, deflation in the context of saline implants) or silent (ie, silicone implants). In regard to the former, it is recommended that removal or replacement of the device occur within 1 month to avoid contraction of the pocket. In regard to the latter, it is recommended that women with silicone implants undergo screening MRIs at 3 years following primary surgery, and then every 2 years thereafter in order to detect silent rupture. At this point, it is uncertain who will bear the burden for the cost of these MRIs. Regardless, when rupture has been detected (via characteristic radiographic findings such as the linguini sign, subcapsular lines, teardrop sign, keyhole sign, noose sign), the implant should be removed and/or replaced. Consequences of silicone rupture are mainly local in nature, due to the fact that the majority of ruptures are intracapsular (ie, remain within the boundaries of the scar tissue capsule surrounding the implant). Local breast complications may include breast hardness, change in shape or size, and breast pain. Rare but reported symptoms due to extracapsular rupture have included granuloma formation, nerve injury, tissue breakdown, and lymphadenopathy. Currently, the scientific data, including several large epidemiologic studies, fails to find any connection between silicone implants and connective tissue, rheumatologic diseases, or cancer.

Capsular Contracture

The formation of scar tissue encapsulating a breast implant is a normal physiologic process. However, when that capsule becomes excessively thickened and/or contractile in nature, and adversely affects the breast shape and/or is symptomatic; it then becomes pathologic (ie, Baker grade III/IV). The incidence of capsular contracture represents the largest single complication associated with breast augmentation, and constitutes the most frequent cause for reoperation. Its incidence has been as high as 50% in some series, depending on the grade and severity of symptoms as outlined by the Baker classification.

Class I—Breast is soft and looks natural (ie, none)
Class II—Breast looks normal, but is firm to palpation (ie, mild)
Class III—Breast both feels looks and feels abnormal (ie, moderate)
Class IV—Breast is hard, painful, and looks distorted (ie, severe)

The onset of capsular contracture is usually within the first year; however, it may occur at any time. There exist a myriad of inciting factors implicated in causing capsular contracture; however, the majority of them can be grouped into one of two categories: infectious or due to hypertrophic scar formation.

Infectious theories are supported by the fact that *S epidermidis* has been shown to be significantly associated with capsular contracture, and in a prospective study found to be present in 90% of implants removed for this reason.[8] Additionally, numerous other bacterial agents have been implicated, indicating a possible polymicrobial cause. Low-level colonization is thought to occur secondary to skin level contact (especially at the nipple) or via insertion of the implant through transected glandular tissue. These concerns have led to the widespread usage of antibiotic irrigation (eg, bacitracin/cefazolin/gentamicin solution) of the implant pocket and an emphasis on strict sterile technique.[9]

A second leading hypothesis deals with the introduction of non-infectious material as a nidus for capsule formation; with subsequent inflammation and fibroblast proliferation, leading to collagen deposition and contracture formation. Inciting agents include blood, seroma, and powdered glove residue. This hypothesis is supported by early evidence showing a high rate of capsular contracture following complications of hematoma.

Efforts to combat capsular contracture have driven both refinements in surgical technique, as well as implant design. For example, while early silicone implants were notorious for their high rate of capsule formation attributed to gel bleed, successive generations of both silicone and saline implants have demonstrated progressively lower rates. Accordingly, a host of additional factors have been thought to be beneficial in regards to inhibiting capsule formation. Following the low rates found with polyurethane-coated implants, textured implants have been reported to reduce capsular contracture; although this benefit appears to be negated when implants are placed in a submuscular position. There is some evidence that smaller implant sizes (<350 cc) have a reduced incidence of contracture. Additionally, many surgeons recommend postoperative pocket massage and displacement exercises. Finally, as a general recommendation, atraumatic tissue dissection, combined with meticulous hemostasis, has been advocated in contrast to more blunt techniques. Modalities that have not been found to have a significant effect regarding capsule formation include the use of prolonged systemic antibiotics nor the use of surgical drains within the implant pocket.

While prevention is the best method of treatment, techniques for dealing with capsular contracture initially consisted of closed capsulotomy. This method was frequently complicated by uncontrolled capsular tears, resulting in asymmetry and hematoma formation. Additional complications included implant rupture with possible silicone extrusion into surround tissues, resultant chronic inflammation, and siliconomas. This technique has been largely replaced by open capsulotomy/capsulectomy, with the goal of total capsulectomy. Further adjuncts include implant exchange due to concerns of biofilm development and repositioning of the implant to a new surgical site (ie, subglandular to subpectoral or dual plane). Unfortunately, no medical modality (eg, leukotriene inhibitors, NSAIDs, steroids) has been proven to be of any benefit in the prevention or treatment of capsular contracture.

Aesthetic Complications

Aesthetic complications consist of issues regarding size, malposition, asymmetry, and contour irregularities (both dynamic and static). Other than capsular contracture, this category of complications accounts for the highest rates of reoperation following augmentation. According to manufacturers' core study data, implant malposition alone was responsible for 13.6% of reoperations

(Allergan); while in a separate study, request for size/ style change accounted for 14.7% (Mentor). When all combined, these various issues are not only a major source for reoperation, but are also likely preventable; and therefore represent a failure in preoperative planning and education. This is most likely due to mismatches in patient physical characteristics and/or patient desires with the overall surgical plan. It cannot be overemphasized that implant augmentation beyond the physical limitations of the patient's breast habitus place the patient at significant risk for these complications.

Malposition and asymmetry are again often due to ignoring the specific limitations of the patient's breast. This may include violation of the native inframammary fold, resulting in inferior displacement of the implant; overdissection of the lateral pocket, resulting in lateral displacement; division of the sternal origins of the pectoralis muscle, resulting in symmastia; and an overall mismatch between the native breast and underlying implant, resulting in a double-bubble deformity. This latter problem is commonly seen following disruption of the inframammary fold with inferior displacement of the implant, often in conjunction with situations of constricted or tuberous breasts. Additional contour issues include the so-called "Snoopy" deformity, occurring when recurrent, ptotic, native breast tissues hangs over the end of a superiorly displaced implant. In regard to issues of wrinkling and rippling deformities transmitted through the skin, this is most often due to volume underfill associated with saline and textured implants. The opposite is true of "scalloping" along the implant edge, which is indicative of saline implant overfill. Finally, implant placement in a thin and/or athletic individual, in a submuscular position in order to prevent particular aesthetic complications, may instead result in implant deformities associated with pectoralis muscle contraction. Correction of these various issues revolves around recognizing the anatomical basis for the deformity; correcting the surgical error; and/or implementing changes in implant size, pocket dimensions, and/or location using a combination of techniques. A final word needs to be said regarding reoperation for size change following primary augmentation. As previously stated, every effort must be made to accurately assess the patient's desires for final breast size, within the context of what their native tissues can accommodate. This complication should clearly be viewed as avoidable in nature and therefore represents inadequate patient preparation and education or a lack of rapport between patient and surgeon. Regardless, this should prompt a review of one's approach to patient consultation and preoperative preparation.

Local Complications

Local issues include nipple complications (10.4%), hypertrophic scarring (6.7%), hematoma (2.6%), changes in breast sensation (2.2%), seroma (1.6%), and infection (<1%). Additionally, depending on the study, there

appears to be variable amount of what is labeled "chronic breast pain" following augmentation, ranging from 1.7% to 11.4%.

While it is tempting to treat issues of postoperative fluid collections conservatively, hematomas and seromas predispose the patient to more complex issues of infection, capsular contracture, and asymmetry; and should therefore be treated immediately upon diagnosis.

In regard to infection, while rates are low, the impact on the patient can be severe due to the possibility of reoperation and/or implant removal. While *S epidermidis* species are ubiquitous within the breast due to the presence of the lactiferous ducts, *Staphylococcus aureus* species are responsible for the majority of implant related infections. Attempts to prevent infection have been outlined previously, but also include the use of closed filling systems when using saline implants. Treatment of associated infections is geared toward aggressive and prompt management, using a combination if intravenous antibiotics, surgical irrigation and debridement, capsulectomy, and implant exchange. Explantation, healing, and delayed reimplantation is the most conservative approach and is always an option in cases of severe infection, implant exposure, and/or abscess.

Uncommon Complications

Uncommon complications associated with breast augmentation include galactorrhea, late hematoma, Mondor disease, and neoplasm. Mondor disease represents inflammation and subsequent upper abdominal wall venous thrombosis, presenting as a tender, palpable cord, usually located inferior to the inframammary fold. Treatment includes anti-inflammatories, with self-resolution over a few weeks.

While several large, epidemiologic studies have failed to show any increased risk of breast cancer following augmentation, it must be recognized that the development and diagnosis of masses within the breast will become an ever-increasing issue. Inherent within this problem are the limitations of breast imaging associated with implants and the evolving strategies currently available for diagnosis and treatment. Current recommendations include the use of open biopsy versus fine-needle or core biopsy, due to the presence of the implant. Treatment following a diagnosis of breast cancer usually involves mastectomy. Breast conservation therapy is currently not recommended due to several issues. Intrinsically, most patients have limited native breast tissue to begin with. Therefore, obtaining clear margins may be difficult, and the resulting defect following lumpectomy can be substantial and often associated with significant asymmetries. Adjuvant radiation therapy, as a component of breast conservation therapy, has been shown to incur a high rate of complications, foremost among them being capsular contracture (up to 65%). And surveillance and imaging following conservation therapy is even further hampered by the presence of capsule formation around the implant.

● OUTCOMES ASSESSMENT

Despite the plethora of issues surrounding breast augmentation, including patient desires, education, preoperative planning, and potential complications; patient satisfaction following augmentation mammaplasty remains high, averaging 95%. Psychosocial and quality of life assessments have shown mixed results. Similar to other cosmetic surgery patients, women seeking breast augmentation report a higher rate of body image issues, psychiatric disease, and suicide than the general population. However, quantitative improvements following augmentation have been found in the areas of body image, concern over weight, and sexual attractiveness.

REFERENCES

1. American Society of Plastic Surgeons. *Report of the 2010 Plastic Surgery Statistics*. APS National Clearinghouse of Plastic Surgery Procedural Statistics. http://www.plasticsurgery.org/Media/Statistics.html.

2. Miglioretti DL, Rutter CM, Geller BM, et al. Effect of breast augmentation on the accuracy of mammography and cancer characteristics. *JAMA*. 2004;291:442.

3. Tebbetts JB. Dual plane breast augmentation: Optimizing implant-soft-tissue relationships in a wide range of breast types. *Plast Reconstr Surg*. 2006;118(7 Suppl):81S.

4. Tebbetts JB, Adams WP. Five critical decisions in breast augmentation using five measurements in 5 minutes: The high five decision support process. *Plast Reconstr Surg*. 2006;118(7 Suppl):35S.

5. Mentor Corporation. Bodylogic System. http://www.mentor wwllc.com/global/physician-information/bodylogic.htm.

6. Cunningham B. The Mentor Core Study on silicone MemoryGelb breast pmplants. *Plast Reconstr Surg*. 2007;120 (7 Suppl 1):19S.

7. Spear SL, Murphy DK, Slicton A, et al. Inamed silicone breast implant core study results at 6 years. *Plast Reconstr Surg*. 2007;120(7 Suppl 1):8S.

8. Pajkos A, Deva AK, Vickery K, et al. Detection of subclinical infection in significant breast implant capsules. *Plast Reconstr Surg*. 2003;111:1605.

9. Adams WP, Rios JL, Smith SJ. Enhancing patient outcomes in aesthetic and reconstructive breast surgery using triple antibiotic breast irrigation: Six-year prospective clinical Study. *Plast Reconstr Surg*. 2006;118(7 Suppl):46S.

chapter 47

Congenital Breast Deformities

S. Alex Rottgers, MD / *Derek Fletcher, MD* / *Angela Song Landfair, MD* / *Kenneth C. Shestak, MD*

● INTRODUCTION

Aesthetically "normal" breasts are of great importance for young women because their perception of femininity and sexual identity. Morphological deformities of the breast can cause issues with wearing clothes, psychological stress, depression, peer rejection, and psychosexual dysfunction, particularly in adolescent females. Many of these deformities lend themselves to reconstruction during or after breast development is complete.

In addition, abnormalities of breast development can carry with them serious implications for the medical, functional, and psychological well-being of the patient. Congenital breast deformities may be associated with abnormalities of other organ systems (genito-urinary) which should be sought out for treatment.

As the breast constantly evolves over time and revisions may be required in the future following initial surgery, the timing and method of reconstruction should be determined only after a detailed discussion with the young patient and her family to understand her expectations and to best ensure that they together understand the realities and limitations of a proposed procedure. This is central to the process of informed consent and is the foundation of the doctor–patient relationship.

Pediatric breast deformities can be divided into hyperplastic, hypoplastic, and post-traumatic defects. Each represents various pathologies and a spectrum of disease which warrant consideration on a case-by-case basis. Treatment goals should focus on accurate diagnosis and appropriate timing and technique selection that will optimize the cosmetic outcome and best satisfy the psychological needs of the patient.

● EMBRYOLOGY AND DEVELOPMENT

Breast development is initiated between the 5th and 7th week of gestation. At this time, the mammary lines form as bilateral linear condensations of ectoderm extending from the axillary areas to the groin region, which invaginate and come to lie below the ectodermal surface forming the mammary ridges. In most instances, only a small focus of mammary tissue overlying the thoracic region in the area of the fourth intercostal space persists and will go on to form the true breast, while those foci in the other areas promptly regress. This tissue continues to divide and thicken; and by the 8th gestational week, ectoderm has invaded into the underlying mesenchyme in a branching patter. At 16 weeks of gestation, 15 to 25 epithelial branches have formed, but canalization has not begun. It is during the third trimester, under the influence of placental sex hormones (mainly estrogen and progesterone) that these epithelial branches are canalized, and primitive breast ducts begin to form. At 32 weeks, differentiation of the parenchyma into lobules begins. The nipple-areola complex begins to form and is completed in the early postnatal period. Branching and canalization continue after birth and through early childhood.[1,2]

Breast development is relatively quiescent throughout childhood. Further breast growth and maturation is subsequently initiated at the time of thelarche. With the increased growth at thelarche, the breast progresses through a series of morphological stages, as described by the Tanner classification. A Tanner stage 1 breast is prepubertal, with no appreciable breast parenchyma and slight nipple elevation. At thelarche, the breast progresses toward Tanner stage 2 with enlargement of the nipple-areola complex and elevation of the breast/nipple as a small mound. Tanner stage 3 describes a breast with further enlargement and a smooth transition between the breast and areola without separation of their contours. As the breast continues to enlarge toward Tanner stage 4, the nipple and areola enlarge more and project as a secondary mound above the breast contour. Finally, at the final Tanner stage 5, the breast achieves its mature size and form. The areola has receded and forms a continuous contour with the surrounding breast.[3] Most females have achieved full breast maturity by age 16 to 18 years; however, the evolution of the breast form continues as a lifelong process based on changes in body habitus, pregnancy, and other factors.

HYPOPLASTIC DISORDERS

Various conditions result in hypoplasia or aplasia of the breast. Hypoplasia in the form of mild asymmetry, constricted breast deformities, and mild presents of Poland syndrome is much more common than aplasia of the breast. Both the constricted breast deformity and Poland syndrome will be discussed in detail below.

Terms used to describe breast aplasia include athelia (isolated absence of the nipple-areola complex), amasia (absence of breast parenchyma), and amastia (absence of both breast tissue and the nipple-areola complex).[1] Although this nomenclature would suggest otherwise, athelia and amasia do not seem to occur without the other. For a comprehensive description of amastia, the reader is referred to description by Trier.[4]

HYPERPLASTIC DISORDERS

Hyperplastic disorders include the excess development of mammary tissue in its normal anatomic location as well as the development of breast tissue or nipple-areola structures in locations remote from the normal thoracic distribution. Treatments require simple observation, excision, or breast reduction techniques. Accurately diagnosing and assessing the degree of deformity is essential, along with counseling the patient and family.

Virginal Hypertrophy

Virginal hypertrophy of the breast is a rare condition that results in excessive, rapid, and often nonyielding proliferation of breast tissue. The etiology is unclear, but pathologic evaluation seems to suggest an abnormal sensitivity of the glandular tissue to circulating estrogen is the cause in the setting of normal levels of this hormone. The condition may be unilateral or bilateral. Patients often exhibit a rapid onset of breast hypertrophy only months after the initiation of breast growth that quickly becomes symptomatic with the typical signs of macromastia (shoulder and neck pain, bra strap grooving, and

rashes) along with tender breast parenchyma, thinned skin, striae, and dilated veins. They will generally present because of the rapid progression.

Treatment is ultimately surgical. Breast reduction techniques are standard as a first-line therapy, and goals should be to first achieve an improved breast size and symptom relief. Improved symmetry in asymmetric cases of hypertrophy is also important. Some patients still require repeated breast reduction operations, and mastectomy may be considered in refractory cases.[5] Pharmacologic therapy in the form of medroxyprogesterone acetate, dydrogesterone, tamoxifen, and bromocriptine has been used but side effects have limited their use.[1,5]

Giant Fibroadenoma

Like virginal hypertrophy, giant fibroadenomas results from abnormal sensitivity of the breast tissue to normal hormonal levels. This entity is a discrete benign tumor which enlarges rapidly and causes asymmetric enlargement of the breast.[5] Treatment is also surgical excision. This is accomplished through breast reduction techniques with a pedicle design and excision pattern that incorporates the mass into the resection specimen and positions the pedicle in the location of the greatest amount of normal breast tissue to preserve breast fullness. Concurrent matching procedures on the contralateral breast or delayed revision mastopexy/augmentative procedures may be needed to achieve symmetry. Timing for surgery is driven by the rate of tumor growth. Excision may be necessitated prior to completion of breast development to limit the distortion of the breast and better achieve an aesthetic result.

The differential diagnosis for fibroadenoma includes cystosarcoma phyllodes, which can be difficult to differentiate on pathology preoperatively or even on frozen sections. Because the incidence of phyllodes tumor is less than 1.3%, treatment should include simple excision of the mass followed by consideration for mastectomy or adjuvant therapy if the diagnosis of phyllodes tumor is made with consultation of surgical oncology or pediatric surgery is recommended.

Polythelia and Polymastia

Polythelia, presence of accessory nipples, is a common pediatric abnormality and has reported incidence as high as 5.6%.[1,4] Polymastia, the development of supernumerary breast tissue, with or without a nipple or areola is much less common. Both are presumed to arise from an incomplete regression of the mammary ridge during embryonic development, leaving residual mammary tissue along the "milk line" between the axilla and pubic region. Polymastia most often occurs with axillary breast tissue.[1] Supernumerary breast tissue may also be removed surgically with placement of closed suction drains.

Gynecomastia

Although usually seen by plastic surgeons in its most severe form, gynecomastia is by far the most common pediatric breast deformity occurring in up to 65% of pubescent males.[1] Gynecomastia is a clinical term denoting enlargement of the male breast such that it is female like. It is most often related to proliferation of ductal epithelium, as no true acnicar development occurs. Most often, it is idiopathic in its etiology, but the proliferation can be a symptom of an underlying pathologic process. "Physiologic" gynecomastia is common during three periods of a male's lifespan. Neonates often exhibit small enlargement of the breast bud and may secrete colostrum transiently as a response to maternal estrogens. As stated above, the fluctuating hormonal milieu of early puberty produces gynecomastia in up to 65% of males between age 14 to 16 years, and declining androgen production seen in later life can lead to a relative estrogen excess and to the development of gynecomastia. If other signs of pubertal development are present, a normal history and physical should suffice for evaluation; but in the absence of normal pubertal development, a more extensive evaluation is needed to elucidate the etiology. In most males, pubertal gynecomastia is mild and transient.[1]

While gynecomastia may be considered normal in these age groups, a history and physical examination should be performed to look for common causes such as testicular cancer, pituitary tumors, adrenal tumors, liver disease, paraneoplastic syndromes, Klinefelter syndrome, thyroid disease, renal failure, myotonic dystrophy, HIV, and the use of marijuana, alcohol, anabolic steroids, and medications known to cause gynecomastia.[1] The most common etiology of gynecomastia in patients older than age 40 years is drug induced.

When significant gynecomastia persists for 2 years beyond puberty, surgery is often indicated to re-create a more normal chest contour and nipple location with limited scaring. The first procedures described for gynecomastia focused on subcutaneous mastectomy through periareola or various other incisions.[6,7] This likely is still the best approach in cases of dense fibrous tissue that is located in a subareola plane. Others have advocated the use of ultrasound-assisted liposuction as the standard first-line approach, followed by secondary excision only for a marked residual deformity. The ideal approach in most cases is a combination of these, with direct periareola excision of the central, fibrous breast buds followed by liposuction to contour the periphery. Severely redundant skin may be excised primarily with a periareola or vertical skin excision, but we believe that the significant elasticity of youthful skin often allows and produces adequate retraction of skin excess, such that in most cases primary skin excision is not warranted. If the skin envelope redundancy persists beyond 6 to 12 months postoperatively, excision can then be undertaken.[6,7] Care must be taken during resection, not to over-resect tissue to avoid a contour indentation "dishing" or nipple retraction. Regardless of technique used, postoperative care involves use of closed suction drains following excision, prolonged compressive garment application (for at least 6 weeks), twice daily deep tissue massage instituted at 1 week postoperative, and abstinence from heavy exercise for 1 month. These adjuncts aid in tissue re-draping, reduce edema, and limit formation of seroma and hematomas.

● AN APPROACH TO CONGENITAL AND DEVELOPMENTAL BREAST ASYMMETRIES

Both hypoplastic and hyperplastic breast disorders represent a spectrum of disease. Often patients present with bilateral manifestations of breast hypoplasia, breast constriction, and hyperplasia. Significant breast asymmetries can result from variable expressions of these. The key to achieving an outcome that both the patient and surgeon are pleased with is to first identify these bilateral and asymmetric abnormalities preoperatively. The surgeon must understand what the patient perceives as abnormal about her breasts, which breast she like better, and what their goals of treatment are. The key is to educate the patient that the goal is improvement of her breast symmetry and contour, rather than perfection. Perfection is always striven for, but in reality is never achieved. Managing patient expectations preoperatively is a key to success in this area of surgery. Significant improvements almost always occur, and if patients understand the limits of surgery before the procedure, they are generally pleased with their result.

If the surgeon can accurately identify which breast bothers the patient or if both are problematic, then he or she can begin to formulate an operative treatment plan. In our experience, the best results in cases of breast asymmetry are achieved in cases where a patient has a smaller, but aesthetically pleasing breast, which they want the larger breast to match. A single-staged reduction or mastopexy can improve symmetry, correct ptosis in the larger breast, and avoid the potential problems of implant-based reconstruction/augmentation. This limits the number of variables at play (eg, issues inherent with implant placement) and increases the predictability of the final outcome.

The operation should be designed based on the amount of resection needed to match the contralateral breast volume, the distance which the nipple must be transposed to achieve symmetry, the degree of ptosis, and the experience/comfort the surgeon has with various pedicle techniques. This is illustrated by the patient in case 1 (Figure 47-1). She presented at age 17 with unilateral right breast hypertrophy. She liked the size of her opposite left breast and did not wish to have surgery on it.

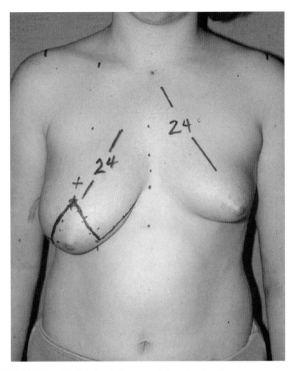

● FIGURE 47-1. An 18-year-old patient with developmental breast asymmetry with unilateral right breast hyperplasia. The plan is for unilateral right breast reduction with 5-cm nipple transposition. A total of 365 g of tissue was resected from the right breast.

She underwent an inferior pedicle breast reduction with a Wise pattern skin excision. She is shown 5 years postoperatively (Figures 47-2 and 47-3A,B) with excellent shape and symmetry of the breasts.

In most cases, the clinical scenario is not so straightforward or simple however. In our experience, most surgical corrections involve bilateral surgery. Differential reductions, mastopexies, augmentations, and most frequently combinations of these must be employed to achieve the most harmonious balance between the breasts when combinations of hypoplasia and hyperplasia coexist. Careful consideration of each breast and each breast abnormality within the context of the patient's expectations is paramount. This includes explaining the details of surgery, such as incision placement, anticipated recovery and the potential surgical, cosmetic complications that may occur including the inherent risks of breast implants specifically focusing on capsular contracture, implant failure, and unplanned additional surgery. It must also be mentioned that the breast appearance will most likely change with weight fluctuation, pregnancy, and aging; regardless of what procedures are undertaken, all are important elements of an informed consent that centrally involves the patient and her parents.

Timing for reconstruction must also be addressed with the patient and her family. As the breast is constantly developing and evolving in form, it is best to delay

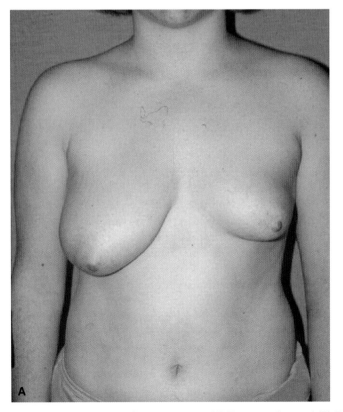

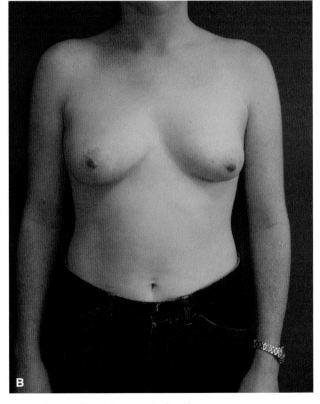

● FIGURE 47-2. (A) Preoperative and (B) 5-year postoperative anteroposterior view showing maintenance of symmetry.

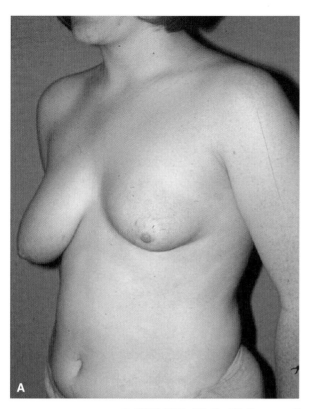
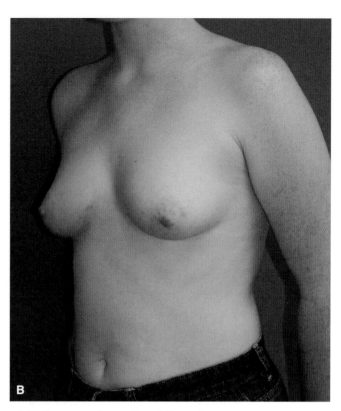

● **FIGURE 47-3.** (A) Preoperative and (B) 5-year postoperative oblique view.

treatment in very young patient. It is most often ideal to delay reconstruction until the patient has finished growing and her breasts are mature (patients who are older than 16 years of age).

We employed this strategy in the patient shown in case 2 (Figure 47-4A,B). She was seen at age 15 with a combination of right breast hypoplasia with breast constriction and left breast hypertrophy. The best approach

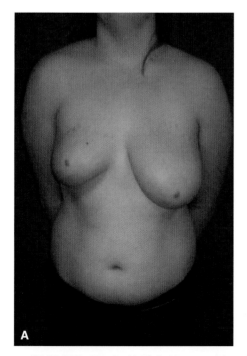
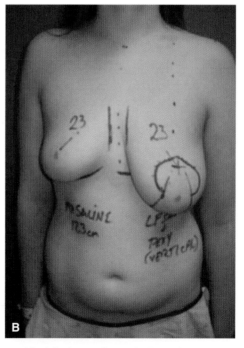

● **FIGURE 47-4.** (A,B) A 16-year-old patient with right breast hypoplasia and left breast hyperplasia. The plan is for a partial retropectoral placement of a 360-cc, moderate profile, saline implant and left vertical reduction of 335 g.

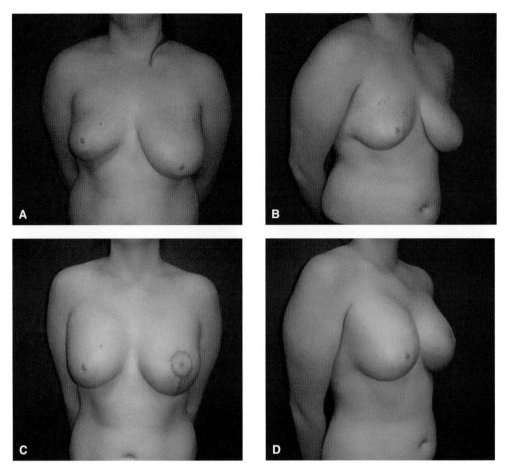

● **FIGURE 47-5.** (A,B) Preoperative and (C,D) 4-month postoperative views showing improved breast symmetry with bilateral breast surgery.

was to wait until the summer prior to her senior year in high school, at which time she underwent a periareola augmentation/mastopexy on the right side with the partial subpectoral placement of a saline implant and a left vertical mastopexy. She is shown at 4 months following surgery (Figure 47-5) with much improved overall breast symmetry.

In cases of more severe deformities in a setting of a patient who appears to be mature (physically and psychologically) at an age younger than 16 years, earlier surgical intervention can be considered. When surgical procedures are undertaken in these younger patients, future revisions are likely to be more common.

Another approach to this problem is placement of a standard tissue expander followed by immediate expansion to correct for the current asymmetry. If patients are young and likely to have continued maturation of their breasts, this expander can be left with subsequent adjustments made to the volume over a period of months to years. The ultimate exchange for a permanent prosthetic can be made when the patient has fully matured, and she desires the completion of her reconstruction. The senior author (KCS) first encountered this strategy when two postmastectomy patients were lost to follow-up after placement of their tissue

expander and subsequent expansion. The patients did not return for placement of their permanent prosthesis until years later. In the interim, they had no complications and exhibited an aesthetic breast contour that was appealing. In the past, we have considered the use of Becker adjustable breast implants (currently no longer available) but experienced difficulty finding the expander port, and fear of implant injury has lead us to favor the use of expanders with magnetized injection ports and robust metallic backstops.

Placement of a breast reconstruction tissue expander should not be considered definitive reconstruction, but it offers a means for a young patient to have her emotional and social concerns centered around a significant breast asymmetry addressed in a timely manner in a way that can be adjusted as she continues to grow and limits the risks of compromising her ultimate outcome once she has reached maturity.

● **TUBEROUS BREAST DEFORMITIES**

Tuberous breast deformity describes a spectrum of aberrant breast morphology first reported by Rees and Aston.[8] The term "tuberous breast" refers to the similarity in shape of affected breasts to a tuberous plant root. Since its original description in 1976, multiple authors have reported similar anomalous breast deformities under various monikers, including "Snoopy" breast, constricted breast, tubular breast deformity, lower pole hypoplastic breast, narrow-based breast, herniated areola complex, domed nipple, and nipple breast.

Clinical Features

Tuberous breast deformity describes a broad spectrum of aberrant breast shape that presents during adolescent breast development. The degree of deformity varies on a continuum from mild to severe. Affected breasts demonstrate a constellation of findings, each with variable degrees of contribution to the deformity as a whole. These findings are listed above.

The key features of tuberous deformity are lower pole skin envelope deficiency in the vertical and horizontal dimensions, parenchymal hypoplasia, and constriction of breast development in the lower pole. Pseudo-herniation of the nipple-areola complex is a common but not constant feature of tuberous breast deformity, occurring in 40% to 50% of cases. However, breasts that are more severely affected and/or asymmetric tend to demonstrate greater degrees of nipple-areola complex involvement, including enlargement of the areola and herniation of underlying parenchyma into the nipple-areola complex.

There is no consensus in the literature regarding what degree of deformity predominates. Either unilateral or bilateral breast involvement may occur, although reports in the literature vary as to which presentation is more common. While the incidence of tuberous breast deformity among the general population is not known, it is much more common than previously anticipated.

Etiology

The definitive etiology of tuberous breast deformity is unknown; however, the theory proposed by Grolleau et al. seems to most aptly fit the clinical picture.[9] They proposed anomalous superficial fascial adhesions between the dermis and the underlying muscular plane. The adhesions restrict normal development of the breast parenchyma and overlying skin envelope in the lower pole. The restriction favors, instead, growth of the breast away from the chest wall, leading to formation of tuberous shape and enlargement of the areola as the breast develops during adolescence. Mandrekas et al. hypothesized that the deformity results from a combination of an abnormal constricting fibrous ring surrounding the periphery of the nipple-areola complex and a normal superficial fascial window beneath the areola.[10] Because the ring density is highest in the lower pole, the developing adolescent breast is unable to expand inferiorly and is forced to grow away from the chest wall toward the superficial fascial window beneath the areola. It is the degree of superficial fascial aberrancy that determines the degree of severity of the deformity.

Classification

The broad spectrum of deformity and inconsistent nomenclature used to describe tuberous breasts lead to the formation of several classification systems. Grolleau classified the deformity into three subtypes based on the degree and location of the breast base constriction and subareola skin deficiency.[9]

Type I: lower medial quadrant deficiency
Type II: lower medial and lateral quadrant deficiency
Type III: deficiency of all four quadrants

Aesthetic reconstruction of the tuberous breast poses a challenge to the plastic surgeon. The broad spectrum in aberrant breast shapes requires a systematic approach to consistently achieve satisfactory outcomes. Once the diagnosis is established, every effort must be made to accurately analyze the deformity. Careful consideration as to the severity of deformity, presence or absence of asymmetry, and the quantification of the various morphological elements contributing to the deformity should be measured and noted. This includes discrepancies in inframammary fold level, the nipple to fold distance, the suprasternal notch to nipple distance, the breast and chest base width dimensions, the patient's torso dimensions and an estimate of her native breast tissue, and any asymmetries of the parenchyma. Once the deformity has been accurately classified, the patient (and her parents) should be engaged in a thorough discussion regarding the various elements of her deformity, the challenges and limitations of operative intervention, possible complications, and appropriate expectations regarding outcome.

The goals of surgery are to restore volume to the hypoplastic breast(s), expand the lower pole by releasing the tethering fibrous attachments or bands between the breast parenchyma and deep fascial and pectoralis muscle and also between the breast parenchyma and skin, and where necessary, reduce the areola size and recess the herniated breast tissue. This is best accomplished with an infra-areola incision which provides direct access for the release of the constricting fibrous bands and for placement of an implant into the subpectoral space. The incision can be easily converted to a periareola incision when needed. Saline implants are currently mandated for reconstruction in the United States for patients younger than 22 years. They offer the advantage of mild adjustability in this population where native breast volume asymmetry is so prevalent. There must be an increase in the base dimensions of the breast in terms of both width and height.[9,10,11] In the vast majority of cases, the procedure can be carried out in a single stage with a period of preliminary tissue expansion (a two-staged procedure is reserved for only the most severe cases).

A typical patient is illustrated in case 3 (Figure 47-6). This adolescent female presented at age 17 with severe bilateral breast hypoplasia and a Grolleau type 3 constriction of both breasts with significant hypoplasia

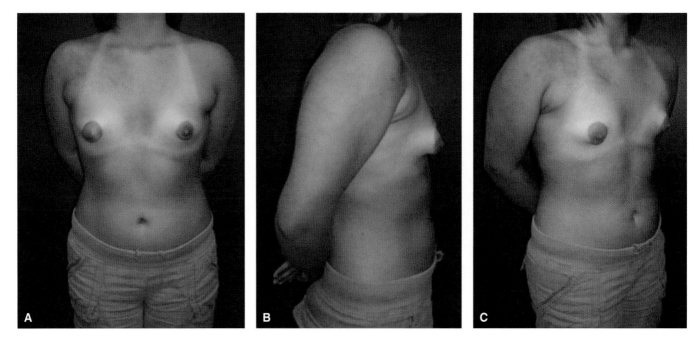

● **FIGURE 47-6.** (A–C) Preoperative view of 18-year-old female with Grolleau type III bilateral breast constriction.

and pseudo-herniation of breast tissue through the areola. The surgical plan entailed the partial retropectoral placement of 330 cc of moderate profile, smooth-surfaced, saline implants, using a dual plane approach incorporated with a periareola mastopexy with Gore-Tex sutures. The 24-month, postoperative, follow-up evaluation demonstrates (Figure 47-7) the patient to have an excellent improvement in breast appearance from the standpoint of volume, contour, and nipple-areola appearance.

In summary, key features of treatment include:

- Assessment of unique features associated with each individual deformity
- Restore mammary base dimensions and re-position inframammary fold
- Release of constricting bands between the breast parenchyma and the deep fascial/muscle tissue and bands between the parenchyma and overlying skin

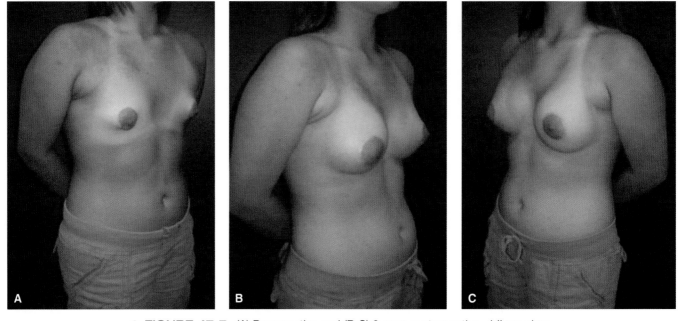

● **FIGURE 47-7.** (A) Preoperative and (B,C) 2-year postoperative oblique view.

- Placement on a prosthetic implant in the subpectoral space using dual plane approach
- Reduce herniated breast tissue and reduce and control the size of the areola through a periareola mastopexy incision
- Balance breast asymmetry with bilateral procedures

POLAND SYNDROME

Pathognomonic of Poland syndrome is the agenesis of the sternocostal head of the pectoralis major muscle. In addition, there are varying degrees of accompanying anomalies of the upper limb and ipsilateral thorax prominently including various degrees of ipsilateral breast hypoplasia in women. Although named after the anatomist Alfred Poland, the thoracic component of the disease was originally described by Lallemand in 1826, and the association with complex syndactyly was made by Floriep in 1839. These initial findings were later reiterated by Poland in 1841 at Guys Hospital in London.[12]

The incidence of Poland syndrome is estimated at 1:30,000 to 1:100,000 live births, with the majority of cases being of sporadic inheritance. The incidence is higher in men than for women at 3:1, and the right side is often more affected than the left by 3:1. The most common presenting deformities seen by the clinician are limb anomalies in both females and males and ipsilateral hypomastia in females. However, many men remain undiagnosed unless they seek treatment for hand anomalies which are most commonly a shortened upper arm, forearm, or fingers, termed brachysymphalangism along with ebbing of the ipsilateral fingers in the form of syndactyly. The frequency of hand abnormalities in the Poland syndrome patient ranges between 13.5% and 56%.[13,14]

Breast deformity in the female is highly variable, ranging from mild hypoplasia to aplasia. The typical breast deformity is marked by deficient parenchyma, a high inframammary fold, and a malpositioned and underdeveloped nipple-areola complex. Indeed 14% of breast aplasia may be accounted for by Poland syndrome. It is important to note that in 20% of cases, there are associated skeletal deformities leading to contour and rotational anomalies of the chest wall. Ribs can be deformed and/or hypoplastic, particularly second through fifth ribs. Poland syndrome is sometimes referred to as "acropectoral renal field defect" due to a high incidence of renal anomalies. The most common anomalies include duplication of the collecting system of unilateral renal agenesis. In very atypical cases, the patient can present with unilateral renal agenesis or dextrocardia in left-sided Poland syndrome. Associations between Poland syndrome and malignancy have been documented. Breast hypoplasia does not preclude development of breast carcinoma. The most commonly associated syndromes are Mobius and Klippel-Feil syndromes.[13,14]

Etiology

The etiology of Poland syndrome remains unknown. The most popular current theory is the subclavian artery supply disruption sequence, a vascular compromise event that occurs during critical 6th and 7th weeks of pregnancy. This event would coincide with fetal breast development between weeks 5 to 7 of gestation, which begins as bilateral thickening of the ectoderm along the mammary line, then partially involutes shortly thereafter. The remaining thickened mammary line forms the mammary ridge. Reduction in blood flow at crucial periods or hypoplasia of internal thoracic artery could lead to disruption in pectoralis major development, where hypoplasia of the branches of brachial artery during development could lead to symbrachydactyly.

Clinical Classification

The Foucras classification, which classifies the Poland syndrome patient into mild, moderate, and severe categories, adequately describes clinical findings based on degrees of thoracic deformity.[13]

Grade I is a minor deformity consisting of pectoralis major hypoplasia and moderate breast hypoplasia, resulting in breast asymmetry in women but only slight chest wall asymmetry in men. Nipple-areola is present, but often smaller and elated. No skeletal abnormalities should be found in a grade I patient.

Grade II is a moderate deformity with marked pectoralis major aplasia, hypoplasia of other chest wall muscles, moderate rib deformity, and marked chest wall deformity in men and women. Breast tissue is severely hypoplastic or absent and the nipple-areola is hypoplastic or absent. In men, grade II is best addressed with a customized chest wall implant or a latissimus dorsi flap, with or without autologous fat injections. In women, a latissimus dorsi flap with tissue expansion and implant may be effective. Adjunct autologous fat transfers can improve symmetry. Chest wall muscles affected may include the adjacent muscles to the pectoralis major, including the serratus latissimus dorsi and external oblique.

Grade III is a severe deformity with aplasia of breast and pectoralis major as well as aplasia of other chest wall muscles, major bone and cartilage anomalies with rib aplasia and sternal deformity, and major chest wall deformity in men and women. In both men and women, the treatment often involves several stages. Complicating the reconstructive ladder, grade III patients also often have absent or severely hypoplastic latissimus dorsi muscles. Free flaps may be the best options, such as contralateral free latissimus dorsi with an implant or abdominal tissue-based reconstructions. Primary skin expansion may often be necessary. Outcomes are often less than satisfactory and serial fat injections can help balance the soft tissue defect.

Treatment

Surgical therapy of Poland syndrome focuses on improving function of the affected limb and improving chest wall appearance. The chest deformities of Poland syndrome rarely cause functional problems, except in the most severe cases. Indications for reconstruction of the thorax include chest wall depression, inadequate protection of the mediastinum, or paradoxical movement of chest walls during respiration. Hand anomalies should be corrected prior to 1 year of age to maximize functional outcomes.

In most cases, surgery for Poland syndrome is for the correction of breast aplasia or hypoplasia in females. In the absence of severe chest wall anomalies, waiting until after puberty affords the best chance of balancing asymmetry.

The challenges to aesthetic breast reconstructions in the patient with Poland syndrome include tight and unforgiving skin envelope, deficient subcutaneous tissue, high inframammary fold, nipple-areola complex malposition or absence, and adequacy of recipient vessels if free flap reconstruction is desired. Often, a variety of treatment of modalities described below must be combined to produce optimal results.

Expander and Implant Reconstruction

Grade I and many grade II patients may be treated with implants. A single-stage correction with a submuscular implant can produce suitable results. For implant reconstruction to be successful, the patient must have adequate soft tissue thickness on the affected side to cover and camouflage the implant. The tight skin envelope, high and tight inframammary fold, and soft tissue deficiency can prove challenging for reconstruction with implant alone. A tissue expander may be utilized in a subpectoral position if there is enough pectoralis major muscle present in the superior and medial position. With expansion of the superior pole of the chest, the nipple-areola complex will descend to a more symmetric position[14] (see below). Implants are frequently used in Poland syndrome but, as with their use in other locations, they are not without drawbacks and morbidity.

Autologous Tissue Transfer

Pedicled latissimus dorsi myocutaneous flap reconstruction, with or without an accompanying implant, has been considered a mainstay of treatment in patients with moderate to severe chest wall deficiency and breast agenesis or hypomastia. The potential benefits are ease of harvest, replacement of pectoralis major with similar tissue, and relative ease compared with microsurgical reconstruction.[15]

This strategy was used in the patient depicted in case 4 (Figure 47-8). She presented at age 19 with a right unilateral Poland syndrome with severe breast hypoplasia, including a superiorly malpositioned nipple-areola complex and absence of the anterolateral axillary fold. There was a deficiency of anterior chest wall and breast skin. The plan was for a two-stage reconstruction with the initial step being slow, gradual expansion of the breast and chest wall

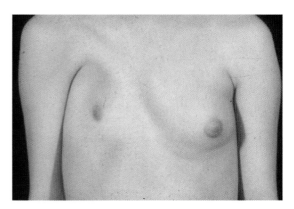

● **FIGURE 47-8.** A 19-year-old patient with unilateral Poland syndrome with severe breast hypoplasia, skin envelope deficiency, and superior nipple malposition. *(Used with permission of Julian J. Pribaz, MD.)*

skin (Figure 47-9). Subsequent to this, the patient underwent removal of the expender along with harvest of the right latissimus dorsi muscle flap through limited back and high axillary incisions. The latissimus dorsi flap was inset (Figure 47-10) to the parasternal area and to the inframammary region through inframammary incision used for the tissue expander placement. A 260-cc saline implant was placed beneath the latissimus dorsi flap. The patient is shown 3 years following the second stage of the reconstruction (Figure 47-11) with a marked improvement in the appearance of her breasts.

The greatest potential limitation of this operation is that the latissimus dorsi can be deficient or absent in the more severe forms of Poland syndrome, leading to

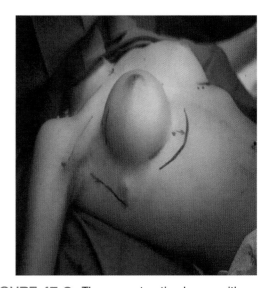

● **FIGURE 47-9.** The reconstruction begun with subcutaneous tissue expansion of the upper and lower aspect of the skin envelope to increase quantitative dimension of skin envelope in an attempt to lower nipple-areola position. *(Used with permission of Julian J. Pribaz, MD.)*

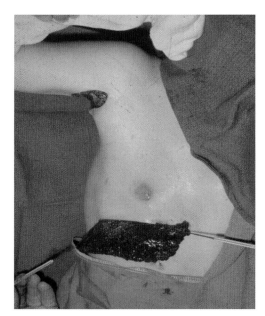

● FIGURE 47-10. The subcutaneous tissue deficit and anterior axillary fold was reconstructed with the right latissimus dorsi muscle fixed to skin of the lower breast and parasternal region. A 260-cc, moderate profile, smooth saline implant was placed beneath the latissimus dorsi muscle. (*Used with permission of Julian J. Pribaz, MD.*)

In addition, other free tissue transfer options include the deep inferior epigastric artery perforator (DIEP), the superior gluteal artery (SGAP), and superficial inferior epigastric artery (SIEA) flap for the treatment of moderate-to-severe Poland syndrome with breast hypoplasia or aplasia. Longaker published a series of nine patients who underwent free tissue transfer for Poland syndrome chest wall reconstruction.[16]

There is a high incidence of anomalies in vasculature arising from the subclavian vessels in Poland syndrome. Preoperative imaging such as ultrasound or CT angiogram is recommended to determine patency and flow in the thoracic vasculature, particularly the internal mammary vessels.

Autologous Fat Transfer by Injection

Coleman's technique of lipostructure is desirable due to low invasiveness and mobility. Pinsolle and colleagues[17] used autologous fat injections in a series of eight patients (mean age, 25 years), using fat harvested from abdominal or trochanteric areas, with fat necrosis occurring in one patient. They noted that fat injection can be used in conjunction with other procedures, and is especially useful in filling the subclavicular hollowing seen in even the mildest cases of patients with Poland syndrome.[17]

At this particular time, serial fat transfers can optimize outcome when used as a touch-up procedure after the definitive reconstruction. Fat transfers can deliver a modest amount of tissue and are best used as adjuncts to tissue expander, implant, and autologous tissue reconstructions. However, we would predict and anticipate that autologous adipose injections will play a substantially larger role in the breast reconstructions performed in patients with breast hypoplasia accompanying Poland syndrome and also in the correction of other congenital and developmental breast deformities in the years and decades ahead.

inadequate tissue bulk or deficient vascular supply. In addition, the harvest of latissimus dorsi flap may decrease function in an upper extremity that may already have decreased function compared with the contralateral extremity. The plastic surgeon must carefully examine the status of the latissimus dorsi muscle in every patient.

Transverse rectus abdominis myocutaneous (TRAM) flaps have been used frequently in patients with Poland syndrome. Pedicled TRAM flaps may encumber the young, active patient by virtue of possible abdominal morbidity. Free TRAM flaps have been utilized successfully.

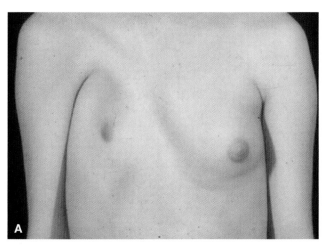
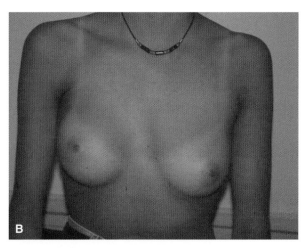

● FIGURE 47-11. (A) The preoperative and (B) 3-year postoperative appearance of the patient is illustrated. (*Used with permission of Julian J. Pribaz, MD.*)

REFERENCES

1. Latham K, Fernandez S, Iteld L, Panthaki Z, Armstrong MB, Thaller S. Pediatric breast deformity. *J Craniofac Surg.* 2006;17(3):454–467.

2. Bickley LS. *Bates' Guide to Physical Examination and History Taking.* 8th ed. Lippincott Williams & Wilkins; 2003.

3. Trier WC. Complete breast absence. *Plast Reconstr Surg.* 36:430–439.

4. Sadove AM, van Aalst JA. Congenital and acquired pediatric breast anomalies: a review of 20 years' experience. *Plast Reconstr Surg.* 115:1039–1050.

5. Ryan R, Pernoll M. Virginal hypertrophy. *Plast Reconstr Surg.* 1985;75:737–742.

6. Rohrich RJ, Ha RY, Kenkel JM, Adams WP. Classification and management of gynecomastia: defining the role of ultrasound-assisted liposuction. *Plast Reconstr Surg.* 111: 909–923.

7. Hammond DC. Surgical correction of gynecomastia. *Plast Reconstr Surg.* 124(1s):61e–68e.

8. Rees T, Aston S. The tuberous breast. *Clin Plast Surg.* 1976;3:339.

9. Grolleau JL, Lanfrey E, Lavigne B, Chavoin JP, Costagliola M. Breast base anomalies: treatment strategy for tuberous breast deformities and asymmetry. *Plast Reconstr Surg.* 1999;104:2040.

10. Mandrekas AD, Zambacos GJ, Anastasopoulos A, Hapsas Dimitrios, Lambrinaki N, Ioannidou-Mouzaka L. Aesthetic reconstruction of the tuberous breast deformity. *Plast Reconstr Surg.* 2003;112:1099.

11. Meara JG, Kolker A, Bartlett G, et al. Tuberous breast deformity: Principles and practice. *Ann Plast Surg.* 2000;45:607.

12. Poland A. Deficiency of the pectoral muscles. *Guy's Hospital Reports.* 1841;VI:191–193.

13. Foucras L, Grolleau-Raoux JL, Chavoin JP. Poland's syndrome clinical series and thoraco-mammary reconstruction. *Ann Chir Plast Esthet.* 2003;48(2):54–66.

14. Urschel HC Jr. Poland syndrome. *Semin Thorac Cardiovasc Surg.* 2009;21(1):89–94.

15. Hester TR Jr, Bostwick J III. Poland's syndrome: correction with latissimus muscle transposition. *Plast Reconstr Surg.* 1982;69:226–233.

16. Longaker MT, Glat PM, Colen LB. Reconstruction of breast asymmetry in Poland's chest-wall deformity using microvascular free flaps. *Plast Reconstr Surg.* 1997;99:429–436.

17. Coleman SR, Saboeiro AP. Fat grafting to the breast revisited: safety and efficacy. *Plast Reconstr Surg.* 2007;119(3): 775–785; discussion 786–787.

chapter 48

Acellular Dermal Matrix in Aesthetic Revisionary Breast Surgery

G. Patrick Maxwell, MD, FACS / *Allen Gabriel, MD, FACS*

● INTRODUCTION

Breast augmentation is the most common aesthetic procedure performed in the United States and perhaps in the world. As plastic surgeons, we strive to achieve perfection and continue to improve our surgical techniques to achieve the aesthetic breast form. Despite advances in implant technology and surgical techniques, undesired outcomes are encountered, leading to revisionary surgeries. In preparing for a revisionary breast augmentation, one must understand patients' goals and expectations and evaluate the probability of their accomplishment, as well as the risk/benefit ratio. When a decision is made to move forward, the goal should be to plan and execute the most precise and efficient surgical correction. To achieve this goal, one must understand the problem(s) and variables involved, and then look for new solutions.

In the past, our options were limited to working with only native tissues that were available to us for these procedures. With the advent of acellular dermal matrices (ADM), the indications and the spectrum of correcting secondary deformities has improved.

It is estimated that over 300,000 primary breast augmentations were performed in the United States in 2009, and therefore there are now over 3 million women with augmented breasts in this country.[1-3] Based on current data, between 15% and 30 % of these women, will have a reoperation within 5 years of their initial procedure.[1-3] Unfortunately, this rate climbs to 35% in patients with prior history of revisionary breast augmentation.[4] As procedures become more complex in nature and number, new techniques and solutions are required of surgeons who perform these challenging operations to improve long term patient outcomes.

Capsular contracture has historically been the most common complication of aesthetic and reconstructive breast surgery and remains the primary reason for most revisionary surgeries.[2,3,5,6] While increasing data suggest capsular contracture can be minimized in primary augmentation by technical detail, including precise, atraumatic, bloodless dissection, appropriate antibiotic breast pocket irrigation, and minimizing any points of contamination during the procedure,[4,7] treatment of an established capsule remains even more challenging than the application of these techniques alone.

With the enforcement of FDA restrictions on silicone gel implants in the early 1990s, American surgeons were forced to use saline implants.[1] Prior to the 1992 "moratorium," the majority of silicone gel implants were placed in the subglandular position; saline implants (due to their palpability) began to be placed under the muscle in an effort to conceal the untoward contour irregularities of these implants.[8] As the number of these implants were of larger volumes, many patients experienced thinning of breast parenchyma and the overlying soft tissue, whether the implants were in subglandular or subpectoral positions. The thinned tissues in turn can lead to long-term complications, such as palpability, rippling, implant extrusion, double bubble, "Snoopy" deformity, symmastia, "bottoming out," and implant malposition.[1,8,9]

Hence, implant malposition and concerns with ptosis or skin stretch are the next most common causes for aesthetic revisionary surgery following capsular contracture.

These are more frequently associated with larger volume saline implants, but can be a result of planning decisions, surgical technique, or effects of time (gravity) with silicone gel implants as well. Historically, our options for revision and improvement have included replacing saline implants with gel implants, capsulorrhaphy, use of capsular flaps, or performing a site change operations. The site change principle, described in the mid-1980s, combined total or partial capsulectomy with conversion to a different pocket (generally a subglandular to subpectoral site change) for the replacement implant.[10] While site change procedures have been successful, none of these procedures alone have resulted in complete resolution of the described complaints.

As change was necessary to improve clinical outcomes in this population of breast revision patients, application and development of newer techniques and technologies were pursued. Many breast revisions require creation of a new pocket for the new implant. Because many patients have had implants in multiple pockets, and as the majority of implants in revisionary patients today are already in the subpectoral position, we developed (in 1991) the "neopectoral pocket" concept to create a new pocket in the subpectoral-precapsular space.[11] Initially developed for double-bubble problems (inferior malposition), this concept was also applied to symmastia (medial malposition), capsular contracture, ptosis, and conversion of round to anatomical-shaped implants (demanding a snug, hand-in-glove fit). The detailed operative technique of creation of the neopectoral pocket has been described in a previous publication.[8] For patients presenting with implants in the subglandular position, a subpectoral site change is utilized.

Notwithstanding the importance of the site change concept, the most important addition to our clinical armamentarium has been the utilization of acellular dermal matrix (ADM), as a regenerative construct, to help solve these challenging clinical presentations.[12] The successful use of ADMs has been reported in a range of clinical settings, including abdominal wall repair, hernia repair, facial and eyelid surgery, cleft palate repair, soft tissue augmentation, tendon repair, ulcer repair, vaginal sling repair, and breast reconstruction.[13-23] While its use in reconstructive expander and implant breast surgery has become a standard of care, its use in aesthetic revisionary breast surgery has evolved more slowly,[24-26] and has only recently gained widespread adaption.[24]

● PATIENT SELECTION

The use of ADM can be categorized into four distinct indications based on the underlying clinical presentation: (1) coverage of implant lower pole (usually for revision mastopexy), (2) implant stabilizer (usually for malposition correction), (3) tissue thickener (usually superomedially or inferiorly), and (4) treatment of capsular contracture (which may be technically similar to lower pole cover or superior-medial thickening) (Figure 48-1).

The important concept and technique of lower pole coverage is perhaps the most frequently used role for ADM. It is employed when performing soft tissue and skin envelope alterations in reoperative surgery (revision mastopexy with augmentation). As many patients with previously placed implants develop laxity, sag, or tissue thinning over time, mastopexy or revision mastopexy over the replacement implant is required to achieve the aesthetic breast form. If the existing implant is subglandular, a subpectoral (subpectoral-fascial) pocket is created (after capsule treatment), the new implant inserted in the newly created subpectoral pocket, and the lower portion of the implant covered with ADM. This allows a circumvertical or inverted T mastopexy to be safely performed without underlying muscle, as the ADM separates the skin closure from the implant. If the existing implant is already subpectoral, a neopectoral site change is carried out, and the ADM utilized similarly. If there has been a previous implant in both the subglandular and subpectoral pockets, lamellar separation (dissecting the pectoralis muscle from its superficial and deep scarred attachments) may be necessary (Figure 48-2). ADM is considered to be the outer layer of the underling implant (to which it is intimately engaged by proximity of placement), and may also require suture stabilization. Thus, the ADM may be tacked to the inferior border of the pectoralis major above and to Scarpa fascia or deep fascia below (at the level of the inframammary fold). Parachute pull-out sutures may alternatively be used to re-drape the ADM. When there is lamellar scarring requiring lamellar separation, the remaining pectoralis muscle may be "window shaded" up in the pocket, requiring lower muscle inferior pull following its release. This lower pole coverage situation is best achieved by suturing of the ADM along the entire length of the lower pectoral border, draping it over the implant inferiorly, and securing it (under more tautness) at or near the inframammary fold. This application is similar to the reconstructive model, as a pectoral muscle extension (Figure 48-3). In all instances, an adequate environment, cover and stability over the nonmuscle-covered portion of the implant (lower pole) by the ADM, allows the skin envelope to be safely lifted and tightened (mastopexy), assuming adequate respect for the vascularity to the re-draped tissue, as well as compliance with all sound surgical principles (Figures 48-4, 48-5, and 48-6).

Regarding the desired biomechanical properties of the desired ADM, rapid revascularization is required to conformability of the ADM to re-drape over the surface of the implant (intimate engagement of surface contours). If the patient had capsular contracture a more compliant material may be desired. If the patient had more laxity or stretch deformity, a more taut material might be preferable.

ADM also allows the surgeon an enhanced control in maintaining implant position in a newly created "neo" pocket or for reinforcement after capsulorrhaphy in various forms of implant malposition correction. Inferior malposition (double bubble), medial malposition (symmastia), or

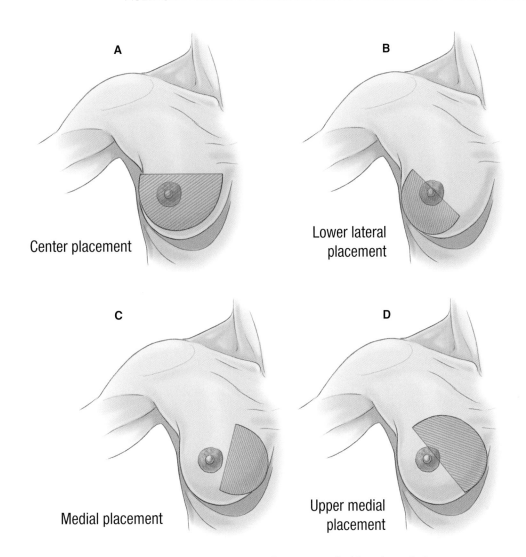

● **FIGURE 48-1.** Placement of ADM at various anatomical locations during revisionary surgery based on distinct indications with underlying clinical presentation.

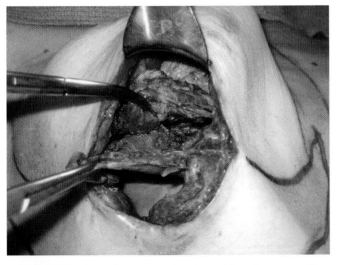

● **FIGURE 48-2.** Intraoperative view of lamellar separation.

lateral malposition are generally treated by capsulorrhaphy or site change (the authors' preference). In a certain percentage of patients, the tissue is strong enough to support this correction with a new pocket and appropriate suturing alone. A number of these patients, however, will have thin tissue, previous scar, or problematic bony contour slopes, such that reinforcement of the site change (ie, neo-pectoral pocket of appropriate dimensions in the correct location with old pocket obliteration) with ADM is highly advised to reinforce or buttress the corrected implant position (Figures 48-6, 48-7, and 48-8). These materials are sutured in appropriate position with proper purchase to achieve support. The biomechanical properties of ADM for this indication are strength and tautness to maintain implant stabilization.

The concept of ADM as a tissue thickener is an extension of second-stage breast reconstruction where expander-

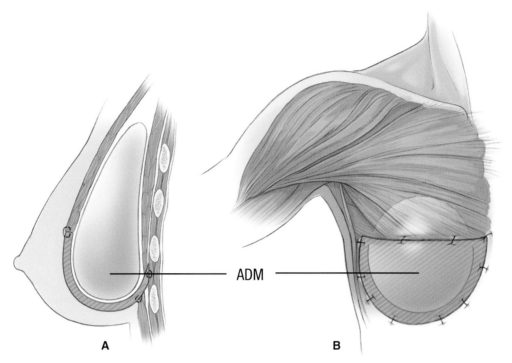

ADM

A   B

● **FIGURE 48-3.** Interposition of regenerative matrix between implant and skin closure. This is similar to the "reconstructive model."

to-implant conversion is facilitated by a superomedial placement of an extra-thick ADM, to enhance soft tissue cover of the implant and give a better visual and palpable confluence of chest to breast form.[27] In aesthetic revisions, this is also most frequently applied to upper pole (or superomedial area) to thicken tissue, minimize visibility of traction rippling, camouflage implant edges, and enhance cleavage. An extra-thick allograft material is generally used and appropriately trimmed. It is draped over the implant (intimate engagement on its deep surface) and in contact with existing capsule or new/neo pocket on its superficial surface. Parachute 2-0 Prolene sutures with Keith needles are used in the ADM corners, and interspersed on the medial side to facilitate placement and re-draping. The suture ends are tied to themselves externally, under no tension, and covered with a Tegaderm for 7 to 10 days. This same application is occasionally used laterally or inferolaterally for implant visibility or palpability, and inferiorly to "thicken" a very thin cutaneous cover (Figures 48-7 and 48-8). The key to success is proper pocket alteration with incorporation of the extra-thick ADM providing bulk, yet revascularization and cellular repopulation.

Even though the presenting problem may be capsular contracture, additional deformities may be identified following detailed analysis from skin envelope to chest wall as noted above. This can include thinned tissue over an encapsulated implant, malposition of the encapsulated implant, or stretched deformity, "Snoopy" deformity, or ptosis over an encapsulated implant. If the encapsulation is in the subglandular position, a total capsulectomy

with site change to the subpectoral position is usually performed. If the encapsulation is in the subpectoral position, a neopectoral pocket with partial anterior capsule excision and residual capsule obliteration, or total (perhaps partial) capsulectomy is performed. In these cases, the ADM is again selected for rapid revascularization, conformability to the implant, and performance. The technique is most frequently similar to the lower pole cover concept, but may be closer to a medial thickener, or malposition reinforce, depending on the presenting problem (Figures 48-9 and 48-10). There is an increasing body of documentation that the coupling of the ADM to the implant will further reduce the incidence of capsular contracture.[12,24] If capsular contracture is the only clinical diagnosis, then we recommend for the placement of the ADM at the lower or middle poles.

● **PATIENT PREPARATION**

ADM is utilized as an adjunct to the sound surgical principles necessary to diagnose and treat the underlying cause(s) necessitating the revisionary aesthetic breast surgery. Clinical data shows the four main indications (drivers) for revisionary surgery are capsular contracture, implant malposition, ptosis, and implant visibility or palpability.[24–26] Each patient must be individually evaluated regarding concerns, goals, knowledge of previous surgical and implant specifics, and careful evaluation of her breasts—dimensions, quality/quantity of overlying soft tissue, and scarring (critical in planning surgery and

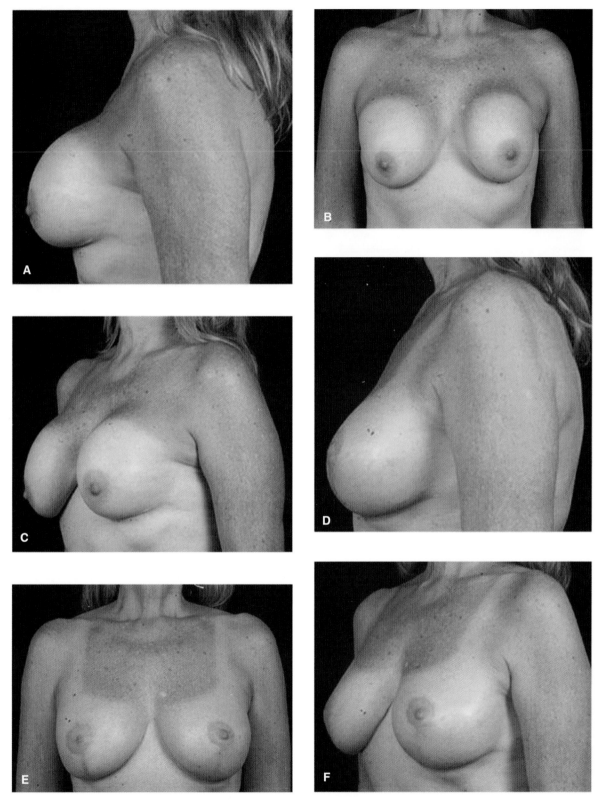

● **FIGURE 48-4.** (A–C) Preoperative views of a 37-year-old woman who had undergone breast augmentation. (D–F) Thirty-two months after revision augmentation/ mastopexy (inverted T), which included the development of neopectoral pocket, lower pole coverage with ADM, and replacement of implants with form stable, highly cohesive gel anatomic implants.

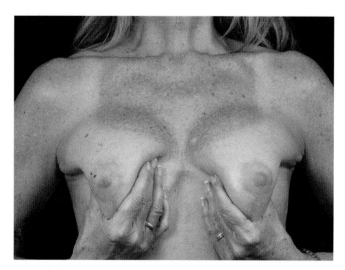

● **FIGURE 48-5.** Patient as seen in Figure 48-4 demonstrating the softness of implants 32 months following the treatment of her capsular contracture and ptosis.

maintaining necessary vascularity to manipulated tissues). As always, appropriate candidate selection is important for achieving successful outcome, and high-risk patients (eg, smoker and those with body mass index >35) should be discouraged to have elective surgery.

Despite the apparent complexity of a given clinical presentation, there are five underlying basic components, which may be the cause, or contribute to the cause, of the problem: the skin, soft tissue, capsule, implant, and chest wall. These underlying components must be carefully and systematically analyzed from outside in, or inside out, until all layers involved are evaluated. The main drivers for reoperative surgery mentioned above should always be kept in mind as these five components are evaluated. We have learned from our revisionary and reconstructive breast experience that one or more of these components and layers may need to be addressed, in addition to the use of ADM. Such surgical manipulations may include skin envelope reduction, fat injection, lamellar separation, capsulectomy. Capsulotomy and site change of the replacement implant. In order to help plan for the surgery, some general principles can be followed.

● **TECHNIQUE**

For patients whose original implants were subglandular, a pocket change to a subpectoral plane and lower pole coverage with ADM is generally performed. For those patients whose original implants were subpectoral, a neopectoral pocket with the addition of ADM is generally performed. For patients who do have adequate breast tissue, a subfascial pocket may be utilized with ADM coverage or support as indicated.

The surgical techniques used are based on the preoperative findings and the indications as described above. The ADM should be conformed to, and in intimate contact

with, the outer surface of the implant (like a hand in a glove). The appropriate pocket is created whether it is a neopectoral, subpectoral, or subfascial.[8,11] Three to five half-mattress, stabilizing "parachute" sutures are placed between the skin and ADM to stabilize the tissue and place it in the desired location. Sizes selected are normally in the 6 to 8 × 10 to 16 cm range (depending on size of implant), rectangle or contour shapes, and trimmed as needed. Seroma formation should be prevented in all breast revisions, to further revascularization and cellular repopulation of the ADM, so drains are always recommended.

The use of acellular dermal products have been popularized in both breast and abdominal wall reconstructions.[13–23] In reconstruction cases, ADMs have been used to replace tissue, extend existing tissue, or act as a supplement. In aesthetic revisions, the ADM essentially becomes an outer conforming, regenerative layer around the implant. They have been used to correct implant rippling and displacement, ptosis, and capsular contracture.[25,26,28] ADMs are used as an alternative to other autologous tissue methods of coverage and provides camouflage, thus decreasing rippling, and increasing soft tissue padding.[29] In addition to all the indications described previously, we have also used ADMs as a mode of treatment for capsular contracture.[24] Breast capsular contracture is similar to lamellar scarring in the eyelids. At the cellular level, capsular contracture is most likely caused by any process that produces increased inflammation, which in turn leads to the formation of deleterious cytokines within the periprosthetic pocket. Consequently, in addition to the many techniques described for treating and preventing capsular contracture,[4,5,8,30–36] the addition of ADM is believed to be another modality in fighting the evolution of the capsule. An ADM can counteract the inflammatory process, adding more tissue in-growth availability and controlling the interface of the pocket by providing a regenerative layer between device and native tissue.

The rising demand for the use of ADM coupled with good outcomes in breast reconstructions has spurred tremendous interest in its use for aesthetic breast surgery patients. In the past, revisionary surgeries were generally performed with a total capsulectomy, removal of the implant from the subglandular plane, and placement of a new implant in the subpectoral position.[5,8,10] This is a fairly simple procedure, involving a change in implant placement from over the muscle to under the muscle. More recently, it has become necessary to perform revisionary surgery on volume-depleted or severely scarred breasts. In correcting these deformities as described in the indication section, in addition to the site change operation, ADMs can provide additional coverage where the repair is performed.

● **COMPLICATIONS**

Numerous complications are possible with revisional breast surgery, including malposition and recurrent rippling and capsular contracture—the same complications which

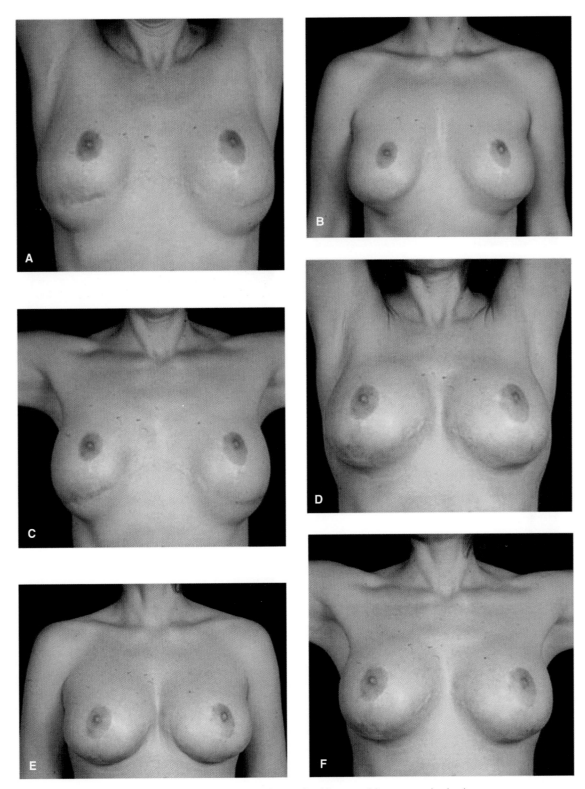

● **FIGURE 48-6.** (A–C) Preoperative views of a 49-year-old woman who had undergone augmentation/mastopexy. (D–F) Thirty months after revision augmentation/ mastopexy (inverted T), which included the development of neopectoral pocket, lower pole coverage and reinforcement of inferior and lateral walls with ADM and replacement of implants form stable, highly cohesive gel anatomic implants. Successful correction of inferior and lateral malposition was achieved.

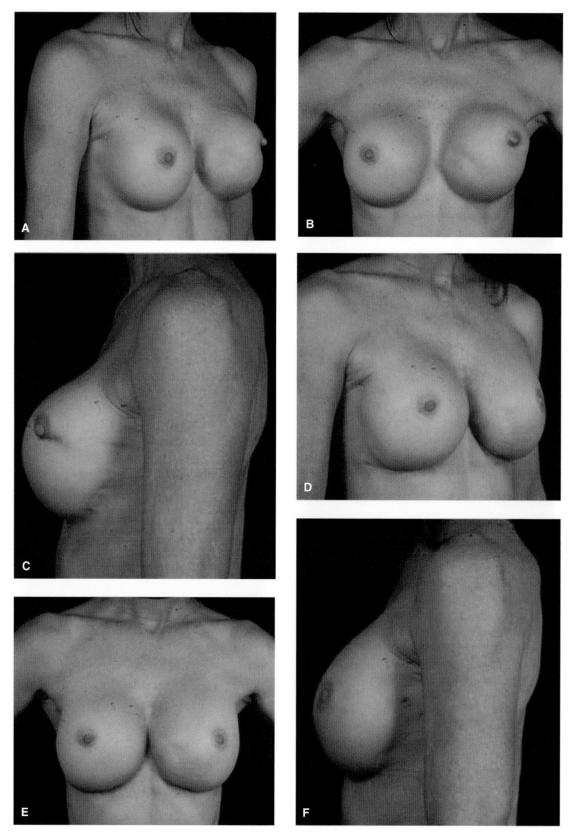

● **FIGURE 48-7.** (A–C) Preoperative views of a 38-year-old woman who had undergone multiple previous revision augmentations. (D–F) Twenty-six months after revision augmentation through inframammary fold incision, which included the development of neopectoral pocket, lamellar separation, lower pole coverage with ADM, and replacement of implants with textured gel implants.

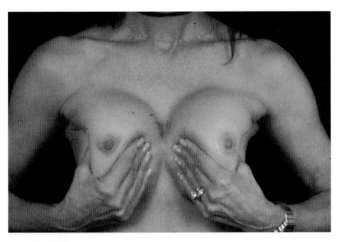

● **FIGURE 48-8.** Patient as seen in Figure 48-7 demonstrating the softness of implants 26 months following the treatment of her implant malposition, lamellar scarring, and tissue thinning.

necessitated the original reoperation. The use of ADM may add a potentially higher rate of infection and/or seroma formation.[37] The dermis takes time to revascularize and may not ward off infection as well as the body's own tissues. Scientific review will determine whether this is true or not.

A challenge that is continually faced in aesthetic revisionary surgery is the cost of these products and their affordability by the patient. This should be balanced against the possible cost of performing another surgical revision due to failure of the planned procedure. Therefore, as surgeons continue to report outcome data using ADMs in revisionary aesthetic breast surgery and compare it to the outcomes without use of ADMs, a new picture may emerge. No doubt, the coming years will be exciting as we further define the issues, advance the science, and our understanding of it via evidence-based medicine, for the benefit of our patient population.

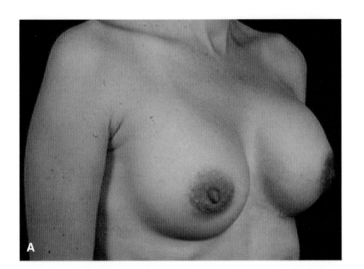

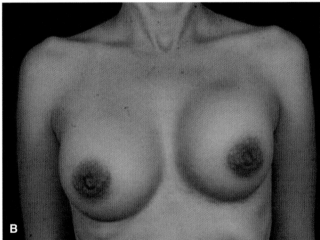

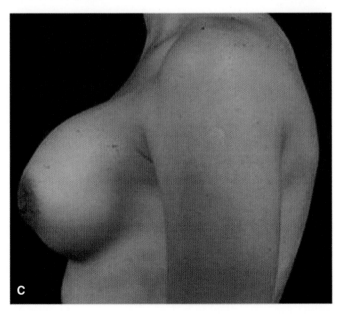

● **FIGURE 48-9.** (A-C) Preoperative views of a 45-year-old woman who had undergone multiple previous attempts at correction of capsular contracture.

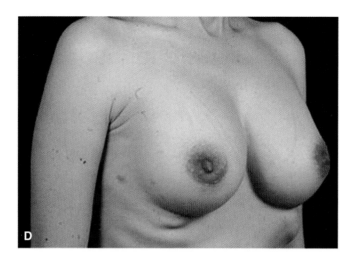

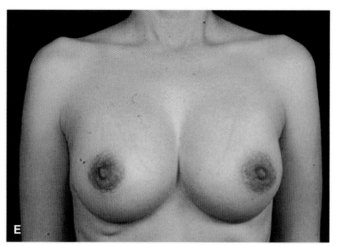

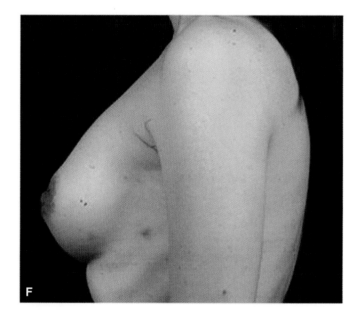

● FIGURE 48-9. (*continued*) (D-F) Twenty-two months after revision augmentation through inframammary fold incision which included the development of neopectoral pocket, lower pole coverage with ADM, and replacement of implants with higher-profile, lower-volume textured gel implants.

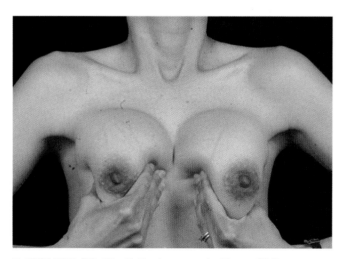

● FIGURE 48-10. Patient as seen in Figure 48-9 demonstrating the softness of implants 22 months following the treatment of her capsular contracture.

● OUTOMES ASSESSMENT

A recent published series of 78 consecutive patients who underwent revisionary breast augmentation/mastopexies with ADMs was one of the largest series to date to address the use of ADM in revisionary aesthetic breast surgery.[12] Of the 78 patients, 56 patients had their original implants in the subpectoral position, and 22 had them in the subglandular position. Complications included two patients (2.5%) requiring reoperation, one for a hematoma and the other for an implant malposition (Table 48-1). Presenting clinical signs are listed in Table 48-2 and the type of operation performed is listed in Table 48-3. As expected, the majority of complaints were due to "implant hardening." Of 78 patients, 77 (99%) were assessed as having soft implants with a Baker I level of capsule contracture at final follow-up; one patient (1%) had a Baker II contracture. No patient had a Baker III or Baker IV classification postoperatively (Table 48-4).

TABLE 48-1. Complications

Complication	No. of Patients
Hematoma	1
Seroma	0
Implant malposition	1
Implant rupture	0
Infection	0
Total	2

TABLE 48-3. Augmentation vs Augmentation/Mastopexy

	No. of Patients
Augmentation	49
Augmentation/mastopexy	29
Total	78

TABLE 48-2. Presenting Clinical Signs

Clinical Signs	No. of Patients
Capsular contracture	56
Implant exposure	2
Rippling	7
Implant malposition	5
Bottoming out	4
Symmastia	4
Total	78

TABLE 48-4. Preoperative and Postoperative Baker Classification in All Patients

	% of Patients	
	Preoperative	Postoperative
Baker I	6.4	97.4
Baker II	20.5	2.6
Baker III	64.1	0
Baker IV	9.0	0

Currently, we have performed over 200 revisionary augmentations with ADM. As the results continue to be satisfactory both to surgeon and patient, we continue to exploit new concepts and new techniques to improve outcomes, minimize risks while enhancing patient safety, purse efficiency, and lower costs. We are now seeing product differentiation in outcome assessment, thus we are carefully documenting these findings to report in peer-reviewed literature.

REFERENCES

1. Maxwell GP, Gabriel A. The evolution of breast implants. *Clin Plast Surg.* 2009;36(1):1–13, v.

2. Spear SL, Murphy DK, Slicton A, Walker PS. Inamed silicone breast implant core study results at 6 years. *Plast Reconstr Surg.* 2007;120(7 Suppl 1):8S–16S; discussion 17S–18S.

3. Cunningham B, McCue J. Safety and effectiveness of Mentor's MemoryGel implants at 6 years. *Aesthetic Plast Surg.* 2009;33(3):440–444.

4. Adams WP Jr, Rios JL, Smith SJ. Enhancing patient outcomes in aesthetic and reconstructive breast surgery using triple antibiotic breast irrigation: six-year prospective clinical study. *Plast Reconstr Surg.* 2006;117(1):30–36.

5. Spear SL, Carter ME, Ganz JC. The correction of capsular contracture by conversion to "dual-plane" positioning: technique and outcomes. *Plast Reconstr Surg.* 2006;118(7 Suppl):103S–113S; discussion 114S.

6. Cunningham B. The Mentor Core Study on Silicone MemoryGel Breast Implants. *Plast Reconstr Surg.* 2007;120(7 Suppl 1):19S–29S; discussion 30S–32S.

7. Adams WP Jr. Capsular contracture: what is it? What causes it? How can it be prevented and managed? *Clin Plast Surg.* 2009;36(1):119–126, vii.

8. Maxwell GP, Gabriel A. The neopectoral pocket in revisionary breast surgery. *Aesthet Surg J.* 2008;28(4):463–467.

9. Maxwell GP, Gabriel A. Possible future development of implants and breast augmentation. *Clin Plast Surg.* 2009;36(1):167–172, viii.

10. Maxwell GP, Tebbetts JB, Hester TR. Site change in breast surgery. Presented at: American Association of Plastic Surgeons. St. Louis, MO; 1994.

11. Maxwell GP, Birchenough SA, Gabriel A. Efficacy of neopectoral pocket in revisionary breast surgery. *Aesthet Surg J.* 2009;29(5):379–385.

12. Maxwell GP, Gabriel A. Use of the acellular dermal matrix in revisionary aesthetic breast surgery. *Aesthet Surg J.* 2009;29(6):485–493.

13. Bindingnavele V, Gaon M, Ota KS, Kulber DA, Lee DJ. Use of acellular cadaveric dermis and tissue expansion in postmastectomy breast reconstruction. *J Plast Reconstr Aesthet Surg.* 2007;60(11):1214–1218.

14. Breuing KH, Warren SM. Immediate bilateral breast reconstruction with implants and inferolateral AlloDerm slings. *Ann Plast Surg.* 2005;55(3):232–239.

15. Breuing KH, Colwell AS. Inferolateral AlloDerm hammock for implant coverage in breast reconstruction. *Ann Plast Surg.* 2007;59(3):250–255.

16. Cothren CC, Gallego K, Anderson ED, Schmidt D. Chest wall reconstruction with acellular dermal matrix (AlloDerm) and a latissimus muscle flap. *Plast Reconstr Surg.* 2004;114(4):1015–1017.

17. Garramone CE, Lam B. Use of AlloDerm in primary nipple reconstruction to improve long-term nipple projection. *Plast Reconstr Surg.* 2007;119(6):1663–1668.

18. Glasberg SB, D'Amico RA. Use of regenerative human acellular tissue (AlloDerm) to reconstruct the abdominal wall following pedicle TRAM flap breast reconstruction surgery. *Plast Reconstr Surg.* 2006;118(1):8–15.

19. Kim H, Bruen K, Vargo D. Acellular dermal matrix in the management of high-risk abdominal wall defects. *Am J Surg.* 2006;192(6):705–709.

20. Nahabedian MY. Secondary nipple reconstruction using local flaps and AlloDerm. *Plast Reconstr Surg.* 2005;115(7):2056–2061.

21. Patton JH Jr, Berry S, Kralovich KA. Use of human acellular dermal matrix in complex and contaminated abdominal wall reconstructions. *Am J Surg.* 2007;193(3):360–363; discussion 363.

22. Salzberg CA. Nonexpansive immediate breast reconstruction using human acellular tissue matrix graft (AlloDerm). *Ann Plast Surg.* 2006;57(1):1–5.

23. Spear SL, Parikh PM, Reisin E, Menon NG. Acellular dermis-assisted breast reconstruction. *Aesthetic Plast Surg.* 2008;32(3):418–425.

24. Maxwell GP, Gabriel A, Perry LC. Role of Acellular Dermal Matrix in Inflammation. Unpublished 2009.

25. Duncan DI. Correction of implant rippling using allograft dermis. *Aesthet Surg J.* 2001;21(1):81–84.

26. Baxter RA. Intracapsular allogenic dermal grafts for breast implant-related problems. *Plast Reconstr Surg.* 2003;112(6):1692–1696; discussion 1697–1698.

27. Maxwell GP. ADM in revisionary breast surgery. Annual Meeting of the American Society of Plastic Surgeons; 2009.

28. Colwell AS, Breuing KH. Improving shape and symmetry in mastopexy with autologous or cadaveric dermal slings. *Ann Plast Surg.* 2008;61(2):138–142.

29. Gamboa-Bobadilla GM. Implant breast reconstruction using acellular dermal matrix. *Ann Plast Surg.* 2006;56(1):22–25.

30. Gancedo M, Ruiz-Corro L, Salazar-Montes A, Rincon AR, Armendariz-Borunda J. Pirfenidone prevents capsular contracture after mammary implantation. *Aesthetic Plast Surg.* 2008;32(1):32–40.

31. Ma SL, Gao WC. [Capsular contracture in breast augmentation with textured versus smooth mammary implants: a systematic review]. *Zhonghua Zheng Xing Wai Ke Za Zhi.* 2008;24(1):71–74.

32. Scuderi N, Mazzocchi M, Rubino C. Effects of zafirlukast on capsular contracture: controlled study measuring the mammary compliance. *Int J Immunopathol Pharmacol.* 2007;20(3):577–584.

33. Weintraub JL, Kahn DM. The timing of implant exchange in the development of capsular contracture after breast reconstruction. *Eplasty.* 2008;8:e31.

34. Wiener TC. Relationship of incision choice to capsular contracture. *Aesthetic Plast Surg.* 2008;32(2):303–306.

35. Wong CH, Samuel M, Tan BK, Song C. Capsular contracture in subglandular breast augmentation with textured versus smooth breast implants: a systematic review. *Plast Reconstr Surg.* 2006;118(5):1224–1236.

36. Zimman OA, Toblli J, Stella I, Ferder M, Ferder L, Inserra F. The effects of angiotensin-converting-enzyme inhibitors on the fibrous envelope around mammary implants. *Plast Reconstr Surg.* 2007;120(7):2025–2033.

37. Chun YS, Verma K, Rosen H, et al. Implant-based breast reconstruction using acellular dermal matrix and the risk of postoperative complications. *Plast Reconstr Surg.* 2010;125(2):429–436.

chapter 49

Physical and Radiologic Evaluation of the Hand

Bradley A. Hubbard, MD / Matthew J. Concannon, MD

● INTRODUCTION

A consistent and thorough hand examination is an essential tool for hand surgeons, emergency room physicians, and primary care physicians alike. In every situation and with every patient, a complete hand examination should be performed. This will prevent missed injuries and guide therapeutic intervention if other abnormalities exist. To the well-practiced physician, this can be performed swiftly, usually under 5 minutes, thus there is no advantage in performing a more limited examination.

● HISTORY

A critical component in the evaluation of the patient with a hand problem or injury is their history. Issues such as the patient's age, sex, hand dominance, and the presence of other medical problems are important to note. In addition, it is important to specifically inquire about issues that are particularly germane to hand problems: Is the patient a diabetic? Is he a smoker? Does she have arthritis? Has he previously been injured or had problems with his hand in the past? When evaluating injuries, have the patient describe exactly how the injury occurred. Have the patient characterize the pain or problem and how long it has troubled them. This type of information can provide understanding into the etiology of the problem and furnish clues as to their solution.

Knowledge of the patient's occupation and hobbies can give a sense of how they use their hand. For example, a construction worker uses his hands in a different way than a touch typist, and has different needs that must be considered. Hobbies that are an important part of the patient's life (such as playing musical instruments) can give insight into the impact of the injury and the most appropriate treatment options.

● OBSERVATION

Spend a moment looking at the hand. Remove all dressings, splints, or packing. Practice this skill with all patients as it can be especially valuable in the unconscious, mentally challenged, or pediatric populations, where communication is difficult or impossible.

Notice whether the skin is calloused, indicating someone involved in manual labor, or if it is soft. In a trauma situation, examine the wounds. Are they "sharp" or is it a stellate "crush type" of injury, which would imply much deeper and widespread tissue damage. Evaluate the color of the hand. This can give clues to vascular status, force of injury, and potential occult damage to the underlying tissue.

Examine the resting finger and hand position; at rest, the fingers fall into a normal "cascade" (Figure 49-1A). Division of the flexor tendons will result in an abnormal posture at rest (Figure 49-1B). Fractures of the phalanges may result in finger rotation or produce an angular deviation (Figure 49-1C).

Examine the musculature of the hand, particularly at the first web space and the thenar eminence. Is there evidence of muscle atrophy? The elderly have a certain degree of muscular atrophy as a natural result of aging, but atrophy can also be evidence of an underlying neural problem,

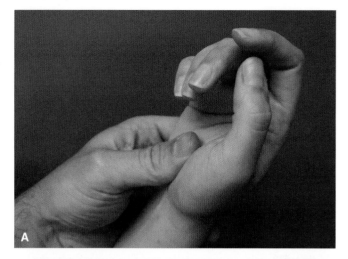

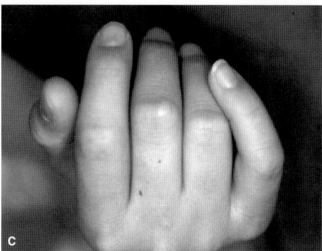

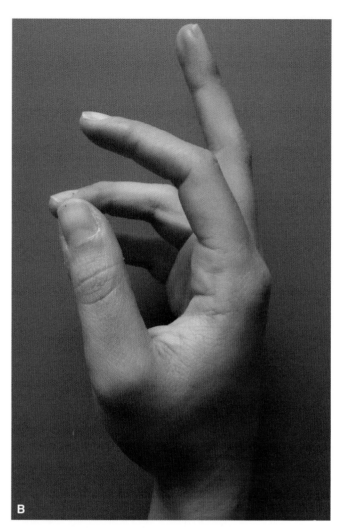

● **FIGURE 49-1.** Observation of finger position at rest. (A) Normal cascade. (B) Middle finger tendon disruption. (C) Osseous injury causing rotational deformity.

such as longstanding nerve compression (eg, carpal tunnel or cubital tunnel syndrome).

● **VASCULAR EXAMINATION**

There are many ways to assess the vascular status of the hand or digit. A word of caution should be interjected about severely angulated fractures, dislocations, or finger torsion. These misalignments can often cause ischemia or venous congestion without true vascular injury and should be reduced prior to formal vascular examination.

After assessment of its color, the radial and ulnar arteries can often be palpated at the volar wrist. If too swollen for adequate palpation, a Doppler probe can be used to analyze the blood flow not only in these arteries, but also as far distally as the volar pulp at the distal phalanx.

If (after visual inspection and Doppler exam) there is some question as to the vascular status, pinprick of the affected part with a 22-gauge needle may be helpful. After pinprick of the finger, both the color and the quality of

the blood expressed can help determine if a vascular problem exists. A completely ischemic part will not bleed at all, whereas one with venous congestion will bleed quite briskly with very dark (almost black) colored blood. Normal perfusion is indicated by moderately brisk bleeding of bright red blood.

The Allen test is used to confirm the adequacy of perfusion to the hand by either the radial or ulnar arteries alone. This is performed by compressing both the radial and ulnar arteries at the wrist and then asking the patient to repetitively make a fist until the hand is exsanguinated. The radial artery is released while maintaining compression on the ulnar artery and the perfusion to the fingers is assessed. The test is repeated except this time the ulnar artery is released and the radial artery is compressed. In a normal test, the fingers should be perfused and pink within 6 seconds. The clinical observation of inadequate or absent revascularization correlates with reduced digit blood pressure.[1]

The Allen test should always be performed prior to any planned manipulation of these vessels (such as radial artery line placement) to avoid the potentially devastating consequences of distal ischemia if the artery becomes injured or thrombosed. If the thumb and index finger do not show a good blush of reperfusion after release of the ulnar artery (while still occluding the radial artery), it is likely that inadequate crossover perfusion from the ulnar side of the hand exists, and any cannulation or manipulation of the radial artery should be avoided to prevent possible ischemic loss.

● SENSORY EXAMINATION

The major nerves to the hand and forearm provide sensory information as well as transmitting motor impulses, and therefore nerve function can be analyzed using both sensory and motor tests. This can be very useful to exploit, because it can help distinguish a tendon injury from a nerve injury if a patient is unable to perform a particular action. Unfortunately, a proper motor examination can be difficult to perform in the acute setting due to pain. Patients will often be unwilling to move or claim they are unable to move the affected part, but after proper anesthesia no underlying injury is found. Therefore, it is standard in our practice to perform the sensory examination, then anesthetize the area prior to testing the motor function.

Testing for sensation is relatively straightforward; however, it is important to realize that the border areas between nerve distributions are not precisely consistent from individual to individual, with extensive crossover. Therefore, it is helpful to know which areas are purely innervated by only the ulnar nerve, median nerve, or radial nerve. The autonomous sensory zones include the following: the volar aspect of the small finger—ulnar nerve; the volar aspect of the index finger—median nerve; the dorsal aspect of the first web space—radial sensory nerve (Figure 49-2).

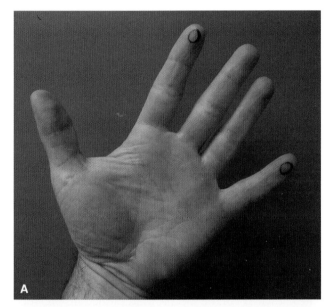

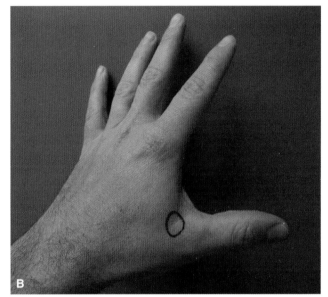

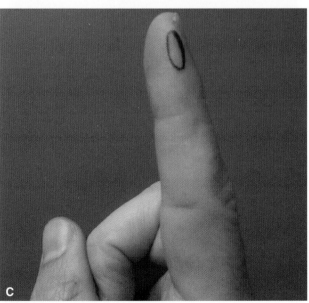

● **FIGURE 49-2.** Areas without sensory nerve overlap. (A) Ulnar nerve—small fingertip; median—index finger tip. (B) Radial nerve—first web space. (C) Digital nerve—lateral aspect of finger tip (index finger radial digital nerve distribution pictured).

Quite commonly the digital nerves need to be assessed in patients who have sustained lacerations or other injury to their hands or fingers. One method to evaluate this function is to test moving two-point discrimination (m2PD). Ideally, a caliper is utilized, starting with the points approximately 5 to 6 mm apart. The points of the calipers are lightly brushed across the radial or ulnar aspect of the finger being examined, as there is a great deal of crossover in the pulp. The patient (with eyes closed) is asked to discern whether they feel one or two points moving across their finger. m2PD of 3 to 5 mm in most people is considered normal. But, it is wise to test the unaffected side and compare. If the patient cannot distinguish between "one" versus "two," the distance between the caliper points is increased until the patient can reliably distinguish the difference. m2PD of greater than 15 mm correlates with a lack of protective sensation and is considered abnormal and suspicious for nerve injury.

Other methods for quantitative sensory testing include static two-point discrimination, monofilament testing, light touch, etc. The moving two-point method is preferable in our practice because it is easy to perform and reproduce.

The sensory examination is often impossible in a noncommunicative patient or a pediatric patient. Additionally, you might have reason to question the reliability of an emotionally distraught or malingering patient. In these situations there are several further useful tests. The quickest, but not always appropriate, test is to apply a pinprick to the fingertip as the associated pain will usually elicit a reaction. If this is not appropriate or the results are equivocal, place the affected digit in warm water. Asking the patient to state if they sense hot or cold will often elicit an honest response. If the examination continues to be equivocal or questionable, leave the digit in the water for several minutes. A fingertip with intact digital nerves will prune, while a dennervated tip will not. In the examination of a chronic nerve injury, sensory and sympathetic denervation of a fingertip will result in a smooth, soft, and dry tip.

● MOTOR EXAMINATION

When examining a patient there can be many reasons why an action (ie, finger flexion) cannot be done.

1. Tendon or muscle is cut *or*
2. Nerve to that muscle is cut or damaged *or*
3. Joint dislocation, fracture displacement, or tendon subluxation place the musculotendinous unit at a mechanical disadvantage *or*
4. Patient cannot follow commands *or*
5. Patient does not want to move the part (either due to pain or secondary gain)

Part of the art of medicine is to try to distinguish these entities. As discussed previously, it is often helpful and our standard practice in the traumatic setting to infiltrate the injured part with a local anesthetic prior to examining the hand for possible tendon, muscle, and motor nerve injuries after the sensory examination has been completed. The use of local anesthesia is often inevitable and patients are usually pleased to finally have pain relief. It is helpful to be facile with digit and wrist blocks in this situation. Nerve blocks proximal to the site of injury are often more effective (lack of dilution from traumatic edema), require fewer needle sticks, and less medication. While waiting for the local anesthesia to take effect, we use this time to review the radiographs as well as prepare for subsequent wound irrigation, exploration, repair, and/or splinting.

In a chronic injury or other situations where local anesthesia is unnecessary, "place and hold" tests can be used if the patient is unable to actively move the affected part. Simply place the finger or hand in the position of maximal excursion of the muscle you are testing, and ask the patient to hold it in that position. If they are able to do so, then the tested musculotendinous unit and its nerve are intact. This is usually less painful for the patient to execute than moving the finger actively. In the cases of tendon subluxation (radial sagittal band rupture or laceration) place and hold tests should relocate the extensor tendon and allow the patient to demonstrate normal function. Reduction of dislocated joints or badly displaced fractures will similarly allow the musculotendinous units to perform normally.

In the sedated, unconscious, or noncommunicative patient, an adequate motor examination is often impossible. However, in these situations examining for a tenodesis effect can be useful (Figure 49-3). The tenodesis effect is demonstrated by passively ranging the wrist from flexion to extension and observing for passive finger extension to flexion, respectively. Any deviation from the normal cascade should alert the examiner to the possibility of a tendon laceration. The evaluation of a motor nerve injury is often delayed because it requires patient cooperation.

Motor Nerve Tests

The knowledge of the specific motor functions provided by each nerve can help verify that the major nerve is intact. Our typical examination involves asking the patient to quickly perform several simple motions, in the following order: wrist pronation (median), finger extension (posterior interosseous nerve), forearm supination (musculocutaneous, median, posterior interosseous nerve), composite fist (median, ulnar), finger crossover test (deep motor branch of the ulnar), make an OK sign (anterior interosseous), and palmar thumb abduction (recurrent branch of the median). Any abnormality in those tasks should be followed by a more complete examination of the affected nerve. A thorough knowledge of the muscle innervation is important for both injury localization as well as to later evaluate the progression of recovery.

Relevant Anatomy

Ulnar Nerve. After traveling through the cubital tunnel the ulnar nerve innervates the flexor carpi ulnaris (FCU)

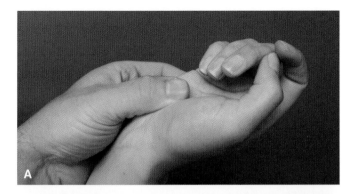

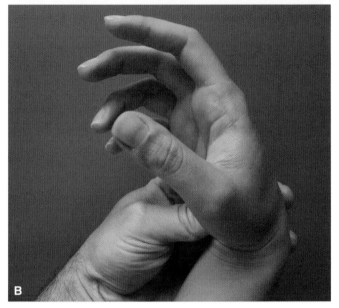

● **FIGURE 49-3.** Tenodesis effect on finger cascade. (A) Passive extension of the wrist. (B) Passive flexion of the wrist.

and flexor digitorum profundus (FDP) of the ring and small fingers. Seventy-five percent of the population has dual innervation (median and ulnar) to the long finger FDP.[2] The dorsal sensory branch exists 8 cm proximal to the wrist crease. After the ulnar nerve passes through Guyon canal, the deep branch innervates the hypothenar muscles, the interosseous muscles, the small and ring finger lumbrical muscles, the adductor pollicus, and the deep head of the flexor pollicus brevis (the superficial head is innervated by the median nerve). An ulnar nerve injury will result in weakness of the above muscles. Acutely, the patient will demonstrate a Wartenburg sign (paradoxical abduction of the small finger keyed to the unopposed pull of the extensor digiti quinti, or EDQ), and a Froment sign (flexion of the thumb interphalangeal [IP] joint due to substitution by the flexor pollicus longus [FPL] during key pinch in the presence of a paralyzed adductor pollicus). In a low ulnar nerve injury, clawing will develop because of the loss of the balancing effect of the lumbrical muscles, resulting in the unopposed pull of the extensor tendons which hyperextend the metacarpophalangeal (MCP) joint and the flexor tendons which hyperflex the IP joints. Clawing does not occur in

a high ulnar nerve injury due to paralysis of the long flexor tendons.

Median Nerve. The median nerve sequentially innervates the palmaris longus, the flexor carpi radialis (FCR), and the flexor digitorum superficialis (FDS) before entering and innervating the pronator teres. The median nerve then gives off the anterior interosseous nerve branch, which continues distally to innervate the FDP for the index and middle fingers, the FPL, and the pronator quadratus. The median nerve travels superficially in the distal forearm giving off the palmar cutaneous branch 5 cm proximal to the wrist crease. In the wrist, the recurrent motor branch innervates the thenar musculature. Motor branches to the lumbrical muscles to the index and middle fingers arise distal to this. Take note that an anterior interosseous nerve injury will result only in motor deficits resulting paralysis of the profundus tendon to the index and the FPL, easily demonstrated by inability to gesture OK. A complete median nerve injury will result in weakness of some or all the above listed muscles, which can be tested individually (see next section). When asked to make a fist, patients with high median nerve injuries will form a Benedictine or papal sign (extended thumb and index finger).

Radial Nerve. The radial nerve passes over the lateral humeral epicondyle with the profunda brachii artery and its radial collateral branch. It innervates the brachioradialis and the extensor carpi radialis longus (ECRL) before dividing into the superficial (sensory) and the deep (motor) branches. The deep branch innervates the extensor carpi radialis brevis then passes through and innervates the supinator, emerging as the posterior interosseous nerve (PIN). The PIN immediately innervates the extensor carpi ulnaris (ECU), then continues down the forearm innervating the extensor digitorum communis (EDC), the EDQ, the abductor pollicus longus (APL), the extensor pollicis brevis (EPB), the extensor pollicis longus (EPL), and the extensor indicis proprius (EIP). The radial nerve and the posterior interosseous nerve, are responsible for wrist and MCP extension, and can be quickly and easily assessed by testing these functions. The inability to extend either the wrist or the MCP joints should raise suspicions of a radial nerve/PIN injury. Remember that the ulnar innervated intrinsic muscles of the hand can provide extension of the fingers at the IP joints, especially when the MCP joint is held in extension.

● **MUSCULOTENDINOUS UNITS**

Each muscle of the arm and hand can be individually tested. This can provide insight into the function and integrity of each specific muscle, its tendon, as well as to confirm the adequacy of its innervation. In the following section, the specific testing maneuvers will be discussed for each muscle.

Dorsal Forearm and Hand

The extensor carpi radialis brevis functions is one of the primary wrist extensors. Since it inserts into the base of the third metacarpal, its function is tested by having the patient forcefully extend their wrist with their fingers slightly flexed, while the examiner's hand rests lightly over the index and long metacarpals. Remember that other muscles can act to extend the wrist, such as the ECRL and ECU. However, if the ECRL or ECU were the only muscle participating in wrist extension, the hand would also radially or ulnarly deviate, respectively. The fingers and thumb are lightly curled to eliminate the possible weak participation by the EDC, EIP, EDQ, and EPL.

The APL and EPB tendons form the volar border of the anatomic snuff box. The tendon of the APL can be easily palpated while having the patient forcefully abduct the thumb metacarpal in the frontal plane. The EPB is tested by having the patient put their palms and thumbs together and abduct the thumbs away from the hand while maintaining contact.

The EPL tendon forms the dorsal aspect of the anatomic snuff box and is tested by having the patient forcefully extend the thumb IP joint against resistance. Alternatively, the EPL can be tested by having the patient rest their palm flat and attempt to lift the entire first ray off the examination table (ie, thumb retropulsion).

The EDC travels across the dorsal aspect of the hand to all of the fingers, except the fifth which may be absent in 29% to 60%. The EDC has a common muscle belly and its function can be evaluated by having the patient extend their MCP joints against resistance or extend the IP joints with the MCP joints flexed. When evaluating the EDC for possible injury (such as in a dorsal hand laceration), one should have a high degree of suspicion for occult EDC transections. Proximal injuries can be easily missed due to the pull from the adjacent junctura tendinae; even if the EDC to the long finger is completely transected, the patient may be able to weakly extend the finger due to the action of the juncturae from the index and ring. In addition, independent MCP extension can be accomplished via the EIP and EDQ in the index and small fingers, respectively. During exploration and/or repair, the EIP and EDQ are usually found ulnar to their respective finger's EDC tendon at the distal extensor retinaculum and at the MCP joint.[3]

Another reason to have a high index of suspicion for tendon injury in dorsal hand wounds is because the soft tissue of the dorsum of the hand is very thin, making the extensor tendons more susceptible to injury. If the MCP is being extended by an adjacent junctura, it is usually a weaker extension than in the uninjured digits. In addition, the patient will often complain of pain while attempting this maneuver. If there is any question as to the status of the tendons in this circumstance, the best thing to do is to explore the wound.

The EIP can be selectively tested by having the patient forcefully extend the index MCP joint while keeping the remainder of the fingers flexed. By flexing the other fingers, the EDC is eliminated from participating in index finger MCP joint extension. Similarly, the EDQ can also be selectively tested by having the patient forcefully extend the MCP joint of the small finger while keeping the other fingers flexed into a fist.

The ECU functions as both a wrist extensor and an ulnar deviator, and can be selectively isolated by having the patient forcefully extend and ulnarly deviate their wrist. The examiner can palpate the tendon just distal to the ulna on the dorsal-ulnar aspect of the wrist during this maneuver.

Volar Forearm and Hand

The pronator teres functions to both pronate the forearm and flex the elbow, and can be tested by extending the elbow and having the patient forcefully pronate their forearm. By extending the arm at the elbow, the muscle is put on maximal stretch, giving it a mechanical advantage over the pronator quadratus, which also functions to pronate the arm. However, pronation could be achieved through function of the pronator quadratus in this position; it is difficult to completely isolate the pronator teres while testing its function.

The pronator quadratus can be selectively isolated by flexing the elbow and then asking the patient to forcefully pronate their arm. By flexing the elbow, the examiner eliminates participation from the pronator teres by placing it at a mechanical disadvantage.

The FCR and FCU are the primary flexors of the wrist. The FCR tendon can be palpated immediately radial to the palmaris longus tendon (if present) with forceful flexion of the wrist with the fingers cupped. The palmaris longus tendon (which can act as a weak wrist flexor) can also be palpated with the same maneuver, although it may be absent in up to 20% of patients. Palpation of the palmaris longus tendon may be more obvious if the patient opposes the thumb to the small finger during wrist flexion (Figure 49-4). The FCU can be easily palpated at the volar wrist by asking the patient to flex and ulnarly deviate their wrist.

The FDS deserves special consideration in examination of the hand. Having the patient simply flex their fingers does not rule out injuries to the superficialis, since this action could also be performed by the FDP. To specifically isolate the FDS (which flexes the middle phalanx), the adjacent fingers are held in full extension by the examiner, and the patient is asked to flex the finger in question (Figure 49-5). This maneuver prevents the FDP from flexing the finger and isolates the FDS for evaluation. The FDS of each finger has its own muscle belly and flexes independently. The FDP is blocked because it has a common muscle belly, eg, the FDP of one finger cannot function independently of the other fingers. The exception to the rule is that in 85% of patients the FDP to the index will have independent motion and may

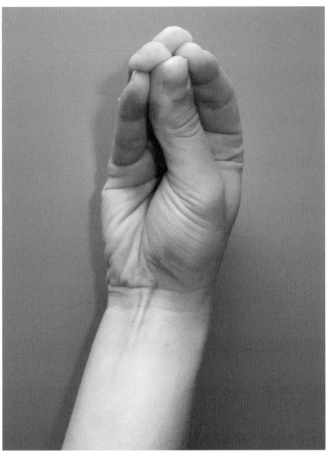

● **FIGURE 49-4.** The palmaris longus tendon is tested by actively flexing the wrist with common pinch of all fingers to the thumb.

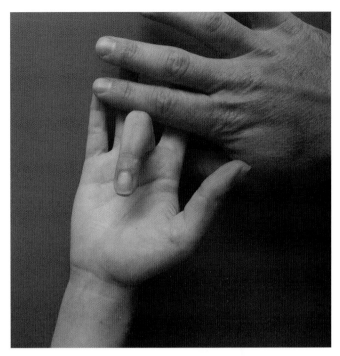

● **FIGURE 49-5.** The flexor digitorum superficialis is tested by extending the adjacent digits and asking the patient to flex the finger being examined.

and paradoxical IP joint extension which is known as a quadrigia effect (Figure 49-6).

The thenar musculature (abductor pollicis brevis, opponens pollicis, and flexor pollicis brevis) can be tested by having the patient forcefully abduct the thumb from

mask a FDS injury. If suspected, wiggle the distal phalanx during this test as its motion should be supple.

To further confuse the examiner, there are many anomalous nerve and tendon connections between the small and ring finger FDS muscles. Using the above examination to test the FDS to the small finger, approximately 34% of the population will be unable to flex the proximal interphalangeal (PIP) joint. If only the index and long finger are held in extension, approximately 16% of the population will be unable to flex the small finger PIP joint. Thus, approximately 16% of the normal population does not have a FDS to the fifth finger.[4]

The FDP of each digit can be tested by asking the patient to flex their distal interphalangeal joint with the middle phalanx held in extension by the examiner. Similarly, the FPL can be evaluated by having the patient flex the thumb IP joint against resistance. In 15% of the normal population, the FPL and index finger FDP will have simultaneous contraction, referred to as the Linburg-Comstock sign due to tendinous interconnections. An interesting examination finding will occur if the FDP is lacerated distal to the lumbrical origin. When asked to make a fist the FDP tendon will pull strongly on the lumbrical origin, which will cause MCP joint flexion

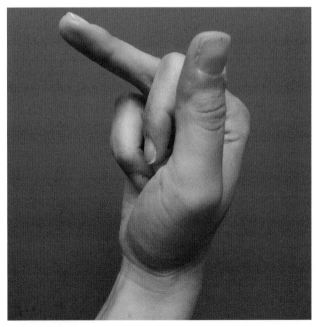

● **FIGURE 49-6.** If the profundus tendon is lacerated distal to the lumbrical origin, MCP joint flexion and paradoxical IP joint extension can be seen when the patient is asked to make a fist.

the plane of the palm (ie, abductor pollicis brevis action) and pronate it across to oppose to the small finger or the examiner's finger (opponens) or flex at the MCP joint (flexor pollicis brevis). The adductor pollicis can be tested by having the patient forcefully bring the thumb adjacent to the index finger, although the Frohman test is more reliable.

The volar interossei muscles can be tested by having the patient forcefully adduct their fingers. By placing your fingers between the patient's, the examiner can gauge the strength of the adduction. The dorsal interossei can be tested by having the patient forcefully abduct their fingers.

● RADIOLOGIC EXAMINATION

Introduction

Acute osseous trauma of the phalanges and metacarpals are seen most frequently in young men, but is still the most common fracture in any age, sex, or ethnicity.[5] When evaluating a hand injury, the diagnosis can usually be obtained with history and physical examination alone. However, in any setting, other than simple lacerations, there should be a low threshold for obtaining a standard three-view radiographic examination.

The nature of the fracture pattern is determined by the direction and the degree of the force applied, whereas the displacement or angulation of the fracture segments are the result of deforming forces from intrinsic or extrinsic musculotendinous units. Transverse fractures result from forces perpendicular to the long axis of the bone or three-point bending loads. Axial loading produces oblique fractures, the degree of which is directly related to the magnitude of axial strain. Spiral fractures result from axial loading with rotational stress. The majority of proximal phalanx fractures have volar angulation, whereas metacarpal fractures are dorsally angulated. This results from to the strong pull of the intrinsic muscles, not the injuring force.

Classification

Fractures in the hand can be classified by multiple means: location, articular involvement, angulation, displacement, and nature (greenstick, transverse, oblique, spiral, or comminuted). The most important distinction for treatment in the proximal and middle phalanges is articular involvement. Metacarpal fractures, alternatively, are best subdivided for management by anatomic location and digit involved.

Imaging

Standard three-view radiographs include posteroanterior, lateral, and oblique views. This series is usually sufficient to diagnose most fractures and dislocations of the metacarpal and phalangeal bones. It is often helpful with isolated digital injuries to obtain three views of the involved digit alone.

The posteroanterior view is perhaps the most useful view. It should be read in a systematic fashion, much like the physical examination. One approach is to start at the top, checking the phalanges, then the metacarpals, and so on. Check the edges of the bone, making sure the cortical edges are smooth. Any sharp defects are indicative of fracture. Also, confirm that the joint spaces appear roughly equal in size. This view is particularly helpful in the evaluation of the bases of the metacarpals and proximal phalanges. The bases of the second through fifth MCP joints should form an M configuration, the loss of which implies dislocation.

The lateral view is obtained with the fifth ray adjacent to the cassette. Superimposition can be minimized by fanning the fingers. This view is important in classifying the angulation or rotational displacement of fractures and diagnosing dislocations. The oblique view is taken with the hand rotated 45 degrees, or half-way between the previous views. This view allows for good visualization of the first and second MCP joints.

Additional Imaging/Special Views

An oblique view of the thumb is obtained through the posteroanterior view of the hand. A true posteroanterior view of the thumb, called a Roberts view (Figure 49-7A), is preferable when a thumb fracture is suspected. This is performed by hyperpronating the forearm and placing the back of the thumb against the x-ray cassette.[6] A Brewerton view (Figure 49-7B) is rarely necessary, but can be helpful in visualizing the metacarpal heads, hook of the hamate and the fourth and fifth carpometacarpal (CMC) joints. The Brewerton view may also show erosions of the metacarpal heads and the bases of the phalanges. The hand is in the anteroposterior position with the palm facing upward. The MCP joints are flexed to 45 degrees with the phalanges in contact with the film. The tube is angled 20 degrees from the ulnar side to the head of the third metacarpal.[7] Computed tomography, magnetic resonance imaging, three-phase bone scans, and ultrasound are rarely necessary in the acute setting.

● OSSEOUS INJURIES

Metacarpal Fractures

Intra-articular fractures of the first metacarpal base commonly occur in two patterns: the Bennett fracture and Rolando fracture (Figure 49-8A,B). The Bennett fractures make up approximately one third of all fractures involving the thumb. They are characterized by an oblique fracture line at the base of the metacarpal with the proximal-ulnar fragment (smaller fragment) held on the trapezium by the

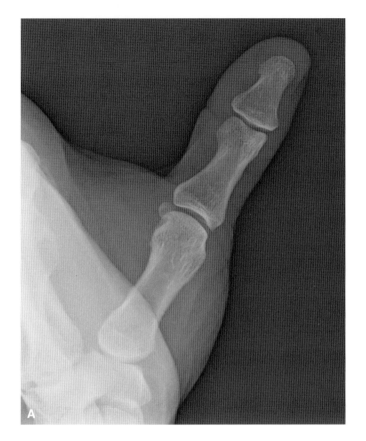

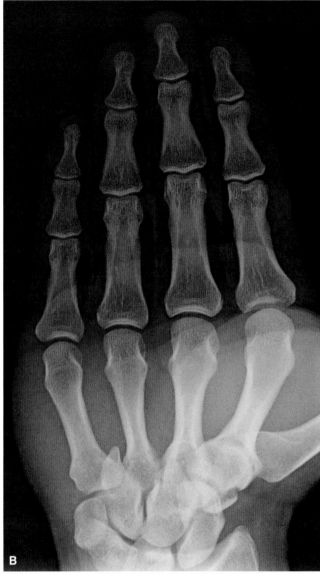

● **FIGURE 49-7.** Commonly used additional hand plain films. (A) Roberts view. (B) Brewerton view.

volar oblique ligament or "beak ligament" and the distal-radial fragment (majority of the metacarpal) pulled proximally and radially by the force of the APL. The Rolando fracture is much less common. It is characterized by a Y- or T-shaped fracture-dislocation of the base of the first metacarpal. The extrinsic muscle forces typically displace the distal metacarpal fragment dorsally. Extra-articular fractures comprise the approximately 35% of first metacarpal bone fractures.

Metacarpals 2 to 5 can be subdivided based on the relative stability of the respective CMC joints. The index and long CMC joints are relatively motionless and an extensor lag will develop with very little angulation as opposed to the more ulnar CMC joints.

A fracture of the metacarpal neck is the most common fracture of the metacarpal bones. It usually involves the fifth and occasionally the fourth metacarpals and is characterized by a transverse fracture with volar angulation.

A fifth metacarpal neck fracture, or so-called boxer's fracture, is most commonly caused by striking an object with a closed fist.

Fractures of the metacarpal midshaft and base are less common than neck fractures. Midshaft oblique and spiral fractures can be associated with shortening and a loss of the knuckle prominence. Small rotational deformities in the metacarpal shaft will rotate the orientation of the MCP joint and can cause significant finger scissoring with flexion. Only 5 degrees of rotational deformity will result in nearly 1.5 cm of fingertip overlap.[8]

Basilar fractures are rare, except with the fifth metacarpal. The "baby Bennett" or "reverse Bennett" fracture is characterized by an oblique intra-articular fracture with proximal and ulnar displacement of the distal metacarpal fragment (Figure 49-9). As in a Bennett fracture, the displacement is due to the strong pull of the extrinsic muscles.

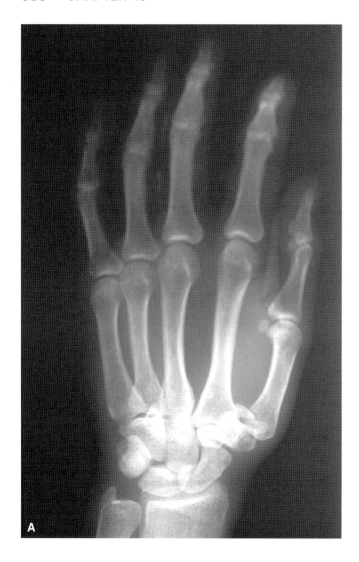

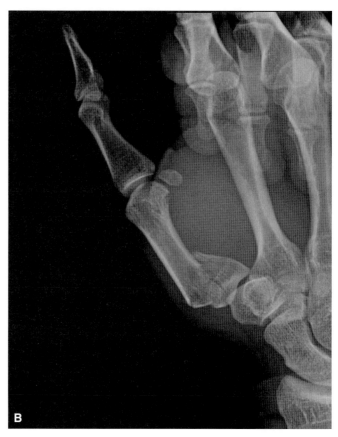

● **FIGURE 49-8.** Fracture dislocation of thumb proximal phalanx. (A) Bennett fracture. (B) Rolando fracture.

Proximal Phalanx Fractures

Fractures of the proximal phalanx should be considered by location: base, midshaft, and head. Oblique intra-articular fractures should inspire further physical examination to ensure the associated collateral ligament is intact. Oblique and spiral midshaft fractures are commonly associated with shortening or rotation, although the rotational deformity will not produce finger tip overlap or scissoring to the same extent as metacarpal fractures. Transverse fractures can be relatively stable, but often volar angulation will be seen due to the pull of the intrinsic muscles on the proximal segment. Fractures of the head of the proximal phalanx can range from small chip fractures to complete involvement of one or both condyles.

Middle Phalanx Fractures

The incidence of middle phalanx is similar to that of proximal phalanx fractures. The classification of these fractures can be thought of in the same ways as the proximal phalanx. Little angulation is tolerated due to impingement of the flexor sheath volarly and the relatively fixed length of the extensor mechanism from the insertion on the middle phalanx to the insertion on the distal phalanx.

Distal Phalanx Fractures

Distal phalanx fractures are usually the result of crush injuries. Soft tissue injury to the nail bed is commonly associated with subungual hematoma (usually involving >80% of the nail bed). Nonarticular and tuft fractures are usually comminuted, but minimally displaced. Fractures at the base of the distal phalanx are complicated by the forces exerted from the terminal tendon dorsally and the FDP volarly. A mallet fracture is an oblique fracture of the dorsal cortex, including the terminal tendon insertion. A "jersey finger" is an FDP tendon avulsion. The avulsed FDP tendon is occasionally associated with a bone fragment. Depending on the fragment size the fragment can become lodged at the distal edge of the A2 or A4 pulley.

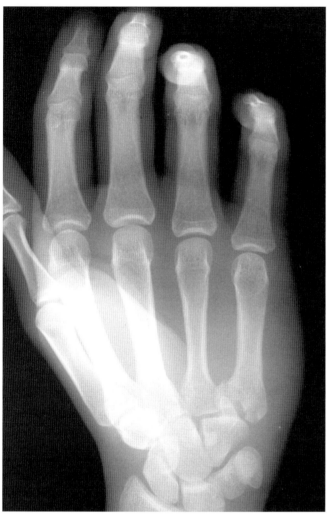

● FIGURE 49-9. Fracture-dislocation of the fifth metacarpal base, a "reversed" Bennett fracture.

● LIGAMENTOUS INJURIES

Thumb

Because of the physical differences in the joints and supporting ligaments, the thumb and fingers will be again discussed separately. Pure dislocation of the basal or CMC joint of the thumb is rare. The joint stability results from the strong volar oblique ligament. Dislocation forces on the thumb CMC joint will result in the Bennett fracture-dislocation as previously described.

Pure dislocations at the MCP joint of the thumb can occur, but are quite rare. These dislocations are dorsal and include injury to the volar plate. The extent of the injury is variable depending on the extent of accessory and true collateral ligament damage. In its most severe form, the proximal phalanx lies dorsal and parallel to the metacarpal, the so-called bayonet deformity.

Ulnar collateral ligament damage at the thumb MCP, the so-called skier's or gamekeeper's thumb, is relatively common. It is diagnosed when there is greater than 40 degrees of MCP joint instability while applying a radial

stress to the proximal phalanx, or 20% or more angulation than the unaffected thumb. A Stener lesion is a name that has been applied to the ruptured proximal portion of the ulnar collateral ligament that has displaced dorsal to the adductor aponeurosis.[9] Stener lesions can be caused by excessive ulnar angulation of the thumb MCP joint during the injury or by the overzealous examining physician. This can occasionally be detected on radiographs if a bone fragment is associated with the avulsed ligament (Figure 49-10).

Dislocations at the thumb IP joint are incredibly rare because the simple hinge joint is quite resistant to radial or ulnar stress. Dislocations are dorsal and the torn volar plate usually remains attached distantly and does not impair reduction.

Fingers—Metacarpophalangeal Joint

Metacarpophalangeal joints in the fingers can be either subluxed or truly dislocated. In subluxations, the joint is hyperextended 60 to 90 degrees and easily reducible. Subluxations are more likely in the middle and ring fingers, whereas true dislocations are more common in the index finger and to a lesser degree the small finger.[10] True dislocations are usually dorsal and closed reduction is nearly impossible.

When the index finger proximal phalanx dislocates dorsally, it slides proximally on the metacarpal head. The flexor tendons wrap around the ulnar neck and the lumbrical tendon wraps around the radial neck of the metacarpal.

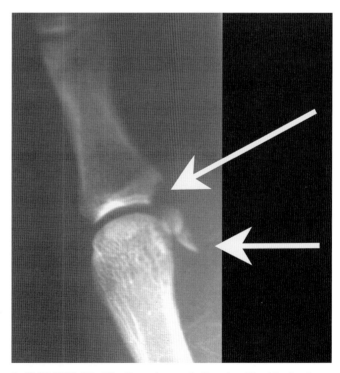

● FIGURE 49-10. Gamekeeper's thumb with chip fracture off the proximal phalanx base (*top arrow*), demonstrating a Stener lesion (*bottom arrow*).

This effectively creates a "noose" that will tighten with attempted reduction. In the small finger a similar "noose" is formed by the abductor digiti quinti ulnarly and the flexor tendons radially. Volar dislocations are rare, but equally difficult to reduce in a closed fashion. However, volar dislocations are made irreducible due to the interposition of the dorsal capsule.

Isolated injuries to the MCP joint collateral ligament complex of the fingers will present as swelling and pain around the affected joint. The radiographic examination will be normal. A radial collateral ligament injury of the small finger is a more severe injury and will be unstable due to the pull from the abductor digiti minimi.

Fingers—Proximal Interphalangeal Joint

The collateral ligaments, volar plate, and extensor mechanism encircle the PIP joint. For a significant dislocation to occur, at least two of these structures must be disrupted. Dorsal dislocations are the most common and are characterized by both volar plate and collateral ligament disruption. Frequently, the volar plate will be connected to a bone fragment from the middle phalanx base. Multiple fracture-dislocation grading systems, ie, Hastings, have been created based on the joint stability and size of the bone fragment (percentage of fractured joint surface).[11] For fragments less than 30% of the joint surface, a stable closed reduction is usually possible. For larger fragments or unstable joints, an open reduction is usually necessary.

Volar dislocations of the PIP joint are notoriously difficult to reduce. The head of the proximal phalanx will become entrapped between the central slip and lateral band of the extensor mechanism. Finger traction will tighten the extensor tendon, making attempted closed reduction difficult if not impossible.

Owing to the support of the strong collateral ligaments, FDP, and terminal tendon insertions, distal interphalangeal dislocations are rare. Dislocations at this joint are usually caused by open lacerations of one or more of the supporting structures.

REFERENCES

1. Gelberman RH, Blasingame JP. The timed Allen test. *J Trauma*. 1981;21(6):477–479.

2. Bhadra N, Keith MW, Peckham PH. Variations in innervation of the flexor digitorum profundus muscle. *J Hand Surg Am*. 1999;24(4):700–703.

3. Celik S, Bilge O, Pinar Y, Govsa F. The anatomical variations of the extensor tendons to the dorsum of the hand. *Clin Anat*. 2008;21(7):652–659.

4. Tan JS, Oh L, Louis DS. Variations of the flexor digitorum superficialis as determined by an expanded clinical examination. *J Hand Surg*. 2009;34(5):900–906.

5. Hove LM. Fractures of the hand. Distribution and relative incidence. *Scand J Plast Reconstr Surg Hand Surg*. 1993;27(4):317–319.

6. Robert P. Bulletins et mémoires de la société de radiologie de médicale de France. 1936;24:687.

7. Lane CS. Detecting occult fractures of the metacarpal head: the Brewerton view. *J Hand Surg Am*. 1977;2(2):131–133.

8. Manktelow RT, Mahoney JL. Step osteotomy: a precise rotation osteotomy to correct scissoring deformities of the fingers. *Plast Reconstr Surg*. 1981;68(4):571–576.

9. Stener B. Displacement of the ruptured ulnar collateral ligament of the metacarpophalangeal joint. *J Bone Joint Surg Am*. 1962;44B(4):869–879.

10. Calfee RP, Sommerkamp TG. Fracture-dislocation about the finger joints. *J Hand Surg Am*. 2009;34(6):1140–1147.

11. Hastings H 2nd, Carroll C 4th. ent of closed articular fractures of the metacarpophalangeal and proximal interphalangeal joints. *Hand Clin*. 1988;4(3):503–527.

chapter 50

Soft Tissue Reconstruction of the Upper Extremities

Elvin G. Zook, MD / Srdjan A. Ostric, MD

● PATIENT EVALUATION AND SELECTION

Conditions affecting the nail bed can be categorized within the three major categories of trauma, infection, and tumors. Nail bed trauma is by far the most common of these conditions, and to some extent, because of a lack of knowledge in this subject by many practitioners, treatment of secondary deformities of the fingertip is also common. In all cases, proper treatment of the fingertip and nail bed is predicated on a complete understanding of the anatomy.

The fingertip is defined as the portion distal to the insertion of the flexor and extensor tendons on the distal phalanx. The perionychium includes the nail fold, nail bed, and nail plate, and is unique to primates. All the components of the hand are present in this compact area, including flexor and extensor tendon insertions, nerve, vessels, and bone (Figure 50-1).

The nail, a complex structure with many functional roles, helps stabilize the fingertip during pinch and allows one to interface with the world. Without a nail plate, two-point discrimination increases by a factor of 2. In addition, there is a high number of immunological factors concentrated in the hyponychium.

In evaluating an acute nail bed injury, it is important to establish the nature of the injury (eg, crush, laceration, avulsion). It is equally important to obtain a complete history and physical examination, with particular focus on factors such as age, hand dominance, general health of the patient, and the nature of the patient's employment, as all these factors will guide the selection of a particular treatment.

A complete examination of the injury is necessary to determine whether the nail plate should be removed.

It is clear that when the nail plate is fractured or avulsed, there is often a nail bed laceration which must be repaired. A fracture of the tuft or bending of the nail plate may injure the nail bed, but may not overcome the force needed to break the nail plate. In general, a fracture of the tuft is associated with a nail bed injury and the nail plate will have to be removed. If there is no tuft fracture, it has been our experience that a subungual hematoma of greater than 50% requires a removal of the nail plate, inspection, and repair of the nail bed. If less than 50%, the subungual hematoma may be drained with the disposable cautery devices in the emergency room (ER) or a heated paperclip at home.

● PATIENT PREPARATION

Preparing a fingertip for surgical intervention, whether it is for tumor, trauma, or infection, is guided by standard principles. Oftentimes, except in the case of small children, nail bed injuries are addressed within an ER setting. In most cases, the whole hand or arm should be prepped to allow the surgeon sterile access either to the volar or dorsal surface.

The finger is anesthetized by performing a digital nerve block with 1% lidocaine. Several reports have discussed the utility and the safety of a solution with epinephrine, as it can aid with hemostasis and lengthen the duration of analgesia; however, if the patient has a risk of vascular compromise, plain lidocaine will suffice. A flexor tendon sheath block can be delivered intrathecally with an injection just proximal to the A1 pulley in the palm, but this can be quite painful, especially if the patient has not received sedation. In this case, we

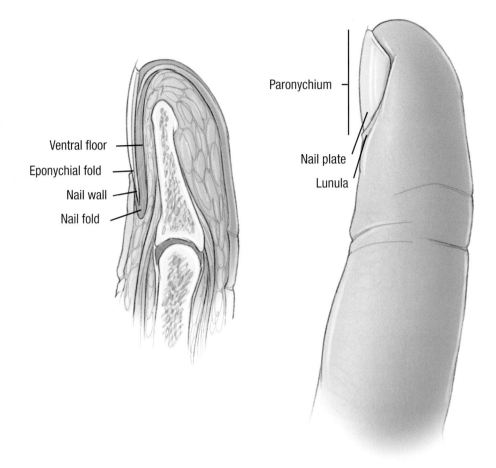

Ventral floor
Eponychial fold
Nail wall
Nail fold

Paronychium
Nail plate
Lunula

● FIGURE 50-1. Germinal matrix where nail production begins. Sterile matrix has been referred to as the road bed for the nail. The nail plate is not adherent to the nail at a point distal to the sterile matrix, therefore, disruption of the sterile matrix, or improper treatment may result in nonadherence of the nail plate. Eponychium is in the dorsal roof covering for the germinal matrix. Hyponychium refers to the area where the nail separates from the nail bed. Paronychium is at the junction of the nail bed and skin at the sides of the tip. The perionychium includes the nail bed, hyponychium, paronychium, and eponychium.

prefer to anesthetize the dorsal skin at the metacarpophalangeal level, then infiltrate in the web spaces, as this tends to be less painful for the patient. A 27- or 30-gauge needle is used for infiltration, and in general, 4 to 6 cc are necessary to obtain satisfactory analgesia.

Tourniquet control can be achieved with a Turnicot; however, these are not always available in ER settings, and because they are rolled on the fingers to help exsanguinate the finger, they should not be used in the presence of infection to avoid spreading the infection proximally. Therefore, we prefer to use a 1-inch Penrose that is placed circumferentially at the base of the affected finger. It is tightened and clipped with a hemostat, making sure that there is no rolling of the Penrose to minimize possible damage to neurovascular bundles. The presence of a large hemostat will help to remind the surgeon to remove the tourniquet at the end of the case.

Generally, 5-0 nylon sutures are used for skin, while 7-0 chromic sutures are preferred for the nail bed, although in the case of small children, a 5-0 chromic suture may also be used for the skin. Fractures are reduced with two small Kirschner (K-) wires, rather than one, to help prevent axial rotation of the fracture segment; and in smaller children, or smaller facture segments, when a 28-gauge K-wire is too large, a Keith needle has been used with success. Loupe magnification is highly recommended.

● TECHNIQUES

Infections

Paronychia. Paronychia are infections of the nail fold specifically, and are the most common infection of the hand. The most common causative agent is *Staphylococcus aureus* or *Pseudomonas*, although a variety of organisms can be involved depending on the patient's health and exposure.

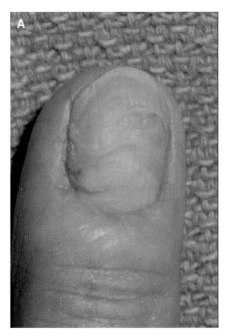 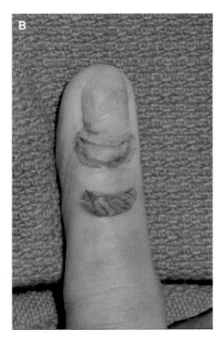 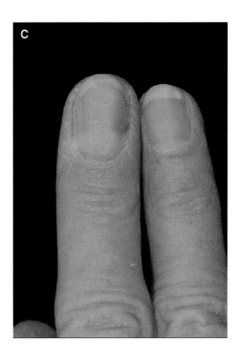

● FIGURE 50-2. Example of the treatment for a chronic paronychia. (A) Infection on the undersurface of the dorsal roof of the nailfold. (B) Full thickness section of the dorsal roof removed to eliminate infected tissue. (C) Post healing, visible nail slightly longer but has normal appearance.

An incision and drainage is the mainstay of treatment. After the area has been prepared and the area infiltrated with a digital block, pus can be expressed by entering the sulcus of the nail plate and the eponychial fold and raising it with a fine elevator, such as the Kleinert-Kutz. Sometimes the infection can spread to the subungual space. In this case, at least a portion of the nail plate should be removed to ensure adequate drainage. An incision through the eponychial fold is not necessary and should be avoided, as necrosis of the flap tips can ensue with nail fold scarring and a resultant nail deformity. Prompt care is vital because these infections have the potential to spread or become chronic paronychiae.

Chronic paronychiae, which have been present for several months, or even years, are commonly caused by mixed gram-negative organisms or fungi. Treatment consists of marsupialization, which consists of excision of a full-thickness, arc-shaped wedge of skin that is allowed to heal secondarily (Figure 50-2).

Felons. Felons are closed space infection of the finger pulp. They tend to involve the thumb and index fingers most frequently, and they typical present with pain. There are numerous small vertical septa which serve to attach the skin to the periosteum, providing stability to the finger pulp. These septa are unyielding and in the presence of infection, with an increase in pressure, pain ensues. After a few days, if the felon is left untreated, the septae will eventually erode, and the pain will often diminish, falsely giving the impression that the condition is getting better, when it is actually getting worse.

Once again, incision and drainage is the mainstay of treatment, and several incisions have been suggested in the treatment of felons. Small longitudinal incisions over the maximal area of tenderness on the pad are preferred. A "fish mouth" incision should be avoided, as this incision will often result in skin necrosis and a painful deformed fingertip. Likewise, transverse or high lateral incisions may jeopardize the neurovascular bundle or devascularize the fingertip (Figure 50-3).

A differential diagnosis should always include herpetic whitlow. These painful, whitish, vesicular lesions are caused by the herpes simplex virus (HSV-1 in 60% of case and HSV-2 in 40% of cases). Oftentimes, these lesions occur in small children secondary to finger and thumb sucking or health care workers who have direct exposure to saliva (ICU nurses, etc). In the case of HSV-2 (genital herpes), herpetic whitlow is caused by autoinoculation. In all cases, the treatment is conservative, and the patient is placed on an antiviral medication. These lesions should not be drained, especially in small children, as there are case reports of viral encephalitis ensuing after drainage of these lesions (Figure 50-4).

Trauma

Healing by Secondary Intention. Following a fingertip amputation, if there is enough soft tissue coverage or if only a small portion of bone needs to be removed to achieve primary closure, secondary healing is the simplest and easiest method of treatment for the practitioner. In children, who have a high capacity for healing, this may

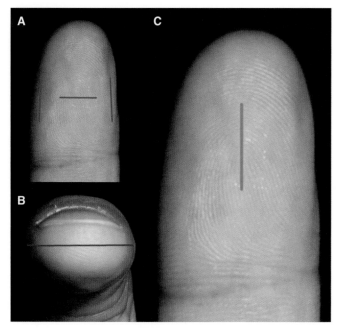

● FIGURE 50-3. Lateral and transverse incisions (A) are not recommended for felon drainage, as risk of neurovascular compromise is high. Likewise, a "fish mouth," or even hemi "fish mouth" (B) incisions carry the risk of a creating a painful scar at the fingertip. (C) A small, longitudinal incision over the infection is best tolerated.

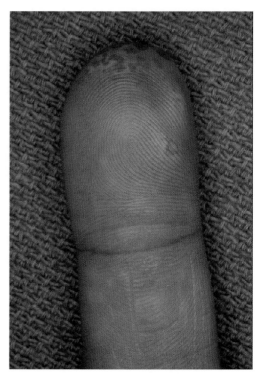

● FIGURE 50-4. An example of an herpetic whitlow, which can easily be mistaken for a paronychia or felon. However, incision and drainage is contraindicated.

also be a suitable option. In larger wounds (>1 cm), healing may take upward of 3 to 4 weeks, which may result in an unnecessary and unacceptable delay of return to work. In addition, as the wound bed contracts, this will cause the nail to hook to varying degrees.

A scar will not always provide stable soft tissue coverage, and depending on the particular requirement of the patient, secondary healing may be an unsuitable option. In this case, a glabrous split or full-thickness skin graft may be harvested from the hypothenar or proximal phalanx area. Likewise, if nonglabrous skin is used, a variety of donor sites are available from the ipsilateral arm or the groin.

Nail Bed Laceration. When there is suspicion of a nail bed laceration (eg, subungual hematoma/tuft fracture, avulsion of the nail from the eponychium or paronychium), the nail plate should be removed to inspect the nail bed. The most sensitive physical finding for a nail bed laceration is a tuft fracture, and a subungual hematoma that is greater than 50% of the nail bed will have a nail bed laceration about two thirds of the time. Oftentimes, these crushing injuries will result in complex stellate lacerations. In either case, removal of the nail will reveal the injury, and the nail bed should be repaired meticulously under loupe magnification with 7-0 chromic sutures.

Salvage of All Usable Parts. In an amputation, when the specimen is available, a determination must be made by the surgeon whether it possible to replace this part.

Unless the amputation is proximal, microsurgical reconstruction is usually not a reasonable option. At this point, management is predicated on the level of the amputation in addition to the functional needs of the patient.

In an amputation distal to the lunula, the decision whether to use a cap graft or a composite graft must be made. In general, composite grafts do not survive in older patients, especially if a smoking history is present, and are not replaced. In children, the opposite is generally true. However, some recent retrospective studies have shown a rate of salvage in some individuals that might sway some to attempt this.[1]

A cap graft can be used for coverage of the amputated fingertip. The amputated specimen is trimmed down essentially to its dermal surface, removing all fat and bone. This is easily done with a combination of sharp scissors and a scalpel. Once this has been performed, "tailor tacking" of the graft can be performed with a small incision down the midline of the graft, which is lengthened and the excess trimmed to achieve a well-contoured graft. A bolster may be fashioned with nonabsorbable stitches; however, if the graft is sewn on meticulously and a stable dressing is applied that is not too tight, then a bolster is not always necessary.

Of note, when the amputation occurs at or proximal to the level of the lunula, and the amputated specimen cannot be replaced, the residual germinal matrix needs to be ablated to prevent the formation of a nail horn.

When multiple fingers have been injured, all usable parts should be used to reconstruct the fingertips, even if the tissues are not derived from the same finger. This type of selective reattachment should be guided by the particular needs of the patient; however, restoration of the thumb index pinch is valuable for most daily activities.

Microsurgical Reconstruction. A wide variety of micro-surgical procedures have been described for the finger-tip, ranging from toe or partial toe transfer to arterialized venous skin flaps. Although they have been described by many practitioners in the United States, they are not routinely performed, except perhaps in the case of thumb reconstruction where not only restoration of coverage is important but also sensibility. In Eastern cultures, these flaps tend to be performed more commonly, and they can be a valuable reconstructive option for the carefully selected patient.[2]

Nail Bed Avulsion. Approximately 15% of all nail bed injuries are avulsions. There are two major types of avulsion, and they each must be addressed in specific ways in order to prevent a secondary nail deformity.

The first of these is avulsion distal to the eponychial fold. Originally, the recommendation was to separate the nail bed from the nail plate and replace the nail bed; however, we found that procedure too disruptive to the avulsed nail bed, and have since then simply sewn the avulsed nail plate and nail bed as one unit with favorable results.

Avulsion of the nail and attached nail bed from the eponychial fold must be exposed by reflecting the eponychial fold with incisions 90 degrees to the eponychial fold. Only in this way is possible to optimize visualization and thereby meticulously repair the germinal matrix so as to avoid a nail deformity (Figure 50-5). The nail should be removed to allow replacement of the germinal matrix back into the nail fold.

Free Graft of the Nail Bed. If the avulsed nail bed is not salvageable, it must be replaced with a free graft, either a split-thickness sterile matrix or a full-thickness graft of the germinal matrix. When ER facilities are adequate, this may be done with a graft from the great toe. If bone is visible, a graft should be attempted in any case, as an avulsion injury can leave enough periosteum for survival of the graft. However, if bare bone is exposed, we have found that in the case of small grafts, they will survive on the basis of plasmatic imbibition from the edges of the nail bed, until the graft revascularizes.

Burns. Until recently, burns of the fingertips have gone largely untreated. However, they create a characteristic deformity of the nail. As the dorsal skin of the hand contracts it will cause the eponychial fold to retract and evert. Treatment of this deformity is very similar to treatment of burn scar contractures elsewhere in the body. The contracture is released sharply proximal to the eponychial fold, allowing the correction of the eversion. The defect is then grafted with a full thickness graft.

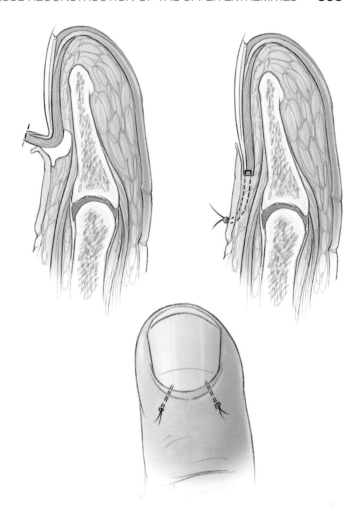

● **FIGURE 50-5.** Epopnychial avulsion accounts for approximately 15% of nail bed avulsions. Proper repair mandates that exposure be obtained through incisions in the eponychial fold at 90 degrees, so that the base may be inset properly with mattress stitches.

Favorable results of this procedure have recently been described in a recent study.[3]

V-Y Advancement

Atasoy-Kleinert Flap. This classic V-Y volar advancement flap is highly reliable and very useful for dorsal oblique fingertip amputations. The flap may only be advanced about 1.0 to 1.5 cm, and it is necessary to have enough relatively uninjured palmar tissue to create and advance this flap. Once the V is designed based on the palmer distal interphalangeal (DIP) crease, and the incision has been made through the skin, a combination of careful blunt and sharp dissection should be used to disrupt the vertical septa in the finger pulp to allow advancement of the flap. Care should be taken to avoid excessive tension for two reasons: (1) necrosis of the flap and (2) tension on the distal attachment of the flap this will tend to a hook nail, creating a bothersome and unsightly secondary deformity that is difficult to correct.

Kutler V-Y Flap. This flap is a bilateral lateral V-Y advancement flap from the sides of the tip, similar to the volar advancement flap. The main disadvantages of this flap include possible disruption of the neurovascular bundle resulting in hypersensitivity. The flaps also do not as readily advance as the volar V-Y flap; however, a good indication for this flap is an oblique amputation of the fingertip with more soft tissue on the sides.

Thenar Flap. Thenar flaps provide durable coverage for the index and the long fingers. In the classic description a proximally based flap is created on the thenar eminence. Although modifications have been described, thenar flaps often leave painful scarring or an anesthetic skin graft in the palm because the donor site cannot be closed primarily.

A modification of this procedure proposed by Russell et al. in 1981, presents a solution to some of the disadvantages of the standard thenar flap. The metacarpophalangeal (MCP) crease flap is a radially based flap that is designed between the two creases at the thumb volar MCP and can be closed primarily, leaving a fine-line scar. This flap must be harvested with great care to identify and protect the neurovascular bundles on the thumb, as they are superficial and subject to injury (Figure 50-6).

Cross-Finger Flap. When there is insufficient pulp for the volar V-Y advancement flap, the cross-finger flap can be used. This flap is harvested from the dorsum of the finger adjacent to the injured finger. A flap is elevated over the middle phalanx in a plane superficial to the peritenon of the extensor mechanism, to allow skin grafting of the donor site. The flap is then turned 180 degrees like a book page, and it is sewn into the adjacent fingertip defect. The flap is then divided in 2 to 3 weeks. Although this flap has the possibility of restoring sensation to the injured fingertip, it has several drawbacks. The donor site must be skin grafted, and being a two-stage procedure, the immobilization of the fingers results in joint stiffness, especially in a noncompliant patient who will not engage in active range of motion exercises. Although stiffness may be overcome in children, it is then often necessary to pin the proximal interphalangeal (PIP) joint to prevent flap separation. This flap should not be used in an older patient population, or those with preexisting conditions that predispose them to joint stiffness (eg, arthritis).

Reversed Homodigital Flap. As our understanding of anatomy has increased, so has our ability to treat nail bed injuries with more advanced procedures intended to restore not only contour to the finger pulp, but sensation as well.

When there is a fingertip amputation, tissue from the same finger can be utilized by creating a distally based flap along the midlateral line distal to the web space. The

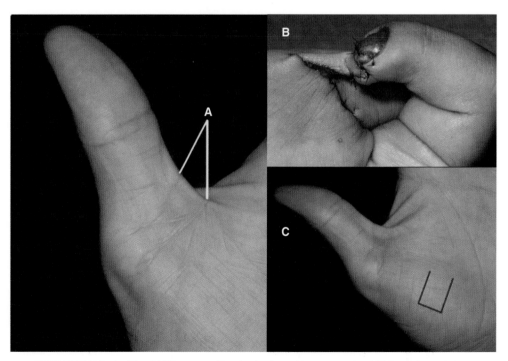

● FIGURE 50-6. The MCP crease flap is designed between the MCP crease of the thumb and the first thumb crease distal, which is consistently 1.5 to 2.0 cm in width (A). The radially based flap (B) is highly reliable, and offers the distinct advantage of primary closure in a natural crease in the hand. The thenar flap (C) has several modifications, but oftentimes cannot be closed primarily, resulting in a unaesthetic of painful scar.

reversed digital artery flap can provide durable tissue without invading the palm or another digit, and can be transferred as a single stage procedure.

● ANATOMY

There are palmar vascular plexuses located at the MCP joint, the PIP joint, and the finger pulp, as well as dorsal vascular plexus at the nail fold, that provide an extensive communication between the two digital arteries. The blood supply to this island flap is from retrograde flow through the digital artery after having crossed through the vascular plexuses at the middle and distal phalangeal level after the proximal ipsilateral artery is transected and ligated. A dorsal branch of the proper digital nerve can be incorporated into the flap design, which then requires neurorrhaphy to the distal stump of the severed digital nerve. Venous outflow is initially from retrograde flow in the venous plexuses in the perivascular fat surrounding the digital arteries until local venous anastomoses are established. A skin flap corresponding to the fingertip defect is outlined along the radial or ulnar side of the proximal phalanx. The ulnar side of the index and radial side of the small are used to avoid scars on the outside of the border digits. A midlateral incision extends from the flap to the midpoint of the middle phalanx ensuring the incision does not cross the

neutral axis of the PIP joint. The skin flap is incised and elevated with the digital artery and a surrounding cuff of subcutaneous tissue to ensure venous drainage. After flap elevation the tourniquet is released. A microvascular clamp is applied to the digital artery proximal to the flap. Bleeding from the tip of the flap and viability of the digit is ascertained prior to dividing the artery. Donor sites up to 2 × 3 cm can be closed primarily, otherwise a full-thickness skin graft from the volar wrist or elbow crease is applied.

A branch of the dorsal sensory nerve can be included in this flap; however some studies have not included it with similar results as they believe the flap become neurotized eventually.

The main arguments against the use of this flap are the necessity of skin grafting the donor site and the sacrifice of the digital artery. And since this is a reversed flap, venous drainage is dependent on a circuitous communicating and collateral bypass route, which may pose a risk for venous engorgement of the flap.

The Thumb

Special attention must be given to the thumb. Its importance in hand function can not be underestimated, and as a result, several distinct methods of reconstruction have been developed to treat the thumb specifically (Figure 50-7).

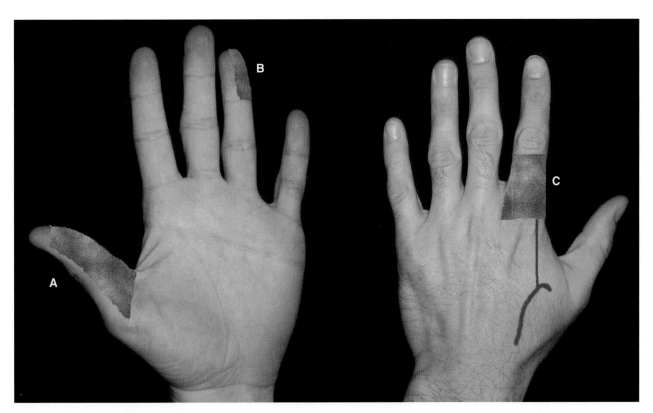

● **FIGURE 50-7.** The three most commonly used local flaps for thumb reconstruction include the (A) Moberg advancement flap, (B) the Littler neurovascular island flap, and (C) the "kite" or Foucher flap.

Moberg Advancement Flap. This classic flap, also known as the rectangular volar advancement flap, has been described as a method for reconstruction of thumb defects of approximately 1.5 to 2.0 cm distal to the interphalangeal joint. The major limitation of this flap is its limited transposition which usually requires interphalangeal joint flexion to provide adequate soft tissue coverage, although it can provide near-normal sensation to the thumb tip. This flap, based on both neurovascular bundles, is raised to the MCP crease, superficial to the flexor pollicis longus sheath. There are several flap variations that can be used to lengthen the distance of this flap will advance, including raising the flap as an island flap, and skin grafting proximally, extending the incisions past the MCP crease, or excising Burrow triangles at the base. Advancing the flap more than 2 cm carries the risk of an interphalangeal joint contracture, which may or may not be functionally limiting, depending on the degree of the contracture and also the functional needs of the patient. This flap cannot be used on the finger, as it will cause joint contractures, and has the potential to disrupt the blood of the dorsal skin distal to the PIP, which is dependent on the volar neurovascular bundles.

Littler Method. Littler described this flap in the late 1950s as a neurosensory flap for thumb reconstruction as an option for larger thumb defects when a Moberg flap cannot be used. This flap is a neurosensory island flap based on the nonopposition side of the ring finger (the long finger can also be used as well) which is elevated and transposed along with the skin and neurovascular bundle and sutured into the volar aspect of the thumb. The donor site defect is then skin grafted. Although in the classic description only skin and subcutaneous tissue are used, unpublished reports have described a composite variation of this flap that includes bone. This can be useful if multiple fingers have been injured, and the opportunity exists to use an injured finger for reconstruction of the thumb tip.

Although it can provide sensation to the tip of the thumb, one of its major drawbacks is that cortical reorientation does not occur, especially in older patients, which can be disturbing to some individuals. Also, this flap sacrifices one of the neurovascular bundles to a finger, so the circulation to that finger must be assessed before the flap is placed on the thumb.

First Dorsal Metacarpal Artery Flap. Initially described by Foucher in the late 1970s, the term "kite flap" has also been used to describe this flap. This flap, much like the Littler neurovascular island flap, can provide sensation to the base of the thumb, but once again, cortical reorientation may be a problem. This flap is a neurovascular island flap that is raised from the dorsum of the index finger proximal phalanx. It is based on the ulnar branch of the first dorsal metacarpal artery which

itself arises from the radial artery where it pierces the two heads of the first dorsal interosseous muscle in the first web space. When the flap is harvested, the plane of dissection is superficial to the peritenon and index finger and includes the fascial layer of the first dorsal interosseous muscle to ensure the arterial pedicle is included. A superficial vein and branches of the radial sensory nerve are harvested with the flap is well.

Secondary Nail Deformities/Complications

Although any condition may result in a nail deformity, the most common cause of a nail deformity is the inappropriate treatment of a nail bed trauma.

Pincer Nail (Trumpet Nail). This deformity is characterized by an excessively curved and distorted nail in the transverse dimension. Zook et al. presented a series of 49 patient in 2005, where the paronychial folds were dissected laterally off the distal phalanx periosteum and either alloderm or autograft dermis was used to elevate the paronychial fold with good results (Figure 50-8).

Split Nail. A split nail results from a scar in the sterile or germinal matrix. The scar is generally oriented longitudinally, although a transverse scar may cause a split nail, but it is more likely to result in nonadherence of the nail. In any case, treatment is centered on replacement of the scar. For a narrow scar, minimizing the scar with re-excision can help correct the deformity. The addition of multiple z-plastys for a longitudinal scar is also very helpful. However, for wide scars, a sterile matrix graft should be used. Relaxing incisions to help advance the nail bed have been described, but in our experience, this has not produced a satisfactory outcomes.

A sterile matrix graft can be obtained from the adjacent portion of sterile matrix or the toes, and tends to satisfactorily correct the deformity. For a distal split nail, successful treatment has also been described for placement of a thin piece (0.20-inch) of silicone sheeting between the nail and the nail bed.

Tumors

Glomus Tumor. Subungual glomus tumors are benign lesions of the glomus apparatus, which is responsible for thermoregulatory control. The glomus apparatus contains an afferent vessel, a Sucquet-Hoyer canal, and multiple shunts in the glabrous skin of the hand and beneath the nail beds.

A patient with a glomus tumor often presents with the classic triad of cold hypersensitivity, paroxysmal pain, and exquisite pinpoint pain. The pain is not usually relieved with salicylates, and can help differentiate a glomus tumor from other conditions.

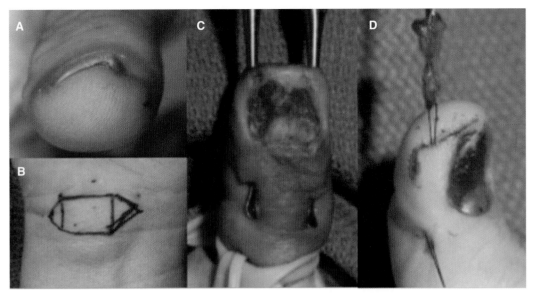

● FIGURE 50-8. The pincer nail, or trumpet nail deformity (A) causes a characteristic deformity. A dermal autograft (B) can be obtained from a variety of locations. Homograft dermis has also been used with success. After tunnels are made which elevate the lateral nail bed (C), the dermis can be pulled through most easily with a suture (D).

Physical findings of a glomus tumor include painful subcutaneous nodules in the subungual region. Sometimes, a nail deformity is present, and/or it is discolored with a bluish tinge. Approximately 75% of glomus tumors are found in the hand with about two thirds of these in the fingertip. Multiple tumors may exist and should be looked for. Pain can be elicited by the examiner with light touch or cold exposure. Imaging of glomus tumors includes MRI, which delineates a dark, well-defined lesion on T1-weighted images and a bright lesion on a T2-weighted image.

Treatment of the glomus tumor involves surgical excision. Once the nail plate is removed and the eponychial fold is reflected, if necessary, a small, longitudinal incision is utilized to extract the glomus, which will most often "shell out" easily. A bilenticular incision is not necessary, as the redundant nail bed will conform over time without excess once the glomus has been removed. The recurrence rate can be as high as 20%, and thus, the matrix should be carefully examined and any suspected remnant of the tumor removed (Figure 50-9).

DIP Ganglion. The DIP ganglion or mucous cyst is not as common as the typical volar or dorsal wrist ganglions, but it does occur with some frequency. It is frequently treated in the same manner as other ganglions of the hand with cyst excision and as a result often reoccurs. These ganglions usually present as cystic lesion off the midline on the dorsum of the distal phalanx over or just distal to the DIP joint. The patient may give a history of intermittent spontaneous drainage, sometimes through the eponychial fold. The ganglion will often but not invariably communicate with the DIP joint, and although there are studies which have shown lack of reflux back into the joint, it is still not a wise idea to aspirate these for refilling is almost certain.

The most effective method of treatment actually does not involve treatment of the ganglion itself per se, but its root cause which is an osteophyte of the DIP joint most commonly due to osteoarthritis.

A T-shaped incision, which can be extended into an H-shaped incision if necessary, is utilized. Care must be taken to not violate the extensor mechanism, as it can be lacerated upon entering the wound. Once the lateral edge is elevated the dorsal joint osteophytes are rongeured away and the ganglion itself is simply drained, not excised. Recurrence rates are extremely low in my experience with this technique (Figure 50-10).

Subungual Pigmented Lesions. Subungual lesions of the nail bed are not uncommon, and as a result, they must be investigated carefully to rule out the possibility of melanoma. Melanomas of the hands and feet tend to have a poorer prognosis as they are often mistaken for other benign conditions, such as viral warts, and appropriate treatment is often delayed. Therefore, it is wise when evaluating these lesions to obtain a careful history that includes when the patient first noticed this lesion, how the lesion has changed over time, sun exposure and family predisposition to melanoma, and to carefully examine, and *re-examine*, these lesions when necessary.

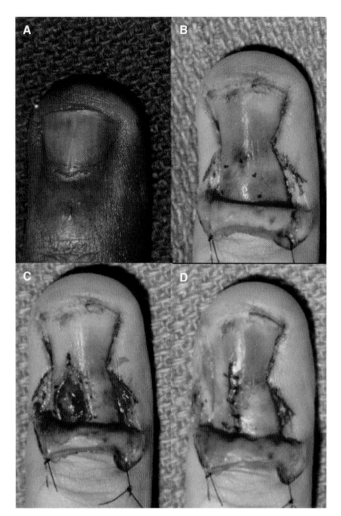

● **FIGURE 50-9.** The glomus tumor can often be difficult to visualize clinically (A), but once its presence has been confirmed, the eponychial fold is reflected back (B), and a longitudinal incision is used to extract the glomus (C). The nail bed is then sutured back together without trimming excess (D), as the nail bed will contract and recontour over time.

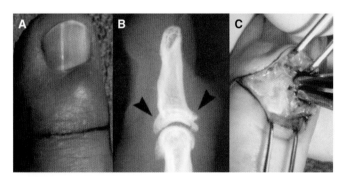

● **FIGURE 50-10.** The DIP ganglion is accessed through an H-shaped incision (A), and although the ganglion can cause a nail deformity, it is important to understand that the osteophytes in the DIP joint (B) are ultimately responsible for these changes. Therefore, they must be debrided (C) taking care not to injury the extensor mechanism.

In many cases, the patient may not recall a history of direct trauma to the nail, and in these cases, it is useful to use the technique of scratching the nail plate proximal and distal to the pigment spot and observing if the lesion advances with nail growth. If the scratches move with the nail it is a subungual hematoma secondary to trauma. If the scratches move away from the pigment and there is a suspicion of melanoma, the lesion should be biopsied. Removal of the nail plate is not always necessary; and in some instances, once the nail plate is removed, the exact location of the lesion may be difficult to determine. For this reason, some method of marking the lesion prior to nail plate removal is helpful. If a melanoma is subsequently diagnosed, then it should be staged and treated accordingly with the appropriate resection, which in many cases is an amputation at the adjacent joint.

For less aggressive tumors, such as some well-differentiated squamous cell carcinomas, judgment should be exercised as to the extent of the resection in order to maximize function. For instance, a professional musician's finger might be treated differently than that of a retired octogenarian. In any case, clear margins are a must, and if the lesion extends to involve the bone, an amputation at the adjacent joint is most likely necessary. More importantly, clinical suspicion for a tumor must be present, as studies have revealed that the average time from first observation to diagnosis to treatment is approximately 4 years (Figure 50-11).

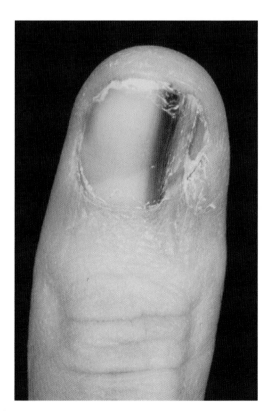

● **FIGURE 50-11.** Patient with an example of a nail streak which should be treated with biopsy.

REFERENCES

1. Lille S, Brown RE, Zook EG, Russell, RC. Free nonvascularized composite nail grafts: an institutional experience. *Plast Reconstr Surg*. 2000;105:2412–2415.

2. Endo T, Kojima T, Hirase Y. Vascular anatomy of the finger dorsum and a new idea for coverage of the finger pulp defect that restores sensation. *J Hand Surg*. 1992;17A:997–932.

3. Donelan MB, Garcia JA. Nailfold reconstruction for the correction of burn fingernail deformity. *Plast Reconstr Surg*. 2006;117:2303–2308.

SUGGESTED READING

Brown RE, Zook EG, Russell RC. Fingertip reconstruction with flaps and nailbed grafts. *J Hand Surg*. 1999;24A:345–351.

Brown RE. Acute nail bed injuries. *Hand Clin*. 2002;18(4): 561–575.

Foucher G, Braun JB. A new island flap from the dorsum of the index to the thumb. *Plast Reconstr Surg*. 1979;63:344–349.

Gingrass MK, Brown RE, Zook EG. Treatment of fingernail deformities secondary to ganglions of the distal interphalangeal joint. *J Hand Surg*. 1995;20;502–505.

Jebson PJ. Infections of the fingertip. Paronychias and felons. *Hand Clin*. 1998;14:547–555.

Russell RC, Casas LA, Management of fingertip injuries. *Clin Plast Surg*. 1989;16(3):405–425.

Russell RC, Van Beek EG, Wavak P, Zook EG. Alternative hand flaps for amputations and digital defects. *J Hand Surg*. 1981; 6:399–405.

Sommer N, Neumeister MW. Tumors of the perionychium. *Hand Clin*. 2002;18(4):673–689.

Zook EG, Chalekson CP, Brown RE, Neumeister MW. Correction of pincer nail deformities with autograft or homograft dermis: modified surgical technique. *J Hand Surg*. 2005; 30(2):400–403.

Zook EG, Russell RC. Reconstruction of a functional and aesthetic nail. *Hand Clin*. 1990;6(1):59–68.

chapter 51

Fractures of the Hand and Wrist

Jeffrey M. Jacobson, MD / Walter B. McClelland, Jr., MD / James P. Higgins, MD

● PATIENT EVALUATION AND SELECTION

The hand and wrist are integral components of nearly all human pursuits, including work, leisure, and activities of daily living. This level of involvement makes injuries to these structures common and long-term disability devastating. Hand and wrist injuries pose special intellectual and technical challenges for upper extremity surgeons, requiring a knowledge of complex regional anatomy, strict adherence to good surgical technique, and a full understanding of rehabilitation methods and goals.

The patient evaluation begins with an accurate diagnosis through a complete history and physical examination, and adequate imaging studies. For most injuries of the hand and wrist, an x-ray evaluation is sufficient for diagnosis and treatment decisions. For injuries distal to the carpus, appropriate x-ray views generally include posteroanterior, lateral, and oblique views of the hand, as well as lateral views of an injured digit. For injuries to the carpus, posteroanterior, lateral, and oblique views should be obtained. Special x-ray views are available for a variety of suspected injuries and should be utilized when appropriate. If questions exist as to whether a certain finding is pathologic or native to the patient, images of the contralateral extremity can be obtained for comparison. In certain circumstances, elaborated below, advanced imaging modalities may be necessary to confirm or further evaluate a suspected injury. Because many injuries to the hand and wrist involve load transmission throughout the upper extremity, care must be taken to evaluate and rule out concomitant injury to the forearm, elbow, or shoulder.

The first determination in the management algorithm is classifying an injury as stable or unstable. Stable injuries are ones in which length, alignment, and rotation are expected to be maintained throughout fracture healing and may or may not require an initial reduction or formal immobilization. Unstable injuries are more apt to require operative stabilization and should be followed closely if attempts are made to treat them nonoperatively. A fracture initially felt to be stable may reveal itself to be unstable by loss of reduction on serial x-rays. In certain circumstances, even stable injuries warrant operative intervention. Some examples would include open fractures, fractures with significant soft tissue injury, and fractures necessitating early rehabilitation to improve functional outcomes.

The primary goal of treatment is the timely restoration of function through acceptable bony alignment, length, and rotation while maintaining adjacent joint range of motion. Although individual patient circumstances and fracture characteristics must be considered on a case-by-case basis, there are certain general principles that tend to guide treatment planning. Optimal outcomes will be achieved if the treatment method is tailored to the unique clinical situation, and the surgeon is facile with the technical aspects of the surgery and the integrated rehabilitation plan. Once a treatment plan is formulated, it should then be discussed with the patient to establish realistic goals and expectations for acute care, rehabilitation, and long-term functional outcome.

Concepts regarding fracture management of the hand and wrist are varied, and guidelines for treatment of these fractures are specific to the mechanism of injury, natural history of the untreated fracture, relative stability of reduction, proximity or involvement of joints, and morbidity of operative techniques.[1,2] Given the breadth of injury types and fixation options, an exhaustive review is beyond the scope of this text. Instead, this installment will address management and operative techniques of the more common fractures by anatomic location.

● PATIENT PREPARATION

Fracture fixation of the hand and wrist can typically be accomplished with a limited amount of additional supplies. The patient should be placed supine on the operative table with the affected extremity extended on an arm board. Care should be taken to avoid excessive shoulder abduction to prevent traction injury to the brachial plexus. A nonsterile tourniquet should be applied to the upper portion of the patient's arm, even if tourniquet control is not anticipated during the case. A lead hand or other hand positioning device can assist in maintaining the hand and wrist in the desired position during the case, freeing the first assistant to take part in other portions of the procedure.

A C-arm should be available to evaluate the adequacy of reduction and appropriate placement of hardware. Ideally, this should enter the surgical field from the end of the arm table to avoid the surgeon or assistant having to move while obtaining fluoroscopy. Loupe magnification can be helpful during dissection to identify and protect important soft tissue structures. If concomitant neurovascular repair or reconstruction is necessary, a microscope may provide better visualization than loupes alone.

Regarding anesthesia, many cases may be managed with either local or regional anesthetic. This can be combined with sedation as necessary. In the setting of lengthy or complicated procedures, or if the patient is difficult to sedate by lesser means, general anesthesia may be required. These decisions should take into account the length and type of the procedure, health status of the patient, and skill level and preferences of the anesthesiologist.

The most common implant utilized during fracture fixation of the hand and wrist is the Kirschner wire (K-wire). It comes in a variety of sizes, with .035″, .045″, and .054″ being the most commonly used in hand and wrist surgery. Wires smaller than .035″ provide inadequate stability for bony fixation, and those larger than .054″ can be overwhelming for work on small tubular bones.

A modular hand tray is also of great value, providing specialized bone reduction forceps, as well as plate and screw systems ranging from 1.0 to 2.4 mm in size. While plates have typically been preferred for fractures proximal to the metacarpophalangeal (MCP) joint, newer low profile designs have expanded the use of these implants to the proximal and middle phalanx. Plates are typically of greatest benefit in transverse fractures, fractures with significant comminution, or long fractures that involve the majority of a given segment. In oblique fractures, screws can provide stable fixation with less soft tissue dissection and implant bulk. When screws alone are used, a balance must be achieved between orienting perpendicular to the fracture to maximize compression and orienting perpendicular to the long axis of the bone to neutralize shear forces.[3] In general, given the increased dissection required for implantation, plates should be applied only when less invasive implants provide inadequate reduction or stability.

The final implant category is variable pitch headless compression screws. These implants provide compression across a fracture or potential space without use of a lag technique. These implants have revolutionized the fixation of scaphoid fractures in particular and are widely used in other forms of intercarpal stabilization. Suture anchors are another useful implant in the repair and reconstruction of the hand and wrist. However, given that their use is primarily for soft tissue injuries, their use will not be further described here.

In general, a surgeon must strive to employ minimally invasive techniques while achieving maximal stability of the construct. Additional dissection may cause further insult to the tenuous soft tissue structures of the hand and digit, whereas more rigid stabilization allows earlier rehabilitation and motion without concern for loss of fixation.

● TECHNIQUES FOR FRACTURES OF THE HAND

Fractures of the Distal Phalanx

Distal phalanx fractures are generally encountered as extra-articular tuft and shaft fractures related to crush injuries. Intra-articular fractures are also common and result from avulsion fractures of the terminal extensor tendon ("mallet finger") or flexor digitorum profundus tendon ("jersey finger"). Tuft fractures are often associated with an injury to the specialized nail elements, which must be fully evaluated and appropriately managed to avoid a chronically deformed or painful nail. The bony injury is often adequately managed with irrigation and a short period (1–3 weeks) of splint immobilization, which should not include the proximal interphalangeal (PIP) joint. Not infrequently, these fractures will fail to unite, resulting in a fibrous union. It bears mentioning that if the nail plate is removed to decompress a subungual hematoma or repair a nail bed laceration, the tuft fracture should now be considered open, and treatment should include a short course of oral antibiotics.

If the fracture is diaphyseal with more sizeable fracture fragments, consideration can be given to K-wire stabilization, particularly if the fragments are displaced. A single 0.28- or 0.35-inch longitudinal pin is usually sufficient and may be advanced across the distal interphalangeal joint for added stability, if necessary.

Extra-Articular Fractures of the Proximal and Middle Phalanx

Diaphyseal and meta-diaphyseal fractures of the proximal and middle phalanx come in a variety of forms, and management decisions are often based on subtle nuances. Many of these fractures are reducible and stable and can be treated in a nonoperative fashion with 3 to 4 weeks of buddy taping and/or splinting. Proximal phalangeal shaft fractures are often angulated apex volar due to the pull of the intrinsic muscles and the action of the extensor mechanism, whereas their middle phalanx equivalents can be angulated in any direction dictated by the injury mechanism and fracture location.

Certain fracture patterns more commonly require greater intervention. Spiral oblique fractures may require open treatment due to their tendency to foreshorten and rotate. Transverse midshaft fractures require particularly close monitoring as they tend to angulate over time.

Surgical treatment of many of these fractures is often adequately performed with K-wires. In the case of spiral oblique fractures, interfragmentary screw fixation can provide fracture compression while eliminating the concern of pin tract infection (Figure 51-1), provided the fracture line is at least 1.5 times the diameter of the bone. Regardless of technique, fracture management of the phalanges carries a great risk of motion loss. Operative techniques are aimed at avoiding the tendon adhesions that accompany excessive soft tissue dissection. Particular caution is exercised in surgical approaches or hardware placement in or about the PIP joint, as it is the greatest contributor to the digit's composite range of motion.[4]

Condylar Fractures of the Proximal and Middle Phalanx

Condylar fractures of the phalangeal head are typically unstable and require surgical intervention. Despite the small size of the bony fragment, fixation with a single K-wire is typically inadequate for unicondylar fractures. Therefore, multiple K-wires or 1.0 to 1.5 mm lag screws should be utilized.[5] For bicondylar or comminuted fractures, treatment options range from open reduction and internal fixation (ORIF), to traction/external fixation, to primary arthrodesis. Regardless of the form of fixation, patients should be counseled about the high likelihood of motion loss postoperatively. An oblique x-ray can be very useful in evaluation of the fracture.

Pilon Fractures of the Proximal and Middle Phalanx

Pilon fractures refer to phalangeal base fractures associated with an axial-loading mechanism (Figure 51-2). They are associated with varying degrees of articular depression and splaying of the articular fragments. They pose a difficult treatment dilemma for upper extremity surgeons, with a high rate of residual articular incongruity and motion loss postoperatively. While conservative management has been described, these injuries are typically best treated with traction/dynamic external fixation or ORIF with or without bone grafting.[6]

Fracture-Dislocations of the PIP Joint

The PIP joint is the dominant contributor to digit motion. Thus, ongoing derangement in this area is a significant risk factor for poor clinical outcomes and low patient satisfaction. Although lateral and volar dislocations occur, they are far less frequently encountered than dorsal dislocations. When these injuries occur as fracture-dislocations, the evaluation must include an assessment of the size of the volar fragment and the stability of the joint following reduction. When the fracture fragment represents 40% of the articular surface or less, the collateral ligaments' insertion on the middle phalanx is maintained and the joint tends to remain stable following reduction. Beyond 40%, the collateral ligament insertion is typically contained in the volar fracture fragment, resulting in persistent instability following reduction.

In the case of a stable injury, the joint is initially immobilized with a dorsal blocking splint in a position of stable flexion (typically 15–30 degrees) for 1 to 2 weeks.

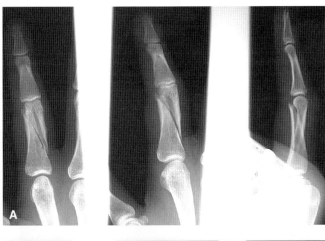
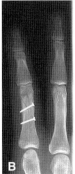
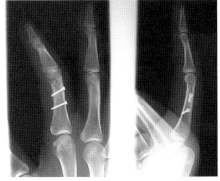

● **FIGURE 51-1.** (A) A spiral oblique fracture of the proximal phalanx. The fracture shortening and apex volar angulation would result in an unsatisfactory clinical result if treated conservatively. (B) Stabilization using two 1.5-mm compression screws restores the alignment anatomically.

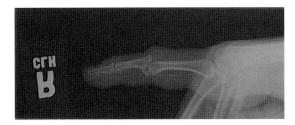

● **FIGURE 51-2.** A pilon fracture of the index finger middle phalanx. Note the articular widening and central depression resulting from the axial load mechanism. This patient required open reduction internal fixation to reduce the articular incongruity.

Full-finger flexion allowed by PIP extension is initially blocked. The digit is gradually extended within the range of stability over the next 2 to 4 weeks. Early commencement of supervised hand therapy is critical in these injuries to prevent excessive stiffness. If initial immobilization of the PIP joint beyond 30 degrees is required for joint stability, then the risk of flexion contracture is too great and surgical intervention should be considered.

In unstable or irreducible PIP joint fracture-dislocations, open reduction with or without fixation is indicated. The risk of open management through wide exposure of these fractures is a significant loss of motion, so minimally invasive techniques should be employed when feasible. Fracture fragments can often be manipulated with joystick K-wires to set the stage for percutaneous pinning with dynamic or static external fixation. Postoperatively, there is a premium on early active motion to take advantage of the anatomic reduction and fracture stability.

Perhaps the most challenging fracture of the hand is the unstable PIP fracture dislocation with severe comminution and impaction of the volar lip of the middle phalanx. Adequate reduction of these fractures is difficult to obtain and often impossible to maintain without reestablishing the stability afforded by the volar base of the middle phalanx. In the absence of a large enough fragment to achieve adequate fixation, three modes of surgical management have been proposed.

1. Dynamic external fixation with volarly directed force on the middle phalanx: This combination of effects is achieved by a "force coupling" fixation technique, which prohibits dorsal translation of the joint while permitting active flexion. The ultimate joint stability relies on a combination of bone callous, fibrocartilage, and scar tissue that forms during this period of provisional stabilization (Figure 51-3).

2. Volar plate arthroplasty: An open volar approach to the joint is used to remove impacted fragments. The volar lip of the middle phalanx is recreated with advancement of the volar plate on its proximal attachments.

3. Osteochondral autografting: This technique takes advantage of the anatomic similarities in the biconcave articular surface of the base of the proximal phalanx and the distal surface of the hamate. By harvesting and transplanting the dorsal majority of the hamate's articulation with the ring finger and small finger metacarpal, articular congruency is restored, allowing early motion with minimal donor site morbidity (Figure 51-4).[7]

Fracture-Dislocations of the MCP Joint

MCP joint dislocations are much less common in the adult than their PIP counterpart due to the relatively sturdy ligamentous housing of the MCP articulation. When these dislocations do occur, the vast majority are dorsal dislocations affecting the vulnerable border digits. Patients present with pain, an inability to flex the MCP joint, and a posture of mild hyperextension at the MCP joint with slight flexion of the distal joints. In the case of a subluxated joint, closed reduction is generally possible with dorsally applied pressure to the base of the proximal phalanx. Axial distraction should be avoided as it may encourage the volar plate to interpose itself in the joint and make closed reduction impossible. In the case of a true dislocation, the volar plate is often already interposed, requiring an open reduction.

Fractures of the articular surface of the proximal phalanx are generally treated with internal fixation. Metacarpal head fractures, while rare, can generally be treated in a nonoperative manner unless a large portion of the articular

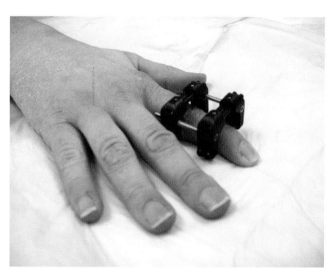

● **FIGURE 51-3.** Dynamic ex-fix device used for indirect reduction of a middle phalanx base fracture. Stable reduction by ligamentotaxis allows early motion as the fracture unites.

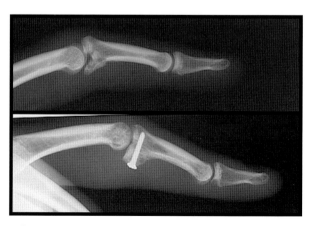

● **FIGURE 51-4.** Pre- and postoperative imaging of a hemi-hamate reconstruction for a middle phalanx condylar base fracture. Volar plate arthroplasty was contraindicated due to the size of the articular surface involved, while the degree of comminution precluded direct reduction and stabilization.

surface is involved or there is greater than 1 mm of articular incongruity. Even in this setting, severe comminution may preclude operative intervention if hardware purchase is expected to be limited.

Metacarpal Fractures of the Digits

Metacarpal fractures can be considered in three subsets: (1) fractures of the metacarpal neck, (2) fractures of the metacarpal diaphysis, and (3) metacarpal base fractures and carpometacarpal (CMC) dislocations.

Fractures of the metacarpal neck occur commonly and most frequently affect the fourth and fifth metacarpals. The increased mobility of the ulnar carpometacarpal joints leaves these metacarpals vulnerable to off-axis loading when the metacarpal head strikes an unyielding object. While it is agreed that the reduction of these apex-dorsally angulated fractures must correct any rotational deformity, there exists significant controversy about the acceptable postreduction angulation.

Reduction of a "boxer's fracture" is reliably effected by use of the Jahss maneuver, in which the MCP is flexed 90 degrees and a dorsally directed force is applied to the metacarpal head through manual pressure on the proximal phalanx (Figure 51-5). If a stable reduction can be achieved, immobilization in an ulnar gutter splint for 4 to 5 weeks followed by protected return to motion is appropriate. Even with a significant degree of angulation, patients can function well in the absence of rotational deformity. They may notice a flattening of the dorsal knuckle or a prominence of their metacarpal head in their palm during grip, but range of motion is typically quite satisfactory given the compensatory motion of the CMC joint.

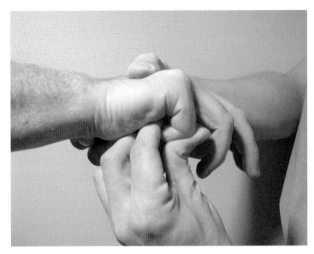

● FIGURE 51-5. Clinical photograph of the Jahss maneuver for reduction of metacarpal neck fractures. Applying force to the head of the proximal phalanx allows a greater lever arm and more force generation to assist in reduction.

If the patient demonstrates malrotation or an inability to extend the MCP joint to neutral position, or if a stable reduction cannot be maintained, surgical intervention is recommended. In these cases, soft tissue dissection should be minimized to avoid the formation of mobility-limiting scar tissue. While various methods of treatment have been described, the authors' preference is to treat the vast majority of these in a closed fashion. We avoid plating and collateral recess pin techniques when possible to minimize joint stiffness and employ transmetacarpal pinning and limited incision intramedullary "bouquet" pinning techniques more commonly (Figure 51-6).[8]

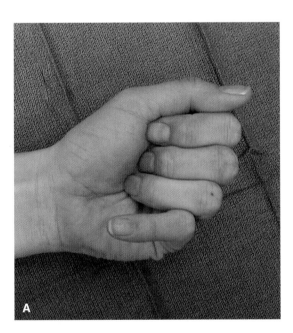
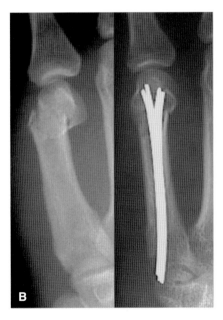

● FIGURE 51-6. (A) Clinical photo demonstrating significant malrotation through a small finger metacarpal neck fracture. (B) Pre- and postoperative demonstrating fracture reduction and stabilization using the bouquet pinning technique. Increasing the number of intramedullary pins greatly increases the construct rigidity.

Fractures of the metacarpal diaphysis are treated based on the fracture characteristics, with the greatest emphasis placed on malrotation. Most isolated shaft fractures without malrotation can be treated in a closed fashion. Spiral fractures, open fractures, and multiple metacarpal fractures are usually treated with operative fixation due to increased difficulty with rotational control. Particular caution is exercised for the border digits, which may demonstrate more rotational instability than their central counterparts. Closed fractures of the central digits may remain stable, even in the setting of spiral fracture pattern or comminution, due to the stability afforded by the intermetacarpal ligament and interossei attachments to the surrounding uninjured metacarpals. If a stable reduction cannot be obtained, operative treatment must be pursued with fixation appropriate to the fracture pattern. Transverse diaphyseal fractures are usually treated with plate fixation, whereas more oblique and spiral fractures are treated with interfragmentary screw fixation if possible (Figure 51-7).

Metacarpal base fractures are most frequently seen in the fourth and fifth digits and are often associated with fractures of the neighboring carpal bones. These fractures can best be visualized on an oblique supination radiograph and can be missed on standard anteroposterior and lateral views. They are generally treated by ORIF to reestablish the preinjury anatomy of the CMC joints and prevent recurrent dorsal and ulnar subluxation of the metacarpal bases. If a dorsal dislocation is encountered, CMC pinning is indicated given the typical instability associated with this injury.

Metacarpal Fractures of the Thumb

The thumb metacarpal is most susceptible to injury at its base, fracturing much less commonly in its diaphysis. Extra-articular fractures are treated in a similar fashion to metacarpal diaphyseal fractures. Because the thumb derives most of its utility and function from its wide range of motion at the CMC joint, intra-articular fractures at the metacarpal base are potentially morbid injuries if not appropriately treated.

Bennett fractures are intra-articular fractures of the base of the thumb metacarpal produced by an axial load sustained by a flexed joint. The fracture line splits the articular surface, leaving an undisplaced smaller articular fragment on the volar ulnar surface attached to the anterior oblique ligament of the CMC joint. The larger portion of the articular surface, which includes the remainder of the thumb ray, is displaced dorsally, proximally, and radially with the intact metacarpal shaft due to the unopposed pull of the abductor pollicis longus.

While some authors advocate closed treatment of these fractures if the articular step-off is less than 1 mm, these fractures are unstable due to the effects of the surrounding musculature on the distal metacarpal and are best treated with closed reduction and percutaneous

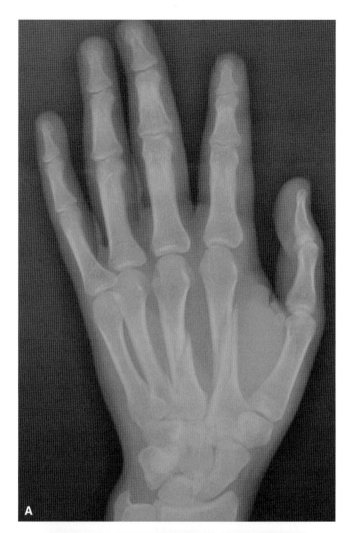

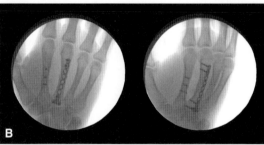

● **FIGURE 51-7.** (A) Preoperative imaging demonstrating spiral fractures of the index and middle finger metacarpal with shortening and rotational malalignment. (B) Fixation using two techniques. The index finger reduced easily and demonstrated stability with three interfragmentary compression screws. The middle finger had an additional nondisplaced fracture line extending distally, necessitating bridge plate fixation.

pinning or ORIF. Percutaneous pinning is often selected if an anatomic closed reduction can be achieved and the volar-ulnar fragment is too small to provide purchase for screw fixation. If an adequate closed reduction cannot be achieved, and/or if the fracture fragment is large enough to accommodate rigid internal fixation, open treatment is considered.[9]

Rolando fractures can vary from a three-part intra-articular T or Y fracture to a severely comminuted variant that defies fragment characterization. Since restoration of the articular anatomy is the most important goal in treatment of these fractures, they are almost always best treated in an open fashion. If plating or screw fixation is achieved, patients are started on supervised motion shortly after surgery. If pin fixation alone is utilized, 5 to 6 weeks of thumb spica splinting is required. If fracture severity or comminution mandates the use of external fixation, a longer period of immobilization may be necessary to allow fracture consolidation.

● TECHNIQUES FOR FRACTURES OF THE CARPUS

Fracture management for each of the carpal bones will be described with more detailed discussion dedicated to those of greater clinical relevance (See Table 51-1).

Scaphoid Fractures

Scaphoid fractures are one of the most common fractures of the upper extremity and comprise more than 75% of all carpal bone fractures. The classic mechanism of injury is axial loading with wrist hyperextension, commonly sustained during a fall on an outstretched hand. Wrist extension greater than 90 degrees and radial deviation at the time of compressive loading places the scaphoid at greatest risk of fracture.[10] Approximately 70% of scaphoid fractures occur through the midportion, commonly referred to as the waist. The remainder are divided between the distal pole (10%–20%), the proximal pole (5%–10%), and the tubercle (5%) (Table 51-1).

The blood supply to the scaphoid is derived from the radial artery through both volar and dorsal branches.

TABLE 51-1. Relative Incidence of Fractures of the Carpal Bones

Bone	Number	Percentage of Total
Scaphoid	5036	78.8
Triquetrum	880	13.8
Trapezium	144	2.3
Hamate	95	1.5
Lunate	92	1.4
Pisiform	67	1.0
Capitate	61	1.0
Trapezoid	15	0.2
	6390	

These branches pierce the cortex at the distal pole and dorsal ridge, respectively, and feed the bone in a retrograde fashion. This anatomic finding makes fractures of the proximal pole at increased risk for nonunion. Plain film radiographs should be obtained, including posteroanterior, lateral, and oblique views. A "scaphoid view," a posteroanterior radiograph with the wrist in extension and ulnar deviation, can be invaluable by providing a profile view of the scaphoid waist. A clenched fist view can be added if concern for a scapholunate ligament injury exists. Nondisplaced fractures are not always immediately visible on plain films. If the clinical suspicion is high for a scaphoid fracture, one of the following two treatment plans is employed. The first option involves empirically immobilizing the patient in a thumb spica splint or cast and repeating the x-rays 2 to 3 weeks postinjury. Marginal resorption will typically occur at the fracture site over this time, rendering the fracture line more visible. The second option involves the use of advanced imaging modalities, including CT scan, MRI, and bone scan. While all can be used to accurately diagnose acute fractures of the scaphoid, MRI is our preferred method, since it allows visualization of the surrounding soft tissue structures, an assessment of the vascularity of the proximal pole, and detection of the subtle edema pattern of an occult fracture.[11]

Acute nondisplaced scaphoid fractures can be successfully treated both operatively and nonoperatively. The method by which conservative care is undertaken is a matter of much debate, with no consensus in the literature regarding length of immobilization, appropriate position of the immobilized wrist, or casting technique. Our protocol involves a short-arm thumb spica cast with the wrist in neutral position until the patient's clinical examination and radiographs demonstrate evidence of bony union (typically 12–16 weeks for a waist fracture). A CT scan can be obtained if union is in question to look for evidence of bone bridging the fracture site. In cases of undisplaced waist fracture, the decision to proceed with cast immobilization for a prolonged period of time should take into consideration the patient's physical demands, social situation, and handedness.

If a patient is unable or unwilling to tolerate 12 to 16 weeks of immobilization, or if the fracture involves the proximal pole, percutaneous or mini-open screw fixation is appropriate. With the development of cannulated variable pitch screws, stabilization of these fractures can be achieved in a reliable and minimally invasive fashion (Figure 51-8). This form of treatment allows a shorter period of immobilization and a more rapid return to activities. In addition, there is some data to suggest that screw fixation decreases the time to union, although this has not been consistently borne out in the literature.

In general, any acute scaphoid fracture that is comminuted or displaced more than 1 mm, or is associated with concomitant ligamentous injury of the wrist, is best managed with an open reduction and stabilization.

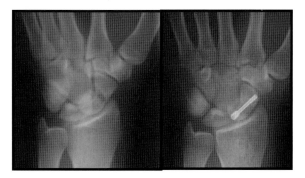

● **FIGURE 51-8.** Scaphoid waist fracture stabilized with a differentially threaded screw. Note the compression across the fracture site. This screw was implanted through a minimally invasive approach, limiting additional trauma to the fragile blood supply of the scaphoid.

Approaches to the scaphoid can be made either volarly or dorsally. A volar approach is best used for distal pole fractures, or in the presence of a flexion or "humpback" deformity of the scaphoid, allowing access to the distal pole for reduction. A dorsal approach is preferable for proximal pole fractures, or in the setting of concomitant ligamentous injury to the wrist, such as a trans-scaphoid perilunate injury.

Additionally, any scaphoid fracture that fails to unite, either through failure of appropriate therapy, patient neglect, or missed diagnosis, is likely to require surgical intervention. Given the absence of connection to the proximal carpal row when the fracture is distal to the insertion of the dorsal intercarpal ligament, the distal pole tends to progressively flex in the setting of a non-union, resulting in the aforementioned "humpback" deformity. This will often require a structural bone graft placed volarly to extend the distal fragment. Bone grafts can take the form of vascularized or nonvascularized, depending on the length of nonunion and vascularity of the proximal pole. For this reason, an MRI may be of value for preoperative planning. The most convenient site for nonvascularized structural graft is the ipsilateral distal radius. Local pedicled vascularized bone grafts may be obtained from the volar and dorsal radius, while increasing interest has been given to free bone flaps from the medial femoral condyle.

Scaphoid nonunion occurs in approximately 5% to 10% of fractures, with a higher incidence in fractures of the proximal pole. If left uncorrected, these injuries lead to a predictable progression of carpal degeneration known as a scaphoid nonunion advanced collapse. This can result in significant pain, stiffness, and functional loss. Surgical salvage procedures to treat this disorder are limited (ie, proximal row carpectomy, scaphoid excision/midcarpal fusion, scaphoid distal pole excision) and have significant drawbacks. For this reason, much effort is directed at successful identification and treatment of these fractures acutely.

Fractures of the Triquetrum

Fractures of the triquetrum come in three types. Dorsal cortical fractures occur through a variety of mechanisms, including avulsion, shear, and impaction. These fractures can often be treated conservatively with 4 to 6 weeks of immobilization. However, given the insertion of the dorsal intercarpal and dorsal radiotriquetral ligaments in this area, care must be taken to rule out an associated carpal instability. In the absence of carpal instability, these fractures typically result in pain free recovery and remain asymptomatic, even if resulting in nonunion.

Fractures of the triquetral body can occur in isolation or in conjunction with perilunate injuries. If in isolation, they are typically non-displaced and can be treated conservatively with 4 to 6 weeks of immobilization.

Volar cortical fractures, like their dorsal counterparts, can be an indication of carpal instability through disruption of the palmar ulnar triquetral ligaments or the intercarpal lunotriquetral ligament. Given the location of these injuries, they are often missed on initial x-ray evaluation, and advanced imaging should be pursued based on physical exam and clinical suspicion.

Fractures of the Trapezium

As with the triquetrum, fractures of the trapezium tend to come in three forms. Marginal trapeziometacarpal fractures typically result from acute instability of the thumb CMC joint. Treatment decisions are directed to the subluxation/dislocation, with the marginal fracture rarely needing to be addressed directly.

Fractures of the trapezium body result from force transmission longitudinally through the thumb metacarpal or through thumb hyperextension. In displaced fractures, the fracture line tends to extend into the distal articular surface, and care must be directed at restoring articular congruity to prevent post-traumatic arthrosis. A CT scan may provide useful information about the fracture pattern or articular alignment.

Trapezial ridge fractures can be divided into two types and typically result from direct injury or avulsion of the flexor retinaculum. Type I injuries occur at the base and typically heal with immobilization. Type II injuries, representing the trapezial tip, often go on to nonunion and can be excised if symptomatic. These injuries typically require a CT scan, carpal tunnel x-ray view, or a Betts view (thumb extended/abducted, hand pronated, hypothenar eminence resting on plate, beam directed at scaphotrapeziotrapezoidal joint for detection).

Fractures of the Hamate

The most recognizable fractures of the hamate are those involving the hamular process, or hook of the hamate. These are common injuries in club/racquet sports, such as golf, tennis, squash, and baseball. Patients typically present with deep ulnar-sided wrist pain. Because the hook of the

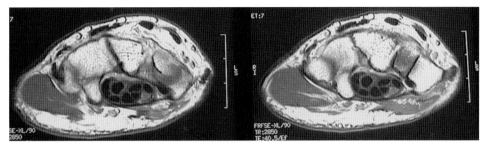

● **FIGURE 51-9.** MRI of a 28-year-old golfer with chronic ulnar-sided wrist pain. This nondisplaced hook of the hamate fracture was successfully treated with immobilization and activity modification.

hamate acts as a pulley for the flexor tendons in ulnar deviation, resisted small finger flexion in this position should elicit pain. If clinical suspicion exists, these injuries can often be better elucidated on a carpal tunnel x-ray view, CT scan, or MRI (Figure 51-9).

The treatment of acute hook fractures involves immobilization. Due to the poor blood supply of this region nonunion is a common sequelae. If symptomatic, these injuries may be addressed with a hook excision or ORIF with or without bone grafting. The former option results in limited functional loss and prevents a host of potential complications that may accompany ORIF. Given the position of the hook of the hamate in Guyon canal, fractures can result in nerve injury to the ulnar nerve or ulnar artery. In a chronic setting, flexor tendon rupture can result from friction against the fractured surface.

Fractures of the body of the hamate are typically oblique and tend to extend radial to the hook of the hamate. They are often stable and respond well to a short period (4–6 weeks) of immobilization. If intra-articular, they commonly exit between the facets of the ring finger and small finger metacarpals. In the setting of significant displacement or CMC instability, open reduction and K-wire stabilization may be required.

Fractures of the Lunate

Fractures of the lunate have been catalogued by Teisen and Hjarbaek, who described five different types of fracture in a series of 17 patients.[12] Because of the important ligaments and nutrient vessels that attach to the palmar pole, fractures of this region should be fixed to prevent the development of carpal instability or avascular necrosis. Like the scaphoid, the blood supply of the lunate is somewhat tenuous, and avascular necrosis can result. This should not be confused with Kienbock disease, or idiopathic avascular necrosis of the lunate.

Fractures of the Pisiform

Fractures of the pisiform most commonly result from a direct blow to the hypothenar space but have been described after repetitive trauma. A CT scan or special x-ray views, such as a supination oblique or carpal tunnel view, may be necessary for their diagnosis. Because almost half of all pisiform fractures occur in conjunction with other upper extremity injuries, they are often missed during the initial survey. Late sequelae of pisiform fractures include nonunion and pisotriquetral arthritis. In this instance, pisiform excision provides fairly predictable relief without significantly compromising wrist function. Because of the proximity of the pisiform to Guyon canal, careful evaluation of ulnar nerve function must accompany any documented injury.

Fractures of the Capitate

Fractures of the capitate are often nondisplaced and localized to the body. They are said to represent approximately 1% of all carpal fractures, but with the increased use of MRI for evaluation of the scaphoid, the incidence of these injuries is increasing. If a capitate fracture is diagnosed, a careful examination of the stability of the wrist must ensue, as 50% of capitate fractures are associated with concomitant ligamentous and bony injury.[13]

The proximal portion of the capitate is completely intra-articular, resulting in limited blood supply. Waist fractures, therefore, can lead to nonunion and avascular necrosis of the proximal pole. Even with treatment, whether by bone grafting, midcarpal fusion, or excision arthroplasty, persistent symptoms are common.

Fractures of the Trapezoid

Fractures of the trapezoid are the least common of all carpal fractures due to the stout ligamentous protection provided by its relationship to the trapezium, capitate, and index metacarpal. Fractures are typically the result of an indirect force directed through the index metacarpal and can be associated with carpometacarpal or axial pattern dislocations. Basic fracture principles apply to these injuries, with large or displaced fractures requiring stabilization and small or nondisplaced fractures being adequately treated by conservative means.

● COMPLICATIONS

Fractures of the hand and wrist are susceptible to the same complications as fractures in other areas of the body. Malunion is a common complication that often results from delayed presentation or closed treatment of displaced fractures. While significant deformity can be tolerated in the some settings (ie, small finger metacarpal neck fractures), it is less acceptable in the phalanges or carpal bones. Therefore, it is paramount for treating physicians to understand the kinematics of the hand and wrist to determine what constitutes an adequate reduction.

Nonunion can occur in many locations, but are most frequently encountered in open fractures with significant soft tissue stripping, or in areas known to have poor blood supply, such as the scaphoid. Treatment can consist of stabilization (in the setting of failed conservative care), nonvascularized bone grafting, or vascularized bone grafting. As previously discussed, the distal radial metaphysis is a good source of local nonvascularized autograft for nonunions of the hand and wrist.

Avascular necrosis is a rare complication that can result either from the initial injury or from surgical treatment. As with nonunions, this is typically of concern in areas of known poor vascularity. Care must be taken by the surgeon intraoperatively to respect the soft tissue envelope and avoid further vascular insult during surgical stabilization. Avascular fragments in the hand typically require excision, with management of the remaining void based on size and location of the defect. Avascular fragments of the carpus may also be treated with excision, but should be considered for vascularized bone grafting. The longevity of the condition and status of the surrounding articulations are important factors in assessing salvage options.

In fractures treated surgically, hardware complications, including loss of fixation, symptomatic hardware, and hardware failure, are introduced as possible complications. Surgeons must ensure stable constructs with tolerable hardware, using low-profile designs and counter-sinking where appropriate. Infection can also result from injuries treated in an open fashion, so pre-operative antibiotics should be administered whenever implant use is anticipated.

The most frequently battled complication of hand and wrist fracture management is stiffness. An excellent radiographic result may belie a poor functional result. Consideration of the benefits of aggressive fracture management (stable fixation, anatomic reduction, early mobilization) must always be weighed against the risks of soft tissue and joint contracture and stiffness.

● OUTCOMES ASSESSMENT

Given the broad range of injuries presented in this chapter, and the significant variability that can be associated with each, it is difficult to make definitive statements about patient outcomes. However, several general principles do apply. In the hand, long-term satisfaction is strongly related to rotational alignment and joint motion. With that in mind, some tolerance of angular malalignment is acceptable, while tolerance of rotational malalignment is extremely limited. Treatment decisions should always include a consideration for rehabilitation of the injured hand. Typically, the most minimally invasive solution that will still allow early motion is the best choice.

Regarding the carpus, it is essential to recognize that many seemingly isolated injuries may be part of a broader injury pattern. Therefore, care must be taken to assess the overall alignment and stability of the wrist when an injury is identified. The anatomy of the carpus makes complete evaluation by standard x-rays difficult, so a treating physician must have a full understanding of specialized x-ray views and know when to apply them. A low threshold for advanced imaging will also help avoid missing injuries.

REFERENCES

1. Amadio PC, Moran SL. Fractures of the carpal bones. In: Green DP, Hotchkiss RN, Pederson WC, Wolfe SW, eds. *Green's Operative Hand Surgery.* 5th ed. Philadelphia: Churchhill Livingstone; 2005:711–768.

2. Stern PJ. Fractures of the metacarpals and phalanges. In: Green DP, Hotchkiss RN, Pederson WC, Wolfe SW, eds. *Green's Operative Hand Surgery.* 5th ed. Philadelphia: Churchill-Livingstone; 2005:277–341.

3. Steel WM. The A.O. small fragment set in hand fractures. *Hand.* 1978;10:246–253.

4. Strickland JW, Steichen JB, Kleinman WB. Phalangeal fractures: Factors influencing digital performance. *Orthop Rev.* 1982;11:39–50.

5. Weiss AP, Hastings H. Distal unicondylar fractures of the proximal phalanx. *J Hand Surg Am.* 1993;18:594–599.

6. Stern PJ, Roman RJ, Kiefhaber TR, McDonough JJ. Pilon fractures of the proximal interphalangeal joint. *J Hand Surg Am.* 1991;16:844–850.

7. Williams RM, Hastings H, Kiefhaber TR. PIP Fracture/Dislocation Treatment Technique: Use of a Hemi-Hamate Resurfacing Arthroplasty. *Tech Hand Up Extrem Surg.* 2002;6:185–192.

8. Foucher G. "Bouquet" osteosynthesis in metacarpal neck fractures: a series of 66 patients. *J Hand Surg.* 1995;20A: S86–S90.

9. Timmenga EJ, Blokhuis TJ, Maas M, Raaijmakers EL. Long-term evaluation of Bennett's fracture. A comparison between open and closed reduction. *J Hand Surg.* 1994;19:373–377.

10. Kozin SH. Incidence, mechanism, and natural history of scaphoid fractures. *Hand Clin.* 2001;17:515–524.

11. Gaebler C, Kukla C, Breitenseher M, Trattnig S, Mittlboeck M, Vecsei V. Magnetic resonance imaging of occult scaphoid fractures. *J Trauma.* 1996;41:73–76.

12. Teisen H, Hjarbaek J. Classification of fresh fractures of the lunate. *J Hand Surg Br.* 1988;13:458–462.

13. Shah MA, Viegas SF. Fractures of the carpal bones excluding the scaphoid. *J Am Soc Surg Hand.* 2002;2:129–140.

chapter 52

Management of Hand Infections

Suhail Kanchwala, MD / Benjamin Chang, MD, FACS

● GENERAL PRINCIPLES

Infections of the hand can lead to significant patient morbidity, including pain, disability, lost time, and productivity at work. The sequelae of acute and chronic hand infections can be devastating to the patient. In addition, infections in the hand can be the presenting symptom in a number of systemic illnesses. As a result, the prompt and accurate diagnosis of surgical infections in the hand is critical for minimizing disability and facilitating a rapid recovery (Table 52-1).

Early surgical intervention plays a critical role in the treatment of hand infections. Evaluation of a hand infection should include an assessment of depth of infection, presence of pus, degree of erythema, and range of motion of the affected digits. In addition, a thorough medical history should be obtained with emphasis on those factors that affect the ability of the patient to ward off infection (diabetes, HIV, immunosuppression).

The anatomy of the hand, with numerous fascial compartments, allows the inflammatory response to infection itself to become pathogenic. For example, excessive swelling in the hand can result in increased pressure on tendons in the fingers and palm leading to ischemia and tendon necrosis.

Early infections in the hand, regardless of location, can be managed initially by a period of rest, elevation, antibiotics, close observation, and splinting in the safe position. For those infections that have progressed or whose initial presentation indicates the presence of an abscess (ie, fluctuance and drainage), the definitive treatment must include adequate surgical drainage and debridement of devitalized tissues. In those cases where there may be a delay in taking the patient to the operating room for debridement, the abscess cavity should be aspirated to reduce compartment pressures and the risk of tendon and neurovascular structure injury.

Empiric antibiotics that are designed to cover the most likely pathogens for each type of infection should be started after wound cultures have been obtained. However, antibiotics are not a substitute for adequate surgical drainage and debridement. Infections in the hand are often polymicrobial—a critical consideration when making a selection of empiric antibiotic therapy.[1] All wounds that are a result of exposure to soil, animals, or the oral cavity (ie, human bite wounds) should be appropriately treated with tetanus prophylaxis.

Surgical intervention in patients with hand infections can often be performed using regional anesthetic techniques. However, the infiltration of local anesthesia directly into an area of cellulitis or infection is ill-advised. For example, fingertip infections can be managed with digit blocks, but deep space infections of the hand should be drained under either general anesthesia. The use of the operative tourniquet is crucial to avoid excessive bleeding which can impair visualization. When using the tourniquet with infection, the extremity should be exsanguinated by elevation and gravity, rather than the use of an elastic band to avoid the potential spread of the infection (Figure 52-1).

● ACUTE PARONYCHIA

Paronychia, or runaround infections of the fingertip, are infections of the soft tissue fold surrounding the nail plate, typically with staphylococcal species. Risk factors for paronychial infection include hangnails, nail biting, manicures, and poor hand hygiene. Hallmarks of paronychial infection include pain, swelling, and erythema in the perionychium.

TABLE 52-1. Common Hand Infections, Usual Offending Organisms, and Appropriate Therapeutic Regimens

Condition	Most Common Offending Organisms	Recommended Antimicrobial Agents	Comments
Paronychia	Usually *Staphylococcus aureus* or streptococci; *Pseudomonas*, gram-negative bacilli, and anaerobes may be present, especially in patients with exposure to oral flora	First-generation cephalosporin or anti-staphylococcal penicillin; if anaerobes or *Escherichia coli* are suspected, oral clindamycin (Cleocin) or a beta-lactamase inhibitor such as amoxicillin-clavulanate potassium (Augmentin)	Incision and drainage should be performed if infection is well established. If infection is chronic, suspect *Candida albicans.* Early infections without cellulitis may respond to antibiotics alone.
Felon	*S. aureus*, streptococci	First-generation cephalosporin or anti-staphylococcal penicillin	Incision and drainage should be performed if infection is well established.
Herpetic whitlow	Herpes simplex virus types 1 and 2	Supportive therapy	Antivirals may be prescribed if infection has been present for <48 hours. For recurrent herpetic whitlow, suppressive therapy with an antiviral agent may be helpful. Consider antibiotics if secondarily infected. Incision and drainage are contraindicated.
Pyogenic flexor tenosynovitis	*S. aureus*, streptococci, anaerobes	Parenteral first-generation cephalosporin or antistaphylococcal penicillin *and* penicillin G *or* Parenteral beta-lactamase inhibitor such as ampicillin-sulbactam (Unasyn) Use ceftriaxone (Rocephin) or a fluoroquinolone if *Neisseria gonorrhoeae* is suspected	Early surgical assessment is suggested. *N gonorrhoeae* or *C albicans* should be suspected in sexually active or immunecompromised patients. Incision and drainage with catheter irrigation of the sheath should be performed if no improvement within the first 12 to 24 hours of conservative therapy.
Human bite, clenched-fist injury	*S. aureus*, streptococci, *Eikenella corrodens*, gram-negative bacilli, anaerobes	Parenteral first-generation cephalosporin or antistaphylococcal penicillin *and* penicillin G *or* Beta-lactamase inhibitor such as ampicillin-sulbactam or amoxicillin-clavulanate potassium *or* Second-generation cephalosporin such as cefoxitin (Mefoxin)	Prophylactic oral antibiotics should be used if outpatient therapy is chosen. Wounds should be explored, copiously irrigated, and surgically debrided. Hospitalization and parenteral antibiotics often are indicated.

Initial management of paronychial infections include warm soaks and oral antibiotics. When paronychial infections lead to abscess formation within the eponychial fold or under the nail plate, surgical drainage is necessary. When performing an incision and drainage of a paronychia, it is important to angle the blade away from the nail bed to avoid inadvertent damage to the nail bed and subsequent ridging of the nail.

When the area of abscess formation is under the nail plate it is important to remove the nail to allow adequate drainage of the abscess. Again, the key to the prevention of nail abnormalities following successful drainage is to minimize the trauma to the nail bed (Figure 52-2).

● HERPETIC WHITLOW

Commonly confused with paronychial infections, herpetic infections of the hand typically involve the fingertip and soft tissues surrounding the nail plate. While herpetic infections may mimic bacterial infections

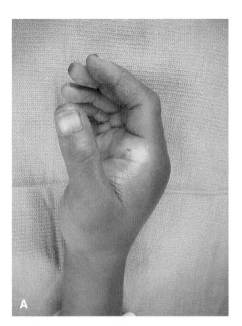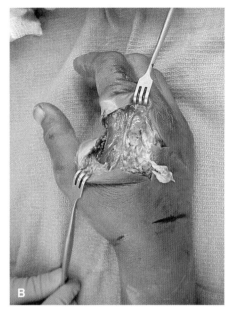

● **FIGURE 52-1.** (A) A patient with large subcutaneous abscess in the first web space. (B) Wide surgical debridement is essential.

of the hand in many ways, they can usually be distinguished from bacterial infections by an adequate history and examination.

Herpetic infections in children and health care workers (dentists, respiratory therapists, etc.) are most often the result of viral inoculation from the oropharynx by the herpes simplex virus type 1 (HSV-1). In adults, however, HSV-2 predominates and is most often due to inoculation from genital herpes. Herpetic infections typically have an

incubation period of 2 weeks, after which patients experience pain and mild swelling in the affected digit. Following this period, small 1–2 mm vesicles erupt in the affected digits. These vesicles then coalesce to form large bullae. A Tzanck smear test is diagnostic.[2]

The management of herpetic hand infections does not involve surgery unless there is bacterial superinfection. In fact, surgical intervention in cases of herpetic whitlow because of a misdiagnosis can lead to systemic

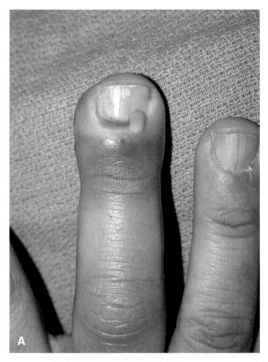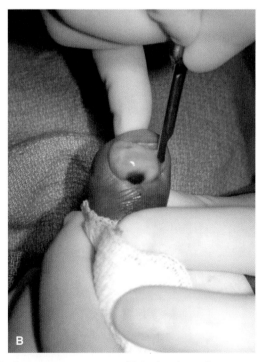

● **FIGURE 52-2.** (A) An acute paronychia in the emergency room. (B) Incise through most fluctuant region.

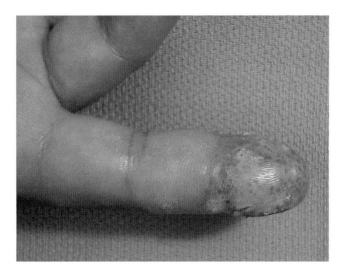

● FIGURE 52-3. Herpetic whitlow.

spread.[3] Viral infection of the hand can lay dormant in the nervous system for many years and then reactivate (Figure 52-3).

Chronic paronychia is a distinct clinical entity from acute paronychia. Chronic inflammation of the soft tissues surrounding the nail plate can lead to repeated episodes of erythema, pain, and drainage from the infected region. Patients who have repeated exposure to water (waiters, dishwashers, etc) are at highest risk for development of this chronic inflammation. *Streptococcus pyogenes*, *Staphylococcus epidermidis*, and *Candida* are the most common causes of chronic paronychia.

The treatment of chronic paronychia involves the excision of a minimum 3 mm wide crescent of skin and subcutaneous tissue parallel to the eponychial fold running the entire width of the finger. This procedure is referred to as eponychial marsupialization. The wound is then left open for drainage and the patient is placed on a regimen of hand soaks in a variety of solutions such as dilute povidone-iodine. The warm soaks are continued until the inflammation/drainage has ceased. Nail irregularities caused by chronic paronychia can be treated by the removal of the entire nail.[4] As long as the eponychial fold is appropriated stented, the nail should regrow without abnormalities assuming the paronychia has been treated appropriately.

● **FELON**

A felon is an infection in the soft tissue pulp on the volar aspect of the fingertip. The distal finger pad is an anatomically distinct structure from the rest of the finger. Numerous fibrous septae attach the dermis of the distal finger pad directly to the underlying bone, allowing the fingertip to be used for essential functions such as grasp. If a significant number of these septae are disrupted during draining of a felon, a mobile, nonfunctional fingertip can result.[5]

Surgical management of the felon requires antibiotics and adequate incision and drainage. In order to preserve fingertip sensibility and perfusion, we advocate the use of a volar incision, directly over the point of maximal fluctuance. Incisions should not be carried over the joint flexion crease to minimize postoperative contracture (Figure 52-4).

● **PYOGENIC TENOSYNOVITIS**

Pyogenic tenosynovitis is a closed space infection of the flexor tendon sheath of the fingers or thumb. The most common cause of this infection is penetrating injury to the proximal interphalangeal or distal interphalangeal joint on the volar surface. The flexor tendon sheath can

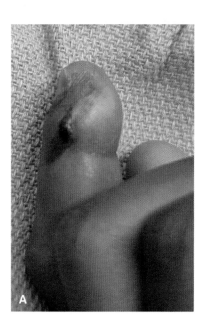
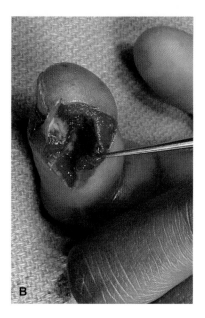

● FIGURE 52-4. (A) Felon. (B) All necrotic tissue must be excised.

be compromised by foreign bodies or even teeth (as in the case of a human or animal bite). Rarely, pyogenic tenosynovitis is spread to the fingers from a distant source, such as disseminated gonorrheal infection. The most common organisms cultured from patients with pyogenic tenosynovitis are *Staphylococcus aureus* and beta-hemolytic streptococcal species.

Pyogenic tenosynovitis can be extremely disabling because infections in the tendon sheath interrupt the normal gliding mechanism of the flexor tendons. Late recognition and treatment of this disorder can result in fibrosis, or tendon necrosis and permanent loss of function.

Hallmarks of this infection include the following clinical signs that were initially postulated by Kanavel:[6]

1. Semi-flexed finger position
2. Symmetrical enlargement of the whole digit
3. Excessive tenderness limited to the course of the flexor tendon sheath
4. Pain on passive extension of the finger

The management of pyogenic tenosynovitis involves adequate drainage and irrigation of the tendon sheath. A variety of drainage procedures have been advocated. There is a consensus that copious irrigation of the tendon sheath with minimized exposure of the tendon itself through carefully placed incisions leads to fewer postoperative complications secondary to adhesion formation within the flexor sheath (Figure 52-5).[7]

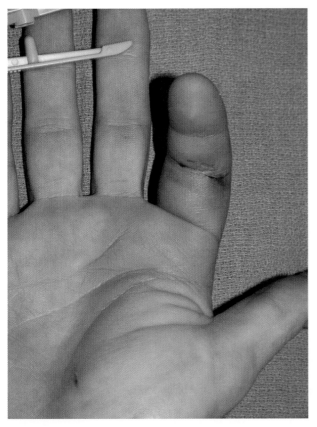

● **FIGURE 52-5.** Pyogenic flexor tenosynovitis.

● **DEEP SPACE INFECTIONS**

Deep space infections of the hand can be broken down into three general regions: the palmar, thenar, and Parona spaces. The thenar eminence is the most common region for deep space infections to occur. These occur most commonly as direct puncture wound to the region or from nearby infection of the tendon sheath.

Deep space infections in the hand have decreased in frequency as a result of earlier management of localized infections in the hand (eg, pyogenic tenosynovitis of the fingers) and treatment with antibiotics.

Management includes incision and drainage of the region. Placement of the incisions depends on the locations of the abscesses: middle space infections—curvilinear from distal palmar crease to hypothenar eminence; thenar—curvilinear along thenar crease (avoid recurrent branch of median nerve).

● **COLLAR BUTTON ABSCESS**

Commonly seen in laborers, collar button or web space abscesses are hand infections beneath palmar calluses that localize to one of the three web spaces. Since the dorsal skin is more compliant than the palmar skin, swelling and fluctuance from collar button abscesses are often greater dorsally. Complete drainage of these abscesses often requires incisions both dorsally and on the palmar surface.[8] The failure to recognize the extent of the infection on the palmar surface can lead to incomplete drainage and spread of the infection to the deep palmar space. It is important to avoid damage to the web itself to avoid contractures postoperatively.

● **RADIAL AND ULNAR BURSA INFECTIONS**

Knowledge of the anatomy of the radial and ulnar bursae of the hand are critical to understanding the development of bacterial infections in this region. The radial bursa is the proximal extent of the flexor sheath of the thumb, while the ulnar bursa includes the flexor sheath of the little finger and just the sheath of the second to fourth metacarpal flexor tendons in the palm. The Parona space (the potential space between pronator quadratus and the flexor tendons) serves as a bridge between the radial and ulnar bursae and allows the formation of "horseshoe" abscesses. When draining abscesses in the Parona space, it is particularly important to avoid injuring the median nerve and its palmar cutaneous branch.

● **HUMAN BITES**

Human bite injuries can lead to some of the most complex of all the common hand infections. Typically, human bite injuries occur through clenched fist injuries where the patient's fist strikes an opponent's tooth, piercing the metacarpophalangeal joint. The initial puncture wound may look innocuous but leads to a septic joint in days. Most of these infections are polymicrobial and have a wide range of possible pathogens due to the high number of bacterial species present in the human mouth.[9] Skin flora and *Eikenella* species are the most common organisms isolated. Additionally, this patient population is often noncompliant and there is also a significant delay in seeking medical attention.[10]

The management of human bite injuries includes admission, x-rays to evaluate foreign bodies and fractures, exploration in the operating room, and empiric antibiotics. Superficial abrasions and infections can be managed with antibiotics and close observation. If the extensor mechanism has been penetrated, or the depth of penetration cannot be determined, the wound should be explored in the operating room.

The management of animal bites (eg, dog and cat) is quite similar to that of human bites. Prophylaxis with tetanus is paramount. Dog and cat bites tend to be less polymicrobial than human bites; and cat bites have a high likelihood of *Pasteurella multocida* infection. Of the two, cat bites are more likely to become infected because the puncture wound is small and seals quickly.

● SEPTIC ARTHRITIS

Finger joint infections are typically the result of the spread of infection from local tissues and less commonly the result of hematogenous spread to the joint spaces. Symptoms of a septic joint include swelling, fluctuance, and warmth which is usually held in slight flexion and have pain on even slight passive movement of the joint.

Joint aspiration is an important diagnostic tool and will typically reveal a purulent/cloudy fluid:

1. Gram stain >50,000 WBC
2. >75% polymorphonuclear cells
3. Fluid glucose ≤40 mg

Once pus is identified in the joint, it is a surgical emergency. Rapid and adequate irrigation and debridement is essential to minimize the cartilage and joint destruction that can result from septic arthritis. Cultures should be obtained prior to starting antibiotics, and empiric therapy initiated, based on the Gram stain results.

● OSTEOMYELITIS

Osteomyelitis of the hand is typically the result of penetrating trauma or open fractures in the hand. The degree of damage to the soft tissues overlying the affected bone plays a significant role in the development and pathogenesis of osteomyelitis. Direct spread from a soft tissue infection such as pyogenic tenosynovitis is a rare cause of osteomyelitis.

The diagnosis of osteomyelitis can be made after a thorough history identifying risk factors as well as radiographic analysis starting with x-rays and often including nuclear medicine imaging (bone scan, tagged white blood cell scan) as well as magnetic resonance imaging of the hand.

The management of osteomyelitis depends on the severity of the presenting complaint/disability and the duration of infection. Early infections with minimal complaints may be cautiously managed with intravenous antibiotics alone. However, most often, in order to achieve adequate resolution of the infection, surgical debridement is mandated.[11] When a sequestrum is present, curettage of all necrotic bone is essential and the wound should be packed open. Should a bone defect be present after debridement, reconstruction should only be considered after clearance of infection (Figure 52-6).

● NECROTIZING FASCIITIS

Necrotizing fasciitis is a limb and potentially life-threatening infection that is often caused by minor of trauma to the affected extremity. Hallmarks of necrotizing fasciitis in the upper extremity include bright, shiny skin, nonpitting edema, poorly demarcated redness, and skin discoloration and necrosis. Patients who are diabetic or immunocompromised have a much higher risk of contracting necrotizing fasciitis. A single organism is found

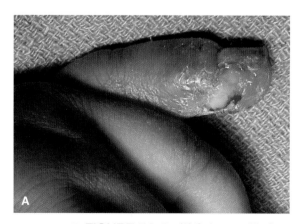
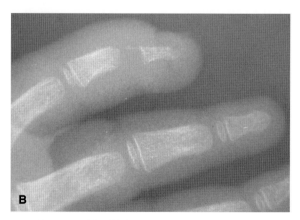

● **FIGURE 52-6.** (A) Osteomyelitis from untreated paronychia. (B) Note the resorbed distal phalanx epiphysis.

as the causative agent in nearly 50% of cases, most often group A beta-hemolytic streptococcal species (occasionally *S aureus*).[12]

Because the mortality of this infection can be as high as 40%, early and aggressive surgical intervention and debridement is mandatory. Early empiric treatment with broad-spectrum antibiotics, even before cultures have been obtained, can significantly decrease the morbidity of this infection. Depending on the degree of infection and soft tissue damage, multiple debridements and even amputation may be necessary.

● IV DRUG ABUSE

The direct inoculation of bacteria into the subcutaneous tissues by IV drug use can lead to the rapid formation of abscesses. In addition to the introduction of bacteria, the injectate itself can lead to local tissue necrosis. The most common causative agents are staphylococcal and streptococcal species. These infections are polymicrobial and present many challenges to treatment.

Appropriate management involves rapid and adequate debridement and antibiotic therapy. Repeated debridements may be necessary. Despite adequate drainage, recurrent abscesses are not uncommon. Large abscesses can be effectively drained through multiple small incisions along the periphery of the cavity. Penrose drains are threaded through these incisions, across the cavity, to maintain drainage until purulence resolves (2–3 days) (Figure 52-7).

● NOSOCOMIAL INFECTIONS

Due to the enhanced vascularity of the hand, postoperative infections are quite rare. The routine use of prophylactic antibiotics in clean, routine hand cases is not recommended. The most common causative organism for hand infections secondary to surgery is *S aureus*. Routine use of perioperative antibiotics is recommended for those operations involving bone or joint spaces.

● TREATMENT OF RESISTANT ORGANISM INFECTION

There has been a dramatic increase in the number of patients who are admitted to hospital with nosocomial methicillin-resistant *S aureus* (MRSA) wound infections in the past decade. This trend has been seen in the outpatient setting as well. Karanas et al. reported a case series of four patients with community-acquired MRSA hand infections who had no previous risk factors for MRSA infection (eg, diabetes, IV drug use, catheter-related infections).[13] The emergence of resistant organisms will predictably play a large role in the management of future infections.

The increase in resistant infections underscores the importance of routine wound culture prior to initiating antibiotic therapy, whenever possible, to guide antibiotic therapy. Many institutions publish hospital-specific guidelines for empiric antibiotic coverage which accounts for individual drug resistance patterns.[14,15] These guides should be consulted prior to the initiation of empiric antibiotic therapy.

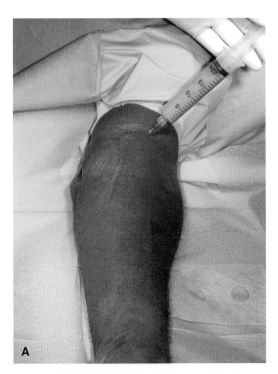
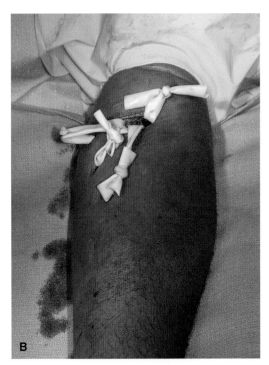

● **FIGURE 52-7.** (A) Large subcutaneous abscess from intravenous drug abuse. (B) The use of multiple small incisions and Penrose drains to manage a large loculated abscess.

REFERENCES

1. Wright PE II. Hand infections. Canale ST, ed. *Campbell's Operative Orthopedics*. 9th ed. St. Louis, MO: Mosby; 1998.

2. Louis DS, Silva J Jr. Herpetic whitlow: herpetic infections of the digits. *J Hand Surg*. 1979;4(1):90–94.

3. Clark DC. Common acute hand infections. *Am Fam Physician*. 2003;68(11):2167–2176.

4. Grover C, Bansal S, Nanda S, et al. En bloc excision of proximal nail fold for treatment of chronic paronychia. *Dermatol Surg*. 2006;32(3):393–398; discussion 398–399.

5. Connolly B, Johnstone F, Gerlinger T, Puttler E. Methicillin-resistant Staphylococcus aureus in a finger felon. *J Hand Surg Am*. 2000;25(1):173–175.

6. Kanavel, AB. *Infections of the Hand; A Guide to the Surgical Treatment of Acute and Chronic Suppurative Processes in the Fingers, Hand and Forearm*. Philadelphia: Lea & Febiger; 1912.

7. Boles SD, Schmidt CC. Pyogenic flexor tenosynovitis. *Hand Clin*. 1998;14:567–578.

8. Brenman, S. Hand infections and related extremity injury. In: Georgiade GS, Georgiade NG, Riefkohl R, Barwick WJ, eds. *Textbook of Plastic, Maxillofacial and Reconstructive Surgery*. Baltimore, MD: Williams & Wilkins; 1987: 1222–1223.

9. Chuinard RG, D'ambrosia RD. Human bite infections of the hand. *J Bone Joint Surg*. 1977;59a(3):416–418.

10. Zubowicz VN, Gravier M. Management of early human bites of the hand: a prospective randomized study. *Plast Reconstr Surg*. 1991;88:111–114.

11. Dormans JP. Hand infections. In: Pediatric Orthopaedics and Sports Medicine. Philadelphia: Mosby; 2004.

12. Bisno AL, Stevens DL. Streptococcal infections of skin and soft tissues. *N Engl J Med*. 1996;334(4):240–245.

13. Karanas YL, Bogdan MA, Chang J. Community acquired methicillin-resistant Staphylococcus aureus hand infections: case reports and clinical implications. *J Hand Surg Am*. 2000;25(4):760–763.

14. Moran GJ, Krishnadasan A, Gorwitz RJ, et al. Methicillin-resistant S. aureus infections among patients in the emergency department. *N Engl J Med*. 2006;355(7):666–674.

15. Bug Drug Web site. http://www.uphs.upenn.edu/bugdrug/.

chapter 53

Compressive Neuropathies in the Upper Extremity

David J. Slutsky, MD

● INTRODUCTION

A neuropathy may be defined as any disorder that results in abnormal nerve function. Neuropathies can be generalized and are as such frequently associated with a number of systemic disorders such as diabetes, hypothyroidism, alcoholism, vitamin B12 deficiency, and lead poisoning. The neuropathy may be focal or restricted to a specific anatomical location. Many of these focal neuropathies arise due to nerve compression, although traction plays a significant role.

In early nerve compression, the symptoms are of a vascular nature. Fluid shifts that occur with limb position result in endoneurial edema. The absence of lymphatic drainage from the endoneurial space makes the clearance of edema slow. The edema cuts off the blood supply by pinching off the arterioles which course through the perineurium obliquely. This impairs the ATP-dependent ion exchange pump. This ultimately results in a reversible metabolic conduction block, which leads to paresthesia. Chronic compression leads to inflammation and secondary fibrosis, which disrupts this gliding layer, ultimately leading to nerve tethering. Any compressive neuropathy therefore frequently has a component of traction neuropathy as well. Traction alone can cause conduction block.

● NERVE ANATOMY

Median Nerve

The median nerve contains the nerve root fibers from C6-T1 and arises from the medial and lateral cords of the brachial plexus. In the upper arm, it lies lateral to the axillary artery but crosses medial to it at the level of the coracobrachialis. At the elbow, it travels in front of the brachialis and behind the bicipital aponeurosis. At distal part of the cubital fossa, the motor branches of the median nerve consistently collect into three fascicular groups. There is an anterior group (to the pronator teres and flexor carpi radialis [FCR]), middle group (motor to the flexor digitorum superficialis [FDS] and hand intrinsics; sensory to the thumb, index, and middle fingers), and a posterior group (to the anterior interosseous branch). The nerve and artery pass through the antecubital fossa underneath the lacertus fibrosis and gives off branches to the palmaris longus, FCR, FDS, and rarely the flexor digitorum profundus (FDP). The nerve then dives between the deep and superficial heads of the pronator teres to which it supplies one to four branches. The fibrous arch of the pronator teres lies 3.0 to 7.5 cm below the humeral epicondylar line. The fibrous arch of the superficialis arch lies 6.5 cm below the humeral epicondylar line. The median nerve enters the forearm deep to the fibrous arch of the FDS and emerges beneath the radial side of the muscle belly of the middle finger superficialis where it is quite superficial and near the palmaris longus tendon. The anterior interosseous nerve (AIN) is the largest muscular branch that emerges from the median nerve. It innervates the FDP to the index and middle fingers, the FPL, and the pronator quadratus. The terminal portion also provides sensory innervation to the carpal joints. The AIN arises from the median nerve on the dorsoradial surface about 5 to 8 cm distal to the medial epicondyle. The AIN travels between the FDS and FDP, and then passes dorsally in the interval between the flexor pollicus longus

(FPL) and FDP, giving off two to six branches to each of these muscles. The nerve reaches the anterior surface of the interosseous membrane and travels with the anterior interosseous artery where it passes deep to the pronator quadratus which it also innervates. It ends by sending sensory afferent branches to the intercarpal, radiocarpal, and distal radioulnar joints.

The carpal tunnel is open-ended proximally and distally, but behaves like a closed compartment physiologically and maintains its own distinct tissue fluid pressure levels. It is a fibro-osseous canal that is bounded by the concave arch of the carpal bones dorsally, and the flexor retinaculum palmarly. The hook of the hamate, triquetrum, and pisiform form the ulnar border, while the radial border consists of the scaphoid, trapezium, and the fascial septum overlying the FCR. The flexor retinaculum consists of three zones: a proximal zone that is continuous with the deep forearm fascia, a central zone which is composed of the transverse carpal ligament (TCL), and a third zone which consists of the aponeurosis between the thenar and hypothenar muscles. The median nerve at the wrist has approximately 30 fascicles. The motor recurrent branch often consists of two fascicles, which are situated in a volar position, with the various sensory groups in the radial, ulnar, and dorsal positions. The motor branch can be separated from the main trunk without harm for up to 100 proximal to the thenar muscles. The sensory fibers travel within the common digital nerves to the thumb, index and middle, as well as the communicating branch to the third web space.

Median nerve compression neuropathies in the distal arm and forearm are extremely uncommon when compared with carpal tunnel syndrome (CTS). The more proximal of the median nerve compression neuropathies is the pronator syndrome. The syndrome is classically associated with any of four potential areas of compression: the ligament of Struthers, the lacertus fibrosis, the aponeurotic fascia of the superficial, or deep head of pronator teres or the FDS arch. Both carpal tunnel syndrome and AIN entrapment should be excluded. The nerve may be compressed by the ligament of Struthers, which is rarely associated with a supracondylar process. It spans the supracondylar process and medial epicondyle and creates an arcade that contains the median nerve and brachial artery. The ligament of Struthers has also been described in the absence of an associated supracondylar process. In the forearm, the median nerve can be compressed by the pronator teres, the FDS arch or the bicipital aponeurosis. Rare causes of compression include a persistent median artery, the Gantzer muscle (accessory head of the FPL), and the palmaris profundus.

Isolated AIN palsy accounts for less than 1% of all upper extremity peripheral neuropathies. It is still uncertain as to whether this syndrome is due to inflammation or compression (Figure 53-1). The AIN may be compressed by fibrous bands from the deep (most common) or superficial head of the pronator teres, the fibrous arcade of the FDS, enlarged bursae or tumors, aberrant or thrombosed

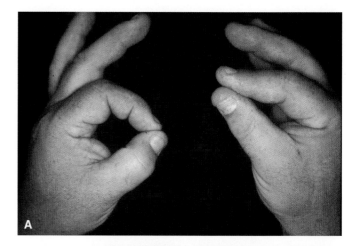

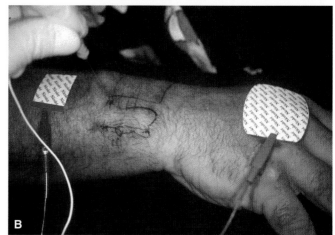

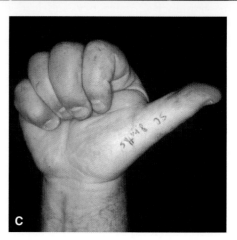

● **FIGURE 53-1.** Anterior interosseous nerve compression. (A) Inability to perform the OK sign. (B) Needle placement during EMG of the pronator quadratus. (C) Clinical photo at 8 months showing active flexion of the distal phalanx of the index but no active thumb IP joint flexion. (*Copyright David J. Slutsky, with permission.*)

vessels, an accessory bicipital aponeurosis, and fractures of the forearm and distal humerus.

In the carpal canal, there are two potential sites of compression anatomically. The first is at the proximal edge of the TCL, where compression may be produced by acute wrist flexion. This accounts for the positive Phalen test (wrist flexion test) in CTS. The second is adjacent to the hook of the hamate, where an hourglass deformity of the median nerve may be seen. In this case, the patient will have a positive median nerve compression (Durkan test) but a negative Phalen test. Compression within the carpal tunnel may also result from any lesion that takes up space within the canal, such as flexor tenosynovitis, hematoma, palmar carpal dislocation, distal radius fractures, tumors, and ganglia. Although many cases have been attributed to a nonspecific synovitis, synovial biopsies typically fail to show evidence of inflammation. They do reveal edema and vascular sclerosis, which may be secondary to compression rather than the primary event.

Ulnar Nerve

The ulnar nerve contains the nerve root fibers from C8-T1 and arises from the medial cord of the brachial plexus. It provides the motor supply to the hypothenar muscles, the ulnar two lumbricals, the interosseous muscles, the adductor pollicus, flexor carpi ulnaris (FCU) and the profundus to the ring and small fingers. Its sensory distribution includes the palmar surface of the small and the ulnar half of the ring finger as well as the dorsoulnar carpus. It lies medial to the axillary artery and continues distally to the mid-arm where it pierces the medial intermuscular septum The superior ulnar collateral artery often accompanies the nerve. At the elbow, it lies between the medial epicondyle and the olecranon where it is covered by the Osborne ligament. It enters the forearm between the two heads of the FCU covered by a fibrous aponeurosis (the cubital tunnel). It runs deep to the FCU until the distal forearm.

The ulnar tunnel or the Guyon canal is approximately 4 cm in length, which begins at the proximal edge of the carpal transverse ligament and ends at the fibrous arch of the hypothenar arch. It is bounded medially by the pisiform, and radially by the hamate hook. The floor consists of the carpal transverse ligament and the roof consists of the continuation of the deep forearm fascia, ie, the volar carpal ligament. The ulnar nerve has 15 to 25 fascicles at the wrist. It can be clearly divided into a volar sensory component and a dorsal motor component. At the wrist, the ulnar nerve passes over the TCL, medial to the ulnar artery, through the Guyon canal. The deep motor branch is given off at the pisiform and passes underneath a fibrous arch to lie on the palmar surface of the interossei. It crosses the palm deep to the flexor tendons, to terminate in the adductor pollicus and ulnar head of the flexor pollicis brevis.

The ulnar nerve may be compressed anywhere from 10 cm proximal to 5 cm distal to the medial epicondyle. Ulnar nerve compression at the elbow is second only to median nerve compression in the carpal tunnel as the most common neuropathy in the upper limb. Five potential sites for compression have been described. The most proximal site is the arcade of Struthers (different than the ligament of Struthers), a fascial band that courses obliquely over the ulnar nerve in the upper arm. The second site is at the medial epicondyle when a cubitus valgus deformity is present. The third site is a fibro-osseous tunnel at the olecranon bounded anteriorly by the medial epicondyle, laterally by the olecranon and ulnohumeral ligament, and covered by a fibroaponeurotic band. Compression at this site can be caused by lesions within the groove such as tumors (Figure 53-2), conditions outside the groove such as external compression or anomalous muscles, and conditions that predispose the nerve to displace from the groove. The fourth site is between the two heads of the FCU muscle. The floor of the passageway through FCU is the medial collateral ligament

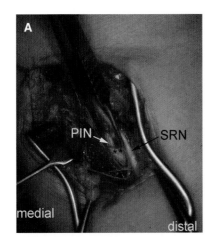 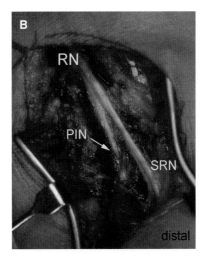

● **FIGURE 53-2.** Anterolateral approach to PIN decompression. (A) Anterior approach with a view of the proximal volar forearm demonstrating the arcade of Struthers (*). SRN, superficial radial nerve. PIN, posterior interosseous nerve. (B) After release of the arcade. Note the normal appearance of the PIN. RN, radial nerve. (*Copyright David J. Slutsky, with permission.*)

of the elbow and the roof is a fibrous band (Osborne ligament, arcuate ligament) that is a continuation of the fibroaponeurotic covering of the epicondylar groove. At the elbow, the ulnar nerve contains about 20 fascicles, including the motor branches to the forearm muscles. The fascicles within a nerve are not uniformly affected by compression. Those on the periphery of a nerve sustain greater injury than centrally placed fascicles. The motor fascicles to the FCU and the intrinsics are centrally located, whereas the sensory fibers are superficially located. The usual sites of compression in cubital tunnel syndrome are superficial to the nerve (Osborne ligament, arcade of Struthers). The internal topography of the ulnar nerve at the elbow explains the relative sparing of the FCU and FDP because their motor fibers lay deep within the nerve. The intrinsics are often uninvolved until the late stages of compression for similar reasons whereas the superficially located sensory fibers are more susceptible to early compression.

The Guyon canal may be divided into three zones. In zone 1, nerve compression leads to mixed motor and sensory symptoms. In zone II, symptoms are purely sensory; and in zone III, symptoms are purely motor and restricted to muscles innervated by the deep ulnar motor branch. Two sites of entrapment distal to the abductor digiti minimi have also been described. In these cases, the abductor digiti minimi will be preserved while there is weakness and wasting of the intrinsics.

Radial Nerve

The radial nerve contains contributions from C5–C8 spinal roots and arises from the posterior cord of the brachial plexus. The nerve runs medial to the axillary artery. At the level of the coracobrachialis, it courses posteriorly to lie in the spiral groove of the humerus. In the lower arm, it pierces the lateral intermuscular septum to run between the brachialis and brachioradialis. Opposite the head of the radius, there are some fibrous bands from the joint's capsule and immediately distal to this, the nerve is regularly crossed by several prominent veins, the "leash of Henry." It divides 2 cm distal to the elbow into a superficial radial nerve (SRN) and a deep motor branch, the posterior interosseous nerve (PIN). It gives off branches to the, extensor carpi radialis longus (ECRL) and brevis (ECRB), brachioradialis and anconeus before giving off the PIN branch. The PIN continues on between the superficial and deep head of the supinator muscle, to exit on the dorsal forearm. After it emerges from the distal border of the supinator, the PIN sends branches to the extensor digitorum communis (EDC), extensor carpi ulnaris, extensor digiti quinti, extensor pollicus longus and brevis, and the extensor indicis proprius (EIP) in descending order, although there may be considerable variation. The radial sensory nerve exits from under the brachioradialis approximately 5.0 cm proximal to the radial styloid and bifurcates into a major volar and a major dorsal branch at a mean distance of 4.2 cm proximal

to the radial styloid. It then moves distally where it supplies sensation to the dorsum of the thumb, the first web space and the dorsoradial aspect of the carpus, extending up to the index and middle fingers.

Entrapment of the PIN at the elbow can result in two separate clinical syndromes. Although the same nerve is compressed, the clinical presentation may be different and merely represents two ends of the spectrum of PIN compression. The PIN is said to be a motor nerve, but it also contains sensory nerve branches from which the pain from radial tunnel compression is derived. The different clinical presentation may reflect the internal fascicular topography of the radial nerve. Pain symptoms predominate with nerve compression secondary to superficial structures and motor paralysis occurs from compression from below due to lesions arising from the radiocapitellar joint. As it travels distally through the radial tunnel, the PIN may potentially be entrapped by fibrous bands anterior to the radiocapitellar joint, the radial recurrent leash of vessels, the fibrous edge of the ECRB, the proximal border of the supinator, ie, the arcade of Frohse or the distal edge of the supinator muscle.

● PATIENT SELECTION

Median Nerve Compression

The patient with median nerve compression will typically complain of numbness and paresthesia along the nerve's distribution. Clinical symptoms of pronator syndrome include forearm pain as well as distal median paresthesia. Symptoms are typically precipitated by activity, especially repetitive elbow flexion/extension and forearm pronation/supination. Nocturnal paresthesias are not common as they are with CTS. Numbness and tingling may also involve the thenar area supplied by the palmar cutaneous branch, which takes off proximal to the carpal transverse ligament and is not compressed in CTS.

Phalen and Durkan tests will be negative in pronator syndrome unless CTS coexists. There may be a positive Tinel sign over the proximal nerve as well as a firm and tender pronator teres and tenderness along the median nerve in the proximal forearm. Manual compression of the median nerve over the pronator teres for 30 seconds (ie, pronator compression test) may elicit paresthesia in the median nerve distribution. Pain or paresthesia produced by resisted forearm supination in combination with resisted elbow flexion beyond 120 degrees suggests compression at the bicipital aponeurosis. Paresthesia resulting from resisted forearm pronation, while the elbow is slowly extended from full flexion, is indicative of compression between the two heads of the pronator teres. Resisted proximal interphalangeal (IP) joint flexion of the middle finger producing paresthesia in the radial three digits and/ or pain over the FDS arch is consistent with entrapment under the fibrous origin of the FDS. These tests are, however, neither specific nor sensitive.

Anterior interosseous nerve syndrome (AINS) must be differentiated from a brachial plexus neuritis (Parsonage-Turner syndrome) in which there is usually no history of trauma. The pain symptoms may be unrelated to the motor findings, and can appear spontaneously or following a viral illness or vaccination. By contrast, the patient with AINS will usually have a history of trauma or repetitive injury. Complaints will include vague, aching pain in the proximal forearm, which occurs at rest and is exacerbated by activity. The patient can have difficulty with writing and pinching activities, and they may have sensory abnormalities in the median nerve distribution.

AINS is characterized by loss of function of the FPL and FDP to the index and sometimes the long finger and the pronator quadratus. Sensibility is unaffected. Inability to make an "O" sign during attempted tip pinch results in extension of the index finger at the distal IP joint with compensatory increased flexion at the proximal IP joint. The thumb hyperextends at the IP joint with increased flexion of the metacarpophalangeal joint. The pronator quadratus can be tested by resisted pronation with the elbow flexed to relax the pronator teres. AINS can be incomplete, with either weakness or absence of the FPL or FDP of the index finger alone with normal pronator quadratus function. All of the profundus tendons may be innervated by the AIN, with subsequent weakness of all the fingers. The hand intrinsic muscles may be affected if there is a coexisting Martin-Gruber anastomosis. This is where C8-T1 motor fibers destined for the hand intrinsics travel in the median nerve. They then cross over to the ulnar nerve, usually through connections in the AIN (91%). If the FDS is also innervated by the AIN (30%), patients may present with weakness in this muscle also. One must differentiate between AINS and rupture of the FDP or FPL, which may occur from rheumatoid arthritis, Keinböck disease, and scaphoid nonunion. The integrity of these tendons can be assessed by observing the tenodesis effect of the FPL and the index FDP. This causes passive thumb IP and index distal interphalangeal flexion with passive wrist extension.

Initially symptoms of CTS occur at night due to a combination of wrist flexion during sleep and fluid shifts that occur with the horizontal position, which increases the carpal canal pressure. With early compression the symptoms are intermittent, and the edema is reversible. As the symptoms progress, they become more frequent during the day and are precipitated by gripping and pinching activities as well as those tasks requiring repetitive wrist flexion. CTS represents a constellation of signs and symptoms in which no one test absolutely confirms its diagnosis. A positive Tinel sign may be present over the median nerve at the wrist, and produces paresthesia in the thumb and radial 2.5 digits. The Phalen test consists of subjective paresthesia in the median nerve distribution with passive wrist flexion for 1 minute. This is best performed with the elbows extended because simultaneous wrist and elbow flexion may reproduce ulnar nerve symptoms as well. Direct compression of the nerve or the Durkan test is thought to be more sensitive.

Ulnar Nerve Compression

The patient with ulnar nerve entrapment presents with complaints of numbness and/or tingling in the small and/or ring finger. Symptoms can range from mild numbness in the ring and little fingers to severe pain on the medial aspect of the elbow with dysesthesia radiating distally into the hand. In chronic cases, patients may complain of a loss of dexterity with fine manipulation tasks. Symptoms are provoked by repetitive or sustained elbow flexion activities. The ulnar nerve is palpated for enlargement or subluxation during elbow flexion. There may be a positive Tinel sign at the epicondylar groove or over the proximal FCU. An elbow flexion test is performed and consists of placing the elbow in full flexion with a hyperextended wrist, while manual pressure is applied to the nerve for 1 minute. The test is considered positive when paresthesia and/or numbness occur in the ulnar nerve distribution of the hand. False-positive results occur in approximately 10% of patients. There may be a sensory deficit involving all or part of the ulnar nerve distribution, including the dorsoulnar carpus. When intrinsic muscle weakness is severe, there is often clawing of the ring and little fingers. One may see a positive Froment sign (flexion of the IP joint of the thumb with side pinch), a positive Jeanne sign (hyperextension of the metacarpophalangeal joint of the thumb), and paradoxical abduction of the small finger due to a paralyzed third palmar interosseous (positive Wartenberg sign). Extrinsic weakness may involve the FDP to the little finger and ring finger. Weakness of the FCU rarely occurs.

Patients with distal ulnar nerve entrapment may present with complaints of numbness and tingling of the small and/or ring finger sparing the dorsoulnar aspect of the hand. The patient may give a history of repetitive trauma to the hypothenar eminence as seen with automobile mechanics, martial artists, and Kodo drummers. A history of Raynaud symptoms should alert one to the possibility of ulnar artery thrombosis. There are no characteristic findings of ulnar tunnel entrapment per se. A Tinel sign may be present at the wrist but not the elbow unless there is an associated cubital tunnel entrapment. Intrinsic atrophy may also occur in chronic compression, but the FCU and the FDP are not affected. There should be a negative Tinel sign at the elbow and a negative elbow flexion test. If there is an associated ulnar artery aneurysm there may be a palpable thrill and an audible bruit. With ulnar artery thrombosis, the Allen test will be positive for ulnar artery occlusion. With an associated fracture of the hook of the hamate, there will be localized tenderness in the palm, 1 cm radial and 1 cm distal to the pisiform. Ancillary testing such as ultrasound, CT, angiography, and MRI may be employed to aid in the diagnosis of these associated entities.

Radial Nerve Compression

In the arm region, radial nerve palsy often occurs in association with some form of unconsciousness. In "Saturday night" palsy, an obtunded patient sits with his arm over a chairback or rests his head on the lateral surface of his arm. Alternatively, the radial nerve can be compressed in the groove between the brachialis and forearm muscles when one person rests her head on the middle third of the arm of another ("Honeymooner's" palsy). The patient will typically present with a wrist drop and an inability to extend the fingers, thumb, or wrist. In addition, the brachioradialis will be affected along with variable involvement of the triceps. They will also have diminished sensation over the dorsum of the first web space.

The presenting complaint in radial tunnel syndrome (RTS) is proximal forearm pain often coexisting with lateral epicondylitis, with neither sensory nor motor loss. The patient often gives a history of performing repetitive pronation/supination activities, such as using a screwdriver. The symptoms of RTS often coexist and overlap those of lateral epicondylitis. A number of provocative tests have been described, including resisted extension of the middle finger, which tenses the ECRB and entraps the nerve, tenderness over the supinator muscle and pain with resisted supination. None are pathognomonic for this condition however. A diagnostic local anesthetic block of the PIN, which produces a temporary wrist drop is useful if the pain is completely relieved.

In PIN syndrome, the presenting symptoms are weakness and/or paralysis of the extensor muscles, which result in a wrist or finger drop. There may be a history of a fall onto an extended and pronated arm, although many cases are spontaneous, especially if due to an underlying lipoma, ganglion, or rheumatoid nodule arising from the radiocapitellar joint. The patient will demonstrate variable weakness or paralysis of the extensor pollicus longus, EIP, EDC, and extensor carpi ulnaris. Motor function of the ECRB/L should be preserved because they are innervated before the PIN dives between the two heads of the supinator muscle. The patient will hence extend their wrist in radial deviation.

The SRN can be injured in the distal forearm or at the wrist by tight bracelets or watchbands, handcuffs, radius fractures, lacerations, venous cutdown, and blunt trauma. The SRN may also be entrapped as it exits the fascia between the tendons of the brachioradialis and ECRB. In patients with entrapment of the SRN, the presentation may include a history of compressive or crushing forearm injuries, work activities requiring frequent pronation and wrist hyperextension, and associated illnesses, such as diabetes. Patients may complain of altered sensibility over the dorsoradial aspect of the hand and dorsoradial cutaneous pain with ulnar flexion of the wrist or with gripping and pinching. The physical examination may demonstrate alteration in touch perception, moving two-point discrimination >15 mm, static two-point discrimination (s2PD) more than 5 mm difference versus the contralateral first web space, a positive Tinel sign over the course of the nerve, and aggravation of the patient's symptoms with forced forearm pronation and wrist ulnar flexion.

● PATIENT PREPARATION

Electrodiagnostic Studies

Ancillary tests include nerve conduction studies (NCSs) and quantitative sensory testing. These cannot replace a detailed history and thorough examination of the upper limb, but they can provide a means for staging the degree of neuropathy and for ruling out more generalized disorders that may masquerade as a focal neuropathy. A recording electrode will detect activity in the largest myelinated fibers first, since these fibers conduct at the fastest rates and have a lower depolarization threshold than the small unmyelinated nerves. Large fibers are also more vulnerable to compression and ischemia than are small fibers.

Latency and conduction velocity depend on the time that transpires from stimulation of the nerve to the first recording. If only a fraction of the large thickly myelinated fibers remain and transmit impulses, the recorded latency and conduction velocity remains normal because the recording electrode mostly detects the fastest fibers. The electrical conduction in smaller, thinly myelinated or nonmyelinated nerves is much slower and hence not usually detected in a routine NCS. Large myelinated and small unmyelinated fibers can be affected differently. The large myelinated nerves undergo segmental demyelination, and the small unmyelinated nerves undergo degeneration and regeneration. An NCS only tests the faster conducting fibers. This explains the paradox of the patient who has established carpal tunnel syndrome but shows normal on electrodiagnostic studies. It is the worst fascicles that produce symptoms, but it is the best fascicles that account for the normal nerve conduction studies.

The presence of fewer nerve fibers reduces the size of the electrical charge, leading to smaller amplitudes. When there is sensory or motor loss, there is usually degeneration of nerve fibers. Despite the restoration of neural blood flow following nerve decompression, remyelination of the axon is often incomplete, which accounts for persistently abnormal nerve conduction, even though the patient may be without symptoms.

Quantitative sensory testing is reportedly more sensitive than the NCS, as only 25% of the large myelinated nerve fibers need to be conducting normally in order to yield a normal nerve conduction test. With nerve degeneration it is more difficult to distinguish two points from one point. Static and moving two-point discrimination typically test the innervation density. Threshold tests would include vibrometry and Semmes-Weinstein monofilament testing. Vibrometry is relatively insensitive to early changes and is not commonly used. Semmes-Weinstein testing involves placing nylon filaments of varying thickness on the skin until the filament is seen to deflect. The test is repeated with varying diameter filaments until the threshold is determined. An abnormal Semmes-Weinstein test is consistent with nerve demyelination.

Median Nerve Testing

NCSs are rarely diagnostic for pronator syndrome. There may be prolongation of the distal median sensory latencies as well as reduced amplitude of the compound motor action potential (CMAP) to the abductor pollicis brevis. There may be slowing of forearm conduction but this can be misleading since reduced forearm velocity is seen up to 20% to 30% of the time when there is a markedly delayed distal median motor latency due to severe CTS. Needle stimulation of the median nerve in 1 cm increments while recording from the abductor pollicis brevis may identify an area of focal conduction block near the pronator teres muscle. Nerve conduction studies during provocative maneuvers such as elbow flexion, forearm pronation, and middle finger flexion against resistance do not increase the yield. The electromyography (EMG), however, may be of some value since membrane instability may be seen in the median-innervated muscles, including the pronator teres, FCR, and FDS.

Shoulder girdle and upper limb EMG in AINS should be performed to rule out a brachial plexitis. In this case, there will be membrane instability in the proximal limb muscles. The most appropriate technique involves recording the CMAP from the pronator quadratus. Side-to-side comparative latencies are helpful in establishing the diagnosis. EMG testing of the pronator quadratus and FPL muscles should demonstrate signs of membrane instability. Quantitative sensory testing should be entirely normal since the condition only affects a motor branch. Any abnormalities are due to nonrelated causes conditions.

The nerve conduction study can yield useful information in carpal tunnel syndrome, but the severity of the preoperative nerve conduction deficit does not provide significant data for prediction of the final outcome or return to work after carpal tunnel release (CTR). There are some caveats for NCSs in CTS. First, sensory abnormalities usually occur before motor abnormalities. In other words, the distal sensory latencies often slow before the distal motor latency. This is not surprising since 94% of the axons in the median nerve at the wrist level are sensory. The sensory nerve axons are larger than the motor axons and hence more susceptible to compression. If the distal motor latency is abnormal in the presence of normal sensory nerve action potentials (SNAPs), extra care must be taken to rule out anterior horn cell disease or a 8 radiculopathy, although isolated recurrent motor branch compression has been reported. Second, the nerve conduction studies may not return to normal following decompression due to retrograde fiber degeneration or incomplete remyelination, even in the presence of a full clinical recovery.

Ulnar Nerve Testing

On quantitative sensory testing, s2PD testing remains normal in mild cases. With more severe and/or longer standing median nerve compression, the s2PD becomes abnormal (ie, >5 mm) in variable combinations of the thumb, index, middle, and radial ring finger. Loss of protective sensation occurs when the s2PD is >15 mm, and >25 mm correlates with complete anesthesia. Two-point discrimination is relatively insensitive in picking up changes as compared with testing using the pressure-specified sensory device (PSSD) devised by Lee Dellon. In CTS testing of the index finger, pulp may initially show an abnormal s2PD pressure threshold. With progression, the surgeon sees a widening of the s2PD distance, followed by an abnormal s1PD threshold. A prospective side-by-side comparison of NCS and PSSD testing was undertaken in 60 patients (86 tests) with clinical signs and symptoms of CTS (D. J. Slutsky, unpublished data). Eleven of these patients then underwent a CTR and were tested again at 6 months. Clinical improvement was gauged by relief of symptoms, absent provocative tests and at least a 1.04 improvement in the Brigham CTS questionnaire. Both the NCS and PSSD were roughly comparable in terms of sensitivity and specificity. When combined, however, 80/86 cases of CTS were detected, including 14 patients who had symptoms of CTS but negative clinical signs.

Ulnar motor studies are more popular than ulnar sensory studies. The distal motor latency is determined by recording from an electrode placed over the midpoint of the abductor digiti minimi while stimulating the ulnar nerve 8 cm proximally (S1). Normal values include a distal motor latency less than or equal to 3.6 ms and amplitude greater than 4.0 mV. Alternatively, the latencies can be measured from the first dorsal interosseous (FDI), which then assesses conduction through the deep motor branch of the ulnar nerve. The FDI to abductor digiti minimi latency should not exceed 2.0 ms. The ulnar nerve is then stimulated 4 cm distal to the medial epicondyle (S2). By subtracting the latency for S1 from S2 and measuring the intervening distance, the forearm conduction velocity is obtained. Ulnar nerve conduction across the cubital tunnel is calculated by stimulating the nerve at S3, which is 12 cm proximal to S2, and subtracting the latencies. Most labs measure conduction with the elbow flexed between 90 and 135 degrees. Normal forearm NCV is greater than 48 m/s. Across the cubital tunnel the NCV should be greater than 45 m/s. More than 10 m/s of slowing between the above and below elbow NCV is abnormal. Amplitude drops of greater than 20% are a more sensitive indicator of conduction block or axonal loss.

Ring electrodes are placed on the small finger and the ulnar nerve is stimulated 14 cm proximally. Recordings are also taken from the ring finger after stimulation of both the ulnar and median nerves. This allows for comparison of the ulnar to the median SNAPs. Normal peak sensory latencies are less than or equal to 3.5 ms and less than 0.5 ms median-ulnar difference. Mixed palmar orthodromic studies can be elicited by stimulating the ulnar nerve in the fourth web space and recording over the ulnar nerve at the wrist 8 cm proximally. This measures the sensory nerve conduction through Guyon canal. Normal values are less than 2.2 ms.

Combining ulnar motor and sensory techniques adds useful information in complex cases, where clinical examination fails to localize the lesion. Conduction to the dorsal cutaneous branch of the ulnar nerve can be measured. This test is relatively insensitive for detecting proximal ulnar nerve compression, since it is abnormal in only 55% of patients with cubital tunnel syndrome. Electromyography demonstrates axonal degeneration in muscles. Because these changes are seen in chronic neuropathies, EMG is not as useful as conduction times for the diagnosis of early nerve compression. When muscle abnormalities are noted, they are usually initially seen in the intrinsic muscles, generally the first dorsal interosseous, followed in frequency by the muscles in the hypothenar eminence. On quantitative sensory testing, PSSD testing shows an abnormal s2PD in the ring and small finger initially, followed by increased s1PD. Abnormal s2PD may also be seen over the ulnar dorsum of the hand.

The usual nerve conduction studies are inadequate at assessing distal ulnar nerve entrapment. Short segment incremental studies is a sensitive and specific way to assess the deep motor branch since focal conduction abnormalities also tend to be normalized over the distance between the abductor digiti minimi and the FDI. The ulnar nerve is stimulated in 1 cm increments from 3 to 4 cm proximal and distal to the wrist crease. Abnormal values include a greater than 0.5 ms jump or a greater than 120% drop in amplitude. When this is combined with FDI conduction and interosseous-latency differences, the diagnostic yield increases. On quantitative sensory testing, the s2PD to the small finger is the first to go, followed by an abnormal s1PD. The dorsoulnar carpus should remain normal unless there is an associated C8-T1 radiculopathy.

Radial Nerve Testing

With palsy of the radial nerve, the NCS typically demonstrates the absence of the superficial radial SNAP. Motor recordings are more difficult since no muscle is sufficiently isolated from other radially innervated muscles. A surface electrode over the EIP results in a volume conducted response from the adjacent radial innervated muscles, which makes side-to-side amplitude comparisons difficult. Radial nerve recordings using needle electrodes in the EIP are more common as a result, which makes it difficult to approximate the degree of axonal loss by assessing the amplitudes. The EMG, however, is quite useful and permits a relatively accurate localization of the lesion. In a spiral groove lesion, for example, all three heads of the triceps should be normal, with denervation of the brachioradialis and all muscles distal to it. With quantitative sensory testing, the patients will have an abnormal s2PD and possibly s1PD over the dorsum of the first web.

In both radial tunnel and PIN compression, sensory testing over the dorsum of the first web space should be normal unless there is a superimposed C6 neuropathy. Some authors have postulated that RTS reflects a dynamic entrapment of the PIN. If the ECRB develops a fibrous edge, the PIN can be entrapped by a scissoring action between this edge and the arcade of Frohse during repetitive forearm supination and pronation. This can lead to intermittent PIN compression. Differential latency testing is based on this premise. Across elbow radial motor nerve conduction is performed with the elbow extended and the forearm positioned in neutral, pronation, and supination for 30 seconds. The testing is then repeated. An abnormal latency difference of greater than 0.30 ms is indicative of radial tunnel entrapment.

Compression of the PIN does not affect the superficial radial SNAP, which should be normal. The CMAP of PIN innervated muscles may show a drop of conduction velocity or amplitude, but this is difficult to assess with surface electrodes. Needle EMG is the best technique for localization, especially with partial lesions. In acute denervation decreased recruitment, increased insertional activity and fibrillation potentials plus/minus positive sharp waves are present. In chronic lesions seen after 3 to 6 months, decreased recruitment may still be seen along with giant motor unit potentials and polyphasia due to peripheral axonal ingrowth.

On quantitative sensory testing, patients with SRN compression will have an abnormal s2PD and possibly 1PS over the dorsum of the first web space. With electrodiagnostic studies, the distal radial sensory latency may be normal even in the presence of abnormal forearm conduction. This commonly occurs with nerve entrapment due to segmental conduction velocity slowing. In more advanced cases, slowing or a complete block of the distal SRN occurs. If the response is absent, it is difficult to localize the lesion.

● TECHNIQUE

Pronator Syndrome

The hallmark of treatment for pronator syndrome consists of activity modification and NSAIDs. Steroid injections are of no benefit. Immobilization in an above elbow splint with the elbow flexed 90 degrees with slight forearm pronation and wrist flexion for 4 to 6 weeks may relieve pressure and traction on the median nerve.

Although the majority of patients will respond to nonoperative therapy, failure to improve is an indication for surgical release. The procedure is performed under tourniquet control. An anteromedial incision is made crossing the antecubital fossa, starting 5 cm above the elbow flexion crease. The medial antebrachial cutaneous nerve is isolated as it runs with the basilic vein. The median nerve is identified proximal to the elbow, next to the brachial artery, and it is traced distally, resecting the ligament of Struthers if present. The nerve is followed through the two heads of the pronator teres where branches from the anterior bundle (FCR, pronator teres fascicles) are given off. Both the superficial head of the pronator teres and the FDS can be divided and tagged for later repair if better exposure is needed. The posterior (AIN branch) and the middle (intrinsic, sensory) bundles pass deep to the superficialis arch, which is also incised. Epineurotomy or internal neurolysis is of no benefit. Subcutaneous transposition of the median nerve is also not recommended. Postoperatively, the arm is placed in an above elbow splint for comfort with the elbow flexed 90 degrees, the forearm in midpronation and the wrist in slight flexion. Gentle elbow range-of-motion exercises are begun after the first week, unless it is necessary to protect the reattachment of the pronator teres and/or FDS insertions. Resistive activities are avoided until 6 to 8 weeks postoperatively.

If there is no improvement either clinically or by EMG studies 4 to 6 months after onset, surgical exploration is indicated. Even though return of function has been reported up to 18 months after onset of symptoms, expectant treatment is less predictable than surgical intervention. The surgical approach for AIN palsy is essentially the same as for pronator syndrome. A microscopic interfascicular neurolysis of the AIN up to the elbow should be considered in cases where there is no obvious compression site because hourglass-like fascicular constrictions that are not discernible through the intact epineurium have been reported. The arm is placed in a bulky, above-elbow plaster splint that maintains the elbow at 90 degrees of flexion, the forearm in 45 degrees of pronation, and the wrist in slight flexion for comfort.

Nonoperative therapy for CTS includes splinting the wrist in a neutral position, steroid injections, and management of any underlying systemic diseases. Steroid injection offers transient relief to 80% of patients, but only 20% will be symptom-free 12 months later. Those most likely to benefit from conservative management have had

symptoms for less than 1 year, only intermittent numbness, normal two-point discrimination, less than 1 to 2 ms prolongation of distal motor and sensory latencies, and no motor findings. Forty percent of this group will remain symptom free for longer than 12 months.

A failure of nonoperative treatment is an indication for surgical release. The procedure is performed under tourniquet control. A 3- to 5-cm incision is made in the palm parallel to the thenar crease and inline with the ring finger axis in order to protect the palmar cutaneous branch of the median and ulnar nerves (Figure 53-3A–B). Tenotomy scissors are used to spread down to the palmar aponeurosis. This is divided exposing the transverse carpal ligament. The TCL is divided from distal to proximal. This procedure can also be performed through a mini-incision technique. A hemostat may be used to protect the median nerve. The skin is retracted and the deep flexor retinaculum is divided under direct vision for an additional 2 cm. The nerve and tendons are retracted to the radial side and the floor of the canal is inspected for any masses. The recurrent motor branch is inspected and decompressed separately, if necessary. Postoperatively, finger motion may begin immediately, which also aids in median nerve excursion. A below elbow splint is applied for comfort for the first week, followed by desensitization and progressive strengthening.

In advanced cases of median nerve compression, internal neurolysis and epineurotomy have both been described. Their efficacy has not been supported by clinical studies and they are no longer advocated. Small finger numbness due to coexistent Guyon canal compression often improves after CTR alone, since MRI studies have demonstrated an increase in the volume of Guyon canal after a CTR. Routine tenosynovectomy does not provide better results than CTR alone and is mostly recommended with associated proliferative tenosynovitis from some other cause, such as rheumatoid arthritis or granulomatous infection.

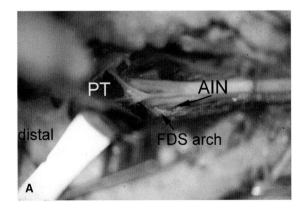 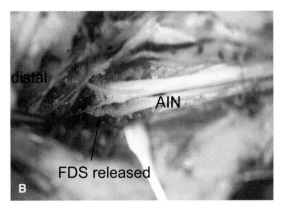

● **FIGURE 53-3.** (A) Anteromedial approach to the median nerve. Note the fibrous border of the sublimus muscle. PT, pronator teres; AIN, anterior interosseous nerve; FDS, flexor digitorum sublimus. (B) Following release of the sublimus arch. (*Copyright David J. Slutsky, with permission.*)

Ulnar Nerve

Most acute or subacute cases of distal ulnar nerve entrapment resolve by activity modification with avoidance of activities that require repetitive elbow flexion and avoiding external pressure from leaning on their medial elbow or forearm. Alterations can sometimes be made in the workplace, such as positioning a computer keyboard so that the operator's elbows are not acutely flexed. When symptoms are severe and have persisted for weeks, temporarily immobilizing the elbow in approximately 35 degrees of flexion and the wrist in neutral may provide relief. Patients are instructed to wear the splint day and night for 3 to 4 weeks. NSAIDs can be helpful but corticosteroid injections around the nerve are ineffective.

In patients with recurring symptoms, surgery is often necessary. In the absence of muscle weakness, the timing for surgery is totally dependent on the severity of symptoms. Muscle wasting and weakness are an indication for surgery. Surgery can be divided into two groups of procedures: decompression without transposition of the ulnar nerve and decompression with transposition of the nerve. The procedures are performed under axillary block or general anesthesia using a tourniquet.

To perform a subcutaneous anterior transposition, a 5-cm posteromedial incision is made over the medial epicondyle. Branches of the medial antebrachial cutaneous nerve are identified and protected. The deep fascia overlying the proximal ulnar nerve is divided as well as any associated ligament of Struthers. The fascia over the nerve is released sequentially; first in the upper arm, followed by the fibroaponeurotic covering of the epicondylar groove, then Osborne ligament at the cubital tunnel, and finally, the fascia where the nerve passes between the two heads of the FCU. A 1-cm segment of the medial intermuscular septum is resected where it attaches to the epicondyle to prevent a secondary site of compression, taking care to prevent injury to fragile veins medial to the septum. Articular branches to the elbow are divided but motor branches to the FCU should be preserved. A vessel loop is placed around the nerve, which is then gently transposed anterior to the medial epicondyle along with the superior ulnar collateral vessels (Figure 53-4). A 1-cm-wide medially based flap of fascia from the common flexor origin can be turned down and sutured to the proximal skin edge to prevent posterior subluxation of the nerve. The patient uses a sling for comfort postoperatively and is started on progressive elbow extension as tolerated.

To perform submuscular transposition, a slightly larger incision is made and the nerve is decompressed in a similar fashion. A z-plasty lengthening of the common flexor origin is preserved and the nerve is transposed deep to the muscle. Care must be taken to divide the fibrous attachment of the FDS to the humeral epicondyle to prevent secondary impingement while avoiding injury to the medial collateral ligament of the elbow. The ulnar nerve is now positioned onto the bed of the brachialis muscle and it is important to ensure that its path from the proximal end

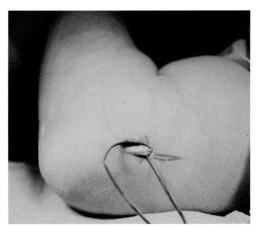

● **FIGURE 53-4.** Mini-incision approach to a subcutaneous anterior transposition of the ulnar nerve (vessel loop). (*Copyright David J. Slutsky, with permission.*)

of the operative field to the distal end is relatively straight. The flexor-pronator mass is then repaired with 2-0 nonabsorbable sutures. Postoperatively the elbow is immobilized at 90 degrees for 4 weeks, allowing elbow flexion but no extension. The elbow is then gradually extended over the ensuring 2 to 4 weeks.

The mainstay of treatment for distal ulnar nerve palsy is activity modification. Bicyclists should avoid riding in the crouch position with their hands low on the handlebars, because this is a recognized precipitant of symptoms, and change their hand position frequently. Automobile mechanics, martial artists, and Kodo drummers should avoid repetitive percussion on the ulnar border of their palm. Wrist splinting and cortisone injections have no role in this condition. The presence of a mass-occupying lesion mandates surgical treatment, as does a failure to respond to conservative measures. Surgically, the ulnar nerve is identified proximal to the distal wrist crease between the FCU and the flexor tendons through a curving incision which crosses the wrist obliquely, and bisects the interval between the pisiform and the hook of the hamate. The ulnar nerve is followed distally as the volar carpal ligament is released. The fibrous arch of the hypothenar muscles is incised and the floor of the canal is explored for masses, fibrous bands, or anomalous muscles. With entrapment in the palm, the deep motor branch is followed distally as it traverses the palm lying on the interosseous fascia, deep to the flexor tendons and superficial palmar arch. The dissection is completed as the motor branch ends in the muscle belly of the adductor pollicus (Figure 53-5A–C).

Radial Nerve

For the majority of patients with radial nerve palsy, nonoperative treatment is the mainstay. A nonadvancing Tinel sign combined with failure to improve within 6 months are indications for exploration. With severe compression, surgical treatment may be necessary and

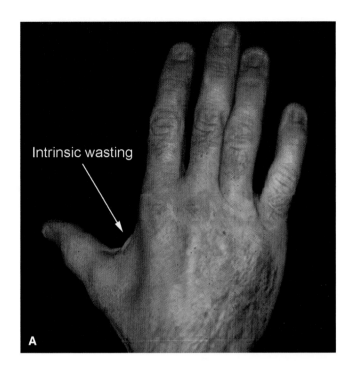

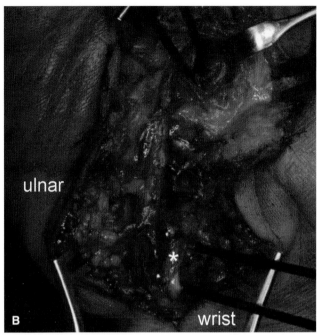

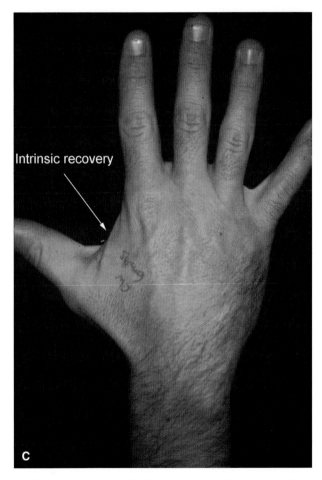

● **FIGURE 53-5.** (A) Dorsal preoperative photograph of attempted index finger abduction. Note the marked wasting of the first, second and third dorsal interossei. (B) Intraoperative view following an ulnar nerve decompression in Guyon canal as it splits into a superficial sensory branch (*white asterisk*) and deep motor branch (*) which passes under the hypothenar arch. (C) Six months after operation. Note the normal bulk of the dorsal interossei and the active index finger abduction. (*Copyright David J. Slutsky, with permission.*)

can include nerve exploration with neurolysis or nerve grafting. In delayed treatment, nerve transfers using redundant sublimus fascicles from the median nerve to the PIN may be considered if 12 months has elapsed, as there may be insufficient time for nerve ingrowth following a nerve graft, but the motor endplates are still viable. If more than 18 months have passed, then tendon transfers should be considered since the muscle can no longer be reinnervated. A 6- to 8-cm incision is made over the posterolateral aspect of the midhumerus. The radial nerve is identified in the spiral groove and followed distally through the intermuscular septum. Any obvious areas of nerve constriction or loss of the normal striations (bands of Fontana) should undergo an epineurolysis. The use of intraoperative nerve stimulation will help differentiate a neuroma in continuity from nonviable nerve tissue. In the former case, an internal neurolysis is justified as compared with excision and grafting. Postoperative management including immediate elbow mobilization is instituted following nerve decompression or neurolysis. Nerve grafting may require temporary elbow splinting for 4 weeks but it is preferable to insert a graft of sufficient length to allow early elbow extension.

The majority of RTS cases will resolve with activity modification. In the early stages above elbow splinting with the elbow flexed to 90 degrees and the forearm in supination will relieve the dynamic compression and allow the inflammatory response around the PIN to subside. PIN gliding exercises will help maintain nerve excursion and consist of simultaneous elbow extension, forearm pronation, wrist flexion, and ulnar deviation. In many instances, the treatment that is instituted for a coexisting lateral epicondylitis will also resolve the symptoms of radial tunnel compression as well. Operatively, the volar approach to the radial nerve is through an 8-cm anterolateral incision under tourniquet. The muscular fascia is divided and the intermuscular interval between the brachialis and brachioradialis is developed with blunt dissection. Recurrent branches from the radial artery must be ligated to gain access to both nerve branches. The radial nerve is identified proximal to the elbow and followed distally. At the level of the radial head, the radial nerve gives off branches to the ECRB and brachioradialis, which should be protected. It then divides into the superficial radial nerve branch which travels distally under the brachioradialis. The PIN continues distally crossed by the radial recurrent vessels, which are ligated. The proximal border of the supinator muscle (the arcade of Frohse) is divided along with the superficial head of the supinator. The PIN disappears from view at this point as it penetrates the dorsal extensor compartment. If there is a suspicion of distal entrapment a separate dorsal approach to the PIN is necessary. This can be accomplished by extending the incision distally and dorsally. The PIN nerve is then approached through a dorsolateral approach, developing the plane between the ECRB and the EDC. At this level, the PIN contains motor fibers only, hence separate fascicle identification is unnecessary. The

distal border of the supinator is delineated and divided. A combined approach can also be performed through a dorsolateral incision.

Posterior Interosseous Nerve

Unless preoperative imaging studies reveal a lesion compressing the PIN, most are treated with observation and serial EMG studies. A wrist splint may be used for comfort. Lesions that show no signs of recovery after 6 months are candidates for exploration. The surgical treatment of PIN compression is identical to that of radial tunnel decompression. Postoperatively, elbow motion and PIN gliding exercises are instituted after an initial period of splinting for comfort.

For distal sensory symptoms due to SRN compression, release is again advised. The nerve is accessed via a 2-cm incision made just proximal to the radial styloid. The nerve is identified as it exits from underneath the tendon of the brachioradialis. The overlying fascia is split while care is taken not to disturb the nerve.

● OUTCOMES

Surgical decompression for pronator syndrome generally yields good results. Olehnik et al. reported improvement in 77% of their patients following decompression of the median nerve in the proximal forearm with 33/36 patients returning to work.[1] A clinical series by Johnson et al[2] and Hartz and co-workers[3] reported improvement in 92% of patients. Patients with normal NCS seem to fare better than patients with abnormal studies, which may be related to the severity of the compression. Clinical improvement may be seen for up to 1 year following surgery but recovery is often incomplete.

Open median nerve decompression leads to symptomatic relief in the majority of patients with CTS. After open carpal tunnel release, patients typically regain their preoperative baseline grip strength within 3 months, and pinch strength within 6 weeks. Ketchum did a comparison of open CTR, CTR with flexor tenosynovectomy, and tenosynovectomy alone.[4] He noted a significant decrease in pillar pain and earlier return to work in the isolated synovectomy group. Several endoscopic methods to release the carpal tunnel have been introduced in an effort to decrease postoperative morbidity. Although a slightly earlier return to work has been demonstrated, pillar pain has not been reduced. Endoscopic carpal tunnel release shortens this period by 2 weeks on average. Mini-incision open techniques have also been described.

As in CTS, the patient's clinical findings and response to conservative measures should be a major determinant in the surgical decision-making with distal ulnar entrapment. Patients who have paresthesiae only, with no motor or sensory abnormalities (McGowan Stage I), can still benefit from an in situ release of the ulnar nerve, even if the NCS are normal. The results are largely determined by the preoperative degree of compression. When there are constant symptoms, demyelination is present and recovery may take 6-8 months. Residual sensory complaints are common. Even though intrinsic wasting rarely recovers in an adult, prevention of further denervation is crucial.

Early reports of RTS decompression were generally optimistic. Rinker et al. reported 80% good or excellent results in his series of 109 decompressions.[5] A more recent review by Sotereanos et al. however found good results in only 11/28 patients, with many patients experiencing residual symptoms.[6] The results were worse in patients receiving workers compensation.

Kline et al reported their experience with 45 surgically treated posterior interosseous nerve entrapments, tumors, or injuries over a 27-year period.[7] Most muscles innervated by the PIN achieved Grade 3 or better functional outcomes. They generally found that the PIN entrapment or injuries responded well to PIN release and/or repair.

Dellon and MacKinnon reported on a group of 51 patients with complaints related to entrapment of the superficial sensory branch of the radial nerve.[8] Seven (37%) of 19 patients treated with nonoperative modalities after a mean of 28 months from the onset of symptoms or their injury were improved. Of the 32 patients treated with surgery there was excellent subjective improvement in 37%, good subjective improvement in 49%, and fair subjective improvement in 6%, and 8% were not improved.

● COMPLICATIONS

The complications for each procedure are similar. They include wound problems related to infection, skin healing, tender scars due to injured cutaneous nerves, hematoma and iatrogenic injury due to rough nerve handling, and/or retraction. These can be minimized by meticulous hemostasis, gentle nerve handling, and precise surgical technique. Stiffness can occur and is minimized by early joint mobilization. The incidence of residual symptoms are predicated by the preoperative degree of nerve injury.

REFERENCES

1. Olehnik WK, Manske PR, Szerzinski J. Median nerve compression in the proximal forearm. *J Hand Surg Am.* 1994;19: 121–126.

2. Johnson RK, Spinner M, Shrewsbury MM. Median nerve entrapment syndrome in the proximal forearm. *J Hand Surg Am.* 1979;4:48–51.

3. Hartz CR, Linscheid RL, Gramse RR, et al. The pronator teres syndrome: compressive neuropathy of the median nerve. *J Bone Joint Surg Am.* 1981;63:885–890.

4. Ketchum LD. A comparison of flexor tenosynovectomy, open carpal tunnel release, and open carpal tunnel release with flexor tenosynovectomy in the treatment of carpal tunnel syndrome. *Plast Reconstr Surg.* 2004;113:2020–2029.

5. Rinker B, Effron CR, Beasley RW. Proximal radial compression neuropathy. *Ann Plast Surg.* 52:174–180; discussion 2004;181–183.

6. Sotereanos DG, Varitimidis SE, Giannakopoulos PN, et al. Results of surgical treatment for radial tunnel syndrome. *J Hand Surg Am.* 1999;24:566–570.

7. Kim DH, Murovic JA, Kim YY, et al. Surgical treatment and outcomes in 45 cases of posterior interosseous nerve entrapments and injuries. *J Neurosurg.* 2006;104:766–777.

8. Dellon AL, Mackinnon SE. Radial sensory nerve entrapment in the forearm. *J Hand Surg Am.* 1986;11:199–205.

chapter 54

Replantation and Revascularization

Bradon J. Wilhelmi, MD, FACS / *Scott M. Schulze, MD*

● INTRODUCTION

Microsurgical reattachment of a severed or amputated body part represents the culmination of plastic and reconstructive surgery. Replantation or revascularization of these injured body parts offers a result that is usually superior to any other type of reconstruction. The decision to attempt a replantation or revascularization and the techniques involved in replantation of amputated parts are often extremely challenging.

The replantation of these parts involves more than microsurgery, as successful repair of bony and tendinous injuries must be performed as well.

Thousands of severed body parts have been reattached since the first replant was performed over 50 years ago, which have preserved a measure of hand function superior to that of an amputation. Malt performed the first replantation on May 23, 1962, at Massachusetts General Hospital on a 12-year-old boy who had sustained a transhumeral amputation of his right arm in a train accident.[1] The repair included fixation of the humerus using a Kuntscher nail in addition to a repair of the brachial artery, the brachial veins, as well as the median, ulnar, and radial nerves. At 11 months, the patient had protective sensation to his hand and early intrinsic function but required a wrist arthrodesis and tendon transfers for elbow and shoulder flexion.[2] Technologic advances and the use of the operating microscope have enabled surgeons to replant other body parts, including the thumb, fingers, ear, scalp, facial parts, and genitalia.[3-27]

● PATIENT EVALUATION AND SELECTION

Not all amputees benefit from or are candidates for replantation.[28] The decision to replant a severed part is influenced by many factors, including the importance of the part, the level of injury, the expected return of function, and the mechanism of injury.[29-31] Replantation is indicated for thumb amputation at any level, multiple finger amputations, single-digit amputations distal to the flexor superficialis insertion, and amputations through the carpus, wrist, and the distal forearm (Figure 54-1).[32-36] Above elbow replantation should be attempted for elbow preservation, even though the chance for nerve recovery is low. If subsequent nerve regeneration is inadequate after upper arm replantation, a revision amputation at the mid-forearm level can then allow for a below elbow prosthesis.[32] A below elbow prosthesis with a gravity-activated grip is more functional than an above elbow prosthesis. Less functional recovery is expected for replantations at certain levels, including amputations proximal to the flexor superficialis insertion within zone II of the fingers and at the muscle belly and elbow level.

Amputations in zone II proximal to the sublimus insertion are relatively contraindicated since the patient is often left with marked finger stiffness with minimal or no functional benefit and require prolonged rehabilitation that significantly delay return to work.[4] There are cultural differences, however, that justify replantation. In many Asian societies, it is important to have five digits because a common form of punishment for criminals in some countries is to amputate a finger. Replantation of zone II finger amputations have been justified in Japan, so that patients can avoid being confused with Japanese mafia members (Yakuza) who have amputated their fingers as a symbol of devotion to their mob bosses.

Perhaps, the most predictive indicator for success with replantation is the mechanism of injury. O'Brien has demonstrated significantly higher success rates with replantation of guillotine versus avulsion amputations.[31] It may be unrealistic to expect to successfully replant severely crushed and mangled body parts. Avulsion injuries with traction along the neurovascular bundles create intimal tears and disruption of small branches to the skin. Small hematomas in the skin along the course of the neurovascular bundle

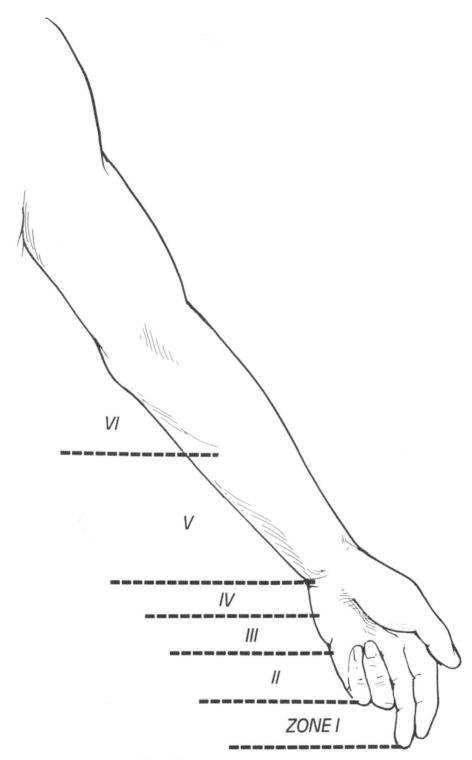

● FIGURE 54-1. Levels of replantation.

are known as the "red line" sign. It heralds an injury to the neurovascular bundle. Replantations of amputated digits that exhibit the red line sign are often fraught with failure because even though the anastomosis may be patent there is no flow of arterial blood to the skin. Another indication of injury to the vessels of an amputated digit is the "ribbon" sign. The ribbon sign is an indication of torsion and stretch on a vessel. The vessel resembles a ribbon that has been stretched and curled for decoration on a wrapped gift. Vessels that have the ribbon sign will often thrombose due to the damage to the intima. When a replantation is attempted in digits with the ribbon sign, vein grafting proximal and distal to this zone of injury is necessary. If this intimal injury extends distal to the trifurcation of the

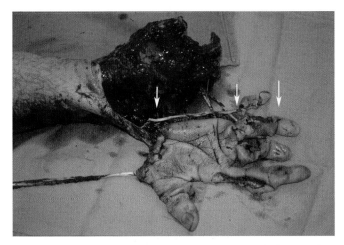

● FIGURE 54-2. This patient degloved hand in log crusher splitter, resulting in multilevel neurovascular and bone injuries.

digital artery, vein grafting distal to the zone of injury is not possible, which precludes an attempt at replantation.

Two other relative contraindications to replantation include multiple level injuries (Figure 54-2) and mentally unstable patients. The only absolute contraindication to replantation exists when associated injuries or preexisting illness prevent a prolonged and complex operation. In this circumstance, temporary ectopic implantation of the amputated part has been described for preservation of the amputated extremity before eventual elective replantation later.[6,37,38]

● PATIENT PREPARATION

Replantation of arms, hands, digits, or even fingertips has become common in various institutions. Physicians, paramedics, and patients are informed regarding the possibility of replantation of amputated body parts. Because of this, it is common for the patient to bring the part to the emergency room. Even if not replantable, this amputated part can provide a valuable tissue source for reconstruction. The amputated part should be wrapped in a saline-moistened gauze sponge and placed in a sealed plastic bag which is kept on ice. The amputated part should not be placed directly on ice because this can result in frostbite damage to the vessels.[39] The part should not be immersed in water because this has been demonstrated by Urbaniak et al. to make digital vessel repair more difficult and less reliable, because of cob webbing of the intima.[40,41] Bleeding vessels in the stump should not be clamped. Hemostatic control of the stump can be achieved with a compressive dressing and elevation.

The recommended ischemia times for reliable success with replantation are 12 hours of warm and 24 hours of cold ischemia for the digits, and 6 hours of warm and 12 hours of cold ischemia for major replantations with large amounts of muscle. Reports of successful replantation after longer ischemia times do exist however.[7,42–45] Minimizing ischemia time is more critical in replantation levels that

are proximal to the digits. In such cases, a temporary arterial shunt to the amputated limb may be beneficial.[6,37,38]

Before surgery, radiographs of the amputated parts and the stump should be performed to determine the levels of injury and suitability for replantation. Both parts should be photographed for documentation. An informed consent should be obtained, discussing the pros and cons with the patient and family regarding the failure rates, length of rehabilitation, and realistic expectations of sensation, mobility, and function. The preoperative preparation of the patient should also include consideration for prophylactic antibiotics, updating the patient's tetanus, fluid resuscitation to prevent hypotension, warming the patient to prevent hypothermia and vasoconstriction/spasm, Foley insertion for volume monitoring, and protection for pressure points during an expected long operation.

● TECHNIQUE

Preparation of the Amputated Part

The preparation of the amputated part can be initiated before the patient is brought to the operating room. This preparation is performed on a back table under sterile conditions in the operating room. The use of a microscope assists with the assessment of the digital vessels. Signs of arterial damage should be noted, including the telescope, cobweb, and ribbons signs, or terminal thrombosis, which would require resecting the damaged section of the vessel and harvesting a vein graft. This vein graft should be harvested prior to osteosynthesis to minimize warm ischemia time. If the amputated part is grossly contaminated, it should be cleansed gently with normal saline irrigation and foreign material should be removed. Care must be taken not to further injure the digital vessels or soft tissue. The neurovascular structures of the fingers are exposed with bilateral longitudinal incisions in the midaxial line instead of volar zig-zag incisions which could complicate amputation stump skin viability should the replant fail. Dorsal incisions may be required to expose the dorsal veins. Once these neurovascular structures have been identified, labeling with 9-0 nylon sutures or hemoclips can facilitate and expedite identification at the time of coaptation.

Many surgeons prefer to shorten the bone to avoid the potential need for arterial, venous, and nerve grafts later. The tagged neurovascular structures are gently relocated during the bone shortening, which can usually be safely performed with a rongeur. Approximately, 5 to 10 mm of bone shortening may be necessary for tension-free vessel repairs. The bone shortening should be performed on the amputated part if possible to retain length should the replant fail. Bone can be resected on the stump side for the fingers, but not for the thumb where length preservation is more critical, or if the amputation level is near the joint on the amputated part. Hand function is compromised with thumb loss proximal to the interphalangeal (IP) joint. If the amputation level is through the joint, fusion in the functional position is required. Primary implant arthroplasty has been described in replantation but there is an increased risk for infection.[46] Retrograde Kirschner (K-) wires or intraosseous wires can then be placed through the bone on the amputated part.

Preparation of the Stump

Usually there is enough time before the patient is transported to the operating room for preparation of the amputated part. Alternatively, a second team can be recruited to begin the preparation of the stump. The neurovascular structures are identified, isolated, and tagged on the stump side under tourniquet control. Before the arterial anastomosis, the tourniquet is deflated to assess inflow pressure by the spurting of blood from the proximal artery.[47] If the spurt is inadequate, additional proximal vessel shortening is required. Furthermore, in preparing the stump, exposure of the proximal flexor tendon for placement of a core suture is easier at this point than after bone fixation.

The order for repairing the various structures is individualized. The sequence of repairing the bone, extensor, veins, dorsal skin, artery, nerve, and flexor is preferred, as it efficiently allows for repairing all the dorsal structures before the volar structures, to reduce warm ischemia time.[31] If the warm ischemia time is unusually long, the artery can be repaired earlier.

Osteosynthesis

Techniques of osteosynthesis vary: many surgeons prefer crossed K-wires, because they are quick and safe. However, union rates have been reported to be better with intraosseous wires, either in combination with a K-wire or as 90-90 wires.[8,48] Ninety-ninety wires consist of two intraosseous wires placed perpendicular to each other.

Extensor Tendon Repair and Dorsal Vein Repair

After the osteosynthesis, the hand is pronated and the extensor tendon is repaired next. If the amputation is at the proximal phalanx level, it is important to repair the lateral bands to prevent loss of extension at the IP joints. Next, the dorsal veins are repaired. At least two veins should be repaired in finger replantations, especially for replantations proximal to the proximal IP joint. Dorsal veins are preferred because they are larger and do not interfere with subsequent repair of volar structures (Figure 54-3). If the injury is very distal, arterial repair first may be required, because the veins become smaller and more difficult to identify, and may be easier to locate by back bleeding. If a dorsal vein cannot be located in the amputated part, creation of an arterial venous communication can be considered to avoid venous compromise. Because veins stretch easier than arteries, vein grafts are rarely needed for venous repairs. Once the dorsal structures have been repaired, the dorsal skin is loosely approximated with a few small-caliber, simple interrupted sutures.

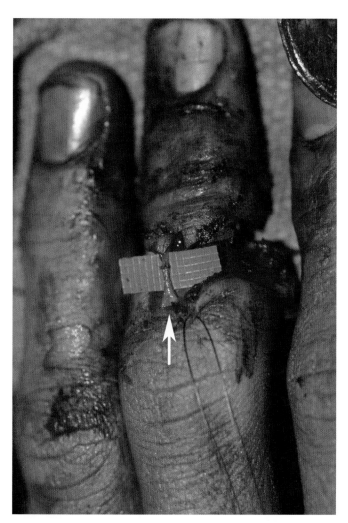

● **FIGURE 54-3.** An example of a dorsal vein repair with 10-0 nylon suture in simple interrupted fashion over the previously repaired extensor tendon.

Digital Artery Repair

The hand is then supinated to repair the injured volar structures. At least one digital artery is repaired. Several anastomotic techniques have been described. One described technique of microvascular repair involves applying a microvascular approximating clamp then placing the first two sutures at 10 o'clock and 2 o'clock, then at 12 o'clock; and then the vessel is turned 180 degrees and additional simple interrupted sutures are placed in sequence. The last two or three sutures are tied at the end to avoid catching the back wall with the final sutures, which would lead to vessel thrombosis. After the completion of the digital artery repairs, the tourniquet is deflated and the clamps are removed. The patency of the arterial anastomosis can be assessed using a patency test or flicker test and checking the capillary refill of the replanted part and bleeding after pinprick. If arterial flow seems inadequate, one should confirm that the patient has adequate blood pressure and volume, and that the tourniquet actually has been deflated. Bathing the vessel with papaverine, lidocaine, magnesium sulfate, and warm irrigation has been described to counteract the vasospasm.[9] The hand can even be placed in the dependent position to increase inflow pressure with gravity.[49] **The surgeon would allow at least 10 minutes observation time for resolution of vasospasm before manipulating the anastomosis with a "milk test" to demonstrate patency. It is accomplished with two vascular forceps. The first forceps is placed just distal to the anastomosis. The second forceps is used to milk blood away from the distal aspect of the first forceps, and is closed leaving a flat, collapsed vessel. The first forceps is then released. Distention of the vessel distal to the anastomosis confirms that the anastomosis is open.** If the milk test is abnormal or if petechiae of the measles sign or ballooning of the sausage sign is encountered, suspect thrombosis and redo the anastomosis.[47,50] Frequently, in redoing the anastomosis, further vessel resection is necessary. If the additional vessel resection places the vessel repair under tension, an interposition vein graft is required. Also, a second artery should be repaired as a safeguard measure.

Digital Nerve Repair

Located superficial and volar to the digital arteries, the digital nerves are coapted next. This can be performed before or after the tourniquet has been deflated. The epineurial nerve repair technique is preferred and can be achieved with as few as three sutures. A nerve conduit or graft is required if one is unable to repair the nerve primarily. Of the upper extremity nerve graft donors, the posterior interosseous nerve is preferred over the medial antebrachial nerve because this avoids a donor sensory deficit, but it only yields a small 1-cm graft and is only suitable at the distal interphalangeal level. Alternatively, a vein graft or polyglycolic acid conduit can be used for small defects of 2 cm or less.

Flexor Tendon Repair

At this point, the flexor tendon is repaired, tying the previously placed proximal and distal core sutures. Performing the tendon repair later permits finger extension, giving better exposure for the microsurgical repair of the digital arteries and digital nerves.

Arterial Interposition Vein Graft

Common indications for arterial interposition vein grafts include thumb replantations, ring avulsions, segmental artery loss, or the need to extend outside the zone of injury because of intimal trauma.[51-53] Potential vein graft harvest sites for distal digit replantations include the palmar forearm and wrist. The wrist is preferred by many because the volar wrist veins match the digital vessel caliber (Figure 54-4).[5,54-56] The leg or contralateral arm may be used to harvest vein grafts for major

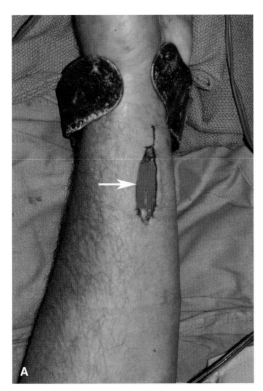 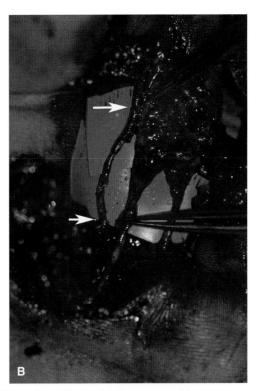

● **FIGURE 54-4.** (A) Harvesting a vein graft from the volar distal forearm provides an appropriate size match for a proper digital artery defect. (B) Notice the size match of a vein graft harvested from the palmer distal forearm being used to interpose this arterial defect between the two forceps.

replantations of the hand, forearm, or multiple fingers, with a second team working simultaneously. Vein grafts must be reversed for arterial interposition because of valves within the veins.

Thumb Replantation

In the thumb, the ulnar digital artery is usually of larger caliber than the radial digital artery.[57,58] Arterial revascularization in thumb replantation is therefore more reliable when based on the ulnar digital artery. This vessel is difficult to expose for the microsurgical anastomosis, however, and requires extreme arm pronation or supination, which can result in having to work at different levels of microscopic focus. This situation can be avoided by either repairing the ulnar digital artery before the osteosynthesis or by using an arterial interposition graft.

If the amputation level is distal to the metacarpophalangeal (MCP) joint and the proximal end of the ulnar aspect digital artery is well exposed, a primary arterial anastomosis can sometimes be performed without the need for a graft. **A technique that has been described to optimize exposure of the ulnar digital artery during the microanastomosis involves performing the microanastomosis before the osteosynthesis.**[10,11] The bone shortening and retrograde K-wires are placed first. The ulnar digital artery and nerve are then repaired with the hand in supination, before the osteosynthesis, which provides a better angle for the microscope and exposure for the anastomosis without having to work in and out of the field of focus. The bone ends are then aligned and the osteosynthesis is carefully completed. The digital artery clamps are left in place until the extensor tendon and dorsal veins are repaired. The flexor tendon core sutures are now tied. Then, digital artery and vein clamps are carefully removed to establish arterial inflow and venous outflow.

When the thumb has been amputated at or near the MCP joint and the proximal ulnar digital artery has retracted and is difficult to expose, a vein graft can be used from the ulnar digital artery distally to the radial artery in the snuffbox, end to side (Figure 54-5). Interposition vein grafting of the thumb has been shown to increase survival rates for thumb replantation two- to threefold. In using this vein graft to the radial artery technique for replantation for the thumb, the vein graft is repaired to the distal ulnar artery first on the back table, which provides a flat surface for the microsurgery (Figure 54-6). The vein graft is then carefully pulled through the subcutaneous tunnel to the radial artery in the snuffbox. The digital nerves also can be repaired at this point with better exposure before the osteosynthesis. Then, the osteosynthesis is carefully performed by passing the previously placed K-wires retrograde through the proximal bone. At this point, the extensor tendon and dorsal veins are repaired. The vein graft is then repaired end to side to the radial artery in the snuffbox. In performing thumb replant procedures one should have a low threshold for shortening the

bone to avoid tension on the digital nerves. This provides the best chance for return of sensation, which is critical to thumb function. Bone shortening or IP fusion should be considered for the thumb because these patients achieve useful motion of the thumb through the MCP and basilar joints and this obviates the need for repairing the flexor pollicis longus.

Multiple Finger Replantations

In multiple finger replantations, the finger with the best chance for successful replantation, best expected recovery, and best contribution to function should be repaired first. If all the fingers are injured at the same level and with the same chance for success, the authors prefer to repair the middle finger, then index finger, then ring finger, and finally the small finger (Figure 54-7). If the index finger is stiff or insensate, the patient will bypass this to use the middle finger. When all the fingers are stiff, the index finger can actually impede the function and opposition of the other fingers to the thumb. **Because it is essential to minimize ischemia time with multiple digit replantations, each finger is replanted separately.** The amputated fingers should be brought to the operating room as soon as possible, where the digital vessels, nerves and tendons can be identified and tagged with sutures or clips, to save time and minimize ischemia. The order for repairs can be improvised with multiple replantations. Initially, the osteosynthesis, extensor tendon, one dorsal vein, and one digital artery can be repaired for each finger to minimize overall ischemia time. Another dorsal vein, the digital nerves and flexor tendon core suture can be repaired later, once the blood flow to the fingers has been reestablished.

Major Limb Replantation

The order of the replant procedure is modified for major replantations of the hand and upper extremity. **Early use of arterial shunting has been described to minimize muscle ischemia time.**[6,38,49] It is critical to minimize warm ischemia time to less than 4 hours to avoid muscle necrosis. Intravenous tubing or carotid shunts can be used to infuse and return blood to and from the amputated part (Figure 54-8). Fasciotomies are required with major limb replantation and can be performed during the shunting reperfusion to save time. Bone shortening may avoid the need for nerve and vein grafting and allow for soft tissue closure over the repairs. With humeral level replantations, the brachial artery and brachial venae commitante are repaired. The ulnar, median, and radial nerves are repaired. The skin is lightly re-approximated. Skin grafts are usually required for definitive closure. These upper extremity replantations may require several operating room debridements at 48-hour intervals to remove devascularized nonviable muscle at the amputation level. Amputations at this level often denervate the biceps muscles and later require latissimus or pectoralis muscle transfers to provide for active elbow flexion.

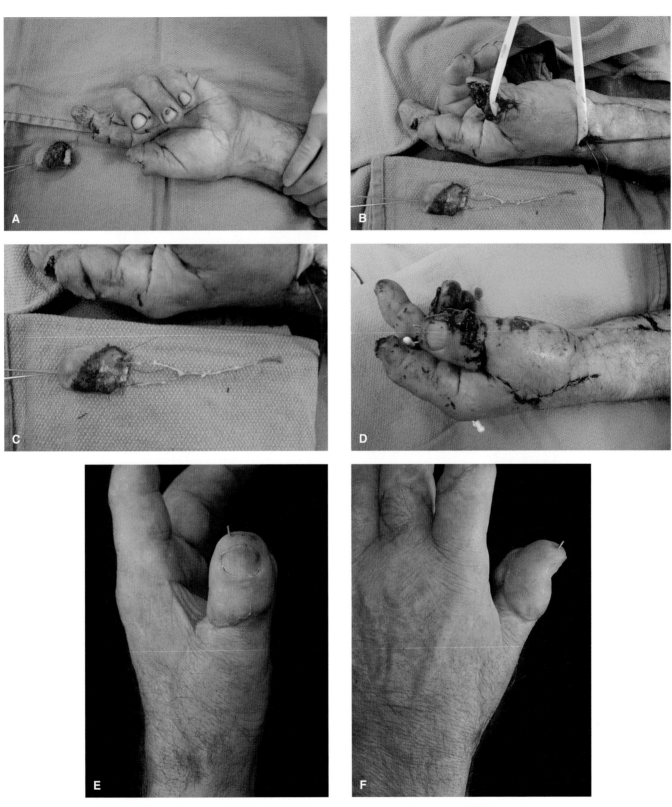

● **FIGURE 54-5.** This patient had his thumb amputated by a saw. (A) There was an oblique flap that obstructed the view of the ulnar digital artery. A digital artery graft was therefore used. (B) The vein graft was harvested from the distal volar wrist. (C) The graft was reversed and repaired to the ulnar digital artery on the back table, which provided a uniform field of focus and flat resting surface for the microsurgery. Then the proximal end of the vein graft was carefully passed into the snuffbox. The ulnar digital nerve was repaired. (D) Then the osteosynthesis was completed in retrograde fashion passing K-wires distal to proximal. Then the radial digital nerve and two dorsal veins were repaired. The flexor and extensors did not require repair as the IP joint was fused. (E, F) These photos demonstrate the thumb replant after suture removal at 8 weeks post replant.

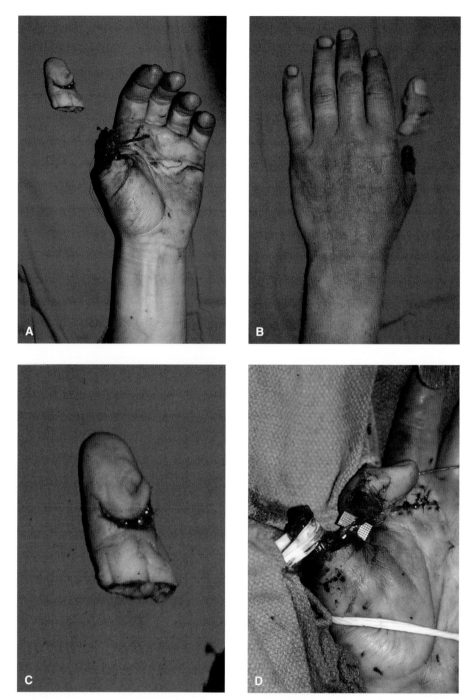

● FIGURE 54-6. (A, B) This patient amputated his thumb with a rope in a boating accident. The replantation actually involved repairs at two levels. First K-wires were placed in the amputated part. (C) The structures were identified on the back table and the bone was shortened. Repairs were performed on the amputated part first on the back table. Two dorsal veins, the ulnar aspect digital artery and nerve, were repaired in the amputated part with the microscope on the back table. (D) The ulnar aspect digital artery of the amputated part was repaired to the proximal end of the ulnar aspect digital artery on the stump side with the microscope before osteosynthesis to avoid the struggle for exposure often requiring extreme hand pronation. The digital nerve was repaired. The osteosynthesis was performed carefully passing the K-wires distal to proximal.

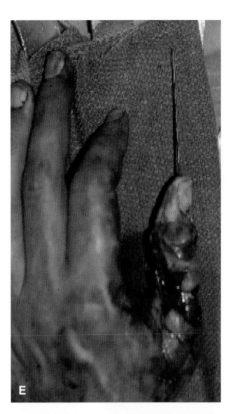

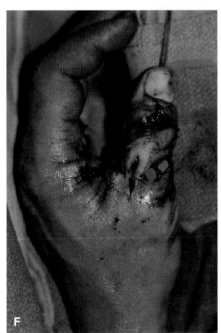

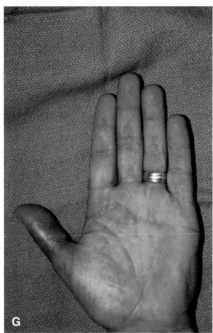

● FIGURE 54-6. (*continued*) (E, F) The amputated part, extensor pollicis longus
tendon, and two dorsal veins were repaired to the stump, before removing digital artery
clamps proximal and distal to the microanastomosis. Leaving the clamps maintains
hemostatic control and better exposure for the vein repairs. Lastly, the flexor pollicis
longus tendon core sutures are carefully tied and the skin is loosely approximated.
(G) This photo shows survival of the thumb replant at 12 weeks postoperative.

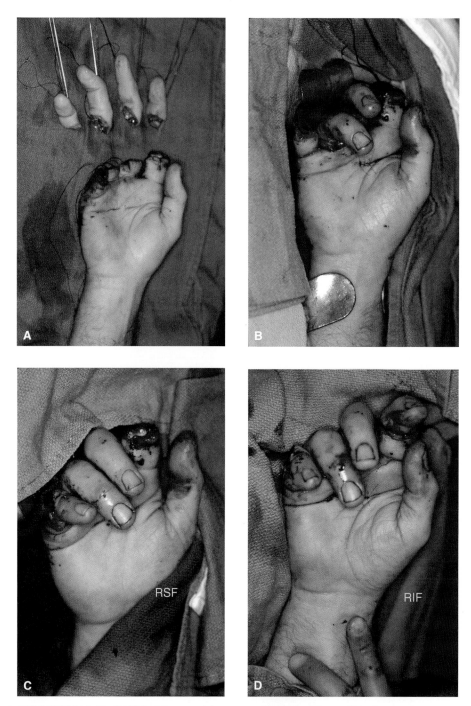

● **FIGURE 54-7.** (A) This 50-year-old man amputated all four of his fingers in a printing press at work. (B–D) Each finger is replanted separately to minimize warm ischemia time. Two dorsal veins and one digital artery were repaired for each finger in the dorsal and volar sequence described by **O'Brien**.[31] The fingers were replanted in order of functional importance. We repaired this patient's index finger last because the amputation level was the proximal interphalangeal level and would be less functional. All four replantations survived.

Hand Replantation

In performing hand replantations, the vessels, nerves, and tendons are identified and tagged and K-wires are placed in the retrograde fashion into the amputated part. This can be done prior to the patient being transported to the operating room, at the back table, shortening operative time. Similarly, the ischemia time can be minimized by shunting, during which fasciotomies can and should be performed prophylactically. **The most time-consuming component of a hand replant is tendon repairs. The exposure**

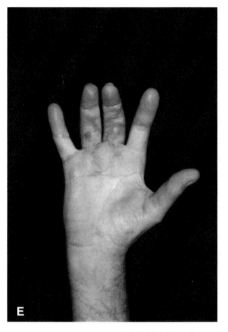
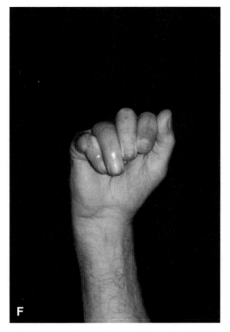
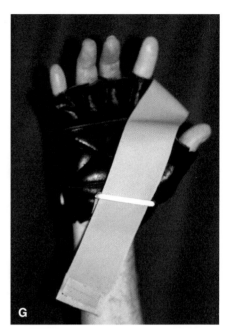

● **FIGURE 54-7.** (*continued*) (E, F) He did require a tenolysis procedure and correctional osteotomy of index finger to regain greater than 50% total active motion. (G) He even created this glove, which he uses to help lift weights.

of the proximal flexor tendon ends can be optimized by placing a longitudinal incision up the midportion of the forearm. Also, tagging of the proximal and distal flexor tendon ends before the osteosynthesis can facilitate the repair of the flexor tendons later. It is important to understand the stacked array of the flexor tendons with the middle and ring flexor digitorum sublimis tendon volar to the index and small finger superficialis flexors. Replantation of hand amputations at the wrist level may necessitate bone shortening with a proximal row carpectomy to avoid nerve and vein grafts. Overall, the ulnar and radial arteries, four veins, median, ulnar, and superficial radial nerves are repaired as well as many tendons as possible. At least the four flexor digitorum profundus tendons, flexor carpi radialis, flexor carpi ulnaris, four extensor digiti communis tendons, extensor carpi ulnaris, extensor carpi radialis, extensor pollicis longus, and flexor pollicis longus should be performed. In general, replantations at this level can achieve very good results.

● **COMPLICATIONS**

Postoperative care has traditionally included warming the patient's room to avoid vasospasm and positioning the extremity at the heart level to minimize edema but not compromise arterial or venous flow. Anticoagulation is generally not needed. Several investigators recommend the routine use of aspirin and dextran with replantation[31,59,60] and therapeutic heparin for crush avulsion injuries.[49,59]

Depending on the mechanism of injury, antibiotics may be continued. Patients are encouraged to abstain from smoking and caffeine use for 1 month.[61,62] The replanted part is monitored by checking color, capillary refill, tissue turgor, and temperature. Sympathetic blocks have been described for high-risk replantations after crush avulsion injuries.[47] Venous insufficiency is considered to be the most common cause for replantation failure. Venous congestion should be suspected with rapid capillary refill, increased tissue turgor, or bleeding of wound edges.[59] Treatment of venous congestion includes removal of tight dressings and sutures and increasing elevation to promote venous drainage with gravity. Leeches are also effective at treating venous congestion in replantation. Nail plate removal and application of a heparin-soaked sponge to the nail bed has been described for distal replantations when a vein cannot be repaired and the patient refuses leeches.[63] Operative revision can be considered, but is less successful than re-exploration for arterial insufficiency. Arterial insufficiency is suggested by decreased capillary refill, tissue turgor, and temperature. Treatment of arterial insufficiency includes removal of potentially constricting dressing and tight sutures, decreasing extremity elevation to promote inflow with gravity, and sympathetic blockade. Finally, early operative intervention can be considered if there is no improvement with the above measures. Re-exploration to correct arterial insufficiency has been reported to be successful in 50% of return visits.[31,59] **The most common complication of a digit replant is cold intolerance. The**

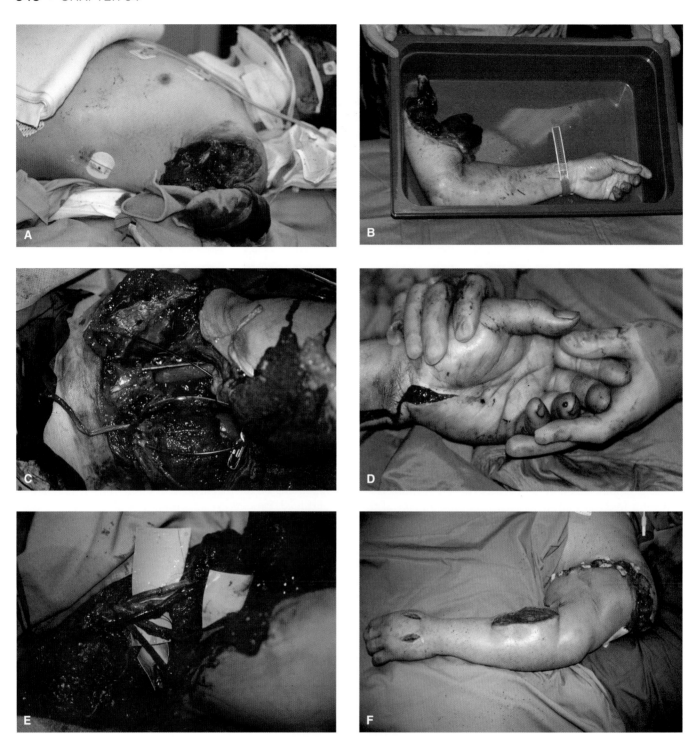

● FIGURE 54-8. (A, B) This 40-year-old man amputated his left arm in a rollover car accident. His amputated arm was found in a ditch, 30 feet in front of him and his upside-down car. The arm was brought to the operating room before the patient was extensively irrigated. Neurovascular structures to be repaired were identified and labeled. The humerus was shortened enough to allow for skin approximation over the repairs. (C) Then, osteosynthesis was performed with a 4.0 compression plate. The use of carotid shunts to and from the amputated part minimized the total ischemia time to 3 hours. (D) During this shunting reperfusion, forearm and hand fasciotomies were performed. (E) Then, the brachial artery was repaired. Then, the median, ulnar and radial nerves were coapted. (F) At 48-hour intervals for 2 weeks, he returned to the operating room for debridement of portion of the triceps, distal deltoid, and biceps muscles and skin edges.

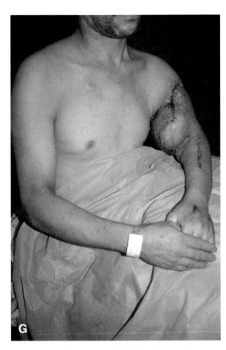

● **FIGURE 54-8.** (*continued*) (G) At 2 months post-operatively, he did not have any open areas or evidence of nerve regeneration. He later required a muscle transfer with latissimus dorsi for active elbow flexion.

most common complication of a major limb replant is systemic infection from devitalized muscle. If leeches are required, patients need to be prophylactically treated with antibiotics active against *Aeromonas hydrophila*, which is endogenous to the leech gut.

● OUTCOMES AND ASSESSMENT

The overall success rates for replantation approach 80%. In reviewing a number of retrospective reports with large patient numbers, these success rates range from 54% to 82%. The Overall, success rates are significantly higher for replantations of guillotine (77%) versus crush amputations (49%).[31,59] Several studies have demonstrated that approximately 50% achieve two-point discrimination less than 10 mm.[64-68] Glickman reviewed 12 series of digit

replantations conducted between 1977 and 1989. Of the 327 fingers and 87 thumbs successfully replanted, overall mean two-point discrimination was 12 mm in fingers and 11 mm in thumbs.[69] In general, younger patients with distal guillotine amputations experienced better return of sensation. Several studies have determined the average replant to achieve 50% of normal function (ie, 50% total active motion and 50% grip strength).[66,70-72] Return of function was worse for zone II injuries and for patients of advanced age. Russell published the largest review of major limb replantations and found 11/24 achieved greater than 50% total active motion, and 19/24 patients were satisfied with the function and appearance of their replanted part.[35]

Jupiter showed the function of replanted digits could be significantly improved with tenolysis procedures.[73] In his review, the total active motion of 37 replanted digits was significantly improved ($P < 0.001$) with tenolysis and no digits were lost.[73]

● SUMMARY

With the evolution of microsurgical techniques, replantation has become a common approach to the treatment of amputation and devascularizing injuries, potentially providing superior results to other reconstructive options. Replantation and revascularization should be attempted for thumb, multiple digit, hand, wrist, and upper arm injuries. Techniques which allow for optimizing microsurgical exposure, back table microsurgery, rituals for preparation, techniques for minimizing ischemia times, and avoiding the need for grafts can maximize success rates and functional return for amputation and devascularizing injuries. Patient satisfaction rests on their level of expectation as defined and explained in the preoperative discussion and informed consent. Studies have demonstrated patients can be expected to achieve 50% function and 50% sensation of the replanted body part. Initially, all that was amputated was replanted, as surgeons adopted the philosophy of George C. Ross (1843-1892): "Any fool can cut off an arm or leg but it takes a surgeon to save one." However, more than 50 years after the first replant in 1962, we recognize the ultimate goal—not merely to preserve all living tissue through nonselective replantation, but rather to preserve one's quality of life by improving their function and appearance.

REFERENCES

1. Malt RA, McKhann CF. Replantation of severed arms. *JAMA.* 1964;189(10):716–722.

2. Malt RA, Remensnyder JP, Harris WH. Long term utility of replanted arms. *Ann Surg.* 1972;176(3):334–342.

3. Tsai TM. Experimental and clinical application of microvascular surgery. *Ann Surg.* 1973;181(2):169–177.

4. Urbaniak JR, Roth JH, Nunley JA. The results of replantation after amputation of a single finger. *J Bone Joint Surg Am.* 1985;67A(4):611–619.

5. Van Beek AL. Kutz JE, Zook EG. Importance of the ribbon sign indicating unsuitability for the vessel in replanting a finger. *Plat Reconstr Surg.* 1973;61(1):32–38.

6. Godina M, Bazec J, Baraga A. Salvage of the mutilated upper extremity with temporary ectopic implantation of the undamaged part. *Plast Reconstr Surg.* 1986;78(3):295–299.

7. Chiu HY, Chen MT. Revascularization of digits after thirty-three hours of warm ischemia time a case report. *J Hand Surg.* 1984;9A(1):63–67.

8. Lister G. Intraosseous wiring of the digital skeleton. *J Hand Surg Am.* 1978;3(5):427–435.

9. Swartz WA, Brink RR, Buncke HJ. Prevention of thrombosis in arterial and venous microanastomosis by using topical agents. *Plast Reconstr Surg.* 1976;58(4):478–481.

10. Caffee HH. Improved exposure for arterial repair in thumb replantation. *J Hand Surg Am.* 1984;10A(3):416.

11. Shafiroff BB, Palmer AK. Simplified technique for replantation for the thumb. *J Hand Surg Am.* 1981;6(6):623–624.

12. Kutz JE, Sinclair SW, Rao V, Carler A. Cross hand replantation: preliminary case report. *J Microsurg.* 1982;3:251–254.

13. Sixth People's Hospital. Replantation Surgery in China. Report of the American replantation mission to China. *Plast Reconstr Surg.* 1973;52(5):476–489.

14. Baudet J. Successful replantation of severed ear parts. *Plast Reconstr Surg.* 1973;51:82.

15. Chen CW Chien YC, Pao YS. Salvage of the forearm following complete traumatic amputation: report of a case. *Chin Med J.* 1963;82:632.

16. Chen ZW, Zen BF. Replantation of the lower extremity. *Clin Plast Surg.* 1983;10(1):103–113.

17. Cohen BE, May JW Jr. Successful clinical replantation of an amputated penis by microneurovascular repair: case report. *Plast Reconstr Surg.* 1974;59:276–279.

18. Gayle LB, Lineaweaver WC, Buncke GM, et al. Lower extremity replantation. *Clin Plast Surg.* 1991;18(3):437–447.

19. Kleinert HE, Kasdan ML. Anastamosis of digital vessels. *J Ky Med Assoc.* 1965;63:106–108.

20. Komatsu S, Tamai S. Successful replantation of a completely cut-off thumb. *Plast Reconstr Surg.* 1968;42:375–376.

21. Lu M. Successful replacement of avulsed scalp. *Plast Reconstr Surg.* 1967;43:231.

22. Nahai F, Hayhurst JN, Silibian AH. Microvascular surgery in avulsive trauma to the external vascular surgery in avulsive trauma to the external ear. *Clin Plast Surg.* 1978;5:423.

23. Nahai F, Herteau J, Vasconez LO. Replantation of entire scalp and ear by microvascular anastomoses of only one artery and vein. *Br J Plast Surg.* 1978;31:339.

24. Norman JJ. Survival of large replanted segment of upper lip and nose. *Plast Reconstr Surg.* 1976;58:623.

25. Serafin D, Kutz JE, Kleinert HE. Replantation of completely amputated distal thumb without venous anastomosis. *Plast Reconstr Surg.* 1973;52(5):579–582.

26. Walton RL, Beahm EK, Brown RE, et al. Microsurgical replantation of lip: a multi-institutional experience. *Plast Reconstr Surg.* 1998;102(2):358–368.

27. Wilhelmi BJ, Kang RH, Movassaghi K, et al. First successful replantation of face and scalp with single-artery repair: Model for face and scalp transplantation. *Ann Plast Surg.* 2003; 50(5):535–540.

28. Wilhelmi BJ, Lee WPA, Pagensteert GI, et al. Replantation of the mutilated hand. *Hand Clin.* 2003;19(1):89–120.

29. Buncke HJ, Alpert BS, Johnson-Giebink R. Digital replantation. *Surg Clin North Am.* 1981;61(2):383–392.

30. Kleinert HE, Juhala CA, Tsai TM, Van Beek A. Digital replantation selection, technique, and results. Symposium on replantation and reconstructive microsurgery. *Orthop Clinics North Am.* 1977;8(2):309–318.

31. O'Brien B. Replantation surgery. *Clin Plast Surg.* 1974;1(3): 405–426.

32. Brown RW. The rational selection of treatment for upper extremity amputations. *Orthop Clin North Am.* 1981;12(4): 843–948.

33. May JW Jr, Toth BA, Gardner M. Digital replantation distal to the proximal interphalangeal joint. *J Hand Surg Am.* 1982;7(2):161–165.

34. Meyer VE. Hand amputations proximal but close to the wrist joint: prime candidates for reattachment. *J Hand Surg Am.* 1985;10(6 Pt 2):989–991.

35. Russell RC, O'Brien BM, Morrison WA, et al. The late functional results of upper limb revascularization and replantation. *J Hand Surg Am.* 1984;9A(5):623–633.

36. Vanstraelen P, Papini RP, Sykes PJ, Milling MA. The functional results of hand replantation. The Chepstow experience. *J Hand Surg Br.* 1993;18(5):556–564.

37. Bajec J, Grossman JA, Gilbert D, Williams MM. Upper extremity preservation before replantation. *J Hand Surg Am.* 1987;12(2):321–322.

38. Chernofsky NA, Sauer PF. Temporary ectopic implantation. *J Hand Surg Am.* 1990;15(6):910–914.

39. Hayhurst JW, O'Brien BM, Ishida H, Baxter TJ. Experimental digital replantation after prolonged cooling. *Hand.* 1974;6(2):134–141.

40. Usui M, Ishii S, Muramatsu I, Takahata N. An experimental study on replantation toxemia. The effect of hypothermia on an amputated limb. *J Hand Surg Am.* 1978;3(6):589–595.

41. VanGeisen PJ, Seaber AV, Urbaniak JR. Storage of amputated parts prior to replantation an experimental study with rabbit ears. *J Hand Surg Am.* 1983;8(1):60–65.

42. May JW Jr. Digit replantation with full survival after 28 hours cold ischemia. *Plast Reconstr Surg.* 1981;67(4):566.

43. May JW Jr, Hergrueter CA, Hanson RH. Seven digit replantation digit survival after 39 hours cold ischemia. *Plast Reconstr Surg.* 1986;78(4):522–523.

44. Wei FC, Chen HC, Chuang CC. Three successful digital replantation in a patient after 84,86,94 hours cold ischemia time. *Plast Reconstr Surg.* 1988;82(2):346–350.

45. VanderWilde RS, Wood MB, Zeng-gui S. Hand replantation after 54 hours of cold ischemia a case report. *J Hand Surg Am.* 1992;17A(2):217–220.

46. Wray RC, Young VL, Weeks PM. Flexible inplant arthroplassty and finger replantation. *Plast Reconstr Surg.* 1984;74:97.

47. Gallico GG. Replantation and revascualrization of upper extremity. In: McCarthy JG. *Plastic Surgery.* Vol 7. 3rd ed. Philadelphia: WB Saunders; 1990:4355–4383.

48. Whitney TM, Lineaweaver WC, Buncke HJ, Nugent D. Clinical results of bony fixation methods in digital replantation. *J Hand Surg Am.* 1990;15(2):328–334.

49. Goldner RD, Urbaniak JR. Replantation. In: Hotchkiss RN, Pederson WC, Kozin SH, Green DP, eds. *Green's Operative Hand Surgery.* Vol 1. 4th ed. New York: Churchill Livingstone; 1999:1139–1155.

50. Acland R. Signs of patency in small vessel anastomosis. *Surgery.* 1972;72(5):744–748.

51. Comtet JJ, Willems P, Mouret P. Ring injury with bilateral rupture of the digital arteries without skin damage. *J Hand Surg Am.* 1979;4(5):415–416.

52. Schlenker JD, Kleinert HE, Tsai TM. Methods and results of replantation following traumatic amputationj of the thumb in sixty–four patients. *J Hand Surg Am.* 1980;5(1):63–70.

53. Earley MJ, Watson JS. Twenty-four thumb replantation. *J Hand Surg Br.* 1984;9(1):98–102.

54. Beimer E. Vein grafts in microvascular surgery. *Br J Plast Surg.* 1977;30:197–199.

55. Buncke HJ, Alpert B, Shah KG. Microvascular grafting. *Clin Plast Surg.* 1978;5(2):185–194.

56. Urbaniak JR, Evans JP, Bright DS. Microvascular management of ring avulsion injuries. *J Hand Surg Am.* 1981;6(1):25–30.

57. Parks BJ, Arbelaez J, Horner RL. Medical and surgical importance of the arterial blood supply of the thumb. *J Hand Surg Am.* 1978;3(4):383–385.

58. Hamilton RB, O'Brien BM, Morrison A, MacLeod AM. Survival factors in replantation and revascularization for the amputated thumb 10 years experience. *Scand J Plast Reconstr Surg.* 1984;18:163–173.

59. O'Brien BM, Miller GD. Digital reattachment and revascularization. *J Bone Joint Surg Am.* 1973;55(4):714–723.

60. Tamai S. Twenty years' experience of limb replantation—review of 293 upper extremity replants. *J Hand Surg Am.* 1982;7(6):549–556.

61. van Adrichem LN, Hovius SE, van Strik R, van der Meulen JC. The acute effect of cigarette smoking on microcirculation of a replanted digit. *J Hand Surg Am.* 1992;17(2):230–234.

62. American Society for Surgery of Hand. *The Hand: Primary Care of Common Problems.* 2nd ed. New York: Churchill Livingstone; 1990:61.

63. Gordon L, Leitner DW, Buncke HJ, Alpert BS. Partial nail plate removal after digital replantion as an alternative method of venous drainage. *J Hand Surg Am.* 1985;10(3):360–364.

64. Gelberman RH, Urbaniak JR, Bright DS, Levin LS. Digital sensibility following replantation. *J Hand Surg Am.* 1978;3(4):313–319.

65. Poppen NK, McCarroll HR, Doyle JR, Niebauer JJ. Recovery of sensibility after suture of digital nerves. *J Hand Surg Am.* 1979;4(3):212–216.

66. Tark KC, Kin YW, Lee YH, Lew JD. Replantation and revascularization of hands clinical analysis and functional results of 261 cases. *J Hand Surg Am.* 1989;14(1):17–26.

67. Zumiotti A, Ferriera MC. Replantation of digits factors influencing survival and functional results. *Microsurgery.* 1994;15:18–21.

68. Yamauchi S, Nomura S, Yoshimura M, et al. A clinical study of the order and speed of sensory recovery after digital replantation. *J Hand Surg Am.* 1983;8(5):545–549.

69. Glickman LT, Mackinnon SE. Sensory recovery following digital replantation. *Microsurgery.* 1990;11(3):236–242.

70. Matsuda M, Shibahara H, Kato N. Long-term results of replantation of 10 upper extremities. *World J Surg.* 1978;2:603–612.

71. Scott FA, Howar JW, Boswick JA. Recovery of function following replantation and revascularization of amputated hand pars. *J Trauma.* 1981;21(3):204–214.

72. Wei CC, Qing QY, Jia YZ. Extremity replantation. *World J Surg.* 1978;2:513–524.

73. Jupiter JB, Pess GM, Bour CJ. Results of flexor tendon tenolysis after replantation in the hand. *J Hand Surg Am.* 1989;14(1):35–44.

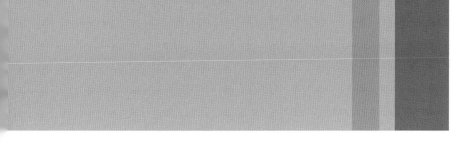

chapter 55

Tendon Transfers

Paul A. Martineau, MD, FRCSC / Thomas Trumble, MD

● BACKGROUND

The indications for tendon transfer are to replace functional motor loss in cases where nerve, tendon, or muscle repair is impossible or unlikely to succeed, to augment diminished and functionally insufficient muscle power, or to restore the delicate balance between the flexor and extensor systems of the hand.

Muscle Physiology

The physiologic parameters of the injured muscle being replaced as well as those of the muscle to be transferred must be taken into account when designing a tendon transfer. The more closely the muscle and tendon to be transferred approximate the physiologic parameters of the muscle being replaced, the more likely the tendon transfer is to succeed.[1]

Muscle Force. Muscle force is proportional to the cross-sectional area of the muscle. In essence, this represents the summation of the force generated by each individual muscle fiber participating in a contraction.

Excursion. Excursion is proportional to the fiber length of the muscle. As a practical guideline, the excursion of different muscles can be estimated using the 3-5-7 rule. Muscles attaching at the level of the wrist have approximately 3 cm of excursion; motor units attaching at the level of the metacarpophalangeal (MCP) joint have 5 cm of excursion; and motor units attaching at the level of the finger tips have 7 cm of excursion.

Work. Work produced by a muscle is proportional to the volume of the muscle. Work integrates muscle excursion and force to produce work capacity.

Muscle Fiber Geometry. Muscle fiber geometry can influence the previously mentioned physiologic parameters. For example, muscle length is proportional to muscle fiber length in spindle-shaped muscles. However, pennate muscles generate more power with shorter fiber length and less excursion because they are made up of a converging pattern of muscle fibers.

Blix Curve. The relationship between muscle length and force was described by Magnus Blix. The Blix curve combines the length tension curves of a muscle being passively stretched and undergoing active contraction. The Blix curve was subsequently modified by Brand to take into account the energy stored by stretching the fiber length of antagonistic muscles (Figure 55-1).[1] The curve reflects the normal function of a muscle, as it would function in a clinical setting with an antagonistic muscle.

● PRINCIPLES OF TENDON TRANSFERS

In 1922, Starr published the principles of tendon transfer surgery.[2] These principles are so frequently reiterated, that their importance may be forgotten. However, these principles remain essential to successful tendon transfers. They can be paraphrased into the following key principles:

1. One muscle, one function: if a muscle is asked to perform more than one task, it will only move the joint which has the tightest attachment.
2. The tendon transfer should have as straight a line of action as possible, and the directions should parallel that of the muscle fibers of the damaged or paralyzed muscle that is to be replaced.

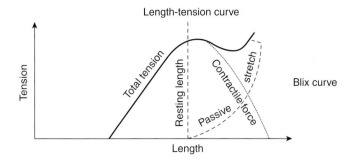

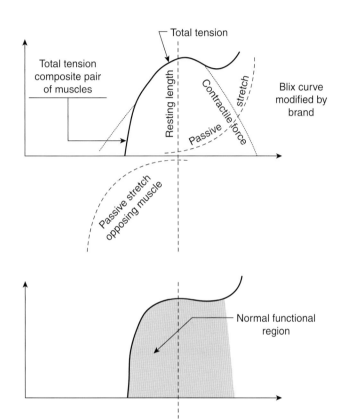

● FIGURE 55-1. The Brand modification of the Blix curve integrates the active contraction and the elastic recoil of the Blix curve as well as the elastic curve of the opposing muscle subtracted from the active output of the primary muscle. *(Redrawn from Trumble TE. Principles of Hand Surgery and Therapy. Philadelphia: WB Saunders; 2000.)*

3. It is important to try to use a muscle that has excursion equal to or greater than that of the injured motor unit. However, it may not always be possible to replace the excursion of some muscles such as flexor digitorum profundus (FDP) due to its tremendous excursion.

4. The muscle should have the capacity of generating a force of contraction similar to that of the injured muscle. Replacing a strong motor with a weak one can result in poor functional outcome.

5. The tenodesis action of the wrist should be preserved. A wrist arthrodesis should only be combined

with tendon transfers as a measure of last resort. The normal tenodesis effect of the wrist passively extends the fingers with the wrist maximally flexed and passively flexes the fingers with wrist extension. The tenodesis effect enhances the function of tendon transfers and even allows many tendon transfers to work statically, even though they do not actively contract.

6. Power versus positional muscles: even though some motors may be quite strong, their main function may be only to provide position. For example, the thumb abductor pollicis brevis (APB) is predominantly a positional muscle to set the thumb in opposition. Once the thumb is placed in this position of opposition for grasping objects, the powerful flexor and adductor muscles then take over to provide the power pinch and grip. Therefore, occasionally even fairly weak motors can be used as transfers to replace the function of positional muscles.

7. Correction of contracture: maximum passive range of motion of the joints must be achieved before any tendon transfer is attempted because no tendon transfer will move a stiff contracted joint.

8. Expendable donor motor for transfer: the harvesting of a donor for transfer must not result in unacceptable loss of function.

9. The effect of the tendon is determined by two variables: tension of the tendon and the moment arm or perpendicular distance of the tendon from the axis of rotation.

10. Tendon transfers should not pass through areas of scar tissue or beneath skin grafts.

11. Synergism between the transferred motor and the original motor may facilitate rehabilitation.

● TENDON TRANSFERS FOR RADIAL, MEDIAN AND ULNAR NERVE PALSIES

Tendon transfers are divided according to the specific motor nerve they are designed to replace. Tendon transfers are then classified into those to reconstruct high (elbow) level injuries to nerve or low (wrist) level injuries to nerve. They can be further subdivided into transfers for single nerve injury or combined nerve injuries.

Radial Nerve Palsy

Low Radial Nerve Palsy. Low radial nerve palsy occurs as a result of injury to the posterior interosseous nerve. Functional loss incurred as a result of this injury includes the loss of finger extension as well thumb extension. These patients maintain active wrist extension albeit with radial deviation of the wrist due to the paralysis of the extensor carpi ulnaris and the unopposed action of the extensor carpi radialis longus (ECRL) and brevis (ECRB). Patients with complete radial nerve palsy have a wrist drop, in addition to having the loss of function of the posterior interosseous nerve innervated motors.

There exist multiple potential options for tendon transfers to reconstruct low radial nerve palsies. The three most common transfers are the Brand, Jones and Boyes transfers.

Technique

Brand Tendon Transfer

Wrist extension	Pronator teres-ECRB
Thumb extension	Palmaris longus-extensor pollicis longus (EPL)
Finger extension	Flexor carpi radialis (FCR)-extensor digitorum communis (EDC)

A longitudinal incision is made along the radial aspect of the forearm. The wrist extensors are retracted radially and the pronator teres is detached from the radius taking a strip of periosteum to provide additional length for the tendon weave. Two passes using a Pulvertaft weave technique provide the maximal amount of strength with a minimal amount of bulk at the repair site. The proper tension is applied to the pronator teres to ECRB transfer site to allow for neutral resting position of the wrist in the flexion/ extension plane with the forearm suspended (Figure 55-2). It is important to note that the transfer of pronator teres to ECRB for wrist extension will produce some degree of radial deviation concurrently with

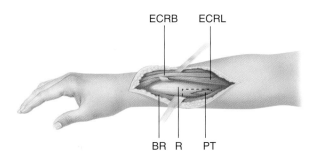

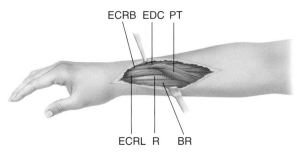

● **FIGURE 55-2.** An incision along the radial border of the forearm allows for exposure of the pronator teres (PT) after the extensor carpi radialis brevis (ECRB) and longus (ECRL) have been retracted dorsally. The pronator teres is woven into the ECRB to reestablish wrist extension. BR, brachioradialis; EDC, extensor digitorum communis; R, radius. (*Redrawn from Trumble TE. Principles of Hand Surgery and Therapy. Philadelphia: WB Saunders; 2000.*)

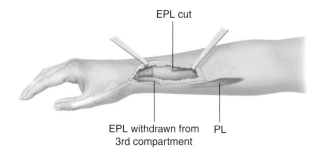

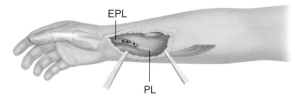

● **FIGURE 55-3.** The extensor pollicis longus tendon is transected proximally while the palmaris longus is transected distally. A Pulvertaft weave is performed securing the palmaris longus to the extensor pollicis longus to reestablish thumb interphalangeal joint extension. (*Redrawn from Trumble TE. Principles of Hand Surgery and Therapy. Philadelphia: WB Saunders; 2000.*)

extension since the ECRB is attached to the radial side of the long finger metacarpal. In order to obtain pure wrist extension, the insertion of the ECRB has to be centralized to the dorsum of the metacarpal.

The palmaris longus to EPL transfer is performed after detaching the palmaris longus from its insertion onto the palmar fascia via a small transverse incision at the level of the distal wrist crease. After dividing the insertion of the palmaris longus, the tendon is mobilized and brought out through a dorsal radial incision. The EPL is identified after the third dorsal compartment is released using a dorsal midline incision. The EPL is divided as far proximally as possible, at its musculotendinous junction, and the sheath of the third dorsal extensor compartment is released such that the tendon may be displaced toward the palmar side of the thumb (Figure 55-3). The proper tension for the transfer is determined by pulling the palmaris longus musculotendinous unit out to full length with traction and marking the underlying tissues with an indelible marker. Next, the palmaris longus musculotendinous unit is allowed to passively retract and this new length is marked. Finally, the EPL tendon is secured to the palmaris longus using a Pulvertaft weave at approximately half the resting length of the palmaris longus tendon. This should result in the palmaris longus to EPL transfer being placed in sufficient tension to bring the interphalangeal (IP) of the thumb to neutral position with the wrist having previously been set in neutral position by the transfer of pronator teres to ECRB.

The FCR to EDC transfer is then performed to provide finger extension. The FCR is identified and detached at the level of the distal wrist crease. It is transferred to the dorsal aspect of the distal forearm (Figure 55-4). In similar fashion

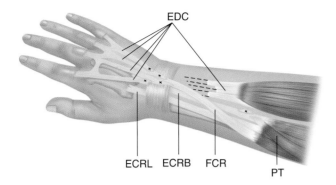

Brand transfer

● **FIGURE 55-4.** The flexor carpi radialis tendon is transferred dorsally and split into two tails so that it can be attached in a side-to-side fashion to all four of the finger extensor tendons. The extensor digiti minimi to the small finger is used as a recipient tendon in this transfer because the extensor digitorum communis to the small finger is frequently absent. (*Redrawn from Trumble TE. Principles of Hand Surgery and Therapy. Philadelphia: WB Saunders; 2000.*)

to the transfers for wrist extension and thumb extension, the tension must be adjusted for the FCR to EDC transfer to provide finger extension. The tension should be set with the fingers fully extended with the wrist at neutral extension, taking care to ensure that all the fingers are in the same amount of extension. The tension must be set in the wrist extensor (pronator teres to ECRB) transfer prior to setting the tension for the finger extension transfer. The extensor digiti minimi should be included with the tendons of EDC because 80% of patients lack a separate tendon of the EDC to extend the small finger. The FCR is split longitudinally and placed on either side of the digit extensor tendons such that they can be sutured together using a mattress stitch in a sandwich configuration technique. Although the sandwich technique is not quite as strong as the Pulvertaft technique, it does allow for more accurate alignment of the digits to avoid having the fingers extending to different degrees and creating scissoring or extensor lag. In cases of irreversible nerve injury, we recommend cutting the digit extensors at the level of the musculotendinous junction to perform an end-to-end tendon transfer instead of a side-to-side transfer.

Jones Tendon Transfer

Wrist extension	Pronator teres-ECRB
Thumb extension	Palmaris longus-EPL
Finger extension	Flexor carpi ulnaris (FCU)-EDC

The only difference between the Jones and Brand transfers lies in the use of the FCU to the digit extensors as opposed to the FCR. Similar to the Brand transfer described above, the tension must first be set in the tendon transfer for wrist extension. The pronator teres to ECRB and palmaris longus to EPL transfers are performed and adjusted and then the FCU is exposed and

detached through a distal incision centered over the pisiform. The FCU tendon is brought out through a separate incision on the ulnar border of the forearm at the junction of the distal and middle thirds of the forearm. The finger extensor tendons are identified using a dorsal midline incision. The FCU is passed into this midline incision and sutured to the EDC using a sandwich technique. Many surgeons are reluctant to sacrifice the FCU to provide finger extension because it is the most powerful motor in the wrist.

Modified Boyes Tendon Transfer

Wrist extension	Pronator teres-ECRB
Thumb extension	Palmaris longus-EPL
Finger extension	Flexor digitorum superficialis (FDS) IV-EDC

The original Boyes tendon transfer used the long finger FDS III for finger extension and the ringer finger FDS IV for extension of the thumb and the index finger.[3] The FDS IV was split and one half was transferred to the EPL and one half to the extensor indicis proprius (EIP) in order to attempt to achieve independent thumb and index finger extension.

The modification of the Boyes tendon transfer presented here takes into consideration Starr's principle that one transferred motor cannot provide two independent functions. Therefore, the modified Boyes transfer does not attempt to combine thumb extension and index finger extension. The palmaris longus to EPL transfer as described for the Brand transfer is used to provide thumb extension with minimal added morbidity, whereas FDS IV is used to provide finger extension (FDS IV to EDC). The FDS IV is used rather than FDS III for restoring finger extension because FDS III plays an important role in power grip activities. FDS IV provides more than ample power for extension of all four fingers. The wrist extension pronator teres to ECRB transfer is performed as described previously. FDS IV is harvested through a transverse incision at the distal palmar crease. A longitudinal incision is made along the dorsum of the distal forearm and the FDS IV is then transferred to the EDC using a sandwich technique.

Rehabilitation After Tendon Transfers for Radial Nerve Palsy. A long arm splint is used to maintain the elbow at 90 degrees of flexion, the wrist at 15 to 20 degrees of extension and the MCP joints in 30 degrees of flexion with the proximal interphalangeal (PIP) joints in complete extension. Two weeks after surgery, the patient is placed in a below elbow splint and hyperextension exercises of the MCP joints that allow PIP flexion are begun to prevent digit stiffness. At 4 weeks, the plaster splint is removed and the patients are started on finger flexion exercise with a dynamic extension splint, which is worn for an additional 2 to 3 weeks. The dynamic splint holds the wrist in 30-degree extension and provides finger and thumb extension.

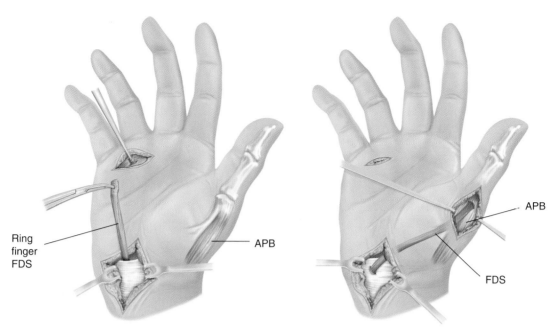

● FIGURE 55-5. The tendon transfer of the flexor digitorum superficialis of the ring finger to the abductor pollicis brevis reestablishes thumb opposition. (*Redrawn from Trumble TE. Principles of Hand Surgery and Therapy. Philadelphia: WB Saunders; 2000.*)

Median Nerve Palsy

Low Median Nerve Palsy. Low median nerve injuries are common because of the exposed position of the median nerve in the distal forearm. The major functional deficit resulting from a low median nerve palsy involves the loss of thumb opposition. Opposition of the thumb is a complex motion involving abduction, flexion, and pronation. The goal of tendon transfers in this setting are mainly to reconstruct the course of the fibers of the APB.[4] With respect to the APB, it is important to understand that the vector of the APB intersects the pisiform. Therefore, tendon transfers that are distal to the pisiform result in more thumb flexion than opposition, whereas transfers proximal to the pisiform provide more thumb palmar abduction. The two most commonly used tendon transfers to compensate for the loss of thumb opposition include the use of EIP or FDS IV as donor motors. However, of the two, the FDS IV tendon transfer more closely approximates the line of pull of the APB.

Technique

FDS IV Tendon Transfer for Opposition. The FDS IV tendon is harvested through a transverse incision at the level of the distal palmar crease. This tendon transfer requires a pulley near the pisiform to recreate the line of pull of the APB muscle. The pulley can be created by fashioning a hole in the palmar fascia just radial to the pisiform. An alternate technique for creation of a pulley involves the use of the FCU to make a tendon loop. A distally based slip of the FCU tendon is mobilized and sutured back onto itself to fashion the pulley.

A separate curvilinear incision is made over the radial aspect of the thumb at the site where the APB inserts onto the base of the proximal phalanx. The FDS IV tendon is then passed through the pulley that has been created and tunneled through the subcutaneous tissue across the palm. The FDS IV is then inserted through the APB tendon and sutured back upon it (Figure 55-5). Although the transfer of one half of the FDS tendon is classically described, we have used the complete FDS tendon to the APB with favorable results.

EIP Transfer for Thumb Opposition. This popular transfer is performed by transferring EIP around the ulnar side of the forearm to the APB. A curved incision is made over the dorsum of the index finger MCP joint. A second incision is made over the dorsum of the wrist and the EIP tendon is withdrawn through this incision. A third incision is made over the ulnar border of the forearm. Finally, an incision over the APB insertion on the radial side of the thumb MCP joint is prepared and the EIP is passed through a subcutaneous tunnel across the palm from the ulnar side of the forearm to the incision on the thumb. The ulna functions as the pulley in this tendon transfer. The EIP tendon is woven through the insertion of the APB and secured with horizontal mattress sutures (Figure 55-6). A strip of the extensor hood mechanism must be included with the harvested EIP if the tendon is to supply enough length to complete the transfer.

Palmaris Longus Transfer for Opposition. The Camitz palmaris longus tendon transfer for opposition provides mostly palmar abduction because the vector of the

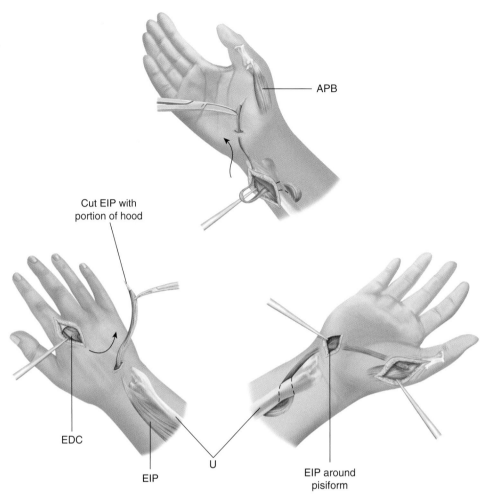

APB

Cut EIP with portion of hood

EDC

EIP

U

EIP around pisiform

● **FIGURE 55-6.** Transferring the extensor indicis proprius (EIP) around the ulnar border of the forearm to the abductor pollicis brevis (APB) provides opposition of the thumb. It is important to remove the EIP tendon elongated by a strip of the extensor hood mechanism to provide adequate length to reach the insertion of the APB. EDC, extensor digitorum communis; U, ulna. (*Redrawn from Trumble TE. Principles of Hand Surgery and Therapy. Philadelphia: WB Saunders; 2000.*)

palmaris longus is proximal to the pisiform. This transfer has been used effectively in patients who have had paralysis of the APB as a result of long standing carpal tunnel syndrome.[5] The use of an extended carpal tunnel incision provides excellent exposure to mobilize the palmaris longus tendon with a strip of palmar fascia to provide sufficient length for the transfer. The palmaris longus tendon is then passed through a subcutaneous tunnel to an incision over the radial border of the thumb MCP joint where it is sutured into the ABP insertion.

Abductor Digiti Minimi (ADM) Transfer for Opposition. The Huber transfer is occasionally used for adults with low median nerve palsy, but its main use lies in reconstruction of the congenital hypoplastic thumb.[6]

A longitudinal incision is made along the ulnar border of the hand. Since the neurovascular bundle to the ADM enters proximally, the muscle can be mobilized over nearly its entire length. A second incision is made over the radial border of the thumb MCP joint to expose the insertion of the APB. The tendon of the ADM is inserted into the ABP tendon after having been passed through a subcutaneous tunnel.

Rehabilitation After Tendon Transfers for Low Median Nerve Palsy. After tendon transfers for thumb opposition, the hand is immobilized in a thumb spica cast that maintains the thumb in a position of opposition for 4 weeks with the wrist held in flexion for the FDS IV and the palmaris longus tendon transfers. The wrist can be maintained in neutral position for the EIP tendon transfer. Wrist position does not have an effect for the ADM transfer. After 4 weeks of immobilization in plaster, the patient is placed in a removable splint and begins active thumb opposition exercises. Strengthening exercises are started 2 months after surgery.

High Median Nerve Palsy

High median nerve injuries involve a loss of flexion of the index finger, long finger and thumb due to the paralysis of the FDP to fingers II and III and the flexor pollicis longus (FPL). However, since the FDP to the long finger receives dual innervation from the median and ulnar nerve, patients usually maintain some flexion of the long finger albeit weaker than in the ring finger.

When the ulnar nerve is intact, side to side transfer of the index and long finger FDP to the FDP of the ring and small fingers is a simple and effective way of restoring flexion. In cases of combined high median nerve palsy and ulnar nerve injury, a transfer of the ECRL can provide flexion for all four digits. In both isolated high median palsy and combined median and ulnar palsies the transfer of brachioradialis is useful as a transfer to the FPL for thumb IP joint flexion.

Technique

Side-to-Side Transfers of FDP IV and V to FDP II and III. A longitudinal incision on the volar aspect of the distal forearm provides sufficient exposure of the profundus tendons. The FDS tendons are retracted radially along with the median nerve to expose the FDP tendons. Transverse sutures locking the four FDP tendons together are performed with care taken to make sure that the fingers are correctly positioned with the normal flexion arcade.

ECRL to all Four Fingers. An incision is made that curves proximally from the radial aspect of the distal third of the forearm to the mid aspect of the volar wrist crease. A separate transverse incision is necessary over the second dorsal compartment near the base of the index finger metacarpal in order to transect the insertion of the ECRL. The ECRL tendon is then transposed to lie parallel to the fibers of the FDP.

Brachioradialis to FPL. The brachioradialis to FPL transfer can be added to either of the aforementioned tendon transfers to restore digit flexion. The BR is sharply elevated from its insertion onto the radial border of the radius after releasing the first dorsal compartment underneath which the BR inserts. The tendon can then be split and sutured to the FPL using a Pulvertaft weave.

Rehabilitation After Tendon Transfers for High Median Nerve Palsy.
Patients are splinted for 4 weeks following a thumb opposition transfer with the thumb held in its position of opposition during the period of immobilization. When tendon transfers for digit flexion are added, the wrist is immobilized in neutral position with the MCP joints held in flexion and the IP joints blocked in extension using a dorsal block splint. A program of passive digit range of motion exercises can be used during the period of immobilization of the hand and wrist to prevent stiffness of the IP joints. Active flexion exercises are started 4 weeks after surgery, beginning with place and hold exercises with the wrist in flexion. At 6 weeks, the patients are allowed to begin wrist extension and active finger flexion.

Ulnar Nerve Palsy

The ulnar nerve innervates the majority of the hand intrinsic muscles, which provide the fine control for gripping and pinching activities.

Low Ulnar Nerve Palsy. The functional deficits resulting from a low ulnar nerve injury include clawing, loss of power pinch and persistent abduction of the small finger. The paralyzed muscles following ulnar nerve palsy include the dorsal and palmar interossei, the lumbricals to the ring and small finger, the adductor pollicis, and the hypothenar muscles.

Correction of Clawing. With the loss of intrinsic function, clawing occurs because of unopposed action of the extrinsic muscles supplying primary extension at the MCP joints and flexion of the distal interphalangeal and PIP joints. Clawing produces a roll-up deformity of the hand that makes it difficult to grasp objects of different diameters.

In a low ulnar nerve palsy, the index and middle fingers do not demonstrate clawing because the lumbricals to these two fingers are innervated by the median nerve. Clawing does not occur in a high ulnar nerve palsy because the FDP to the small and ring fingers are also paralyzed with this injury. Therefore, the imbalance between the extrinsics and intrinsics muscles seen in low ulnar nerve palsy does not occur. However, patients with high ulnar nerve palsy lack the ability to flex the distal interphalangeal joints of their small and ring fingers to complete grasping functions.

Technique

Transfer of FDS IV to the Lateral Bands or Proximal Phalanges of the Small and Ring Fingers. This tendon transfer is very effective for patients who have and isolated low ulnar nerve palsy. A Brunner incision is used to expose the FDS IV tendon at the level of its insertion onto the middle phalanx with a radially based flap such that the same approach can be used to expose the lateral band on the radial side of the finger. If the tendon is to be inserted onto the base of the proximal phalanx, then a smaller Brunner incision is required to expose the FDS tendon and a separate incision can be made at the level of the distal palmar crease in order to retrieve the FDS tendon from the ring finger proximal to the fibro-osseous sheath. The FDS tendon is then split longitudinally. The tails are passed deep to the neurovascular bundles, but palmar to the transverse intermetacarpal ligaments in order to reconstruct the pull of the lumbrical muscles. One tail is passed to the ring finger and the other tail is passed to the small finger. The tendons can then be woven into the lateral bands with enough tension to produce MCP joint

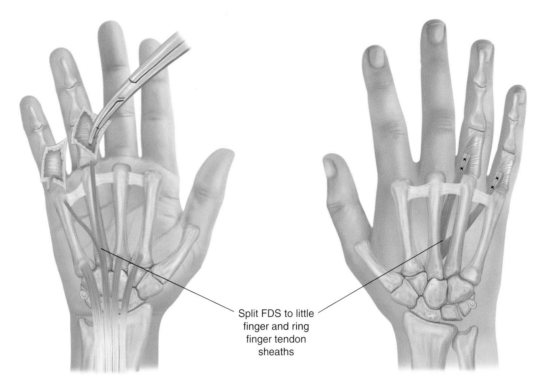

Split FDS to little
finger and ring
finger tendon
sheaths

● **FIGURE 55-7.** The flexor digitorum superficialis tendon transfer to the lateral bands of the small and ring finger corrects the claw deformity. (*Redrawn from Trumble TE. Principles of Hand Surgery and Therapy. Philadelphia: WB Saunders; 2000.*)

flexion and PIP joint extension (Figure 55-7). Although some authors recommend attaching the tendons to bone, attachments to the lateral bands have been successful in the senior authors' experience.

Zancolli Lasso Procedure. Zancolli recommended a modification of the FDS to intrinsic transfer that would function as a static tenodesis to provide MCP joint flexion. This technique is particularly useful in patients who have paralysis of muscles other than those affected by the ulnar nerve palsy.

The Zancolli modification procedure is performed in a manner very similar to the FDS to intrinsic transfer described above, except that the slips of the FDS are passed through the interval between the A1 and A2 pulleys. The lasso is made by suturing the tendon slip back onto itself in order to provide MCP joint flexion that allows the patient's extrinsic extensor tendons to direct their force to the PIP joint rather than the MCP joint. This tenodesis produces a fixed MCP joint contracture for the ability to grasp both small and large diameter objects.

Brand Tendon Transfer of the ECRB to the Intrinsics. The Brand tendon transfer for the intrinsics can be performed to all four digits in patients who have combined clawing involving all the fingers, such as in a C8-T1 plexus injury or combined low median and low ulnar nerve palsies. The Brand intrinsic tendon transfer is also valuable when there has been trauma involving the flexor tendons because the surgeon can avoid the area of scar tissue

and the uncertainty of whether the transferred tendons will glide.

The ECRB is identified using a small transverse incision over the third metacarpal. A second incision is made proximal to the extensor tendon retinaculum such that the ECRB can be withdrawn through the proximal incision. This tendon transfer does require elongating the ECRB using a tendon graft such as the palmaris longus or the plantaris tendon passed through the distal end of the ECRB tendon. By folding the graft, a two-tailed extension of the ECRB is fashioned to transfer to both the small and ring finger. By splitting each tail further into half, a separate tendon slip can be transferred to all four digits. A transverse incision is made at the level of the distal palmar crease to allow the slips of the tendon grafts to be passed in a dorsal to palmar direction to bring them out through the palm. The tendon grafts are then passed palmar to the transverse intermetacarpal ligament to reconstruct the line of pull of the lumbrical muscles. Longitudinal midaxial incisions are made over the radial aspect of the digits receiving the tendon transfer. The tendon transfers are passed through small incisions in the lateral bands making sure that the insertion site distal and dorsal enough to produce MCP joint flexion as well as PIP joint extension (Figure 55-8).

Rehabilitation After Tendon Transfer to Correct Clawing. The patient is placed in a plaster splint that maintains the MCP joints in 70 degrees of flexion and the PIP joints in an extended position. The wrist is

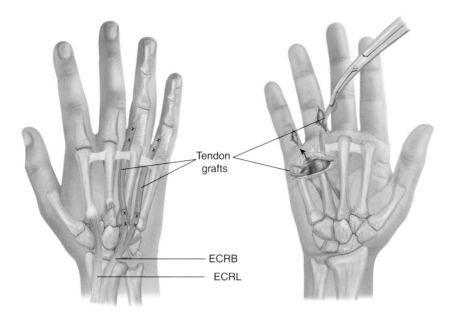

● **FIGURE 55-8.** The Brand tendon transfer to the intrinsics uses a tendon graft that connects the extensor carpi radialis brevis (ECRB) tendon to the lateral bands of the small and ring fingers. The ECRB tendon provides enough power for a four-tailed graft and can be used to reestablish intrinsic function to all four digits when combined nerve injuries have produced a complete intrinsic paralysis to the hand. *(Redrawn from Trumble TE. Principles of Hand Surgery and Therapy. Philadelphia: WB Saunders; 2000.)*

maintained in slight flexion when the FDS tendon was used and in slight extension when the ECRB tendon was used. The splint is maintained for 4 weeks and then a removable hand-based splint that blocks the MCP joints in 30 to 40 degrees of flexion is worn. The hand-based splint is worn for an additional 4 weeks to prevent the tendon transfer from stretching out. Eight weeks after surgery the patients can be started on gentle strengthening exercises.

Reconstruction of Power Pinch. Power pinch occurs by the combined action of the adductor pollicis and the first dorsal interosseous. The adductor pollicis originates from the index and long finger metacarpals and inserts on the thumb metacarpal and functions to pull the thumb toward the index finger. The first dorsal interosseous muscle arises from the thumb and index metacarpals and attaches to the radial side of the base of the index finger proximal phalanx to create a powerful scissors-type action that pulls the index and thumb towards one another.

Patients with low ulnar nerve palsy compensate for the loss of these muscles by using EPL. EPL is a secondary adductor of the thumb but lacks substantial pinch power. To achieve additional power and to place EPL under the greatest tension, patients use FPL concomitantly. Hence, the result is that patients develop a hyperflexion of the IP joint of the thumb known as the Froment sign.

Technique

ECRB to Adductor Pollicis with Tendon Graft. The Smith transfer is an excellent transfer for reconstructing power pinch, partly because wrist extension is a synergistic action to power pinch. This transfer spares the FDS so it can be used for other tendon transfers such as to correct concomitant clawing. The downside of this tendon transfer is that it does require a tendon graft, which has the potential for stretching out or forming adhesions.

The ECRB is identified through a transverse incision over the base of the third metacarpal. A separate transverse incision is made proximal to the retinaculum of the extensor tendons. The ECRB is released from the third metacarpal and brought out through the proximal incision. A tendon graft from palmaris longus or plantaris is obtained and sutured into the distal end of the ECRB using a Pulvertaft technique.[7] A third incision is made over the ulnar aspect of the thumb MCP joint. A curved clamp is used to pass the tendon graft around the second metacarpal to the third incision over the ulnar aspect of the thumb. The second metacarpal becomes the pulley for this tendon transfer. The tendon graft is woven through the adductor pollicis so that the thumb lies gently along the radial border of the index finger with the wrist in neutral position with the ECRB tendon at 50% of its maximum length (Figure 55-9). As a check on tension of the transfer the thumb should abduct as the wrist goes into flexion and adduct against the index as the wrist moves into extension.[7]

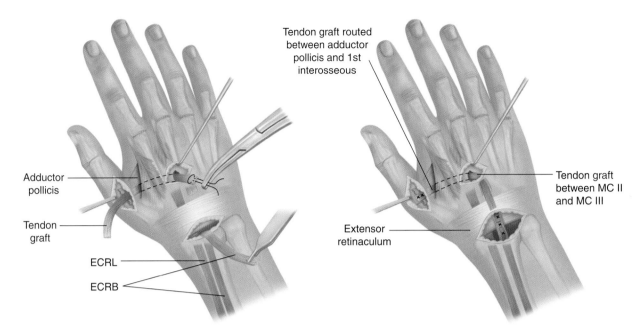

Adductor pollicis

Tendon graft

ECRL

ECRB

Tendon graft routed between adductor pollicis and 1st interosseous

Tendon graft between MC II and MC III

Extensor retinaculum

● **FIGURE 55-9.** In low ulnar nerve palsy, the ECRB tendon can be transferred to the adductor pollicis to restore pinch. The tendon graft passes around the second metacarpal, using it as the pulley for the tendon transfer. ECRB, extensor carpi radialis brevis; ECRL, extensor carpi radialis longus; MC, metacarpal. (*Redrawn from Trumble TE. Principles of Hand Surgery and Therapy. Philadelphia: WB Saunders, 2000.*)

FDS IV to the Adductor Pollicis. This is a good transfer for isolated low ulnar nerve palsies. The FDS IV provides the necessary strength for power pinch and can easily be directed along the course of the adductor pollicis fibers. When muscles other than those innervated by the ulnar nerve have been paralyzed or when a high ulnar nerve lesion has occurred, the surgeon may want to consider sparing the function of the FDS IV particularly for use in other tendon transfers.

The FDS IV tendon is harvested through a transverse incision at the level of the PIP joint flexion crease of the ring finger in order to obtain as much length as possible for transfer. A second incision is made at the level of the distal palmar crease and the distal end of the FDS tendon is retrieved from this incision. The insertion of the adductor pollicis is identified using a longitudinal incision along the ulnar border of the thumb MCP joint. The FDS tendon is passed subcutaneously just palmar to the flexor tendons and neurovascular bundles. The tendon is secured to the tendon of the adductor pollicis with a Pulvertaft technique. The tension is adjusted so that the thumb lies just along the index finger with the FDS tendon at 50% of its resting length.[8]

Rehabilitation After Tendon Transfer to Reconstruct Power Pinch. Patients are placed in a short arm splint that maintains the thumb against the index finger. With the ECRB tendon transfer, the wrist is maintained in slight extension; whereas with the FDS tendon transfer, the wrist is maintained in slight flexion. Four weeks after surgery, a removable hand-based splint is made holding the thumb in

adduction. The patient is started on gentle active exercises. Gentle resistive exercises are started 8 weeks after surgery and strengthening exercises are begun 10 to 12 weeks after surgery.

High Ulnar Nerve Palsy. The major functional deficits in high ulnar nerve palsy include the inability to fully flex the small and ring fingers due to paralysis of the FDP and loss of power pinch. Clawing is not a significant factor in high ulnar nerve palsy. Tendon transfers for high ulnar nerve palsy include transfers to the adductor pollicis to reconstruct power pinch as well as transfers to reestablish the function of the FDP to the small and ring fingers.

Tendon Transfers to Reconstruct Power Pinch. Tendon transfers can be used as described for reconstruction of power pinch in low ulnar nerve palsy. The senior author's preference is to use the ECRB to the adductor pollicis as described by Smith, since the FDS IV–based transfers to the adductor pollicis decrease the strength of flexion of the ring finger, which is particularly apparent in the setting of loss of FDP function in this finger associated with high ulnar nerve palsy. The transfer of EIP to the adductor pollicis is a transfer that is the "mirror image" of EIP opponens tendon transfer, but the EIP is a relatively weak motor that does not produce substantial pinch strength.

Tendon Transfers to Reestablish Function of the FDP IV and V. The side-to-side transfer of the index and middle finger FDP to the small and ring finger FDP can be performed in a manner analogous to the tendon transfers for high median nerve palsy. For patients with an intact median nerve, this is the preferred transfer.

Tendon Transfers for Small Finger Abduction. The interosseous muscles are the primary muscles providing abduction and adduction of the fingers. Although loss of finger adduction function decreases the patients overall hand dexterity, this is not a functional loss of high priority for reconstruction. Reconstruction of clawing and loss of power pinch remain much more significant functional losses. The tendon transfers to the intrinsics are designed to correct the abduction of the small finger by performing the transfers to the lateral bands to the radial side of the digits. For patients with persistent abduction of the small finger despite tendon transfers to the intrinsics or in patients with an isolated problem of small finger abduction, the ulnar

portion of the extensor digiti minimi can be transferred to the radial side of the small finger.

● COMPLICATIONS

In all tendon transfers, the main problem is in achieving ideal tension. The surgeon also wants to avoid stretching out the tendon transfers during the rehabilitation phase while still allowing early motion to prevent adhesions. Additional surgery to adjust the tension of the tendon transfer can be helpful in patients who have lost function because the transfer has stretched out. If adhesions form, a tenolysis may be of benefit to the patient. Finally, it must be explained to the patient that they can never achieve the same function that they had with the original muscle tendon units and that the tendon transfers offer a compromise that should improve their overall hand function.

REFERENCES

1. Brand PW, Hollister AM. *Clinical Mechanics of the Hand.* 3rd ed. St-Louis, MO: Mosby; 1999.
2. Starr CL. Army experiences with tendon transference. *J Bone Joint Surg Am.* 1922;4:2–3.
3. Chuinard RG, Boyes JH, Stark HH, et al. Tendon transfers for radial nerve palsy: use of superficialis tendons for digital extension. *J Hand Surg Am.* 1978;3:560–570.
4. Cooney WP, Linscheid RL, An KN. Opposition of the thumb: an anatomic and biomechanical study of tendon transfers. *J Hand Surg Am.* 1984;9:777–786.
5. Braun RM. Palmaris longus tendon transfer for augmentation of the thenar musculature in low median palsy. *J Hand Surg Am.* 1978;3:488–491.
6. Littler JW, Cooley SG. Opposition of the thumb and its restoration by abductor digiti quinti transfer. *J Bone Joint Surg Am.* 1963;45:1389–1396.
7. Smith RJ. Extensor carpi radialis brevis tendon transfer for thumb adduction–a study of power pinch. *J Hand Surg Am.* 1983;8:4–15.
8. Hamlin C, Littler JW. Restoration of power pinch. *J Hand Surg Am.* 1980;5:396–401.

chapter 56

Congenital Hand Anomalies

Brian A. Pinsky, MD / Jaimie T. Shores, MD

● INTRODUCTION

Approximately 1% to 2% of neonates are born with congenital malformations, and 10% of these children have involvement of the upper extremity. Most anomalies are inherited through genetic transmission or sporadic mutations, and relatively few are due to environmental exposure or teratogens. Congenital hand anomalies have both aesthetic and functional implications. Research and experimentation in upper limb embryology has led to an improved understanding of the molecular mechanisms behind these abnormalities. The most widely accepted classification system was developed by Swanson in the 1960s. This system divides limb anomalies into seven categories according to the failed developmental process: failure of formation, failure of differentiation, duplication, overgrowth, undergrowth, constriction band syndromes, and generalized skeletal abnormalities.

● EMBRYOLOGY

Upper limb development begins at 4 weeks after fertilization and is complete at approximately 8 weeks with the presence of all upper limb structures. The expression of sonic hedgehog protein by the notochord initiates limb bud formation. The limb bud is an outgrowth of somatic and lateral plate mesoderm into the overlying ectoderm. Three distinct signaling centers have been identified that control the process of limb growth and differentiation. The timing and interaction of these signaling centers are essential to normal limb development.

The apical ectodermal ridge (AER) is located between the dorsal and ventral layers of ectoderm and controls proximodistal development, as well as interdigital necrosis. Members of the fibroblast growth factor family are involved in cell signaling from the AER.[1] The zone of polarizing activity (ZPA) is situated along the posterior aspect of the developing limb and controls the anteroposterior limb axis. Sonic hedgehog protein is the primary signaling molecule of the ZPA and orchestrates radial and ulnar orientation of the upper limb. Defects in ZPA signaling result in a mirror-image duplication. Finally, the wingless-type signaling center controls dorsal and volar axis development. Wingless-type proteins cause the underlying mesoderm to develop dorsal characteristics.[7]

● PATIENT EVALUATION

Many congenital hand anomalies are sporadic and occur in isolation. However, certain upper extremity malformations are associated with developmental errors in other organ systems that can range from mild to life-threatening. Radial longitudinal deficiency is associated with other congenital syndromes in up to 44% of affected newborns.[8] Radial longitudinal deficiency is often seen in patients with Holt-Oram syndrome (atrial septal defects, arrhythmias), VACTERL association (*v*ertebral anomalies, *a*nal atresia, *c*ardiac abnormalities, *t*racheoesophageal fistula, *r*enal agenesis, and *l*imb defects), Fanconi anemia (pancytopenia developing between 5 and 10 years of age), and thrombocytopenia-absent radius syndrome.[7]

All patients with suspected radial deficiency require skeletal radiographs, a renal ultrasound, echocardiogram, and a complete blood count. Early diagnosis with chromosomal breakage studies is essential for patients suspected of Fanconi anemia prior to the onset of pancytopenia. This maximizes the amount of time available to find a suitable bone marrow donor. Bone marrow transplantation is the only known cure for the once fatal disease. These patients are often small in stature with feeding difficulties.

Ulnar deficiencies are associated with other musculoskeletal malformations but not anomalies in other organ systems.[7] These patients should have a general skeletal x-ray, but do not require an extensive multisystemic workup.

TABLE 56-1. Classification of Thumb Hypoplasia

Type	Findings	Surgical Procedure
I	Generalized reduction in size, skeletal/soft tissue components all present	Usually no treatment
II	Absence of thenar/intrinsic muscles	Huber transfer (opponensplasty)
	Narrowing of web space	Web space deepening/release
	UCL insufficiency	UCL reconstruction
III	Type II plus:	IIIA: Reconstruction
	Extrinsic muscle/tendon abnormalities and skeletal abnormalities	IIIB: Ablation and Pollicization
	A: Stable CMC joint	
	B: Unstable CMC joint	
IV	*Pouce flottant* or floating thumb	Pollicization
V	Complete absence of thumb	Pollicization
Five-fingered hand	All digits within same plane of hand	Pollicization

CMC, carpometacarpal; UCL, ulnar collateral ligament.

Modified Blauth classification, adapted from: Abdel-Ghani H, Amro S. Characteristics of patients with hypoplastic thumb: a prospective study of 51 patients with the results of surgical treatment. J Pediatr Orthop B. 2004;13:127–138.

Treatment of these conditions involves a coordinated, multidisciplinary team approach. Proper diagnosis allows for referral to the relevant specialists and appropriate family counseling.

Transverse Deficiency

Transverse deficiencies are also known as congenital amputations. The etiology is thought to involve a disruption of the AER or fibroblast growth factor proteins.[6] The malformation is named for the anatomic level at which the amputation occurs. This can range from aphalangia to complete amelia. The most common congenital amputation occurs at the proximal third of the forearm and is called the below-elbow defect.[6]

Referral to pediatric rehabilitation medicine or pediatric orthopedics is important to have the patient evaluated for prosthetic use early. Most rehabilitation centers use the standard of having the child "fit to sit," meaning fitting of a child with a passive prosthesis by 6 months of age (the approximate age of sitting up) with graduation to a more active device by 12 to 15 months of age.[3,10]

Radial Longitudinal Deficiency

Radial longitudinal deficiency represents a spectrum of hypoplasias of the forearm, wrist, and thumb. These can range from mild hypoplasia to complete absence of radial structures known as the "radial club hand." The malformation is more common in males, more common on the right side, and 40% to 60% occur bilaterally. As previously mentioned, radial (preaxial) deficiencies are associated with malformations in other organ systems that may be life-threatening and must be worked up appropriately.

The skeletal abnormalities are the most obvious; however, they are associated with deficiencies of the accompanying muscles, nerves, joints, and vessels.[8] Classification is based on the severity of the deformity. Complete absence of the radius results in an ulna that is short and radially bowed, with the hand medially bent and displaced due to poor support of the wrist.[8]

Thumb hypoplasia is defined by the Blauth classification (Table 56-1), which takes into account thumb size, depth of first web space, intrinsic and extrinsic muscle deficiency, and joint stability.[6] The thumb accounts for 40% of overall hand function.[8] Grade IV represents the classic *pouce flottant* or floating thumb in which the remnant digit is nonfunctioning and attached by a skin bridge containing only neurovascular structures without any bone, tendon, or musculature.[8]

Reconstruction depends on anatomic deficiency and functional use. The goal is to create a stable digit for pinch, grip, and prehension.[7,11] Deficient thenar musculature is treated with either an abductor digiti minimi transfer (Huber opponensplasty) or ring finger flexor digitorum sublimis opponensplasty. Metacarpophalangeal joint instability is treated with capsular tightening or reinforcement with the transferred tendon during opponensplasty. A narrow first web space is treated with local tissue rearrangement including a four-flap z-plasty.[8] Children with grade IIIB or higher hypoplasias lack a stable thumb carpometacarpal joint. These patients are not candidates for thumb reconstruction and are treated with ablation and pollicization (Figure 56-1).

Forearm radial dysplasias are similarly classified based on severity of anatomic deficiency. The most common presentation is the Bayne and Klug classification type IV, which presents as complete absence of the radius. The ulna is

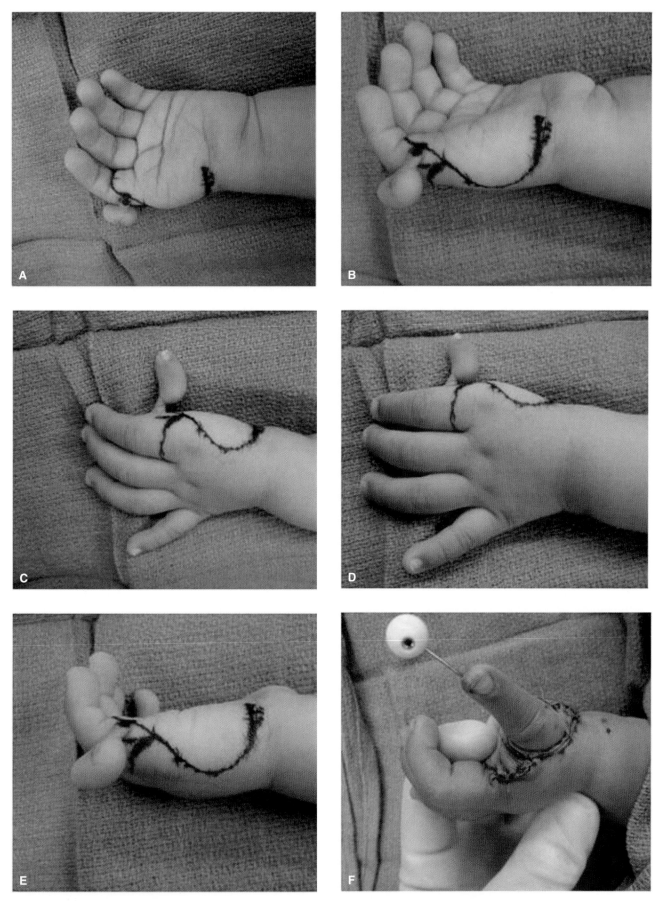

● **FIGURE 56-1.** Type IV thumb hypoplasia (*pouce flottant*) with surgical markings for pollicization (A–E) and immediate postoperative result (F).

bowed secondary to the tethering effects of the shortened and fibrotic radial musculature and soft tissues. Forearm length averages 60% of the contralateral normal side, and the relative shortening remains constant throughout growth.[8] Radial longitudinal deficiencies are also associated with proximal radioulnar synostosis and congenital radial head dislocation.

Forearm reconstruction involves both surgical and nonsurgical techniques. Initial management consists of serial splinting and stretching to lengthen the tight radial soft tissues. The goal is to achieve passive correction of the wrist deformity prior to surgical intervention. Surgical realignment of the wrist on the distal ulna is achieved through centralization or radialization.[8] These techniques involve aligning the distal ulna with either the middle or index metacarpal, tightening or reinforcement of the ulnar wrist capsule, and transfer of the radial soft tissue structures. The extrinsic muscles are transferred ulnarly to balance the radial deforming forces. Ulnar osteotomies may be necessary to correct any additional angular deformity. Nonsurgical management is chosen in cases of older children with established patterns of functional compensation and in cases of severe, bilateral elbow extension contractures.[8] In these patients, the flexed position of the wrist and radial hand deviation allow for movement of the hand to the face.

Central Deficiency

Central longitudinal deficiencies are malformations of the central rays of the hand (index, middle, and ring fingers).[6] These are commonly known as cleft hand, lobster claw, and split hand-foot malformation.[6] There are two distinct types of central deficiencies, typical and atypical. Each type has unique clinical features and separate embryologic etiologies. In fact, many authors suggest that they are better classified in different categories of congenital malformations.[7]

The typical cleft hand has a V-shaped deformity (Figure 56-2), usually to the level of the metacarpal, with varying degrees of long ray absence.[7] This results from a fusion of the digital rays rather than a failure of development. Inheritance is X-linked dominant with incomplete penetrance. Typical cleft hand is often bilateral with associated foot anomalies, such as split hand-split foot. Cleft lip and palate, along with border digit syndactyly, is also seen with typical cleft hand.[7]

In contrast, atypical cleft hand has a U-shaped appearance with a shallower cleft that often contains rudimentary digital elements.[6] Atypical cleft hand is a type of symbrachydactyly caused by necrosis of mesenchymal tissue with failed attempts at regeneration.[6,7] It is generally sporadic and unilateral without foot involvement. Symbrachydactyly can range from short, connected fingers to complete absence of the central rays. Symbrachydactyly is often seen in Poland syndrome along with absence of the sternal portion of the pectoralis major muscle and other associated chest wall abnormalities.[6,7] This is due to vascular disruption of the developing upper limb in utero.

Reconstruction can involve both functional and aesthetic concerns. The first web space may require deepening for improved function with z-plasty or other local flaps. Central reconstruction may involve soft tissue rearrangement and ulnar transposition of the index ray. However, most children will adapt to their deficiency without significant intervention.

Ulnar Deficiency

Ulnar deficiency involves the postaxial border of the limb and is significantly less common than radial deficiency[6,7] The radius undergoes progressive bowing with lateral hand deviation.[5] Nearly half of all patients with ulnar deficiency have associated musculoskeletal abnormalities, such as clubfoot, spina bifida, and proximal femoral focal deficiency.[6] However, ulnar deficiency is not associated

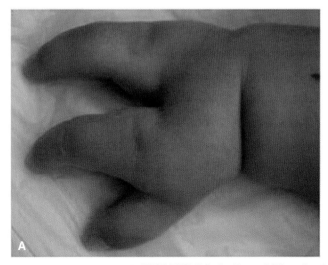
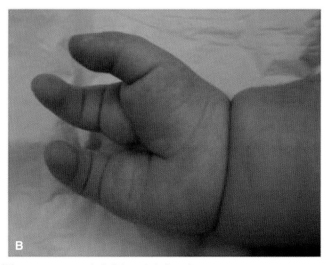

● **FIGURE 56-2.** Dorsal (A) and volar (B) appearance of cleft hand deformity.

with the systemic malformations seen in radial longitudinal deficiencies. Therefore, a complete skeletal radiographic survey is needed without any systemic workup.

Ulnar deficiency is often misdiagnosed as a radial deficiency. Thumb hypoplasia is often seen in ulnar deficiencies. The radius often develops ulna-like characteristics, including radiohumeral fusion that results in a proximal radius that appears similar to an ulna.[7]

● FAILURE OF DIFFERENTIATION

Syndactyly

Syndactyly is one of the most common congenital anomalies of the hand and can occur in up to 1:2000 live births.[6] Syndactyly is defined by the degree of interconnection between two or more adjacent digits. Simple syndactyly involves connections of only skin and soft tissue, and complex syndactyly involves a fusion of both bone and soft tissue. Complete syndactyly occurs when the digits are fused along the entire length to the fingertip, and an incomplete syndactyly involves only a proximal connection. Complicated syndactyly describes a bizarre collection and orientation of normal skeletal elements and may be associated with various syndromes.

Syndactyly may be inherited as autosomal dominant with variable expressivity and incomplete penetrance, and is associated with an abnormality on chromosome 2.[7] However, the vast majority of syndactyly are sporadic mutations. Some specialized types of syndactyly are characteristic of certain developmental syndromes. Symbrachydactyly is seen in up to 14% of patients with Poland syndrome.[6] Acrosyndactyly is associated with constriction band syndrome (Figure 56-3). These patients often have truncated digits due to congenital amputations, deep transverse grooves, small residual web space clefts, or sinuses with distal connections between digits.[6] A constriction band around the lower extremity is also commonly seen.

Apert syndrome, also known as acrocephalosyndactyly, is associated with multiple suture craniosynostosis, maxillary hypoplasia, hypertelorism, proptosis, developmental delay, and complex syndactyly.[6,7] Apert hand patterns are defined according to the position of the thumb and have been described as spade like, spoon like, mitten like, rosebud like, and hoof like.[7]

Reconstruction of digit syndactyly involves separation of the digits using some variant of zig-zag skin flaps, creation of a web space with a local skin flap, and coverage of any remaining defect with a skin graft. A variety of techniques have been described, and most involve a dorsal proximally based web space flap (Figure 56-4). Full-thickness skin grafts should be used to decrease the rate of contracture and are most often harvested from the groin or instep of the foot. Surgery is most often done at approximately 1 year of age; however, border digits should be released at 6 to 9 months to prevent growth disturbance secondary to tethering from the adjacent, shorter digit. Only one side of a finger should be released in a single procedure to prevent

arterial compromise and finger necrosis. Complicated syndactyly in patients with functional compensation is often left alone to avoid disrupting established patterns of function.

Clinodactyly

Clinodactyly presents as an angular deformity of a digit in the radioulnar plane, most commonly seen in the fifth digit distal phalanx. This is secondary to an abnormally shaped articular surface of the middle phalanx.[6] X-rays will often show a bracketed epiphysis of the middle phalanx or a triangular-shaped delta phalanx. The angulation is usually radial toward midline and has little functional consequence. Most cases are mild and require no treatment. In severe forms of angulation greater than 25 degrees, correction can be performed with a closing wedge osteotomy or physiolysis.[7] Most corrections are for more aesthetic than functional concerns.[6] Inheritance is usually autosomal dominant. Clinodactyly is seen in up to 79% of patients with Down syndrome.

Camptodactyly

Camptodactyly is a flexion contracture of the proximal interphalangeal joint most commonly seen in the fifth finger. It is usually painless and gradually progressive.[6] The true etiology is unknown; however, it has been attributed to tightness of the skin and underlying fascia, or abnormal insertion of the lumbrical or flexor digitorum superficialis tendons.[4] Most patients have no functional deficit. Camptodactyly is bilateral in approximately two thirds of cases.[7]

Three types of camptodactyly have been identified. Type I is present at birth, affects males and females equally, and is usually seen only in the small finger. Type II is acquired and presents in preadolescent females. Type III often involves severe contractures of multiple digits and is associated with many developmental syndromes, including arthrogryposis.[7]

Asymptomatic patients do not require treatment. Symptomatic patients with severe contractures (60–90 degrees) are initially treated with serial splinting. Surgical outcomes are unpredictable.[4] Surgical intervention addresses mostly imbalance of the flexor, extensor, and intrinsic forces with the flexor digitorum sublimis and lumbrical tendons.[2]

Arthrogryposis

Arthrogryposis is a disorder of stiff and immobile joints most commonly due to a motor unit defect between the anterior horn cells of the spinal cord and its effector muscle. Decreased fetal movement in utero can result in joint contractures. The disorder can present on a spectrum from mild and localized (to the hand), to generalized involving both the upper and lower extremities.[6] Classically, these patients present with symmetric, rigid joints, and

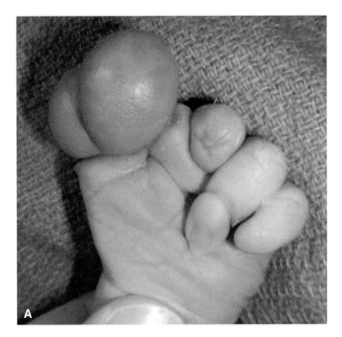
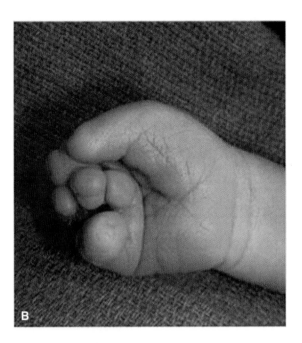
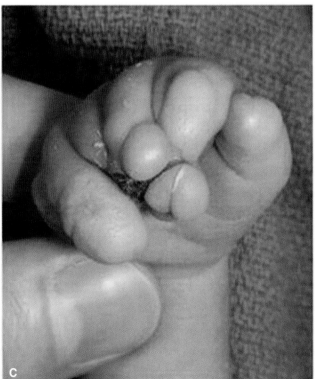

● FIGURE 56-3. Amniotic band syndrome of bilateral hands with digit amputation, bands of the ring finger and thumb (A) and acrosyndactyly (B, C).

decreased musculature.[6] Treatment is directed at overcoming severe contractures with therapy and substituting for absent muscle units.

Trigger Thumb

Pediatric trigger thumb presents with the thumb either locked in a flexed position at the interphalangeal joint or as intermittent, painful catching of the interphalangeal joint.[4]

This is secondary to constriction of the thumb A1 pulley and nodular thickening of the flexor pollicis longus tendon (Notta's node). Studies have shown that the triggering is not present at birth.[4,6] Pediatric trigger thumb is typically sporadic and bilateral. Nonsurgical management is initially recommended, including stretching, as 30% to 50% will resolve spontaneously within 1 year.[4,6] Some hand surgeons recommend surgical release of the A1 pulley at age 1 year, as the results are satisfactory with minimal morbidity.

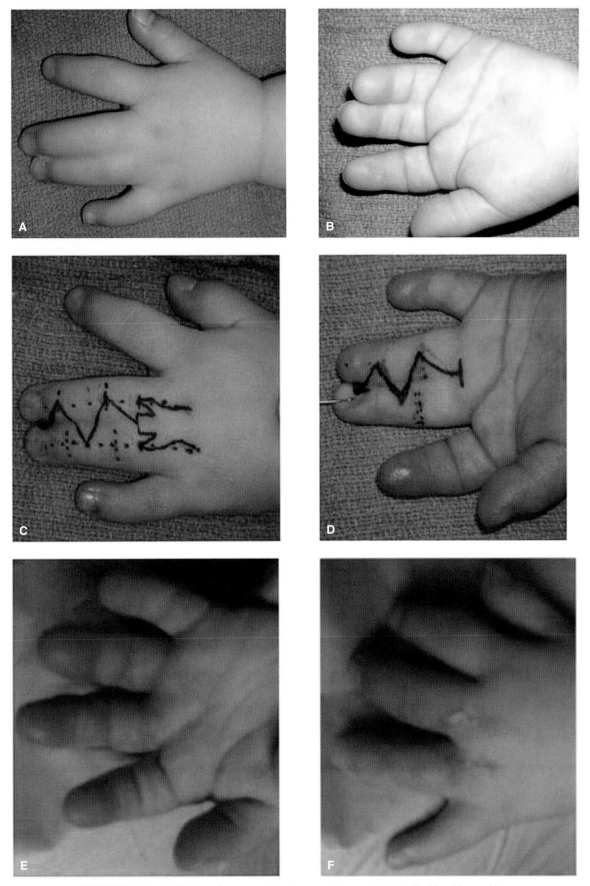

● **FIGURE 56-4.** Third web space simple complete syndactyly (A, B), with markings for reconstruction using the trilobed flap repair method (C, D); 1-year postoperative results (E, F).

Radioulnar Synostosis

Radioulnar synostosis is a rare condition resulting from a fusion of the proximal radius and ulna likely due to an embryologic failure of separation.[4] The forearm becomes fixed in a pronated position with limited rotational movement. It can be isolated or associated with a radial head dislocation.[6] It is frequently associated with other congenital syndromes, such as Apert syndrome, Carpenter syndrome, trisomy 13 or 21, and fetal alcohol syndrome. Diagnosis is often delayed until the child participates in more complex activities such as eating or catching a ball. In addition, shoulder and wrist movements can partially compensate for lack of forearm rotation. Severe fixed pronation may require a rotational osteotomy through the fusion mass to place the hand in a more favorable position.[4]

● DUPLICATION

Radial (Preaxial) Duplication

Polydactyly is a relatively common malformation with distinct ethnic differences. Radial polydactyly is much more prevalent in white and Asian populations.[6] These include thumb duplications, triphalangeal thumb, and index finger duplications. Thumb duplications are usually sporadic and unilateral malformations. The accepted classification system is the Wassel classification (Table 56-2), which divides the duplicated digit according to the number of bones and joints affected from distal to proximal. More than half of the cases seen have duplicated distal and

proximal phalanges with a common bifid metacarpal articulation corresponding to a Wassel type 4 duplication.[6] The duplicated thumbs are usually hypoplastic and share some degree of all components including neurovascular bundles, tendons, and soft tissue.

Reconstruction of the duplicated thumb involves using components of each digit to construct a thumb that is properly aligned and functional[6] (Figure 56-5). When both digits are of similar size and degree of development, a technique such as the Bilhaut-Cloquet procedure can be used that combines slightly more than half of each hypoplastic thumb. This procedure is often complicated by residual nail deformities with occasional epiphysiodesis, and is a more often discussed but rarely used surgical technique. Otherwise, the less developed digit is often excised while maintaining the tendons and adjacent ligaments to either reconstruct or augment the remaining digit's tendons or collateral ligaments. The metacarpal head may need to be partially excised and the digit centralized. Most commonly, the ulnar digit is maintained due to its dominance and to avoid the need to reconstruct the ulnar collateral ligament. The radial collateral ligament should be preserved and reconstructed on the ulnar duplicate when the radial duplicate is ablated, and vice versa.

Triphalangeal Thumb

In this malformation, the thumb presents with an extra phalanx. The clinical presentation can be highly variable. If the extra digit is an abnormally shaped delta phalanx between the proximal and distal phalanx, it is often excised

---

TABLE 56-2. Classification of Thumb Duplication

Type	Level of Duplication	Surgical Procedure
I	Bifid distal phalanx	Historically: Bilhaut-Cloquet procedure Most commonly: ablation of nondominant digit keeping lateral border of ablated digit for closure
II	Duplicate distal phalanges	Historically: Bilhaut-Cloquet procedure Most commonly: ablation of nondominant digit keeping lateral border of ablated digit for closure. IP joint centralization and chondroplasty of proximal phalanx head
III	Bifid proximal phalanx	Usually ablate radial thumb and retain ulnar thumb. Reconstruct RCL and centralize extrinsics
IV	Duplicate proximal and distal phalanges	Usually ablate radial thumb and retain ulnar thumb. Reconstruct RCL and centralize MCP joints and extrinsics
V	Bifid metacarpal	Resection of thumb metacarpal head/neck and digit. Retain ulnar digit if possible. Centralize metacarpal head and neck if necessary
VI	Duplicate metacarpals, proximal and distal phalanges	Resection of a metacarpal and a digit. Consider excision of ulnar metacarpal and radial digit with transfer of ulnar digit on top of radial metacarpal (on-top-plasty) if ulnar metacarpal impinges upon index metacarpal and radial metacarpal has best placement and movement
VII	Triphalangeal thumb	Dependent on individual anatomy, may require multiple stages

IP, interphalangeal; RCL, radial collateral ligament; MCP, metacarpophalangeal.

Adapted from Wassel HD. The results of surgery for polydactyly of the thumb. A review. Clin Orthop. 1969;125:175–193.

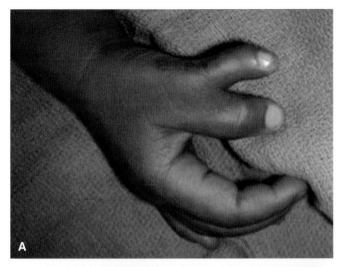

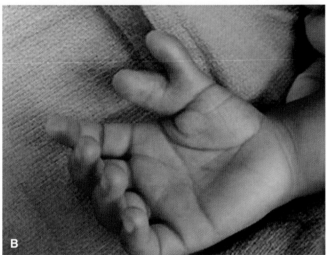

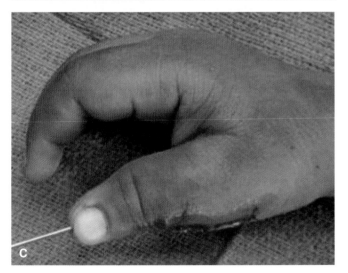

● FIGURE 56-5. Wassel type IV thumb duplication with preoperative (A, B) and immediate postoperative views (C).

TABLE 56-3. Classifications of Ulnar (Postaxial) Polydactyly

Stelling and Turek[a]	Type 1: Floating appendage linked by a narrow skin bridge
	Type 2: Partial duplication of the digit with skeletal elements, single metacarpal
	Type 3: Complete duplication of the metacarpals and phalanges
Temtamy and McKusick[b]	Type A: Well-formed duplicate with skeletal elements, may articulate with fifth metacarpal or duplicate metacarpal
	Type B: Rudimentary, poorly duplicated remnant, usually narrowly based on a small skin stalk

[a]Data from Stelling F. The upper extremity. In: Fergusun AB, ed. Orthopaedic Surgery in Infancy and Childhood. Baltimore, MD: Williams & Wilkins; 1963:304–308.

[b]Data from Temtamy SA, McKusick VA. The Genetics of Hand Malformations. New York: Liss; 1978:364.

Central Polydactyly

This rare type of polydactyly often presents with syndactyly and can be difficult to diagnose. Reconstructed digits are often stiff or deviated. Ring finger polysyndactyly has been attributed to a mutation of the *HOXD13* gene on chromosome 2.[6,8]

Ulnar (Postaxial) Polydactyly

Ulnar polydactyly involves the fifth digit and is 10 times more common in the African American population. Inheritance is autosomal dominant with variable penetrance.[7] Two major classification systems exist, with the Temtamy and McKusick system being most commonly used (Table 56-3). The supernumerary digit ranges from a well-developed, fully formed extra digit (type A) to a small, rudimentary narrowly based digital remnant (type B).[6,7] Type B digits can be ligated at the base with a suture at the bedside. The digit will turn gangrenous and autoamputate. The most common complication is a residual bump or nubbin on the ulnar aspect of the hand.[7] These digits may, alternatively, be treated in the operating room to remove the residual ulnar nubbin that can be left after ligation. Type A digits require formal operative excision with reconstruction of the fifth finger ulnar collateral ligament.[7]

● UNDERGROWTH

Undergrowth generally refers to thumb hypoplasia, which may occur alone or in conjunction with other abnormalities such as radial longitudinal deficiency.

early. Later presentations are treated by the combination of one joint arthrodesis and wedge osteotomy. The thumb may function like an index finger without opposition (the five-fingered hand).[6] This is treated with pollicization.

● OVERGROWTH

Macrodactyly

Macrodactyly is a condition describing overgrowth of all structures within the affected digit. This must be distinguished from overgrowth secondary to isolated bone growth or vascular malformations (hemangioma, venous malformation, etc). Additionally, macrodactyly has been described in several syndromes, including neurofibromatosis, Beckwith-Wiedemann syndrome, Klippel-Trenaunay-Weber syndrome, and Proteus syndrome.[7]

Two types of macrodactyly have been described: static and progressive. Static macrodactyly is present at birth and subsequent growth is commensurate with the rest of the child. Progressive macrodactyly is more common and describes growth of the affected digit out of proportion with the rest of the body.[6] The condition is usually unilateral and may affect more than one digit. Although the etiology is unknown, overgrowth tends to correspond to a neurogenic distribution, most commonly the median nerve.

Progressive growth leads to stiffness, deviation, and loss of function. The growth continues until physeal closure at skeletal maturity. Treatment ranges from digit shortening, debulking, epiphysiodesis, and nerve stripping to amputation. Severe overgrowth isolated to a single digit is often treated with amputation. Symptomatic treatment often results in scarred and stiff digits.

● CONSTRICTION RING SYNDROME

Constriction ring syndrome is also known as amniotic band syndrome or Streeter syndrome. This sporadic syndrome is a result of external compression of the affected part by fibrous bands stemming from rupture of the amnionic membrane. The clinical manifestations of the annular band can range from minor cosmetic external compression, to distal lymphedema and congenital amputation (Figure 56-4).

The extremities are involved in a majority of cases of constriction ring syndrome. Acrosyndactyly refers to a coalescence of the distal digits with residual proximal web space clefts or sinuses. In these cases, the amniotic band occurred after digit separation was complete. Severe tight bands cause lymphedema and vascular compromise resulting in congenital amputations distal to the band.[6] Classically, these cases have a tapered appearance of the bone at the point of amputation.

Treatment of the constriction rings involve complete release of the band along with the skin, subcutaneous tissue, and fascia circumferentially with interposed flaps, most often a z-plasty or w-plasty. Surgical release can usually be performed electively unless the band is severe enough to cause acute neurovascular compromise at birth. In these cases, early release is recommended. Constriction rings may also result in varied clinical presentation such as clubfeet and facial clefting.

● FUTURE DIRECTIONS

Advances in imaging technology, including 3-dimensional ultrasound, have improved the prenatal diagnosis of upper extremity congenital anomalies. This is important given the potential association with severe malformations in other organ systems. The presence of an upper extremity malformation on ultrasound can lead to the ultimate diagnosis of a developmental syndrome.[9] This allows for improved parent counseling and the development of early treatment plans. This may eventually pave the way for in utero surgical techniques to treat these malformations.

REFERENCES

1. Al-Qattan MM, Yang Y, Kozin SH. Embryology of the upper limb. *J Hand Surg Am.* 2009;34:1340–1350.

2. Foucher G, Lorea P, Khouri, et al. Camptodactyly as a spectrum of congenital deficiencies: a treatment algorithm based on clinical examination. *Plast Reconstr Surg.* 2006; 117(6):1897–1905.

3. Gaebler-Spira D, Uellendahl J. Pediatric limb deficiencies. In: Molnar GE, Alexander MA, eds. *Pediatric Rehabilitation.* Philadelphia: Hanley & Belfus; 1999:333–350.

4. Goldfarb CA. Congenital hand differences. *J Hand Surg Am.* 2009;34(7):1351–1356.

5. Jones NF, Hansen SL, Bates SJ. Toe-to-hand transfers for congenital anomalies of the hand. *Hand Clin.* 2007;23:129–136.

6. Linder JM, Pincus DJ, Panthaki Z, Thaller SR. Congenital anomalies of the hand: an overview. *J Craniofac Surg.* 2009; 20(4):999–1004.

7. Kozin SH. Upper-extremity congenital anomalies. *J Bone Joint Surg Am.* 2003;85:1564–1576.

8. Maschke SD, Seitz W, Lawton J. Radial longitudinal deficiency. *J Am Acad Orthop Surg.* 2007;15:41–52.

9. Paladini D, Greco E, Sglavo G, et al. Congenital anomalies of upper extremities: prenatal ultrasound diagnosis, significance, and outcome. *Am J Obstet Gynecol.* 2010;202(6):596. e1–e10.

10. Shaperman J, Landsberger SE, Setoguchi Y. Early upper limb prosthesis fitting: when and what do we fit. *J Prosthet Orthot.* 2003;15:11–17.

11. Thatte MR, Mehta R. Treatment of radial dysplasia by a combination of distraction, radialization, and a bilobed flap—the results at 5-year follow-up. *J Hand Surg Eur Vol.* 2008;33(5):616–621.

chapter 57

Brachial Plexus

Julia K. Terzis, MD, PhD, FACS, FRCS(C) / *Zinon T. Kokkalis, MD*

● INTRODUCTION

Brachial plexus palsy in the adult population represents a devastating injury, which has dramatically increased during the last few years. These patients face significant long-term functional disability because of their paralyzed extremity, socioeconomic hardship, psychological distress, and a prolonged recuperation time. Surgical attempts to reconstruct the injured brachial plexus began in the early twentieth century which led to a number of pioneering surgeons to develop procedures for functional motor and sensory restoration to the paralyzed upper limb.

Brachial plexus palsy can be described as a severe neurological dysfunction of the upper extremity. Although this ailment has affected mankind for centuries, little progress had been achieved in the management of this type of palsy until recently reconstructive strategies, developments, and outcomes have drastically evolved in the past few decades. This progress has led to increasingly successful and more aggressive microsurgical techniques, such as nerve grafting, vascularized ulnar nerve transfer, motor and sensory nerve transfers, and functioning free muscle transplantation, which are now commonly used in reconstruction of the injured brachial plexus.

Historical Review

The literature on posttraumatic brachial plexus palsy began with devastating circumstances and much pessimism. Careful examination of Homer's *Iliad* reveals perhaps the first description of a brachial plexus injury: "Ἕκτωρ αὐερύοντα παρ᾽ ὦμον .... ῥῆξε δέ οἱ νευρήν· νάρκησε δὲ χεὶρ ἐπὶ καρπῷ"[1] (Hector struck him with that jagged rock right on the shoulder, where the collar bones divide the neck from chest, an especially vulnerable spot. The rock broke the bowstring and numbed his hands and wrists).[2]

In the early nineteenth century, Thorburn[3] was the first to report his intraoperative results and direct repair of the brachial plexus. His findings were related to a woman patient who was injured at work by a mill machine. Despite undergoing a neuroma resection and primary nerve repair, there was no recovery of neurologic function at her 4-year follow-up. The first case of neurotization was reported in 1903 by Harris and Low.[4] Because of the complex surgery and poor functional outcomes, brachial plexus injuries were looked upon with pessimism and surgery was rarely recommended.

During World War II, numerous brachial plexus injuries were encountered, which forced many medical centers in Europe to institute treatment for these lesions. In 1947, Seddon[5] introduced the concept of using long nerve grafts in the reconstruction of traction injuries. Seddon's modest outcomes,[6] led to search for suitable extraplexus donors to be used as motor donors for avulsion plexopathies. Transfer of the intercostals nerves were reported by Yeoman and Seddon in 1972;[7] the ipsilateral cervical plexus was reported by Brunelli in 1984;[8] the spinal accessory nerve by Kotani in 1971[9] and Allieu in 1984;[10] the contralateral C7 root by Gu et al. in 1991;[11] the selective contralateral C7 technique by Terzis in 1992;[12] and most recently, the ulnar nerve fascicles to musculocutaneous nerve transfer by Oberlin et al. in 1994.[13] All of these transfers represented significant improvements in the microsurgical management of brachial plexus injuries.

Epidemiology and Classification

Young men are most commonly involved in as many as 90% of the cases, but individuals of any age and of either gender can be affected. Despite improvements in the management and in the initial trauma resuscitation, there has also been a dramatic rise in the frequency of adult brachial plexus palsies due to high-velocity motor vehicle and motorcycle accidents. In our series of 204 patients[14] with posttraumatic brachial plexus injuries, motor vehicle accidents were responsible for the majority of the cases (59%). In other studies,[15] this number has been reported to be as high as 84%. The overall incidence in multitrauma patients secondary to motor vehicle accidents ranges from 0.67% to 1.3% of motor vehicle accidents and increases to 4.2% for victims of motorcycle accidents.[16]

Other common causes include pedestrian–vehicle accidents, snowmobile accidents, industrial accidents, gunshot or knife wounds, and other penetrating injuries.[15,17] Lower-velocity injuries, such as bicycling injuries, skiing, or falling from a height, have also been encountered and reported to have a reciprocal correlation with brachial plexus injuries.[18] Nontraumatic lesions include tumors of the brachial plexus, compression, and irradiation. Kim et al.[19] reported the largest series of brachial plexus lesions in the literature and analyzed the causes involved in 1019 operative brachial plexus injuries during a 30-year period. The majority of the injuries were due to stretch/contusions (50%) and the next most common traumatic lesions were penetrating and were due to gunshot wounds (12%) and lacerations (7%). Nontraumatic lesions causing damage to the brachial plexus were tumors (16%) and thoracic outlet syndrome (16%).

Mechanisms of Injury

There are three major mechanisms of injury implicated with brachial plexus:[20]

1. The brachial plexus may be crushed between the clavicle and the first rib. This results from direct trauma to the neck and upper extremity and is associated with other organ system injuries, depending on the severity of the trauma.
2. Compression of the brachial plexus by adjacent structures that have been injured, such as bone fragments or hypertrophic callus from a clavicle fracture, hematoma, or pseudoaneurysms from vascular lesions.
3. Traction to the brachial plexus combined with neck flexion toward the contralateral side and/or hyperextension of the arm can also result in brachial plexus injury. Caudal traction of the arm will usually damage the upper roots and trunks, and traction in a cephalic direction will most likely damage the lower plexus.

Following a traction injury, the nerve may rupture, be avulsed at the level of the spinal cord, or be significantly stretched but remain in continuity.[21] Root injuries can be differentiated based on the location of the lesion relative to the dorsal root ganglion (DRG). Pre- or supraganglionic injuries occur proximal to the DRG, whereas post- or infraganglionic injuries occur distal to the DRG. Avulsion of one or more nerve roots, which

changes the lesion from a post- to a preganglionic injury, is common, occurring in approximately 70% of severe brachial plexus stretch avulsion injuries[19] (Figure 57-1). Traction forces to the spinal nerve are transmitted to the rootlet and the epidural sac, resulting in a tear of the sac and the presence of a pseudomeningocele on cervical myelography.[22]

All of the above mechanisms can coexist simultaneously and portend a poor prognosis. The velocity and degree of the impact on the brachial plexus and the position of the arm and shoulder in relation to the neck and the trunk at the time of the injury will influence the degree and severity of the injury and will dictate the ultimate prognosis. The incidence of associated injuries varies, but are also frequent. In most reports, concomitant injuries after motor vehicle and/or motorcycle accidents often include closed head injuries, chest wall injuries (hemopneumothorax or rib fractures), vascular injuries to the subclavian or axillary vessels, shoulder dislocation, intra-abdominal injuries, and fractures of the clavicle, scapula, and long bones.[16]

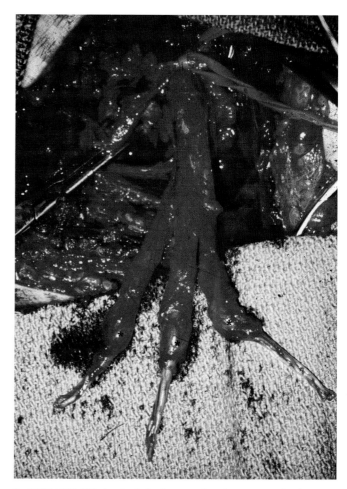

● **FIGURE 57-1.** A clinical example of a preganglionic injury (root avulsion). In this patient, three nerve roots (C7, C8, and T1) are avulsed. The dorsal root ganglia (DRG) are clearly seen (*).

PATIENT EVALUATION

Patients with a brachial plexus injury are usually admitted to the emergency unit with multiple injuries and are often medically sedated. Potentially life-threatening associated injuries take precedence and are treated initially. Arm paralysis is often noted after the patient is awakened. The initial evaluation is usually performed by a physician who is not experienced with this type of injury. Evaluation by a surgeon specializing in brachial plexus should be performed early on so that a management strategy can be established. A detailed history is essential for determining the mechanism of injury and arriving at a correct diagnosis.

Physical Examination

A systematic clinical examination of a patient with a brachial plexus injury is important for the proper diagnosis and decision making. The examination usually commences with an inspection of the involved upper extremity, trunk, and neck regions. Any scars are noticed. Passive and active joint range of motion is documented.

An examination of the upper extremity muscle strength as compared with the contralateral normal side is then carried out. Manual muscle testing starts off by observing signs of muscle atrophy, palpation of the tone of each muscle group, and gauging muscle strength against resistance. The British Medical Research Council muscle grading system[23] can be used to record the examiner's results on a plexus chart. In this classification, M0 = no muscle contraction, M1 = a flicker of contraction, M2 = gravity assist, M3 = strength against gravity, M4 = strength against resistance and M5 = normal strength. In our center, we use the British Medical Research Council grading system, expanded further with intermediate grades of + and − (eg, M3−, M3, M3+).[14]

The sensory examination is performed on the arm, the forearm, and the hand; and includes light touch appreciation, two-point discrimination, testing of vibratory sense, and joint position sense (proprioception). Patients should also be examined for the presence or absence of a Horner syndrome, which consists of miosis, upper eyelid ptosis, and anhydrosis (Figure 57-2). A positive Horner sign signifies a partial or complete avulsion of the C8 and/or T1 roots. The vascularity of the upper extremity should also be examined. Involvement of the subclavian vessels carries a poor prognosis for neurological recovery.

The presence of a Tinel sign, which can be elicited by tapping over the supraclavicular area, is important, as it can differentiate between a root avulsion and root rupture. The patient is asked to identify the area in which a tingling sensation is perceived. If the Tinel sign reproduces tingling along the course of the involved root, the root is considered to be in continuity with the spinal cord and it is assessed as a rupture. The absence of a Tinel sign in the supraclavicular area carries a morbid prognosis, as it signifies a global avulsion plexopathy.

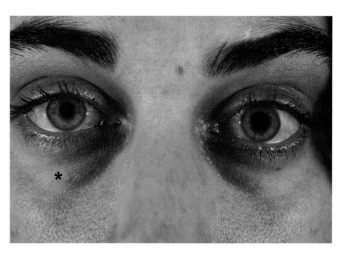

● **FIGURE 57-2.** A patient with a right Horner syndrome (the asterisk identifies the injured side): miosis (small pupil), upper eyelid ptosis, and anhydrosis (absence of facial sweating on the affected side). A positive Horner sign implies disruption of the sympathetic supply to the ipsilateral eye and face through the lower roots (C8 and T1) and is a strong indicator of avulsion of these roots.

Pain Management

Pain following an avulsion injury to the brachial plexus represents the most significant impediment to rehabilitation. Pain management is indicated in patients with unbearable pain. A detailed history of pain and its characteristics (location, onset, duration, frequency, and intensity) should be obtained. Furthermore, the amount and need for analgesic medication should be ascertained. Some patients are given all classes of analgesic agents, including opioids, tricyclic antidepressants, and antipsychotic drugs; but some pain is difficult to treat.

Patients are asked to grade their pain from 1 to 10. The pain is commonly described as continuous, burning, and compressing and is usually located in the hand. Patients with debilitating pain have poor outcomes. For this reason we recommend that these patients undergo dorsal root entry zone (DREZ) lesioning first, before proceeding with the formal brachial plexus reconstruction. This consists of radiofrequency thermocoagulation of the dorsal root entry zone, which includes the central segment of the dorsal rootlets, the tract of Lissauer, and the five dorsal-most layers of the dorsal horn where the primary sensory afferent pathways terminate.

Relief of pain allows the patient to focus on extremity rehabilitation postoperatively. The technique was introduced in 1979 by Nashold and colleagues,[24] who demonstrated good pain relief in 54% of 39 patients (average follow-up, 34 months, range, 14 months to 10 years). In a study by Samii et al., 75% of 49 patients experienced significant pain reduction (average follow-up, 10 years).[25] The long-term efficacy of this procedure strongly indicates that pain after brachial plexus avulsion originates from the deafferented, ie, disrupted (and gliotic), sensory fibers of the dorsal horn.[26] In a retrospective study of 204 patients, we found that early exploration and reconstruction of the brachial plexus afforded good pain relief in the majority of the patients. The senior author (JKT) documented that for all types of lesions, the mean pain score after nerve reconstruction was significantly lower ($P < 0.05$) than it was before surgery;[14] and for avulsion injuries, the mean pain score postoperatively was reduced up to 30% as compared with the preoperative value.

Electrophysiologic Studies

Electrophysiologic studies are of considerable assistance in the preoperative and intraoperative evaluation of the brachial plexus injury. Needle electromyography and nerve conduction studies can be employed for the study of location, number, and pathophysiology of lesions affecting the brachial plexus.

Electromyography. Three weeks after the injury, after the nerve has undergone Wallerian degeneration, needle electrodes are inserted into a muscle to record the electrical activity of individual or groups of motor units. Denervated muscle fibers demonstrate a reduction in the number of motor unit potentials as well as signs of denervation, which include spontaneous involuntary waveforms such as fibrillation potentials and positive sharp waves. If there is peripheral reinnervation from intact motor units through peripheral sprouting, there will be polyphasic motor unit potentials of increased amplitude and prolonged duration.[27] In cases of neurapraxic lesions, the presence of an increased number of motor unit potentials and decrease in the number of fibrillation potentials correlate with a good prognosis for spontaneous recovery. Needle electromyography of the paraspinal muscles, which are innervated by the dorsal rami of the spinal roots, should also be routinely performed; fibrillation potentials in these muscles provides strong evidence of avulsion of the corresponding roots.[28]

Nerve Conduction Studies[29]

Sensory. The presence of sensory nerve action potentials (SNAPs) can be used to differentiate between a pre- and postganglionic lesion. These are low amplitude (50–100 μV) waveforms that are recorded directly off the sensory nerves after electrical stimulation. If the SNAPs are normal but there is a clinical loss of sensation, this implies that there is an avulsion of the sensory spinal roots from the spinal cord with preservation of the DRG where the sensory neurons reside. Even though the sensory axons are intact which results in a normal measured SNAP, there is a disruption of the afferent sensory pathways which leads to subjective loss of sensation and signifies a preganglionic lesion. If the injury is distal to the dorsal root ganglion, the sensory action potentials are absent. Clinically the upper extremity is still anesthetic because

the sensory axons have been disconnected from their cell bodies.

Motor. A mixed or pure motor nerve is stimulated at several sites along the nerve. The summated electrical response of muscle fibers innervated by the motor axons is called the compound action potential which produces a large amplitude waveform (>4 MV) that is typically biphasic in appearance with large amplitude and longer duration.

Lamina Test. Electrical stimulation is applied to each exiting spinal nerve root to determine if the patient perceives any sensation in the dermatome innervated by this root. A positive response would be strong evidence against a nerve root avulsion.

Specialized intraoperative techniques such as motor evoked potentials could be an effective means for investigating the functional status of anterior motor roots and motor fibers in exposed spinal nerves;[30] however, technical artifacts impair their reliability and they require an increased operative time.

Radiological Studies

After a brachial plexus injury, plain x-rays can reveal any coexisting fractures of the cervical spine, shoulder, chest, ribs, clavicle or upper extremity. A clavicle fracture should raise the suspicion of trauma to the underlying brachial plexus. A fracture of the scapula may imply an injury to the suprascapular nerve. Rib fractures may indicate an injury to the underlying intercostals nerves which may exclude their use as donors for nerve transfers. An inspiratory and expiratory chest x-ray or fluoroscopy is performed to evaluate the integrity of the phrenic nerve. A finding of an elevated hemi-diaphragm preoperatively implies an injury to the phrenic nerve which is often associated with an upper plexus lesion and lessens the surgeon's ability to use multiple ipsilateral intercostals nerves as donors. This information is fundamental for any preoperative planning.[31]

A first rib fracture may denote damage to the overlying brachial plexus and be associated with a vascular injury. Patients who have undergone an interposition vein graft or those that are scheduled for free muscle transfers should undergo angiography and a Duplex scan of the upper extremity to evaluate vessel patency. If vascular inadequacy is reported, vascularized nerve grafts will be required. If the arterial flow is insufficient, consultation with a vascular surgeon is needed prior to brachial plexus reconstruction. Current imaging studies may demonstrate traumatic meningoceles, deformity of nerve roots sleeves, dural scars and nerve root avulsions. The combination of a cervical myelogram, introduced by Murphey et al.[32] in 1947, and computed tomographic (CT) myelography are considered the best methods to examine the ventral and dorsal rootlets and rule out avulsions (Figure 57-3). CT myelography is best performed at least 1 month after injury to allow the pseudomeningocele

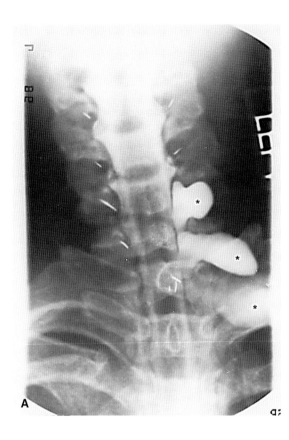
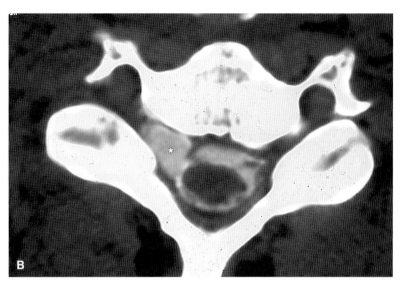

● **FIGURE 57-3.** Multiple root avulsions are clearly seen by plain myelography. A preoperative myelogram shows three large pseudomeningoceles (*) at C7, C8, and T1 levels (A). Excellent visualization of an avulsed root (*) can be afforded by high-resolution CT myelography in an axial section (B).

to fully develop and seal. One should consider that the presence of a pseudomeningocele is strongly indicative of a nerve root avulsion; however, avulsed roots can exist in the face of a normal myelogram.[33] Presently, CT myelography has been proven to have a 95% sensitivity and 98% specificity.[34] Combining these two imaging techniques (CT myelography) improved the resolution and gave a more accurate categorization of the level of nerve root injury.[35]

Magnetic resonance imaging (MRI) has been used to study the cervical cord in an effort to visualize all portions of the brachial plexus and predict any root avulsion. MRI can also reveal large neuromas on T1-weighted imaging and increased signal intensity on T2-weighted imaging. It can also detect any associated inflammation or edema. An MRI should not be used as a routine imaging tool for avulsion plexopathies because of the insufficient contrast between the subarachnoid space and the neural structures, a problem caused mainly by the cerebrospinal fluid pulsation.[36] A recent retrospective study, however, comparing MR imaging to CT myelography of 175 cervical roots in 35 patients indicated the sensitivity of detection of the cervical nerve root avulsion was the same (92.9%) with both modalities.[37]

In contrast to conventional MRI, the more enhanced MRI myelographic techniques are just T2-weighted MRI sequences that emphasize the contrast between the spinal cord and roots and the adjacent cerebrospinal fluid. MR myelography is noninvasive, relatively quick, requires no contrast medium, provides imaging in multiple projections,

and is comparable in diagnostic ability to the more invasive, time-consuming techniques of conventional myelography and CT myelography.[38] Gasparotti et al.[39] opined that conventional MRI can be supplanted by three-dimensional MR myelography. In three-dimensional MRI with a constructive interference in steady state (CISS) technique demonstrated 89% sensitivity, 95% specificity, and 92% diagnostic accuracy.[39]

● **MANAGEMENT**

Open Injuries

The timing of surgery for open and closed injuries is different. The indications for acute surgical intervention include the following: concomitant vascular trauma, open injuries after sharp laceration, and crush or contaminated open wounds. In general, brachial plexus injuries associated with open wounds are infrequent and require early exploration, as with any open wound. Devitalized tissue should be debrided and bony fractures stabilized, and any associated vascular injuries should be repaired on an emergency basis. A clean nerve transection can be repaired primarily by an end-to-end coaptation. In crush or contaminated open wounds, after the debridement, tagging the divided nerve ends with sutures or approximating them, if possible, is advisable for later nerve repair. Emergency nerve grafting procedures are not routinely performed. Reexploration and nerve reconstruction is planned after at least 3 weeks, when the zone of injury can be clearly defined and repair to relatively healthy tissue can be accomplished.

Gunshot wounds involving the brachial plexus do not always transect all the brachial plexus elements, but may contuse, bruise, or stretch neural tissue. Acute exploration is recommended for suspected major vascular interruption or vascular injury presenting as a pseudoaneurysm. Gunshot wounds may result in lesions in continuity and these may cause an incomplete loss of function of the involved plexus element(s). Some of these injuries may show some recovery spontaneously with time, although more often, they may not.[40] Plexus elements that are not in continuity should be repaired within a few weeks (Figure 57-4). Gunshot wounds induced plexopathies can be associated with severe pain and autonomic disturbances, usually localized to the hand. Sympathetic

blocks followed by cervical sympathectomy may offer some relief if a pharmacological approach has failed.

Closed Injuries

The majority of patients with brachial plexus lesions have closed traction injuries. The optimal time for reconstruction may have been the subject of controversy in the past, but currently the consensus is that delays of longer than 3 months after injury diminish the chances of functional recovery.[14,41,42] Prolonged denervation invites muscular atrophy, fibrosis, and joint stiffness which mitigate against successful functional recovery. Thus, physical therapy and slow electrical pulse stimulation[43] should be instituted as soon as possible to prevent soft tissue contractures and to maintain the bulk of the denervated muscles. However,

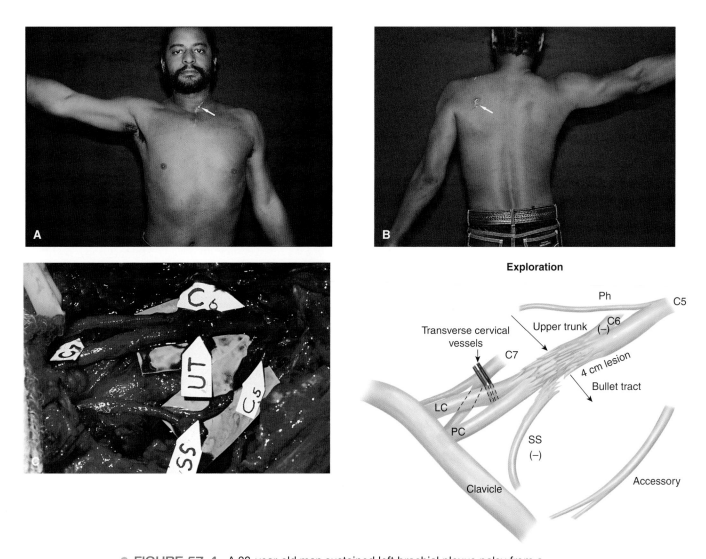

● **FIGURE 57-4.** A 28-year-old man sustained left brachial plexus palsy from a gunshot injury to the neck (arrow). The patient could not abduct his shoulder or flex his elbow (A). Note the bullet exit wound (*arrow*) on the patient's back (B). Two weeks after the injury, an exploration of the left brachial plexus revealed that the bullet tract had penetrated most of the upper trunk (UT) and completely transected the suprascapular (SS) nerve (C).

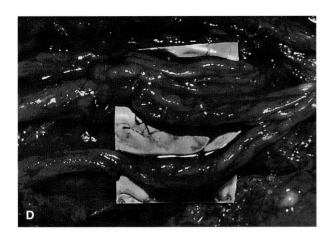

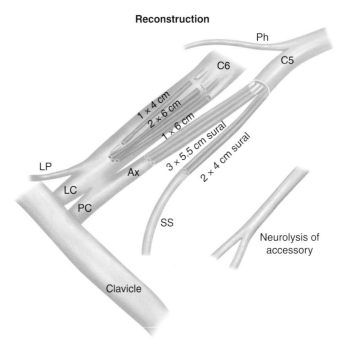

Reconstruction

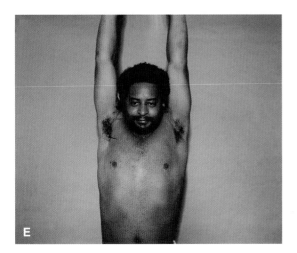

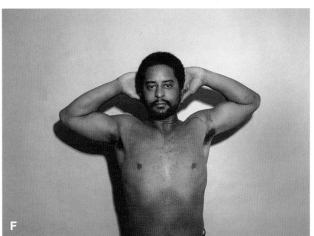

● **FIGURE 57-4.** (*continued*) Plexus reconstruction was performed with interposition sural nerve grafts as follows: C5 root to the SS nerve and posterior cord (axillary); and part of C6 to the lateral cord (LC). Neurolysis was also performed on the accessory nerve (D). Five years after surgery, he has excellent shoulder abduction (E) and excellent external rotation and elbow flexion (F). Note the return of symmetrical muscle bulk.
(*Part A–D: From Terzis JK, Vekris MD, Soucacos PN. Outcomes of brachial plexus reconstruction in 204 patients with devastating paralysis. Plast Reconstr Surg. 1999:104(5):1221–1240.*)

most patients have surgery much later usually because of delayed referral to a specialized center. Other patients undergo late operations either because they have other severe associated injuries initially or they have a severe pain syndrome.[44] We believe that aggressive early reconstruction within 6 weeks to 3 months after injury offers the most rewarding results.[14]

Surgical Exploration

The complex reconstructive surgery of the injured brachial plexus demands light general anesthesia, using sufentanil, and an avoidance of any kind of paralytic drugs, so that intraoperative electrophysiologic studies can be performed. The patient is placed in the supine position with a soft roll along their vertebral spine and under the neck (Figure 57-5). The affected upper extremity is abducted on an arm board. The sterile field includes bilateral upper extremities, both sides of the neck up to the mandible, the anterior and posterior chest to the midline, and bilateral lower extremities. The surgery is executed simultaneously by two teams: the main team explores the injured plexus to define the extent and the type of injury, and the second team harvests nerve grafts from both lower extremities, under 4× wide field loupe magnification.

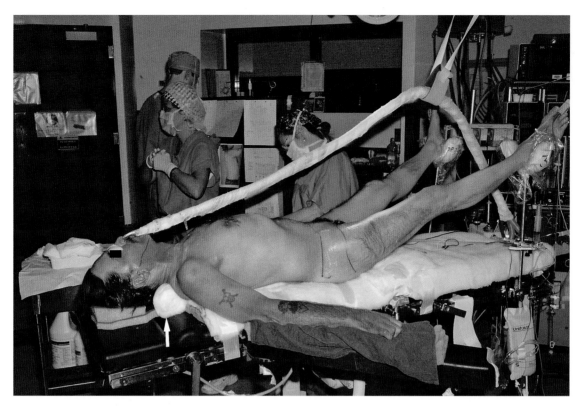

● **FIGURE 57-5.** Positioning of patient for plexus reconstruction. Under general anesthesia the patient is placed in the supine position with a soft roll along the vertebral spine and a separate roll under the neck (*arrow*). The affected upper extremity is placed on an arm board.

A combined supraclavicular and infraclavicular approach is used in the majority of patients (Figure 57-6). For exposure of the supraclavicular plexus, the incision is made parallel to the posterior border of the sternocleidomastoid muscle, then turns laterally over the clavicle and a posteriorly based triangular flap is raised. The supraclavicular sensory nerves and the external jugular vein are preserved. The sternocleidomastoid muscle is retracted medially and the phrenic nerve is identified on the anterior border of the anterior scalene muscle. The phrenic nerve is traced cranially to its C4-C5 origins and it is stimulated with a direct current stimulator at 0.5, 1.0, or 2.0 mA amplitude to verify its integrity, and the movements of the diaphragm are recorded. A rule of thumb is that if neural tissue is normal it will always respond to a 0.5 mA stimulus. If the amplitude of stimulation has to be raised intraoperatively to obtain a peripheral muscle contraction the involved nerve segment is in the injury zone. The dissection proceeds in a caudal direction to expose the C5, C6, and C7 spinal nerves (Figure 57-7). The dorsal scapular, long thoracic, and suprascapular nerves are identified and exposed. As the C7 root is approached, the transverse cervical vessels and omohyoid muscle are isolated and retracted. The C8 and Tl roots are identified superior to the first rib and posterior to the subclavian artery and vein. On left-sided exposures, special care should be taken to avoid injury to the thoracic duct.

For exposure of the infraclavicular plexus, the previous incision continues along the deltopectoral groove to the anterior axillary fold. The cephalic vein is circumferentially dissected and preserved. The humeral insertion of the pectoralis major and the coracoid insertion of the pectoralis minor are tagged and divided for later reapproximation. Then the muscles are raised medially and the infraclavicular plexus is exposed (Figure 57-8). The lateral cord is encountered first, and is traced distally to the exit of the musculocutaneous nerve and the lateral cord contribution to the median nerve. The posterior cord is found posterior and lateral to the lateral cord. Proximodistal dissection leads to the origin of the axillary and radial nerves. Some surgeons perform a clavicular osteotomy to gain better exposure. We do not carry out clavicular osteotomy, due to the risk of a compressive osseous callous on the underlying nerve repairs. Furthermore, bone healing in the clavicle is capricious and malunions or nonunions can result. We routinely connect the supraclavicular and infraclavicular exposures by means of subclavicular blunt dissection.

During the brachial plexus exploration, electrophysiologic studies are performed as soon as each nerve is exposed and before it is manipulated. This is especially useful in lesions in continuity, because a decision has to be made to proceed either with neurolysis or resection and interposition nerve grafting.

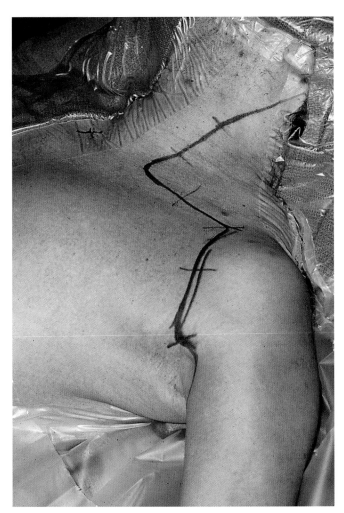

● **FIGURE 57-6.** Standard skin incision for exposure of the supraclavicular and infraclavicular plexus. The incision parallels the posterior border of the sternocleidomastoid muscle and angles over the clavicle into the deltopectoral groove.

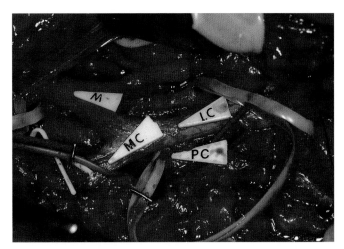

● **FIGURE 57-8.** Exposure of the infraclavicular plexus. LC, lateral cord; PC, posterior cord; MC, musculocutaneous nerve; M, median nerve.

Sensory motor differentiation is accomplished with frozen nerve biopsy studies which can be simultaneously performed for carbonic anhydrase histochemistry (for sensory axons)[45] or cholinesterase staining (for motor axons). These are taken routinely at the level of the spinal root to assess the integrity of the neural tissue versus scar and to ascertain the presence or absence of dorsal root ganglion cells. Proximal root tissue that is found to contain ganglion cells or scar tissue with no evidence of myelinated nerve fibers is not used as a proximal donor for nerve repair. According to Malessy et al.,[46] the intraoperative frozen-section examination is of potential value in decision making. If less than 50% myelin is present, the use of C5-C6 stumps in a grafting procedure aiming at biceps muscle reinnervation should be abandoned in favor of a nerve transfer procedure. This observation warrants further investigation.

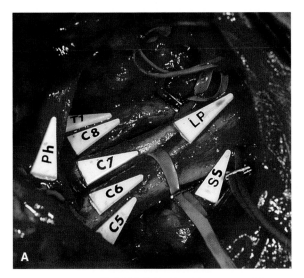

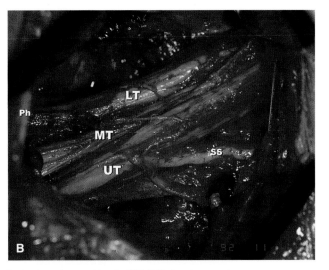

● **FIGURE 57-7.** Exposure of the supraclavicular plexus. Roots (C5-T1), trunks, and divisions are exposed (A). In this patient, neurolysis of the entire supraclavicular plexus was performed (B). UT, upper trunk; MT, medial trunk; LT, lower trunk; SS, suprascapular nerve; Ph, phrenic nerve.

Neurolysis

Upon completion of the exploration, the level, type, and extent of the injury has been ascertained. Neurolysis, nerve grafting, and nerve transfers are surgical options for restoring distal functions. Neurolysis is used when the explored elements of the plexus are hard to palpation, with thickened epineurium but in continuity. Neurolysis is performed to decompress the neural tissue and to examine the integrity of the perineural sheath of individual fascicles. Each neural segment is electrophysiologically tested prior to performing a microneurolysis. Data obtained from such recordings facilitate the decision making whether to perform a microneurolysis alone or resection of part of or the entire injured nerve. Longitudinal epineurotomies and interfascicular neurolysis are performed under high-power magnification under the operating microscope. Bulging of the entrapped fascicles strongly indicates that microneurolysis is effective and bodes for a favorable prognosis. If proximal stimulation of the nerve produces no distal muscle contraction and microneurolysis reveals a loss of perineurial continuity of the individual bundles, the injured segment is resected to healthy tissue both proximally and distally and the defect is bridged with nerve grafts.

Nerve Grafting

Nerve grafting is the gold standard technique for overcoming nerve gaps resulting from the resection of an injured nerve segment. The resected nerve stump must be intraoperatively evaluated for any remaining healthy nerve fascicles and the degree of scarring.[47] While excising a partially ruptured lesion, one has to be careful not to downgrade the existing function by resecting intact fascicles and convert it to a complete one. Various grafts can be used to bridge the gap or bypass the fibrotic area.

The donor nerves available for grafting are the following in order of preference: sural, saphenous, medial brachial, medial antebrachial cutaneous, and superficial radial. The donor nerve of choice has been the sural nerve, which can provide up to 45 cm of useful graft material from each leg. The sural nerve is usually harvested through three or four small incisions on the posterior aspect of the leg. Prior to placement of the grafts, attention is paid to ensuring an adequate vascularization of the underlying bed. Saphenous nerves are also harvested, usually at a second stage, and used as long interposition nerve grafts primarily as cross chest nerve grafts for connection with the contralateral C7 root. One can obtain up to a 63 cm graft from each lower extremity. In cases of C8 and T1 avulsion, the ulnar nerve can be used as a vascularized nerve graft. The theoretical advantage of a vascularized nerve graft is the ability to provide immediate intraneural perfusion in a poorly vascularized bed and to reconstruct large nerve gaps.[48] The vascularized ulnar nerve is based on the superior ulnar collateral artery and vein (Figure 57-9). The distal and proximal portions of the nerve must survive on the superior

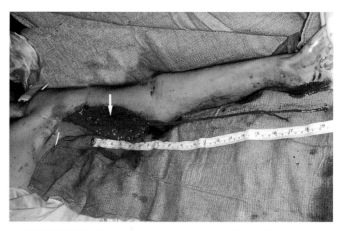

● **FIGURE 57-9.** Harvesting the vascularized ulnar nerve using a longitudinal incision from the medial upper arm to the wrist. The vascularity of the ulnar nerve is based on the superior ulnar collateral artery and vein (*arrow*). Fifty-six centimeters of vascularized trunk graft can usually be obtained.

ulnar collateral vessels and survive transfer even if placed in a scarred bed.[49,50]

Although nerve allografts also provide a boundless source of nerve graft material, they still need immunosuppression to prevent allograft rejection hence this requires further study.[51]

Nerve Transfers

The transfer of a functional but less important nerve to a distal denervated but higher priority target is called neurotization or nerve transfer procedure.[18,52] In these reinnervation procedures, it is important to anticipate the functional result and the possible resulting deficit from the donor nerve. The number of myelinated axons available in possible donors is important for nerve transfers and the recovery of muscle function.[53] Also, the use of distal motor nerve transfers provides donor motor fibers that are very close to the target muscle. One or more nerve transfers are usually performed for shoulder, elbow, and hand functions. Options include intraplexus and extraplexus sources. Neurotizations may be performed for motor or sensory recovery (Figure 57-10).

Intraplexus Neurotization. Intraplexus transfers are far more reliable than extraplexus ones and are superior to the musculotendinous transfers in reconstruction of simple functions such as elbow flexion, shoulder abduction, or wrist extension.[54] Intraplexus donor options include the undamaged roots or available branches or fascicles of functioning donors. In C5-C6 root avulsions, reconstruction of the shoulder and elbow function can be achieved by means of the ipsilateral C7 root[55,56] which can be sacrificed for higher priority targets. Then, the distal targets innervated by the C7 root can be neurotized with extraplexus motor donors.[18] Other potential donors include the medial

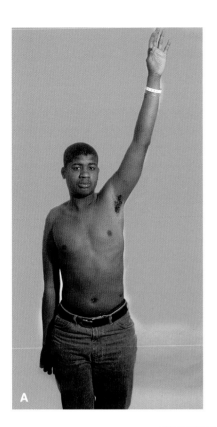
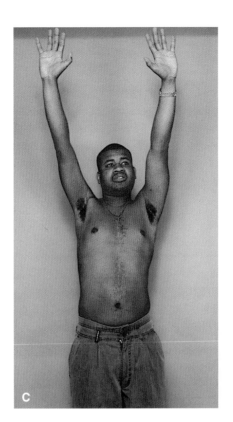
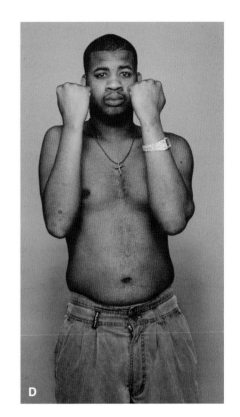

Exploration

C2
C3
Acc
C4
C5 - Avulsion
C6 - Avulsion
● C5
● C6
○ C7
Ax
R
MC
M

B

Reconstruction

C2
C3
Acc
C4
SS
Ax
MC
Left LP

● **FIGURE 57-10.** An 18-year-old man sustained right brachial plexus palsy secondary to a motor vehicle accident. Preoperative evaluation revealed an upper plexus injury (loss of shoulder abduction, external rotation, and elbow flexion) (A). Six months after the injury, an exploration of the right brachial plexus revealed C5 and C6 root avulsions. Plexus reconstruction was performed with interposition sural nerve grafts as follows: C3 and C4 motor roots to the axillary nerve (AX); and contralateral lateral pectoral (LP) to the musculocutaneous nerve (MC). End-to-end coaptation of the distal accessory (Acc) to the suprascapular (SS) nerve was also performed (B). Three years postoperatively, he demonstrates excellent shoulder abduction (C) and full elbow flexion (D). (*Part A, B: From Terzis JK, Kostopoulos VK. The surgical treatment of brachial plexus injuries in adults. Plast Reconstr Surg. 2007;119(4):73e–92e.*)

pectoral nerve[57] or the thoracodorsal nerve[58] to the musculocutaneous nerve. Leechavengvongs et al.[59] reported excellent results with the long head of the triceps branch transfer to the axillary nerve, achieving an average shoulder abduction of 124 degrees in his series. Furthermore, for upper brachial plexus injuries, excellent results were validated by several authors with the Oberlin technique[13,60,61] in which a single redundant ulnar nerve fascicle (innervating the flexor carpi ulnaris) is transferred to the biceps branch of the musculocutaneous nerve in the medial arm to restore elbow flexion. They also noted that hand and ulnar nerve function, was not compromised during a long-term follow-up period. The key aspect of the procedure is to reinnervate the biceps branch of the musculocutaneous nerve close to its motor entry into the muscle. Elbow flexion function can be further augmented (especially in cases of delayed surgery) by concomitantly reinnervating the brachialis muscle by using a graft from the medial pectoral nerve[62] or a fascicle of the adjacent median nerve.[63]

Extraplexus Neurotization. In global root avulsions where intraplexus donors are not available, reconstruction is carried out by using only available extraplexus donors. Global avulsion of the brachial plexus carries the worst prognosis among all types of plexus lesions. The prime goal is to restore shoulder stability, elbow flexion, and hand sensation. Extraplexus neurotization is the transfer of a nonbrachial plexus nerve to distal plexus elements for neurotization of a higher priority target. Options include the distal spinal accessory nerve, the ipsilateral intercostal nerves, the phrenic nerve, and motor branches of the cervical plexus (C3-C4).

The distal part of the spinal accessory nerve is used as donor to preserve upper trapezius function. It is synergistic with the suprascapular nerve, and direct repair is usually possible. In our series, 81% of the distal spinal accessory to the suprascapular nerve transfers were carried out directly, without the need for an interposition nerve graft. The outcomes were good and excellent in 79% of the patients for the supraspinatus muscle and 55% for the infraspinatus muscle.[64] In our series, concomitant neurotization of the axillary nerve yielded improved outcomes in shoulder abduction function, as compared with repair of only the suprascapular nerve.[65] The accessory nerve has also provided reliable results when used with an interposition graft to the biceps.[66]

Intercostal nerves have yielded acceptable results, especially for reconstruction of the axillary, triceps, or musculocutaneous nerve.[67,68] Intercostal nerves are challenging and time consuming to harvest, and each one has approximately 1200 axons. When neurotization of the musculocutaneous nerve is planned, which is composed of approximately 6000 fibers, at least three intercostal nerves need to be used for this neurotization to yield an acceptable result.[14,52] Intercostal nerves may also be used to innervate a free muscle transplant.[18,69] in addition, their sensory branches may be used separately for sensory neurotization of the anesthetic hand.

Other options for motor donor nerves for reconstruction include the phrenic nerve and the contralateral C7 root. The phrenic nerve is considered to be a good motor donor, with approximately 800 axons, but the risk of potential long-term respiratory consequences should be considered.[18,52,70] The senior author has used the proximal phrenic nerve for neurotization only if the patient presents with a paralyzed diaphragm preoperatively. In cases where all the ipsilateral intercostals are to be used for neurotization procedures, the senior author's preference is to perform an end-to-side coaptation between the phrenic nerve and a nerve graft, thereby preventing denervation of the ipsilateral diaphragm. The phrenic nerve can be directly coapted to the suprascapular nerve, or used with an interposition nerve graft to the axillary or musculocutaneous nerve.[71]

The preliminary results of the contralateral C7 transfer have been encouraging.[72,73] The contralateral C7 transfer can be extended and enhanced by using a vascularized ulnar nerve graft in patients with C8-T1 avulsions, and the median nerve is the most common recipient. In our series, median nerve neurotization yielded mostly protective sensibility and some return of the grasp in selected patients.[50] A selective contralateral C7 technique was introduced by the senior author.[12] Using microdissection techniques, selective neurectomies deprive only certain components of the C7 divisions (anterior division destined for the pectoralis major and posterior division for the latissimus dorsi and triceps) and rarely the entire root. The functional motor and sensory donor deficit is minimal and recovers by 6 months. Neurotization of single motor nerve using the selective contralateral C7 technique, such as the musculocutaneous, triceps branch, and axillary nerve, yielded useful function in the majority of patients.[50]

The restoration of hand sensibility is of prime importance in global plexopathies and can be achieved by neurotization of the median nerve from sensory intercostal nerves or from the supraclavicular sensory nerves. A vascularized ulnar nerve graft to the median nerve from either intraplexus ipsilateral donors (Figure 57-11) or from the contralateral C7 root has been used to restore both sensory protection and some finger flexion.[48] Poor results are caused by the long distances involved and the long denervation time. To avoid misdirection, selective neurotization of specific fascicles of the median nerve in the arm has been proposed.[74] Nevertheless, in patients with complete brachial plexus palsy, discriminatory sensibility is rarely restored, but protective sensibility is useful for patients with completely anesthetic hands.[75]

Free Muscle Transplantation

Free functioning muscle transfer for brachial plexus paralysis management[76,77,78] is a reconstructive option for patients who have sustained complete brachial plexus avulsions, for late cases,[79] or when the restored muscle

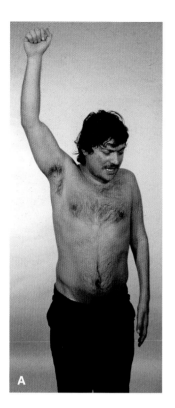
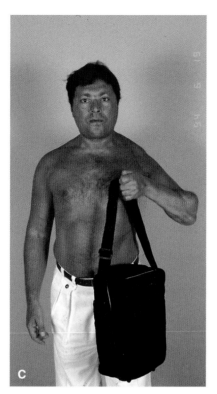
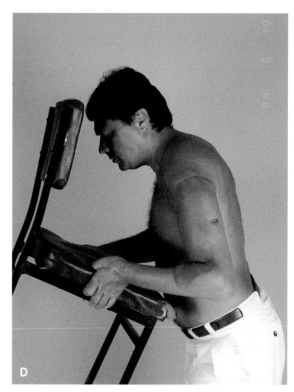

Exploration

Reconstruction

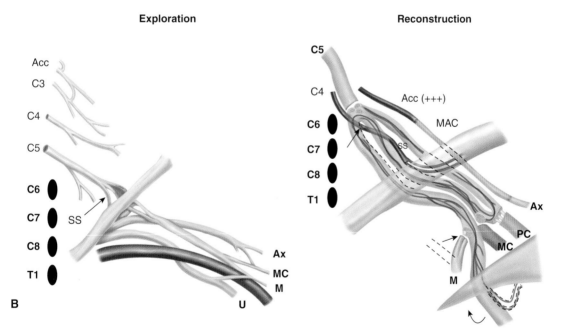

● **FIGURE 57-11.** A 32-year-old man sustained a global left brachial plexus paralysis following a motorcycle accident. Preoperatively, he presented with a totally flail, anesthetic arm with severe, intolerable pain (A). The patient underwent an exploration of his supraclavicular and infraclavicular left brachial plexus 6 months after the injury. The intraoperative diagnosis was rupture of C5 root and avulsions of C6 to T1 roots. Plexus reconstruction included: accessory (Acc) to axillary nerve (AX) with interposition nerve graft; direct neurotization of C4 motor branch to suprascapular (SS) nerve; and C5 to musculocutaneous (MC), median (M), and posterior cord (PC) by means of a vascularized ulnar nerve graft. The patient also underwent secondary procedures such as wrist fusion, free gracilis muscle transfer for finger extension, and free latissimus dorsi transfer for posterior deltoid and triceps muscle substitution (B). Six years after the injury, he has strong elbow flexion and finger flexion through the median nerve neurotization. The patient is able to lift easily his shoulder bag or a chair and he is currently pain free (C, D). *(Part B: From Terzis JK, Vekris MD, Soucacos PN. Outcomes of brachial plexus reconstruction in 204 patients with devastating paralysis. Plast Reconstr Surg. 1999:104(5):1221–1240.)*

function after primary plexus reconstruction is deemed inadequate.[14,18] Currently, free muscle transfers are performed routinely for restoration of elbow flexion[80,81] or elbow extension and for reanimation of the hand.[82–84]

Free muscle transfer of the contralateral latissimus dorsi or the gracilis are the treatment of choice when muscles from the ipsilateral side are not strong enough to support elbow flexion. In our center, the latissimus dorsi and the rectus femoris muscles are considered the optimal muscles to provide elbow flexion or elbow extension. The transferred muscles are neurotized either directly from local motor donors (ie, intercostal nerves) or by banked nerves from ipsilateral motor donors, such as the accessory nerve or cross-chest nerve grafts from the contralateral anterior or posterior divisions of the C7 root. With such a transfer, a functional outcome of at least M3 strength (antigravity) can be achieved in the majority of cases (78%).[85]

For hand reanimation, the gracilis muscle can also be transferred to the forearm for finger flexion or extension or to substitute intrinsic muscle function.[14,18] Electrophysiologic assessment of the free muscle transfer can reveal contractions as early as 3 to 4 months, and a full range of contraction can be expected at approximately 6 to 12 months. Transplantation of the gracilis muscle for finger flexion at the optimal resting tension, along with early aggressive passive motion exercises, allow for grip strength of 50% of normal.[86]

Secondary Procedures

Additional procedures can be performed to facilitate and augment specific functions in late cases where the muscle targets have degenerated or when primary reconstruction has not yielded satisfactory results. These include tendon transfers, pedicled muscle transfers, joint fusions, and a variety of osteotomies.[87] A common tendon transfer for the shoulder is the transfer of the clavicular and acromial insertion of the trapezius with or without fascia lata to the deltoid insertion on the humerus to enhance shoulder abduction and reverse shoulder subluxation.[14,18] We do not advocate shoulder arthrodesis as a therapeutic modality, because it permits only a limited range of abduction and has a high incidence of complications.[88]

The restoration of elbow flexion can be enhanced by pedicled muscle transfer procedures. A variety of donor muscles can be used: the latissimus dorsi,[14] the sternoclavicular part of the pectoralis major, the long head of the triceps, and the Steindler flexorplasty using the flexor-pronator musculature.[89] In patients with no wrist function, arthrodesis of the wrist can improve comfort or appearance and stabilize the wrist for hand use.[14,90] In our center, wrist fusion is usually performed simultaneously with a free muscle transfer for hand reanimation. This allows a far more accurate setting of tension in

the transferred muscle and thus further improvement of hand function.

Postoperative Management

Complications of plexus reconstruction are rare and include mainly localized wound infection and, very rarely, pneumothorax during intercostal nerve harvesting. For the latter, primary closure of the pleural defect can usually be accomplished, but, occasionally, placement of a chest tube may be necessary. Seroma formation after intercostal nerves or latissimus dorsi muscle harvesting, as a result of the extensive dissection, has been observed at times and can be treated with needle aspiration and compression dressing.

After the completion of surgery, the patient's upper extremity is immobilized in a custom-made shoulder and elbow brace that keeps the arm abducted 45 degrees with the elbow flexed (Figure 57-12). Usually, the patient remains in the brace for 3 to 8 weeks depending on the procedure followed by an arm sling. Physical therapy begins at 6 weeks postoperatively and involves slowly increasing the passive range of motion (ROM) at the different joints of the upper limb. Ultrasound, slow electrical pulse stimulation, and massage are added for rehabilitation to specific muscles. Self-ROM exercises are stressed to avoid stiffness in the joints of the hand. The first follow-up visit is arranged at 3 and then at 6 months after surgery. In cases of severe plexopathies with multiple avulsions, ipsilateral reconstruction takes place in the first procedure, followed 3 months later by the selective contralateral C7 technique. After 1 year, the patient is evaluated fully for return of function and plans for secondary reconstruction are made at that time. Although rehabilitation is time consuming and many patients end up losing their motivation,

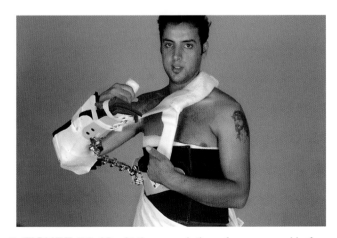

● **FIGURE 57-12.** At the completion of surgery and before extubation, a custom-made brace is applied to the patient's upper extremity. This brace keeps the arm abducted 45 degrees and in anterior flexion, with the elbow flexed.

this therapeutic process is mandatory as it eventually leads to better physical and psychological outcomes.

OUTCOMES

To compare overall results from various large series, we must consider the different group of patients, injuries, surgeons, treatments, and grading scales. The prognosis is highly dependent on the level and extent of injury. The surgical repair is more effective for patients who sustain infraclavicular lesions or for supraclavicular lesions when at least two roots can be used for motor donors.[91] Kim et al.[41] stated that repairs were best for injuries located at the C5, C6, and C7 levels, the upper and middle trunk; conversely, results were poor for injuries at the C8 and T1 levels, and/or for the lower trunk.

In our series[14] of 204 brachial plexus reconstructions it was shown that intraplexus donors, when they are available, resulted in the strongest power, regardless of the muscle target. However, some of the extraplexus donors gave consistently superior results when they neurotized specific targets directly. Direct neurotization of the suprascapular nerve from the distal accessory nerve yielded comparable results to repair with intraplexus donors. Overall, in our series, 79% of patients achieved good and excellent shoulder abduction (muscle grade, +3 or higher), and 55% of patients achieved good or excellent shoulder external rotation after reinnervation of the suprascapular nerve.[64] The best results were seen when direct neurotization of the suprascapular nerve from the spinal accessory nerve or neurotization by the C5 root was carried out. Concomitant neurotization of the axillary nerve yielded improved outcomes in shoulder abduction and external rotation function.[65]

Merrell et al.,[92] in a meta-analysis of the English-language literature regarding neurotizations for restoration of the shoulder and elbow function, suggest that interposition nerve grafts should be avoided whenever possible when performing nerve transfers. Better results for restoration of elbow flexion have been obtained with direct intercostal to musculocutaneous transfers than with spinal accessory nerve transfers, which requires a nerve graft; and direct spinal accessory to suprascapular transfers appear to have the best outcomes for return of shoulder abduction. The use of intercostal nerves to directly neurotize the musculocutaneous nerve continues to be a standard approach in the reconstruction of severe plexus lesions. Direct neurotization is equally effective and less demanding than transfers involving interposition nerve grafts. Different studies have reported good function of the biceps (M3+ and higher) after neurotization with intercostals for 64% to 87% of patients.[67,68]

In the grim scenario of global avulsion, the addition of a contralateral C7 transfer with an interposition vascularized

ulnar nerve graft directed to the median nerve or the musculocutaneous nerve, good results can be expected in almost 60% patients.[14,93] Alternatively, some lower sensory intercostal nerves or cervical plexus elements can be directed to the sensory portion of the median nerve. With this transfer strategy, the majority of the patients will recover protective sensation. In cases of lower root involvement, it is a smart strategy to leave banked nerves at the elbow level either from ipsilateral donors or from the contralateral C7 root by using the selective contralateral C7 technique[12] for future free muscle transplantation for hand reanimation. The reconstruction of these devastating and time-consuming injuries usually involves multiple stages of reconstruction with an extended postoperative course of intensive physical rehabilitation. Pain management should be addressed early and the denervation time should be minimized to improve the prognosis. Despite the complexity of the surgical procedures and the extended recovery period, brachial plexus palsy has considerably evolved with improved functional outcomes, allowing the patient to lead a productive and satisfying life.[15]

CONCLUSION

The surgical management of these severe injuries demands a deep understanding of the brachial plexus and comfort with the current available techniques which can lead in the evolvement of further reconstructive strategies and improved prognosis. Radiographic and electrophysiologic studies are of great assistance in a preoperative and intraoperative evaluation, contributing to a more thorough study of root avulsion of the brachial plexus. Use of novel extraplexus donor nerves, selective neurotizations, and free muscle transfers are all modern surgical procedures that can offer satisfactory outcomes even in multiple avulsion injuries. Nerve grafting or nerve transfer is more rewarding when the distal coaptation is near the muscle target. The current trend is toward targeting the donor nerves for specific muscles directly; the more specific the target, the less misdirection of the donor fibers and, therefore, the muscle target reinnervation is maximized.

Future developments will attempt to apply neuroscience research dealing with neurotrophic growth factors to accelerating the regeneration "clock." Avulsed root reimplantation into the spinal cord may be assisted by a better understanding of the neuronal pools of flexor versus extensor musculature, thus avoiding the "paralyzing" co-contractions. Stem cell manipulation may restore the loss of the motor neurons that follows proximal injuries and lead to a new era of upper limb functional rehabilitation. Finally, distal target atrophy and loss may be prevented from implanted "micropacemakers" that will maintain the muscle by a volley of stimuli until the regenerating axon makes the critical distal connection.

REFERENCES

1. Homer. Ιλιάδα. Ραψωδία Θ΄. "Οι Τρώες έχουν επιτυχίες στην μάχη" (verse: 325–330). 8th century BCE.

2. Homer. The Trojans have success. *The Iliad*. Book Eight. Translation by Ian Johnston, Malaspina University-College, Nanaimo, BC, Canada.

3. Thorburn W. A clinical lecture on secondary suture of the brachial plexus. *Br Med J*. 1900;1(2053):1073–1075.

4. Harris W, Low VW. On the importance of accurate muscular analysis in lesions of the brachial plexus and the treatment of Erb's palsy and infantile paralysis of the upper extremity by cross-union of nerve roots. *Br Med J*. 1903;2:1035.

5. Seddon HJ. The use of autogenous grafts for the repair of large gaps in peripheral nerves. *Br J Surg*. 1947;35(138):151–167.

6. Seddon HJ. Nerve grafting. *J Bone Joint Surg Br*. 1963;45: 447–461.

7. Seddon HJ. *Surgical Disorders of the Peripheral Nerves*. Edinburgh, UK: Churchill Livingstone; 1972.

8. Brunelli G, Monini L. Neurotization of avulsed roots of brachial plexus by means of anterior nerves of cervical plexus. *Clin Plast Surg*. 1984;11:149–152.

9. Kotani T, Toshima Y, Matsuda H, et al. Postoperative results of nerve transposition in brachial plexus injury. *Seikei Geka*. 1971;22(11):963–966.

10. Allieu Y, Privat JM, Bonnel F. Paralysis in root avulsion of the brachial plexus. Neurotization by the spinal accessory nerve. *Clin Plast Surg*. 1984;11(1):133–136.

11. Gu YD, Zhang GM, Chen DS, et al. Cervical nerve root transfer from contralateral normal side for treatment of brachial plexus root avulsions. *Chin Med J (Engl.)* 1991;104(3): 208–211.

12. Terzis JK, Kokkalis ZT. Selective contralateral C7 transfer in posttraumatic brachial plexus injuries: a report of 56 cases. *Plast Reconstr Surg*. 2009;123(3):927–938.

13. Oberlin C, Béal D, Leechavengvongs S, et al. Nerve transfer to biceps muscle using a part of ulnar nerve for C5-C6 avulsion of the brachial plexus: Anatomical study and report of four cases. *J. Hand Surg Am*. 1994;19:232–237.

14. Terzis JK, Vekris MD, Soucacos PN. Outcomes of brachial plexus reconstruction in 204 patients with devastating paralysis. *Plast Reconstr Surg*. 1999;104(5):1221–1240.

15. Choi PD, Novak CB, Mackinnon SE, Kline DG. Quality of life and functional outcome following brachial plexus injury. *J Hand Surg Am*. 1997;22(4):605–612.

16. Midha R. Epidemiology of brachial plexus injuries in multitrauma population.*Neurosurgery*. 1997;40:1182–1189.

17. Kandenwein JA, Kretschmer T, Engelhardt M, Richter HP, Antoniadis G. Surgical interventions for traumatic lesions of the brachial plexus: a retrospective study of 134 cases. *J Neurosurg*. 2005;103(4):614–621.

18. Terzis JK, Papakonstantinou KC. The surgical treatment of brachial plexus in adults. *Plast Reconstr Surg*. 2000;106(5):1097–1122; quiz 1123–1124.

19. Kim DH, Murovic JA, Tiel RL, Kline DG. Mechanisms of injury in operative brachial plexus lesions. *Neurosurg Focus*. 2004;16(5):E2.

20. Coene LN. Mechanisms of brachial plexus lesions. *Clin Neurol Neurosurg*. 1993;95 Suppl:S24–S29.

21. Moran SL, Steinmann SP, Shin AY. Adult brachial plexus injuries: mechanism, patterns of injury, and physical diagnosis. *Hand Clin*. 2005;21(1):13–24.

22. Yeoman PM. Cervical myelography in traction injuries of the brachial plexus. *J Bone Joint Surg Br*. 1968;50(2):253–260.

23. Medical Research Council. Results of nerve suture. In: Seddon HJ, ed. *Peripheral Nerve Injuries*. Special Report Series, No 282. London: Her Majesty's Stationery Office; 1954:10–11.

24. Friedman AH, Nashold BS Jr, Bronec PR. Dorsal root entry zone lesions for the treatment of brachial plexus avulsion injuries: A follow-up study. *Neurosurgery*. 1988;22(2): 369–373.

25. Samii M, Bear-Henney S, Ludemann W, et al. Treatment of refractory pain after brachial plexus avulsion with dorsal root entry zone lesions. *Neurosurgery*. 2001;48:1269–1277.

26. Sindou MP, Blondet E, Emery E, Mertens P. Microsurgical lesioning in the dorsal root entry zone for pain due to brachial plexus avulsion: a prospective series of 55 patients. *J Neurosurg*. 2005;102(6):1018–1028.

27. Harper CM. Preoperative and intraoperative electrophysiological assessment of brachial plexus injuries. *Hand Clin*. 2005;21(1):39–46, vi.

28. Balakrishnan G, Kadadi BK. Clinical examination versus routine and paraspinal electromyographic studies in predicting the site of lesion in brachial plexus injury. *J Hand Surg Am*. 2004;29(1):140–143.

29. Terzis JK, Dykes RW, Hakstian RW. Electrophysiological recordings in peripheral nerve surgery: A review. *J Hand Surg Am*. 1976;1(1):52–66.

30. Turkof E, Millesi H, Turkof R, et al. Intraoperative electroneurodiagnostics (transcranial electrical motor evoked potentials) to evaluate the functional status of anterior spinal roots and spinal nerves during brachial plexus surgery. *Plast Reconstr Surg*. 1997;99(6):1632–1641.

31. Chuang ML, Chuang DC, Lin IF, et al. Ventilation and exercise performance after phrenic nerve and multiple intercostal nerve transfers for avulsed brachial plexus injury. *Chest*. 2005;128(5):3434–3439.

32. Murphey F, Hartung W, Kirklin JW. Myelographic demonstration of avulsing injury of the brachial plexus. *Am J Roentgenol Radium Ther*. 1947;58(1):102–105.

33. Hashimoto T, Mitomo M, Hirabuki N, et al. Nerve root avulsion of birth palsy: comparison of myelography with CT myelography and somatosensory evoked potential. *Radiology*. 1991;178(3):841–845.

34. Walker AT, Chaloupka JC, de Lotbiniere AC, et al. Detection of nerve rootlet avulsion on CT myelography in patients with birth palsy and brachial plexus injury after trauma. *AJR Am J Roentgenol*. 1996;167(5):1283–1287.

35. Amrami . KK, Port JD. Imaging the brachial plexus. *Hand Clin*. 2005;21(1):25–37.

36. Volle E, Assheuer J, Hedde JP, Gustorf-Aeckerle R. Radicular avulsion resulting from spinal injury: Assessment of diagnostic modalities. *Neuroradiology*. 1992;34(3):235–240.

37. Doi K, Otsuka K, Okamoto Y, et al. Cervical nerve root avulsion in brachial plexus injuries: magnetic resonance imaging classification and comparison with myelography and computerized tomography myelography. *J Neurosurg.* 2002;96 (3 Suppl):277–284.

38. Nakamura T, Yabe Y, Horiuchi Y, Takayama S. Magnetic resonance myelography in brachial plexus injury. *J Bone Joint Surg Br.* 1997;79(5):764–769.

39. Gasparotti R, Ferraresi S, Pinelli L, et al. Three dimensional MR Myelography of traumatic injuries of the brachial plexus. *AJNR Am J Neuroradiol.* 1997;18(9):1733–1742.

40. Kim DH, Murovic JA, Tiel RL, Kline DG. Penetrating injuries due to gunshot wounds involving the brachial plexus. *Neurosurg Focus.* 2004;16(5):E3.

41. Kim DH, Cho YJ, Tiel RL, Kline DG. Outcomes of surgery in 1019 brachial plexus lesions treated at Louisiana State University Health Sciences Center. *J Neurosurg.* 2003;98(5):1005–1016.

42. Bentolila V, Nizard R, Bizot P, Sedel L. Complete traumatic brachial plexus palsy. Treatment and outcome after repair. *J Bone Joint Surg Am.* 1999;81(1):20–28.

43. Liberson WT, Terzis JK. Contribution of clinical neurophysiology and rehabilitation medicine in the management of brachial plexus palsy. In: Terzis JK, ed. *Microreconstruction of Nerve Injuries.* Philadelphia: Saunders; 1987:555–570.

44. Dubuisson AS, Kline DG. Brachial plexus injury: a survey of 100 consecutive cases from a single service. *Neurosurgery.* 2002;51(3):673–682.

45. Carson KA, Terzis JK. Carbonic anhydrase histochemistry: A potential diagnostic method for peripheral nerve repair. *Clin Plast Surg.* 1985;12(2):227–232.

46. Malessy MJ, van Duinen SG, Feirabend HK, Thomeer RT. Correlation between histopathological findings in C-5 and C-6 nerve stumps and motor recovery following nerve grafting for repair of brachial plexus injury. *J Neurosurg.* 1999;91(4): 636–644.

47. Millesi H. Nerve grafting. In: Terzis JK, ed. *Microreconstruction of Nerve Injuries.* Philadelphia: W.B. Saunders; 1987: 223–237.

48. Terzis JK, Skoulis TG, Soucacos PN. Vascularized nerve grafts. A review. *Int Angiol.* 1995;14(3):264–277.

49. Terzis JK, Breidenbach WC. The anatomy of free vascularized nerve grafts. In: Terzis JK, ed. *Microreconstruction of Nerve Injuries.* Philadelphia: W.B. Saunders; 1987:101–116.

50. Terzis JK, Kostopoulos VK. Vascularized ulnar nerve graft: 151 reconstructions for posttraumatic brachial plexus palsy. *Plast Reconstr Surg.* 2009;123(4):1276–1279.

51. Mackinnon SE, Doolabh VB, Novak CB, Trulock EP. Clinical outcome following nerve allograft transplantation. *Plast Reconstr Surg.* 2001;107(6):1419–1429.

52. Chuang DC. Neurotization procedures for brachial plexus injuries. *Hand Clin.* 1995;11:633–645.

53. Gutowski KA, Orenstein HH. Restoration of elbow flexion after brachial plexus injury: the role of nerve and muscle transfers. *Plast Reconstr Surg.* 2000;106(6):1348–1357.

54. Narakas AO, Hentz VR. Neurotization in brachial plexus injuries: Indications and results. *Clin Orthop Relat Res.* 1988;(237):43–56.

55. Terzis JK. Ipsilateral C7 for reconstruction of lateral and posterior cord on obstetrical brachial plexus paralysis. Presented at: XIII International Symposium on Brachial Plexus Surgery. Paris; January 24–26, 2002.

56. Gu YD, Cai PQ, Xu F, et al. Clinical application of ipsilateral C7 nerve root for treatment of C5 and C6 avulsions of the brachial plexus. *Microsurgery.* 2003;23(2):105–108.

57. Samardzic M, Grujicic D, Rasulic L, Bacetic D. Transfer of the medial pectoral nerve: Myth or reality? *Neurosurgery.* 2002;50:1277–1282.

58. Richardson PM. Recovery of biceps function after delayed repair for brachial plexus injury. *J Trauma.* 1997;42(5): 791–792.

59. Leechavengvongs S, Witoonchart K, Uerpairojkit C, Thuvasethakul P. Nerve transfer to deltoid muscle using the nerve to the long head of the triceps, part II: a report of 7 cases. *J Hand Surg Am.* 2003;28(4):633–638.

60. Teboul F, Kakkar R, Ameur N, et al. Transfer of fascicles from the ulnar nerve to the nerve to the biceps in the treatment of upper brachial plexus palsy. *J Bone Joint Surg Am.* 2004; 86-A(7):1485–1490.

61. Leechavengvongs S, Witoonchart K, Uerpairojkit C, et al. Nerve transfer to biceps muscle using a part of the ulnar nerve in brachial plexus injury (upper arm type): a report of 32 cases. *J Hand Surg Am.* 1998;23(4):711–716.

62. Tung TH, Novak CB, Mackinnon SE. Nerve transfers to the biceps and brachialis branches to improve elbow flexion strength after brachial plexus injuries. *J Neurosurg.* 2003;98(2):313–318.

63. Liverneaux PA, Diaz LC, Beaulieu JY, Durand S, Oberlin C. Preliminary results of double nerve transfer to restore elbow flexion in upper type brachial plexus palsies. *Plast Reconstr Surg.* 2006;117(3):915–919.

64. Terzis JK, Kostas I. Suprascapular nerve reconstruction in 118 cases of adult posttraumatic brachial plexus patients. *Plast Reconstr Surg.* 2006;117(2):613–629.

65. Terzis JK, Kostas I, Soucacos PN. Restoration of shoulder function with nerve transfers in traumatic brachial plexus palsy patients. *Microsurgery.* 2006;26(4):316–334.

66. Waikakul S, Wongtragul S, Vanadurongwan V. Restoration of elbow flexion in brachial plexus avulsion injury: Comparing spinal accessory nerve transfer with intercostals nerve transfer. *J Hand Surg Am.* 1999;24(3):571–577.

67. Malessy MJ, Thomeer RT. Evaluation of intercostal to musculocutaneous nerve transfer in reconstructive brachial plexus surgery. *J Neurosurg.* 1998;88(2):266–271.

68. Nagano A. Intercostal nerve transfer for elbow flexion. *Tech Hand Up Extrem Surg.* 2001;5(3):136–140.

69. Chuang DC. Nerve transfers in adult brachial plexus injuries: My methods. *Hand Clin.* 2005;21(1):71–82.

70. Gu YD, Wu MM, Zhen YL, et al. Phrenic nerve transfer for brachial plexus motor neurotization. *Microsurgery.* 1992;13(5):287–290.

71. Songcharoen P, Wongtrakul S, Spinner RJ. Brachial plexus injuries in the adult. Nerve transfers: The Siriraj Hospital experience. *Hand Clin.* 2005;21(1):83–89.

72. Waikakul S, Orapin S, Vanadurongwan V. Clinical results of contralateral C7 root neurotization to the median nerve

in brachial plexus injuries with total root avulsions. *J Hand Surg Br.* 1999;24(5):556–560.

73. Gu Y, Xu J, Chen L, et al. Long term outcome of contralateral C7: A report of 32 cases. *Chin Med J (Engl).* 2002; 115(6):866–868.

74. Zhao X, Lao J, Hung LK, et al. Selective neurotization of the median nerve in the arm to treat brachial plexus palsy. Surgical technique. *J Bone Joint Surg Am.* 2005;87 Suppl 1 (Pt 1):122–135.

75. Ihara K, Doi K, Sakai K, et al. Restoration of sensibility in the hand after complete brachial plexus injury. *J Hand Surg Am.* 1996;21(3):381–386.

76. Chuang DC. Functioning free muscle transplantation for brachial plexus injury. *Clin Orthop Relat Res.* 1995;(314): 104–111.

77. Manktelow RT, Zuker RM. The principles of functioning muscle transplantation: Application to the upper arm. *Ann Plast Surg.* 1989;22(4):275–282.

78. Terzis JK, Sweet RC, Dykes RW, Williams HB. Recovery of function in free muscle transplants using microneurovascular anastomoses. *J Hand Surg Am.* 1978;3(1):37–59.

79. Barrie KA, Steinmann SP, Shin AY, et al. Gracilis free muscle transfer for restoration of function after complete brachial plexus avulsion. *Neurosurg Focus.* 2004;16(5):E8.

80. Bishop AT. Functioning free-muscle transfer for brachial plexus injury. *Hand Clin.* 2005;21(1):91–102.

81. Akasaka Y, Hara T, Takahashi M. Free muscle transplantation combined with intercostal nerve crossing for reconstruction of elbow flexion and wrist extension in brachial plexus injuries. *Microsurgery.* 1991;12(5):346–351.

82. Doi K, Muramatsu K, Hattori Y, et al. Restoration of prehension with the double free muscle technique following complete avulsion of the brachial plexus. Indications and long-term results. *J Bone Joint Surg Am.* 2000;82(5):652–666.

83. Doi K, Sakai K, Fuchigami Y, Kawai S. Reconstruction of irreparable brachial plexus injuries with reinnervated free-muscle transfer. Case report. *J Neurosurg.* 1996;85(1): 174–177.

84. Doi K, Hattori Y, Kuwata N, et al. Free muscle transfer can restore hand function after injuries of the lower brachial plexus. *J Bone Joint Surg Br.* 1998;80(1):117–120.

85. Chung DC, Carver N, Wei FC. Results of functioning free muscle transplantation for elbow flexion. *J Hand Surg Am.* 1996;21(6):1071–1077.

86. Manktelow R. Functioning muscle transplantation to the arm. In: Terzis JK, ed. *Microreconstruction of Nerve Injuries.* Philadelphia: Saunders; 1987:267–281.

87. Berger A, Brenner P. Secondary surgery following brachial plexus injuries. *Microsurgery.* 1995;16(1):43–47.

88. Yuceturk A. Palliative surgery: tendon transfers to the shoulder in adults. In: Gilbert A, ed. *Brachial Plexus Injuries.* London: Martin Dunitz; 2001:116–122.

89. Liu TK, Yang RS, Sun JS. Long-term results of the Steindler flexorplasty. *Clin Orthop Relat Res.* 1993;(296):104–108.

90. Sedel L. Repair of severe traction lesions of the brachial plexus. *Clin Orthop Relat Res.* 1988;(237):62–66.

91. Sedel L. The results of surgical repair of brachial plexus injuries. *J Bone Joint Surg Br.* 1982;64(1):54–66.

92. Merrell GA, Barrie KA, Katz DL, Wolfe SW. Results of nerve transfer techniques for restoration of shoulder and elbow function in the context of a meta-analysis of the English literature. *J Hand Surg Am.* 2001;26(2):303–314.

93. Gu YD, Chen DS, Zhang GM, et al. Long term functional results of contralateral C7 transfer. *J Reconstr Microsurg.* 1998;14(1):57–59.

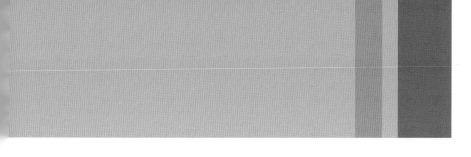

chapter 58

Dupuytren's Disease

Andrew J. Watt, MD / *James Chang, MD*

● INTRODUCTION

A Dupuytren contracture is a progressive disease of the palmar and digital fascial structures of the hand, characterized by nodular thickening and subsequent contracture. Deformity occurs primarily at the metacarpophalangeal (MCP) and proximal interphalangeal (PIP) joints resulting in functional disability. The disease process presents a formidable challenge to hand surgeons because of distortion of the native anatomy and the recalcitrant nature of the underlying pathologic process.

Early descriptions of Dupuytren's disease attributed the hand contractures to flexor tendon involvement. Dupuytren himself did not dispel this belief until 1831 when he described the disease process as affecting the aponeurotic tissue of the palm, sparing the flexor tendons themselves.[1] The etiology and pathogenesis of Dupuytren's disease remained a matter of both speculation and incidental correlation. It has been only over the past 25 years that surgeons and scientists have begun to unravel the underlying mechanisms that contribute to the development of the disease. Despite these advances, our current understanding of the disease process remains incomplete.

Dupuytren's disease belongs to the overarching category of benign superficial fibromatoses and, as such, is closely related to Peyronie disease (penile fibromatosis) and Lederhosen disease (plantar fibromatosis). Histologically, the affected tissue is characterized by nodular rests of myofibroblasts surrounded by dense collagen. Molecular analysis reveals a preponderance of type III collagen, which is not typically observed in mature palmar fascia, and increased concentrations of prostaglandins, as well as several subtypes of transforming growth factor beta.[2,3] The presence of CD-3+ T cells has also been noted raising the question of immunologic involvement. The exact role of these factors in the pathogenesis of Dupuytren's disease as well the underlying diathesis remain a matter of supposition at the current time. Despite this ambiguity in the underlying cause of Dupuytren's disease, the course of disease progression has been well described. In 1959, Luck described the pathogenesis of Dupuytren contracture in pathologic terms consisting of *proliferative, involutional,* and *residual* phases. The disease process progresses from an early proliferative phase with the formation of myofibroblast-rich nodules in the palmar and digital fascia. These nests of myofibroblasts actively deposit disorganized type III collagen. The myofibroblasts reorganize, differentiate, and align along the lines of tension during the involutional phase. During the residual phase, contraction occurs with the development of thickened cords of diseased fascia.[4] The cumulative effect is transformation of the normal fascial bands to fibrotic, diseased cords.

● EPIDEMIOLOGY

The overall incidence of Dupuytren's disease varies according to the population studied, with published rates ranging between 2% and 42%.[5] The incidence is highest among individuals of northern European ancestry. The disease is rare in individuals of African or Asian descent; however, there are isolated populations in Japan and Taiwan that maintain a disease incidence comparable to that of northern Europeans. Men are 6 times more likely to develop Dupuytren's disease than are women.[6] The disease onset is primarily in the fifth decade of life for men, and the sixth decade for women. Bilateral disease occurs in 59% of affected men and 43% of affected women.

Population studies support an autosomal dominant inheritance pattern with variable penetrance. Among male relatives with an affected proband, 68% develop the disease at some point in their lifetimes.[5] Associations with repetitive trauma, alcohol abuse, hepatic disease, diabetes mellitus, smoking, chronic obstructive pulmonary disease,

HIV, and malignancy (paraneoplastic manifestation) have been proposed.[7-9] Patients with Dupuytren's disease clearly demonstrate an increased incidence of both penile and plantar fibromatosis.

● PATIENT EVALUATION AND SELECTION

Patient Presentation and Diagnosis

Patients may present with findings that encompass the spectrum of the disease progression, and the diagnosis is made based on the history and clinical examination. The earliest sign of the disease may consist of a puckering of the dermis overlying the flexor tendon just distal to the distal palmar crease. This pit, or dimpling of the skin, corresponds with the attachment of the longitudinal fibers of the palmar aponeurosis as they insert into the overlying dermis. As the disease progresses and the underlying aponeurosis becomes increasingly fibrotic, a discrete nodule or nodules become distinctly palpable overlying the flexor tendon. Gradually, over the course of years, MCP joint contracture develops, followed, in more severe cases, by PIP joint contracture. With severe contracture of the palm, maceration of the skin may also occur at the distal palmar crease (Figure 58-1).

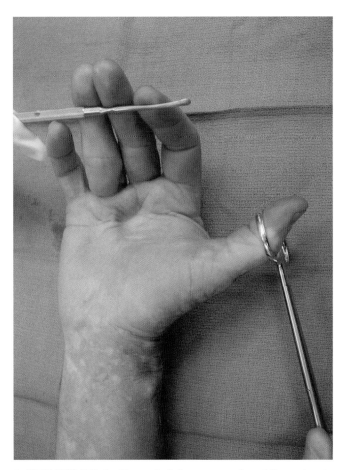

● **FIGURE 58-1.** Characteristic appearance of Dupuytren's disease.

Nodules and contraction may occur throughout the palmar and digital fascia; however, particular regions of the fascia are prone to disease. The ring finger is most commonly affected, followed in prevalence by the small finger, thumb, middle, and index fingers. The presence of nodules is paramount to the diagnosis of Dupuytren's disease. These nodules are firm to palpation and may be tethered to the overlying dermis. Nodules in the palm are principally located at the distal palmar crease, and nodules in the digital fascia occur in proximity to the PIP joint. Over time, the nodules involute, leaving chordal structures in the residual phase of the disease process. Although patients may initially present with a painful palmar nodule, it is important to note that this pain will typically subside over time.

Patients may also present with Garrod nodules, or knuckle pads, located dorsally over the PIP joints. Garrod nodules may be associated with a higher likelihood of bilateral hand involvement; however, their presence does not suggest stage or severity of disease, nor do they result in any functional limitation themselves.[10] The presence of knuckle pads, however, is not necessarily associated with a higher incidence of concomitant fibromatoses, including Peyronie and Lederhosen diseases.

The diagnosis of Dupuytren's disease is based solely on the history and physical examination. The characteristic progression from nodule to fibrotic cord with contracture of the affected palm and digits is pathognomonic for Dupuytren's disease. The history is often significant for an insidious onset with progressive contracture and disability developing over the course of years. Hand radiographs are generally unnecessary to rule out dystrophic calcific component or osseous involvement unless clinical suspicion is high that an underlying arthritis exists. The differential diagnosis may include camptodactyly, traumatic scars, Volkmann ischemic contracture, intrinsic joint arthrosis, locked trigger finger, and spastic digital contracture. These diagnoses may be separated based on the history and physical examination.

Surgical Indications and Contraindications

The primary objective of treatment in patients with Dupuytren's disease is correction of the deformity, thereby reducing disability and restoring hand function. It therefore follows that the degree of joint contracture and, more importantly, the extent of functional disability are the primary indications for intervention. Although promising interventional treatments, including enzymatic lysis of diseased tissue with collagenase and percutaneous needle aponeurotomy, are emerging, the contemporary treatment remains primarily surgical. The presence of a nodule alone is not sufficient to justify surgical intervention. The commonly accepted surgical indications include greater than 30 degrees of MCP joint contracture, and any degree of PIP joint contracture, as these degrees of contracture are commonly cited as functionally limiting.[11]

Surgical intervention for a MCP joint contracture is not urgent since the collateral ligaments are taut in MCP joint flexion, and this position is protective with respect to joint motion. Surgical intervention may therefore be delayed without compromising the functional outcome. In contrast, a PIP joint contracture requires an early surgical release because they are more resistant to correction. A long-standing PIP joint contracture precipitates articular changes with a loss of subchondral bone and a fixed flexion contracture of the joint. In an effort to preserve functional PIP joint motion, surgery is indicated with any degree of contracture. Additional indications for operative intervention include a first web adduction contracture, an unremitting tenosynovitis secondary to a palmar nodule overlying the A1 pulley, and palmar contracture resulting in maceration at the distal palmar crease.

Few contraindications to surgery exist beyond those considerations that would preclude regional or general anesthesia. Poor operative candidates include those patients with long-standing PIP joint contracture and documented underlying articular changes. These patients may require a PIP joint arthroplasty or joint fusion in more severe cases. Even in patients without notable articular changes, full PIP extension is difficult to achieve. In addition, patients who describe pain as their primary symptom and patients who smoke are poor operative candidates.

● PATIENT PREPARATION

Preoperative Considerations

Patient preparation consists of preoperative evaluation and counseling combined with a discussion of the operative choices. The preoperative evaluation should include a comprehensive history and physical examination in addition to a thorough hand examination. Although rare, patients should be evaluated for Dupuytren diathesis as well. Dupuytren diathesis refers to a predisposition to bilateral early onset disease, typically before the age of 40 years, rapid progression, ectopic manifestations, including dorsal knuckle pads, and penile as well as plantar fibromatosis. Clinicians may also choose to document disability with hand-specific questionnaires such as the DASH Outcome Measure or Michigan Hand Outcomes Questionnaire as a reference for postoperative comparison. Operative correction of Dupuytren's disease can be performed with an infraclavicular or axillary block for analgesia, and may be supplemented with local anesthetic and sedation. Anticoagulant and antiplatelet agents should be held at least 7 days prior to surgery in an effort to reduce the incidence of postoperative palmar hematoma. Ideally, patients who smoke should undergo a smoking cessation program prior to surgery. The critical component of patient preparation involves a discussion of the postoperative course, potential complications, and expected outcomes. Most importantly, the hand surgeon should discuss the progressive and persistent nature of the disease process, emphasizing that surgical intervention remains a method of temporizing the disease progression and improving hand function rather than providing a cure for Dupuytren's disease.

Operative Considerations

Patients should be positioned supine with the affected extremity supinated and abducted on a hand table. A surgical tourniquet should be placed on the arm, and the arm exsanguinated with an Esmarch wrap. The extremity should be prepped circumferentially, and a sterile lead hand may be utilized to obtain digital extension with adequate exposure of the palm.

The choice of the operative technique for the correction of Dupuytren contracture is the subject of much debate and is dependent on the individual surgeon's training and an understanding of the progression of the disease process. Operative techniques range from fasciotomy to subcutaneous fasciectomy, limited fasciectomy, regional fasciectomy, radical fasciectomy, and dermatofasciectomy (Table 58-1). The latter techniques differ primarily in the extent of palmar dissection.

A fasciotomy consists of disruption of the diseased cords, which may be performed either percutaneously or through limited incisions overlying the diseased cords. A fasciotomy does not address the nodular component of the disease process. A subcutaneous fasciectomy minimizes the palmar dissection by relying on disruption of the continuity of the palmar aponeurosis and includes resection of discrete Dupuytren nodules. These procedures involve limited dissection minimizing the risk of postoperative complications including hematoma; however, outcomes data show that postoperative correction of joint contracture is not maintained at 3 years.[12] The majority of surgeons reserve these

---

TABLE 58-1. Surgical Options for the Treatment of Dupuytren's Disease

Surgical Technique	Description
Fasciotomy	Division of diseased cords without excision
Local fasciectomy	Removal of segment of diseased cord
Regional fasciectomy	Removal of all diseased fascia as well as local region of grossly normal tissue
Radical fasciectomy	Removal of the entire palmar and digital fascia
Open palm technique (McCash[14])	Division of the palmar aponeurosis without closure of the skin deficit created
Dermatofasciectomy	Removal of the diseased fascia as well as the overlying skin. Closure typically obtained with the use of a full-thickness skin graft

operations for elderly patients with systemic disease who may poorly tolerate a more extensive operation.

Limited fasciectomy removes a portion of the diseased aponeurosis, disrupting continuity of the diseased tissue and resecting aponeurotic tissue associated with the affected digits. This procedure is a compromise between removal all of the diseased aponeurosis, so that recurrence cannot take place, and local excision. Limited fasciectomy limits palmar dissection while effectively addressing the underlying pathology.

Regional fasciectomy is appropriate for the majority of patients upon primary presentation and has become the standard of care for most hand surgeons. Regional fasciectomy consists of removal of *all* of the diseased aponeurosis coupled with resection of a margin of normal palmar aponeurosis. All nodules are resected and digital dissection is performed to address proximal and distal interphalangeal contracture. This procedure limits the risk of disease recurrence while avoiding the morbidity of a radical palmar dissection.

In a radical fasciectomy one strives to remove the entire palmar aponeurosis in an effort to prevent palmar recurrence. This operation is effective in minimizing palmar recurrence; however, the incidence of palmar hematoma increases with the extent of dissection. Given that disease recurrence is typically digital rather than palmar, most hand surgeons reserve radical fasciectomy for patients with Dupuytren diathesis and those with recurrent disease.

Dermatofasciectomy involves resection not only of the aponeurosis, but also the overlying skin with placement of a full-thickness skin graft. Dermatofaciectomy is commonly reserved for patients with recurrent palmar disease.

The specific operative approach is determined by the extent of palmar skin involvement, the presence of MCP and PIP joint contracture, and the digit involved.

OPERATIVE TECHNIQUE

Anatomy

Proper surgical intervention for Dupuytren's disease requires a detailed understanding of both the normal palmar and digital fascial anatomy, which by convention are termed bands, as well as the pathologic progression of the involved fascial structures, which are termed diseased cords. The diseased cords are the result of pathologic change in the normal fascial structures and therefore their anatomic configurations and relationships are predictable (Table 58-2). In addition, the surgeon must consider that the disease process is itself both visible, as discrete nodules, and microscopic, in apparently grossly normal tissue. Consequently, the treatment includes a resection of both involved and potentially involved fascial structures.

Affected structures include the palmar aponeurosis and its digital extensions (pretendinous bands) as well as the digital fascia, natatory ligament, Grayson ligament, spiral

TABLE 58-2. Diseased Cords in Dupuytren's Disease

Diseased Structure	Anatomic Origin	Clinical Significance
Palmar Cords		
Pretendinous cord	Pretendinous band	MCP joint flexion contracture
Vertical cord	Vertical fibers of McGrouther or septa of Legueu and Juvara	Causes painful triggering
Palmodigital Cords		
Spiral cord	Pretendinous band, spiral band, lateral digital sheet, Grayson ligament	Displaces the neurovascular bundle medially and superficially (spiral nerve)
Natatory cord	Natatory ligament (distal fibers)	Web space adduction contracture
Digital Cords		
Central cord	Pretendinous cord (digital extension)	PIP joint flexion contracture
Retrovascular cord	Retrovascular band of thomine	PIP and DIP joint flexion contracture; prevents full correction of PIP joint contracture
Lateral cord	Lateral digital sheet (often closely associated with pretendinous and natatory cord)	PIP and DIP joint flexion contracture; displaces neurovascular bundle medially
Abductor digiti minimi cord	Abductor digiti minimi tendon	PIP joint flexion contracture
Thumb and First Web Space Cords		
Proximal commissural cord	Proximal commissural ligament	First web adduction contracture
Distal commissural cord	Distal commissural ligament	First web adduction contracture
Thumb pretendinous cord	Pretendinous band	MCP joint flexion contracture

MCP, metacarpophalangeal; PIP, proximal interphalangeal; DIP, distal interphalangeal.

A

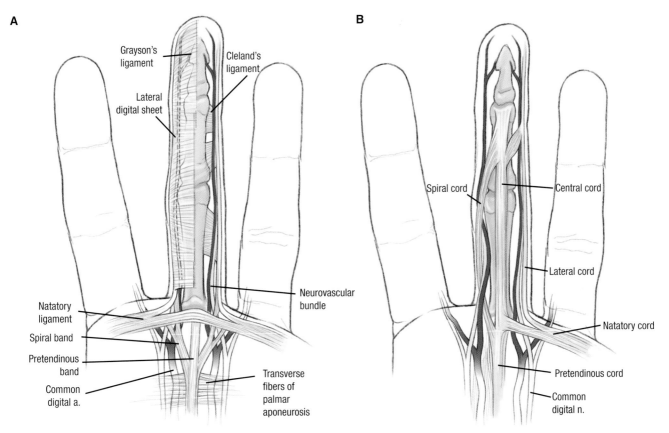

Grayson's
ligament

Cleland's
ligament

Lateral
digital sheet

Neurovascular
bundle

Natatory
ligament

Spiral band

Pretendinous
band

Common
digital a.

Transverse
fibers of
palmar
aponeurosis

B

Spiral cord

Central cord

Lateral cord

Natatory cord

Pretendinous cord

Common
digital n.

● **FIGURE 58-2.** (A) Palmar and digital fascial structures involved and spared by
Dupuytren's disease. Involved structures include the pretendinous band, spiral band,
natatory ligament, lateral digital sheet, and Grayson's ligament. Spared structures include
Cleland's ligament and the transverse fibers of the palmar aponeurosis. (B) Formation
of the spiral cord from the pretendinous band, spiral band, lateral digital sheet, and
Grayson's ligament. Note the spiral cord displaces the neurovascular bundle medially,
superficially and proximally. (*From Mcfarlane RM. Patterns of the diseased fascia in the fingers in
Dupuytren contracture. Plast Reconstr Surg. 1974;54:31–44, with permission.*)

band, and retrovascular fascia (Figure 58-2). The superficial transverse palmar ligament is predominantly spared; however, involvement at its radial extent as it inserts into the base of the thumb may occur, resulting in adduction contracture of the first web space. Cleland ligaments are spared in the disease process.

The operative approach and extent of dissection is determined by the extent of palmar skin involvement, and the degree of MCP and PIP joint contracture. Successful operative intervention is predicated on an understanding of which disease components contributes to contracture at these locations. Palmar skin contracture results from involvement of the palmar aponeurosis itself, and is corrected with a partial or complete palmar aponeurectomy. MCP joint contracture results solely from involvement of the pretendinous bands, and is likewise addressed with a palmar aponeurectomy and excision of the diseased pretendinous cords. Several anatomic components contribute to PIP joint contracture. The digital fascia gives rise to the pretendinous and lateral cords. The pretendinous, spiral, and lateral bands coalesce with Grayson ligament to form

the pathologic spiral cord (Figure 58-2), and the retrovascular fascia forms the retrovascular cord.[13] Each of these pathologic cords, either alone or in combination, result in PIP joint contracture. They must be excised to prevent progression or recurrence of contracture.

Adduction contracture of the thumb as well as abduction contracture of the small finger deserve special attention and are addressed uniquely. Akin to contracture of the fingers, an adduction contracture of the thumb results from involvement of the pretendinous band and the natatory ligament; however, involvement of the radial aspect of the superficial transverse ligament of the palm as it inserts into the skin at the base of the thumb coupled with the formation of proximal and distal commissural cords results in an adduction contracture of the first web space. This situation is unique as the superficial transverse ligament of the palm is spared throughout the remainder of its course. These structures lie superficial to the neurovascular bundle and resection remains straightforward. Dupuytren's disease also characteristically results in an abduction contracture of the small finger. The pretendinous, spiral, and retrovascular cords all contribute to flexion contracture; however, it is the lateral cord, coursing along the ulnar aspect of the small finger that contributes to the abduction.

Incision

The diseased digital and palmar fascia may be approached through a variety of incisions, either separately or in conjunction (Figure 58-3). The diseased aponeurosis may be approached through a transverse palmar incision. This incision begins in the distal palmar crease at the ulnar aspect and ends in the proximal palmar crease on the radial aspect. The transverse palmar incision provides access to the entire palmar aponeurosis and may be modified according to the segment of the aponeurosis to be resected. Alternatively, longitudinal incisions are useful for digital exposure and may be extended into the palm for exposure of the aponeurosis. A longitudinal incision with z-plastys at the flexion creases or a zig-zag Bruner-type incision both provide excellent exposure. Closure with a

Y-V advancement flap provides for additional length and is particularly useful in patients with significant contracture in which a relative deficiency of skin exists upon correction of the contracture. A contracture of the first web space is best approached through a T incision combined with a z-plasty to prevent scar contracture

Dissection

After the skin is incised, it is sharply dissected off the cord in the palm region. Proximal to the MCP joint, the digital neurovascular structures are safe, deep to the cord itself and are therefore protected. With the cord skeletonized, the digital nerves and arteries may be identified and traced distally. All abnormal tissue is excised, including the involved vertical fibers of Legueu and Juvara. Once the palmar aponeurosis and pretendinous cords have been disrupted, the MCP joints will extend without constraint. In the finger, meticulous care is exercised in order to avoid damage to a medially and superficially displaced neurovascular bundle resulting from the presence of a spiral cord (Figure 58-4). The presence of a spiral cord should be suspected in all patients; however, clues to its presence include a PIP joint contracture accompanied by prominence of the skin just proximal to the proximal digital crease.

Surgical correction of PIP joint involvement requires a digital dissection with resection of the central, lateral, spiral, and retrovascular cords. It is safest to incise distal to the cord, within normal tissue, in order to safely identify the digital neurovascular structures. Once the digital arteries and nerves have been identified, it is possible to trace the neurovascular bundles proximally and distally. Dissection is also carried laterally, exposing the lateral cord in a distal to proximal fashion in order to protect the displaced neurovascular structures. The lateral cord is derived from the lateral digital fascia and is markedly adherent to the dermis. Fibers of the lateral cord extend distally to the

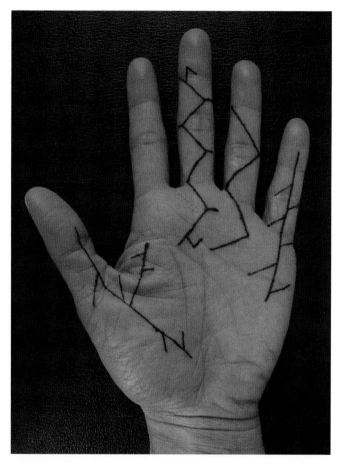

● **FIGURE 58-3.** Incisions utilized in surgery for Dupuytren's disease. The thenar contracture is addressed throught a T incision with z-plastys at the flexion creases. The middle finger demonstrates a modified Bruner incision with Y-V advancement. The ring finger demonstrates a traditional Bruner incision. The small finger demonstrates a longitudinal incision with z-plastys at the flexion creases.

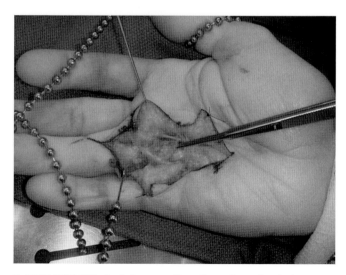

● **FIGURE 58-4.** Intraoperative dissection of spiral cord. Note displacement of the neurovascular structures proximimally, medially, and superficially.

distal phalanx and, in severe cases of Dupuytren's disease, are responsible for a distal interphalangeal joint contracture. The dissection must therefore be carried distally to its insertion on the lateral aspect of the distal phalanx. Attention is then turned to the spiral cord which is in proximal continuity with the pretendinous cord, travels deep to the neurovascular bundle, and spirals superficially to insert at the base of the middle phalanx.

Contracture of the thumb and the small finger are addressed similarly. An adduction contracture of the thumb is not uncommon and is addressed with resection of the pretendinous cord, natatory ligament, and the radial extent of the superficial transverse ligament of the palm as it inserts into the dermis at the base of the thumb. An abduction contracture of the small finger is addressed with both palmar and digital dissection as described for the index, middle, and ring fingers. In addition, the muscle belly of the abductor digiti minimi is exposed and its insertion into the ulnar lateral band is excised.

Wound Closure

The method of closure varies according to tissue availability as well as the incision itself. Transverse incisions may be left open and allowed to heal via secondary intention, as advocated by McCash[14] or a full-thickness skin graft may be used to achieve durable closure. If sufficient tissue exists to achieve primary closure of the transverse incision, sutures may be used to approximate the wound edges. For digital closure, longitudinal incisions are closed with z-plastys at the flexion creases. Zig-zag Bruner-type incisions are amenable to primary closure by incorporating a Y-V advancement flap for increased length. The surgical wound should be closed with 5-0 nylon or absorbable sutures.

Postoperative Care

Postoperative care is based on the maintenance of finger extension and early mobilization in an effort to prevent early recurrent contracture and joint stiffness. Postoperatively, patients should be placed in a volar splint with the MCP and PIP joints in extension. This splint is removed on postoperative day 5. At that time, the wound is also examined for signs of infection or dehiscence. The patient is begun on an active range of motion regimen, and is provided with a night-time extension splint which is worn for 4 to 6 weeks. The sutures are removed on postoperative day 20, allowing for adequate wound healing.

● COMPLICATIONS

Complications in the surgical treatment of Dupuytren's disease may be categorized as operative, early and late. Operative complications most commonly involve damage to the neurovascular bundle as a consequence of their medial and superficial displacement by a pathologic spiral band. Experienced surgeons have reported rates of arterial and nerve injury less than 0.4% and 2.3%, respectively.[15]

Damage to the neurovascular bundle may be avoided by maintaining a high suspicion in all patients and particularly in those patients with PIP joint contracture. Dissection between the distal palmar crease and proximal digital crease should be directed at identifying and preserving the neurovascular bundles. A nerve or vascular laceration should be repaired should it occur. The surgeon should be particularly vigilant during reoperation for recurrent contracture as the digit may be supplied by a single digital artery. Digital ischemia is addressed intraoperatively by (1) minimizing compression from skin closure and dressings; (2) infiltrating agents (papaverine, lidocaine) to decrease vasospasm; (3) decreasing extension of the digit to prevent unaccustomed stretch on the digital vessels; and lastly, (4) microsurgical exploration and repair as necessary.

Early complications include infection, hematoma, skin necrosis, and postoperative flare reaction. Postoperative wound infection typically occurs in 1% to 4% on patients, but has been reported to be as high a 9.5%.[15] This high incidence is likely attributable to bacterial overgrowth within the macerated distal palmar crease as well as to the tenuous blood supply to the palmar flaps. Another common complication of palmar dissection is postoperative hematoma which often results in palmar skin necrosis if not identified and evacuated. The reported incidence in populations undergoing a variety of surgical techniques is 2%; however, the risk with radical fasciectomy is significantly higher.[15] The risk of palmar hematoma may be minimized by obtaining hemostasis with the tourniquet deflated, prior to application of the final dressing, and by minimizing palmar dissection. Some authors advocate application of a pressure dressing; however, this intervention is unnecessary if meticulous operative hemostasis is obtained. The incidence of palmar hematoma may also be reduced with the use of the open palm technique of McCash.[14] Postoperative flare reaction may also occur, consisting of significant pain, swelling, and joint stiffness, characteristically occurring in the third to fourth week following surgery. Flare reaction is significantly more common in women and its incidence is further increased with concomitant procedures, including carpal tunnel release.[15,16] For this reason, multiple procedures should not be performed at time of operation for Dupuytren's disease. This syndrome may be a precursor of complex regional pain syndrome, and the incidence is minimized with the use of axillary or infra/supraclavicular regional anesthesia.

Late complications include complex regional pain syndrome, scar contracture, and disease recurrence or, more appropriately, disease progression. Complex regional pain syndrome refers to a syndrome characterized by pain, allodynia, and hyperalgesia disproportionate to the extent of inciting injury accompanied by evidence of vasomotor instability. This syndrome includes both reflex sympathetic dystrophy and causalgia. The incidence of complex regional pain syndrome in patients undergoing fasciectomy for Dupuytren's disease ranges between 4.5% and 40%, and varies on the choice of anesthetic.

Regional analgesia provides the lowest postoperative incidence, with comparable results achieved with intravenous regional anesthesia accompanied by clonidine. The highest reported incidence occurs with general anesthesia.[17] For this reason, infraclavicular or axillary block should be considered the anesthetic method of choice when operating for Dupuytren's disease. Scar contracture occurs with longitudinal digital incisions with a reported incidence of a 1% in the literature. The risk of contracture may be minimized by using z-plastys at the flexion creases, or Bruner incisions. Prolonged postoperative stiffness is reported in 10% of patients.[18] The most common complication of Dupuytren's disease is recurrence. The incidence of recurrence varies with technique and ranges between 32% and 40% with open techniques,[19,20] and is reported to be as high as 58% with percutaneous transection of the diseased cords.[20] In general, recurrence may be minimized with appropriate digital dissection coupled with more extensive palmar dissection. The benefits of more extensive dissection must, however, be weighed against higher incidence of wound complications. Recurrence does not invariably require additional surgery. Rodrigo and colleagues[21] found that 15% of patients required reexcision following disease recurrence.

● OUTCOMES ASSESSMENT

Numerous studies exist demonstrating the effectiveness of digital and palmar fasciectomy in restoring MCP and PIP joint extensions. Extension at the MCP joint may be reliably restored to within 15 degrees of normal irrespective of the extent preoperative contracture. PIP extension, in contrast, is adversely affected by both the degree and duration of contracture, but may be reliably corrected to within 30 degrees of normal. Restoration of form may be reliably achieved in all but the most severe cases of contracture; however, restoration of function remains the primary objective of surgical intervention in Dupuytren's disease. Despite an extensive body of literature, few studies have been undertaken to demonstrate that restoration of form improves hand function, and no studies exist effectively quantifying patient satisfaction with postoperative outcomes. Sinha and colleagues[22] have objectively studied the correlation between pre- and postoperative deformity with functional outcome. They objectively demonstrated that an increasing hand deformity at the MCP and PIP joints correlated with increasingly poor hand function. They further showed that hand function was most dependent on the degree of deformity at the PIP joint. With the establishment of this correlation, they showed that surgical correction of deformity results in a significant improvement in hand function, and is particularly dependent on the correction of PIP joint deformity. Operative outcomes are tempered by the high incidence of disease recurrence despite the best available surgical management. Therefore, a role for novel therapies as well as adjuvant treatment exists. Ongoing efforts are gradually elucidating the underlying biochemical mechanisms underlying Dupuytren's disease, and will likely provide unique therapeutic targets to supplement or even replace operative therapy.

REFERENCES

1. Dupuytren G. Permanent retraction of the fingers produced by and affectation of the palmar fascia. *Lancet.* 1834;2: 222–225.

2. Kloen P, Jennings CL, Gebhardt MC, et al. Transforming growth factor-beta: possible roles in Dupuytren's contracture. *J Hand Surg Am.* 1995;20(1):101–108.

3. Kloen P. New insights in the development of Dupuytren's contracture: a review. *Br J Plast Surg.* 1999;52(8):629–635.

4. Luck JV. Dupuytren's Contracture. A new concept of the pathogenesis correlated with the surgical management. *J Bone Joint Surg (Am).* 1959;40(4):635–664.

5. Ling R. The genetic factor in Dupuytren's disease. *J Bone Joint Surg (Br).* 1963;45:709–718.

6. Wilbrand S, Ekbom A, Gerdin B. The sex ratio and rate of reoperation for Dupuytren's contracture in men and women. *J Hand Surg Am.* 1999;24B:456–459.

7. Liss GM, Stock SR. Can Dupuytren's contracture be work related? Review of the evidence. *Am J Ind Med.* 1996;29(5): 521–532.

8. Burge P, Hoy G, Regan P, Milne R. Smoking, alcohol, and the risk of Dupuytren's contracture. *J Bone Joint Surg Br.* 1997; 79:206–210.

9. Leslie BM. Palmar fasciitis and polyarthritis associated with malignant neoplasm: a paraneoplastic syndrome. *Orthopedics.* 1992;15(12):1436–1439.

10. Caroli A, Zanasi S, Marcuzzi A, et al. Epidemiology and structural findings supporting the fibromatous origin of dorsal knuckle pads. *J. Hand Surg Br.* 1991;16:258–262.

11. Hueston JT. Current state of treatment of Dupuytren's disease. *Ann Chir Main.* 1984;3(1):81–92.

12. Colville J. Dupuytren's contracture: the role of fasciotomy. *Hand.* 1983;15(2):162–166.

13. McFarlane RM. Patterns of diseased fascia in the fingers in Dupuytren's contracture. *Plast Reconstr Surg.* 1974;54: 31–44.

14. McCash CR. The open palm technique in Dupuytren's contracture. *Br J Plast Surg.* 1964;17:271–280.

15. Bulstrode NW, Jemec B, Smith PJ. The complications of Dupuytren's contracture surgery. *J Hand Surg Am.* 2005; 30(5):1021–1025.

16. Zemel NP. Dupuytren's contracture in women. *Hand Clin.* 1991;7(4):707–711.

17. Nissenbaum M, Kleinert HE. Treatment considerations in carpal tunnel syndrome with coexisting Dupuytren's disease. *J Hand Surg Am*. 1980;5(6):544–547.

18. Reuben SS, Pristas R, Dixon D, et al. The incidence of complex regional pain syndrome after fasciectomy for Dupuytren's contracture: a prospective observational study of four anesthetic techniques. *Anesth Analg*. 2006;102(2):499–503.

19. Au-Yong IT, Wildin CJ, Dias JJ, Page RE. A review of common practice in Dupuytren surgery. *Tech Hand Up Extrem Surg*. 2005;9(4):178–187.

20. Foucher G, Medina J, Navarro R. Percutaneous needle aponeurectomy: complications and results. *J Hand Surg Br*. 2003;28(5):427–431.

21. Rodrigo JJ, Niebauer JJ, Brown RL, et al. Treatment of Dupuytren's contracture: long-term results after fasciotomy and fascial excision. *J Bone Joint Surg Am*. 1976;58:380–387.

22. Sinha R, Cresswell TR, Mason R, Chakrabarti I. Functional benefit of Dupuytren's surgery. *J Hand Surg Br*. 2002;27(4):378–381.

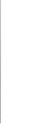

chapter 59

Rehabilitation of the Injured Hand

Michele A. Leadbetter, OTL, CHT / James P. Higgins, MD

● INTRODUCTION TO HAND THERAPY

Hand injuries can be physically and emotionally challenging and require a highly skilled level of supervision and guidance. Therapists provide a critical link between the patient and the surgeon, mitigate potential problems, and serve as patient advocates and educators. Hand therapists help promote the best surgical outcome by restoring function and reducing disability. The field of hand therapy continues to evolve as hand surgery techniques improve and our understanding of the mechanics and biology of tissue healing expands.

Hand therapy is a specialized form of rehabilitation that is carried out by a licensed physical or occupational therapist trained in the treatment of injures to the hand and upper extremity. Certified hand therapists (CHTs) have studied and demonstrated proficiency in rehabilitation of the hand in order to become nationally certified. Eligibility for the certification examination requires at least 5 years of experience and 4000 hours of practice in hand and upper extremity rehabilitation. Certified hand therapists are required to continue their education and competencies not only in the area of physical therapy and occupational therapy but also in current treatment and research specific to hand rehabilitation.

● EVALUATION/SYSTEMS REVIEW

Upon first meeting the patient, CHTs perform a comprehensive evaluation and systems review to establish a baseline and develop an individualized plan of care. The evaluation addresses the patient's physical, psychological, and psychosocial factors.

Objective measurements and tests are completed the first day, respecting any surgical precautions or contraindications for specific injuries. Not all tests and measurements are appropriate or necessary upon the initial evaluation and prioritization is imperative.

CHTs also take note of the patient's posturing, the passive attitude of the hand, how the patient holds and uses their hand, the color and condition of the skin and nails, how the patient talks about their hand injury and rates pain, as well as their willingness to participate in treatment. Physical, mental, and cognitive comorbidities are also documented. These observations provide valuable information for developing a treatment plan.

Components of the initial evaluation:

1. Active, passive, active assisted range of motion (AROM, PROM, AAROM): Degrees and quality of joint motion are recorded, reasons for limitations are documented (ie, intrinsic, extrinsic, capsular tightness, scar adhesions) (Figure 59-1).
2. Strength testing: Grip and pinch measurements, manual muscle testing
3. Sensory evaluation: two-point discrimination, Semmes-Weinstein monofilaments and functional sensory testing (eg: stereognosis, hot/cold, sharp/dull). Electrical nerve studies are completed in some clinics according to physician's orders.
4. Edema measurements: circumferential and volumetric
5. Wound assessment: stage of healing, size, exudate, color, odor, etc
6. Standardized tests for coordination and dexterity
7. Functional capacity evaluation

In addition to the therapy evaluation findings, it is very important for the surgeon to provide as much information as possible regarding the patient's injury and procedure performed. Factors that will affect the evaluation and treatment plan are:

1. Mechanism of injury and the time elapsed from the injury/surgery

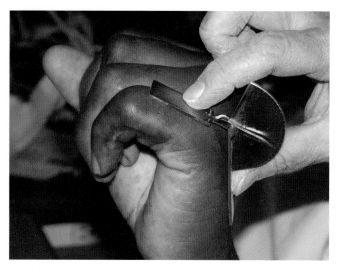

● **FIGURE 59-1.** Tools: digital goniometer.

2. Structures repaired or compromised (ie, pulleys, tendon, digital nerves)
3. Procedure performed, including:
   a. Type, strength, and quality of repair
   b. Method of fixation/stability of fracture
   c. Tension on the repair
   d. Tissue quality/abnormalities

4. Tissue viability/vascular status

These factors can significantly affect the treatment plan and pace. These factors influence the type and position of splints, how much protection is needed, how and when to progress ROM and strengthening, and the rate of improvement expected. The surgeon should communicate any specific precautions or concerns that are identified during the procedure, as well as their own expectations of the outcome. This information, combined with evaluation findings, will assist the therapist in balancing between protecting the stability of the injury and surgery while promoting mobility for function.

● REHABILITATION OF COMMON INJURIES: FLEXOR TENDONS

Flexor tendon injuries are one of the most common injuries to the hand. These injuries present a challenge to surgeon and therapist and require a significant amount of therapy for the patient. Due to the biomechanics of the digital flexors and the tendon excursion necessary for making a fist, it is important to encourage both tendon gliding for function as well as protection of the repaired tendon. Following surgery, the goal of therapy is to promote function and avoid a loss of motion due to rupture or alternatively excessive stiffness and scaring. It is for these reasons that a significant amount of research has been completed to improve surgical technique and postoperative care.

Since the mid 1970s, much research has been done to refine procedures for primary flexor tendon repairs. Through this research it has been demonstrated that tendons heal with increased strength and improved excursion if subjected to early mobilization. The application of controlled stress (ie, motion) has been proven to increase the tensile strength, the collagen organization, and intrinsic healing through synovial exchange. The result is decreased adhesion formation, and a reduced chance of gap formation or rupture at the repair site. Research has also shown that early active mobilization provides greater tendon glide than passive range of motion exercises.[1]

While advances in flexor tendon surgery and rehabilitation have improved outcomes in all zones of flexor musculotendinous injuries, protocols have been evolving with a focus on improvement of injuries in the hand (zones I–V), with particular interest in the most challenging injuries within zone II (the digital flexor tendon sheath) (Figure 59-2).

Traditional immobilization protocols and early PROM protocols such as the Kleinert-Lister Rubber Band Traction, the Modified Kleinert, and the Duran-Houser have largely been replaced with immediate-controlled mobilization protocols. Immobilization for 3 to 4 weeks is no longer the common treatment technique, unless medically indicated.

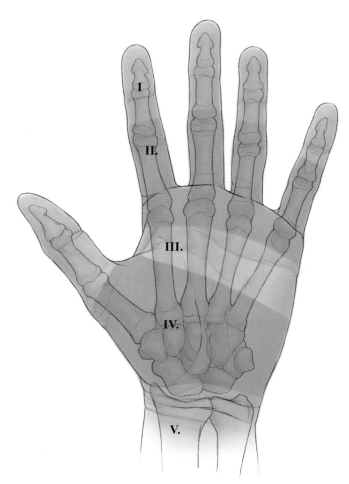

● **FIGURE 59-2.** Flexor tendon zones.

Mobilizing tendons using an early controlled active motion program has now become the standard of care. Exceptions may be made for comorbidities, age, comprehension, or cognitive status.

Early active motion protocols (EAMPs) are largely based on the physiologic phases of wound healing and collagen proliferation. Immobilizing tendon repairs for 3 weeks (into the fibroblastic stage) allows for increased fibroblast and collagen proliferation, and contributes to the formation of adhesions between the tendon and surrounding soft tissue. Initiating early active mobilization at postoperative days 0 to 5 (during the inflammatory phase) has been shown to be the most effective method for limiting adhesions, decreasing work of flexion, and returning the strength and excursion to the repaired tendon.[1,2]

The therapist's ability and confidence using early motion protocols is directly related to improved surgical design, technique, increased number of strands, and type of suture performed. These repairs allow for immediate controlled motion with active "place and hold" exercises and light active contractions within a safe range.[3] According to Strickland, the most favorable outcomes are achieved with a strong suture technique and immediate controlled motion.[1]

Other factors that may influence adhesions and drag on repaired tendons are:

1. Trauma to tendon sheath from injury and/or surgery
2. Tendon ischemia
3. Tendon immobilization
4. Fractures, edema, and wounds
5. Gap formation
6. Tendon sheath/pulley compromise

Different protocols have been created by various centers around the world. Although several specific EAMPs have been described, all EAMPs share the following features:

- Minimum of a four-strand, core suture tendon repair
- Initiation of ROM within the first 3 to 5 days postoperatively[4]
- Edema management and PROM preceding AROM to maintain supple joints
- Cautious limitation of the strength of active muscle contraction
- Reliance on patient compliance and motivation

With most protocols, the dorsal blocking splint is discharged by week 6 and gradual resistive exercises are permitted at week 8. The differences that exist between proposed EAMPs include:

- Splint position (eg, wrist from 30 degrees of flexion to 30 degrees of extension)
- Using multiple splints, rubber band traction versus straps
- Frequency, duration, repetitions, and progression of AROM exercises (Figure 59-3)

Injuries to zones V–VIII may be treated differently based on other additional structures (artery, nerve, wrist flexor muscles), the propensity for adhesion formation, the proximity to the tendon muscle junction, and muscle belly injury. Table 59-1 provides examples of some commonly used EAMPs.

One additional EAMP worth mentioning is the Pyramid of Progressive Force Application, described by Groth.[8] This protocol differs from those previously mentioned by timing the motion exercises based on an individual's biological healing process and speed of their progress. Exercises are progressed based on comparing PROM to AROM during each visit; the less responsive a patient's soft tissue, the faster the program is progressed (Figure 59-4). This protocol does not offer splinting or time parameters.

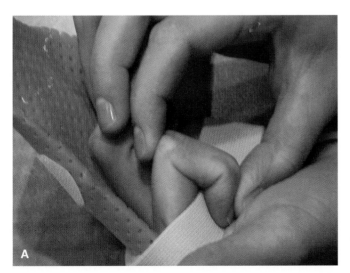
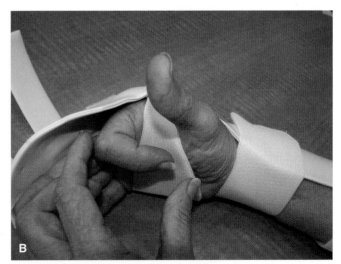

● **FIGURE 59-3.** (A) PROM in dorsal blocking splint and (B) place and hold AROM.

TABLE 59-1. Some Commonly Used EAMPs for Flexor Tendon Zones I–V

Author	Splint Position	Early AROM	Progression
The Curtis National Hand Center (Formby ME. 2004)[2]	Dorsal blocking splint Wrist: neutral MCPs: Flexion 60°–70° IPs: Full extension	Day 0-5: Hourly 1. PROM to prime joints, 10–15 reps 2. Place/hold and AROM 1–3 x to 50% of full PROM arc 3. Increase arc of place/hold as PROM improves	1. Week 3: Increase AROM to full 2. Week 4: Unassisted AROM 3. Modify active reps and sessions depending on AROM progress
The Indiana Hand Center (Cannon and Strickland, 2001)[5] • Uses 2 splints • Static DBS and hinged • Hinged splint used for active tenodesis exercises, weeks 1-4	Dorsal blocking splint Static splint: Wrist: 20°–30° flexion MCPs: 50° flexion IPs: Full extension Hinged splint: Allows full wrist flexion to extension 30° MCPs: 60°, IPs: 0	Day 3: Hourly PROM flexion 15 reps In hinged splint: Hourly 25 reps: 1. PROM digits with wrist extended 30° 2. Gentle active hold flexion 5 seconds 3. Flex wrist and release active fist	1. Week 4: Hinged splint discharged and unrestricted tenodesis exercised are permitted 2. Week 6: Composite extension begins
Short arc motion (Evans and Thompson, 1997)[3,6] • Zones I and II • Limited to repairs with a modified Kessler and epitendinous suture	Dorsal blocking splint Wrist 30°–40° flexion MCPs: 30°–45° flexion IPs: Full extension Zone I: DIP extension block splint 40°–45° flexion Zone II: Dynamic flexion bands with palmar pulley Night: Disconnect dynamic tension bands. IP joints are strapped in full extension	Day 1–3 1. 10–20 reps of PROM to distal palmar crease 2. 10–20 reps of AROM IP extension while holding the MCP flexion with opposite hand 3. 1–3 days postop. Only in therapy, short arc place and hold. Use pinch meter to measure active force. Passive tenodesis exercise	1. Week 3: patient permitted to perform place/hold exercises at home. D/C DIP splint for Zone I repair 2. Progress therapy as per other flexor tendon protocols
Early AROM and dynamic splinting (Silfverskiold and May, 1995)[7] • Uses dynamic tension during the day	Dorsal blocking splint Day: Wrist 30°–40° flexion MCPs: Flexion 50°–70° Dynamic flexion with palmar pulley Splint ends at IP joints Night: Disconnect dynamic tension bands. IP joints strapped in full extension	Hourly, 10 reps 1. Active extension while manually unloading dynamic tension. Then allow dynamic tension to flex digits. 2. When in full passive flexion, gently contract muscle to hold 2–3 seconds	Week 4: Remove splint for unassisted AROM exercises at home

DBS, dorsal blocking splint; AROM, active range of motion; MCP, metacarpophalangeal; IP, interphalangeal; DIP, distal interphalangeal; PROM, passive range of motion; D/C, discharge.

● FLEXOR POLLICIS LONGUS REHABILITATION

The management of lacerations to the flexor pollicis longus (FPL) may be more difficult due to tension from tendon retraction being greater with the FPL than for digital flexor lacerations. Flexor pollicis longus lacerations are most often treated with early PROM or dynamic flexion, and AROM may wait until the 3 weeks postoperative due to less adhesion formation and increased rupture rates. Early AROM for FPL lacerations can be used, yet it has not been shown to significantly improve outcomes.[3,9]

With all tendon rehabilitation, both with early active and immobilization protocols, complications may include adhesion formation, joint contracture, tendon rupture, pulley failure, and tenosynovitis. With associated digital nerve injuries, there are also the possible complications of sympathetic flares and hypersensitivity which can limit functional use of the hand postoperatively.

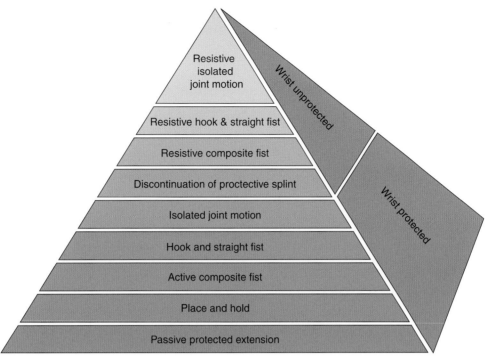

Pyramid of progressive force application

● **FIGURE 59-4.** Progressive force exercises to the intrasynovial flexor tendon injury and repair.[8]

● EXTENSOR TENDONS

The management of extensor tendons presents its own unique challenges because of the complex and intricate anatomy of the extensor tendon system.

The extensor mechanism is a dynamic system involving extrinsic muscles, intrinsic muscles, and their soft tissue connections. Even a minor injury to part of this system can decrease function and alter the mechanics of normal motion.

Treatment for extensor tendon injuries is based on the location, or zone, and severity of the laceration. The level of protection, the splint position, and the ROM permitted have been established from studies measuring the effects that joint position has on tendon gliding.[10] Static splinting generally remains the standard of care for simple extensor tendon injures in zones V–VIII; however, with increased complexity of injuries, patients can benefit from the use of early motion protocols (Figure 59-5).[11] As with primary flexor tendon repairs, early motion protocols for extensor tendon rehabilitation are designed to promote tendon excursion by applying controlled force without compromising the repair. The progression and design of these protocols is based on studies of extensor tendon excursion as it relates to the degree of ROM at individual joints.[10-12] The use of early AROM protocols is dependent on the strength and quality of the repair as well as the level of trauma to the surrounding tissues.

Early motion protocols (Table 59-2) for extensor tendons must be initiated within the first 24 to 48 hours postoperatively with a compliant patient and guided by

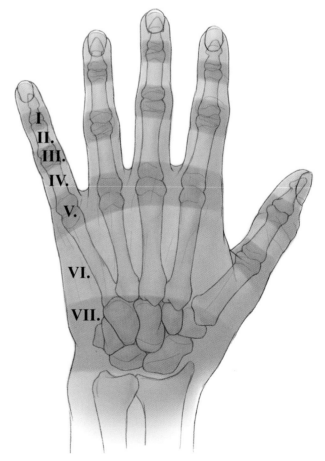

● **FIGURE 59-5.** Extensor tendon zones.

TABLE 59-2. Commonly Used Protocols for Extensor Tendon Zones I–VII

Zone	Splint	Timing Progress	Complications
Zone I and II "Mallet finger" Terminal tendon rupture, avulsion fracture	DIP immobilization 6–8 wk in full extension All proximal joints mobilized	Slow mobilization of the DIP AROM at 6–8+ wk. No early AROM indicated	May require fixation Monitor DIP lag Maceration Night splinting 3–6 mo
Zone III and IV Boutonnière Central slip laceration, rupture, avulsion fracture	PIP extension splint or cast 6 wk, DIP AROM Short arc motion protocol: template splint used to allow limited AROM[10]	Slow mobilization of PIP AROM at 6–8+ wk.	Monitor PIP joint lag for boutonnière Adhesions Night splinting 3–6 mo
Zone III and IV Central slip with lateral band involvement	PIP and DIP extension splint, 6–8 wk in full extension	Slow mobilization of isolated PIP and DIP ROM at 6 wk	Monitor PIP lag for boutonnière Adhesions Night splinting 3–6 mo
Zone V and VI Dorsal hood Sagittal bands Juncturae tendinum	Hand based or forearm based Wrist: 30° extension MCP: extension IPs: free	AROM 3–4 wk, splint 6 wk	MCP deviation MCP extension lag Adhesions
Zone VI and VII	Wrist: 30° extension MCP: extension IPs: free Dynamic MCP extension splint, allow MCP flexion to 40°	AROM 3–4 wk, splint for 6 wk. Limited flexion, assisted extension in dynamic splint until 4 wk	Adhesions very common Extrinsic tightness
Zone VII+ Tendon muscle junction and muscle belly	Wrist: 30° extension possibly long arm splint at 90°	AROM 3–4 wk, splint for 6 wk.	Adhesions very common Extrinsic tightness

DIP, distal interphalangeal; PIP, proximal interphalangeal; AROM, active range of motion; MCP, metacarpophalangeal; IP, interphalangeal.

an experienced hand therapist. Other protocols have been developed using dynamic rubber band traction to allow early tendon glide within a short arc of motion.[12]

Common features of all extensor tendon programs are: any extension lag must be monitored closely and the therapist must adjust the motion and splinting program accordingly, the protective splint is used for 4 to 6 weeks, and occasionally for zone V+, a night interphalangeal (IP) extension splint may be indicated to avoid proximal interphalangeal (PIP) joint contractures. As with flexor tendons, extensor tendon protocols differ in splint position, active and passive ROM, and timing.

Tendon lacerations to the extensor pollicis longus in zones TI are treated similarly to the digits, with IP extension splinting for 6 to 8 weeks. Lacerations in zone TII are splinted in a hand-based splint with metacarpophalangeal (MCP) and IP joints in extension and in full radial abduction. Lacerations in zones TIII and TIV should be splinted with the wrist at 20 to 30 degrees extension and thumb in maximum end range extension and abduction (as compared with unaffected hand). By week 3, AROM to all joints is progressed and by week 6 the splint is discharged. Dynamic protocols can be used and splinting

allows passive flexion of the IP joint, with assisted extension (Figure 59-6).[11,12]

● TENDON TRANSFERS AND FREE MUSCLE TRANSFERS

The body of research for these procedures is small as it relates to hand therapy; however, what has been shown is that given the strength of the weave, early controlled motion can be tolerated and provides improved results with less stiffness and adhesions. According to Brand and Strickland, stiffness and adhesions are the most common cause of disappointment with tendon transfers. Early motion can be beneficial considering the condition of the soft tissue envelope.[7, 13–15] Early motion programs have been described in the literature by various authors for different transfers. Given suitable suture technique, early mobilization of the transfer has been shown to be effective in improving ROM, decreasing adhesions, hastening the motor learning process, and decreasing the time in therapy.[15–17]

The therapist plays an integral part in the preoperative process and can be helpful in preparing the patient for surgery. Preoperative treatment is necessary to resolve joint

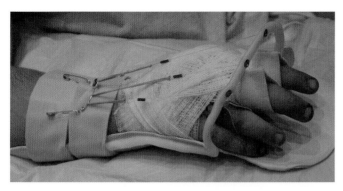

● **FIGURE 59-6.** Dynamic extension splint for complex extensor tendon laceration to allow early motion for tendon gliding.

contracture, maintain joint PROM, strengthen and educate possible donor muscles, and improve soft tissue mobility by minimizing scar tissue and edema. Therapists can also help outline the postoperative plan and assist in setting realistic goals and expectations. If possible, the therapist should observe the surgery to gain a better understanding of the procedure.

Early PROM and/or AROM can be initiated postoperatively between weeks 1 to 3 depending on the surgeon's preference, technique, and the soft tissue status of the transfer route. Typically at week 3 to 4, short but frequent AROM exercise sessions and functional activities are initiated.[16] Biofeedback and electrical stimulation may be beneficial especially when patients are having difficulty activating the transfer. The splint may be discharged by 6 weeks, and at this time any extrinsic or transfer tightness can be addressed with splinting and stretches and very light resistance can begin. As with primary repairs, resistive exercises can be initiated at 8 weeks postoperatively, with the goal to return to work and avocational activities by weeks 10 to 12.

● **NERVE INJURY AND REPAIR**

Hand therapists can be especially valuable following nerve injury and can assist patients in regaining function and minimizing complications. Supervised therapy is aimed at preventing joint stiffness, scar hypersensitivity, allodynia, and chronic regional pain syndrome.

Postoperative treatment is beneficial for many reasons. Often patients will require splinting to protect a nerve repair. The level of tension on a nerve repair postoperatively will determine the position of the splint and level of protection it provides. Splinting may also be indicated to promote function and prevent joint contracture while waiting for muscle reinnervation (Figures 59-7, 59-8, and 59-9). These splints can often be comfortable and low profile to minimize disruption to the patient's daily life. Patients may need these splints for weeks to months following a nerve injury.

As a nerve regenerates, therapy is focused on desensitization, functional sensory reeducation, nerve mobilization, strengthening, ROM, and neuromuscular retraining. Desensitization is a progressive process by which sensory

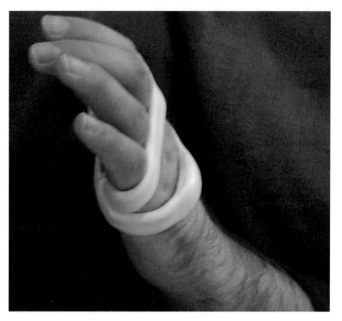

● **FIGURE 59-7.** Ulnar nerve anticlaw splint.

input is introduced to the patient slowly and systematically. As the patient's sensation improves and the painful response to touch diminishes, the noxious stimulus is increased until normal functional sensory awareness is achieved. Sensory reeducation is the next phase and requires a higher level of sensory awareness. It focuses on reeducating the sensory receptors for function, including moving and static touch discrimination, point localization, and object recognition.

Adhesive neuritis may develop from closed traction injuries, open lacerations, or surgical nerve repair/manipulation. Patients may present with significant pain and paresthesias, and may have developed stiffness from avoiding painful motion. Nerve mobilization, or gliding, is a commonly used treatment technique that therapists may use to decrease pain and increase function. Treatment with

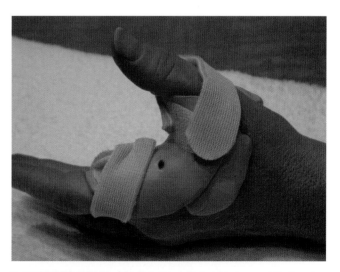

● **FIGURE 59-8.** Medial nerve C-bar to prevent first web space contracture.

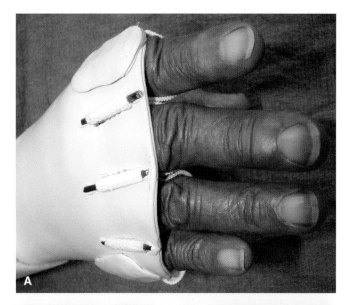

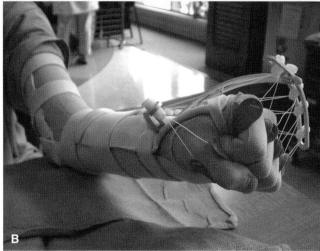

FIGURE 59-9. Radial nerve palsy splints (low profile and with outrigger).

segmental and full length nerve gliding has been shown to be effective in decreasing pain caused by adhesions and inflammation around an injured nerve.

SOFT TISSUE MANAGEMENT: EDEMA AND SCAR

Edema management can be initiated immediately postsurgically and can be effective continuing into the remodeling phase of healing. There are many different techniques used to decrease edema and the selection of which method to use will depend on the stage of healing and tissue quality. Edema management can be as basic as elevation and active pumping or as complicated as manual lymphatic drainage and wrapping. Examples of treatment interventions include:

- Elevation
- AROM (active muscle pumping)
- Massage and manual lymphatic drainage

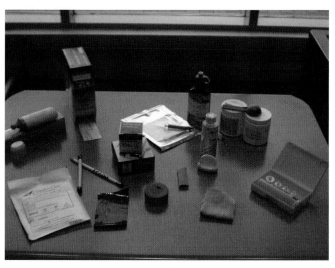

FIGURE 59-10. Scar management products (left to right): massage tools, tape, iontophoresis, scar molds gel pads, Dycem, Coban, gel, and compression sleeves.

- Wrapping (Coban, lymphatic wrapping, string)
- Compression garments (sleeves, gloves, custom or "off the shelf")
- Modalities (ice, electrical stimulation such as high-volt, contrast baths)

Scar management is another critical component of hand therapy. It can be very important for increasing joint and tissue mobility, decreasing adhesions for increased ROM, and decreasing hypersensitivity for improved function. Scar management can also be helpful in restoring and improving the appearance of the injured hand. Through improved cosmesis, patient's may have increased ease of integrating the injured hand back into daily activities.

Studies have demonstrated that pressure and tension on the tissue will decrease the proliferation of collagen formation thus decreasing scar.[18] Examples of treatment intervention for scar management are listed below (Figure 59-10).

- Silicone gel (sleeves and pads)
- Elastomer molds (Figure 59-11)
- Tape
- Compression garments
- Dycem for scar massage/retraction
- Massage tools (vibration and suction)
- ROM
- Casts and splints

FRACTURE MANAGEMENT: HAND AND WRIST

Treatment for patients with fractures about the hand and wrist may vary depending on many factors: the type and location of the fracture, the stability of the fracture or fixation, the mechanism of injury, associated injuries, the patient's age and comorbidities (Table 59-3).

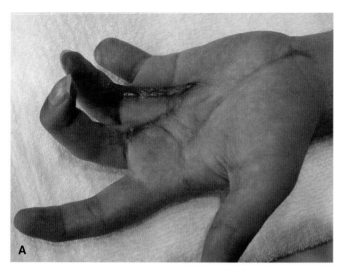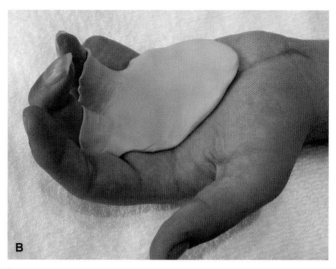

● **FIGURE 59-11.** Elastomer mold for keloid scar before (A) and after application (B).

TABLE 59-3. Treatment for Fractures

Fracture	ROM and Treatment	Splint	Complications
Distal radius ORIF	AROM all unaffected joints (proximal and distal) A/AAROM wrist as allowed Edema management Scar mobilization	At 2–4 wk: Wrist cock-up splint Munster splint or sugar tong to limit rotation with TFC or DRUJ involvement	FPL adhesions (volar plating) Extensor adhesions (dorsal plating) CTS
Distal radius Nonoperative, cast	AROM all unaffected joints (proximal and distal) Edema management to digits	At 4–6 wk: Wrist cock-up splint Munster splint or sugar tong	Digital stiffness Persistent edema Extrinsic tightness CTS
Distal radius Ex-fix, or percutaneous pinning	AROM all unaffected joints (proximal and distal) Edema and scar management Pin care	Protective splinting over ex-fix Wrist splint after hardware removal	Extrinsic tightness Radial sensory nerve irritation CTS Pin site infection
Metacarpal With or without ORIF Percutaneous pinning	ROM PIP/DIP joints ROM MCP and wrist as allowed Edema management Scar mobilization Extensor tendon gliding	Wrist or hand based ulnar or radial gutter MCPs in flexion IP joints in extension	EDC adhesions MCP joint extension contractures PIP joint flexion contractures
Phalanx: proximal and middle With or without ORIF Percutaneous pinning	ROM MCP, PIP, DIP joints as allowed Edema management Scar mobilization	Digital extension splint or gutter with MCPs in flexion IP joints in extension IP joint: 30° flexion with volar plate injury	MCP joint extension contractures PIP joint flexion contractures/extension lag Flexor adhesions
Tuft/distal phalanx With or without percutaneous pinning[19,20]	A/PROM proximal joints Edema management Desensitization	Tip protector or stack splint with DIP in extension	Hypersensitivity at tip or nail bed

ORIF, open reduction and internal fixation; AROM, active range of motion; AAROM, active assisted range of motion; ROM, range of motion; PIP, proximal interphalangeal; DIP, distal interphalangeal; MCP, metacarpophalangeal; TFC, triangular fibrocartilage complex; DRUJ, distal radioulnar joint; IP, interphalangeal; FPL, flexor pollicus longus; CTS, carpal tunnel syndrome; EDC, extensor digitorum communis.

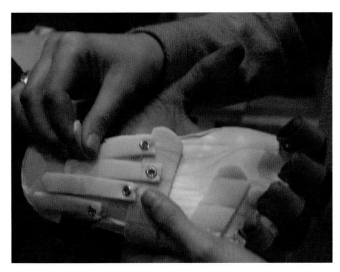

● **FIGURE 59-12.** Splint to resolve intrinsic tightness and interphalangeal joint stiffness.

Regardless of surgical intervention, for all patients with distal radius fractures, common complications can include: median nerve symptoms/carpal tunnel syndrome, extrinsic tightness, distal radioulnar joint instability or triangular fibrocartilage complex injuries, chronic edema and stiffness, and chronic regional pain syndrome. With phalanx and metacarpal fractures,

common complications can include significant joint stiffness, MCP/PIP extension and flexion contractures, PIP extension lag, intrinsic tightness from splint position and edema, extrinsic tightness or adhesions (flexor and extensor), scar, and hypersensitivity particularly when crush injuries occur.

Hand therapists can be helpful in identifying and treating these problems and are particularly critical in preventing stiffness. Using various modalities, ROM, stretching, and scar mobilization techniques, therapy can be beneficial in improving joint and tissue mobility. Patients may also have their protective splints remolded to provide increased stretch or the therapist may choose to fabricate or order a dynamic or static progressive splint to provide low load stretching for tissue elongation. Figure 59-12 shows an example of a static progressive splint to increase digital ROM.

● SUMMARY

Hand therapy has evolved to become a critical component in the treatment of injuries to the hand. Protocols continue to evolve as the understanding of the mechanics and biology of wound healing improves. Communication and coordination of care between the surgeon and therapist is the keystone to enabling hand surgery patients to achieve more rapid and complete return of function.

REFERENCES

1. Strickland JW. Development of flexor tendon surgery: twenty-five years of progress. *J Hand Surg.* 2000;25A: 214–235.

2. Formby ME. Flexor tendon repair. In: Burke SL, Higgins JP, McClinton MA, Saunders RJ, Valdata L, eds. *Hand and Upper Extremity Rehabilitation: A Practical Guide.* 3rd ed. St. Louis, MO: Elsevier; 2004:227–244.

3. Evans RB. Early active motion after flexor tendon repair. In: Berger R, Weiss A, eds. *Hand Surgery.* Philadelphia: Lippincott Williams & Wilkins; 2010:709–735.

4. Halikis MN, Manske PR, Kubota H, Aoki M. Effect of immobilization, immediate mobilization, and delayed mobilization on the resistance to digital flexion using a tendon injury model. *J Hand Surg Am.* 1997;22:464–472.

5. Cannon N, Strickland J. *Diagnosis and Treatment Manual for Physicians and Therapists.* 4th ed. Indianapolis, IN: The Hand Rehabilitation Center of Indiana; 2001.

6. Evans RB, Thompson D. Immediate active short arc of motion following tendon repair. In: Hunter J, Schneider L, Mackin E, eds. *Tendon and Nerve Surgery in the Hand.* St. Louis, MO: Mosby; 1997:362–391.

7. Silfverskiold KL, May EJ. Early active mobilization after tendon transfers using mesh reinforced suture techniques. *J Hand Surg Br.* 1995;20:291–300.

8. Groth GN. Pyramid of progressive force exercises to the injured flexor tendon. *J Hand Ther.* 2004;17:31–42.

9. Elliot D, Moiemen NS, Flemming AF, Harris SB, Foster AJ. The rupture rate of acute flexor tendon repairs mobilized by the controlled active motion regimen. *J Hand Surg Br.* 1994;19:607–612.

10. Evans RB, Burkhalter WE. A study of the dynamic anatomy of extensor tendons and implications for treatment. *J Hand Surg Am.* 1986;11:774–779.

11. Saunders RJ. Management of extensor tendon repairs. In: Burke SL, Higgins JP, McClinton MA, Saunders RJ, Valdata L, eds. *Hand and Upper Extremity Rehabilitation: A Practical Guide.* 3rd ed. St. Louis, MO: Elsevier; 2006:271–292.

12. Carney KL, Griffen-Reed N. Rehabilitation of extensor tendon injury and repair. In: Berger R, Weiss A, eds. *Hand Surgery.* Philadelphia: Lippincott Williams & Wilkins; 2004: 787–778.

13. Trumble TE. Tendon transfers. In: Trumble TE, ed. *Principles of Hand Surgery and Therapy.* St. Louis, MO: Saunders; 2004: 343–360.

14. Brand PW. Mechanics of tendon transfers. In: Hunter JM, Mackin EJ, Callahan AD, eds. *Rehabilitation of the Hand and Upper Extremity.* 5th ed. St. Louis, MO: Mosby; 2002.

15. Germann G, Wagner H, Blome-Eberwein S, Karle B, Wittemann M. Early dynamic motion versus postoperative immobilization in patients with extensor indicis proprius transfer to restore thumb extension: a prospective randomized study. *J Hand Surg Am.* 2001;26:1111–1115.

16. Rath S. Immediate active mobilization versus immobilization for opposition tendon transfer in the hand. *J Hand Surg Am.* 2006;31:754–759.

17. Kozin SH. Tendon transfers for radial and median nerve palsies. *J Hand Ther.* 2005;18:208–215.

18. Evans R, McAcliffe JA. Wound management. In: Hunter JM, Mackin EJ, Callahan AD, eds. *Rehabilitation of the Hand and Upper Extremity.* 5th ed. St. Louis, MO: Mosby; 2002: 311–327.

19. Freeland AE, Torres JE. Extraarticular fractures of the phalanges. In: Berger R, Weiss A, eds. *Hand Surgery.* Philadelphia: Lippincott Williams & Wilkins; 2004:123–137.

20. Duncan SFM, Weiland AJ. Extraarticular distal radius fractures. In: Berger R, Weiss A, eds. *Hand Surgery.* Philadelphia: Lippincott Williams & Wilkins; 2004:247–275.

chapter 60

Reconstruction of the Chest – Congenital and Acquired Anomalies and Defects

Norman H. Schulman, MD, FACS / *Tara Lynn Huston, MD*

The reconstruction of chest wall defects is based on the tissues lost and their respective function. Any repair must consider the underlying thoracic organs as well as the skeletal support and soft tissue coverage. Chest wall defects may be divided into congenital and acquired problems. Most congenital problems are usually nonfunctional and are of concern primarily from an aesthetic point of view. Acquired problems most often follow open-heart surgical procedures, but may also be due to tumor extirpation and trauma. Post cardiac surgery chest reconstruction has evolved into a discipline of its own as not only the sternal deformity must be considered but the co-morbidities of infection, chronic obstructive pulmonary disease, diabetes and the underlying cardiovascular disease. Trauma to the chest often results in rib injuries and only in severe direct trauma, is the sternum ever involved. The ribs and sternum are well vascularized and unless there is severe displacement that requires re-positioning and fixation, healing is generally spontaneous.

Chest wall reconstruction dates back to the eighteenth century when Aimar performed the first recorded resection of osteosarcoma of the ribs in 1778. Airway control with endotracheal tubes and positive pressure ventilation, as well as closed suction systems, were introduced in the late 19th century and thus paved the way for the field of thoracic surgery. A subsequent report in 1898 described resection of a bony chest wall tumor, in which three ribs were included in the specimen.[1] In 1913, Lund performed resection of a sarcoma involving several components of the chest wall.[2]

In 1957, Julian introduced the median sternotomy to gain access to the thoracic cavity.[3] The initial infection rates were high with mortality rates of 70%. Early management consisted of open treatment with granulation and healing by secondary intention. In 1963, Shumaker and Mandelbaum used surgical debridement followed by closed suction irrigation of the sternum. This decreased but did not eradicate the associated mortality.[4] In 1976, Lee improved on this concept of debridement with the addition of transposed omentum in order to bring healthy, vascularized tissue to the mediastinal wound bed.[5] In 1979, P.G. Arnold expanded upon this idea to use muscle flaps, primarily the pectoralis major to promote wound healing.[6] The use of vacuum assisted closure (VAC) therapy in the 1990's for sternal wounds provided a bridge to surgery by improving granulation, reducing bacterial counts, shrinking wound sizes and in some cases resulting in eventual complete healing.[7] In 2006, the Lenox Hill experience with over 14,000 total cardiac patients over a 17-year period was published. The rate of sternal wound infection in this series was 2.3% reflecting present day improvement in thoracic surgery. Of the 336 patients who required secondary closure, the 30-day mortality was 3%, with a morbidity rate of 5%. Either secondary exploration or VAC therapy was required to facilitate complete healing.[8]

The most common congenital anomalies seen are pectus excavatum, pectus carinatum, and Poland syndrome. A few of these deformities may require early intervention as they may lead to severe functional problems during growth and development. Pectus excavatum, a caved-in or funnel shaped chest is the most common congenital chest wall abnormality, which accounts for 90% of the patients with congenital chest wall defects. It occurs in approximately 1 in 300-400 births, with a 3:1 male to female predominance. Even though the etiology is not known, it is thought to be genetic as there is a family history in over one third of the newly diagnosed cases.[9] In its most severe form, it can cause disruption of the placement of the mediastinal structures including the heart, great vessels and bronchi. Pectus excavatum was initially treated using the invasive Ravitch procedure, introduced in 1949, which consisted of sternal detachment and cartilage resection. A small, temporary bar was then inserted underneath the sternum until the cartilage grew back. More recently, the Nuss procedure has been used which places concave steel bars into the chest, below the sternum. The bar is then rotated to a convex position to correct the deformity. Pectus carinatum, or "pigeon chest," is the second most common defect occurring in 5-7% of patients, also more common in males. It rarely requires surgical correction.

Poland syndrome, which consists of the absence of the sternal head of the pectoralis and ipsilateral cutaneous syndactyly, occurs in 1 in 7,000-100,000 live births.[10] It affects males more commonly (3:1) and occurs on the right side of the body twice more commonly than the left. It has been associated with other syndromes, including Möbius syndrome, which is a congenital bilateral facial paralysis and inability to abduct the eyes. Other less common inborn disorders involving defects of the chest wall include cleft sternum, pentalogy of Cantrell, asphyxiating thoracic dystrophy, and spondylothoracic dysplasia.[11]

● PATIENT EVALUATION

A treatment plan is developed during the initial consultation with the plastic surgeon. A detailed history is obtained which includes several key pieces of information. The patient's gender, age, co-morbidities, medications, medical and surgical history, including indications for the cardiac procedure performed (if relevant) are obtained. The details of any prior procedure such as pump time, valve insertion, graft use, or any other prosthetic device or material needed is also ascertained. The patient's use of anti-coagulants is important for timing of reconstruction, as is the current respiratory status.

The initial physical examination should evaluate the chest deformity or wound and any other physical co-morbidities including general body habitus and mental state. A gram-stain with culture and sensitivity of any open or draining wound should be obtained. Antibiotics will rarely cure these post-operative sternal infections but are a vital adjuvant in the success of any attempt at sternal wound reconstruction.

Prior to surgery, all pre-operative studies, scans and medical records should be reviewed. A proper diagnosis and classification of the wound must be made. One algorithm attempts to simplify the classification and treatment (Figure 60-1). Wounds are broken down into three distinct

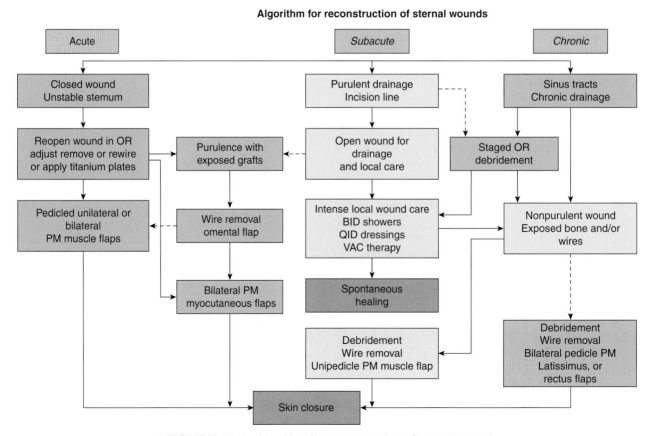

● FIGURE 60-1. Algorithm for reconstruction of sternal wounds.

categories. Acute wounds occur within the first and second weeks of surgery. They can present with open or dehisced skin as well as with or without signs of infection. Sub-acute wounds occur within 2-4 weeks of surgery and are generally marked by infection and purulence. Lastly, chronic wounds occur anytime after the 4th or 5th week and usually present as single or multiple drainage tracts often with positive cultures.[8]

A key part of the pre-operative evaluation is radiologic imaging. Plain chest x-rays are the most important as they provide a baseline condition of the lungs as well as the number, position and condition of the primary fixation devices utilized, usually stainless steel wires, or less commonly titanium bars (or plates) and clasps. Computerized tomography (CT) scans have only occasionally found to be helpful, such as in the discovery of a rare pseudo-aneurysm. The scans may prove useful if the clinical condition of the patient is worse than that indicated by the condition of the wound. In this instance, the CT scan may delineate a deep collection, hidden on physical exam. Contrast material should be avoided as it is not necessary and may be dangerous for patients with pre-existing renal compromise. Spect-CT scans, which combines radio-isotope scanning with computed tomography allows visualization of an abscess or point of inflammation only several millimeters in size.

A team approach is vital to the success of the outcome and must involve co-operation and communication with the cardiothoracic surgery team. This must involve willingness, availability and an ability for the plastic surgeon to work with the cardiac surgeon to participate in all phases of the treatment plan.

● TREATMENT OF THE ACUTE POST CARDIAC SURGERY WOUND

The history and physical should permit categorization of the wound thereby suggesting treatment options. An acute wound occurring within several days to within two weeks of the cardiac procedure must be regarded as a semi-emergent condition requiring early or immediate intervention. These wounds usually represent a dehiscence of the sternum with or without intact skin. Though infection may not be present a large volume of sero-sanguineous fluid in the wound is typical. At greatest risk in a bypass procedure would be exposed freshly placed bypass grafts. Exposure of these grafts risks desiccation and failure therefore they must be protected, kept moist and sealed as soon as possible with well-vascularized tissue.

Omental flaps, delivered from the abdomen superficial to the diaphragm provide well-vascularized tissue, which can readily cover the grafts (Figure 60-2). Muscle flaps may be used but are not as flexible for coverage and may be better utilized in final chest wall closure. General surgeons or plastic surgeons fully trained in general surgery can readily harvest the omentum through an separate, vertical epigastric incision or laparoscopically. With a history of prior abdominal surgery, the open method is preferred as the omentum may not be fully intact and either the right or left segment may have to be obtained on its blood supply. The right-sided blood supply is preferable, as it provides for a flap with the longest reach, to the base of the neck if necessary. Final chest closure is accomplished by using two myocutaneous pectoralis flaps and closing in the midline over the mediastinum.[12]

If sternal rigidity is required, titanium fixation bars (Synthes[R]) that span the two edges of the sternum work well (Figure 60-3).[13] Sternal fixation should not result in tamponade, as closing pressures can be readily controlled by the span of the bars. The bars can be used as bridges and the muscle flaps will not cause mediastinal compression as they are detached on their under surface from the ribs and sternum. In an urgent situation, where time and anesthesia are concerns, the skin can be brought together over the omentum with deep dermal sutures without muscles. To provide infection protection and which later may be revised if necessary.

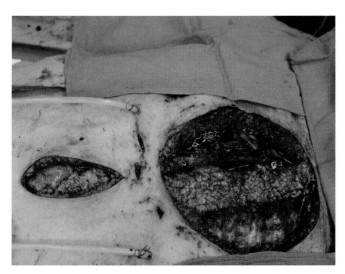

● **FIGURE 60-2.** Omental Inset to Mediastinum.

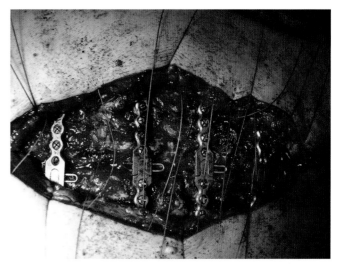

● **FIGURE 60-3.** Titanium bars, screw and release pins. Single layer muscle, dermis closure.

Sub-acute wounds are the most common. They occur 2–4 weeks after surgery and usually present as "sick" patients with fevers, leukocytosis and purulent drainage. Often these patients will have positive blood cultures. These wounds are life threatening, but there is time to prepare the wound properly for definitive therapy. Decompression of the infected wound is performed as soon as possible, either by opening the wound at the bedside under local anesthesia or a more thorough procedure in the operating room, which may include removal of sternal wires. Once adequate drainage and decompression has been achieved, the open wound is prepared for definitive closure. This preparation involves multiple daily dressings of saline or an ultra-dilute solution of povidone (1:100) to prevent wound colonization. If tolerated, it is recommended that the patients take twice daily showers. Once purulent fluid has been cleared, VAC therapy may be used until definitive closure is offered, often a period of 2–7 days. VAC therapy may close some of these wounds, but unless there has been complete wire removal and thorough debridement in the operating room, these wounds require secondary closure, as they may become chronic.

The patient with the now "clean wound" is taken to the operating room for definitive reconstruction. Prior to prepping and draping the wound is re-cultured. Reconstruction is begun by complete excision of all wound edges and wire removal. Blood loss is controlled with the use of two cauterization devices, a Bovie and an argon beam coagulator. Non-viable or infected portions of the sternum are debrided at this time. In the sub-acute wounds, the mediastinum is often healed and adherent to the underside of the sternum, therefore, extra care must be taken to avoid right ventricular tears and absolute paralysis is a must during this part of the procedure. Once debridement has been completed the operative field is copiously irrigated, usually with a pulsatile delivery of at least 2 liters of a broad-spectrum antibiotic solution.[14]

Now a decision must be made for the best closure technique for the particular defect and the particular patient, considering the clinical condition and co-morbidities. As discussed in the opening of this chapter, the introduction of muscle flaps in mediastinal closure has been revolutionary, resulting in a vast improvement in the survival from mediastinitis. The workhorse flap is the uni-pedicled pectoralis major muscle flap. This muscle originates on the clavicle and insets on the sternum, ribs and upper humerus. Its main blood supply arises from the thorcoacromial artery and vein, which should be left intact and never skeletonized. The pedicle can be readily identified arising from the upper medial edge of the pectoralis minor during the dissection of the pectoralis major. If the uni-pedicled pectoralis major muscle is selected, the muscle can be inset from the manubrium to just proximal to the xiphoid if properly mobilized.

The dissection begins with the separation of the skin and fat as a unit from the underlying muscle using cautery dissection technique. The muscle is separated from the sternum and ribs, the pedicle and its blood supply are identified and preserved. The distal end of the muscle is encircled proximal to its humeral attachment, which is just inferior to the cephalic vein. The humeral, sternal, and rib attachments are divided as well as the medial one third of its attachment to the clavicle to provide maximum mobility. The superior medial portion of the pectoralis major may be back cut 3 or 4 cm to fill behind the manubrium if necessary. Closure over the xiphoid can be obtained by approximating the upper medial aspects of both rectus abdominal muscles. Bilateral pectoral major muscles may be used on their separate pedicles if a larger coverage area is required.

The pectoralis muscle is inserted into the mediastinal defect, usually a groove resulting from sternal wound debridement and then suture fixed on all sides. Four large closed suction drains are placed: one in the axilla, one in the muscle bed, one alongside the mediastinal inset (not into the groove defect), and one in the subcutaneous tissue (Figure 60-4). The skin is closed with deep dermal sutures and sealed with staples. This closure minimizes dead space and should be air and water-tight. Suction provided by the drains at 100 mmHg further minimizes dead space, encourages flap adhesion in the wound, and inhibits seroma formation. Absolute hemostasis in a clean wound and continued suction in an airtight closure for 3 to 5 days is the best environment for primary healing.

Chronic wounds occur in the late post-operative period any time after the 4th or 5th week of sternotomy. Although they may present with the same threat as the acute or sub-acute wound, they usually present as persistent local pain with small amounts of drainage from the wound edges. Osteomyelitis of the sternum is common in this group and, after reconstruction, may require long term intra-venous antibiotic therapy. This is not an uncommon sequela to wounds initially allowed to close by VAC therapy alone. These wounds are approached in

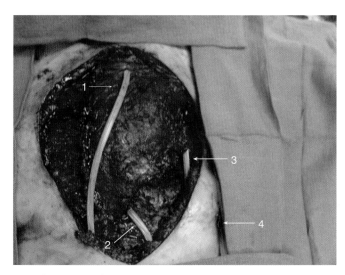

● **FIGURE 60-4.** Unipedicle Pectoralis Major Inset. Drain Arrows: 1. Subcutaneous, 2. Paramediastinal, 3. Muscle bed, and 4. Axillary.

a fashion similar to that of sub-acute wounds mandating thorough debridement of soft tissue and bone and complete foreign body removal, wires, pacing wire remnants, and fixation bars or plates if used.

Other muscles considered are the rectus abdominus and latissimus dorsi muscles. The former are usually secondary options and used only if the ipsilateral internal mammary artery has not been employed as a bypass graft as this forms the superior epigastric artery, which feeds the upper portion of the rectus. Use of the latter is limited as its range is limited and the patient would have to be re-positioned. The latissimus dorsi is a better source as a free flap if other tissues are not available.

The time-tested concept in bone healing by "rigid fixation" is now coming into play in sternal and chest wall reconstruction. This concept, adapted from orthopedic surgery, provides for the most rapid, reliable and strong healing of bones. Titanium spanning bars have been used to achieve rigid fixation and chest wall stability in reconstructed post-sternotomy dehiscence and infections. It is particularly helpful in patients with chronic obstructive pulmonary disease as it not only enhances healing but significantly decreases morbidity and improves breathing as noted by the absence of pain and improved chest wall compliance. Experience is limited in the use of these bars as they are expensive and somewhat difficult to learn to apply, however significant clinical benefits have been documented. If rigid fixation is required then this technique is best. Omentum, as stated earlier, may be used to protect fresh grafts and unless the titanium bars are used as a bridge to hold open the mediastinum to reduce pressure they are not used with omental closures in the otherwise limited capacity of the mediastinum.

CHEST WALL NEOPLASIA

Carcinomas and sarcomas do occur on the musculoskeletal structure of the chest and are uncommon as primary neoplasms. As they occur they are treated accordingly. If extirpation is part of the procedure then reconstruction must be performed to restore form and function, compliance and integrity to the chest wall to allow for normal respiratory effort and unimpeded circulation. Each case must be considered on its own merits, evaluating location of the injury, extent and health and age of the patient. The techniques applied to post cardiac surgery reconstruction are similar and will be elaborately dealt with in the next section.

COMPLICATIONS

Complications are uncommon; however the three, which occur most often are hematoma, seroma and recurrent infection. Hematoma is most closely associated with vigorous early resumption of anti-coagulant therapy, certainly desirable after valve and some forms of bypass surgery. Most cardiac situations can fare well for 72 hours without resumption of anti-coagulation. Consultation with the cardiac surgeon and cardiologist will often permit safe anti-coagulation after reconstruction with low dose aspirin or Heparin (no more than 300 units/hour) in the early postoperative period followed by the institution of Warfarin as early as 48 hours post operative. Clopidogrel and more aggressive Heparin should be withheld for the first 72 hours.

Seroma formation may occur whenever there is the presence of large raw open surfaces such as may exist during muscle and flap mobilization in sternal reconstruction. This is minimized with the liberal use of initial suction drains to continual wall suction of about 100 mmHg. In an average single pedicled muscle flap as many as four large drains are used, commonly 19 French Blake drains and after 72 hours are progressively discontinued as the drainage yield decreases, first subcutaneous, then the muscle bed, then para-sternal and finally axillary. Closed continual wound suction minimizes dead space and helps with early flap adherence.

Recurrent infection in a properly prepared wound is uncommon, occurring about 5% or less. Flaps, with the exception of the omentum, should not be placed in the presence of frank pus. As little as 48 hours of preparation can make a 10-fold difference in the incidence of re-infection. As stated earlier, infected wounds demand decompression and topical therapy of multiple dressings or VAC therapy prior to definitive closure. In the face of acute dehiscence and possibly early infection liberal lavage (pulsatile antibiotic) together with placement of omentum is usually successful in the preservation of acutely uncovered coronary bypass grafts. Re-infected wounds must be re-opened for drainage as all remaining debris and foreign body should have been removed at the reconstruction procedure these wounds will usually heal by secondary intension, commonly aided by VAC therapy. Secondary flap reconstruction is generally not required. However, if not used previously, the omentum may be a good rescue flap as are other muscles such as recti or latissimus.

Although rare, the most feared complication is injury to the underlying cardiothoracic structures. Injury to the bypass graft will result in rapid bleeding which must be managed emergently. Fro this reason, the anatomy of the postoperative heart must be recognized. Bypass grafts, either off the internal mammary artery or saphenous vein, may be close to, and possibly adherent to, the undersurface of the sternum. For this reason, the referring cardiothoracic surgeon should be aware of the procedure and available if needed. Lung injury may result in a persistent and troublesome bronchopleural fistula if not managed correctly. These patients require initial chest tube drainage and observation for cessation of an air leak. In the sub-acute wounds, the mediastinum is often healed and adherent to the underside of the sternum, therefore, extra care must be taken to avoid right ventricular tears and absolute paralysis is a must during this part of the procedure.

● OUTCOMES

Outcomes following chest wall reconstruction have to be analyzed in terms of safety, cost effectiveness and patient benefits. For reconstruction of sternal wound infections, the major variables include time to healing and need for additional surgical procedures. Patients, and their surgeons, want complications managed expeditiously to avoid further hospital stay to return to normal activity. Rigid fixation plates used in selected candidates at the primary procedure has reduced the rate of mediastinitis by 50% and has resulted in earlier and generally pain free hospital discharges.[15]

REFERENCES

1. Parham FW. Thoracic resection for tumors growing from the bony wall of the chest. *Trans South Surg Gynecol Assoc.* 1898;11:223.

2. Lund FB. Sarcoma of the chest wall. *Ann Surg.* 1913; 58:206.

3. Julian OC, Lopez-Belio M, Dye WS, et al. The median sternal incision in intracardiac surgery with extracorporeal circulation: a general evaluation of its use in heart surgery. *Surgery.* 1957;42:753–761.

4. Shumaker HB, Mandelbaum I. Continuous antibiotic irrigation in the treatment of infection. *Arch Surg.* 1963;86:384–387.

5. Lee AB Jr, Schimert G, Shaktin S, Seigel JH. Total excision of the sternum and thoracic pedicle transposition of the greater omentum; useful strategems in managing severe mediastinal infection following open heart surgery. *Surgery.* 1976;80:433–436.

6. Arnold PG, Pairolero PC. Use of Pectoralis Major Muscle Flaps to Repair Defects Anterior Chest Wall, *Plastic Reconstr Surg.* 1979;63:205.

7. Tang AT, Okri SK, and How MP. Vacuum-assisted closure to treat deep sternal wound infection following cardiac surgery. *J Wound Care.* 2000;9:222.

8. Schulman NH. *Plastic Surgery: Clinical Problem Solving.* McGraw Hill Medical; 2009:184.

9. Nuss D, Kelly RE Jr, Croitoru DP, Katz ME. A 10-year review of a minimally invasive technique for the correction of pectus excavatum. *J Pediatr Surg.* 1998;33(4):545–552.

10. Moir CR, Johnson CH. Poland's syndrome. *Semin Pediatr Surg.* 2008;17(3):161–166.

11. Clarkson P. Poland's syndactyly. *Guys Hosp Rep.* 1962;111:335–346.

12. Hugo HE, Sutton MR, Ascherman TK, et al. Single stage management of 74 consecutive sternal wound complications with pectoralis major myocutaneous advancement flaps. *Plast Reconstr Surg.* 1994;93:1433.

13. Sargent LA, Seyfer AE, Hollinger J, et al. The Healing Sternum: A Comparison of Osseous Healing with Wire Versus Rigid Fixation, Walter Reed Army Medical Center; 1992.

14. Schulman NH, Subramanian V. Sternal wound reconstruction: 252 consecutive cases. The Lenox Hill experience; *Plast Reconstr Surg.* 2004;114:44.

15. Song DH, Lohman RF, Renucci JD, et al. Primary sternal plating in high risk patients prevents mediastinitis, *Eur J Cardiothorac Surg.* 2004;26(2):367–372.

chapter 61

Abdominal Wall Reconstruction

Devinder P. Singh, MD / Helen G. Hui-Chou, MD / Ronald P. Silverman, MD, FACS

● PATIENT EVALUATION AND SELECTION

The goal of abdominal wall reconstruction is restoration of the myofascial layer in the anterior trunk. This layer is highly complex and serves multiple functions. First and foremost, it is a protective barrier, holding in place the abdominal viscera. In addition, the abdominal wall musculature contributes to posture, flexion, and rotation of the trunk, respiration, coughing, emesis, defecation, micturation, and parturition. Defects of the abdominal wall can compromise any of these functions, cause pain, or lead to herniation of the viscera. In particular, the risk of visceral incarceration and subsequent strangulation, while rare in larger hernias, cannot be ignored due to the potentially fatal consequences.

Tissue deficit in the abdominal wall can result from a wide variety of causes including congenital, cancer, trauma, burn, and/or infection. The most common cause, however, is iatrogenic: rates of incisional hernias have been reported as high as 11% after laparotomy and even higher in certain subsets of patients (such as open gastric bypass patients).[1] Primary repair of these incisional hernias carries a very high rate of recurrence (reportedly 40%–50%), presumably because of undue tension at the repair site.[2] As a result, the gold standard for initial incisional hernia has become the placement of synthetic mesh to bridge the gap and reduce tension.[3] Laparoscopic hernia repair has improved outcomes but has not overcome issues surrounding the use of synthetic materials, patients with massive defects, or situations where risk for infection at the surgical site exists.

To help stratify patients based on their risk factors for surgical site occurrence, the Ventral Hernia Working Group created a hernia grading system: grade 1 is low risk and includes patients with no history of a comorbid condition or wound infection. Grade 2 includes patients with a comorbid condition, including tobacco use, obesity, diabetes, chronic obstructive pulmonary disease (COPD), and/or immunosuppression. Grade 3 includes patients with potentially contaminated surgical sites, including those with stomas present, violation of the gastrointestinal tract such as enterotomy during hernia reduction, and/or history of wound infection previously healed by secondary intention. Grade 4 is reserved for those patients with an active infection at the hernia site.[4]

In recurrent incisional hernia patients, loss of abdominal wall domain can be profound, and plastic surgeons are now called upon more and more frequently to assist with complex reconstruction in these challenging patients.

● PATIENT PREPARATION

Patient preparation begins with the usual preoperative history and physical examination. Attention should be paid to prior abdominal procedures and the possible use of alloplastic materials. Current symptoms of bowel obstruction and continence should be sought. Physical examination should document the quality of the anterior and lateral soft tissue, the presence and location of any stomas, and the presence of one or more entero-atmospheric fistula. If the bowel is covered with a thin skin graft, an attempt to manually reduce the bowels back in to the abdomen while the patient is supine will help evaluate whether the patient has a loss of domain or not.

Noninvasive imaging such as CT scan or MRI can help define the extent of abdominal wall loss. A thorough survey of images in the axial plane can identify additional smaller areas of herniation or fistulazation in the obese or difficult to manage patient. Furthermore, additional information regarding the potential for loss of domain can be provided.

General anesthesia is a standard approach; as such, preoperative medical and laboratory workup is performed, including perioperative cardiac risk stratification, particularly in patients with limited functional capacity or who otherwise meet indications by clinical history or comorbidity. Additional comorbid conditions, including tobacco use, obesity, diabetes, COPD, and/or immunosuppression, may require additional attention and preoperative interventions to improve reconstructive efforts.

Obtaining informed consent includes counseling patients regarding risks, benefits, alternatives, and indications. This process is a lengthy and complex discussion, and should include mention of observation of the hernia as an alternative to surgery, wound complications, hernia recurrence rates, use of biologic material implant, and the need for urgent operative re-exploration if clinically significant abdominal hypertension develops.

● TECHNIQUE

Success in abdominal wall reconstruction is predicated on a thorough understanding of indications, anatomy, and treatment options. Several questions must be answered by the plastic surgeon, including timing (immediate or staged reconstruction), technique (primary closure, alloplastic closure, autogenous flap closure, or a combination), implant selection (none, synthetic or biologic), and implant location (overlay, interposition, inlay, or underlay).

Anatomy

The abdominal wall can be divided into distinct layers: skin, subcutaneous fat, superficial fascia, deep investing muscle fascia, muscles, transversalis fascia, preperitoneal fat, peritoneum, and viscera. The muscular layer itself may be subdivided into the medially located rectus abdominis muscles, and the laterally located layered triad consisting of external oblique muscles, internal oblique muscles, and transversus abdominis muscles. The midline fusion of bilateral rectus abdominus is the linea alba. The medial and lateral components of each hemi-abdominal wall are separated by the linea semilunaris (the lateral border of each rectus sheath). The fascia surrounding the rectus muscle is known as the rectus sheath and has variable anatomy: superior to the transverse arcuate line, the rectus abdominis muscles fibers are enclosed both anteriorly and posteriorly in its fascial sheath. The anterior component of this sheath is comprised of the external oblique fascia and the superficial layer of internal oblique fascia, whereas the posterior component is composed of the deep layer of internal oblique fascia and the transversalis fascia. In other words, above the arcuate line, the internal oblique contribution splits around the rectus muscle to form the sheath. Inferior to the arcuate line, the rectus abdominis muscles have fascia only on the anterior surface, which is composed of the fused external oblique, internal oblique, and transversalis fasciae. As opposed to the superior abdominal wall, all fascial contributions to the rectus sheath inferior to the

arcuate line are directed superficial to the rectus muscle belly. Posteriorly, one can observe the preperitoneal space directly.

The abdominal wall derives blood supply from a variety of sources, both deep and superficial. The superior epigastric artery, which is the terminal continuation of the internal mammary artery, enters the rectus sheath at the level of the seventh costal cartilage and arises after the takeoff of the musculophrenic artery. The deep inferior epigastric artery, a branch of the external iliac artery, enters the rectus sheath below the arcuate line and gives off perforating blood supply to the muscle and overlying abdominal skin. The deep circumflex branch of the external iliac artery enters the abdominal wall in the region of the iliac crest. Thoracic and lumbar posterior branches of intercostal arteries travel between the internal oblique and transversus layers, and give off direct skin perforators as well. The superficial system is composed of the superficial epigastric artery, superficial circumflex iliac artery, and superficial external pudendal artery; all three originate from the femoral artery.

Nervous supply to the abdomen is particularly important when striving for functional reconstruction. Thoracic and lumbar branches of the intercostal nerves travel between the internal oblique and transversus layers. Knowledge of this location has direct impact on reconstructive decision making.

Timing

Reconstruction can proceed either immediately or in a delayed fashion. Tumor resection and hernia reduction are common indications for immediate single staged reconstruction. Staged or delayed reconstruction is reserved for acute trauma with visceral injury, edematous bowel and elevated compartment pressures, gross fecal contamination, necrotic bioburden, and/or massive infection.

The initial management of an acute loss of abdominal wall domain may be limited in these settings of critical illness, particularly following penetrating trauma. "Damage control" laparotomy with temporary abdominal closure using a negative pressure dressing followed by applying a split-thickness skin graft directly to the bowel, has improved trauma/critical care outcomes.[5] As a necessary consequence, however, the plastic surgeon is faced with increasingly complex, delayed presentations of massive abdominal domain losses (ie, controlled dehiscence with skin graft directly on bowel). Skin grafts provide soft tissue coverage; yet they are not durable or stable, and worse, do not prevent eventration (Figure 61-1). Resultant adhesions can be dense, therefore secondary procedures to excise skin graft and reconstruct the abdominal wall carry a high risk of complication. It is preferable, if possible, to avoid temporary abdominal closure with skin grafting and close the open abdomen during the initial admission, once critical issues have resolved.

expansion of the abdomen carries the same disadvantages as expansion in other areas of the body, including the need for staged reconstruction, risk of peri-prosthetic infection, device failure, erosion, exposure, or extrusion. This option also requires the inconvenience of multiple office visits for the expansion process.

Reliable muscle flaps described for abdominal wall reconstruction include the latissimus dorsi, rectus femoris, and tensor fascia lata muscles. While enabling transfer of bulky healthy, living tissue into the defect, there is significant incumbent donor site morbidity. Furthermore, these flaps rarely replace very large portions of the abdominal wall. Flaps from the thighs cannot reliably reach areas above the umbilicus and conversely latissimus dorsi flaps can only reconstruct a portion of the upper abdominal wall. Delay procedures are a useful adjunct and can increase the territory of these flaps. Free tissue transfers such as the free tensor fascia lata myocutaneous flap or the free anterolateral thigh fasciocutaneous flap have also been described for abdominal wall reconstruction in the most severe cases with massive soft tissue deficits.[9]

Disa et al. have shown in both animal studies and in clinical series that fascia lata can be harvested as a free graft.[10] The graft becomes rapidly vascularized and can be used in contaminated cases. The donor site morbidity of these grafts, though less than for most muscle flaps, is still significant; and its use, along with the use of muscle flaps has generally been abandoned in favor of commercially available biologic grafts.

The most commonly used biologic grafts are composed of acellular dermis. Alloderm and Strattice are composed of human and porcine acellular dermis, respectively, that have been processed to preserve the natural scaffold of the dermal architecture. Both materials have been studied in a variety of applications both in animal models and clinically for use in abdominal wall reconstruction. These biologic materials have gained widespread application. They can be used in temporary abdominal wall reconstruction in critically ill patients or, more commonly, they can offer definitive reconstruction by bridging a fascial defect (inlay or interposition) as well as reinforcing a primary fascial repair (underlay or onlay). They are known to resist infection presumably through revascularization and therefore can be used in many circumstances where synthetic material is undesirable.[11]

Our preferred technique is a combination of bilateral component separation (rectus abdominus muscle flaps) with biologic reinforcing onlay with Strattice mesh. In this powerful technique, we first begin by taking down any intra-abdominal adhesions from the underside of the abdominal wall to prevent tethering of the fascia to the viscera (Figure 61-2). Next, undermining of the skin is performed. Wide undermining of the skin does allow some fascial advancement, but it is not without a cost: the further the undermining, the higher the risk of skin and fat necrosis. We often try to undermine just 1 or 2 cm beyond the rectus to allow for the external oblique

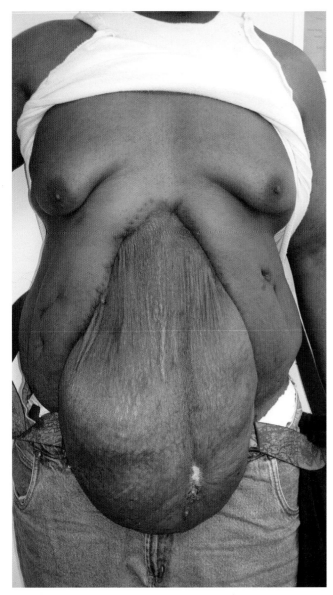

● **FIGURE 61-1.** Appearance of abdominal wall after temporary closure with skin grafting directly to bowel. Eventration and profound loss of domain are present. *(Copyright Devinder Singh, MD.)*

Technique

Reconstructive options for full-thickness abdominal wall defects are numerous and span the reconstructive ladder, including secondary intention and skin grafting, tissue expansion, muscle or fasciocutaneous flaps, fascial grafts, biologic grafts, components separation, free microvascular tissue transfer, and composite tissue allotransplantation.[6,7] Autologous tissue transfer is the treatment of choice for abdominal wall defects when synthetic material is contraindicated.

Tissue expansion has been attempted for most layers of the abdominal wall. It is most often used in the subcutaneous plane when durable soft tissue quantity for coverage is questionable. Placement between the layers of fascia lateral to the rectus muscles has also been reported.[8] Tissue

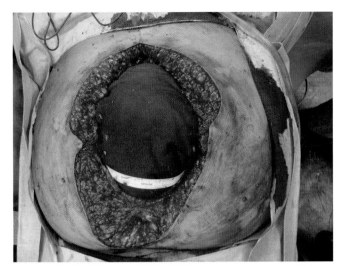

● **FIGURE 61-2.** Massive abdominal loss of domain after lysis of adhesions. (*Copyright Devinder Singh, MD.*)

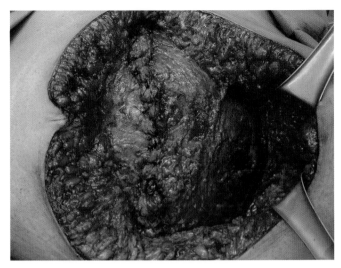

● **FIGURE 61-4.** Close-up of left fasciotomy, demonstrating medial advancement of rectus muscle and lateral retraction of cut external oblique muscle. (*Copyright Devinder Singh, MD.*)

releasing incision and not further unless required for skin closure.

The aponeurosis of the external oblique is then entered and divided lateral to the rectus sheath. The fascia is released superiorly and inferiorly in a vertical direction parallel to the rectus sheath (Figure 61-3). It is important to carry this incision all the way over the costal margin (at this level it is often necessary to divide some of the external oblique muscle fibers in addition to fascia) and several centimeters below the hernia—being careful not to violate the inguinal ligament (Figure 61-4). Dissection in this layer is safe precisely because the neurovascular intercostal bundles lay one anatomic region deeper, in between the internal oblique and transversus layers. This relationship has profound impact on the reconstructive outcome; not only does external oblique fascial release

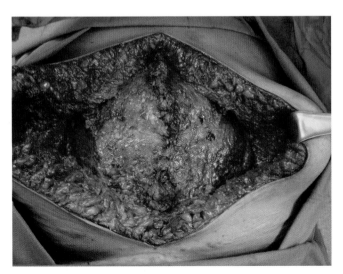

● **FIGURE 61-3.** Primary closure of defect after bilateral separation of components (release of external oblique fascia). (*Copyright Devinder Singh, MD.*)

allow for medialization and primary closure of the rectus abdominus muscles, but it also preserves their innervation and therefore allows for a functional repair.

Useful adjuncts to reduce tension on primary closure with component separation have been described, such as elevation of the posterior sheath from the muscle to allow for some additional advancement. Aggressive dissection and separation along the avascular plane between the external oblique and internal oblique layers can also enable further medial advancement of the rectus muscle flaps. Unilateral medial advancement of up to 5 cm in the epigastrium, 10 cm in the waist, and 3 cm in the suprapubic region is routinely achieved. Component separation is a powerful technique that allows the majority of abdominal defects to close, but close monitoring of intra-abdominal compartment pressures are required. Elevation of the peak airway pressure while utilizing volume control ventilation is a valuable intraoperative guide to determine the presence of excessive intra-abdominal pressure.

It is important to place the relaxing incision within the external oblique fascia rather than in the anterior rectus fascia because there is no posterior rectus fascia below the arcuate line. Postoperatively, the patient will be prone to a bulge in the lower abdomen and recurrence. Similarly, it is important to identify the correct layer of vertical release, to preserve the underlying neurovascular supply to the medialized myofascial flaps. Finally the presence of a stoma is not a contraindication to components separation. Though peristomal scarring in the subcutaneous place can increase the difficulty in exposing the aponeurosis of the external oblique, if the stoma has been correctly delivered through the rectus, it should simply medialize with the muscle flap after external oblique fasciotomy.[12]

Implant Selection

Which implant material to use is a question both controversial and in evolution. Like most, synthetic materials should be avoided in situations where there is active infection, lack of reliable skin coverage, bacterial contamination (such as enterotomy) or substantial comorbidities (such as obesity, diabetes, smoking, immunosuppression, radiation, COPD, and malnutrition), which can place the patient at an increased risk surgical site occurrence. When synthetic material is chosen, it is preferable to use polypropylene mesh due to its excellent incorporation provided that an adequate barrier between the mesh and the bowel can be established. It is important to note that the commercially available synthetic and acellular dermal matrices as well as other types of biologic fascial replacement materials come with varying amounts of data and the field is rapidly evolving. The surgeon should use caution when selecting a product and should base the decision on the best currently available peer-reviewed literature.

Algorithm

Overall, while many reconstructive options exist, one current algorithm for abdominal wall reconstruction involves the use of immediate components separation when this can be accomplished with little to no tension along the suture line. This allows for the reestablishment of an innervated and functional abdominal wall. The suture line is routinely reinforced with a biologic onlay, as well as any areas where the existing fascia has been released (Figure 61-5). When loss of abdominal domain prevents approximation of the rectus muscles despite component separation, the biologic material is placed as a bridging graft instead of

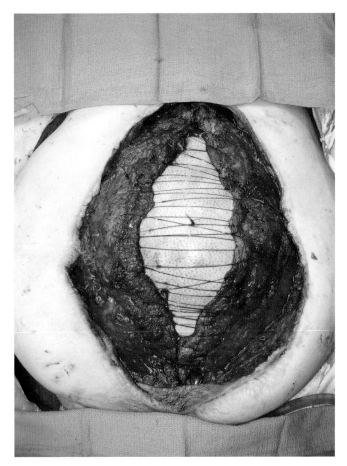

● **FIGURE 61-6.** Demonstration of bridging biologic Strattice mesh in large abdominal defect. Weaving superficial suture further offloads tension and helps to re-approximate myofascial edge to underlying biologic for revascularization. (*Copyright Ronald Silverman, MD.*)

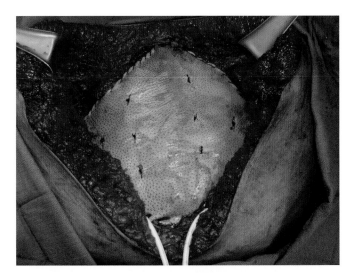

● **FIGURE 61-5.** Demonstration of Strattice biologic mesh reinforcement of abdominal wall closure. Lateral corners are sutured to retracted edges of cut external oblique, reinserting them medially and thereby reconstructing the bilateral donor site. Note quilting sutures and drains to prevent sub-biologic seroma. (*Copyright Devinder Singh, MD.*)

as an onlay reinforcement, taking great care to underlap the existing fascial edges for several centimeters. In these settings, the surgeon should be mindful that the mesh is inset under physiologic tension so that any redundancy or stretch is taken out of the graft to minimize future bulging (Figure 61-6).[11]

● COMPLICATIONS

Postoperative complications include bleeding, scar, pain, deep vein thrombosis/pulmonary embolism, and wound complications. Wound complications are particularly problematic and common, and can include seroma, skin and fat necrosis, and wound infection (Figure 61-7). Hernia recurrence and/or bulging at components separation donor site are distinct possibilities, particularly in cases with multiple previous hernia repairs and significant loss of domain. Visceral injury and abdominal compartment syndrome are particularly devastating complications.

Specifically, to avoid wound complications and exposure of mesh, an attempt is made to minimize the extent of undermining in the skin flaps. Perforator-sparing technique

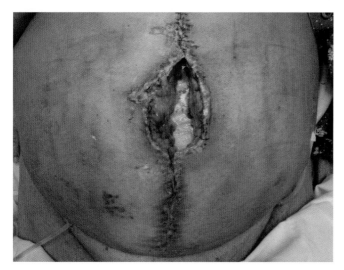

● **FIGURE 61-7.** Typical appearance of surgical site occurrence: wound separation in association with fat and skin necrosis. Visible at base of wound is exposed biologic Strattice mesh. (*Copyright Devinder Singh, MD.*)

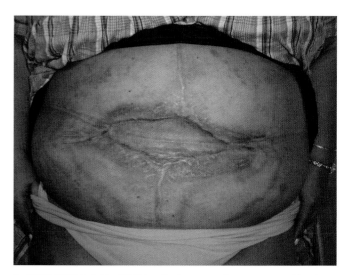

● **FIGURE 61-9.** Well-healed autograft onto wound bed with previously exposed biologic mesh. (*Copyright Devinder Singh, MD.*)

during undermining can improve flap vascularity and healing. Minimal access incision techniques including endoscopic components separation have also been described.[13] Seroma prevention is of particular concern: obliteration of sub-biologic potential space with quilting sutures helps reduce fluid collection and promotes revascularization of the biologic mesh. Sub-biologic fluid collections are most often asymptomatic and found incidentally; management is expectant. Additional maneuvers include the use of submesh closed suction drains, subcutaneous closed suction drains, removal of sub-Scarpa's fat in the undermined area, and quilting or progressive tension sutures from the Scarpa's fascia layer down to the abdominal wall. Subcutaneous fluid collections can often be managed with aspiration and binder compression, or placement of

image-guided drainage catheters. Aggressive debridement of the relatively devascularized skin flaps back to healthy viable tissues helps to further reduce redundancy in skin, minimize dead space and promote better wound healing at the incision (Figures 61-8, 61-9). The use of routine

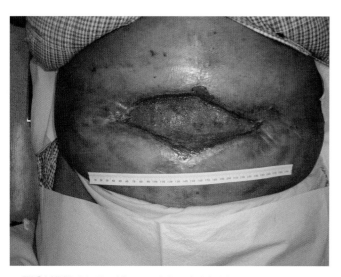

● **FIGURE 61-8.** After excisional debridement and negative pressure wound therapy, evidence of revascularization is evident. (*Copyright Devinder Singh, MD.*)

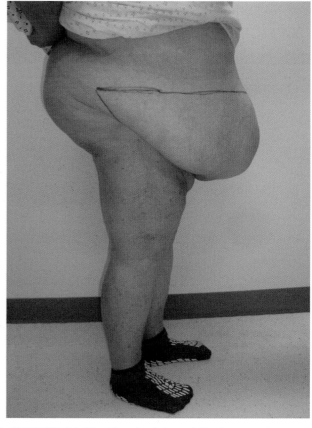

● **FIGURE 61-10.** Massive infraumbilical pannus in association with ventral hernia. (*Copyright Devinder Singh, MD.*)

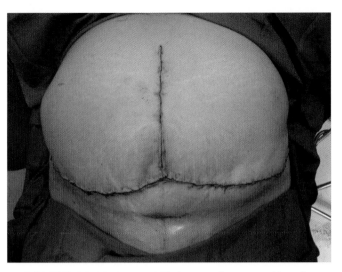

● **FIGURE 61-11.** Inverted-T closure after ventral hernia repair in association with panniculectomy. (*Copyright Devinder Singh, MD.*)

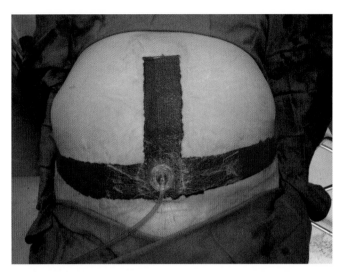

● **FIGURE 61-12.** Incisional wound vacuum-assisted closure applied to closed incision (layer of semipermeable petroleum gauze used to protect skin). (*Copyright Devinder Singh, MD.*)

incisional vacuum-assisted closure (either placed directly on the closed incision with a layer of adaptec to protect skin or segmentally inserted as slender rectangles along the incision) is being investigated as a means to improving wound healing (Figures 61-10, 61-11).[14] Finally, there may be benefit in routine panniculectomy in conjunction with abdominal wall reconstruction; panniculectomy may help to decrease tension on the hernia repair itself (Figure 61-12). Panniculectomy reduces the physiologic burden of ischemic fat and skin. Furthermore, excess pannus may work as a suction ball valve and contribute to seroma production; concurrent pannus removal to reduce seroma formation and subsequent wound complications is also being studied. We utilize a strict abdominal binder protocol post-operatively to minimize further complications after reconstruction. Initially after surgery, use of the binder is avoided to prevent application of any increased pressure and ischemia to abdominal skin flaps. Then, after 1–2 weeks, patients are instructed to wear a loosely applied abdominal binder. Finally, after removal of all indwelling drains, patients are then instructed to wear a very tight abdominal binder to prevent accumulation of seroma fluid.

● OUTCOMES ASSESSMENT

Outcomes from abdominal wall reconstruction vary and depend on technique. Surgeons are usually confronted with complex abdominal defects in patients with many comorbidities including massive obesity or immunosuppression. Even in these high-risk populations, acceptable results have been observed with components separation reinforced with a biologic material as an onlay graft. However, annual follow-up is warranted in order to identify asymptomatic recurrent hernias.

As with standard primary closure alone, hernia recurrence is a distinct possibility and is most likely due to excessive tension on the repair despite component separation. In an effort to reduce the risk for recurrence, placement of a supportive biologic material as an onlay over the repair is recommended. Not only does the onlay position allow for reinforcement of primary closure, but we additionally suture the free edges of the biologic material to the laterally released external oblique fasciotomy, thereby reconstructing the bilateral donor site as well. Any instance where excessive tension is suspected, the fascia should left open (at least partially) and the biologic can instead be used as an inlay fascial replacement to bridge the gap.

REFERENCES

1. Mudge M, Hughes LE. Incisional hernia: a 10 year prospective study of incidence and attitudes. *Br J Surg*. 1985;72:70.

2. Millikan KW. Incisional hernia repair. *Surg Clinic North Am*. 2003;83:1223–1234.

3. Luijendijk RW, Hop WC, van den Tol MP, et al. A comparison of suture repair with mesh repair for incisional hernia. *N Engl J Med*. 2000;343:392–398.

4. Ventral Hernia Working Group, Breuing K, Butler CE, Ferzoco S, et al. Incisional ventral hernias: Review of the literature and recommendations regarding the grading and technique of repair. *Surgery*. 2010;148(3):544–558.

5. Joels CS, Vanderveer AS, Newcomb WL, et al. Abdominal wall reconstruction after temporary abdominal closure: A ten-year review. *Surg Innov*. 2006;13:223–230.

6. Cipriani R, Contedini F, Santoli M, et al. Abdominal wall transplantation with microsurgical technique. *Am J Transplant.* 2007;7:1304–1307.

7. Selvaggi G, Levi DM, Kato T, et al. Expanded use of transplantation techniques: abdominal wall transplantation and intestinal autotransplantation. *Transplant Proc.* 2004;36:1561–1563.

8. Jacobsen WM, Petty PM, Bite D, et al. Massive abdominal-wall hernia reconstruction with expanded external/internal oblique and transversalis musculofascia. *Plast Reconstr Surg.* 1997;100:326–335.

9. Silverman RP, Singh NK, Li EN, et al. Restoring abdominal wall integrity in contaminated tissue-deficient wounds using autologous fascia grafts. *Plast Reconstr Surg.* 2004;113:673–675.

10. Disa JJ, Klein MH, Goldberg NH. Advantages of autologous fascia versus synthetic patch abdominal wall reconstruction in experimental animal defects. *Plast Reconstr Surg.* 1996;97:801.

11. Silverman RP, Li EN, Holton, T, et al. Ventral hernia repair using allogenic acellular dermal matrix in a swine model. *Hernia.* 2004;8:336–342.

12. Maas SM, van Engeland M, Leeksma NG, et al. A modification of the "components separation" technique for closure of abdominal wall defects in the presence of an enterostomy. *J Am Coll Surg.* 1999;189:138–140.

13. Losanoff JE, Richman BW, Jones JW. Endoscopically assisted "component separation" method for abdominal wall reconstruction. *J Am Coll Surg.* 2002;195:288; author reply 288–289.

14. Conde-Green A, Chung TL, Holton L, et al. Incisional negative-pressure wound therapy versus conventional dressings following abdominal wall reconstruction. *Ann Plast Surg.* 2012;68(4) epub ahead of print.

chapter 62

Reconstruction of the Perineum and Genitalia

Aaron T. Pelletier, MD / *Lawrence J. Gottlieb, MD, FACS*

● INTRODUCTION

The perineum is technically defined as the area between the anus and the scrotum in the male, and between the anus and the vulva in the female. Acquired deformities of the perineum and genitalia requiring reconstruction may occur due to trauma, burn injury, necrotizing infection, tumor extirpation, or iatrogenic injury. Congenital deformities such as hypospadias, epispadias, bladder exstrophy, micropenis, vaginal agenesis, or ambiguous genitalia may also warrant similar intervention. Patients with gender dysphoria may seek genital reconstruction to reconcile their body with their psyches.

The goals of reconstructive surgery are to provide stable coverage of wounds, improve appearance and self-image, allow social interaction, and restore sexual function. It is important for surgeons to maintain reconstructive aims in concert with the patient's needs. Often, reconstruction of the genitalia requires a complex approach, best addressed with a multidisciplinary team involving plastic surgeons, urologists, gynecologists, and psychiatrists. The surgeons may then choose from a wide variety of options to best accomplish reconstruction of the specialized tissues of the perineum and genitalia.

Before proceeding with wound closure, bacteriologic control is essential. This requires adequate debridement of all devitalized and infected tissue. Treatment with appropriate topical antimicrobial agents can often assist in decreasing bacterial level to less than 10^5 organisms per gram of tissue. Once this is accomplished, virtually any flap or graft may be employed to provide stable coverage of the perineal wound. For some patients with open wounds, nonoperative treatment, ie, healing by secondary intention, may be appropriate (Figure 62-1).

● PATIENT EVALUATION AND SELECTION

The initial evaluation should begin with a comprehensive history and physical examination to elucidate the nature of the disorder, including the onset and duration of the problem. It is important to determine the patient's reasons for seeking reconstruction, as well as his or her level of expectation. Current and expected urinary and sexual function needs to be defined. For genitalia reconstruction, what does the patient desire in terms of aesthetics and function? Do they wish to have the body part for psychological reasons, with functionality being of secondary importance, or vice versa? The previous medical history, including known comorbidities, smoking history, and cardiovascular health, will determine whether the patient is a medically appropriate candidate for a reconstruction that may require several operations. Previous surgery, especially prior reconstructive attempts, may change the operative approach. The patient's occupation or recreational activities may influence the donor site selection.

In the case of patients with congenital abnormalities, the workup should include chromosomal analysis, endocrine screening, androgen receptor levels, and 5-alpha reductase levels. If it has not previously been done, the genitourinary system should be evaluated with pelvic ultrasound, urography, and CT or MRI as indicated. Patients with congenital adrenal hyperplasia should have a preoperative electrolyte panel drawn, as this condition is associated with hyponatremia and hyperkalemia.

Psychological screening is also very important. Loss or absence of genitalia may be associated with depression, social withdrawal, or other mental illnesses. In the case of transsexuals seeking gender reassignment surgery, formal

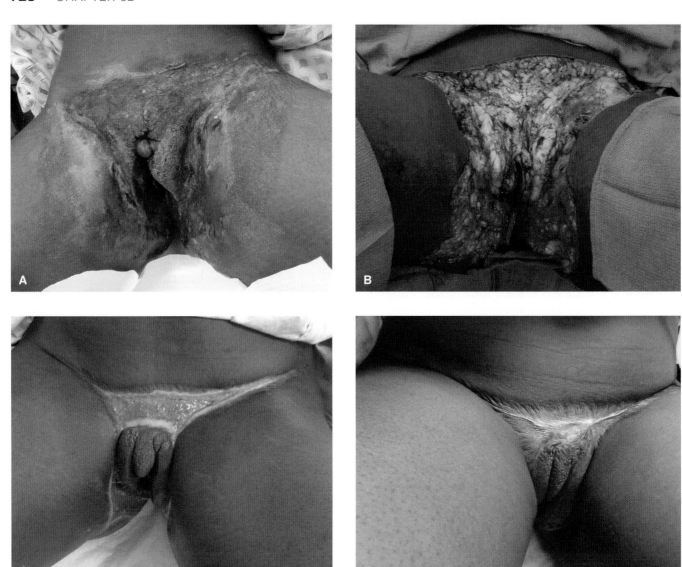

● **FIGURE 62-1.** (A) Extensive hydradenitis of the perineal region of a 26-year-old woman was treated with complete excisional debridement (B) followed by twice daily dressing changes using topical silver sulfadiazine, with weekly physical therapy and hydrotherapy sessions to prevent scar contracture. The wound is over 75% healed at three months (C) and completely healed by 6 months (D).

psychiatric evaluation and treatment is a requirement. Finally, it is important to assess the patient's social support system, including partners as well as family, in order to optimize outcome.

Indications

Patients who have absence, severe deficiency, deformity, or dysfunction of their perineum and genitalia secondary to a congenital malformation, trauma, burns, infection, malignancy, radiation, or iatrogenic injury are potential candidates for reconstruction (Table 62-1). Gender identity disorder patients may become the candidates for genital construction if they meet predetermined psychological and personality guidelines established by the

World Professional Association for Transgender Health, formerly known as the Harry Benjamin International Gender Dysphoria Association.

Contraindications

Elective complex genital reconstruction is inappropriate in patients with major cardiac, vascular, or metabolic diseases. The same is true for those with major psychiatric or psychological problems that would not improve with this procedure. In this instance, close communication with the patient's psychiatrist and/or therapist is invaluable. Consideration must also be given to the patient's level of expectation and ability to deal with potential complications and potentially unsightly donor site scars.

TABLE 62-1. Indications

Congenital deformities
    Ambiguous genitalia
    Micropenis
    Hypospadias
    Epispadias
    Cloacal deformity
    Vaginal agenesis/atresia
Acquired deformities
    Trauma
    Burn
    Infection
    Malignancy
    Radiation
    Iatrogenic
Gender disorders (gender reassignment)

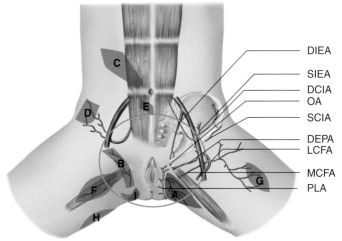

● **FIGURE 62-2.** The pivot points of most loco-regional flaps used for perineal reconstruction are located along the circumference of a 20-cm diameter circle centered over the perineum. (A) V-Y advancement flap, from medial thigh or inferior gluteal area. (B) Pudendal thigh flap. (C) Oblique rectus abdominis myocutaneous (ORAM) or deep inferior epigastric artery perforator (DIEP) flap. (D) Superficial inferior epigastric artery (SIEA) flap or extended superficial circumflex iliac artery (SCIA) flap. (E) Rectus abdominis musculoperitoneal (RAMP) flap. (F) Gracilis myocutaneous flap, shown with vertical skin paddle. (G) Anterolateral thigh (ALT) flap. (H) Gluteal thigh flap. (I) Gluteal fold flap. DCIA, deep circumflex iliac artery; OA anterior branch of obturator artery; DEPA, deep external pudendal artery; LCFA, lateral circumflex femoral artery; MCFA, medial circumflex femoral artery; PLA, posterior labial artery (branch of pudendal artery).

● PATIENT PREPARATION

After thorough evaluation of the patient and development of reconstructive options, a detailed preoperative discussion must specifically reiterate the nature of the problem, the surgeon's understanding of patient desires and expectations, and available options, including risks, benefits, and any other long-term considerations associated with each option. Once the operative plan is chosen and agreed upon by all members of the treating team, informed consent is obtained.

Most perineal and genital defects are amenable to reconstruction using local or regional tissue. The vascular leash of all of the various musculocutaneous, fasciocutaneous, and perforator flaps is along the circumference of a 20 cm diameter circle centered over the perineum (Figure 62-2). Using these options, an appropriate pedicled flap can be selected depending on the size of the defect, the presence of radiation damage, availability of donor tissue, and patient/surgeon preference. Specialized structures such as the urethra, vagina, or penis have additional reconstructive goals which may not be adequately replaced with local or regional tissue and require transfer of distant tissues for optimal results.

Except for minor repairs and revisions, general anesthesia is usually necessary. Patient positioning is completely dependent on the operative plan and may vary from prone, supine, lateral decubitus, frog-leg, lithotomy, jack-knife, or sequential combinations of each. Adequate planning with the entire surgical team is critical to ensure proper positioning of extremities with padding of pressure points to avoid iatrogenic complications. Finally, it is necessary to anticipate and communicate to the patient any special positioning, splinting, or activity limitations that may be required postoperatively to prevent breakdown of suture lines or compromise of any grafts or flaps used in the reconstruction.

● TECHNIQUES: RECONSTRUCTION OF THE PERINEUM AND FEMALE GENITALIA

Except for the use of bowel for vaginal reconstruction, the reconstructive options, armamentarium of flaps, perioperative considerations, and complications are similar for the perineum, vulva, and vagina, and will be discussed together. Perineal defects usually involve adjacent structures and may result following extirpative pelvic surgery, proctectomy, operative treatment of inflammatory bowel disease, radiation treatment, burns, or development of chronic wounds. Perineal wounds are also frequently associated with cavities that require obliteration. Vaginal reconstruction may be required in cases of congenital vaginal agenesis or atresia, for example in Mayer-Rokitansky-Kuster-Hauser syndrome or congenital adrenal hyperplasia. It may also be required after extirpative pelvic surgery for cancer, after trauma or in treatment of male to female transsexuals.

Numerous flaps from the buttock, thigh, or abdomen have been described for perineal and vulvar reconstruction. The choice of technique depends on which tissue is absent, the size or volume of the defect, available donor sites and surgeon's experience, and comfort. The most common flaps used are thin fasciocutaneous flaps based on the pudendal vascular system, abdominal or thigh perforator flaps, or the rectus abdominis or gracilis musculocutaneous flaps. Large defects may require a combination of flaps. Wound closure is usually straightforward. Reconstruction of a functional or aesthetically demanding structure frequently requires multiple operations in a staged fashion.

V-Y Advancement Flap

Advancement of flaps of the medial thigh or inferior gluteal area in a V-Y fashion provides high-quality, well-vascularized, innervated skin for vulvar and perineal defects with very acceptable donor site scars (Figure 62-2A). When designed more posteriorly, the vascular supply of this flap comes from the terminal branches of the superficial perineal artery and may include perforators of the descending branch of the inferior gluteal artery. When the flap is designed more anteriorly, its vascularization is

most likely from perforators of the pudendal, obturator, or medial circumflex femoral systems (Figure 62-3). The versatility and reliability of these flaps have made them the new workhorse for vulvar and perineal reconstruction.[1,2]

Pudendal Thigh (Singapore) Flap

In 1989, Wee and Joseph described the neurovascular pudendal-thigh flap (Figure 62-2B), based on the posterior labial artery, which has rich vascular connections to the deep external pudendal artery, the medial femoral circumflex artery, and the anterior branch of the obturator artery.[3] This flap is elevated in a subfascial plane over the adductor muscles of the thigh, and transposed or tunneled to the vulvar defect or into the vaginal cavity. Monstrey et al. demonstrated that this flap can be safely elevated as an island flap.[4] The donor site in the inguinal crease may be closed primarily and is aesthetically acceptable (Figure 62-4). Although the use

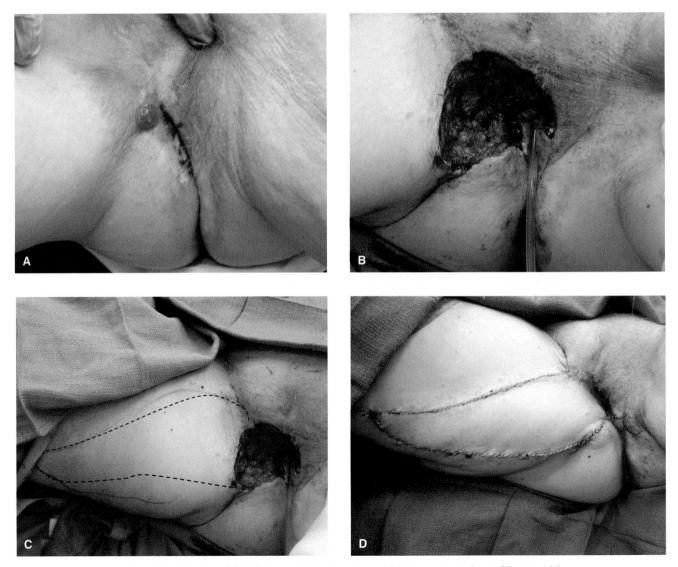

● **FIGURE 62-3.** (A) Painful recurrent squamous cell vulvar cancer in an 85-year-old woman and resultant defect (B) after extirpation. The intraoperative design of a medial thigh V-Y flap (C) and closure following advancement and inset (D).

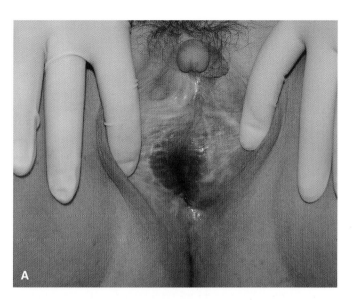

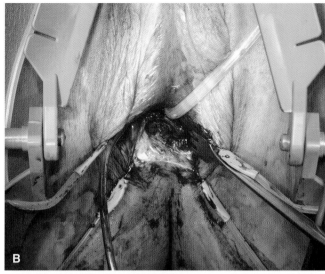

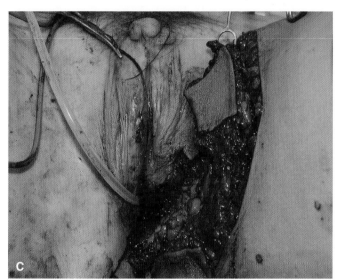

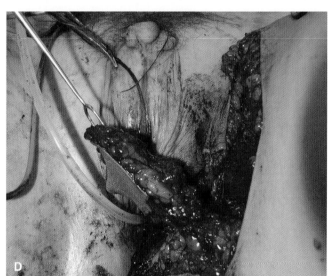

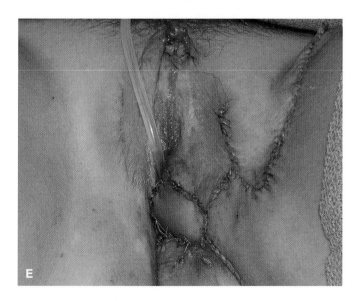

● FIGURE 62-4. (A) Introital stenosis and clitoromegaly in a 10-year-old girl with congenital adrenal hyperplasia requiring incisional release (B). The islandized pudendal flap from the left side is raised (C), transposed (D), and inset to complete the release (E).

of flaps for vaginal reconstruction generally allows the cavity to be maintained without the need for long-term dilators and stents, the pudendal-thigh flaps have been reported to contract somewhat more than other flap reconstructions.

Rectus Abdominis Flap

The inferiorly based rectus abdominis musculocutaneous flap (Figure 62-2C) is excellent for filling large defects with accompanying dead space created by extirpative surgery for cancer.[5] It can also be used for vulvar and vaginal reconstruction. The skin island of a rectus abdominis musculocutaneous flap is most versatile when oriented obliquely on an angle from the umbilicus to the scapula (Figure 62-5A). Not only does it provide a long skin paddle, but this design facilitates abdominal wall donor site closure (Figure 62-5B). The muscle flap alone is a versatile option that can be used to fill the pelvic dead space, close the pelvic floor, or repair intestinal or genitourinary fistulae. The deep inferior epigastric artery perforator or superficial inferior epigastric artery flaps may be used in thin patients requiring less bulk (Figure 62-2D). When performed for complete vaginal reconstruction, it is important to suspend the blind end of the neovagina to the sacral promontory.

Vascularized peritoneum may also be transferred with this flap[6] (Figure 62-2E). The rectus abdominis musculoperitoneal flap has low bulk, and can be useful when dealing with a nonexenterated pelvis in which there is not enough room for bulkier musculocutaneous flaps. Similar in concept to the Davydov procedure, the peritoneum remucosalizes with vaginal mucosa in 2 to 3 months. The rectus abdominis musculoperitoneal flap is best used for partial longitudinal vaginal defects. Unfortunately, when used for circumferential defects of more than two thirds of the upper vagina, there is an increased risk of severe stenosis.

Gracilis Flap

The gracilis muscle and myocutaneous flaps (Figure 62-2F) were popularized for vaginal, vulvar, and perineal reconstruction by McCraw in the mid 1970s.[7] They are useful when the extirpative defect is large, requiring obliteration of dead space. However, the distal skin territory of the longitudinally oriented flap is unreliable. Similarly, the distal third of the gracilis muscle, which is usually the part that is placed in wound cavities, frequently lacks adequate bulk and has marginal blood flow. Wang et al. described a fasciocutaneous thigh flap of almost the same skin island as the gracilis, but with a blood supply which comes from more proximal (medial) perforators of the external pudendal artery.[8]

Anterolateral Thigh Flap

The anterolateral thigh flap (Figure 62-2G) based on the descending branch of the lateral circumflex femoral

artery is a versatile flap that may be customized to accommodate a variety of defects. It may be transferred as a fasciocutaneous perforator flap (Figure 62-6), a vastus lateralis muscle flap, a vastus lateralis musculocutaneous compound flap, or a chimeric flap, including the vastus lateralis and/or rectus femoris muscles. To facilitate the transfer of the lateral circumflex femoral artery flap to the perineum, the flap should be passed beneath the rectus femoris and sartorius muscles, thus creating a direct line from its pivot point as it comes off the profunda femoris vessels to the perineum (Figure 62-7). The main disadvantage of this flap is the visibility of the donor site on the anterior lateral thigh.

Gluteal Thigh Flap

Flaps based on the inferior gluteal artery system allows for a variety of tissue to be transferred to the perineum. The inferior gluteal muscle may be transferred independently or combined with skin as a compound or chimera flap (Figure 62-8). The fasciocutaneous gluteal thigh flap (Figure 62-2H) is based on the descending branch of the inferior gluteal artery. It is associated with the posterior cutaneous nerve of the thigh and has been shown to provide reliable and sensate skin.[9] The point of rotation of this flap is located 5 cm above the ischial tuberosity where the inferior gluteal artery emerges from beneath the piriformis muscle. The central axis of the skin island is midway between the greater trochanter and the ischial tuberosity perpendicular to the gluteal crease. The flap length may extend to within 8 cm of the popliteal fossa. For wounds that have a cavity, a chimera flap consisting of the fasciocutaneous posterior thigh flap as well as a portion of the inferior gluteal maximus muscle can be raised on a single vascular pedicle (Figure 62-9). In this variation, the descending branch of the inferior gluteal artery is separated from beneath the gluteal muscle. A portion of the gluteus maximus muscle is elevated on a separate branch, allowing independent positioning of the muscle and skin.[10] The gluteal thigh flap provides skin coverage and adequate soft tissue bulk and, generally, even when combined with a portion of gluteal muscle, results in no functional deficit at the donor site. Although sensation in this flap is generally considered an advantage, adult patients can have difficulty with cortical reorganization, sensing stimuli of the transferred skin paddle as originating from the posterior thigh.

Gluteal Fold Flap

The gluteal fold fasciocutaneous flap (Figure 62-2I) is a sensate flap with a neurovascular supply similar to that of the pudendal thigh flap. It is designed with the center of the flap situated along the infragluteal crease.[11] This flap may be "islandized" with its proximal portion just medial to the ischial tuberosity, extending laterally for approximately 15 cm in length. The flap may then be transposed anteriorly to reconstruct vulvar defects or posteriorly to

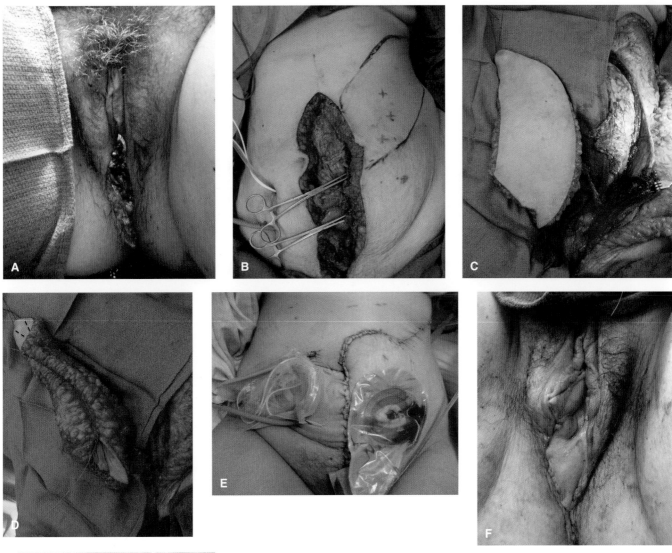

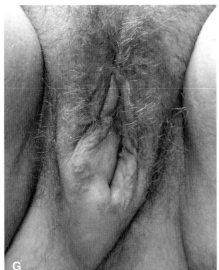

● **FIGURE 62-5.** (A) Resultant perineal and total vaginal defect following pelvic exeneration in a 36-year-old woman with recurrent squamous cell carcinoma of the cervix. (B) Intraoperative skin paddle design of a left oblique rectus abdominis myocutaneous (ORAM) flap. (C) Flap raised on deep inferior epigastric pedicle, leaving inferior portion of rectus abdominis muscle intact for placement of end colostomy. (D) ORAM flap tubed for vaginal reconstruction with markings for non-circumferential introital inset before transfer into pelvis. (E) Primary closure of donor site and laparotomy with placement of ileal conduit and end colostomy. (F) Inset of neo-introitus and perineum and (G) follow-up at three months demonstrates no introital stenosis.

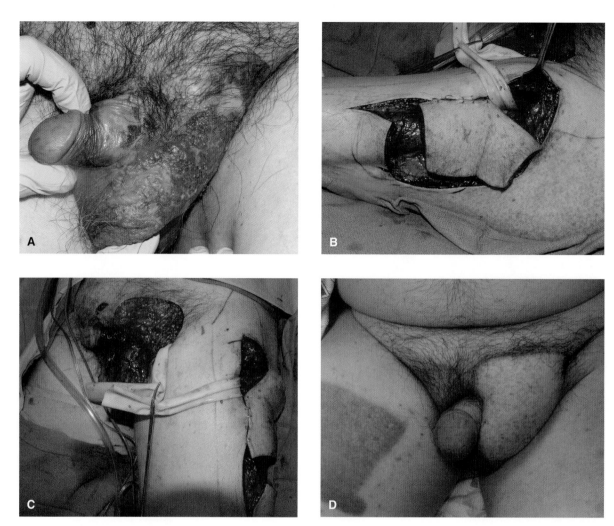

● **FIGURE 62-6.** (A) Squamous cell carcinoma in situ of the penis and scrotum of a 66-year-old man. The left-sided anterior lateral thigh flap (B) based on first septocutaneous perforator of the lateral circumflex femoral system is dissected and a Penrose drain is passed under rectus femoris and sartorius muscles (C) after creation of a tunnel. (D) Flap well healed at postoperative month 6 (penile shaft closed with skin graft).

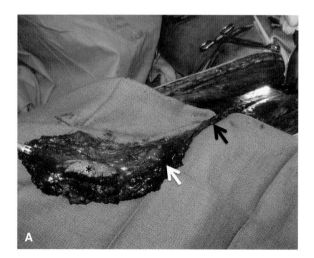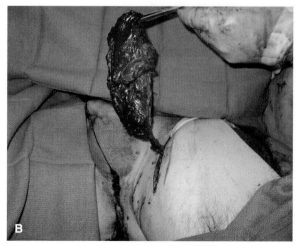

● **FIGURE 62-7.** (A) Vastus lateralis muscle flap (*white arrow*) based on descending branch of the lateral circumflex femoral system (*black arrow*). Small island of skin used as a monitor (*asterisk*). The flap is passed medially under rectus femoris and sartorius muscles (B). Note the improved arc of rotation with its pivot point moved medially.

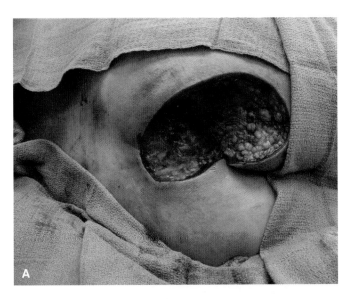

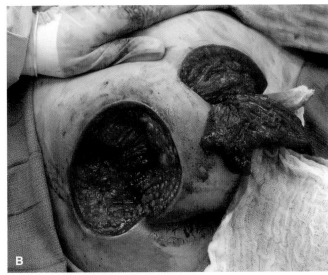

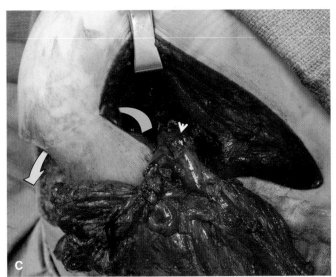

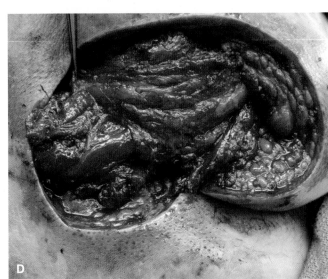

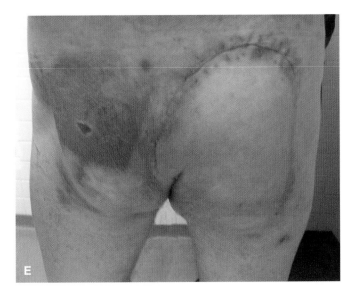

● FIGURE 62-8. A 61-year-old man sustained a large gluteal abscess after 12% burn with inhalation injury. After deep debridement of the abscess (A), an inferior segment of gluteus maximus muscle was harvested through a counter incision (B). The inferior gluteal artery pedicle (*white arrow head*) is shown (C) and the curved white arrow demonstrates path of transfer of this muscle flap. The muscle was secured to fill the defect (D) and the wound was closed with a large fasciocutaneous rotational/advancement flap based on the perforators of the superior gluteal artery. (E) Six months postoperatively he is well-healed with good contour (skin graft of contralateral buttock related to burn injury).

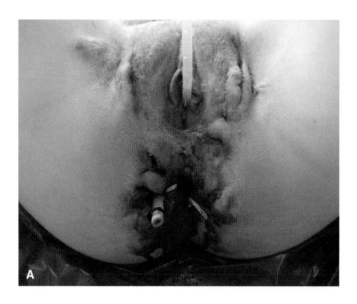

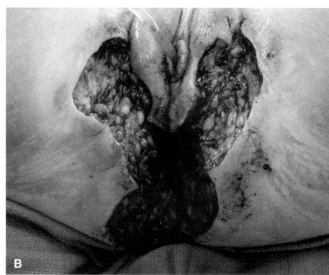

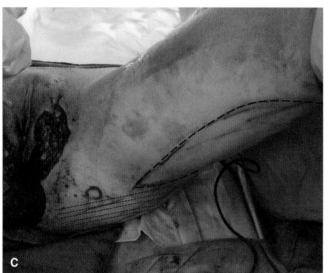

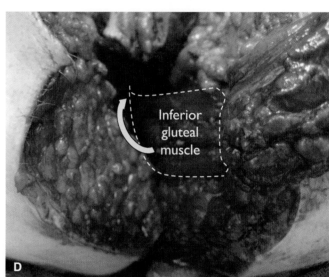

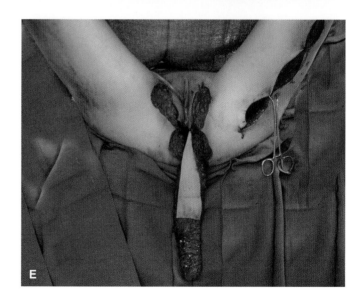

● **FIGURE 62-9.** (A) Severe perianal and perineal Crohn's disease in a 26-year-old woman with multiple fistulae, sinuses, and abscesses. (B) After proctectomy and excision of all involved soft tissue, (C) a chimeric flap was designed using an inferior portion of gluteus maximus muscle and a fasciocutaneous posterior thigh flap, both based on separate branches of the left inferior gluteal artery. (D) Muscle flap transposed into pelvic defect. (E) Posterior thigh flap passed under skin bridge and distal portion de-epithelialized to provide additional bulk for obliteration of defect.

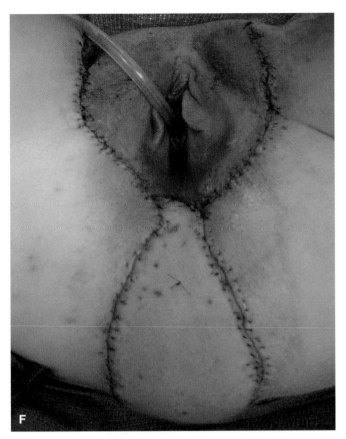
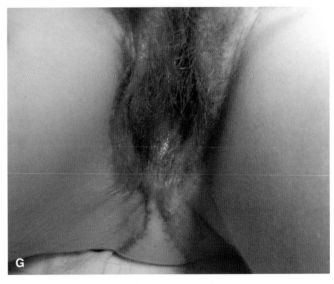

● **FIGURE 62-9.** *(continued)* (F). Inset of posterior thigh flap with primary closure of groin wounds, and (G) well-healed perineal reconstruction 4 months postoperatively.

reconstruct perianal defects (Figure 62-10). The design may be either unilateral or bilateral and may be advanced in a V-Y fashion.[12]

● TECHNIQUES: VAGINAL RECONSTRUCTION

The various methods for vaginal reconstruction may be classified into three categories: stretching techniques, grafting techniques, and flap reconstruction. The choice of technique depends on the amount of vagina absent, size or volume of the accompanying defect, available donor sites, and the patient's acceptance of donor scar. In most developmental abnormalities as well as transgender surgery, the lack of defect precludes most of the bulkier flaps and alternate techniques are preferred. On the contrary, after surgical extirpation, thicker flaps may be preferred so that endopelvic dead space can be filled. Partial defects of the vagina are also common following surgery. Rarely are grafts able to be used in this scenario.

Dilatation or Stretching Techniques (for Vaginal Agenesis)

In patients with vaginal agenesis, the external genitalia are essentially normal. Instead of a vaginal cavity, there

is typically a small pouch or dimple that is 1 to 4 cm in depth. The Frank technique, initially described in 1938, is the only nonsurgical approach to vaginal construction. With the use of graduated dilators pressing on and progressively stretching a severely foreshortened vagina, this technique can increase both depth and caliber. In 1981, Ingram reported his experience using a modified bicycle seat with an integrated dilator that young women would sit on, providing direct pressure on the incompletely developed vagina. This technique works best in compliant, motivated patients who have more depth than just a vaginal dimple.[13,14]

Another dilation technique that has become very popular in Europe is the Vecchietti operation, first described in 1965. It involves the creation of a neovagina via dilatation with a traction device attached to the abdomen. With a combined surgical and dilation approach, a plastic bead with traction sutures attached is placed in the interlabial space. Via a formal laparotomy, a space is made between the urethra/bladder and rectum and the traction sutures are passed extraperitoneally in the abdomen and anchored to a spring traction device placed on the outside of the abdomen. More recently, this has been performed laparoscopically. By applying constant continuous traction, the Vecchietti method creates a functional vagina of 10 to 12 cm length in 7 to 9 days. The vaginal cavity

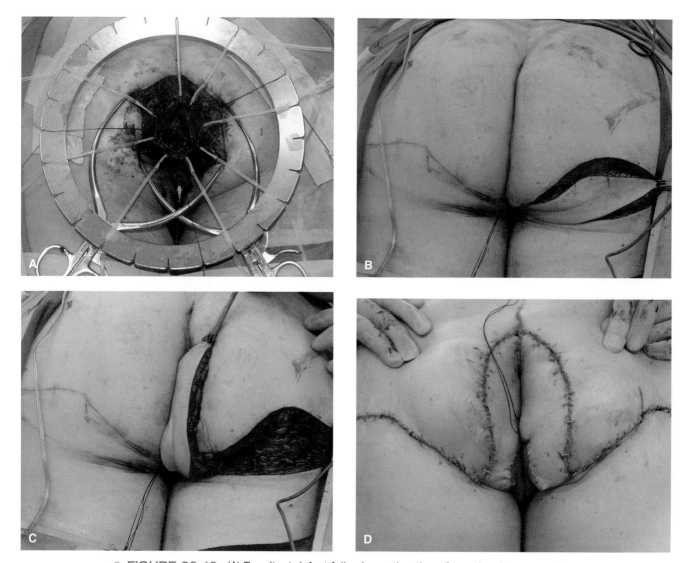

● **FIGURE 62-10.** (A) Resultant defect following extirpation of a perianal squamous cell cancer in-situ in a 55-year-old woman. Bilateral gluteal fold flaps were designed (B) and the right flap is shown transposed into defect (C). Final inset of flaps (D) demonstrates preservation of buttock contour with tensionless closure of donor sites in infragluteal folds.

created must be maintained with vaginal molds for a number of months.[15,16]

Grafting Techniques (for Vaginal Agenesis)

For congenital abnormalities, a simple and often used surgical procedure is utilization of skin grafts to line a cavity dissected in the retrovesical space. Although originally described by Abbe in 1898, McIndoe and colleagues popularized its use four decades later, and the use of skin grafts placed around a stent to create the neovagina is often referred to as the McIndoe procedure. While originally described with the use of split-thickness skin grafts, full-thickness grafts are preferred to decrease contraction of the vaginal cavity. Creating lining with grafts requires long-term (up to 1 year) use of a vaginal mold to prevent contraction and strictures.

Despite this, shrinkage and stenosis are common problems if the patient does not continue intermittent stenting or sexual activity.[17–19]

Locoregional Flaps

Surgical reconstruction of the vagina using local flaps has been reported since the 1800s. These flaps work well when the defect is limited. A number of random and axial pattern skin flaps can be used, taking advantage of the extensive, interconnecting pudendal blood supply. Additionally, flaps incorporating the suprapubic and infraumbilical skin have been described. The thinness and pliability of these flaps as well as inconspicuous donor scars make them attractive options. Williams repopularized vulva flaps in the 1960s and Davydov created vaginas from the peritoneum of Douglas's pouch.[20,21]

Recently, the Davydov technique has been modified with a laparoscopic approach. Flaps of the bladder have also been described. In all cases, the tissue utilized must be mobile, nonirradiated, and nonscarred. Similar to grafting, use of periodic postoperative dilation is necessary to minimize contraction and stenosis.

An alternative option that is excellent for total vaginal reconstruction is to use the previously described ORAM flap. As shown in (Figure 62-5), the skin paddle of the ORAM flap can be tubed to create a neo-vagina. Once passed into the pelvis, care must be taken to perform a non-circumferential inset of the introital region, so as to prevent future stenosis. In addition, the most cephalad portion of the neo-vagina should be secured to the sacral promontory to prevent collapse and/or prolapse.

Intestinal Flap

Reconstruction of the vagina with segments of bowel (initially described by Baldwin in 1904) allows for creation of a cavity that does not require persistent dilation for patency, as well as a mucosa-lined neovagina that creates natural lubrication. The colon or small bowel (usually ileum) may be transferred on a vascular pedicle for vaginal reconstruction.[22,23] This may be performed through an open or laparoscopic approach. A 10- to 15-cm segment of bowel is isolated on its vascular pedicle. It is divided, and a bowel anastomosis is performed to reestablish continuity of the bowel. The proximal end of the pedicled segment of bowel is closed off, and it is then passed into a space that has been dissected between the urethra and rectum. The proximal end is fixed to the sacral promontory to prevent prolapse (Figure 62-11). The distal end is sutured to the vaginal remnant or to perineal skin flaps, with interdigitating flaps to break up a circular suture line and prevent stenosis. Vaginal reconstruction with an intestinal flap provides good patency and satisfactory sexual activity. Patients with this type of reconstruction may complain of excess mucous production. When colon is used there is also the potential to develop diversion colitis. Other diseases of the colon, such as ulcerative colitis or colon cancer have also been reported to occur in colovaginoplasties.[24,25]

Free Jejunal Flap

Due to length limitations of the mesenteric vascular arcade, it is usually necessary to transfer the jejunal segment as a free flap in order to reach the vaginal introitus. A short, second segment of bowel can be externalized for monitoring through an incision required for vascular access. This flap has been shown to have less excess mucous production than other bowel transfers.[26] It is a useful technique for neovaginal reconstruction in late adolescence or early adulthood, providing a single-stage operation with good patient satisfaction. The dimensions of the vaginal cavity are well-maintained, long-term stents and dilators are not required, and natural lubrication is provided for intercourse without mucous hypersecretion or excessive odor.

Postoperative Care

Most patients undergoing vaginal, vulvar, or perineal reconstruction are at high risk for deep venous thrombosis. As such, sequential compression devices and prophylactic anticoagulation should be used perioperatively and continued as appropriate. Patients are placed on pressure relieving mattresses with legs adducted and knees bent. Free flaps are monitored in specialized nursing units for 48 to 72 hours, after which activity is gradually increased. The monitoring segment is removed on postoperative days 7 to 10.

Physical therapy is important for instructing the patient on how to get out of bed without putting pressure on the operative site. Sitting is limited to 5-minute periods on special padding. A Foley catheter is maintained until the patient is ambulating comfortably. Diet is advanced after the return of bowel function. The patient is discharged when tolerating a general diet, ambulating, and pain is controlled on oral medication.

● TECHNIQUE: RECONSTRUCTION OF THE MALE GENITALIA

Hypospadias

Hypospadias is a common congenital anomaly occurring in approximately 1 in 300 newborn males. It is characterized by three anomalies of the penis, including an abnormal ventral opening of the urethral meatus; chordee or an abnormal ventral curvature; and an abnormal foreskin with dorsal hooding and a ventral deficiency. Hypospadias is variable in severity, and the meatal opening may be located anywhere from the ventral glans to the perineum.[27] If the most severe form of hypospadias is associated with an undescended testes, the infant must be evaluated for an intersex state with ambiguous genitalia. The goals of treating hypospadias, and indeed any congenital anomaly of the penis, are to create a straight penis with a continuous urethra with a meatus ending at the tip of the penis, to reshape the glans into a more natural conical configuration, and to achieve penile skin coverage. The resulting penis should enable the patient to void while standing, have an acceptable cosmetic appearance, and be suitable for future sexual intercourse.

The position of the meatus along with the degree of chordee, development of the spongiosum, thinness of urethra, elasticity and thickness of ventral shaft skin, and depth of glanular groove determine the selection of approach to repair. More than 300 different techniques for repair of hypospadias are described, and all are based on standard principles of reconstructive plastic and urologic surgery, which allow for creation of a tubular urethra, correction of chordee curvature, and coverage of the urethral tube with well-vascularized skin flaps that avoid superposition of suture lines. In the twenty-first century, almost all hypospadias repairs are performed by pediatric urologists. Reconstructive plastic surgeons are usually not involved unless there is a severe deformity or the patient

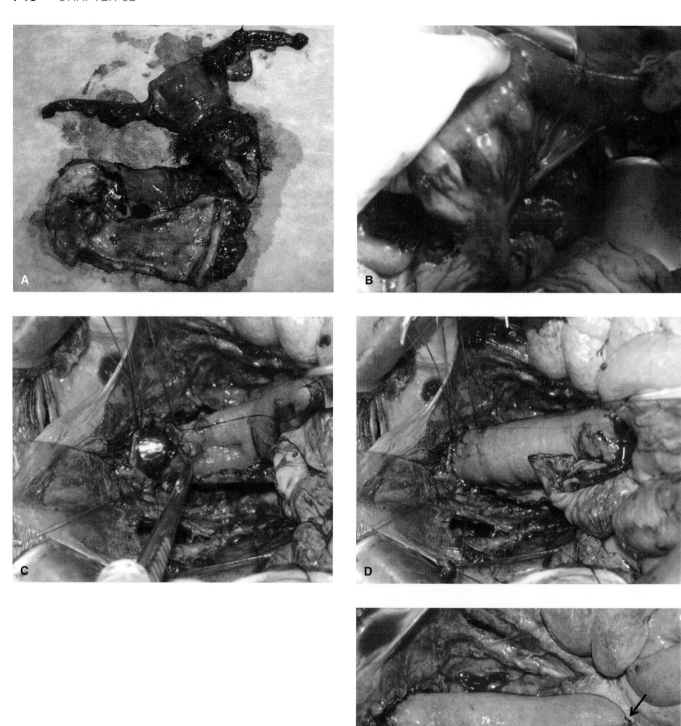

● **FIGURE 62-11.** (A) Surgical specimen from a 66-year-old woman who underwent subtotal vaginectomy, hysterectomy, and bilateral oophorectomy for recurrent colon cancer invading into vagina. (B) Segment of jejunum isolated on its vascular pedicle. (C) The pedicled jejunal flap is secured to the vaginal remnant over a dilator, and the vaginal-jejunal anastomosis (D) is completed. (E) Closed end of jejunum secured to sacral promontory (*black arrow*) to prevent prolapse.

has had repeated complications or failures. Complications include urethrocutaneous fistulae, stricture, meatal dystopia, meatal stenosis, urethral diverticula, hair in the urethra, and persistent curvature. Multiple failed surgeries can lead to a condition with a scarred and dysfunctional penis dubbed the "hypospadias cripple" requiring more complex reconstructive intervention.[28]

Urethral Reconstruction

The male urethra is 17.5 to 20 cm long and extends from the internal urethral orifice in the urinary bladder to the meatus at the end of the penis. It is divided into three portions: the prostatic, membranous, and penile or cavernous urethra. The epithelium of the urethra starts off as transitional cells as it exits the bladder. At the membranous portion it turns into pseudostratified columnar epithelium, then stratified squamous epithelium near the external meatus.

Urethral problems include loss of part or all of the urethra, urethral stenosis and strictures, and urethral sinuses and fistulae. Like hypospadias repair, urologists care for most straightforward urethral problems but a plastic surgeon may be necessary for complicated cases. Injuries involving the urethral meatus may cause stenosis. Mild stenosis can be treated with repeated dilatations. Stenosis unresponsive to dilation may require z-plastys or other interpolations of adjacent skin into the constricting band. Occasionally, persistent strictures require an open approach with urethrotomy and graft placement to widen the lumen. Urethral fistulae may involve the skin, bowel, or vagina. Most urethral fistulae are due to trauma or surgery, especially after radiation. Frequently, these will close with urinary diversion. Persistent fistulae may require operative closure and reinforcement with a nonscarred, nonirradiated local/regional or distant flap. Distal cavernous urethral loss may be repaired using the principles of hypospadias surgery.

Techniques of more proximal cavernous urethral reconstruction continue to evolve. Many methods of restoring urethral continuity and establishing a normal urethral lumen have been devised. Autologous skin or mucosal grafts and local/regional flaps have produced dependable long-term results. The decision regarding which one of the various methods available for urethral reconstruction must be individualized. Factors used in choosing the appropriate option include the location and dimension of the injured or diseased urethra, quality of the urethral bed, availability of local or regional tissue, and quality and availability of distant tissue.

Grafts may be harvested from the oral mucosa, bladder mucosa, or skin. For success, they require a perfect wound bed to achieve a dependable result. Even a small loss of a graft will result in stricture.

Loco-regional flaps of skin or bladder mucosa have the advantage of bringing their own blood supply, thereby not relying on the quality of bed on which they are placed. Scrotal flaps for urethral reconstruction should be avoided because the coarse pubic hair is not tolerated well and leads to urinary stones. Occasionally, a pedicled appendix is used for proximal urethral reconstruction. Injury and scarring from prior surgery or trauma may preclude using local or regional flaps. In addition, reconstructing the proximal male urethra may push the limits of some of these techniques.

When grafts and regional flaps are inappropriate, inadequate or unavailable, free tissue transfers may be the best option. Appendix, tailored intestinal segment, or a long, thin skin flap that is tubed (eg, radial forearm or anterior lateral thigh) may be considered for the treatment of extensive urethral abnormalities when the alternative is chronic supravesical diversion.[29,30]

General Postoperative Care

Again, this is a high-risk population for deep venous thrombosis. As such, sequential compression devices and prophylactic anticoagulation should be used perioperatively and continued as appropriate. If a graft is used for urethral repair, a large bore catheter is left in place for 2 to 3 weeks as a stent. If circumferential replacement with a graft is necessary, then stenting may be required 9 to 12 months. In patients undergoing repair with a flap, a small caliber catheter is used to minimize pressure on the flap. Extensive repairs or reconstruction should have the urine diverted with a suprapubic tube.

Patients undergoing free flap urethral reconstruction are monitored in a specialized unit for a minimum 48 hours. After 2 days of bed rest, gradual mobilization with the assistance of physical therapy begins. The urinary flow remains diverted through the suprapubic tube. When the patient is comfortable with the care of the flap and donor site, he is discharged with the suprapubic tube in place. Three to 4 weeks postoperatively, if healing appears adequate, a retrograde urethrogram is performed. If no fistula is seen, the bladder catheter in the neourethra is removed and the suprapubic tube is clamped, allowing the patient to void. If the patient voids successfully, the suprapubic tube is removed 1 week later.

Penile Reconstruction

The history of total penile reconstruction has paralleled the history of flap development in plastic and reconstructive surgery. The multistage tube pedicle flap reconstruction has given way to the axial pattern skin flaps and muscle flaps. These procedures have subsequently yielded the state-of-the-art neurosensory fasciocutaneous radial forearm free flap.[31] Recently, as knowledge and experience has been gained with various perforator flaps of the lower abdomen and thigh, the popularity of pedicle flaps is starting to reemerge.

Ideally, the reconstructed phallus (or constructed neophallus in transsexuals) should fulfill several criteria to be functionally and psychologically satisfying. It should be aesthetically acceptable with a shaft of adequate length and glans with defined shape and meatus. It should contain a neourethra that can be anastomosed to the patient's residual native urethra. As such, the patient should be able to void while standing. It should have close to normal tactile and erogenous sensitivity, and it should be able to accommodate a stiffener (prosthetic or autologous). The girth should be adequate for sexual function, but not too large to preclude intromission. While multiple techniques have been described to meet these objectives, the authors' preferred method of penile construction is the neurosensory radial forearm free flap.

This flap is a modification of the original radial forearm free flap design described by Chang and Hwang.[32] It incorporates a centrally based T-shaped portion of skin that will make up the neourethral lining in continuity with the neoglans (Figure 62-12A). Two strips of skin,

each 1-cm wide, are de-epithelialized on either side of the neourethral lining from the proximal edge of the flap to within 3-cm of the distal portion (Figure 62-12B). The dimensions of the flap are usually 15 × 17 cm; however, the distal width can be tapered to accommodate a narrower wrist, and the urethral portion may be extended proximally to accommodate a urethral anastomosis in the perineum. This design provides for the maximal dimension of the neophallus, places the urethra over the most hairless and reliable portion of the flap, as well as creates the appearance of a glans. Most importantly, it avoids a concentric suture line at the meatus, decreasing the risk of distal neourethral stenosis.

Preoperatively, an Allen test is performed to assure sufficient vascularization of the hand through the ulnar artery. The flap is outlined on the nondominant volar forearm. The flap, dissected under tourniquet, is based

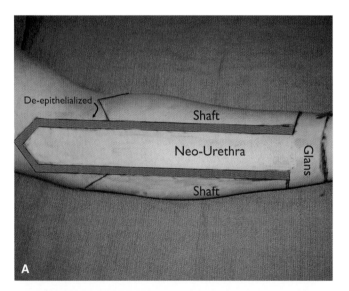

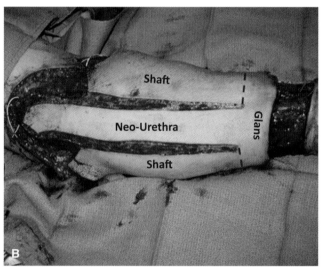

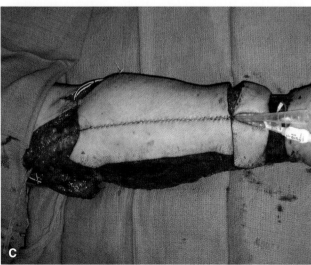

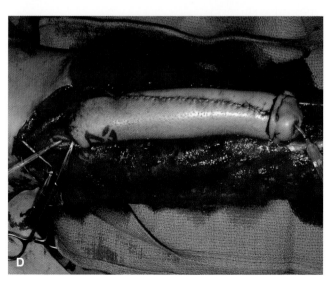

● **FIGURE 62-12.** Neophallus construction with neurosensory radial forearm free flap. (A) Design on forearm. (B, C) Central urethra with flanking de-epithelialized strips enables multiple layer closure for creation of urethral tube. (D) The dorsal side is closed and the neoglans is folded back and secured with mattress sutures.

on the radial artery and its venae comitantes. If necessary, the flap may be based on the ulnar artery. The cephalic vein is also included in the flap and dissection is carried far enough proximally so that the venae comitantes coalesce into a single vein. If this dissection is continued more proximally, the coalesced venae comitantes join the cephalic vein via the profundus cubitalis vein, which is a valveless vein connecting the superficial (cephalic) and deep (venae comitantes) venous systems of the forearm. This added dissection makes it possible for one large caliber vein to drain both venous systems.[33] Additionally, the author creates a distal radial-cephalic arteriovenous fistula to improve the venous outflow. The superficial branch of the radial nerve must be identified and preserved as it pierces beneath the brachioradialis tendon and courses close to the cephalic vein at the wrist. The medial and lateral antebrachial cutaneous nerves are included in the flap and dissected several centimeters proximal to the skin paddle, then tagged and divided.

The neophallus is fashioned while still in continuity with the vascular supply. Full-thickness transverse incisions are then made connecting the distal portion of the centrally placed neourethral skin with the radial and ulnar edges of the flap. The portion of the flap forming the central neourethra is "tubed" over a 12-French silastic urinary catheter and closed in layers (Figure 62-12C). The flap is then turned over and the dorsal skin is closed. The wings of the neoglans are trimmed to the appropriate shape and rolled back on the shaft. The distal portion of the shaft that will be under the rolled-back neoglans is de-epithelialized. The neoglans is then secured in its rolled-back position with full-thickness nylon mattress sutures (Figure 62-12D).

If the patient has a relatively small forearm with a significant amount of subcutaneous fat, then one of the two suture lines on the shaft may not be able to be closed without undo tension. In this situation, the outer layer of the volar suture line may be opened and a full-thickness graft placed, allowing the dorsal suture line to be closed primarily for aesthetic concerns (Figure 62-13).

During flap elevation, a second surgical team prepares the pubic site with recipient vessels and nerves. Approximately, 20-cm of saphenous vein is harvested from the thigh and is left attached to the femoral vein at the fossa ovalis. The divided end of this saphenous vein is then anastomosed to the femoral artery to create a temporary loop arteriovenous fistula. This is allowed to flow for at least 20 minutes until the flap is ready for transfer. The incision used for the saphenous vein harvest is connected to the flap recipient bed incision to prevent compression, torquing, or kinking of the vein grafts.

For reconstruction of a genetic male, a degloving incision is made if a portion of the native phallus exists. If there is no remnant, a W-shaped incision is made over the pubic symphysis. The dorsal penile branches of the pudendal nerve are isolated. If the nerves are not apparent, often in cases of trauma, dissection is continued toward the perineum and the pudendal nerves are identified as they

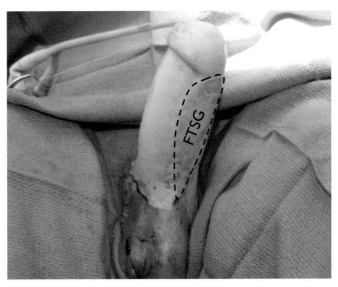

● **FIGURE 62-13.** Full-thickness skin graft (FTSG) placed on ventral surface of neophallus in patients where subcutaneous tissue prevents closure without tension.

emerge from the Alcock canal and travel along the inferior ramus of the pubis.

In transsexuals, inverted V incisions are made in the superior portion of the labia majora and they are retrodisplaced inferiorly for creation of a neoscrotum. The medial aspects of the labia majora are secured together, creating a neoscrotal median raphe. Transsexuals then undergo vaginectomy and an anterior vaginal flap is combined with a portion of the labia minora to fashion a tubed extension of the native urethra. The skin of the clitoris is removed and both clitoral nerves are identified and isolated on vessel loops in preparation for neurorrhaphies to the antebrachial cutaneous nerves of the flap (Figure 62-14).

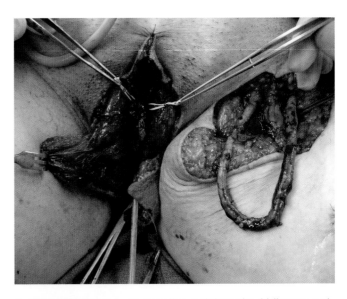

● **FIGURE 62-14.** Neophallus recipient site. Yellow vessel loops around clitoral nerves in female to male transsexuals. Vein loop in left groin.

When both the construct and recipient site preparation are complete, the neophallus is detached from the arm and secured to the recipient site with tacking sutures. The Foley catheter in the neourethra is placed into the bladder and the balloon is inflated. The neourethra is then anastomosed to the native urethra in an end-to-end spatulated fashion in two layers using 4-0 absorbable suture. The saphenous vein loop is divided and the microvascular anastomoses are performed, followed by the epineural neurorraphies. The remaining wounds about the proximal shaft of the neophallus and femoral vessels are closed over closed suction drains.

A suprapubic catheter is placed to allow drainage away from the healing neourethra. The catheter in the neourethra is capped. A thick split-thickness skin graft is applied to the donor site on the arm. A loose dressing is applied to the neophallus and it is supported within a bottomless Styrofoam cup, secured to the lower abdomen with foam tape.

Postoperative Care

Routine free flap monitoring is performed as previously described with mobilization after 48 hours. The Styrofoam dressing is removed and the flap is gently supported with a loose mesh garment. The urinary flow remains diverted through the suprapubic tube. When the patient is comfortable with the care of the flap and donor site, he is discharged with the suprapubic tube in place. Three to 4 weeks postoperatively, if healing appears adequate, a retrograde urethrogram is performed. If no fistula is seen, the bladder catheter is removed and the suprapubic tube is clamped. If the patient voids successfully, the suprapubic tube is removed 1 week later. When adequate protective sensation is gained in the flap, the patient is eligible for insertion of a prosthesis to allow for intromission. Most patients report the ability to achieve orgasm on stimulation of the neophallus within 9 months (Figure 62-15).

Scrotal Reconstruction

The scrotum and vulva are derived from the same embryologic tissue. The differences are that the scrotum descends farther than the vulva and fuses to form the median raphe and the vulva forms the vaginal introitus. In addition, the testicles migrate down to fill the scrotum. Scrotal skin loss may occur secondary to congenital anorchia, Fournier gangrene, burn, traumatic loss, or tumor resection. Reconstruction is guided by what tissue is injured or lost. Small to moderately sized skin defects may be treated conservatively, by allowing the wounds to heal by secondary intention. Common treatment of the surgically or traumatically created defects frequently involves either split-thickness skin grafting or burial of the testes in subcutaneous medial thigh pockets with delayed scrotal reconstruction.

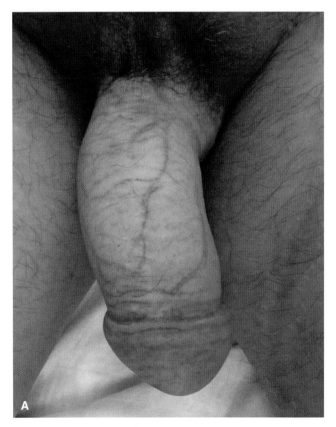
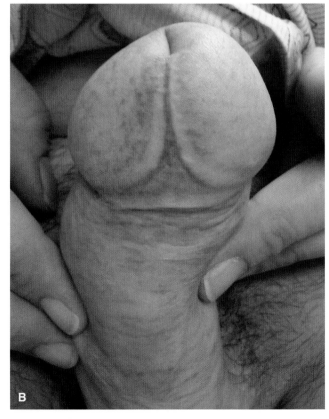

● **FIGURE 62-15.** (A, B) Final neophallus construction (transsexual) after minor revisions, insertion of inflatable prosthesis, and professional tattoo of veins and glans.

When there is a remnant of scrotal skin left, the authors' preferred technique is a two-stage reconstruction with the use of tissue expansion to create the scrotal sac.[34] In the first stage, a small tissue expander is placed beneath the deep Dartos fascia of the residual scrotal or perineal skin at the base of the penis. The expander is then gradually filled to at least a 150-mL capacity over several months. The second stage involves removal of the expander through an inverted V incision at the penoscrotal junction. The testes are mobilized (or testicular prosthesis is inserted) and secured to the inferior portion of the neoscrotal sac as in an orchiopexy. The incisions are then closed in a V-Y fashion, allowing the neoscrotal sac to move inferiorly and to hang in a natural position.

In complete absence of the scrotum, a variety of regional flaps can be used for reconstruction. The appearance of testicles may be created with the fat of a pudendal or medial thigh flap or with the use of silicone prosthesis. Due to the thickness of most fasciocutaneous flaps, it is difficult to recreate the texture of the original scrotum, in addition to problems with color match.

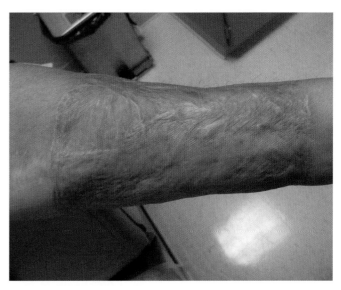

● **FIGURE 62-16.** Forearm donor site closed with split-thickness skin graft.

● COMPLICATIONS

All tissue transfer techniques, whether grafts or flaps, have the inherent potential complication of partial or complete loss with possible infection and resultant contraction and stenosis. All of the techniques have risks of injuring the rectum or urinary tract. The complications of the intra- or transabdominal procedures are similar to any intra-abdominal procedure, including infection, formation of adhesions, and bowel obstruction. Of all the pedicled flaps, the rectus myocutaneous flap seems to have the lowest overall complication rate.[35]

All grafts and flaps are at risk for partial or complete failure. Even a small area of ischemia of the tissue transferred will result in stricture and possible fistula. Most fistulae close spontaneously, those that do not may require secondary surgery. Mild strictures may be amenable to dilatation. Severe but localized strictures may be treated with internal urethrotomy followed by a short period of self-catheterization. Extensive strictures from poor take of a graft or a marginally perfused flap will most likely need revisional surgery.

The most common complications are related to the proximal urethral anastomosis, including sinuses, fistulae, and strictures. Most fistulae close spontaneously. Proximal urethral anastomotic suture line strictures may be treated with internal urethrotomy. One or two neodymium-YAG lasers or cold knife urethrotomies, followed by a short period of self-catheterization, often results in a stabilized widely patent urethra. Occasionally, recurrent proximal urethral suture line complications require surgical correction with local flaps or buccal mucosal grafts. All of our patients were ultimately able to stand to void. Meatal stenosis has not been problematic in these patients since a circumferential meatal suture line is avoided. Urethral

stone formation has not been observed in these patients, despite the hair present on the forearm. It is presumed that the fine hair on forearm skin does not have the same propensity to form stones as that of the thick, coarse hair on scrotal skin. Erosion and extrusion of penile prostheses has been described. It has been found that if prosthesis placement is delayed until protective sensation has returned the risk of prosthetic erosion and extrusion can be minimized.[36]

The greatest drawback of the radial forearm flap is the unsightly donor site (Figure 62-16). The thicker the graft used to close it, the better the aesthetics. Functional disability of the donor extremity has been rare, although the authors have had one patient with a radial nerve palsy that resolved and one patient with postoperative carpal tunnel syndrome that required release. Considering the high quality of penile construction possible with the radial forearm flap, the resultant donor site scar is usually well tolerated by patients. Some patients may not be the candidates for the radial forearm flap, and others may refuse it as a donor site. In these instances, alternative methods of penile reconstruction are possible and should be considered.[37-40]

For vaginal reconstruction, there is no single technique that is successful in all patients. Skin graft techniques are attractive because they are straightforward to perform. The biggest disadvantage is the tendency to contract or shrink over time and long-term use of molds is frequently required. Lining made from skin, whether from grafts or flaps, all have the problem of dryness, desquamation, and the tendency to be malodorous. A common disadvantage of musculocutaneous flaps is excess bulk. Pudendal flaps that are placed through the perineal route for total vaginal reconstruction tend to shorten and or prolapse. To prevent shortening and prolapse of flaps placed transperineally, a simultaneous laparoscopic suspension may be performed to suspend the blind end of the neovagina to the sacral promontory.[41] Patients frequently have sexual dysfunction due to psychological reasons, flap shortening, and difficulty with lubrication.[42]

● OUTCOMES

A successful outcome is achieved if the realistic goals of the surgeon and patient are met. This is best achieved by using a multidisciplinary approach. It should include a preoperative urogenital workup in cases of congenital deformities and psychological counseling for many patients, both pre- and postoperatively. The specific reconstructive option should be tailored to provide the best chance to maintain or restore function, improve quality of life, have acceptable aesthetics, and minimal morbidity. Appropriate follow-up should ascertain functional success as well as emotional health. Outcome measurements should identify whether the urologic, gynecologic, and sexual goals are met. Serial postoperative visits should evaluate the aesthetic appearance of the reconstructed tissues, the regularity and ability to control urine production, the ability to have regular pain-free intercourse if desired, as well as the patient's own satisfaction with the appearance and function of the reconstruction. If all of these outcomes are met, the result may be deemed successful.

REFERENCES

1. Moschella F, Cordova A. Innervated island flaps in morphofunctional vulvar reconstruction. *Plast Reconstr Surg.* 2000;105(5):1649–1657.

2. Salgarello M, Farallo E, Barone-Adesi L, et al. Flap algorithm in vulvar reconstruction after radical, extensive vulvectomy. *Ann Plast Surg.* 2005;54(2):184–190.

3. Wee JT, Joseph VT. A new technique of vaginal reconstruction using neurovascular pudendal-thigh flaps: A preliminary report. *Plast Reconstr Surg.* 1989;83:701.

4. Monstrey S, Blondeel P, Van Landuyt K, et al. The versatility of the pudendal thigh fasciocutaneous flap used as an island flap. *Plast Reconstr Surg.* 2001;107(3):719–725.

5. Tobin GR, Day TG. Vaginal and pelvic reconstruction with distally based rectus abdominis myocutaneous flaps. *Plast Reconstr Surg.* 1988;81:62.

6. Höckel M. The transversus and rectus abdominis musculoperitoneal (TRAMP) composite flap for vulvovaginal reconstruction. *Plast Reconstr Surg.* 1996;97:455.

7. McCraw JB, Massey FM, Shanklin KD, et al. Vaginal reconstruction with gracilis myocutaneous flaps. *Plast Reconstr Surg.* 1976;58:176–183.

8. Vasconez LO, Mathes SJ, Whetzel T, Wang TN. A fasciocutaneous flap for vaginal and perineal reconstruction. *Plast Reconstr Surg.* 1987;80:95–103.

9. Hurwitz DJ, Swartz WM, Mathes SJ. The gluteal thigh flap: a reliable sensate flap for the closure of buttock and perineal wounds. *Plast Reconstr Surg.* 1981;68:521–530.

10. Gottlieb LJ, Jejurikar SS. Management of the persistent perineal wound. In: Michelassi F, Milsom JW, eds. *Operative Strategies in Inflammatory Bowel Disease.* New York: Springer-Verlag; 1999:445–457.

11. Hashimoto I, Nakanishi H, Nagae H, et al. The gluteal fold flap for vulvar and buttock reconstruction: anatomic study and adjustment of flap volume. *Plast Reconstr Surg.* 2001;108(7):1998–2005.

12. Lee, PK, Choi MS, Ahn ST, et al. Gluteal fold V-Y advancement flap for vulvar and vaginal reconstruction: a new flap. *Plast Reconstr Surg.* 2006;118(2):401–406.

13. Lappohn RE. Congenital absence of the vagina-results of conservative treatment. *Eur J Obstet Gynecol.* 1995;59:183–186.

14. Makinoda S, Nishiya M, Sogame M, et al. Non-grafting method of vaginal construction for patients of vaginal agenesis without functioning uterus (Mayer-Rokitansky-Kuster syndrome). *Int Surg.* 1996;81:385–389.

15. Templeman CL, Lam AM, Hertweck SP. Surgical management of vaginal agenesis. *Obstet Gynecol Surg.* 1999;54:583.

16. Veronikis DK, McClure GB, Nichols DH. The Vecchietti operation for constructing a neovagina: indications, instrumentation and techniques. *Obstet Gynecol.* 1997;90(2):301–304.

17. Hojsgaard A, Villadsen I. McIndoe procedure for congenital vaginal agenesis: complications and results. *Br J Plast Surg.* 1995;48:97–102.

18. Alessandrescu D, Peltecu GC, Buhimschi CS, et al. Neocolpopoiesis with split-thickness skin graft as a surgical treatment of vaginal agenesis: retrospective review of 201 cases. *Am J Obstet Gynecol.* 1996;175:131–138.

19. Seccia A, Salgarello M, Sturla M, Loreti, et al. Neovaginal reconstruction with the modified McIndoe Technique: A review of 32 cases. *Ann Plast Surg.* 2002;49(4):379–384.

20. Williams EA. Uterovaginal agenesis. *Ann R Coll Surg Engl.* 1976;58:226–277.

21. Davydov SN. Colpopoiesis from the peritoneum of the uterorectal space. *Obstet Gynecol.* 1969:55–57.

22. Freundt I, Toolenaar TA, Huikeshoven FJ, et al. A modified technique to create a neovagina with an isolated segment of sigmoid colon. *Surg Gynecol Obstet.* 1992;17:11–16.

23. Wesley JR, Coran AG. Intestinal vaginoplasty for congenital absence of the vagina. *J Pediatr Surg.* 1992;27(7):885–889.

24. Kim SK, Park JH, Lee KC, et al. Long-term results in patients after rectosigmoid vaginoplasty. *Plast Reconstr Surg.* 2003;112(1):143–151.

25. Kapoor R, Sharma DK, Singh JK, et al. Sigmoid vaginoplasty: long-term results. *Urology.* 2006;67(6):1212–1215.

26. Emiroglu M, Gultan SM, Adanali G, et al Vaginal reconstruction with free jejunal flap. *Ann Plast Surg.* 1996;36:316–320.

27. Retik AB, Borer JG. Hypospadias. In: Walsh PC, Retik AB, Vaughn ED, Wein AJ, eds. *Campbell's Urology.* 8th ed. Philadelphia: W B Saunders; 2002:2284–2333.

28. van der Werff, JFA, van der Meulen, JC. Treatment modalities for hypospadias cripples. *Plast Reconstr Surg.* 2000; 105(2):600–608.

29. Koshima I, Inagawa K, Okuyama N, Moriguchi T. Free vascularized appendix transfer for reconstruction of penile urethras with severe fibrosis. *Plast Reconstr Surg.* 1999; 103(3):964–969.

30. Bales GT, Kuznetsov DD, Kim HL, Gottlieb LJ. Urethral substitution using an intestinal free flap: a novel approach. *J Urol.* 2002;168(1):182–184.

31. Gottlieb LJ, Pielet RW, Levine LA. An update on phallic construction. *Adv Plast Reconstr Surg.* 1994;(10):267–284.

32. Chang TS, Hwang WY. Forearm flap in one-stage reconstruction of the penis. *Plast Reconstr Surg.* 1984;74(2):251–258.

33. Gottlieb LJ, Tachmes L, Pielet RW Improved venous drainage of the radial artery forearm free flap: use of the profundus cubitalis vein. *J Reconstr Microsurg.* 1993;9:281.

34. Rapp DE, Cohn AB, Gottlieb LJ, et al. Use of tissue expansion for scrotal sac reconstruction following scrotal skin loss. *Urology.* 2005;65 (6):1216–1218.

35. Casey WJ, Tran NV, Petty PM, et al. A comparison of 99 consecutive vaginal reconstructions: an outcome study. *Ann Plast Surg.* 2004;52(1):27–30.

36. Levine LA, Zachary LS, Gottlieb LJ. Prosthesis placement after total phallic reconstruction. *J Urol.* 1993;149:593–598.

37. Khouri RK, Young VL, Casoli VM. Long-term results of total penile reconstruction with a prefabricated lateral arm free flap. *J Urol.* 1998;160:383–388.

38. Sadove RC, Sengezer M, McRoberts JW, Wells MD. One-stage total penile reconstruction with a free sensate osteocutaneous fibula flap. *Plast Reconstr Surg.* 1993;93: 1314–1323.

39. Partridge J, Wille M, Gottlieb LJ, et al. Salvage of end-stage erectile dysfunction using vascularized fibula as autologous implant. *Urology.* 2005;66:188–192.

40. Sengezer M, Öztürk S, Deveci M, et al. Long-term follow-up of total penile reconstruction with sensate osteocutaneous free fibula flap in 18 biological male patients. *Plast Reconstr Surg.* 2004;114(2):439–450.

41. Copcu E, Odabasi AR, Sivrioğlu N, et al Protection of vaginal depth by laparoscopy in vaginal reconstruction with pudendal thigh flaps. *Plast Reconstr Surg.* 2005;115(2):663–664.

42. Scott JR, Liu D, Mathes DW. Patient-reported outcomes and sexual function in vaginal reconstruction: a 17-year review, survey, and review of the literature. *Ann Plast Surg.* 2010;64(3):311–314.

chapter 63

Lower Extremity Reconstruction

Amir H. Tahernia, MD / Lawrence S. Levin, MD, FACS

● INTRODUCTION

Lower extremity defects are encountered following trauma, ablative oncologic procedures, and in the setting of infection. When discussing lower extremity reconstruction, it is helpful to divide the limb into anatomic components: upper leg (thigh to knee), knee, and lower leg (knee to foot). Each area due to its composition and function, presents different reconstructive challenges. The primary goal is to restore form and function of the reconstructed limb. The operative approach must be tailored to each patient, as limb defects arising from trauma will have different reconstructive demands to those following oncologic resection. As such, planning and communication between the ablative and reconstructive team is essential, with goals established early by the clinician and the patient.

● PATIENT EVALUATION

Trauma

Lower extremity injury with open high-energy soft tissue wounds is frequently encountered in trauma centers and often requires the input from reconstructive plastic surgeons. In the setting of severe limb injury, the question of limb salvage versus primary amputation is the most important early decision. Several authors have attempted to use scoring systems to help decide between limb reconstruction and amputation. These include the Mangled Extremity Severity Score, the Limb Salvage Index, and the Predictive Salvage Index. Studies have shown that although these indices may serve as a useful classification of wound severity, they do not reliably predict which limbs should undergo amputation. The primary factors influencing the outcome in leg injuries are the degree of soft tissue damage, the presence or absence of plantar sensation, and the severity of vascular injuries. From this, absolute and relative indications for indications for primary limb amputation have been proposed. Absolute indications include complete disruption of posterior tibial nerve in adults and crush injury with warm ischemia time longer than 6 hours. Relative indications include serious associated polytrauma, severe ipsilateral foot trauma, anticipated protracted course to obtain soft tissue coverage and fracture healing, and massive bone loss.[1]

The most important determinants of outcome after open fractures are wound size, degree of soft tissue damage, and the amount of contamination. The severity of open wounds has been further classified in a landmark paper by Gustillo. Several clinical studies have confirmed the utility of the Gustillo classification as a prognostic tool for recovery of open tibial fractures. Using this classification as a guide, the reconstructive team can determine the appropriate method of limb salvage.

Gustillo Classification of Open Fractures of the Tibia

I—Open fracture with a wound <1 cm
II—Open fracture with a wound >1 cm without extensive soft tissue damage
III—Open fracture with extensive soft tissue damage
IIIA—III with adequate soft tissue coverage
IIIB—III with soft tissue loss and periosteal stripping and bone exposure
IIIC—III with arterial injury needing repair

As with any trauma patient, those who have sustained lower limb injury need to be assessed according to the Advanced Life Trauma Support protocol. Extremity injuries are best treated by a multidisciplinary team that involves orthopedic, plastic, and vascular surgeons. A recent study has shown that this team approach has led to lower complication rates and need for revisional surgery.[2]

Tumor

The objectives of reconstruction of the lower extremity following cancer resection are to provide adequate wound coverage to allow for subsequent adjuvant therapy, to preserve functional capability, and to optimize the aesthetic outcome. As a rule, any extremity that can be preserved with a good potential for function should be salvaged. Currently, there are many effective prosthetic devices, but none of them can replicate the function of the human hand or foot. As a result, surgeons and patients are willing to go to great lengths to salvage affected extremities. Limb salvage rates approach 90% in many studies. This is a testament to technical advances in reconstructive surgery, as well as newer, more effective adjuvant therapies.[3]

Infection

Perhaps the most benign of the three indications, lower extremity wounds due to infectious complications are often the most difficult to manage. Osseous tissues are less vascular than the surrounding soft tissue and thus more resistant to antibiotic therapy, which relies on a healthy blood supply to reach the affected tissues. Management of such injuries requires adequate determination of the offending agent, in this case the specific organism, and precise tailoring of the pharmacologic therapy. Frequent cultures and serial debridements are invaluable in the management of such wounds. Grossly infected bone often needs to be debrided back to healthy tissue in order for the overlying soft tissue to heal. Nowhere is the adage, "Don't put a new roof on a burning building," more true than with bony infection.

● PATIENT PREPARATION

In all three clinical settings, there are instances where preoperative radiographs are indicated. In the instance where a free flap is contemplated, the issue of "zone of injury" as it relates to the vascular status of the affected limb must be addressed. The zone of injury refers to the inflammatory response of the soft tissues that extend beyond the gross wound and results in perivascular changes. These changes include increased friability of vessels and increased perivascular scar tissue, which can contribute to higher anastomotic failures. Therefore, when performing free vascularized bone or soft tissue transfer, it is best to avoid this zone. This is accomplished by extensive proximal dissection of the recipient vessels as well as use of interposition venous conduits. A meticulous clinical examination in combination with Doppler mapping will likely be sufficient to assess the adequacy of recipient vessels for microvascular anastomosis. However, there are times when either CT angiography or formal angiography is necessary to better prepare the reconstructive surgeon. The use of angiography should be determined on a case-by-case basis.

● TREATMENT

Although treatment concepts for the traumatized lower extremity did not change much until the major wars, several early principles of treatment were proposed. Pierre-Joseph Desault (1738–1795) introduced deep incisions for drainage and debridement of devitalized tissue and Louis Ollier (1830–1900) introduced plaster casting for fracture stabilization. By the end of World War I, the concept of treating open wounds with dressings and casts was the mainstay of treatment of lower extremity wounds. Osteomyelitis was a frequent complication and prompted surgeons to perform more aggressive debridement prior to application of a cast.

After World War II, the use of skin grafts for coverage of complicated lower extremity wounds was introduced. Following this period, wound closure was attempted before the appearance of granulation tissue and this led to lower infectious complications. Over the past 40 years, significant advances have been made in the management of soft tissue and skeletal deficiencies. Wounds, which would have resulted in amputation, can now be salvaged with free tissue transfer as well as a variety of local flaps.

Today, wounds can be examined along a spectrum of reconstructive modalities, regardless of the location. Using a "reconstructive ladder" the clinician can formulate an effective approach for coverage based on the existing defect. This is particularly useful in the management of lower extremity defects as management at different levels of the limb mandate different restorative measures (Figure 63-1). The initial management of open fractures consists of emergent debridement of devitalized tissue as well as skeletal stabilization. Thorough debridement is essential prior to any reconstructive endeavor, as any nonviable tissue that remains can lead to failure of the reconstruction.

Timing of Reconstruction

Traditionally, coverage of complicated lower extremity wounds was delayed until the tissue edema had subsided and the wound had stabilized. The issue of delayed versus early reconstruction has been examined closely. In the 1980s, Byrd and colleagues[4] noted that complications were higher if wounds were not covered in the early phase defined as 6 days from the time of injury. Godina demonstrated that with radical debridement and coverage of wounds within 72 hours, the incidence of nonunion and osteomyelitits decreased. Most studies show a significantly lower failure rate in patients in whom free flap reconstruction is performed within 3 days of injury as compared with flaps performed at a later date. Godina[5] noted a failure rate less than 1%, 12%, and 10% when free flaps were performed within 3 days, 3 days to 3 months, and longer than 3 months after injury. It is thought that in the setting of a delayed reconstruction, wounds enter a subacute or chronic phase where

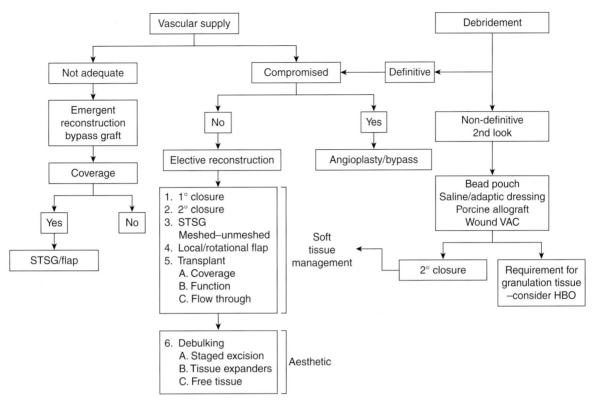

● **FIGURE 63-1.** The reconstructive ladder. STSG, split-thickness skin graft; HBO, hyperbaric oxygen therapy; VAC, vacuum-assisted closure. (*Reprinted with permission from Heller L, Levin LS. Lower extremity microsurgical reconstruction. Plast Reconstr Surg. 2001;108(4):1029–1041; quiz 1042.*)

there is increasing inflammation and bacterial colonization, which may hinder reconstructive efforts. Therefore, the current approach is to perform early coverage with vascularized tissue to reduce complications and lead to shorter hospitalizations.

Methods of Bone Stabilization and Reconstruction

In the setting of lower extremity trauma, bony injury falls into two categories: (1) those with adequate bone stock in need of stabilization and (2) those where significant bone loss has occurred and stabilization with hardware alone would be inadequate. Bone fixation may be of two general types: internal fixation with plates, rods, and/or screws placed within or on top of the bone or external fixation with percutaneous pins held together with hardware outside the leg. Although possible for smaller wounds, casting larger wounds with exposed bone is not an appropriate method of skeletal stabilization.

Plate fixation requires exact opposition and compression of bones by plates and screws. The hardware must be covered with soft tissue. The periosteum is critical for bone healing and one of the problems with use of plate fixation in the setting of trauma is the need for further periosteal stripping prior to plate fixation. This devascularization in addition to what may have been sustained

as a result of the trauma can lead to suboptimal bony union. Several studies have shown increased complication rates, including infection and nonunion, when plates are used in severe leg injuries. As such, for high-energy tibial fractures, the safest choice for skeletal stabilization is external fixation. The advantage of this method is that in addition to providing stability, it is able to hold the bony segments out to their anatomic length, which is of particular importance when a large segment of bone may be missing. The main disadvantages of external fixation are complications associated with hardware, the most common of which is pin tract infection. The longer the pins stay in place, the more chance of infection and this may limit the duration of fixator placement. Ideally, the external fixator should remain until union has occurred, but in certain cases this needs to be balanced with the risk of infection.[6]

Intramedullary nailing of tibial fractures is a method also applied in the management of open tibial fractures. Studies have shown it to result in high union rates and few infections in the setting of low energy wound. In grossly contaminated wounds (Gustillo IIIA or IIIB), intramedullary nailing is associated with increased risk of infection and hardware exposure. In these wounds external fixation is still the best choice for skeletal stabilization.[3]

Complicated lower extremity wounds can be accompanied by significant bone loss mandating reconstruction.

Options for skeletal reconstruction include autogenous bone grafts, vascularized bone transfer (pedicled or free), and the Ilizarov technique. The size of the bony defect will determine the ideal reconstructive approach. For defects of the tibia less than 6 cm, bone grafts have been shown to be an acceptable option assuming there is adequate soft tissue coverage. Although alloplastic bone graft can be used, it is fraught with a relatively high infection rate. As such, cancellous autografts are preferred. The bone grafts are typically placed following placement of antibiotic spacers and 4 to 6 weeks after soft tissue reconstruction to allow for the transferred tissue to further sterilize the wound. An intact fibula facilitates bone grafting, as it may act as a strut to keep the extremity at length.[7,8]

Vascularized bone transfers have been described using iliac crest and scapula but by far the most commonly harvested bone is the fibula. Vascularized bone transfer can be performed based on a preserved vascular pedicle (Figure 63-2) or as a free flap with microvascular anastomosis (Figure 63-3). The fibula can be transferred with or without an overlying skin paddle. The bone has great strength and is able to provide adequate length in many

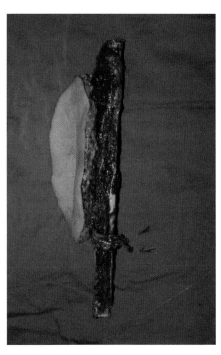

● **FIGURE 63-3.** Harvested free fibular flap with pedicle and skin island.

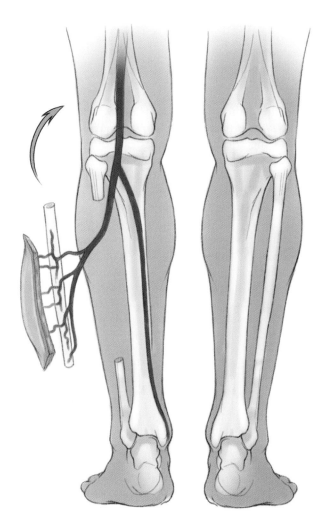

● **FIGURE 63-2.** Arc of rotation of a pedicled fibula osteoseptocutaneous flap.

circumstances. To provide more stability and bulk, the bone may be folded on itself. In doing so, the fracture rates and time to full weight bearing is diminished.[9]

Bone transport or distraction techniques provide an alternative for bony reconstitution. This method was first described by Codvilla[10] and popularized by Ilizarov. This can be used for defects less than 10 cm. The technique requires debridement of the fractured ends with pin placement near the bone ends on either side of the gap. A corticotomy is made high on the tibia and serves as the source of regenerate after the bone is distracted with transfixation pins on an external frame.

Acute shortening of the bone can also be done using the Ilizarov method. This allows for subsequent lengthening with distraction performed at 1 mm/day. Typically a latency period of 7 days where no distraction is performed is followed as protocol. Acute shortening is especially useful in cases of nerve or vascular repair. One of the advantages of the Ilizarov method is that during the distraction period the soft tissue is also transported over the length of the defect, allowing for closure of soft tissue defects without the need for flaps or grafts. Theoretically, no limit exists regarding bone loss that can be filled using this technique. The length and alignment of the bone are maintained throughout treatment, allowing improved extremity function and ambulation. Levin and colleagues[11] have reported on using a combination of distraction with microsurgical free tissue transfer to provide an additional option for extremity reconstruction. Disadvantages of the Ilizarov method include joint deformities, nonunion, and pin site infections.

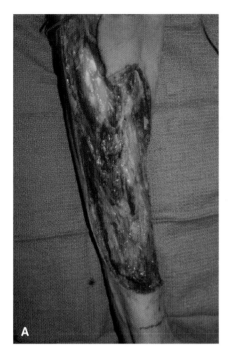
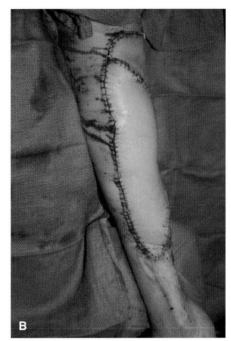
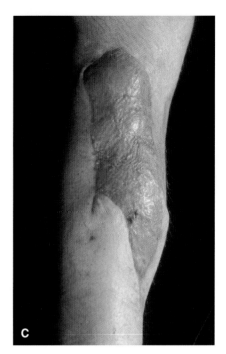

● **FIGURE 63-4.** (A–C) Large posterior calf defect covered with myocutaneous latissimus dorsi flap.

Soft Tissue Reconstruction

With any lower extremity reconstruction, three tenets are essential: (1) adequate preparation of wound bed, including debridement and control of infection prior to coverage; (2) stabilization and management of associated orthopedic injuries; and (3) overall assessment of the patient's suitability for reconstruction and rehabilitation. As a reconstructive adjunct, a vacuum-assisted closure (VAC) device can be used to optimize the wound bed and minimize dressing changes in preparation for reconstruction. In the lower extremity, muscle and fasciocutaneous flaps remain primary choices for soft tissue coverage with free flaps being the first-line for the distal third of the leg. For free flap reconstruction, it is important to anastomose vessels outside the zone of injury and reconstruct the soft tissue first followed by restoration of skeletal support.[12]

In the lower extremity reconstruction, the workhorse flaps for soft tissue coverage are the latissimus, serratus, rectus, and gracilis muscles, and more recently the anterolateral thigh flap has gained popularity. The latissimus dorsi flap has the advantage of a large amount of bulk to fill dead space (Figure 63-4A–C). Over time, the flap loses bulk, which aids in restoring normal contour to the leg. For coverage of massive lower extremity wounds, the latissimus dorsi can be coupled to the serratus anterior using a single thoracodorsal pedicle. The latissimus muscle also has the added advantage of having a relatively long pedicle, anywhere from 9 to 11 cm, allowing for vessel anastomosis to occur well outside the zone of injury. For smaller defects, the gracilis muscle is an ideal choice. The gracilis is relatively easy to harvest with minimal donor site or functional morbidity (Figure 63-5A,B). The anterolateral thigh flap is based on one or two perforators arising from the descending branch of the lateral femoral circumflex artery. It is a fasciocutaneous flap with a large skin paddle (Figure 63-6A,B). The donor site can be closed primarily or skin grafted if a large flap is harvested.

Microvascular Soft Tissue Reconstruction

When confronted with a lower extremity wound where the location of injury and extent of tissue loss mandates free tissue transfer, certain critical considerations need to be made prior to reconstruction. One of the controversial issues is the use of angiography in lower extremity reconstruction. A good clinical examination corroborated with ultrasonography is a reliable enough assessment to proceed with a microvascular anastomosis. There are certain situations where we feel that a vascular road map (formal angiography, CT angiography, or MR angiography) would be a useful tool for preoperative planning. One of these circumstances is the extremity that has undergone a vascular reconstruction at another facility and is then transferred for soft tissue reconstruction. In this situation, one would need to confirm beyond the clinical examination, the reconstructed vascular anatomy of the leg prior to embarking on free tissue transfer. The other clinical scenario where angiography is warranted is in the setting of a Gustillo IIIC wound (associated vascular injury).[13]

With respect to the technical aspects of microvascular anastomosis, the posterior and anterior tibial arteries are the most common recipient vessels. The arterial anastomosis enjoys more success when it is performed in an

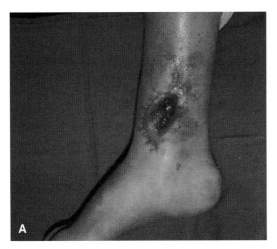
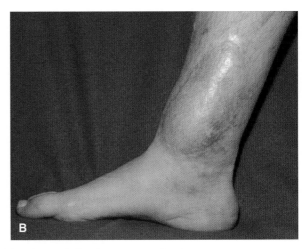

● **FIGURE 63-5.** (A) Patient with exposed hardware following open reduction and internal fixation of the ankle. (B) Postoperative photograph 16 months following debridement and coverage with a free gracilis muscle flap with a split-thickness skin graft.

end-to-side fashion, whereas the venous anastomosis is usually performed end to end to one or preferably both of the venae commitantes. Superficial veins are more prone to spasm and as such are avoided in microvascular reconstruction, except in the situation where supercharging of a flap is desired. In this setting, if the flap has an available venous perforator, an additional venous anastomosis can be done to decrease the potential for venous congestion. Venous congestion is known to be a common cause of early flap failure and mandates a return to the operating room.

The role of microsurgery in the amputee is another area worth mentioning. Once amputation is inevitable,

the main objective of surgery is to preserve a functional stump. Free tissue transfer is a valuable tool in preserving length and restoring contour of the lower limb stump. Parts from the amputated limb such as the calcaneal-plantar unit and classic free flaps such as the latissimus dorsi, scapula, and anterior lateral thigh flaps can be used to achieve stable and rapid rehabilitation of the patient. The "free fillet" flap principle was described as part of "spare part" preservation.[14] This allows for the use of tissue in the absence of additional donor site morbidity. This strategy can be applied on the basis of an immediate use of flaps and a multistaged reconstruction with banking of free flaps.

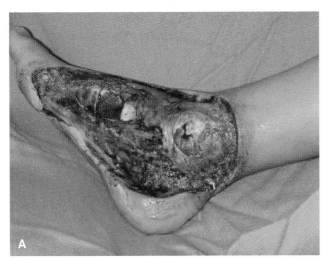
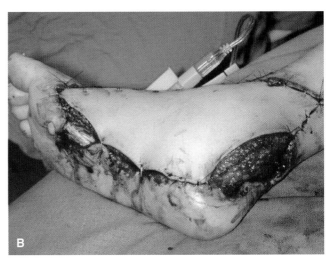

● **FIGURE 63-6.** (A) Patient with a degloving injury to the medial aspect of foot. (B) Wound bed following debridement and coverage with a free anterolateral thigh flap.

Site-specific Soft Tissue Reconstruction

In the thigh, the need for pedicled or free flap reconstruction is minimal. Given the large amount of local muscle and skin, wounds can be closed either primarily or muscle can be covered with a split-thickness skin graft. In cases where the defects are very large or femoral vessels are exposed, a pedicled rectus abdominis muscle (based on the inferior epigastric vessels)—with or without the overlying vertical pattern of skin—can be used. For smaller defects the gracilis (medial femoral circumflex) or tensor fascia lata (ascending branch of the lateral femoral circumflex) can be rotated into the wound.

As a general rule, the area around the knee can be covered with local rotational flaps. Special consideration must be given to preserving the knee extensor mechanism. Techniques have been described where either one or both gastrocnemius muscles (sural artery) have been used for both coverage of knee wounds and restoration of the extensor mechanism. There are instances, however, where free tissue transfer may be necessary due to defect size. An area of particular interest with regard to knee reconstruction is in the setting of a failed knee arthrodesis where a free fibula can be transferred to achieve joint fusion.

For coverage of the defects around the upper third of the tibia, the main rotational flaps include both lateral and medial heads of the gastrocnemius, proximally based soleus (peroneal artery), and tibialis anterior (anterior tibial artery). The medial head of the gastrocnemius allows for a longer advancement as compared with the lateral head. The pedicle is the medial sural artery. Advancement is facilitated by release of the origin of the muscle from the femoral condyle and scoring of the fascia. When harvesting the lateral head of gastrocnemius, care should be taken not to injure the peronreal nerve. The soleus muscle based proximally can be reliably carried to a point about 5 cm above its tendinous insertion. The tibialis anterior is important in dorsiflexion of the foot and is not considered expendable. Nonetheless by maintaining its origin and insertion, the muscle might be raised as a bipedicled flap and transposed to cover a neighboring defect.

For coverage of middle tibial wounds, the soleus and gastrocnemius are the main reconstructive options. Other flaps include the flexor digitorum longus (posterior tibial artery), the extensor digitorum longus (anterior tibial artery), the extensor hallucis longus (anterior tibial artery), and the tibialis anterior (anterior tibial artery). The flexor digitorum longus is a small and its use is reserved for coverage of small defects or in conjunction with other flaps. There is minimal donor site morbidity as the flexor digitorum brevis can supplement toe flexion. The extensor digitorum longus and extensor hallucis longus are also small and are used for coverage of wounds less than 5 cm in diameter. In the setting of large wounds where local flaps are inadequate, free tissue transfer must be considered.

Due to insufficient soft tissue available for transposition, local flaps have a limited role in coverage in the area of the distal leg and ankle. As such, free flaps are the first choice for reconstruction. However, for small defects in this area there are some local muscle and distally based superficial flaps that can be used. Attinger and colleagues[15] have described several of these, including such the medial plantar artery flap. It is important to realize that these are only for small defects and in the right patient they may prevent the use of a free flap. Therefore, a careful evaluation of the wound will allow one to decide on the best course of action. The sural flap as a fasciocutaneous flap has been used in coverage of the lower third of the leg. It is supplied from its distal aspect by perforators from the medial superficial sural artery. Because of the reverse orientation of the flap, venous congestion can compromise flap viability. For this reason, the flap can be supercharged with a microvascular anastomosis performed between the greater saphenous vein within the flap and the lesser saphenous vein. In attempts to redirect blood flow and decrease the risk of flap necrosis and other complications, several authors have described sural flap delay procedures as an additional method for improving flap survival (Figure 63-7A–C).[16,17]

The goal of reconstruction of the foot is functional: to restore weight bearing during ambulation. Important components to achieve this goal include stable and well-contoured bony support, and a sensate and durable plantar surface. The overall soft tissue contour should allow the use of regular foot apparel or a reasonable orthotic device. Otherwise, a normal gait cycle may not be possible. Donor site morbidity should be minimal. Unfortunately, attaining all of these goals in one reconstruction is not always possible. Bulky flaps may be durable but insensate and clumsy. Innervated flaps may offer sensibility with less than optimal durability or donor site morbidity. Cases are therefore individualized to each patient's needs and desires. When embarking on a foot reconstruction, it is critical to assess the potential soft tissue defect, the amount and location of remaining bone, the expected plantar sensation, and the vascular status of the limb after the ablative portion of the procedure. Actual flap choices will be guided by the findings. The vascular supply to the foot is assessed first. If the patient has a history of vascular disease, claudication, or rest pain, or if pulses are not palpable on physical examination, a preoperative arteriogram is obtained. Poorly vascularized distal extremities may best be served by amputation or reconstruction in concert with a revascularization procedure. Bony support of the foot should be addressed next. If the areas of the first metatarsal head and calcaneus are uninvolved, minimal bony work should be required because these are the normal weight-bearing areas. Bony prominences should be recontoured to allow the distribution of forces over as wide an area as possible.

The choice of soft tissue coverage must be individualized for the particular case. Considerations in flap selection include defect size, required bulk, surface durability,

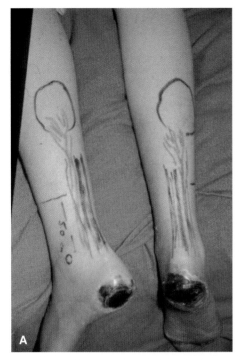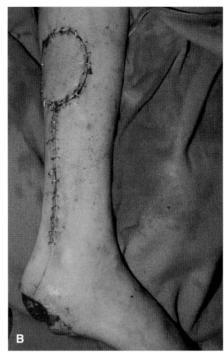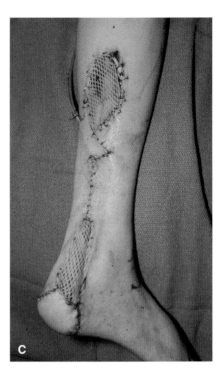

● **FIGURE 63-7.** (A) Patient with bilateral necrotic heel ulcers and planned coverage with bilateral sural artery flap. Flaps are designed with the pivot point of the pedicle 5 cm above the lateral malleolus. (B,C) Delay of the flap is used to decrease the incidence of venous congestion. The flap is elevated and secured back into the wound bed. At 3 weeks, the flaps are re-elevated and transposed into position for coverage of heel wound.

and sensory reinnervation. These considerations should be prioritized because any particular flap rarely can satisfy all possible needs. For skin defects with exposure of vital structures such as tendon, bone, or joint spaces, an innervated free fasciocutaneous flap is preferred. Examples of this type of flap include the radial forearm flap (Figure 63-8A,B) and the lateral arm flap. These flaps provide well-vascularized, thin, pliable soft tissue that facilitates restoration of foot contour with durable sensate skin. This allows patients to wear normal shoes. When larger, more complex defects are anticipated, a muscle free flap is a good choice to fill the dead space and accomplish reconstruction with a healthy pad of tissue. Skin grafting is required, and although no nerves are reanastomosed, patients may be functional from proprioceptive feedback and some protective sensation from the defect bed and surrounding skin. Regardless of the flap procedure performed, patient education in meticulous foot care is imperative. Patients need to inspect their feet frequently and recognize any incipient problems. Special footwear should be prescribed following plantar resurfacing.

Cross-Leg Flaps

Prior to the advent of free tissue transfer, when local tissue was not an option for lower extremity wound coverage, the cross-leg flap was the treatment of choice for

coverage, particularly in the elderly patient. Currently there are limited indications. The patient who is not a free flap candidate and is immobilized for other reasons may be a candidate. Cross-leg flaps are transferred as fasciocutanoeus flaps with a 3:1 length-to-width ratio. A recent analysis of cross-leg flaps by Dawson indicated a high morbidity. In a review of 99 patients local flap necrosis was identified in 40% and infection in 28%.

Soft Tissue Expansion

Although tissue expansion has enjoyed good results in coverage of defects in the chest and head and neck regions, its use in the lower extremities has been associated with high rates of infection and implant extrusion. Its primary use in the lower extremity is to resurface areas of unstable soft tissue or unsightly scar. If used in the lower extremity, expanders are placed in a subcutaneous pocket above the muscular fascia. In the foot and ankle region, the use of expanders is almost always avoided. Proximal placement is associated with higher success rates. It has been shown that lateral expansion of defects has a decreased failure rate when compared with advancement in a longitudinal vector. Overall, the role of tissue expansion in lower extremity reconstruction is limited. Its use should be tailored to patients on an individual basis.

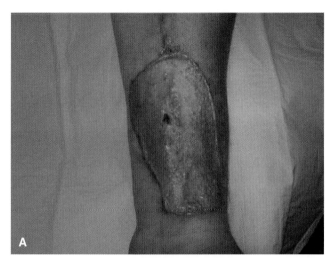 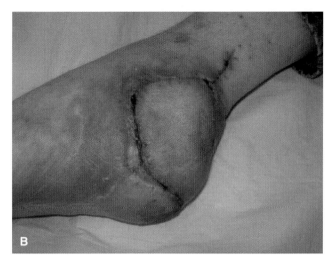

● **FIGURE 63-8.** (A) Donor site in a patient with a nonhealing wound of the heel covered with a free radial forearm flap. (B) Recipient site of the radial forearm free flap 2 weeks after free tissue transfer.

Vacuum-assisted Closure

Over the past decade, VAC devices have improved treatment of open wounds. The device applies continuous subatmospheric pressure causing decreased tissue edema and decreased wound circumference. It has been shown to promote granulation tissue in the wound bed by virtue of increased blood flow and decreased bacterial counts. It is an ideal bridging therapy to definitive reconstruction of the lower extremity. Pribaz et al. showed that for complicated wounds, including Gustillo III defects, VAC can decrease the need for free flap coverage. They demonstrated rapid production of granulation tissue over exposed bone, tendon, and hardware with subsequent coverage with skin grafts or delayed primary closure. Although this study demonstrated encouraging results with VAC and skin graft, negative pressure therapy will not replace the role of vascularized tissue transfer in the management of complex lower extremity wounds.

Oncologic Wounds

Wide tumor resection in the lower extremity can expose neurovascular structures or bone devoid of its periosteum and can require coverage of allografts or internal metal prostheses. Often, the surrounding soft tissues are inflexible and cannot be mobilized to provide adequate wound coverage, especially when local tissues have been previously irradiated. In these cases, creative solutions using distant flaps to restore form and function are required. When amputation is inevitable, preparation of the wound bed for an external prosthesis becomes the main objective of the reconstruction. And most important, it is imperative that the reconstructive plan facilitates a rapid recovery so that patients can quickly receive any required additional adjuvant treatment modalities and resume their activities of daily living.

Surgery is infrequently used alone for treatment of soft tissue sarcomas of the extremities and is often performed between courses of systemic chemotherapy. It is imperative that the surgery, not interfere with the administration of chemotherapy. Previous studies have shown that neoadjuvant chemotherapy does not usually complicate a microsurgical tissue transfer, and similarly, microsurgical tissue transfers do not usually interfere with the subsequent delivery of adjuvant chemotherapy. When compared with the use of local tissues alone or primary wound closure, microsurgical tissue transfer allows for better wound healing when used in association with adjuvant chemotherapy.

Over the last decade, microsurgical techniques have been increasingly utilized to reconstruct bone and soft tissue tumors in the lower extremity. Specifically, with the emphasis placed on limb salvage after compartment resection rather than amputation, microsurgical techniques have allowed the orthopedic oncologist and reconstructive surgeon to work together, resulting in limb preservation. Specifically, in soft tissue sarcoma, where entire compartments are resected, microsurgical transplantation replaces components of both muscle and skin to maintain limb contour and aid in healing. For example, a large anterior compartment resection for a malignancy may expose the tibial cortex. Microsurgery is the only reconstructive option for wound closure. A flap such as the latissimus dorsi muscle could be used to cover the tumor defect. This muscle can also be innervated to assist in dorsiflexion of the foot.[18]

The radiated wound, encountered in the treatment of soft tissue sarcomas, has a high incidence of wound complications after attempted primary closure. Radiated wounds generally have a poor vascular supply, making surgery through these wounds difficult and prone to breakdown. Importing well-vascularized tissue into the wound results in more rapid wound healing and may improve local circulation in radiated areas. For this reason, many centers have adopted the policy that immediate microsurgical reconstruction be performed after tumor extirpation.[19] The results of immediate microsurgical transfers in these cases have been well substantiated and have led to decreased hospital time, decreased costs, decreased morbidity, and increased rate of limb salvage, as well as high patient satisfaction. The traditional treatment for high-grade sarcomas of bone, such as osteosarcoma, was amputation before the advent of free-tissue transfer. Limb salvage surgery has become a viable alternative for many patients due, in part, to the development of more effective perioperative chemotherapy. The success of limb salvage in these patients primarily depends on wide resection margins and the addition of perioperative chemotherapy.

The current management of soft tissue sarcomas or osteogenic sarcomas stresses more conservative resection and limb-sparing operations. Local flaps generally do not provide adequate coverage, and free tissue transfer is often the only option. This type of resection creates complex composite defects of bone and soft tissue that require the use of composite flaps in the reconstructive process, such as an osteocutaneous fibula flap for an intercalary bone defect that also has an accompanying overlying skin defect. A recent study looked at one center's experience with free fibula transfer for long bone defects after sarcoma resection and showed high rates of union and good functional outcomes. Although vascularized fibula flaps may never achieve the native size or shape of a tibia, they can hypertrophy under a mechanical load. This is in contrast to allograft, which can restore size and shape similar to that of resected bone, but essentially acts as a dead spacer for years before bone formation occurs at the graft-host junction. With a lower infection rate and better bony union rate than allograft, reconstruction with a free fibula flap produces a better result than allograft in long bone sarcoma patients who undergo wide en bloc excisions. There are also defects following cancer resection, which large combined soft tissue and skeletal defects. In this setting a double-free flap may be needed to achieve skeletal support with stable soft tissue coverage.[20,21]

Approaching these cases with a multidisciplinary team facilitates the planning of the surgical resection, oncologic treatment, and reconstruction timing. Operative details such as incisions, design of skin flaps, exposure, and preservation of the recipient site vessels should be carefully planned with the ablative surgeon. It is usually possible to establish the soft tissue and bony requirements of the wound early in the operation and to begin the flap harvest concurrent with the tumor resection. If oncologic margins are not predictable, then it is best to complete the resection before beginning dissection of the free flap flaps are indicated to cover neurovascular structures (particularly if radiated), bone devoid of periosteum, and allografts or tumor prostheses that cannot be covered with local tissues. Sometimes blood supply to local flaps may be compromised or vessels may be taken during tumor resection.

Secondary Reconstruction

Patients who undergo secondary reconstruction can be divided into two groups. The first includes those who undergo tumor resection and develop acute wound complications such as skin flap necrosis in the early postoperative period. These patients may require debridement and free flap coverage within the first or second postoperative week. It is safe to let questionable areas demarcate before surgery. Patients who present later with impending allograft or prosthesis exposure should undergo surgery as soon as possible to avoid infection of the implant or allograft.

The second group of patients requires reconstruction several months or years after primary tumor resection. Some of the patients in this group present with chronic unstable soft tissue coverage, wound dehiscence, prosthesis infection, and prosthesis failure or limb growth that compromises soft tissue. Although free tissue transfer adds extra time and technical complexity to the tumor operation, it may also lead to a decrease in amputation rates by decreasing wound complications. In addition, it allows the oncologic surgeon to obtain adequate margins of resection, which may favorably influence amputation rates by contributing to a decrease in local recurrence.

With respect to wound location following tumor extirpation, much of the reconstructive options implemented are based on the same principles and options, which guide lower extremity reconstruction secondary to trauma. In the lower third, although local options exist for small defects, free tissue transfer is often the best choice for both soft tissue and bony reconstruction as needed. In the middle third of leg, the pedicled gastrocnemius based on the sural artery and the soleus muscle based on the peroneal promixally and posteior tibial distally, can be used. For the knee, the gastrocnemius combined with a skin graft has remained a reliable method to reconstruct the knee and popliteal regions. In some situations, a microsurgical tissue transfer around the knee and popliteal region may be needed. A microvascular tissue transfer should be considered when the defects are too large for local flaps, when local tissue flaps are not available due to previous surgery or injury, or when patients have received previous radiation to the local donor sites. An anterior lateral thigh flap, a rectus abdominis muscle flap with a skin graft, a latissimus dorsi muscle flap with skin graft, or a composite latissimus dorsi and serratus anterior muscle flap based on the subscapular system can provide adequate coverage to reconstruct these defects.

Orthopedic Sepsis

Osteomyelitis is now a treatable disease. The classic treatment of osteomyelitis includes thorough debridement of infected bone and necrotic tissue, appropriate antibiotic therapy and, if necessary, subsequent closure of the resultant dead space with well-vascularized tissue. The management of dead space after sequestrectomy relies heavily on the technique of free tissue transfer. Free muscle flaps provide coverage for the debrided bone and soft tissue, obliterate dead space, improve vascularity, and enhance leukocyte function. Advances in skeletal reconstruction and fixation have improved the treatment of patients with osteomyelitis and large (>6 cm) segmental bone defects. In the past, despite successful treatment of osteomyelitis, some patients required amputation due to chronic nonunions. Now, once the bone infection is treated, vascularized bone transplants or bone lengthening using the Ilizarov technique facilitate reconstruction and provide structural stability for limb function.

Local muscles were traditionally used to treat chronic osteomyelitis, and free flaps have been described more recently for this use. Local gastrocnemius and soleus muscle flaps are still used to cover smaller wounds on the upper and middle thirds of the leg, respectively. However, local muscle flaps will not reliably cover defects larger than 25 cm² or those on the distal third of the leg, ankle, or foot. For these defects, free muscle transfers are preferred. The advantages of using the free muscle flaps, such as the latissimus dorsi, serratus anterior, and rectus abdominis, instead of local pedicled muscle flaps, such as the gastrocnemius muscle, are that free flaps provide greater bulk (filling larger wounds), have longer pedicles (increasing flexibility in muscle positioning), and carry larger diameter vessels (facilitating the microanastomoses).

Postoperative Management

Monitoring free tissue transfer is essential to assure transplant success. Many different monitoring devices and techniques have been used with varying levels of success. There is no ideal flap monitoring system, but improving the existing monitoring techniques and a better understanding of the information they give will help improve the salvage rate in cases that develop complications. Clinical evaluation remains the gold standard by which all methods of monitoring need to be compared. This involves observing skin color, temperature, capillary refill, and bleeding characteristics. Changes are often initially subtle and, by the time they are clinically apparent, salvage of the flap may be impossible because of irreversible tissue damage.

One common practice is routine monitoring of patients using an implantable Doppler probe. This is usually done in the intensive care unit for the first 24 hours when postoperative problems most frequently occur after free tissue transfer. With the implantable device, we are able to continuously monitor free flaps and any change in signal prompts an immediate evaluation. The device is usually left in place until the fifth postoperative day.

● COMPLICATIONS

Acute complications occur usually in the first 48 hours and include venous thrombosis, arterial thrombosis, hematoma, hemorrhage, and excessive flap edema. Arterial insufficiency can be recognized by decreased capillary refill, pallor, reduced temperature, and the absence of bleeding after pinprick. This complication can be caused by arterial spasm, vessel plaque, torsion of the pedicle, pressure on the flap, technical error with injury to the pedicle, a flap harvested that is too large for its blood supply, or small vessel disease (due to smoking or diabetes). Management of arterial compromise requires prompt surgical intervention to restore the blood flow.

Pharmacological intervention includes vasodilators, calcium blockers, and anticoagulants for flap salvage presenting with arterial insufficiency. Venous outflow obstruction should be suspected when the flap has a violaceous color, brisk capillary refill, normal or elevated temperature, and produces dark blood after pinprick. Venous insufficiency can occur due to torsion of the pedicle, flap edema, hematoma, or tight closure of the tissue over the pedicle. Venous outflow obstruction can result in extravasation of the red blood cells, endothelial breakdown, microvascular collapse, thrombosis in the microcirculation, and flap death. Given the irreversible nature of the microcirculatory changes in venous congestion that occur even after short periods of time, the surgeon must recognize venous compromise as early as possible. These complications can occur alone or in any combination.

Clinical observation and patient monitoring should alert the surgeon to complications. The surgeon must then decide between conservative and operative intervention. There is frequently little downside but significant benefit to re-exploration in the operating room. However, conservative treatment may be helpful; include draining the hematoma by the bedside and/or release of a few sutures to decrease pressure. In cases of venous congestion, leeches may be helpful if insufficient venous outflow cannot be established, despite a patent venous anastomosis. The leeches inject a salivary component (hirudin) that inhibits both platelet aggregation and the coagulation cascade. The flap is decongested initially as the leech extracts blood and is further decongested as the bite wound oozes after the leech detaches. The donor site should be given the same attention as the recipient site during the postoperative period. Complications of the donor site include hematoma, seroma, sensory nerve dysfunction, and scar formation.

Flap Failure

Occasionally, free flaps fail despite early return to the operating room for vascular compromise. Options for management include the performance of a second free tissue transfer, noting the technical or physiologic details that led to initial failure. Most of the time, free tissue transfers fail due to technical errors in judgment, which can include flap harvest, compromise of the pedicle during the harvest, improper microvascular technique during anastomosis, improper insetting resulting in increased tissue tension and edema, and postoperative motion of the extremity resulting in pedicle avulsion. Although rare, avulsion does occur. The next decision made by the operating surgeon regarding the management of the patient is based on several factors. Obviously, if a patient requires a free flap in the first place, a second free flap should be considered.

If a decision is made not to redo the flap, it could be left in place using the Crane principle in hopes that underlying granulation will be sufficient such that skin grafting can be performed once the necrotic flap is removed. The Crane principle is based on the fact that a local flap or a free tissue transfer that necroses in part or totally can act as a biological dressing or eschar over a wound bed. If there is no infection, then the eschar can be left on the wound bed with hopes that some healing can occur underneath the eschar. This would be in the form of granulation tissue that may form under the eschar. Ultimately, the eschar could be removed and, with an appropriate granulation bed, the wound can be skin-grafted, thus obviating the need for another free tissue transfer. By observing the wound, if such a bed is not produced, then a second flap must be considered. Some prefer not to leave the necrotic flap in place because the flap can become a source of sepsis and further compromise local tissues. Necrotic, nonviable flaps should be removed, and a temporary wound dressing, such as a bead pouch or wound VAC, should be used.[22]

Occasionally, when flaps fail in severely compromised extremities, consideration can be given to amputation in that the morbidity of a second free tissue transfer and perhaps the resultant extremity state renders the extremity less favorable for salvage and more favorable for amputation. If a second free flap is considered, obvious errors that lead to flap compromise need to be recognized. It may be prudent to obtain an arteriogram, evaluate the coagulation profile, and research other issues that lead to failure.

A recent comprehensive study looking at over 580 free flaps performed for lower extremity reconstruction revealed a failure rate of 8.5%.[23] This study spanned over 25 years with 18% of those patients going on to amputation. The remainder was salvaged with secondary free flaps, local flaps, and skin grafting. The most common causes of flap failure included venous thrombosis, infection, and arterial thrombosis. In this study, the researchers noted a significantly higher rate of failures in the first half of the study period with significant improvements in outcome in the latter period. The improved success rate seen in the second half of the study period was attributed to a more critical selection of free flap candidates, improved understanding of the physiology surrounding acute trauma and a more sophisticated multidisciplinary team organization.[24]

● OUTCOMES

The final stage of the reconstructive ladder involves the issue of aesthetic restoration of the limb. Not infrequently, patients are traumatized by scars, skin grafts, and bulky free flaps, and consideration should be given to the psychological comfort of the patient in addressing these issues. The reconstructive ladder could involve the use of staged excision of scars, scar revision, dermabrasion, and tissue expanders to expand the normal skin, recruiting dermal and epidermal elements, followed by transposition of these expanded skin segments to stage out or eliminate unsightly scars. In some instances, even free tissue transplantation can be performed for aesthetic recontouring of limbs, which can be of major psychological benefit to patients and may even allow further reconstruction, if necessary.

REFERENCES

1. Heller L, Levin LS. Lower extremity microsurgical reconstruction. *Plast Reconstr Surg.* 2001;108(4):1029.

2. Zenn M, Levin LS. Microsurgical reconstruction of the lower extremity. *Semin Surg Oncol.* 2000;19(3):272.

3. Pederson W. Limb salvage. *Plast Reconstr Surg.* 1991;1:125.

4. Heitmann C, Levin LS. The orthoplastic approach for management of the severely traumatized foot and ankle. *J Trauma.* 2003;53:379.

5. Godina M. Early microsurgical reconstruction of complex trauma of the extremities. *Plast Reconstr Surg.* 1986; 78(3):285.

6. Levin LS, Aponte RL, Nunley JA. Soft tissue coverage for the foot and ankle. *Foot Ankle Clin.* 1999;8:1.

7. Wei FC, Chen HC, Chuang CC, Noordhoff MS. Fibular osteoseptocutaenous flap: Anatomic study and clinical application. *Plast Reconstr Surg.* 1986;78(2):191.

8. Malizos KN, Nunley JA, Goldner RD, et al. Free vascularized fibula in traumatic long bone defects and in limb salvage following tumor resection: Comparative Study. *Microsurgery.* 1993;14:368.

9. Heller L, Levin LS. Bone and soft tissue reconstruction. In: Bucholz RW, Heckman JD, eds. *Rockwood and Green's Fractures in Adults.* Philadelphia: Lippincott Wilkins & Wilkins; 2001:415–462.

10. Gustillo RB, Merkow RL, Templeman D. The management of open fractures. *J Bone Joint Surg Am.* 1990;72(2):299.

11. Ong SY, Levin LS. Lower limb salvage in trauma. *Plast Reconstr Surg.* 2010;125(2):582.

12. Parrett N, Matros E, Pribaz J. Lower extremity trauma: trends in the management of soft-tissue reconstruction of open tibia-fibula fractures. *Plast Reconstr Surg.* 2006;117(4):1315.

13. Basheer M, Wilson SM, Lewis H, Herbert K. Microvascular free tissue transfer in reconstruction of the lower limb. *J Plast Reconstr Aesthet Surg.* 2008;61(5):525.

14. Levin LS. Microsurgical autologous tissue transplantation. *Tech Orthop.* 1995;10:134.

15. Pinsolle V, Reau AF, Pelissier P, et al. Soft tissue reconstruction of the distal lower leg and foot: Are free flaps the only choice? Review of 215 cases. *J Plast Reconstr Aesthet Surg.* 2006;59(9):912.

16. Follmar KE, Baccarani A, Baumeister SP, et al. The distally based sural flap. *Plast Reconstr Surg.* 2007;119(6):138e.

17. Baumesiter SP, Spierer R, Erdmann D, et al. A realistic complication analysis of 70 sural artery flaps in a multimorbid patient group. *Plast Reconstr Surg.* 2003;11(2):129.

18. Corderio PG, Neves RI, Hidalgo DA. The role of free tissue transfer following oncologic resections in the lower extremity. *Ann Plast Surg.* 1994;33:9.

19. Barwick WJ, Goldberg JA, Scully SP. Vascularized tissue transfer for clusre of irradiated wounds after soft tissue sarcoma resection. *Ann Surg.* 1992;216:591.

20. Hoy E, Granick M, Benevenia J, et al. Reconstruction of musculoskeletal defects following oncologic resection in 76 patients. *Ann Plast Surg.* 2006;57(2):190.

21. Chen CM, Disa JJ, Lee HY, et al. Reconstruction of extremity long bone defects after sarcoma resection with vascularized fibula flap: a 10 year review. *Plast Reconstr Surg.* 2007;119(3):915.

22. Khouri RK, Shaw WW. Reconstruction of the lower extremity with microvascular free flaps: A 10 year experience with 304 consecutive cases. *J Trauma.* 1989;29:1086.

23. Heller L, Kronowitz S. Lower extremity reconstruction. *J Surg Oncol.* 2006;94:479.

24. Culliford AT 4th, Spector J, Blank A, et al. The fate of lower extremities with failed free flaps: a single institution's experience over 25 years. *Ann Plast Surg.* 2007;59(1):18.

chapter 64

Pressure Sores

Lisa C. Moody, MD / Wesley T. Myers, MD / John D. Bauer, MD / Linda G. Phillips, MD

● INTRODUCTION

Pathogenesis

Pressure sores result from ischemia of the soft tissue as a consequence of prolonged pressure, shearing forces, friction, moisture, decreased mobility, decreased sensation, and spasticity. Lindan[1] demonstrated that areas of greatest pressure are found over bony prominences. In the prone position, the knees and chest are the areas of greatest pressure. In the supine position, the buttock, heels, and occiput carry the highest pressure. The ischial tuberosities are at greatest risk for developing pressure sores in the sitting position because pressures can reach as high as 300 mm Hg (Figure 64-1). When external pressure is greater than end-capillary bed pressure (32 mm Hg), there is a decline of blood flow to the tissue and ischemia results. Dinsdale[1] proved that constant pressure of 70 mm Hg applied for 2 hours leads to irreversible ischemia and tissue loss. Muscle is the most sensitive to ischemia and necrosis of muscle can occur before there are overlying skin changes. Shea[1] classified pressure sores based on tissue depth and pathophysiologic changes. Although there have been some modifications over the years, it remains the most accepted pressure sore classification system (Table 64-1). Stage I pressure sores are confined to the epidermis and are defined by acute inflammation and present as an area of nonblanchable erythema. Typically, stage I pressure sores can be reversed by eliminating pressure. Stage II pressure sores have breakdown to the dermis with acute and chronic inflammation and usually possess more defined borders than stage I pressure sores. Wound care and behavioral modification to reduce contributing pathophysiologic factors usually allows stage II pressures to heal without the need for surgical intervention. Stage III pressure sores extend through the subcutaneous fat but do not violate the deep fascia. They can involve fat necrosis caused by thrombosis of small vessels, undermining, and tunneling with thickened epidermal edges in the periphery of the wound. Stage IV pressure sores entail destruction of the deep fascia, muscle, and bony structures and can be complicated by extensive undermining, necrosis of all tissue layers, involvement of the joint, and osteomyelitis.

● PATIENT EVALUATION AND SELECTION

A thorough history and physical examination is imperative in the evaluation of patients presenting for treatment of their pressure sores. Recognition of medical comorbidities, risk factors, and behaviors that contributed to the development of the pressure sore are necessary in order to make changes for optimization of the patient prior to surgery. Diabetes, malnutrition, vitamin deficiencies, spasticity, joint contractures, urinary and bowel incontinence, infection, anemia, smoking, spinal cord injury, and prolonged pressure in the area—all can contribute to development and progression of pressure sores. Spasticity is common among patients with spinal cord injuries and is a contributing factor to pressure sore development and wound dehiscence postoperatively. Higher spinal cord injuries result in an increased incidence of muscle spasticity. Muscle spasticity increases shearing and friction forces and makes transfers more difficult. Patient compliance with lifestyle modification is one of the most important factors to a successful reconstruction. Patient should shift weight every 10 minutes when sitting and every 1 to 2 hours when lying down, keep skin clean and dry, and invest in pressure reducing devices such as air mattresses, air-fluidized beds, and ROHO cushions.

Urinary and bowel incontinence can precipitate the development of pressure sores by sustaining a moist

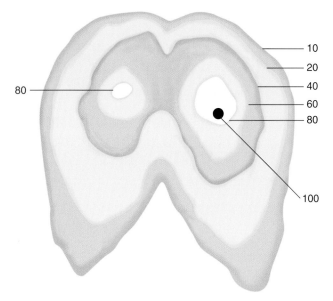

● **FIGURE 64-1.** Pressures over the ischial tuberosities in a patient sitting with the feet supported. (*With permission from Lindan O, Greenway RM, Piazza JM. Pressure distribution on the surface of the human body: Evaluation in lying and sitting positions using a "bed of springs and nails." Arch Phys Med Rehabil. 1965;46:378.*)

environment and leading to skin maceration. Contamination of pressure sores with urine and fecal contents can also lead to wound infection. Pressure sores can be complicated by osteomyelitis of the underlying bone, which is usually polymicrobial. Anemia can be an indicator of poor nutrition or chronic blood loss and should be worked up and corrected.

Contraindications for surgical reconstruction of pressure sores include critically ill patients who are unable to tolerate general anesthesia, sepsis, wound bacterial load greater than 10^5 colony-forming units or the presence of beta-hemolytic streptococci, osteomyelitis, malnutrition, inability of the patient to tolerate prone positioning, failure to control spasticity, and unwillingness of patients to alter behaviors that contributed to the development of pressure sores. Patients who use tobacco products should be counseled regarding smoking cessation. Smoking leads to peripheral vasoconstriction and decreases tissue oxygenation. Continued tobacco use can lead to flap failure.

● **PATIENT PREPARATION**

Stage III and stage IV pressure sores are indications for surgical reconstruction provided that the preoperative evaluation is clear. In diabetics, glucose and hemoglobin A1C levels should be checked and optimized. Hyperglycemia slows wound healing and increases the risk of wound dehiscence and infection. Malnutrition can be assessed by serum albumin, pre-albumin, and transferrin levels. An albumin level greater than 3.5 is a predictor in optimizing wound healing and preventing dehiscence. Vitamin C, vitamin A, copper, magnesium, iron, and zinc are essential for wound healing and should be supplemented when deficiencies exist.

Treatment of muscle spasticity should be implemented prior to surgery. The most common medical treatments for muscle spasms include baclofen, diazepam, and dantrolene. Botulinum toxin is an emerging treatment for spasticity and has been shown to be effective in reducing localized spasticity of the upper and lower limbs with minimal adverse effects. The lasting effects of the botulinum toxin treatment for muscle spasticity are approximately 3 months.[2] A chart review of 28 patients with spinal cord injury receiving botulinum toxin type A (doses 10–119 Units per muscle) demonstrated improvement for 56% of patients in ambulation, 71% of patients in positioning, and 78% of patients in upper-extremity function.[3] A decrease in pain was reported in 83.3% of patients receiving botulinum toxin injections.[3] Splinting and physical therapy can also be beneficial in treating contractures. For those patients who fail medical treatment, surgical alternatives can be explored, and include surgical rhizotomy, amputation, and contracture release.

Wound biopsies should be sent for quantitative tissue cultures preoperatively. Infection is defined as greater than 10^5 organisms and should be treated with appropriate antibiotics prior to surgery. Urinalysis and urine cultures should also be included in the preoperative workup. Paraplegic and quadriplegic patients typically require routine catheterization for urinary retention that predisposes them to urinary tract infections.

If suspected, a workup for osteomyelitis should be instituted. Bone biopsy is the gold standard for diagnosing osteomyelitis. Plain x-rays may demonstrate periosteal

TABLE 64-1. Pressure Sore Stages

	Stage I	Stage II	Stage III	Stage IV
Depth	Limited to epidermis	Through epidermis and into dermis	Extends through subcutaneous fat down to but not through deep fascia	Full-thickness skin loss with damage to deep fascia, muscle, and bony structures
Clinical Signs	Nonblanchable erythema; acute inflammatory response	Mixture of acute and chronic inflammatory response	Fat necrosis, undermining, and tunneling	Extensive undermining and necrosis of all layers of tissue

changes and heterotopic new bone formation, but only have a 54% sensitivity and a 68% specificity.[4] In addition, it can take many weeks for changes to become apparent on x-ray. A negative bone scan rules out osteomyelitis. False-positives on a bone scan can result from trauma, surgery, degenerative joint disease, malignancies, and inflammatory bone conditions. If plain films are normal, the sensitivity and specificity of a bone scan for the diagnosis of osteomyelitis is 94% and 95%, respectively.[4] MRI is an accurate test in the diagnosis of osteomyelitis with a 90% sensitivity and 79% specificity and can detect changes as early as 3 to 5 days.[4] Osteomyelitis is treated with appropriate antibiotics and surgical debridement. Treatment failure is likely to occur without surgical debridement.

In addition to optimizing the patient medically and avoiding pressure at the site of the pressure sore, local wound care can be provided for those with contraindications to surgical interventions. Sharp, enzymatic, and mechanical debridement can be performed at the bedside. Debridement of the pressure sore removes necrotic tissue, decreases the bacterial count, and converts a chronic wound into an acute wound that promotes wound healing and the development of a granulated tissue bed. Daily wound cleansing should be performed with a neutral, nonirritating, nontoxic solution such as mild soap and sterile water. Antiseptic agents such as iodine should be avoided. If infection is suspected, obtain a tissue biopsy and quantitative culture, treat with appropriate antibiotics, and initiate local dressing changes with topicals such as Dakin solution, silver sulfadiazine, or mafenide acetate to decrease the bacterial count. A bacterial count of 10^5 colony-forming units per gram of soft tissue or any level of beta-hemolytic streptococci can impair wound healing.[5] Topical antibiotics should be discontinued once bacterial balance is reestablished. Moist dressings are most appropriate for pressure sores because they promote faster epithelialization than leaving the wound exposed to air. Negative pressure dressings are an alternative treatment that can be used in grades III and IV pressure sores that fail conventional nonsurgical therapy. Negative pressure wound therapy removes exudates and debris, controls bacterial colonization, and promotes tissue perfusion and formation of granulation tissue, but it will not replace large tissue losses.

Once patients are optimized medically, operative planning and preparation can proceed. It is imperative to identify the unique reconstructive needs of each individual. The goal is to provide soft tissue coverage of the pressure sore defect, while maintaining as many options as possible for future use. The recurrence rate of pressure sores has been reported to be as high as 91%.[6] If a patient is ambulatory, a reconstructive procedure should be chosen that will preserve function.

● TECHNIQUE

Surgical interventions for pressure sores include debridement of necrotic tissue and its bursa, ostectomy to decrease bony prominences, and definitive closure of the defect with viable soft tissue. General anesthesia with endotracheal intubation is the most appropriate induction for patients undergoing surgery for pressure sore reconstruction. It is essential to have a definitive airway due to the positioning required for adequate exposure of the operative sites. Succinylcholine should be avoided in the first few months after spinal cord injury.

Prone jack-knife positioning is used for adequate exposure of sacral and ischial pressure sores and lateral decubitus positioning is utilized for adequate exposure of trochanteric pressure sores.

Debridement

Debridement should be performed prior to designing the flap. Once all nonviable tissue is removed, the defect is typically larger than anticipated. The superficial changes of pressure sores can be deceiving in predicting the extent of involvement beneath the surface. In the absence of infection, debridement and reconstruction can be performed in a single operation.

Ostectomy

Bony prominences within the pressure sore are significant contributors to recurrence. Therefore, partial ostectomy is frequently recommended for ischial, trochanteric, and sacral pressure sores. Conversely, total unilateral ischiectomy is contraindicated because it leads to pressure over the contralateral ischial pressure and resultant tissue loss on the contralateral side. Similarly, bilateral total ischiectomies place pressure on the perineum and leads to perineal ulceration and urethral fistulae.

Ischial Coverage

The most common location of pressure sore occurrence is the ischium. Reconstructive options for ischial pressure sores include flaps based on the gluteus maximus muscle, inferior gluteus thigh flap, gracilis flap, V-Y hamstring flap, tensor fascia lata flap (expanded or delayed), and the rectus abdominis flap.

The entire gluteus maximus flap is an excellent first approach for ischial pressure sore coverage because it provides a large skin paddle with large muscle and soft tissue bulk while allowing primary closure of the donor site with minimal tension. In addition, this flap can be re-elevated or rotated for local recurrence and preserves all other local flaps for future use. The inferior gluteus maximus island flap is a good choice for patients who are ambulatory because it preserves function. The blood supply to the inferior gluteus maximus island flap comes from the inferior gluteal artery and venae comitantes with the pedicle running deep to the gluteal muscle, inferior to the piriformis muscle. The inferior gluteus maximus flap originates from the gluteal line of the sacrum and ilium and inserts into the greater tuberosity of the femur and iliotibial band of the fascia lata. The skin paddle should be made as large as possible despite the size of the defect and is centered over the gluteal crease

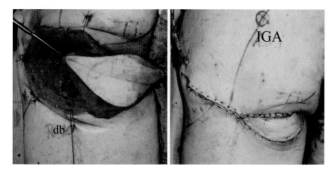

● **FIGURE 64-2.** Inferior gluteus maximus island flap for ischial pressure sore coverage. (*With permission from Scheufler O, Farhadi J, Kovach S, et al. Anatomical basis and clinical application of the infragluteal perforator flap. Plast Reconstr Surg. 2006;118:1389–1400.*)

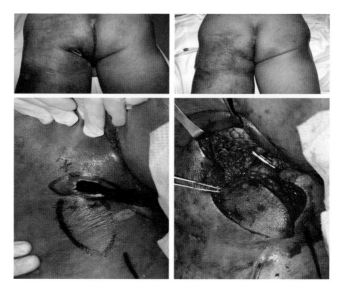

● **FIGURE 64-3.** Inferior gluteus thigh flap for ischial pressure sore coverage. (Above left) Pre-operative view; (above right) 21 months post-op; (below left) flap design (below right) intraoperative view. (*With permission from Kim YS, Lew DH, Roh TS, et al. Inferior gluteal artery perforator flap: a viable alternative for ischial pressure sores. J Plast Reconstr Aesthet Surg. 2009;62:1347–1354.*)

between the ischial tuberosity and the greater trochanter. The medial edge of the skin paddle should abut the lateral edge of the pressure sore. The skin is then incised and the muscle divided distally with several centimeters of muscle exposed beyond the skin island flap. The muscle should then be divided superiorly and laterally to mobilize the inferior half of the gluteus maximus muscle. The muscle is then rotated medially and inset over drains. Lastly, the donor site is closed primarily (Figure 64-2).[7]

The inferior gluteus thigh flap is an effective flap for ischial pressure sore coverage and can be re-advanced in the future should the pressure sore recur. The blood supply to this flap is provided by the descending terminal branch of the inferior gluteal artery. A line drawn perpendicular to the gluteal crease and equidistant between the ischial tuberosity and the greater trochanter marks the central axis of the inferior gluteus thigh flap where the inferior gluteal artery continues down to the posterior thigh. The flap is centered over the posterior thigh and should be less than 12 cm if primary closure is desired. The distal end of the flap can be extended to within 8 cm of the popliteal fossa. Skin incisions are made at the distal end of the flap first. Dissection is carried down to the deep fascia to identify the posterior femoral cutaneous nerve. The posterior cutaneous femoral nerve should be located at the distal tip midline, and confirms that the flap is centered over the vascular pedicle. The descending branch of the inferior gluteal artery is then ligated and the flap is elevated to gluteal crease, rotated into the defect and inset over drains. The donor site is closed primarily (Figure 64-3).[8] The flap does not include muscles, preserving function, but not providing bulk for a large defect.

The gracilis flap is typically a last choice for ischial pressure coverage because these flaps tend to be small (Figure 64-4). The gracilis flap is supplied by the ascending branch of the medial circumflex femoral artery and venae comitantes. The gracilis muscle originates from the pubic tubercle and inserts into the medial condyle of the tibia. The gracilis muscle can be found 2 cm posterior and parallel to a line drawn from the pubic tubercle to the medial

condyle of the femur. The flap should be designed with an 8 × 15 cm skin island centered over the proximal third of the gracilis muscle. A majority of the musculocutaneous perforators supply the skin overlying the proximal third of the gracilis muscle. A small incision is first made over the medial aspect of the knee to identify the tendinous insertion of the gracilis. A suction drain is then positioned around the tendon and upward traction is applied. This allows visualization of the gracilis muscle as it travels proximally and permits confirmation of skin island position over the proximal third of the gracilis. The skin incisions are made and the gracilis muscle is identified superiorly and inferiorly. Temporary sutures may be used to keep the

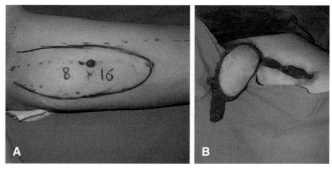

● **FIGURE 64-4.** Gracilis flap for ischial pressure sore coverage. (A) Flap design; (B) elevation of flap. (*With permission from Bagdatli D, Kara IG. Proximally located partial skin-paddle necrosis in the gracilis musculocutaneous flap. J Plast Reconstr Aesthet Surg. 2009;62:424–425.*)

skin island adherent to the muscle. The insertion of the gracilis is then divided and the flap is elevated superiorly while ligating branches of the superficial femoral artery as necessary. The muscle is rotated into the defect and inset over drains.[9]

The V-Y hamstring flap is another option for ischial pressure sore coverage. This myocutaneous flap is based on the biceps femoris, semimembranosus, and semitendinosus. The blood supply to this flap is derived from the perforating branches of the profunda femoris artery. The profunda femoris artery passes through the adductor magnus to enter each of the muscles on their posterior aspect. The semimembranosus, semitendinosus, and the long head of the biceps femoris all originate from the ischial tuberosity. The short head of the biceps femoris originates from the linea aspera of the femur. The biceps femoris is the largest hamstring muscle and travels most lateral to insert into the head of the fibula. The semitendinosus and semimembranosus both travel medial to the biceps femoris and insert into the medial condyle of the tibia. The base of the flap should be designed as the same width of the ischial defect. A V-shaped incision is made from medial and lateral borders of the defect distally. The biceps femoris, semitendinosus, and semimembranosus are divided distal to apex of the skin island. The flap is elevated and the origin of the short head of the biceps femoris is divided at the linea aspera. The origins of the three hamstring muscles are detached from the ischium allowing mobilization of the flap to cover the defect. The flap is inset over drains

and sutured in place (Figure 64-5). The donor site is closed primarily. The V-Y advancement flap can be modified to maintain function of the lower extremity by only utilizing the long head of the biceps femoris for advancement into the defect.

The tensor fascia lata flap is not as reliable in the distal portion of the flap, which is essential for ischial pressure sore coverage. If the tensor fascia lata flap is going to be used for ischial pressure sore coverage, the flap should be delayed or expanded. Delay involves a first-stage incision and primary closure of the periphery of the flap without elevation followed by a second-stage flap elevation and rotation. Lastly, the rectus abdominis flap can be tunneled through the groin for ischial pressure sore coverage.

Sacral Coverage

The V-Y gluteus maximus rotation or advancement flap is the major reconstructive option used for coverage of sacral pressures sores. Both flaps can be advanced past the midline and therefore a contralateral flap can be used. Bilateral gluteus maximus flaps are used for large sacral defects and are usually approximated at the midline. The gluteus maximus flaps provide large bulk and can be re-advanced in the future for recurrence. Ambulatory function can be preserved by solely advancing the superior half of the gluteus maximus muscle instead of performing complete muscle advancement. The blood supply to the V-Y gluteus maximus advancement flap is provided by the superior gluteal

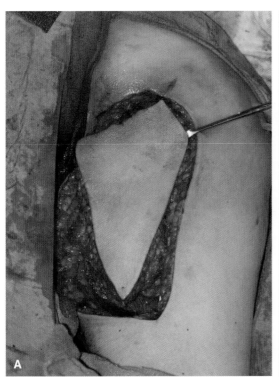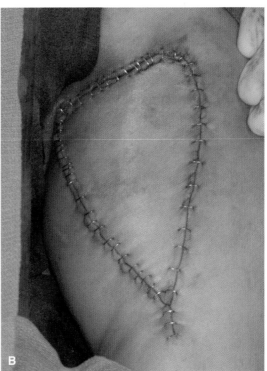

● **FIGURE 64-5.** V-Y hamstring flap for ischial pressure sore coverage. (A) Musculocutaneous flap attached by its vascular pedicles. (B) Flap inset over ischial pressure sore.

artery and the venae comitantes and enters the deep surface of the gluteus maximus at the level of the piriformis muscle. The dominant vascular pedicle enters the muscle at the lateral edge of the sacrum. The gluteus maximus muscle originates from the gluteal line of the ilium and sacrum and inserts in the greater tuberosity of the femur and the iliotibial band of the fascia lata. The superior and inferior boundaries of the muscle are the posterior superior iliac spine and the ischial tuberosity, respectively. The skin island is centered over the medial portion of the muscle and abuts the sacral wound. The skin island should be designed as large as possible to allow for re-advancement should the pressure sore recur. Oblique incisions across the buttocks are made with the base of the triangle abutting the wound and the apex located laterally. The superior and inferior aspects of the gluteus maximus muscle are elevated with blunt dissection and carefully separated from the gluteus medius underneath. The muscle is then divided at the origin. The piriformis muscle is a good landmark for the midportion of the gluteus maximus muscle and identifies the point where the superior and inferior gluteal arteries enter the gluteus maximus. The muscle is elevated over the sacrum and inset over drains into the defect. The muscle is sutured to the contralateral gluteus maximus. The donor site is closed in a V-Y fashion (Figure 64-6).

Trochanteric Coverage

Trochanteric pressure sores usually have extensive bursa formation and undermining despite nominal skin changes.

This is worsened by uncontrolled muscle spasticity and contractures. The most common flaps used for reconstruction of trochanteric pressure sores are the tensor fascia lata (TFL) musculocutaneous flap with or without V-Y modification and the vastus lateralis flap. The V-Y modification provides use of the proximal, more vascularized tissue for coverage. The TFL flap permits elevation of a large skin island despite the size of the muscle. The blood supply to the TFL flap is provided by the lateral femoral circumflex artery, which is a branch of the profunda femoris artery. The lateral femoral circumflex artery enters the tensor fascia lata muscle 10 cm below the anterior superior iliac spine and can have up to three branches that divide the TFL into upper, middle, and lower thirds. The tensor fascia lata originates from the anterior superior iliac spine and inserts in the iliotibial tract of the fascia lata. A line is drawn from the anterior superior iliac spine running anterolaterally to the distal thigh. The posterior portion of the V is drawn from the apex of the anterolateral line to the posterior perimeter of the trochanteric pressure sore. The flap should be large enough to cover the trochanteric defect. The flap is then elevated from the apex progressing proximally. Dissection may continue up to the vascular pedicle. The flap is then rotated superiorly and posteriorly and inset over drains into the defect. The donor site is then closed primarily.[10] The tensor fascial lata flap can be re-elevated and re-advanced in the future for local recurrence. If the TFL has been advanced multiple times, consideration can be given to the vastus lateralis flap (Figure 64-7).

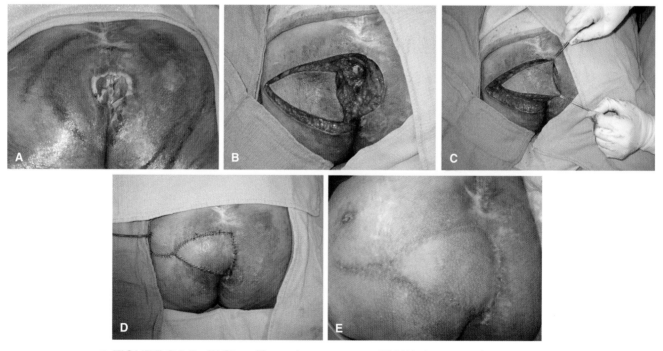

● **FIGURE 64-6.** (A) Stage III sacral pressure sore. (B) V-Y gluteus maximus flap. (C) The musculocutaneous flap is then mobilized to the sacral defect. (D) The musculocutaneous flap is sutured into place with underlying drains. The donor site is closed primarily. (E) Postoperative result.

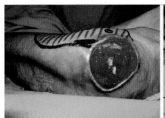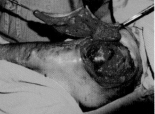
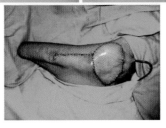

● **FIGURE 64-7.** Tensor fasciae lata perforator flap for trochanteric pressure sore coverage. (*With permission from Ishida L, Munhoz A, Montag E, et al. Tensor fasciae latae perforator flap: minimizing donor-site morbidity in the treatment of trochanteric pressure sores. Plast Reconstr Surg. 2005;116:1346–1352.*)

The vastus lateralis is a muscle flap that must be used in combination with the TFL flap or a split-thickness skin graft because this flap does not have an associated cutaneous territory. In fact, the overlying skin is part of the tensor fascia lata territory. The blood supply to the vastus lateralis is the lateral femoral circumflex artery. The vastus lateralis originates from the greater trochanter, the gluteal tuberosity and the linea aspera and inserts into the lateral border of the patella. An incision is made along a line from the anterior superior iliac spine to the lateral border of the patella. The fascia lata is then incised along the muscle. The vastus lateralis is then separated from the rectus femoris. The origin can then be divided if needed. The muscle is sutured over the defected and covered with a split-thickness skin graft or tensor fascia lata flap. This flap is particularly useful if a girdle stone procedure is performed, as the muscle can be used to obliterate the dead space.

COMPLICATIONS

Long-term sequelae of pressure sores include wound infection, osteomyelitis, septic hip joints, and malignant degeneration of a chronic wound into squamous cell carcinoma. Local wound infections are managed with appropriate antibiotics and local wound care. Osteomyelitis requires appropriate antibiotics and debridement of the involved bone as discussed previously. If the hip joint becomes infected, then proximal femoral head resection (Girdlestone arthroplasty) with soft tissue coverage is recommended for eliminating infection.

Postoperative complications include seroma, hematoma, wound infection, wound dehiscence, flap necrosis, and recurrence. Seromas are usually avoided by placing drains during surgery. Drains should be left in place until output decreases to 20 to 30 mL over 24 hours. If a seroma forms after removal the drains then percutaneous drainage is recommended. Hematomas predispose patients to other complications and should be evacuated immediately. Wound infections should be treated with appropriate antibiotics and local wound care. Wound dehiscence, flap necrosis and recurrence should be treated with local wound care in addition to controlling spasms and optimizing the patient medically. If the pressure sore recurs and becomes large enough, another reconstructive surgery may be necessary.

OUTCOMES ASSESSMENT

Ultimately, a satisfactory outcome is determined by a closed, healed ulcer that does not recur. This apparently simple concept however requires a complex, careful, multidisciplinary approach. Only a combination of medical optimization, nutritional support, control of muscle spasticity and contractures, pressure relief, local wound care and surgical relief will lead to better outcomes and patient and physician satisfaction. Specific metrics for outcome assessment include absence of recurrence, duration until recurrence, and occurrence of surgical or nonsurgical complications.

REFERENCES

1. Bauer J, Phillips LG. MOC-PSSM CME article: Pressure sores. *Plast Reconstr Surg.* 2008;121(1 Suppl):1–10.

2. Sheean G. Botulinum toxin treatment of adult spasticity: a benefit-risk assessment. *Drug Saf.* 2006;29(1):31–48.

3. Marciniak C, Rader L, Gagnon C. The use of botulinum toxin for spasticity after spinal cord injury. *Am J Phys Med Rehabil.* 2008;87(4):312–317; quiz 318–320, 329.

4. Chihara C, Segreti J. Osteomyelitis. *Dis Mon.* 2010;56(1):6–31.

5. Levi B, Rees R. Diagnosis and management of pressure ulcers. *Clin Plast Surg.* 2007;34(4):735–748.

6. Evans GR, Dufresne CR, Manson PN. Surgical correction of pressure ulcers in an urban center: is it efficacious? *Adv Wound Care.* 1994;7(1):40–46.

7. Scheufler O, Farhadi J, Kovach SJ, et al. Anatomical basis and clinical application of the infragluteal perforator flap. *Plast Reconstr Surg.* 2006;118(6):1389–1400.

8. Kim YS, Lew DH, Roh TS, et al. Inferior gluteal artery perforator flap: a viable alternative for ischial pressure sores. *J Plast Reconstr Aesthet Surg.* 2009;62(10):1347–1354.

9. Bagdatli D, Kara IG. Proximally located partial skin-paddle necrosis in the gracilis musculocutaneous flap. *J Plast Reconstr Aesthet Surg.* 2009;62(3):424–425.

10. Ishida LH, Munhoz AM, Montag E, et al. Tensor fasciae latae perforator flap: minimizing donor-site morbidity in the treatment of trochanteric pressure sores. *Plast Reconstr Surg.* 2005;116(5):1346–1352.

chapter 65

Lymphedema

Richard W. Dabb, MD

● INTRODUCTION

Lymphedema is a process of failure of lymphatic drainage resulting in the abnormal swelling of the subcutaneous compartments of the body with protein-rich interstitial fluid. This swelling results in a chronic disability with impaired immunity, susceptibility to infection, impaired wound healing, and subcutaneous fibrosis (Figure 65-1). Regardless of the etiology, it is an exceptionally debilitating clinical problem, which in most cases seems to elude surgical treatment. Of all areas facing the reconstructive surgeon, lymphedema may be the most frustrating and difficult to approach with an anticipation of a successful result.

Interstitial fluid contributes to the nourishment of tissue. Ninety percent of the fluid enters the venous capillaries, the remaining 10%, which is composed of high-molecular-weight protein and water held by osmotic pressure, enter into the lymphatic capillaries. This fluid is transported by pre-collector lymphatic vessels to larger lymphatic vessels and ultimately to the thoracic duct. The superficial lymphatics drain into subdermal channels which parallel the superficial venous system. Other large molecules and particulate matter enter the lymphatic system due to its unique valve-like openings between the cells. Lymphatic drainage is influenced by the contraction of skeletal muscle, arterial pulsation, and contraction of smooth muscle in lymphatic trunks themselves. The lymphatic trunk consists of an endothelial layer, a smooth muscle layer, and a loose adventitial layer. Recent discovery of genes responsible for lymphatic development are adding to a better understanding of both the anatomic development of lymphatics and their pathogenesis.[1] The interruption in the development of the lymphatic system from blood endothelial cells in the evolution of the lymphatic plexus has been now described. The reality, however, is that we know very little about the regional anatomy of lymphatics and are rather unaware of how phenomenally dynamic and complex is the process of lymph flow. Until the recent work of Suami in Melbourne, Australia, there had been no definitive study of lymphatic anatomy for close to 100 years.[2] All anatomic textbook references since then are based on initial anatomic studies performed nearly a century ago. This work shows that there may be, indeed, only two major lymph nodes draining the upper extremity. This could explain the unfortunate cases of lymphedema following sentinel node biopsy.

● PATIENT EVALUATION

Classically, lymphedema has been categorized as "primary lymphedema," which is genetically determined, or "secondary lymphedema" which has been caused by some inciting event. Primary lymphedema may present in several forms. Milroy disease, or congenital hereditary lymphedema comes from an autosomal dominant with incomplete penetrance. It is associated with a genetic mutation on chromosome 5 and may be associated with cholestasis or an intestinal lymphangiectasia secondary to VEGFR3 tyrosine kinase receptor deficiency specific for lymphatic vessels. Meige disease, or lymphedema praecox, usually presents during puberty and constitutes 60% to 80% of all cases of primary lymphedema. This follows an autosomal dominant pattern with association with the *FOXC2* and *VEGFR3* genes. This often presents as a unilateral process and may have associated syndromes such as pulmonary hypertension, cerebrovascular malformations, distichiasis, and the yellow nail syndrome. Lymphedema tarda presents in midlife, and represents 10% of primary lymphedema. It is related to the *FOXC2* gene and the lymphatics show hyperplastic, tortuous vessels with absent or incompetent valves.

Secondary lymphedema is an acquired process. The etiology is usually secondary to destruction of the lymphatic

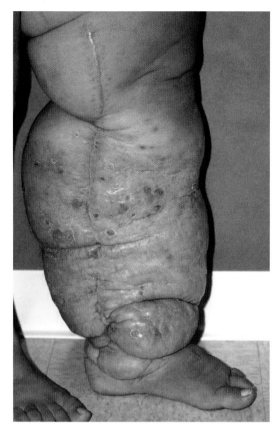

● **FIGURE 65-1.** Chronic lymphedema.

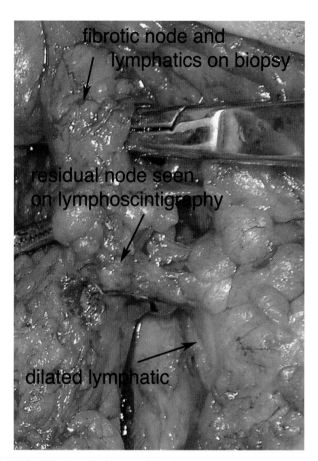

● **FIGURE 65-2.** Residual inguinal node seen on lymphoscintigraphy with fibrosis above and dilatation below. Thirty-year-old woman following radical hysterectomy, node dissection, and radiation.

system by either infectious disease, parasitic or bacterial, or by cancer and its associated treatment. Filariasis is by far the most common etiologic agent of lymphedema worldwide. There are millions of people suffering and due to the infestation with *Wuchereria bancrofti*. Medical therapy centers on the use of anti-helminthics (diethylcarbamazine and Mectizan). Most cases observed in the West are secondary to lymphadenectomy and associated radiation. In addition, lymphedema may develop secondary to metastatic obstruction of lymphatics.

Heffel and Miller[3] present a paradigm concept that lymphedema may present following an insult depending on where one is positioned in the preexisting state of lymphatic anatomy and function. The presentation of secondary lymphedema then is based on one's ability to compensate for trauma and ablation of certain lymphatics depending on one's preexisting location in this paradigm. This concept certainly is consistent with the presentation of a patient with classic spontaneous appearance of lymphedema in midlife following the most minor trauma. However, it may not necessarily apply in all situations, and creates a certain negativity to approach the clinical problem surgically.

With obstructive lymphedema, there is massive dilatation of the lymphatics that remain distal to the injury. This leads to valvular incompetence and has associated progressive fibrosis of the lymphatic walls. Fibrin thrombi accumulate within the lumen of the remaining lymphatics, progressively obliterating lymphatic channels. Spontaneous lymphatic-venous shunts may develop and lymph nodes also become progressively fibrotic (Figure 65-2). The protein-rich fluid causes an increased inflammatory reaction in the subcutaneous tissue. Macrophage activities increased elastic fibers are destroyed along with increasing fibrosis. Fibroblasts migrate into the interstitium and deposit collagen, leading to nonpitting edema. Local immunologic control is suppressed by this process leading to associated chronic infections and possible malignant degeneration with lymphangiosarcoma. Lymphangiosarcoma is quite rare, occurring in less than 0.5% of patients with long-term lymphedema and is usually fatal. As the process progresses, the skin becomes thickened. Ultimately, it takes on a verrucous appearance, develops cracks which leads to further infection. Lymphorrhea may develop.

The process of ablation of lymphatics following proximal trauma has been poorly understood. There are many unanswered clinical questions, such as: Why does a replanted extremity usually not exhibit lymphedema? Why does it take so long for the clinical onset of lymphedema following lymph node ablation? The work of Koshima et al.,[4] showing the progressive proximal to distal fibrosis of lymphatics, may give logic to the selection of appropriate candidates for lymphatic-venous bypass.

● PATIENT PREPARATION

A patient that presents with lymphedema may be managed based upon a treatment algorithm (Figure 65-3). A careful history and physical examination may immediately differentiate between "primary" and "secondary" lymphedema. Patients with true primary lymphedema are referred to physical therapy for careful evaluation and instruction (Figure 65-4).

Conservative therapy needs to be approached at several levels. There needs to be encouragement for a healthy lifestyle, including weight loss, exercise, avoidance of minor trauma, and possibly avoidance of restrictive clothing. The patient is encouraged to carry prophylactic antibiotics and to take them immediately in the presence of the most minor trauma. The use of benzopyrones (Coumarin and flavenoids), agents that effect protein absorption into the vascular system, is controversial. Comfrey, a common weed, has been reported to increase lymphatic flow when prepared as a tea or a wet compress. Occasionally diuretics are indicated. The use of manual compression with low stretch compression bandages and meticulous skin care is encouraged and taught to the patient. Proper fitting compression garments can only be obtained when an optimal result has been obtained by proper wrapping techniques prior to measurement. Endermologie[5] may be effective

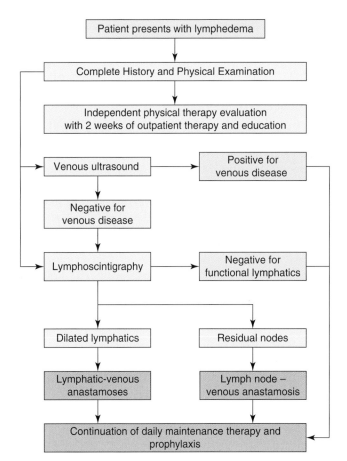

● **FIGURE 65-3.** Treatment algorithm.

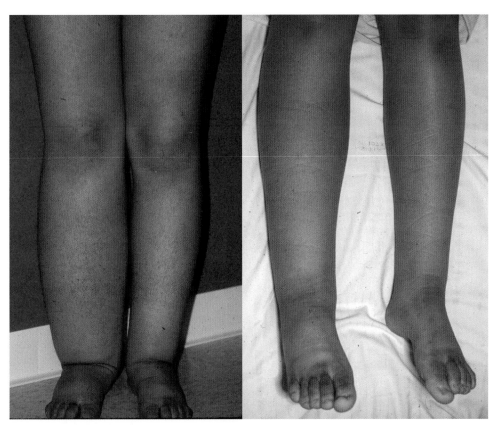

● **FIGURE 65-4.** Congenital lymphedema before and after compression.

to reduce edema and improve the vascularity of the skin. Improvement by conservative modalities of therapy may obviate the need for surgery. Improvement with therapy, however, may also be considered as a positive indicator that one might be a more likely to be a surgical candidate for lymphatic-venous bypass.

The patient with presumed "secondary" lymphedema is referred for venous ultrasound. One must rule out venous insufficiency, prior deep vein thrombosis, and iliac compression disease. If the venous system is competent, the patient is then referred for lymphoscintigraphy. The results of response to therapy, venous ultrasound, and lymphoscintigraphy will dictate the possibility for surgical therapy. The goal of surgery is always presented to the patient as a goal of improvement of their status and not a "cure."

If diagnostic venous ultrasound demonstrates venous insufficiency or venous hypertension, the patient is advised to continue conservative modalities since they are not a candidate for lymphatic-venous anastomosis. Following the venous ultrasound, lymphoscintigraphy is obtained. Patients who are suspected of having lymphedema should not be subjected to lymphangiography. Lymphangiography was the standard for evaluation of lymphatics for many years; however, the inflammatory reaction to the remaining lymphatics may obliterate any remaining vessels. Lymphoscintigraphy, on the other hand, seems to have no deleterious effect on lymphatics. This test helps define the anatomy and patency of lymphatics, dynamics of flow with possible reversal of flow, the severity of an obstructive process, and the presence of residual lymph nodes. If there is no obvious lymphatic activity of the extremity, the pursuit of lymphatic-venous anastomosis is abandoned. Several alternative results from lymphoscintigraphy may be obtained which would encourage the physician to proceed with the procedure. The presence of lymphatics with delayed transit, obstructive lymphedema with dilated lymphatics, and localized areas of obstructive lymphedema are all possible indicators that could benefit from surgery. The presence of a residual lymph node may warrant an attempt at lymph node-venous anastomosis rather than a more distally oriented lymphatico-venous anastomosis.

Prior to lymphatic-venous anastomosis, the patient is encouraged to maximally wrap the extremity and obtain as much result from compression as possible for approximately 2 weeks prior to the surgery. If the patient is unable to do this himself, he is referred to a physical therapist for daily treatment. Immediately prior to surgery, the patient is given an appropriate systemic antibiotic, usually a cephalosporin and an aspirin suppository. One hour prior to anesthesia, technetium sulfur colloid is injected into the web spaces of the involved extremity.

● TREATMENT

The indications for surgery include failed conservative therapy with associated diminishing function, recurrent lymphangitis (more than three episodes a year) and increasing skin changes with lymphedema. Lack of tolerance with the maintenance regimen seems to be the most common reason for a patient to seek a surgical intervention. Surgery should be entertained when the patient understands that continued postoperative conservative management will be necessary, but may be made easier than prior to surgery. A reasonable goal is to continue wraps and compression at night, but to be able to abandon the compression garment during daily activity.

Surgery may be divided into "physiologic" versus "excisional" procedures. Excisional procedures would include sequential liposuction, staged subcutaneous excision, and total subcutaneous tissue and skin excision. These procedures have significant problems with wound healing and certainly have certain indications when a more physiologic approach cannot be obtained.

The Charles procedure involves the excision of all subcutaneous tissue, including muscle fascia and coverage with a skin graft. This procedure has a high morbidity and is usually reserved for the most recalcitrant of cases. The result can be functional, but has significant drawbacks secondary to the skin changes associated with the skin grafts. The Thompson procedure involves the excision of subcutaneous tissue and the burying of de-epithelialized dermal flaps in the muscle. The original goal was to create a lymphatic communication from the subcutaneous tissue to the "uninvolved" muscle compartment. The staged subcutaneous excision originally described by Sistrunk in 1918 and Homans in 1936 was revitalized by Miller in 1998. Seventy percent of Miller's cases showed reasonable results at 8 years. Liposuction as an adjunct to other modalities of treatment has also been suggested. This may be used for proximal reduction of a successful lymphatic venous bypass. The author would prefer to utilize conservative measures when a physiologic operation cannot be a performed.

The concept of local flaps such as omental transposition and entero-mesenteric bridges has been attempted with no demonstrated long-term benefits. It is has occasionally been observed that a free flap, placed in a heavily radiated bed, may also somewhat improve the associated lymphedema. The author's preference of treatment, beyond conservative therapy, is lymphatic-venous or lymph node-venous anastomosis. At the moment, this seems to give the most improvement at the least cost of deformity to the patient. The experience of the author along with Koshima (proposed "supermicrosurgery") has given patients improvement for longer than 5 years.

Lymphatic-Venous Anastomosis

Under general anesthesia, the arm or leg is mapped with a gamma probe looking for dominant lymphatic channels and confirming residual lymph nodes that may have been observed on lymphoscintigraphy preoperatively. Areas are considered for exploration when they have a discreetly higher signal than the surrounding background. Once these areas have been assessed, Lymphazurin

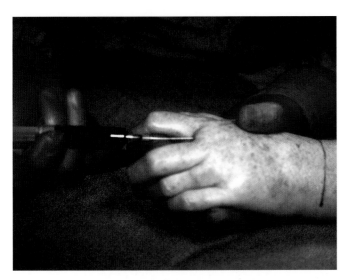

● **FIGURE 65-5.** Injection of lymphazerin dye.

dye is injected into the web spaces of the extremity (Figure 65-5).

Dissection is initiated under the microscope at high magnification through the skin and into the subcutaneous layers. Meticulous dissection follows in the subcutaneous compartment looking for dyed lymphatics that were initially detected by the gamma probe. Potential recipient veins are dissented simultaneously. The dissection process is facilitated by "plucking" the adjacent fat from around these tiny vessels.

Once the appropriate lymphatics and veins are isolated in a region of dissection, the anastomoses are then performed. End-to-side anastomoses are preferred when possible (Figure 65-6). For the smaller lymphatics, a sleeve anastomosis is most frequently used (Figure 65-7). A specialized set of microsurgical instruments and vasodilators (Figure 65-8) are used. Most anastomoses are performed with 11-0 nylon sutures. At least three anastomoses per patient are attempted. Closure of the wound consists of a simple 5-0, subcuticular, polydioxanone suture followed by a skin adhesive. The patient is splinted in a position of function for the first 48 hours. The cases are usually limited to 4 hours of surgery and are performed as an outpatient. Improvement may be observed in the first 24 hours. The patient is instructed to elevate the arm or leg for the first 48 hours, not to wear compression during this period of time, and to restrict vigorous exercise for at least 6 weeks. At approximately 1 week postoperatively, the patient may return to basic maintenance therapy, which includes evening wraps. Most patients are able to abandon their compression garment during the day. The patient is kept on antibiotics for approximately 1 week following surgery.

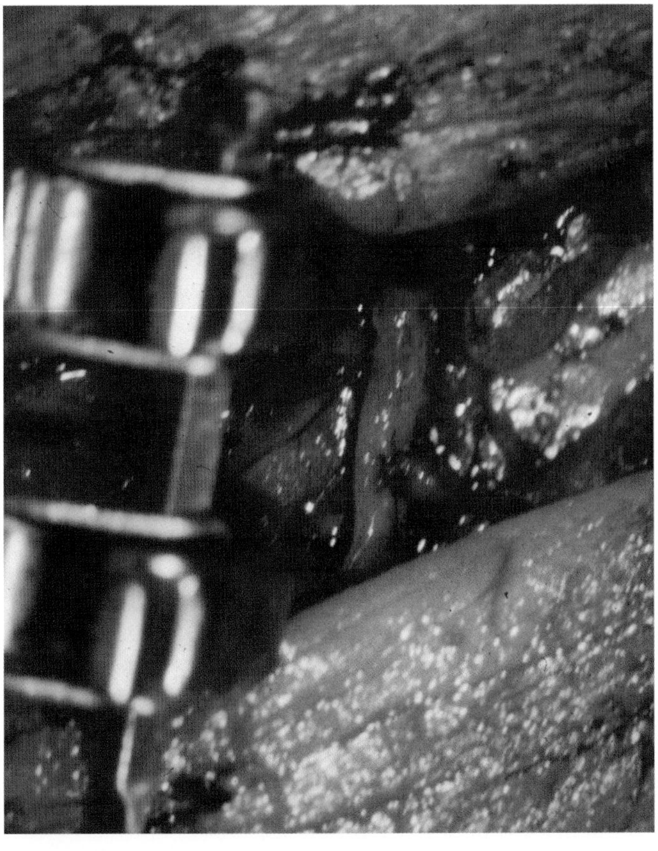

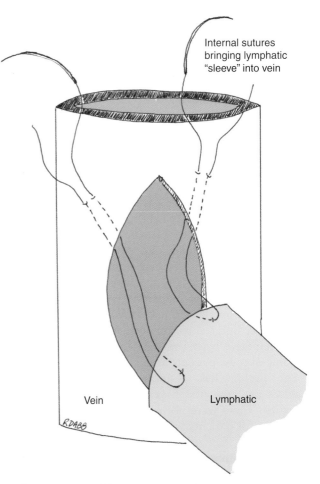

Internal sutures bringing lymphatic "sleeve" into vein

Vein   Lymphatic

RDABB

● **FIGURE 65-6.** Lymphatic venous anastomosis.

● **FIGURE 65-7.** Sleeve anastomosis.

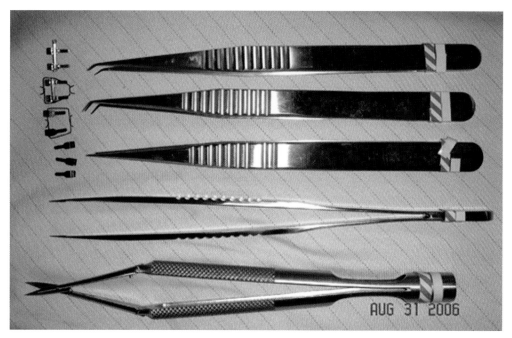

● **FIGURE 65-8.** Instruments for micro-lymphatic surgery.

● **COMPLICATIONS**

Complications may be frequent but are limited to local wound related problems. None of the cases performed by the author experienced immediate postoperative complications. Only one patient experienced worsening of the lymphedema beyond the preoperative status 6 weeks following the procedure.

● **OUTCOMES**

Sequential excision under flaps and lymphatic-venous anastomosis gives the most promising results presently with 70% improvement in long-term results reported. Re-evaluation of the anatomy of the lymphatic system, as described by Suami,[2] and a better understanding of the pathophysiology of the process as shown in the work of Koshima et al.[4] justifies the goal to develop more discreet bypass procedures. The optimal timing of these operations is to be determined. Improved visualization with more exact diagnostic mapping than lymphoscintigraphy or intraoperative gamma probe assessment would significantly improve the outcomes for bypass procedures. There may be a role for robotic surgery with the elimination of tremor. Microsurgical lymph node transfer, stem cell therapy, preemptive bypass may all theoretically change the outcome of these patients in the future.

The author has performed 36 lymphatic-venous bypasses over the past 5 years in the upper and lower extremity. There were no immediate postoperative complications. All patients were evaluated postoperatively at 3 months and then annually. Seventy percent were found to have some improvement in their swelling and discomfort of the extremity. Neurotrophic symptoms, secondary to the swelling, seemed to have significant, immediate

improvement. Two patients experienced an episode of lymphangitis, requiring antibiotics 1 year following surgery. One patient, who underwent a lymph node-venous bypass in the groin, experienced worsening of her lymphedema after initial improvement at 6 weeks. She refused further evaluation or reoperation. It is the author's opinion that measurements of the extremity serve little purpose in judging the merits of the operation because of the significant variation that occurs normally with temperature, amount of activity prior to measurement, and compliance to daily management.

The patients were given a scale from 1 to 10 to rate the procedure as to their level of expectation prior to surgery. Seventy percent of patients favorably related a value of 7 to the procedure at 1 year. They related that they could wrap the extremity for a much shorter period of time at night. Two patients related totally normal function with no need for any maintenance therapy, and rated the procedure a 10. The patient who reported the increased swelling at 5 weeks feels that the procedure should never have been done and that the procedure made her worse.

Not all cases of lymphedema present with the conventional, circumferentially, "swollen extremity." There are cases where a single drainage region of the extremity may be involved, such as a single anatomic compartment. Areas of extensive radiation, such as the abdominal wall, vulva, and breast may be involved in the process and respond to therapy (Figure 65-9). This procedure has the greatest chance of a significant improvement for acquired lymphedema in a properly selected patient. The present success rate may be secondary to being able to better identify functional lymphatics, intraoperatively, with the gamma probe and also related to the emphasis on

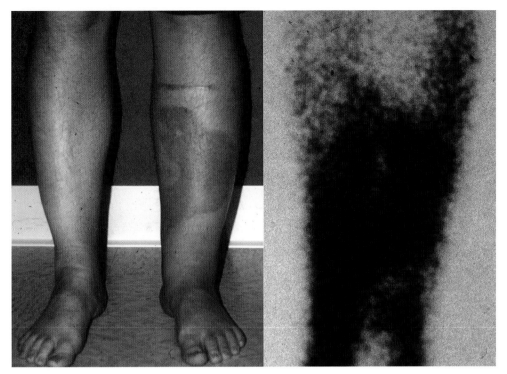

● FIGURE 65-9. Localized lymphedema of the anterior compartment secondary to a "tight" cast. Thirty-six-year-old man with four hospitalizations for lymphangitis in 1 year. Three lymphatic venous anastomosis in the area of involvement gave complete resolution of symptoms for longer than 10 years.

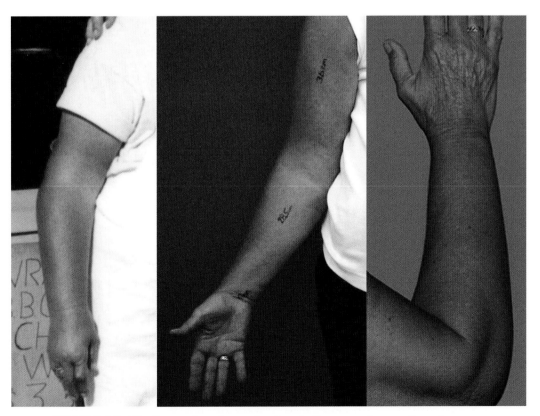

● FIGURE 65-10. Pre- and postoperative lymphatic venous bypass three times at 5 years' post-lymphatic surgery. Sixty-five-year-old woman with 12-year history of lymphedema following radical mastectomy, axillary node dissection, and radiation therapy. She does not wrap or use compression garments.

long-term follow-up with continued maintenance therapy and prophylaxis. When successful, this procedure offers physiologic improvement without the obvious wound-related problems of excisional, debulking procedures.

There seems to be no correlation between duration of onset of lymphedema or whether it is the upper or lower extremity as to clinical improvement following surgery (Figure 65-10).

REFERENCES

1. Alitalo K, Tammela T, Petrova T. Lymphangiogenesis in development and human disease. *Nature.* 2005;438:946–953.

2. Suami H. Mapping the human lymphatic system. Unpublished, Department of Anatomy and Cell Biology, Taylor Lab, University of Melbourne, Australia.

3. Heffel DF, Miller TA. Lymphedema of the extremity. In: Achauer BM, Eriksson E, Guyuron B, et al. *Plastic Surgery, Indications, Operations, and Outcomes.* Philadelphia: Mosby; 2000:4463–4464.

4. Koshima I, Kawada S, Moriguchi T, et al. Ultrastructural observations of lymphatic vessels in lymphedema in human extremities. *Plast Reconstr Surg.* 1996;97:397–405.

5. Campisi C, Boccardo F, Zella H, et al. Techniques in the treatment of peripheral edema: clinical preliminary results and perspectives. *Eur J Lymphol.* 2002;X:35–36.

chapter 66

Foot and Ankle Reconstruction

Mark Warren Clemens, MD / Christopher E. Attinger, MD

● INTRODUCTION

Improvements in surgical technique combined with the introduction of novel wound care modalities has helped reverse the antiquated notion of amputation as the optimal treatment for complex lower extremity wounds. Infection as well as changes in blood supply, sensation, immune status, and biomechanics renders the foot and ankle susceptible to breakdown. Traditionally, the inability to salvage an injured foot usually led to amputation. This carries dramatic sequelae for the amputee because it mandates a lifetime dependence on prosthetic devices or a wheelchair-bound existence. In addition, it shortens life expectancy and places the other limb at increased risk for amputation. Reconstructive surgeons continue to be called upon to address wounds that result from trauma and/or infection. The first task is to convert the existing wound into a healthy wound. Most wounds can then be closed using simple soft tissue techniques such as delayed primary closure, skin grafts, or local flaps. However a significant portion of wounds require more sophisticated techniques that mandate an intimate knowledge of the local angiosomes, arterial blood supply, and flap anatomy. All reconstructions must be biomechanically sound and most require a multiteam approach to avoid recurrent breakdown.

● PATIENT EVALUATION AND SELECTION

A careful medical history should be obtained to evaluate the most likely disease states that directly affect wound healing. Attention should be focused on diseases that may negatively affect arterial inflow into and venous outflow from the wound. Close attention should be paid to the immune system, hematological system, and to nutrition, all of which can affect wound healing. The presence of autoimmune diseases (such as rheumatoid arthritis, pyoderma gangrenosum, systemic lupus erythematosus,

scleroderma, etc) may cause inflammatory wounds that initially require medical management rather than surgical care. Optimizing these wound types with medical management first will then allow wounds to go through the normal stages of healing. It should be noted that the medications used to treat autoimmune diseases (ie, steroids or chemotherapy) can also contribute to poor wound healing. The nutritional status also affects wound healing and should be assessed (optimal is albumin >3.0 g/dL and/or total lymphocyte count >1500). Smoking significantly decreases local cutaneous flow and should be documented and addressed with the patient. Finally, a complete list of medications and drug allergies should be obtained. Given the complexity of various diseases affecting the healing process, multiple medical specialists may be called in to assist in the patient's medical management and help optimize his or her medical condition, so that the wound has a better chance of healing.

● PRINCIPLE ETIOLOGIES OF LOWER EXTREMITY WOUNDS

Before considering wound debridement, the surgeon has to determine the etiology of the wound, any history of previously administered wound therapies, and the patient's overall medical condition. A thorough history should be obtained from the patient, family, friends, emergency medical technicians, and/or referring doctor to help determine the etiology of the wound. In addition, the origin and age of the wound should be determined. If the wound is traumatic in origin, it should be defined in terms of high impact, low impact, repetitive, temperature related, caustic, radiation induced, type of bite, presence of drug abuse, and so on. The patient's tetanus immunization status should be obtained, and the patient should be re-inoculated if revaccination is indicated. In chronic wounds, the age of the

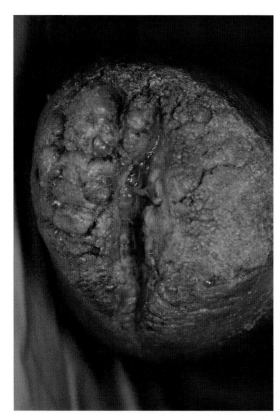

● **FIGURE 66-1.** The chronicity of wounds can be perpetuated by applying a caustic agent to the wound surface. Hydrogen peroxide, alcohol, 10% iodine, etc all negatively affect the healing process. This stump was treated with hydrogen peroxide for 1 year and never healed.

wound is important, because longstanding wounds can be malignant (Marjolin ulcer). Previous topical therapy to the wound should be delineated because certain topical agents can contribute to the wound's chronicity (eg, caustic agents such as hydrogen peroxide, 10% iodine, Dakin solution) (Figure 66-1).

Diabetes is of particular concern to the reconstructive surgeon. Seven percent of all Americans have documented diabetes mellitus and 15% of them eventually develop a foot ulcer during their lifetime. Almost 15% of the health care budget of the United States goes toward management of diabetes, with 25% of diabetic hospital days for the treatment of diabetic foot ulcers. Two thirds of all the major amputations performed per year in the United States are performed in diabetics.[1] With a team approach, more than 97% of these limbs can be salvaged. Salvage not only allows the patient to maintain quality of life but it is also far less expensive for the health care system than major amputations (ulcer $7,500; toe amputation $22,705; foot amputation $42,675; leg amputation $51,280).

Diabetic peripheral polyneuropathy is the major cause of diabetic foot wounds. More than 80% of diabetic foot ulcers have some form of neuropathy present. The neuropathy is a consequence of chronically elevated blood sugars that cause vascular and metabolic abnormalities.

Chronic hyperglycemia leads to the glycosylation of collagen with subsequent loss of elasticity in connective tissues. This is most evident in the Achilles tendon, which looses its flexibility and the foot can no longer dorsiflex beyond neutral. This loss of motion places a high pressure for a prolonged period during the push-off phase of gait both at the arch/midfoot and underneath the metatarsal heads. The excess pressure at the midfoot can lead to Charcot collapse, while at the forefoot it can lead to ulceration at the plantar metatarsal heads. This problem is compounded by concomitant hypoesthesia in neuropathic patient, which robs the patient of the early warning signs of resultant pain.

The surgeon tests the elasticity of the Achilles tendon by evaluating the patient's ability to dorsiflex the supinated foot. If the patient can dorsiflex the foot more than 15 degrees with the leg straight and bent, then the tendon has sufficient plasticity. If the foot can only be dorsiflexed when the leg is bent, then the gastrocnemius portion of the Achilles tendon is tight. If the foot cannot dorsiflex when the leg is straight or bent, then both the gastrocnemius and soleus portions of the Achilles tendon are tight. Open or percutaneous release of the Achilles tendon decreases forefoot pressure in the equinovarus foot during gait sufficiently to allow for healing of plantar forefoot ulcers in an average of 6 weeks (Figure 66-2). The release results in a permanent decrease in push-off forces, which has to been shown to decreasing ulcer recurrence rate fourfold at 7 months and twofold at 27 months (40%). Unless correction of underlying biomechanical abnormalities that led to soft tissue breakdown is part of the treatment plan, debriding and good wound care is usually futile.

Hyperglycemia can also affect the body's ability to fight infection. As a result of this depressed immune state, diabetics are especially prone to streptococcal and staphylococcal skin infections. Deeper infections tend to be polymicrobial, with gram-positive cocci, gram-negative rods, and anaerobes being frequently present on culture. Postoperative complication rates correlate directly with the level of postoperative hyperglycemia.

Up to 60% of diabetics with nonhealing ulcers have concurrent macrovascular disease. The arteries below the popliteal trifurcation are most commonly involved while the smaller arteries of the foot and ankle are often spared. For this reason, distal bypass in the diabetic patient is frequently possible. Noninvasive arterial studies, including ankle-brachial indices, should be performed in every diabetic, and results less than 0.9 should be referred to a vascular surgeon for evaluation. Ankle-brachial indices can be misleading in the diabetic because vascular calcification decreases the compressibility of the vessels. Some therefore feel digital arterial toe pressures greater than 40 mm Hg or tissue oxygen levels (T_CO_2) higher that 40 mm Hg may be more reliable indicators of the quality of blood flow in diabetics. If there is any question, the patient should be seen by a vascular surgeon who is trained in distal revascularization techniques.

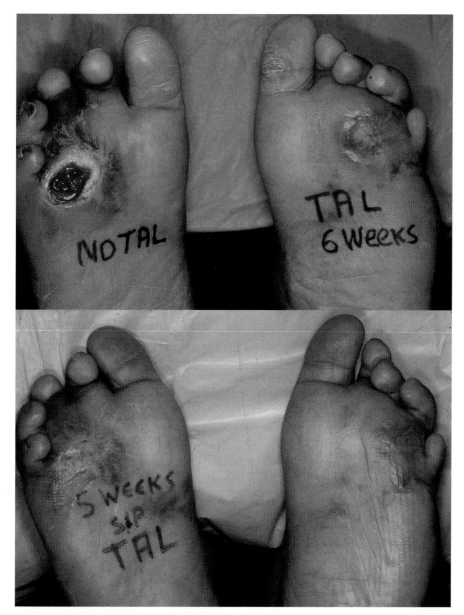

◉ **FIGURE 66-2.** A 39-year-old obese diabetic patient had bilateral lateral plantar metatarsal ulcers secondary to equinovarus deformity (above). Both the gastrocnemius and soleus portions of the Achilles tendon were tight. The left Achilles was released percutaneously, and the left foot healed in 6 weeks with conservative wound care of the ulcer (below). The right forefoot ulcer healed similarly within 5 weeks after Achilles tendon release. Correcting the biomechanical abnormality was all that was required for healing to occur.

Atherosclerotic disease is a common cause of nonhealing foot ulcers, especially when in combination with diabetes. Hypercholesterolemia, hypertension, and tobacco use are major risk factors for atherosclerosis. The etiology of the ischemia has to be diagnosed. If the arteries are not palpable, the Doppler signal over the posterior tibial artery, the dorsalis pedis artery, and the anterior perforating branch of the peroneal artery should be evaluated. A triphasic Doppler signal indicates normal blood flow, a biphasic signal indicates adequate blood flow, and a monophasic signal warrants further investigation. If the quality of flow is questionable, a formal noninvasive arterial Doppler evaluation has to be performed. If the flow is inadequate, the patient should then be referred to a vascular surgeon who specializes in endovascular techniques and in distal revascularizations. Debridement should be delayed in a stable wound with dry gangrene and inadequate blood flow, until blood flow has been corrected (Figure 66-3). Premature debridement of a de-vascularized wound may cause future loss of potentially salvageable tissue. However, immediate debridement is called for when wet gangrene, ascending cellulitis from a necrotic wound, or necrotizing fasciitis

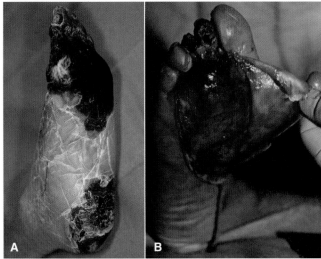
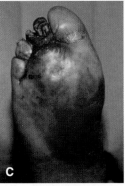

● **FIGURE 66-3.** A patient with dry gangrene and no cellulitis should be evaluated by the vascular surgeon and revascularized before debridement to save a maximal amount of tissue (A). However, if there is wet gangrene, surrounding cellulitis from a necrotic wound base, or necrotizing fasciitis, the wound should be debrided immediately (B, C).

are present (Figure 66-3). Revascularization should follow as soon as possible thereafter. It is important to remember that optimal tissue oxygenation around a wound after bypass surgery takes 6 to 10 days, and with endovascular surgery it can take up to 28 days. Premature wound closure fails to take full advantage of the revascularization.

The connective tissue disorders (eg, systemic lupus, rheumatoid arthritis, and scleroderma) are frequently associated with Raynaud disease that causes distal vasospasm and cutaneous ischemia. More than 60% of these wounds have a coagulopathy associated with them. The treatment of these connective tissue disorders frequently requires immunosuppressive drugs such as steroids or chemotherapy agents as well as anticoagulation regimens. The wound retarding effects of steroids can be partially reversed with oral vitamin A (20,000 U/day every other day while the wound is open) and topical vitamin A.

Venous stasis ulcers are three to four times more prevalent than arterial ulcers and are caused by local venous hypertension. The leg has a superficial and deep venous system connected to one another by perforators. Blood flow is largely due to muscle contracture which compresses the veins while directional flow is due to the presence of unidirectional valves that prevent backflow. The valves become incompetent after thrombus formation or with old age. Surgical treatment of incompetent saphenous or lesser saphenous vein or of incompetent perforators can help relieve the local venous hypertension sufficiently to allow the wound to heal. The mainstay of venous ulcer therapy has been compression therapy accompanied by an exercise regimen that increases venous return to the heart. Chronic ulcers may benefit from aggressive wound debridement and application of cultured skin derivatives.

Wound Evaluation

The wound should be assessed carefully by measuring its size and depth. The area is determined by multiplying the length and width along the two longest axes perpendicular to one another (Figure 66-4). The depth and type of exposed tissue (dermis, subcutaneous tissue, fascia, muscle, and/or bone) should then be established. The wound should be photographed and referenced with patient identification data and a ruler. If cellulitis is present, the border of the erythema should be delineated (Figure 66-5). The physician can then determine before the culture results are available whether the initially prescribed antibiotics and/or initial debridement is successfully addressing the infection. If the erythema has extended beyond the inked boundary, either the antibiotics are inadequate or the wound has been inadequately debrided.

The depth of the wound should be carefully assessed for tendon, joint, or bone involvement. A metallic probe

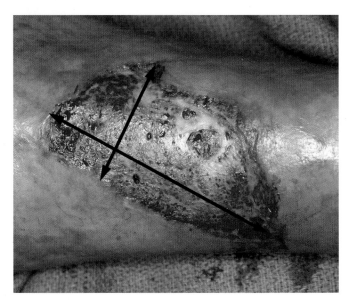

● **FIGURE 66-4.** The wound area is crudely determined by measuring the longest horizontal and vertical axes of the wound that are perpendicular to one another. The product is then recorded. Then the depth of the wound and the type of tissue exposed at the base of the wound are also recorded. A picture of the wound is then taken and remains part of the medical record.

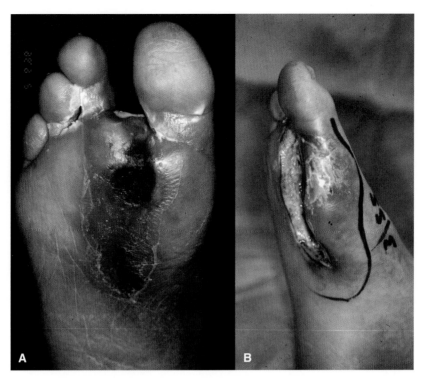

● **FIGURE 66-5.** A gangrenous forefoot with surrounding cellulitis (A) is initially debrided to viable tissue. The border of the erythema around the wound is then delineated with indelible ink (B). The time and date are likewise inscribed. The wound is then checked 4 to 6 hours later. If the erythema recedes, then the debridement and antibiotics chosen were appropriate initial treatment. If the erythema progresses beyond the border, then further debridement is necessary and/or the antibiotics need to be changed.

(Figure 66-6) can be used to assist in evaluating the depth of the wound. If the probe touches bone, there is an 85% chance that osteomyelitis is present and a radiograph should be obtained. It is important to remember that it can take up to 3 weeks for osteomyelitis to be visible on a radiograph. Magnetic resonance imaging is considered the accepted standard in diagnosing osteomyelitis in diabetic foot ulcerations. However, both magnetic resonance imaging and nuclear scans are expensive and unnecessary if the bone is going to be directly evaluated during debridement. These studies are useful if the extent of osteomyelitis in the suspected bone is unclear or if there is suspicion that other bones may be involved. If tendon is involved, the infection is very likely to have tracked along its sheath. The tendon sheath should be checked for bogginess and milked toward the open wound to assess whether there is purulence. If pus appears, then that tendon sheath will have to be opened along the infected track. If the suspicion is strong that a distal infection has spread proximally, the proximal areas where the tendon sheaths are readily accessible should be checked. This can be done with a simple needle aspiration or the strategic placement of a small incision and spreading with a straight clamp to the tendon sheath.

Sensation and motor function must also be assessed. A careful nerve examination is crucial in traumatic sounds

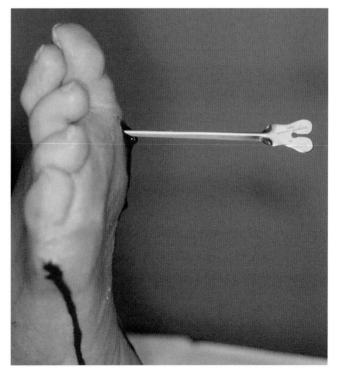

● **FIGURE 66-6.** A metal probe can be very useful for determining whether bone lies at the base of the wound. If bone is palpated, then there is an 85% chance that osteomyelitis is present.

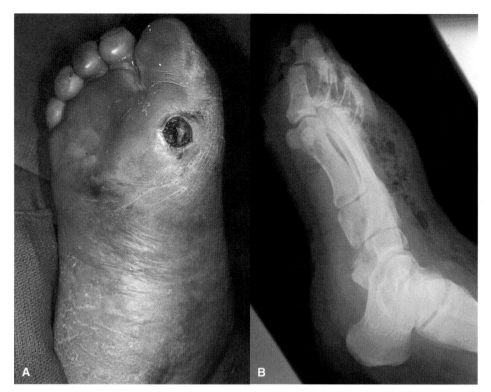

● **FIGURE 66-7.** (A) A diabetic patient with a plantar ulcer rapidly developed a massively swollen and erythematous foot that had crepitus when examined. (B) Radiograph revealed gas both on the plantar and dorsum of the foot. The patient was taken to the operating room immediately for radical debridement. It is important to remember that while the tissue usually involved is at and above the fascial layer, there may be elevated compartment pressure underneath that will also need to be addressed.

and assessing compartment syndrome. This sensory loss impairs patients from realizing damage that occurs due to excessive local pressure from prolonged decubitus position; from tight shoes, clothes, or dressings; from biomechanical abnormalities; or from the presence of foreign bodies.

In the infected wound, it is important to know the source and extent of the infection. Obtaining a radiograph of the affected area lets the physician know whether the bone is involved and whether gas is present in the soft tissue (Figure 66-7). If gas is seen within the tissue planes on the radiograph, then gas gangrene is present and the wound becomes a surgical emergency. This gas is usually a byproduct of anaerobic bacteria (usually *Clostridium perfringens*); it tends to be foul smelling and to travel along the fascial planes. If there is a question of a deep abscess, ultrasound imaging or computed tomography scanning can be very useful.

If the wound is acutely infected with draining purulence, with odor emanating from it and/or with proximally ascending erythema, it needs to be debrided immediately and very aggressively to prevent limb loss or death. The involved compartments of the extremity should be released if there is any question that the compartment pressures are abnormally high. It is important to remember that just because an extremity presents with gas gangrene, it should *not* be summarily amputated, because aggressive

repetitive debridement, with or without hyperbaric oxygen, can often salvage enough of the limb to preserve a functional extremity. Hyperbaric oxygen has been shown to be particularly helpful in the control of anaerobic infections (Figure 66-8).

Aerobic and anaerobic cultures of the wound are obtained during the debridement by taking pieces of deep infected tissue and purulence. A swab or superficial tissue culture is of limited use, because it usually reflects surface flora rather than the actual underlying bacteria responsible for the infection. One should then debride the wound as specified above and start broad-spectrum antibiotics after the deep tissue cultures have been obtained. The antibiotic spectrum can be narrowed as soon as the culture sensitivities become available. It is important to remember that a deep culture may miss up to two thirds of the bacteria species present. Persisting signs of infection may be due to inappropriate antibiotics or undrained purulence or necrotic tissue.

For suspected osteomyelitis, obtain cultures of both the debrided osteomyelitic bone and the normal bone proximal to the area of debridement. When only healthy bone remains at the base of the wound, a one-week course of appropriate antibiotics usually suffices. The exception to a 1-week course of antibiotics after closure is when the surgeon suspects that the bone left behind may still harbor

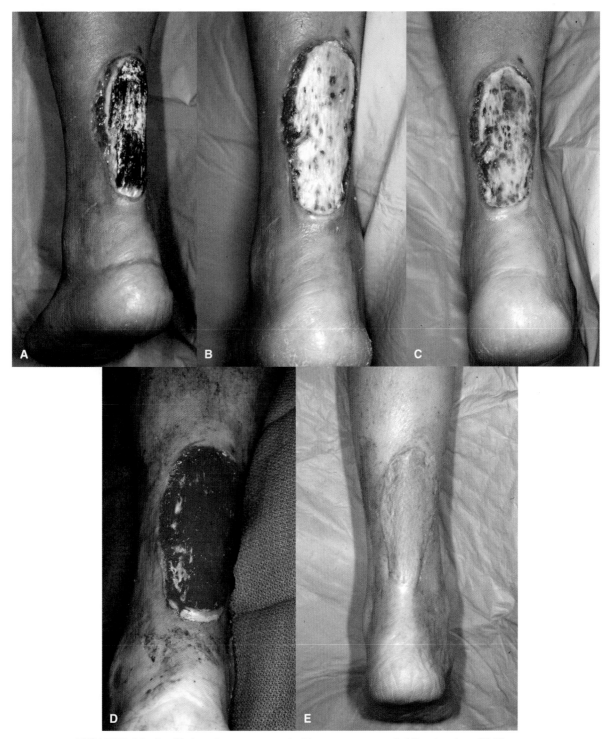

● **FIGURE 66-8.** (A) A patient presented with a gangrenous Achilles tendon. (B) The necrotic tendon was sharply debrided to shiny underlying tendon. Hyperbaric oxygen and topical growth factor therapies were started, and the tendon began to granulate (B, 1 week; C, 2 weeks; D, 3 weeks). The Achilles tendon was then successfully skin grafted and healed completely after 4 weeks (E).

osteomyelitis (eg, calcaneus or tibia). In that case, a longer course of antibiotic therapy is needed. The appropriate antibiotic course is best determined and monitored by an infectious disease physician for treatment as well as for untoward side effects.

The patient's current and anticipated level of activity is important to assess to best determined if the leg should be salvaged and to what degree it should be reconstructed. If the patient is using the leg in any way, including simple transfers, then salvage is usually indicated. However, if the limb is not going to be used, then strong consideration should be given to performing a knee disarticulation or above knee amputation to cure the problem and minimize the risk of recurrent breakdown.

The complexity of the reconstruction depends on the ultimate functional goal. For the younger patient or athlete who can tolerate microsurgery, restoration of normal function is the goal. However, a fancy reconstruction with a marginally functional leg may limit activity more than a below knee amputation with an athletic prosthesis. For the patient who uses the leg simply to transfer, the simplest solution that will achieve that goal should be chosen even if it means sacrificing part of the foot.

● PATIENT PREPARATION AND STAGING

If a wound has responded to aggressive antibiotic therapy, healthy granulation should appear, edema should decrease and neo-epithelialization should appear at the wounds edge. The surgeon may be tempted to proceed to definitive closure after initial debridement of a chronic wound. The complication rate of single-stage closure is high because bacterial identification and clearance may not have been achieved. Studies looking at one-stage amputations (definitive below or above knee amputations) versus two-stage amputations (open ankle guillotine amputation followed by definitively closed below or above knee amputations) yielded a wound complication rate of 21% versus 0%, respectively. It is therefore useful to wait for closure 2 to 3 days after initial debridement until definitive bacterial cultures are known, glycemic control addressed, and nutritional deficits corrected. Whenever closing a wound, it should first be completely re-debrided to ensure that no residual biofilm is present. A double instrument setup, consisting of an additional set of instruments, gloves, gowns, drapes, suction, and Bovie is then used to avoid contaminating the reconstruction of the freshly debrided wound with the just contaminated debriding tools.

Adequate Debridement of Wound

The most important surgical step in treating any wound is to perform adequate debridement to remove all foreign material and unhealthy or nonviable tissue until the wound edges and base consist only of normal and healthy tissue. Only an atraumatic surgical technique (sharp dissection, skin hooks, bipolar cautery, etc) should be used to avoid damaging the underlying healthy tissue (Figure 66-9) that will provide all the necessary ingredients for the future healing process. Damaging the wound edge by crushing or burning may establish a nidus for bacteria to proliferate. This becomes even more apparent when dealing with the severely immunocompromised patient with poor blood flow (ie, the renal failure diabetic patient with peripheral vascular disease).

The goal of surgical debridement is to excise the wound until only normal, soft, well-vascularized tissue remains. Using a simple color scale to guide debridement can be helpful. Debride until the only tissue colors present are red, yellow, and white. Any tissue of any other color (except a blue patent vein) should be removed. The tone of the tissue can also guide the debridement. Getting rid of hard, indurated soft tissue until only normal soft tissue is left is ideal. For tendon, any soft liquefied tissue should be removed until only hard shiny tissue is left. For infected or diseased bone, all soft bone should be removed until only hard bone with punctuate bleeding is left. Although a tourniquet is frequently placed as a precautionary measure, it is preferable to debride the wound without an inflated tourniquet, so that the quality of bleeding at the debrided wound edges can be continually assessed. Bleeding can usually be stopped with gentle pressure with or without topical coagulants. Pinpoint cautery or suture ligation may be necessary. The debrided tissue should be sent for pathologic analysis for a specific diagnosis of osteomyelitis, vasculitis, or cancer. Deep tissue cultures should always be obtained.

For the sensate patient, a regional block allows the health professional to debride aggressively in the office under most circumstances. The wound should be debrided in the operating room if the wound cannot be adequately anesthetized with a regional block or if the debridement will lead to bleeding that may be difficult to control.

Role of Negative Pressure Dressings

Once the wound is clean and adequately vascularized, then it can be covered with a negative pressure dressing. The vacuum dressing applies subatmospheric pressure to a wound via a closed suction mechanism.[2] The subatmospheric pressure decrease edema, removes wound healing inhibitory wound healing factors, increases local blood flow, and alters the cellular cytoskeleton. The combination of these factors stimulates the rapid formation of new tissue. The negative pressure dressing should only be used on clean, debrided wounds. If the wound is ischemic or still has necrotic tissue in it, its use is counterindicated. In the former case, it can cause further necrosis of the wound edges. In the latter case, an infection can develop.

Negative pressure dressings have changed the way wounds are currently being treated.[3] It is an excellent initial dressing after wound debridement because it decreases edema as well as the local bacterial count. It is an excellent temporizer because it allows the reconstructive surgeon time before committing to a definite reconstruction. The reconstructive plans are usually simplified because the dressing shrinks the size of the wound so that most wounds can be closed with a combination of local flaps and skin grafts. Small wounds can heal by secondary intention more rapidly with the application of a vacuum dressing. Most wounds develop sufficient granulation tissue to cover or fill in a defect, so that the wound can then be skin grafted. The area over an exposed fracture or joint can be covered with a local or pedicled flap while the rest of the wound is skin grafted.

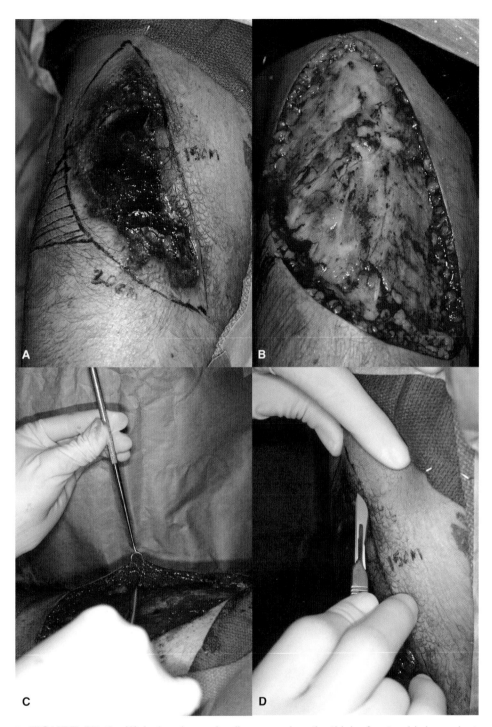

● **FIGURE 66-9.** (A) A chronic, nonhealing wound on the thigh of a steroid-dependent diabetic patient with renal failure. Thorough debridement to healthy bleeding tissue both at the wound edges and base was required to convert this wound to an acute wound, so that it can go on to heal (B). The key in debridement is to avoid damaging the residual tissue by using excellent atraumatic surgical techniques. This means using skin hooks for retraction (C) rather than crushing forceps, and sharp dissection with a knife (D) rather than cautery to minimize damage to the tissue left behind.

● TECHNIQUE

Once the wound is clean, the reconstructive ladder encompasses the following options: (1) allowing the soft tissue defect to heal by secondary intention, (2) closing the wound primarily, (3) applying a split- or full-thickness skin graft, (4) rotating or advancing a local random flap, (5) rotating a pedicled flap, or (6) coverage with a microvascular free flap. The solution is guided by the patient's health, the depth of the wound, the location of the wound, and the surgeon's experience. Useful guidelines suggest simple coverage if there is no tendon, joint, or bone exposed within the wound. For more complex defects that involve exposed vital structures, flaps (local, pedicled, or free) are usually necessary. The exception here is that wounds over the Achilles tendon tolerate skin grafts very well if they develop an adequate granulation bed. In the foot, creative amputations that preserve length are often the most rapid way of obtaining adequate soft tissue envelope with minimal sacrifice of function. Using these criteria, more than 90% of all wounds can usually be closed by simple techniques and less than 10% require flaps.

Because one is dealing with a previously infected wound, deep sutures should be avoided and the wound should be closed with as few non-dissolving monofilament (least reactive) sutures as possible. This minimizes the amount of foreign material within the wound that can potentiate subsequent infection. Closing with vertical mattress sutures creates good tissue eversion along the wound's edge without requiring deeper sutures. Interrupted suture closure allows the surgeon to remove one or two of the overlying sutures when draining an underlying seroma or hematoma.

Delayed Primary Closure

When closing a wound by delayed primary closure, the wound edges have to be freshly debrided and the wound should be closed without tension. Because the leg, ankle and foot consist of a circumferential soft tissue envelope around a boney pillar, it is easy to apply excessive circumferential pressure when a wound is closed too tightly. It is therefore important to check distal arterial pulses pre and post closure to avoid compromising distal blood flow.

Often the skin edges are too far apart to close primarily (ie, post-fasciotomy, post-fracture). Gradual re-approximation of the skin edges is possible by serial operations every 2 to 3 days where the skin edges are approximated up to the point of blanching with horizontal mattress sutures. A vacuum-assisted closure (VAC) can be placed over the remaining soft tissue gap to help decrease the edema and make the surrounding tissue more mobile.

Skin Graft

The skin graft is the simplest of all coverage techniques, with the only prerequisite being a wound with a bed of healthy granulation tissue. The superficial layer of granulation tissue is removed to ensure that there is minimal bacterial contamination within the interstices of the granulation buds. The use of the Versa Jet (a water-based debriding agent) in this setting is ideal because one can precisely adjust the depth of debridement and rapidly establish a smooth and level recipient bed. It also removes all residual biofilm, reducing the risk of infection.

Preferable donor sites include the ipsilateral thigh, leg, or instep. The size of the defect is measured to determine the amount of skin graft needed. The thickness of the harvest is set at 15/1000″, which is an effective compromise between adequate take rate and skin graft contraction. If

the skin at the donor site is flabby or hard to stabilize, the area should be tumesced by injecting sufficient normal saline into the donor site until the entire site is firm. The harvested skin graft can then be meshed (1:1) to allow for a natural egress of the inevitable buildup of underlying fluid or blood but need not be stretched as this may increase healing time. A larger ratio of meshing (ie, 3:1) is often difficult with which to work because it allows the bridges of skin to rotate so that the epidermis faces the wound bed. Spraying the recipient site with topical thrombin just before placing the skin graft helps control bleeding at the recipient site. The graft can be secured to the recipient site using skin clips or absorbable monofilament suture. Although a bolster dressing can be used to stabilize the skin graft over the recipient bed, a VAC is more effective and provides successful skin graft take rates of as high as 95%.[4] The fresh skin graft is first covered with a nonadherent dressing (silicone or Vaseline mesh). A VAC sponge is then placed on top and continuous pressure is applied for postoperative days 3 to 5.

When considering skin grafting over bone, tendon, or joint, creating a neodermis improves the chances of skin graft flexibility and durability. Integra artificial dermis is composed of an overlying removable silicone film (to prevent desiccation) with an underlying dermal matrix of cross-linked bovine collagen and chondroitin sulfate.[5] The dermal layer functions as a dermal template to facilitate the migration of the patient's own fibroblasts, macrophages, lymphocytes, and endothelial cells as well as new vessels. The sheet of Integra is meshed, cut to fit the wound, and affixed to the site with staples or suture. Over the ensuing week(s), a new cell populated dermis is formed. The revascularization process is accelerated three- to fourfold by placing a VAC over the sheet of Integra. Then, the silicone layer can be removed so that a thin skin autologous skin graft (8/1000″–10/1000″) can be placed on it.

For wounds on the weight-bearing portions of the foot (heel, lateral midfoot, under the metatarsal heads), plantar glabrous skin grafts should be considered. These should be harvested from the nonweight-bearing portion of the plantar foot: the instep. The instep is infiltrated with normal saline to create a smooth but firm harvesting surface. The graft is harvested at a thickness of 30/1000″. The instep should be covered with a thin autograft (8/1000″–10/1000″) from the thigh so the donor site can heal without problem. The glabrous skin graft is then inset over the recipient site and sewn in with a 5-0 monofilament suture. Because of its thickness, the graft takes longer to heal and weight bearing should not be allowed until the graft has completely healed. The graft may take up to 6 to 8 weeks to heal but should hold up better than a normal skin graft to the normal wear and tear that occurs with ambulation.

Local Flaps

Local flaps are flaps with unidentified blood supply adjacent to a given defect that are either rotated on a pivot point or advanced forward to cover the defect. They come in various shapes (square, rectangular, rhomboid, semicircular or bi-lobed). They usually consist of skin and the underlying fat or skin, fat, and the underlying fascia. It is important to carefully pre-plan the flap by first accurately determining the size of the defect that needs to be covered after debridement. **Only exposed bone, tendon, nerve, or joint need flap coverage while the rest of the wound can be skin grafted.** This combination of limited local flap and skin graft frequently obviates the need of larger pedicled or free flaps. If correctly designed, a local flap can also improve the surgical exposure of the underlying tissue if corrective bone surgery has to be performed. The harvesting of an appropriately designed flap often improves the exposure of joints, bone or tendons sufficiently to avoid making an extra incision. In addition, local flaps are a very useful mode of reconstruction when trying to close a wound within the confines of an external fixation device.

The ratio of length to width is critical for the survival of the tip of the flap.[6] Because the blood flow to the skin in the foot and ankle is not as developed as in the face, the length-to-width ratio should not exceed a 1:1 or 1:1.5 ratio. The length-to-width ratio of a flap can be increased when one can Doppler out a cutaneous perforator at the base of the planned flap. To ensure adequate tension-free coverage, the flap should be designed in the area where the tissue is the most mobile and a slightly larger pattern should be used than what would anatomically be necessary. A force of 25 mm Hg causes enough venous congestion for flap necrosis unless the tension is released within 4 hours. If the flap remains pale when inset, it should be rotated back into its bed and delayed for 4 to 7 days while it develops more robust blood supply. During that time, a VAC can be placed on the open wound to ensure that no edema develops.

Atraumatic technique is a necessary prerequisite when dissecting the flap (bipolar cautery, sharp dissection rather than cautery dissection, grasping flap with skin hooks rather than pickups, etc.) and when insetting the flap (half buried horizontal mattress or simple vertical mattress stitch with nonreactive suture). The stitches are biased to bring the flap toward the distal edge of the defect. This minimizes tension at the most vulnerable distal of the flap: its distal end.

In order to increase the size of the random flap beyond the 1:1.5 ratio without risking necrosis, the flap should to be delayed for 4 to 10 days. The simplest way to accomplish this is to incise both sides, and undermine the flap. The incisions are then closed. This interrupts vertical blood flow from the underlying muscle or artery to the center of the flap and forces the blood to flow from the base of the flap toward the tip and vice a versa. When the flap has been sufficiently delayed, the tip is incised and the flap is elevated and rotated into position.

Specific Local Flaps

The *rotation flap* is useful on the plantar aspect of the foot where the flap is elevated off the plantar fascia and rotated into position. It can also be used over the plantar forefoot, at both malleoli, and on the dorsum of the foot. If vascular anatomical considerations dictate, the flap can also include underlying fascia and or muscle. The *transposition flap* is the most frequently used option to cover the malleoli or exposed tibial-talar fusion around an Ilizarov frame. The *V-Y flap* is especially useful for defects on the sole of the foot. It depends on direct underlying perforators to stay alive and hence is dissected out by simply cutting through skin fat and fascia without any undermining. Its advancement is limited to 1 to 2 cm, so that if the defect is large, double opposing V-Y flaps should be considered.

Pedicled Flaps

Pedicled flaps have identifiable blood vessels feeding the flap. They can contain various tissue combinations, including cutaneous, fascio-cutaneous, muscle, musculo-cutaneous, osteo-cutaneous, osteo-musculo-cutaneous type flaps, etc. These flaps work well if they were not involved in the initial trauma, infection, or radiation field. Otherwise, the flaps are stiff, difficult to dissect out, and difficult to transfer. In addition, the flap has to be soft and pliable because the vascular pedicle is usually intolerant of any twisting or turning that occurs when the flap is swung into its new position.

These flaps are often more difficult to dissect and have a higher complication rate than a free flap, which can be as high as 30% to 40%. Harvesting a pedicled flap often places a donor site deficit on the foot and ankle that has to be skin grafted. However, pedicled flaps allow the surgeon to perform a rapid operation with a short hospital stay that yields excellent long-lasting results. The anatomy and techniques of dissection are discussed above and in flap anatomy books.[7] It is important to practice these flap on cadaver legs as the dissections are often tedious and can be difficult. The distal reach of the flap often provides insufficient tissue so that it is very important to understand the size limitations of each flap.

Lower Leg and Ankle Flaps: Muscle

The lower leg muscles are poor candidates for pedicled flaps because most of them have segmental minor pedicles as their blood supply (type 4) and therefore only a small portion of the muscle can safely be transferred. The distal portion of some of these muscles can be used to cover small defects around the ankle medially, anteriorly, laterally. For small and proximal defect, the muscle flap can usually be separated from its distal tendon to minimize the loss of function.

The extensor hallucis longus muscle (supplied by the anterior tibial artery) can cover small defects that are as distal as 2 cm above the medial malleolus. The extensor digitorum longus muscle and peroneus tertius muscle (anterior tibial artery) are used for small defects as distal as 2.1 cm above the medial malleolus. The peroneus brevis muscle (peroneal artery) can be used for small defects as distal as 4 cm above the medial malleolus. The flexor digitorum longus muscle (posterior tibial artery) can be used for small defects as distal as 6 cm above the medial malleolus. The soleus muscle (popliteal, peroneal, and posterior tibial arteries) is the only type 2 muscle in the distal lower leg where the minor distal pedicles can be safely detached and the muscle rotated on its intact proximal major pedicles to cover large (10×8 cm) anterior lower leg defects as distal as 6.6 cm above the medial malleolus. It can be harvested as a hemi-soleus for small defects and as an entire soleus for larger defects. The muscles described herein generally have to be skin grafted for complete coverage. In addition, the ankle has to be immobilized to avoid dehiscence and ensure adequate skin graft take. The use of external frames can be very useful with the former and the use of a negative pressure dressing for the latter.

If a larger flap or wider angle of rotation is needed, one of the three major lower leg arteries with the relevant minor perforators has to be taken with the muscle flap. The sacrifice of a major artery should only be considered if all three arteries are open and there is excellent retrograde flow. These flaps are usually harvested distally and therefore the accompanying artery depends on retrograde flow. Because these flaps are larger, the tendon is also taken with the muscle. It is therefore important to tenodese the distal portion of the severed tendon to the tendon of a similar muscle so that the function is not lost. For example, if the distal extensor hallucis longus muscle is harvested, the extensor hallucis longus tendon distal to the harvest should be tenodesed to the extensor digitorum longus so that the hallux maintains its position during gait. Because the loss of the anterior tibial tendon is so debilitating, the distal muscle should not be harvested unless the ankle has been or is being fused.

Lower Leg and Ankle Flaps: Fasciocutanous Flaps

Fasciocutaneous flaps are useful for reconstruction around the foot and ankle although the donor site usually has to be skin grafted.[8] The retrograde peroneal flap is useful for ankle, heel, and proximal dorsal foot defects. Its blood flow depends on an intact distal peroneal arterial-arterial anastomosis with either or both the anterior tibial artery and/or posterior tibial artery. The dissection is tedious and it does sacrifice one of the three major arteries of the leg. A similar retrograde anterior tibial artery flap fasciocutaneous flap (retrograde anterior tibial artery) has been described for coverage in young patients with traumatic wounds over the same areas. Because the anterior compartment is the only compartment of the leg whose muscles depend solely on the anterior tibial artery, only the lower half of the artery can be safely harvested as a vascular leash. The retrograde sural nerve flap (retrograde sural artery) is a versatile neuro-fasciocutaneous flap that is useful for ankle and heel defects. The venous congestion often seen with this flap can be minimized if the pedicle is harvested with 3 cm of tissue on either side of the pedicle with the overlying skin intact. Problems with the venous drainage can be further helped by delaying the flap 4 to 10 days earlier and tying off the proximal lesser saphenous vein and sural artery. The inset of the flap is critical to avoid kinking of the pedicle. The Ilizarov external frame is the safest splint that not only immobilizes the foot and ankle but also keeps all pressure off the site by suspending the area of concern in midair. The major donor deficit of the flap is the loss of sensibility along the lateral aspect of the foot and a skin grafted depression at the posterior calf donor site that may pose a problem if the patient later has to undergo a below knee amputation. The supra-malleolar flap (superior cutaneous branch of the anterior perforating branch of the peroneal artery) can be used for lateral malleolar and heel defects as well as for dorsal foot defects. It can be either harvested with the overlying skin or as a fascial layer that can then be skin grafted. When harvested as a fascial layer only, the donor site can be closed primarily. Small, fasciocutaneous flaps based on individual perforators can also be designed over the row of perforators originating from the posterior tibial artery medially and the peroneal artery laterally. Although the reach and size of these flaps are limited, they can be expanded by applying the delay principle. These flaps have proven to be extremely useful in the closure of soft tissue defects around the ankle in patients in an Ilizarov frame because accessibility to the normal pedicled flaps or to recipient vessels for free flaps is always a problem.

Foot Flaps: Muscle Flaps

The muscle flaps in the foot have a type 2 vascular pattern with a proximal dominant pedicle and several distal minor pedicles and are useful to cover relatively small local defects. The abductor digiti minimi muscle (lateral plantar artery) is very useful for coverage of small mid- and posterior lateral defects of the sole of the foot and the lateral calcaneus. Its dominant pedicle is just distal and medial to its origin off of the calcaneus and it has a thin, distal muscular bulk. The abductor hallucis brevis muscle (medial plantar artery) is larger and can be used to cover medial defects of the mid- and hind foot as well as the medial distal ankle. Its dominant pedicle is at the take-off of the medial plantar artery and its relatively thin, distal muscular bulk can be difficult to dissect off the flexor hallucis brevis muscle. The extensor digitorum brevis muscle (lateral tarsal artery) has disappointingly little bulk but can be used for local defects over the sinus tarsi or lateral calcaneus. The muscle can either be rotated in a limited fashion on its dominant pedicle, the lateral tarsal artery, or in a wider arc if harvested with the entire dorsalis pedis artery. The flexor digitorum brevis muscle (lateral plantar artery) can be used to cover plantar heel defects. Because the muscle bulk is small, it works best if it is used to fill a defect that can be covered with plantar tissue.

Foot Flaps: Fasciocutaneous Flaps

The most versatile fasciocutaneous flap of the foot is the Medial Plantar flap that is the ideal tissue for the coverage of plantar defects.[9] It can also reach medial ankle defects. It can be harvested to a size as large as 6×10 cm, has sensibility, and has a wide arc of rotation if it is taken with the proximal part of the medial plantar artery. It can be harvested on the superficial medial plantar artery (cutaneous branch of the medial plantar artery) or on the deep medial plantar artery (deep branch of the medial plantar artery). It is preferable to harvest the flap with the superficial branch if the artery can be identified by Doppler, because it will minimally disrupt the existing foot vascular blood supply. However, if it is to be harvested with retrograde flow, the flap should be harvested with the deep branch of the medial plantar artery. The lateral calcaneal flap (calcaneal branch of the peroneal artery) is useful for posterior calcaneal and distal Achilles defects. Its length can be increased by harvesting it as an L shape posterior to and below the lateral malleolus. It is harvested with the lesser saphenous vein and sural nerve. Because the calcaneal branch of the peroneal artery lies directly on top of periosteum, there is a great danger of damaging or cutting it during harvest. The dorsalis pedis flap (dorsalis pedis and its continuation, the first dorsal metatarsal artery) can be either proximally or distally based for coverage of ankle and dorsal foot defects. A flap wider than 4 cm usually requires skin grafting on top of extensor tendon paratenon which leaves the dorsum of the foot with less than ideal coverage. The loss of the dorsalis pedis can pose problems unless the collateral circulation is intact. Because the donor site is vulnerable both from a vascular and tissue breakdown perspective, this flap is now rarely used. The filet of toe flap (digital artery) is useful for small forefoot web space ulcers and distal forefoot problems, although the reach of the flap is always less than expected. The technique involves removal of the nail bed, phalangeal bones, extensor tendons, flexor tendons, and volar plates while leaving the two digital arteries intact. A variation of this technique is the very elegant toe lsland flap where a part of the toe pulp is raised directly over the ipsilateral digital neurovascular bundle. The flap is then elevated with its long vascular leash to cover a distal defect. The leash is buried under the intervening tissue.

Microsurgical Free Flap

The microsurgical free flap is the most complex reconstruction that paradoxically enjoys the highest success rate (>95%). Although it is beyond the scope of this chapter to cover the technical aspects of microsurgery, I would refer the reader to many excellent texts[10] that cover the field. However, it is important to mention some of the key points for using this type of reconstruction successfully. The key is to have accessible and open recipient artery and vein(s) to which the flap vessels can be anastomosed. The recipient artery should not be sacrificed by performing an end-to-end anastomosis; instead, an end-to-side

should always be performed. Two venous anastomoses should always be performed whenever possible to ensure adequate outflow. The flap is then carefully tailored to the defect and inset. The better the initial fit, the less likely the need for later revision of a bulky flap. This obviously is very important because the reconstructed foot will have to fit inside a shoe.

The key to choosing the appropriate flap is the distance between the recipient vessel and the existing defect. Harvesting a larger flap and removing normal tissue between the defect and the recipient vessel can decrease that distance. The flaps with longest pedicles are the serratus muscle and the radial forearm flap. Muscle flaps with a skin graft work the best to cover osteomyelitis and defects on the sole of the foot. Good donor muscles include the gracilis from the ipsilateral leg, the rectus abdominus, the serratus, and the latissimus dorsi. The latter should be avoided whenever possible as sacrifice of the latissimus dorsi muscle may affect the patient's ability to crutch walk and will definitely hinder the patient's ability to propel himself in a wheelchair. Muscles should be aggressively trimmed to better fit a given defect as long as the main vascular pedicle remains intact.

Fasciocutaneous and cutaneous flaps work better on the nonweight-bearing portions of the foot (ie, dorsum of the foot, ankle). Flaps that are frequently used include the radial forearm, the lateral arm, the lateral thigh, and the parascapular. The key in choosing the appropriate flap is to match the depth of the defect with the relative thickness of the harvested flap. This can be difficult in obese patients. Trimmed muscle with skin graft or fascial flaps with skin graft may be more appropriate.

● COMPLICATIONS

Once the flap has been successfully raised, it can still fail because of tension at the insetting, inadequate blood flow, twisting of the pedicle, hematoma and/or infection, or coagulopathy. Failure to appropriately evaluate the direction of arterial flow, whether it be antegrade or retrograde, can lead to flap loss. The direction of flow is easily determined with a Doppler by occluding the artery proximally and distal to the location where the artery is being heard. Partial or complete occlusion of the vascular pedicle occurs when the artery and vein feeding the flap are twisted as the flap is placed into the recipient site. This occurs if the base is skeletonized, the vascular pedicle isolated, and the flap is rotated at a sharp angle or if the base is indurated and inflexible (chronic scar tissue, radiation). Proper flap design and donor site selection should prevent this from occurring.

Hematoma creates pressure on the flap which can limit venous return and eventually can lead to flap necrosis. The presence of free blood in the deep space is also cause for concern because the red blood cells themselves release superoxide radicals that can contribute to flap necrosis. Hematoma can be prevented by meticulous hemostasis, topical agents, and closed suction drainage. Postoperatively, it is important to visualize the flap and an occlusive transparent dressing facilitates this. If there is any suspicion of existing hematoma, then the wound should be explored and the hematoma evacuated. If the flap was closed with interrupted sutures, removal of one or two stitches allows for evacuation of the hematoma without risking the disruption of the whole repair. It is important to flush the space with normal saline to get rid of any remaining hemolyzed blood. If the hematoma cannot be removed in this way, the patient should be returned to the operating room for formal evacuation. External pressure by applying a bandage so that it does not allow for normal postoperative soft tissue swelling or too tightly can also impede blood flow.

Infection can damage or destroy a flap by increasing the metabolic demand of the flap so that it outstrips existing blood supply. It is therefore important not to plan a reconstruction before all signs of infection are gone. This means that the skin edges are soft with no surrounding induration or erythema, the pain has diminished, and there are signs of healing (granulation and neo-epithelialization). This may require serial debridements that may take up to 1 month before the wound is ready.

Offloading Techniques

For lower leg wounds, an Unna boot dressing over a skin graft allows the patient to ambulate immediately postoperatively. If a graft or flap is in an area (eg, ankle or distal forefoot) where joint motion could disrupt the graft or flap pedicle, then immobilization with a posterior splint, cast, or external fixator and no weight bearing for 2 or more

week is critical for the reconstruction to take successfully. For heel wounds, the Ilizarov frame is very useful because it immobilizes the ankle as well as suspends the foot in midair so that the patient cannot disrupt a graft or flap. If a flap is on the plantar aspect of the foot, there should be no weight bearing until the flap has matured (usually 6 weeks). For some patients with challenging wounds, a cost-effective alternative to Ilizarov frames such as simple fiberglass or plaster casting may by used.

● SUMMARY

Complex lower extremity reconstructions can only be done effectively by using a team approach which at the minimum includes a wound care team, a vascular surgeon, a foot and ankle surgeon, an infectious disease specialist, an endocrinologist, and a prosthetist. Wounds need to be accurately assessed, debrided, and cultured. The vascular and medical status has to be optimized. The repair is then dictated by how much function of the leg and foot remain postdebridement and how the wound can be closed in the most biomechanically stable construct possible. This may involve skeletal manipulation, tendon lengthening and/or partial foot and leg amputations. Soft tissue reconstruction can be as simple as allowing the wound to heal by secondary intention or as complex as coverage with a microsurgical free flap. More than 90% of the wound can be closed using simple methods from healing by secondary intention to skin grafting. Utilizing the techniques described in this chapter should allow for a stable functional wound closure and decrease the primary and secondary major amputation rate to below 5%.

REFERENCES

1. Wrobel JS, Mayfield JA, Reiber GE. Geographic variation of lower-extremity major amputation in individuals with and without diabetes in the Medicare population. *Diabetes Care.* 2001;24(5):860–864.

2. Argenta LC, Morykwas MJ. Vacuum-assisted closure: a new method for wound control and treatment: clinical experience. *Ann Plast Surg.* 1997;38(6):563–576; discussion 577.

3. DeFranzo AJ, Argenta LC, Marks MW, et al. The use of vacuum-assisted closure therapy for the treatment of lower-extremity wounds with exposed bone. *Plast Reconstr Surg.* 2001;108(5):1184–1191.

4. Scherer LA, Shiver S, Chang M, et al. The vacuum assisted closure device: a method of securing skin grafts and improving graft survival. *Arch Surg.* 2002;137(8):930–933; discussion 933–934.

5. Moiemen NS, Staiano JJ, Ojeh NO, et al. Reconstructive surgery with a dermal regeneration template: clinical and histologic study. *Plast Reconstr Surg.* 2001;108(1):93–103.

6. Hallock GG. Distal lower leg local random fasciocutaneous flaps. *Plast Reconstr Surg.* 1990;86(2):304–311.

7. Masquelet AC, Gilbert A. *An Atlas of Flaps in Limb Reconstruction.* Philadelphia: Lippincott; 1995.

8. Cormack GC, Lamberty BGH. *The Arterial Anatomy of Skin Flaps.* 2nd ed. London: Churchill Livingston; 1994.

9. Acikel C, Celikoz B, Yuksel F, Ergun O. Various applications of the medial plantar flap to cover the defects of the plantar foot, posterior heel, and ankle. *Ann Plast Surg.* 2003; 50(5):498–503.

10. Serafin DG. *Atlas of Microsurgical Composite Tissue Transplantation.* Philadelphia: Saunders; 1996.

chapter 67

Postbariatric Surgery Reconstruction

Jonathan W. Toy, MD, FRCS(C) / *J. Peter Rubin, MD*

● INTRODUCTION

Morbid obesity is an increasing health concern in the United States.[1] The World Health Organization defines overweight as a body mass index (BMI) of 25 to 29.99 kg/m², with obesity beginning at 30 kg/m² (Table 67-1).[2] A rise in bariatric surgical procedures due to the obesity epidemic in the United States has resulted in growing numbers of patients seeking removal of the excess skin and fat that remains following weight loss.[3,4] Massive weight loss may be described as weight loss in excess of 50 pounds. Plastic surgeons have had to modify traditional surgical approaches and techniques in order to appropriately treat the unique deformities found in this emerging patient population.

● PATIENT EVALUATION

Patient evaluation begins with a complete medical history. A distinction must be made in the mode of weight loss. A number of patients have lost weight through gastric bypass or other bariatric procedures, and others have achieved their goals through diet and exercise alone. This has important clinical implications as patients undergoing malabsorptive bariatric surgical procedures are at higher risk of having nutrient deficiencies, including protein, vitamins, and iron.[5] Key information to obtain regarding the patient's weight includes:[6]

- Date of bariatric surgical procedure, bariatric surgeon
- Maximum, lowest, and current weight, and BMI
- If patient has reached his or her weight goal
- If any recent (past 3 months) changes to weight status

Other important information to obtain includes:

- History of past or current tobacco use, nicotine replacement therapies
- Prior surgeries
- Prior pregnancies, plans for future pregnancies
- History of prior deep venous thrombosis, pulmonary embolism, or coagulopathy
- Psychiatric history
- Sequelae of gastric bypass (dumping syndrome, prolonged emesis)
- General medical issues such as cardiac disease or diabetes

Screening for nutritional status is important.[7] Many patients may be nutritionally depleted. Protein intake by history is assessed, and considered adequate if 70 to 100 g of protein per day is reported. Deficiencies in nutrients and vitamins, such as thiamine, folate, B12, and iron are common, which may be represented frequently by anemia.[5,8,9]

A generalized physical assessment of the degree of skin excess, distribution of fat, number and location of rolls, and the quality and elasticity of the remaining skin indicates which areas of the body would benefit from contouring surgery. Scars from prior surgeries are important to document. Ventral hernias and rectus diastasis must be identified and may be reconstructed in conjunction with abdominal contouring procedures. Any asymmetries are pointed out to the patient. A complete set of standardized photographs is taken.

A proper medical workup is essential. Preoperative clearances from internists, psychiatrists, and other

TABLE 67-1. BMI and Obesity Classification

BMI (kg/m²)	Classification
<18.5	Underweight
18.5–24.9	Normal weight
25.0–29.9	Overweight
30.0–34.9	Class I obesity
35.0–39.9	Class II obesity
40.0–49.9	Class III—Morbid obesity
50.0–59.9	Class III—Super obesity
≥60.0	Class III—Super, Super obesity

physicians who care for the patient are the rule. Investigations include a chest x-ray (as indicated), electrocardiogram, complete blood count, coagulation profile, pre-albumin, albumin, pregnancy screen in females of child-bearing age, and a mammogram in accordance with American Cancer Society guidelines (Table 67-2).[10] Preoperative counseling, which explores the patient's goals, expectations, and areas of greatest concern, aids in patient selection and priority when multiple procedures are to be performed. Patients must be made aware of the lengthy scars that occur with large skin resections, and must be willing to trade a better contour with the resultant scar. Education should encompass pre- and postoperative expectations, the length of surgical procedures, as well as the nature and length of recovery following multiple procedures.

TABLE 67-2. Key Points in the Assessment of the Massive Weight Loss Patient

Detailed medical history, including weight loss history
Nutritional screening and assessment
Physical examination
Degree of skin excess
Body fat distribution
Number and location of rolls
Quality and elasticity of skin
Preexisting scars (quality and location)
Abdominal wall defects, hernias
Standardized photographs
Preoperative consultations (internist, psychiatrist, etc)
Chest radiograph
Electrocardiogram
Bloodwork (complete blood count, coagulation profile, pre-albumin, albumin, pregnancy screen)
Mammogram
Additional diagnostic studies as indicated
Patient counseling and education (goals and expectations)

● PATIENT SELECTION

Patients presenting following massive weight loss should be at or around their goal weight, and be weight stable for at least 3 months prior to body contouring surgery. This usually corresponds to a period of 12 to18 months following bariatric surgery. A BMI higher than 35 kg/m² increases the risk of surgical complications.[11,12] Aesthetic outcomes are improved with a lower BMI. In general, a BMI of 25 to 30 kg/m² is ideal. Patients with a high BMI are counseled to further lose weight. A notable exception to this guideline is the patient with the disabling giant pannus, or panniculus morbidus. Such severe soft tissue excesses of the abdomen, which on resection may weigh well over 100 pounds, cause significant functional disability.[9] These patients will generally benefit from the removal of abdominal excess in order to improve ambulation, quality of life, hygiene, and further their weight loss.[13]

Patients with severe medical comorbidities, psychiatric comorbidities, unrealistic expectations, and patients currently using tobacco are preoperatively optimized. Of note, tobacco use has been shown to increase the risk of flap loss, wound infection, and wound dehiscence.[14] These issues are reassessed at the second preoperative visit and surgical management is offered only once improved or resolved.

Severe systemic medical disease that would render general anesthesia dangerous is a contraindication for body contouring surgery. Relative contraindications include active smoking, BMI greater than 35 kg/m², uncorrected coagulopathies, severe disorders that affect wound healing, and any medical disease that places the patient at high risk for surgery.

Psychologic Considerations Following Bariatric Body Contouring

Massive weight loss is considered by many to be a "life-altering event." All patients should be congratulated on their weight loss. Pre- and postoperative counseling as to usual postoperative course is essential, including expectations on recovery, activity, and drain care. Family and social support will aid in the postoperative recovery period.

Prior to bariatric surgery, up to one third of patients are found to have at least one psychiatric diagnosis.[15] Mood disorders, personality disorders, and poor body image are most common. Patients with a history of bipolar disorder and schizophrenia must be offered surgery with caution.[16]

● TREATMENT

Any major body contouring surgery should be performed in a fully accredited ambulatory care facility or hospital.[17] With exposure of large surface areas and prolonged operative times, prevention of hypothermia is crucial. Active warming, beginning in the preoperative period, and continuing through surgery, is important.

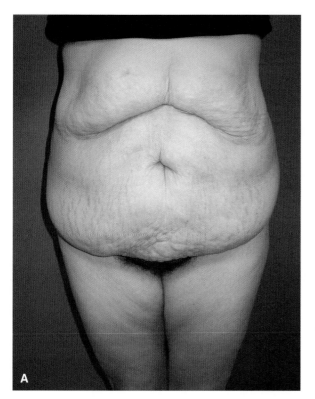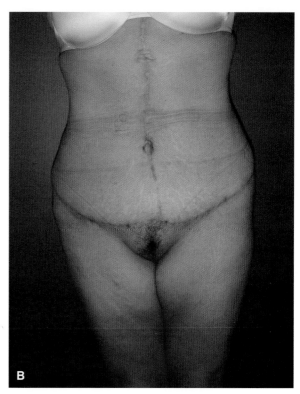

● **FIGURE 67-1.** Fleur-de-lis abdominoplasty. This 38-year-old woman lost 50 kg. Pre- and postoperative views 12 months following fleur-de-lis abdominoplasty, including plication (A,B). Note improved waist definition.

Patient positioning may improve the ease of surgery and prevent untoward complications secondary to pressure. Compression on the eyes must be avoided as blindness has been reported following prone positioning.[18] Neural and vascular compression may occur, especially in the extremities.[19]

Venous thrombosis prevention must be performed, as surgeries are lengthy. Early ambulation, mechanical lower extremity compression devices applied preinduction, and prophylactic chemoprophylaxis may be used.[20]

Length of surgery is an important consideration. Combining multiple body contouring procedures is frequent and can significantly increase operative time. There is no consensus on the time limits for body contouring surgery. However, fewer procedures performed and less operative time generally result in a lower complication rate.

Abdominal Contouring

Along with aesthetic concerns, a hanging abdominal pannus may be symptomatic, causing recurrent intertrigo and infections in skin folds, hindering ambulation, and making intimacy difficult. Following abdominoplasty or panniculectomy after massive weight loss, patients indicate a consistent improvement in body image and subjective quality of life.[21]

A true panniculectomy is a functional operation designed to relieve symptoms related to an overhanging abdominal pannus. It is performed in patients with a higher BMI or more severe medical comorbidities. Skin flap undermining is limited, and the risk of a traditional abdominoplasty is minimized. No plication is performed and the umbilicus is commonly sacrificed in cases requiring large skin and soft tissue resection. Final scar placement must be taken into consideration. The inferior margin for the transverse resection is planned 6 cm superior to the vulvar commissure in women and from the base of the penis in men. In keeping the scar low, its ultimate position will be hidden in most undergarments. Abdominal wall reconstruction for ventral or umbilical hernias may be accessed through the low transverse abdominal incision. In patients with a favorable BMI, more emphasis can be safely placed on aesthetic outcomes. In patients with significant epigastric laxity, a vertical trunk excision may be combined with the low transverse excision, creating a fleur-de-lis type abdominoplasty (Figure 67-1).[22–24] Resuspension of a ptotic pubic region to the anterior abdominal fascia is frequently necessary.

Lower Body Lift/Buttock Contouring

Characteristic findings of the posterior trunk after massive weight loss include buttock deflation and ptosis, skin laxity, and descent of soft tissues in the lateral thighs. Abdominal procedures alone cannot provide contour improvement of the abdomen buttocks and lateral thighs

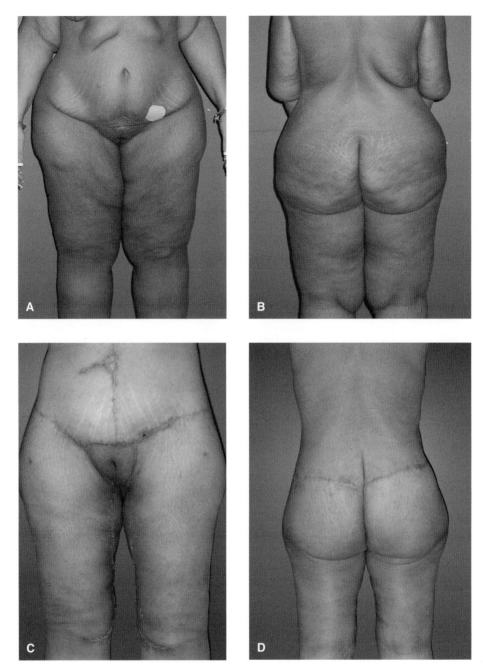

● **FIGURE 67-2.** Lower body lift. A 39-year-old woman status post 45 kg weight loss (A, B). After a, first-stage lower body lift with 9 L debulking liposuction of the thighs, the patient underwent a second-stage vertical medial thigh lift 6 months following initial procedure (C,D).

in a single stage. A number of circumferential procedures have been designed to reshape these areas, including the lower body lift, belt lipectomy, and circumferential torsoplasty (Figure 67-2).[25–28] Circumferential dermolipectomy with careful closure of the strong superficial fascial system, along with buttock augmentation with autologous flaps, have enhanced aesthetic results and the longevity of these procedures.[25,29,30]

The design of the operation is critical in determining overall effects. Planning a resection more superiorly will allow direct excision of flank rolls and emphasizes

the waist. A lower resection will provide a stronger elevation and vertical pull on the lateral thigh area and provides greater control in shaping the buttocks with autologous flaps. Discontinuous undermining of the lateral thigh regions increases flap mobilization during closure.[25]

Medial Thigh Contouring

The lower extremity must be evaluated as two distinct areas. Very rarely can excess tissue in the medial and

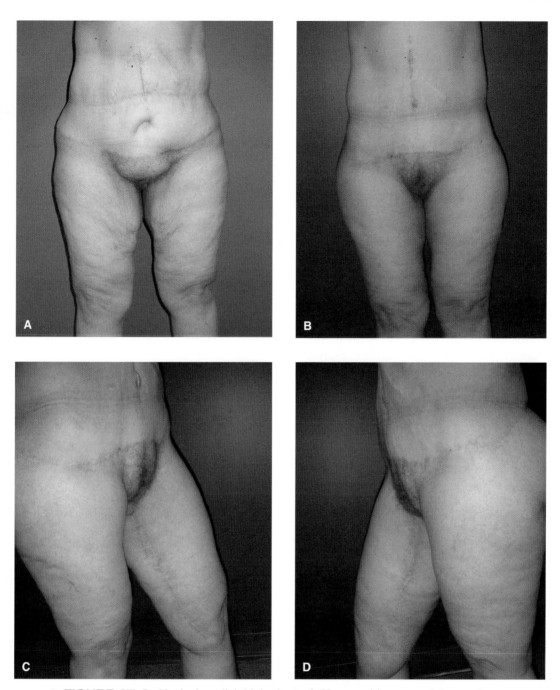

● **FIGURE 67-3.** Vertical medial thigh plasty. A 52-year-old woman status post 60 kg weight loss and prior abdominoplasty. Preoperatively (A). Postoperative views 1 year after revision abdominoplasty and vertical medial thigh lift without having had a lower body lift (B–D). Often, a vertical medial thighplasty will follow a lower body lift as a staged procedure.

lateral thigh areas be treated by a single surgical procedure. Circumferential truncal dermolipectomy procedures create a significant pull on the lateral and posterior thighs, but the medial thighs remain minimally altered.

Choice of procedure in correcting the medial thighs varies depending on the skin and soft tissue excess, as well as the patient's tolerance for scars. In mild cases, a simple, crescenteric transverse medial thigh excision may lift the tissues of the proximal medial thigh, leaving the distal thigh tissues untouched. This technique is reliant on suspension to Colles fascia.[31,32] The advantage is a well-concealed scar. An excisional procedure in a vertical direction allows more direct control over contour and is much more powerful (Figure 67-3).[33] The disadvantage is the visible scar, which may be varied in length. An excision into the groin crease may be added.[34]

Brachioplasty

With massive weight loss, arm deflation leads to varying degrees of upper arm deformity, from minor residual fat deposits to large aprons of skin. The severity of deformity found in these patients requires novel techniques from the norm to correct. Changes in the arm following massive weight loss include laxity and displacement of the posterior axillary fold, residual lipodystrophy of the arm, and loose, hanging skin.

Selection of procedure is dependent on the distribution and amount of remaining fat and the extent of skin excess. In patients with minor skin excess and lipodystrophy, liposuction alone may suffice. In patients seeking improvement in contour with minimal scarring, skin excision limited to the axilla treats the proximal third of the upper arm. A short-scar brachioplasty, with the scar extending down only a portion of the upper arm treats skin laxity more distally but limits incisions. A full-scar brachioplasty with the scar extending distally to the elbow is the only treatment for patients with extreme skin excess (Figure 67-4).[35,36] Brachioplasty excisions may be merged with excisions for upper body lift and mastopexy procedures.

The major disadvantage with a full-scar brachioplasty is poor scar formation. The scar may be red and raised for up to a year postoperatively. Complications include seroma and lymphoceles, paresthesias, neurapraxia of the medial antebrachial cutaneous nerve, and wound dehiscence.[37]

Mastopexy and Upper Body Contouring

Volume deflation, significant ptosis, and flattening of the overall breast shape occur following massive weight loss. The nipple-areola complex is medialized, and lateral chest rolls develop contiguous with the breast. Varying amounts of asymmetry between the breasts is the norm. A significant amount of skin excess occurs, while parenchymal volume may be deficient. Traditional techniques for breast ptosis are usually inadequate for these deformities.[38,39]

Goals in mastopexy after massive weight loss include elevation and repositioning of the nipple-areola complex, breast reshaping, development of a natural and aesthetic curve of the lateral breast, volume recruitment if possible from the lateral thoracic roll, restoration of superior pole fullness, minimization of scar and proper scar placement, and creating a long-lasting result.[40]

The senior author has developed a technique based on an extended Wise pattern that achieves all of the goals of mastopexy following massive weight loss (Figure 67-5). Elevation of the lateral chest excess allows its rotation medially into the breast mound. De-epithelialization of the entire Wise pattern and its elevation as an infero-centrally based dermoglandular pedicle allows parenchymal reshaping with dermal suspension of the reshaped breast mound to rib. The overlying remaining envelope of skin and parenchyma is elevated at approximately 1.5 cm thick and redraped over the newly reshaped parenchymal breast structure.

Other approaches to mastopexy after massive weight loss include the rotation-advancement of a supero-medial pedicle, as well as the simultaneous use of implants for additional parenchymal volume.[41] Choice of technique is dependent on breast morphology, patient desires and expectations, and surgeon preference.

Posterior upper body excess may be addressed with either a circumferential transverse excision (scar placed within bra line), or an excision in the midaxillary line. This procedure may be combined with breast or arm contouring excisions.

Gynecomastia in the Massive Weight Loss Patient

Although male breast enlargement is most commonly related to gynecomastia (benign enlargement of male breast glandular tissue), enlargement following massive weight loss typically is the result of pseudogynecomastia.[42,43] Pseudogynecomastia is characterized by increased subareolar fat without the enlargement of the breast glandular component. Along with varying degrees of skin redundancy in the chest, deflation, prominent lateral chest wall rolls, and medialization and enlargement of the nipple-areola complex are common findings.[42]

Pseudogynecomastia must be differentiated from true gynecomastia. In patients with minimal skin redundancy and good skin elasticity, liposuction may be used. Male breast tissue is classically fibrous and dense. Ultrasound-assisted liposuction techniques are ideal to break up this fibrous tissue. For patients with moderate to severe skin and soft tissue excess, treatment with liposuction alone is not adequate. More aggressive excisional procedures that remove skin and soft tissue, while allowing resizing and repositioning of the nipple-areola complex are required (Figure 67-6). The nipple-areola complex may be repositioned on a thin, inferiorly based dermoglandular pedicle, or as a free nipple graft.[44] Skin excision of the chest may be followed laterally to remove the commonly present lateral thoracic roll.

Staging and Combination Procedures

Unlike many patients presenting for correction of specific areas, the postbariatric patient often presents requesting a number of areas be treated. Factors, including medical status, length of procedure, vectors of tension, surgeon experience and preferences, operative assistance, recovery time, patient desires, and cost to the patient play a role.

Although no consensus exists, many surgeons believe that stages should be separated by a minimum of 3 months. A patient should be back to their preoperative health status prior to a second stage. Regarding maximum operative time, a 7-hour upper limit has been suggested, but there is no evidence to suggest an absolute time limit.[45,46]

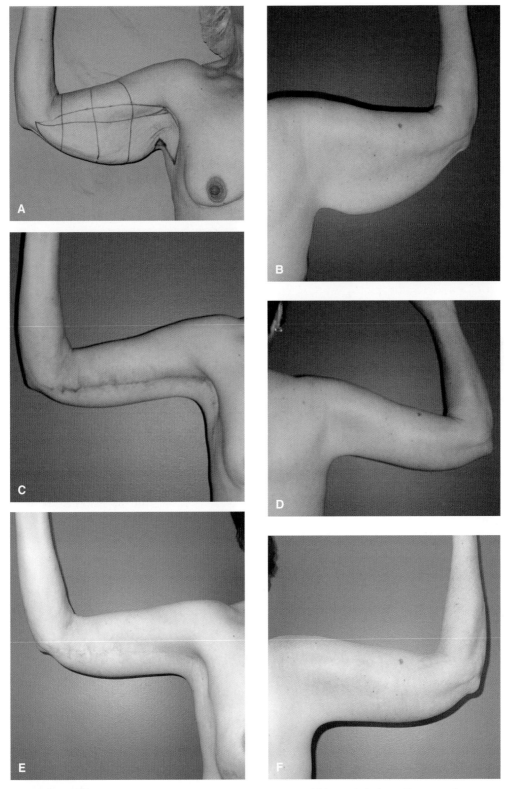

● **FIGURE 67-4.** A 43-year-old woman status post 60 kg weight loss. Preoperative views, including markings for brachioplasty (A,B). Characteristic changes following massive weight loss are seen, including laxity and displacement of the posterior axillary fold with resultant broadening of the attachment of the arm to the chest wall, residual lipodystrophy of the arm, and skin laxity and excess. Postoperative views shown at 4 months (C,D) and 2 years (E,F). Note progression of scar maturation.

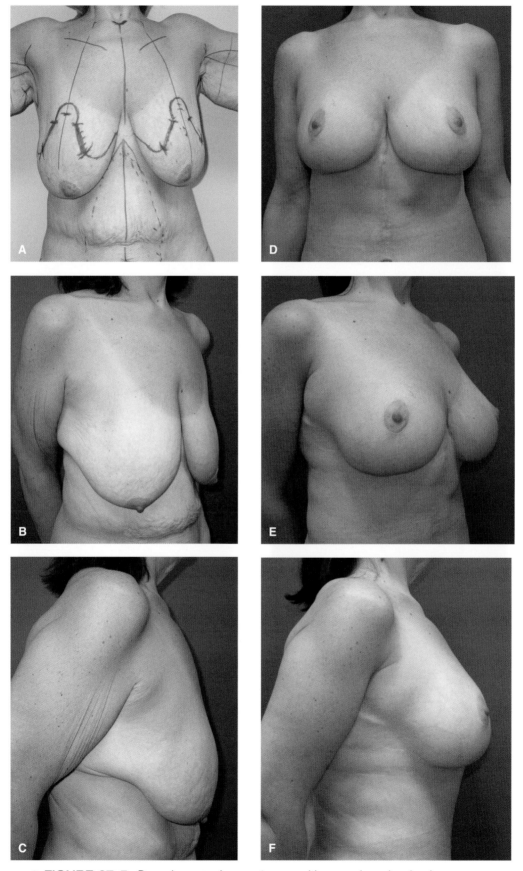

● FIGURE 67-5. Dermal suspension mastopexy with parenchymal reshaping. A 51-year-old woman status post laparoscopic gastric banding after 180 lb weight loss. (A–C) Preoperative views and markings for dermal suspension mastopexy with parenchymal reshaping. (D–F) Postoperative views at 2.5 years.

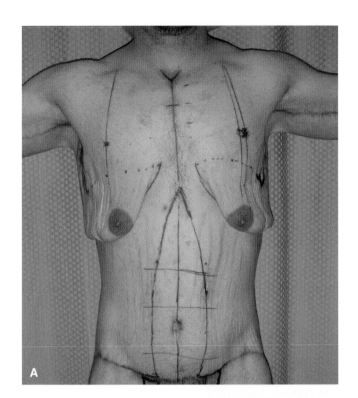
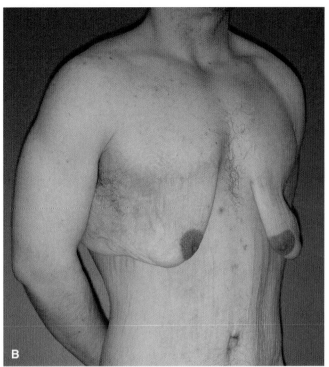
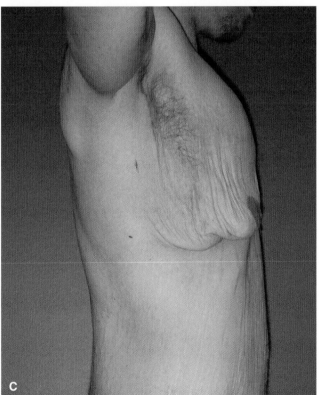

● **FIGURE 67-6.** Excisional gynecomastia with elevation of the nipple-areola complex on a dermoglandular pedicle. A 26-year-old man status post gastric bypass with 250 lb weight loss. (A–C) Preoperative views with markings.

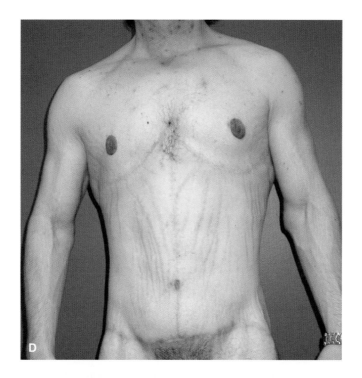

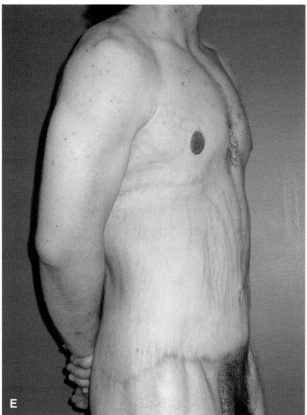

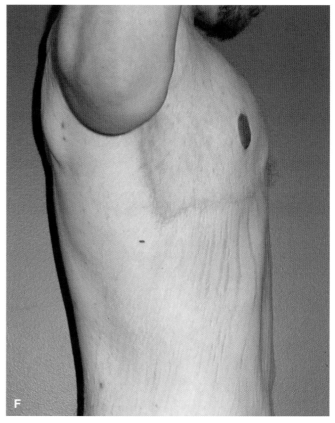

● **FIGURE 67-6.** (*continued*) (D–F) Postoperative views at 1 year following excisional gynecomastia with elevation of the nipple-areola complex on a dermoglandular pedicle, fleur-de-lis component of abdominoplasty, and medial vertical thigh lift as a second stage. The first stage was performed 5 months earlier than the second, involving a lower body lift, panniculectomy, and brachioplasty. Note the marked improvement in chest contour with good positioning of the nipple-areola complex as well as placement of the chest scars at the location of the visual inframammary fold. (*Reprinted with permission from Gusenoff JA, Coon D, Rubin JP. Pseudogynecomastia after massive weight loss: detectability of technique, patient satisfaction, and classification. Plastic Recon Surg. 2008;122(5):1301–1311.*)

When faced with a patient requesting multiple procedures, the order in which they are carried out may vary from patient to patient. Assessing an individual's desires regarding the areas of the body are of priority is a must. This, along with surgeon experience and preferences will help decide the order of procedures. In general, if a lower body lift procedure is considered, the circumferential truncal procedure should be done in the first stage. If multiple procedures are performed in a single stage, opposing vectors of tension should be avoided in a single stage. This will set the foundation for following procedures and may safely be combined with other upper body procedures.

● COMPLICATIONS

The majority of complications from postbariatric body contouring are wound related. Small areas of wound breakdown or dehiscence, along with suture extrusion are common occurrences. Seromas also occur not infrequently and may be treated with serial aspiration, placement of a drain, or injection of a sclerosing agent into the seroma cavity such as doxycycline.[47] The risk of deep venous thrombosis in the postoperative period should be reduced with the appropriate use of prophylactic measures. BMI at the time of surgery may impact complication rates.[48] Three or more procedures in a single stage may increase the risk of blood transfusion and increase the length of postoperative hospital stay.[49] Recurrence of varying amounts of skin laxity may also occur, sometimes requiring revisional surgery.

● OUTCOMES

Despite the fact that complications are not infrequent in patients undergoing postbariatric reconstruction, most patients tolerate the procedures well and are pleased with the outcome. They understand that surgery is primarily reconstructive in nature rather than cosmetic and must be willing to accept the risks of wound dehiscence, seroma formation, and possible systemic complications. Staging the anatomic locations into more manageable surgeries facilitates the postoperative course of each. Patients must also be willing to trade the excess skin and subcutaneous tissue for long and sometimes unsightly scars. Outcomes may be improved by selecting patients with a stable BMI in the 25 to 30 kg/m^2 range and counseling patients who are higher than this level.

REFERENCES

1. Hedley AA, Ogden CL, Johnson CL, et al. Prevalence of overweight and obesity among US children, adolescents, and adults, 1999-2002. *JAMA.* 2004;291:2847–2850.

2. World Health Organization. Global Database on Body Mass Index. BMI classification. 2006. http://apps.who.int/bmi/index.jsp?introPage=intro_3.html. Accessed May 9, 2010.

3. American Society of Plastic Surgeons. 2008 Cosmetic Surgery Trends: 1992, 2007, 2008. 2008. http://www.plasticsurgery.org/Media/stats/2008-ASPS-member-surgeon-cosmetic-trends-statistics.pdf. Accessed April 11, 2010.

4. Trus TL, Pope GD, Finlayson SR. National trends in utilization and outcomes of bariatric surgery. *Surg Endosc.* 2005; 19:616–620.

5. Clements RH, Katasani VG, Palepu R, et al. Incidence of vitamin deficiency after laparoscopic Roux-en-Y gastric bypass in a university hospital setting. *Am Surg.* 2006;72:1196–1202; discussion 1203–1194.

6. Gusenoff JA, Rubin JP. Plastic surgery after weight loss: current concepts in massive weight loss surgery. *Aesthet Surg J.* 2008;28:452–455.

7. Bloomberg RD, Fleishman A, Nalle JE, et al. Nutritional deficiencies following bariatric surgery: what have we learned? *Obes Surg.* 2005;15:145–154.

8. Love AL, Billett HH. Obesity, bariatric surgery, and iron deficiency: true, true, true and related. *Am J Hematol.* 2008;83:403–409.

9. von Drygalski A, Andris DA. Anemia after bariatric surgery: more than just iron deficiency. *Nutr Clin Pract.* 2009;24:217–226.

10. Rubin JP, Nguyen V, Schwentker A. Perioperative management of the post-gastric-bypass patient presenting for body contour surgery. *Clin Plast Surg.* 2004;31:601–610, vi.

11. Matory WE, Jr., O'Sullivan J, Fudem G, et al. Abdominal surgery in patients with severe morbid obesity. *Plast Reconstr Surg.* 1994;94:976–987.

12. Vastine VL, Morgan RF, Williams GS, et al. Wound complications of abdominoplasty in obese patients. *Ann Plast Surg.* 1999;42:34–39.

13. Friedrich JB, Petrov RV, Askay SA, et al. Resection of panniculus morbidus: a salvage procedure with a steep learning curve. *Plast Reconstr Surg.* 2008;121:108–114.

14. Gravante G, Araco A, Sorge R, et al. Wound infections in post-bariatric patients undergoing body contouring abdominoplasty: the role of smoking. *Obes Surg.* 2007;17: 1325–1331.

15. Kalarchian MA, Marcus MD, Levine MD, et al. Psychiatric disorders among bariatric surgery candidates: relationship to obesity and functional health status. *Am J Psychiatry.* 2007;164:328–334; quiz 374.

16. Sarwer DB, Fabricatore AN. Psychiatric considerations of the massive weight loss patient. *Clin Plast Surg.* 2008;35:1–10.

17. Colwell AS, Borud LJ. Optimization of patient safety in postbariatric body contouring: a current review. *Aesthet Surg J.* 2008;28:437–442.

18. Manfredini M, Ferrante R, Gildone A, et al. Unilateral blindness as a complication of intraoperative positioning for cervical spinal surgery. *J Spinal Disord.* 2000;13: 271–272.

19. Shermak M, Shoo B, Deune EG. Prone positioning precautions in plastic surgery. *Plast Reconstr Surg.* 2006;117:1584–1588; discussion 1589.

20. Venturi ML, Davison SP, Caprini JA. Prevention of venous thromboembolism in the plastic surgery patient: current guidelines and recommendations. *Aesthet Surg J.* 2009;29:421–428.

21. Stuerz K, Piza H, Niermann K, et al. Psychosocial impact of abdominoplasty. *Obes Surg.* 2008;18:34–38.

22. Dellon AL. Fleur-de-lis abdominoplasty. *Aesthetic Plast Surg.* 1985;9:27–32.

23. Ramsey-Stewart G. Radical "Fleur-de-Lis" Abdominal after Bariatric Surgery. *Obes Surg.* 1993;3:410–414.

24. Friedman T, Coon D, Michaels JV, et al. Fleur-de-lis abdominoplasty: a safe alternative to traditional abdominoplasty for the massive weight loss patient. *Plast Reconstr Surg.* 2010;125(5):1525–1535.

25. Lockwood T. Lower body lift with superficial fascial system suspension. *Plast Reconstr Surg.* 1993;92:1112–1122; discussion 1123–1115.

26. Aly AS, Cram AE, Chao M, et al. Belt lipectomy for circumferential truncal excess: the University of Iowa experience. *Plast Reconstr Surg.* 2003;111:398–413.

27. Van Geertruyden JP, Vandeweyer E, de Fontaine S, et al. Circumferential torsoplasty. *Br J Plast Surg.* 1999;52:623–628.

28. Carwell GR, Horton CE, Sr. Circumferential torsoplasty. *Ann Plast Surg.* 1997;38:213–216.

29. Song AY, Askari M, Azemi E, et al. Biomechanical properties of the superficial fascial system. *Aesthet Surg J.* 2006;26:395–403.

30. Lockwood TE. Lower-body lift. *Aesthet Surg J.* 2001;21:355–370.

31. Kirwan L. Anchor thighplasty. *Aesthet Surg J.* 2004;24:61–64.

32. Le Louarn C, Pascal JF. The concentric medial thigh lift. *Aesthetic Plast Surg.* 2004;28:20–23.

33. Cram A, Aly A. Thigh reduction in the massive weight loss patient. *Clin Plast Surg.* 2008;35:165–172.

34. Mathes DW, Kenkel JM. Current concepts in medial thighplasty. *Clin Plast Surg.* 2008;35:151–163.

35. Guerrerosantos J. Brachioplasty. *Aesthet Surg J.* 2004;24:161–169.

36. Aly A, Pace D, Cram A. Brachioplasty in the patient with massive weight loss. *Aesthet Surg J.* 2006;26:76–84.

37. Symbas JD, Losken A. An outcome analysis of brachioplasty techniques following massive weight loss. *Ann Plast Surg.* 2010;64(5):588–591.

38. Rubin JP, Khachi G. Mastopexy after massive weight loss: dermal suspension and selective auto-augmentation. *Clin Plast Surg.* 2008;35:123–129.

39. Rubin JP. Mastopexy after massive weight loss: dermal suspension and total parenchymal reshaping. *Aesthet Surg J.* 2006;26:214–222.

40. Rubin JP, O'Toole J, Agha-Mohammadi S. Approach to the breast after weight loss. In: Rubin JP, Matarasso A, eds. *Aesthetic Surgery After Massive Weight Loss.* Philadelphia: Elsevier; 2007:37–48.

41. Losken A, Holtz DJ. Versatility of the superomedial pedicle in managing the massive weight loss breast: the rotation-advancement technique. *Plast Reconstr Surg.* 2007;120:1060–1068.

42. Gusenoff JA, Coon D, Rubin JP. Pseudogynecomastia after massive weight loss: detectability of technique, patient satisfaction, and classification. *Plast Reconstr Surg.* 2008;122:1301–1311.

43. Braunstein GD. Clinical practice. Gynecomastia. *N Engl J Med.* 2007;357:1229–1237.

44. Tashkandi M, Al-Qattan MM, Hassanain JM, et al. The surgical management of high-grade gynecomastia. *Ann Plast Surg.* 2004;53:17–20; discussion 21.

45. Safety considerations and avoiding complications in the massive weight loss patient. *Plast Reconstr Surg.* 2006;117:74S–81S; discussion 82S–83S.

46. Borud LJ. Combined procedures and staging. In: Rubin JP, Matarasso A, eds. *Aesthetic Surgery in the Massive Weight Loss Patient.* Philadelphia: Elsevier; 2007:159–165.

47. Shermak MA, Rotellini-Coltvet LA, Chang D. Seroma development following body contouring surgery for massive weight loss: patient risk factors and treatment strategies. *Plast Reconstr Surg.* 2008;122:280–288.

48. Coon D, Gusenoff JA, Kannan N, et al. Body mass and surgical complications in the postbariatric reconstructive patient: analysis of 511 cases. *Ann Surg.* 2009;249:397–401.

49. Shermak MA, Chang D, Magnuson TH, et al. An outcomes analysis of patients undergoing body contouring surgery after massive weight loss. *Plast Reconstr Surg.* 2006;118:1026–1031.

Index

Page numbers followed by *f* or *t* indicate figures or tables, respectively.